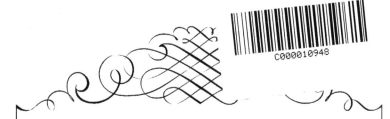
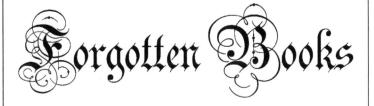
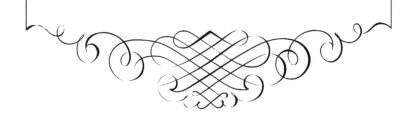

ISBN 978-1-5278-7600-2
PIBN 10923264

1 MONTH OF
FREE
READING

at

www.ForgottenBooks.com

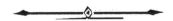

By purchasing this book you are eligible for one month membership to ForgottenBooks.com, giving you unlimited access to our entire collection of over 1,000,000 titles via our web site and mobile apps.

To claim your free month visit:

www.forgottenbooks.com/free923264

English
Français
Deutsche
Italiano
Español
Português

www.forgottenbooks.com

Mythology Photography **Fiction**
Fishing Christianity **Art** Cooking
Essays Buddhism Freemasonry
Medicine **Biology** Music **Ancient
Egypt** Evolution Carpentry Physics
Dance Geology **Mathematics** Fitness
Shakespeare **Folklore** Yoga Marketing
Confidence Immortality Biographies
Poetry **Psychology** Witchcraft
Electronics Chemistry History **Law**
Accounting **Philosophy** Anthropology
Alchemy Drama Quantum Mechanics
Atheism Sexual Health **Ancient History**
Entrepreneurship Languages Sport
Paleontology Needlework Islam
Metaphysics Investment Archaeology
Parenting Statistics Criminology
Motivational

EDITOR'S PREFACE

TO THE

FOURTH AMERICAN EDITION.

THE last American edition of this work was published in 1880, and although less than three years have elapsed, many changes and additions have been found necessary to bring it up to the present state of knowledge upon the subject. As in the previous edition, comparatively few changes have been made in the original text, but it has been found advisable to change the order of some of the chapters. The numerous additions, which will be found throughout every chapter in the book, have been accommodated without increasing the number of pages, by the use of a new and very condensed cut of letter. In the chapter upon Diseases of the Lids, descriptions of Landolt's Method of Blepharoplasty, and of the Editor's Method of Treating Depressed Scars of the Face, have been added. In the chapter on Diseases of the Conjunctiva, the section on the Purulent Conjunctivitis of New-born Children is entirely new, as is also that on Membranous Conjunctivitis; and large additions have been made to the section on Diphtheritic Conjunctivitis. In the section on Chronic Granular Conjunctivitis, the views of Sattler upon the nature of Trachoma have been inserted. No mention has been made of the treatment of obstinate Pannus and Trachoma by the local application of infusions of the Jequirity Bean, owing to the MSS. having been in type before the observations on this subject were published. In the chapter upon the Diseases of the Iris and Ciliary Body, the observations upon the Comparative Physiological and Therapeutical Value of Various Mydriatics are new. In the chapter on Sympathetic Ophthalmia have been embodied Mooren's views as to the optic nerve being the seat of the lesion; as well as the discussion upon the same subject before the London Inter_ national Medical Congress in 1881. Additional observations upon the value of Optico-ciliary Neurectomy will also be found here. In the chapter on Glaucoma, the views of Priestley Smith and Brailey upon the Nature and Causes of Glaucoma have been added. A fuller discussion of the subject of the Removal of Particles of Steel or Iron from the Eye by means of the Magnet will be found in the chapter on Diseases of the Vitreous Humor. In the chapter upon the Diseases of the Optic Nerve will be found a recent contribution of Hughlings-Jackson to the literature of Optic Neuritis in Intracranial Disease. Important additions have also been made to the chapter on Diseases of the Ocular Muscles, with reference to the occurrence of Conjugate Deviation of the Eyes in Bulbar Lesions of the Encephalon.

The Editor has labored earnestly to bring the present edition fully up to the standard of preceding editions, and trusts that the result of his efforts will have the approval of the profession. All additions by the Editor are enclosed in brackets with the letter [B.], and wherever other sources have been borrowed from, full recognition by quotation-marks, name of work, and name of author has been carefully given.

The reading of the proofs and supervision of the press have been confided to Dr. Charles A. Oliver, of Philadelphia, to whom the Editor takes this opportunity of acknowledging his indebtedness.

C. S. B.

New York, *June*, 1883.

PREFACE TO THE SECOND EDITION.

IT has afforded me no small gratification that the first edition of this work should have met with so very favorable a reception, both by the profession at large, and by the British and Foreign Medical Press; and especially that it should have been deemed worthy of being translated into French and German, in both of which languages it will be published in the course of this year.

Stimulated by such encouragement, I have endeavored to render the second edition as complete as possible, and have made numerous additions, incorporating all the important facts elucidated by the most recent researches, so that the work might be brought up to the latest date.

16 SAVILLE ROW, *May*, 1870.

PREFACE TO THE FIRST EDITION.

WITHIN the last few years the want has often been expressed of an English treatise on the diseases of the eye, which should embrace the modern doctrines and practice of the British and Foreign Schools of Ophthalmology, and should thus enable the practitioner and student to keep up with the knowledge and opinions of the present day.

I now venture to lay before the Profession a work which I trust may be deemed, to a certain extent, worthy to meet this desideratum. Whilst I have endeavored to enter fully into all the most important advances which have been lately made in Ophthalmic science, I have not contented myself with simply recording the views of others, but have sought in most instances to make myself practically conversant with them, so that I might be able, from my own experience, to form an independent and unbiassed opinion as to their relative value. The vast and peculiarly favorable opportunities which I have had at Moorfields of studying all phases and kinds of eye disease, as well as the great benefit which I have enjoyed of witnessing the practice and operations of my colleagues, have most materially assisted me in the possibility of doing this.

In preparing this work, I have steadily kept one purpose in view, viz., to make it as practical and comprehensive as possible; and I have, therefore, entered at length into an explanation of those subjects which I have found to be particularly difficult to the beginner. I have, on purpose, occasionally repeated important points in diagnosis and treatment, in order to render each article, to a certain extent, complete in itself, so as to obviate the necessity of the reader having constantly to refer to other portions of the book for explanation or information. Moreover, I have thought that this would prove of great convenience to those who may desire to consult and study certain subjects, without being obliged to peruse the greater portion of the book.

The subjects of "Injuries to the Eye," and of "Congenital Malformations of the Eye," have assumed such considerable dimensions that I have been obliged to treat of them somewhat briefly, and would, therefore, refer the reader who seeks for fuller information to special treatises upon these affections. Of these, I would particularly recommend the following excellent works: "Injuries of the Eye, Orbit, and Eyelids," by Mr. George Lawson;

"Verletzungen des Auges," by Drs. Zander and Geissler; and the "Malformations and Congenital Diseases of the Organs of Sight," by Sir William Wilde.

My best and warmest thanks are due to my colleagues at the Royal London Ophthalmic Hospital, Moorfields, and more especially to Mr. Bowman, for their constant kindness in permitting me to have free access to their cases, and for affording me much valuable information and advice upon all subjects connected with Ophthalmology.

Owing to the great liberality of my friend Dr. Liebreich, and of his publisher, Mr. Hirschwald, of Berlin, I have been able to illustrate this work with sixteen excellent colored ophthalmoscopic figures which are copies of some of the plates of Liebreich's admirable "Atlas d'Ophthalmoscopie."

As very frequent reference is made to certain Ophthalmic periodicals, I have used the following abbreviations:

R. L. O. H. Rep. signifies "Royal London Ophthalmic Hospital Reports," edited by Messrs. Wordsworth and Hutchinson (Churchill).

A. f. O. signifies "Archiv für Ophthalmologie," edited by Profs. Arlt, Donders, and Von Graefe (Peters, Berlin).

Kl. Monatsbl. signifies "Klinische Monatsblätter der Augenheilkunde," edited by Prof. Zehender (Enke, Erlangen).

The following symbols are also frequently employed in the course of the work: $\frac{1}{A}$, means range of accommodation; *r*, punctum remotissimum (far point); *p*, punctum proximum (near point); ∞ (= 0), infinite distance; ', foot; ", inch; "', line.

The test types of Jaeger may be obtained from the Secretary of the Royal London Ophthalmic Hospital, Moorfields, and those of Snellen from Messrs. Williams and Norgate, Henrietta Street, Covent Garden.

16 SAVILLE ROW,
December, 1868.

CONTENTS.

"Verletzun...
formations a...
Wilde.

My best a...
London Op...
Bowman, for ...
to their eas...
upon all subj...

Owing to r...
lisher, Mr. H...
with sixteen ...
some of the pi...

As very freque...
have used the t...
R. L. O. H. I...
edited by Mess...
A. f. O. signif...
Donders, and Voo...
Kl. Monatsbl. ...
edited by Prof. Z...

The following sy...
work: $\frac{1}{A}$, means ...
point); *p*, punctu...
', foot; ", inch; "...

The test types of the...
Royal London Ophth...
Messrs. Williams and ...

16 SAVILLE ROW,
December, ...

Chapter XI.

DISEASES OF THE RETINA.

Chapter XII.

DISEASES OF THE OPTIC NERVE.

Chapter XIII.

AMBLYOPIC AFFECTIONS.

Chapter XIV.

THE ANOMALIES OF REFRACTION AND ACCOMMODATION OF THE EYE.

Chapter XV.

AFFECTIONS OF THE MUSCLES OF THE EYE.

CHAPTER XVI.

THE USE OF THE OPHTHALMOSCOPE.

CHAPTER XVII.

DISEASES OF THE ORBIT.

LIST OF ILLUSTRATIONS.

COLORED OPHTHALMOSCOPIC PLATES.

A TREATISE

DISEASES OF THE EYE.

INTRODUCTION.

In order to avoid unnecessary repetition in the course of this work, I think it advisable to give in this introduction a brief description of some of the more important and frequent modes of examination of the eye, as well as of certain remedies and appliances in common use in ophthalmic practice.

Eversion of the upper eyelid has frequently to be practised if the presence of a foreign body is suspected beneath it, or if certain remedies are to be applied to its lining membrane. Various contrivances have been suggested for facilitating this proceeding, but it is best done in the following manner: The patient being directed to look downwards, the surgeon seizes lightly the central lashes of the upper lid between the forefinger and thumb of his left hand, and draws the lid downwards, and somewhat away from the eyeball. He next places the tip of the forefinger of his right hand on the centre of the lid, about half an inch from its free margin. With a quick movement, the edge of the lid is to be then turned over the tip of the forefinger (which should be simultaneously somewhat pressed downwards). By slightly pressing the margin of the everted lid backwards against the upper edge of the orbit, the whole retro-tarsal fold will spring into view, and the lid

[Fig. 1.]

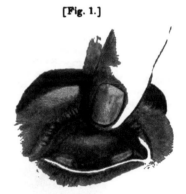

becomes fully everted. [Fig. 1.] In those exceptional cases in which the patient is very unmanageable, and forcibly contracts the orbicularis muscle, it may be necessary to use a probe, or the end of a quill pen or pencil, over which to turn the lid, instead of the forefinger. [Fig. 2.] But as a rule, it is more convenient to employ the latter, as we may not always have a probe at hand, and as anything in the shape of an instrument frightens some patients, whereas we may often succeed in everting the lid with the finger, before they have even time to resist. The surgeon may also stand behind the patient, and steady the head of the latter against his breast, and evert the lid from behind.

oblique or *focal illumination* is in constant requisition for ascertaining the condition of the structures of the anterior half of the eyeball. By its aid we are enabled to examine, with great minuteness, the appearances of the cornea, iris, pupil, lens, and even the most anterior portion of the vitreous humor [and to detect foreign bodies [and delicate exuda-

[Fig. 2.]

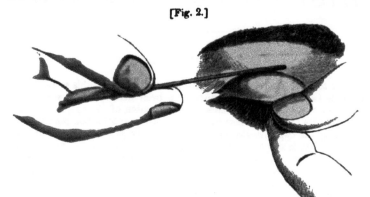

chamber, delicate false membranes in the pupi deposits upon the iris and capsule of the lens, and slight which would often escape the observation of the unthis mode of examination is to be thus conducted: A somewhat in front and to one side of the patient, at a (Fig. 3), and on a level with his eye, the light

Fig. 3.

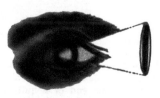

the cornea or the crystalline lens by a strong bi-convex The observer's eye is then to be placed on one to catch the rays emanating from the eye of the light from one portion of the cornea or lens thoroughly, examine its whole expanse and In order to gain a larger image, we may emmagnifying glass [which should be held directly in (Fig. 4.)—H.]. Opacities of the cornea or lens illumination (reflected light) of a light gray or the ophthalmoscope (transmitted light) they will bright red background. the eye with the ophthalmoscope will be found upon the ophthalmoscope.

The mode of ascertaining the degree of intra-ocular tension is as follows: The patient being directed to look slightly downwards, and gently to close the eyelids, the surgeon applies both his forefingers to the upper part of

[Fig. 4.]

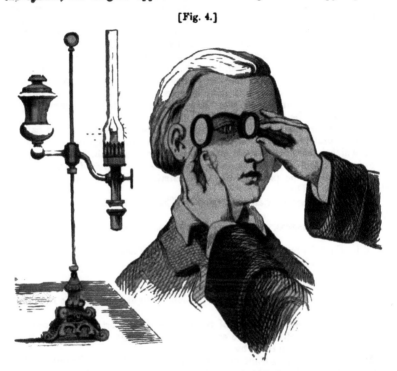

the eyeball behind the region of the cornea [that is, to the sclera; for if the pressure be applied directly to the cornea, the tension seems to be increased.—B.]. The one forefinger is then pressed slightly against the eye so as to steady it, whilst the other presses gently against the eye, and estimates the amount of tension, ascertaining whether the globe can be readily dimpled, or whether it is perhaps of a stony hardness, yielding not in the slightest degree even to the firm pressure of the finger. The beginner will do well to make himself thoroughly conversant with the normal degree of tension, by the examination of a number of healthy eyes, and then, if he should be at all in doubt as to the degree of tension in any individual case, he should test the tension of the patient's other eye (if healthy), or that of some normal eye, so as to be able to draw a comparison between them. If there is much œdema of the lids, or conjunctival chemosis, or if the eyes are small and deeply set, it may be difficult to accurately estimate the degree of tension.[1]

[1] In order, if possible, to estimate the degree of intra-ocular tension with extreme nicety, instruments, termed tonometers, have been devised by Von Graefe, Donders, Dor, etc. It must, however, be admitted that the results obtained by them were not sufficiently accurate to render them preferable to the palpation by the fingers. But more lately Monnik has invented a tonometer, which appears to answer well, and which is constructed on the principle of indicating the depth to which a minute pin, connected

I would call particular attention to the signs which Mr. Bowman has devised for the designation of the different degrees of tension of the eyeball, as they will be found most useful, not only in practice, but also in the reporting of cases, or in the preservation of an accurate record of the state of tension.

Mr. Bowman introduced this subject to the attention of the profession in 1862, in his admirable paper "On Glaucomatous Affections, and their Treatment by Iridectomy," read before the Annual Meeting of the British Medical Association,[1] in which he says, "I have long paid special attention to the subject of tension of the globe, and particularly since it has assumed so much additional importance in the last few years. I have found it possible and practically useful to distinguish nine degrees of tension; and, for convenience and accuracy in note-taking, have designated them by special signs. The degrees may be thus exhibited:[2]

"T represents *tension* ('t' being commonly used for 'tangent,' the capital T is to be preferred). Tn, *tension normal.* The interrogative, ?, marks a *doubt*, which in such matters we may often be content with. The numerals following the letter T, on the same line, indicate the *degree of increased tension;* or, if the T be preceded by —, of *diminished tension*, as further explained below. Thus:

"T 3. *Third* degree, or *extreme tension.* The fingers cannot dimple the eye by firm pressure.

"T 2. *Second* degree, or *considerable tension.* The finger can slightly impress the coats.

"T 1. *First* degree, *slight* but *positive increase of tension.*

"T 1? Doubtful if tension is increased.

"Tn. Tension normal.

"—T 1? Doubtful if tension be less than natural.

"—T 1. First degree of reduced tension. Slight but positive reduction of tension.

"— T 2 ⎱ Successive degrees of reduced tension, short of such consider-
"— T 3 ⎰ able softness of the eye as allows the finger to sink in the coats. It is less easy to define these by words.

"In common practice, some of these may be regarded as refinements; but in accurate note-taking, where the nature and course of various diseases of the globe are under investigation, I have found them highly serviceable, and they have as much precision as perhaps is attainable or desirable.

"It is also to be borne in mind that the normal tension has a certain range or variety in persons of different age, build, or temperament; and according to varying temporary states of system as regards emptiness and repletion. Experience will make every one aware of these varieties, which do not encroach on the above abnormal grades of tension. Medical men may understand how important is this matter of the *degree of tension*, by consid-

with the instrument, is pressed into the sclerotic, and also the force employed to produce the depression. For a further account of it, *vide* "Kl. Monatsbl.," 1868, p. 364, and "Annales d'Oculistique," 1869, p. 68. [Still later a tonometer has been perfected by Snellen and Landolt, on the same principle as Monnik's, which *they* think answers better. With this instrument an impression or depression is made in the sclera with a given definite force, the depth, breadth, and general shape of which in all directions can be accurately measured. A description of the instrument may be found in "Graefe und Saemisch's Handbuch der Augenheilkunde," Bd. iii. p. 192.—B.]

[1] "British Medical Journal," Oct. 11, 1862, p. 378.

[2] "Since this paper was read I have simplified the signs, with the concurrence of my friend, Professor Donders, in order to adapt them for general use. The simplified form has been substituted above."

ering how priceless would be the power of accurately estimating it *by the touch* in the case of various *head affections*."

For the examination of the acuteness of vision [which means the power of distinguishing form.—B.] various test-types are used, more especially those of Jaeger and Snellen. The former do not, however, afford a perfect clue to the acuteness of vision, for a person may be able to read No. 1 of Jaeger with facility and yet not enjoy a normal acuteness of sight. Snellen has, however, devised a set of test-types which fulfil this desideratum. The letters are square, and their size increases at a definite ratio, so that each number is seen at an angle of five minutes. Thus, No. 1 is seen by a normal eye up to a distance of one foot, at an angle of five minutes, No. 2 up to two feet, and so on. These numbers cannot, as a rule, be seen distinctly beyond these distances.[1]

[As commonly used, the term *acuteness of vision* is confined to vision at the centre of the visual field, for the periphery of the retina has only an imperfect power of distinguishing the shape and size of objects.—B.]

Now, if the eye is suffering from any diminution of acuteness of vision, it will require to see the letters under a larger angle than that of five minutes, in order to gain larger retinal images. No. 1 cannot be read at a distance of one foot, but only, perhaps, No. 4 or 5. We may easily calculate the degree of the acuteness of vision thus:

"The utmost distance at which the types are recognized (d) divided by the distance at which they appear at an angle of five minutes (D), gives the formula for the acuteness of vision (V): $V = \dfrac{d}{D}$.

"If d and D be found equal, and No. 20 be thus visible at a distance of twenty feet, then $V = \dfrac{20}{20} = 1$; in other words, there is normal acuteness of vision. If, on the contrary, d be less than D, and if No. 20 is only visible within ten feet, No. 10 only within two feet, No. 6 only within one foot, these three cases are thus respectively expressed:

$$V = \frac{10}{20} = \frac{1}{2}; \quad V = \frac{2}{10} = \frac{1}{5}; \quad V = \frac{1}{6}.$$

d may sometimes be greater than D, and No. 20 be visible at a greater distance than twenty feet. In this case vision is more acute than the normal average." [This condition, as a matter of experience, is not at all uncommon, not only in hypermetropic eyes, but in emmetropic eyes.—B.]

It must, however, be confessed that some patients (more especially amongst the lower classes) often experience a difficulty in fluently reading type composed of these square letters. They have always been accustomed to ordinary type, the letters of which are of unequal thickness, and differ both in dimensions and definition. I, therefore, generally employ Jaeger's test-types for ascertaining the fluency with which small print can be read, and

---

[1] At Professor Longmore's suggestion, Dr. Snellen has given in his second edition of the test-types some tables containing a series of figures and single numbers for the examination of such recruits for the British Army as are unable to read. For further information as to the examination of the sight of recruits, I must refer the reader to Professor Longmore's excellent "Ophthalmic Manual," which I would also recommend to the special notice of the surgeons of the Militia and Volunteer Corps. These test-types may be obtained at Messrs. Williams & Norgate's, Henrietta Street, Covent Garden.

[A selection from the test-types of both Jaeger and Snellen, sufficient for use in ordinary practice, will be found at the end of this volume.—H.]

those of Snellen for testing with accuracy the acuteness of vision [at a distance.—B.].

[Various modifications of these types have been proposed. Dr. John Green, of St. Louis, thinks that the different sizes of types should hold a certain definite relation of size to one another, and thus form an arithmetical series. He also prefers, instead of the "block letters" ordinarily used (**E**), the simpler form (**E**). In making practical use of any of the various forms of test-type, a sheet of card-board, having on it letters of various sizes, should be hung up in a good light, and the number of the smallest size should be less than the number of feet in the available distance. For testing near vision, use is made of the pamphlet test-type, published by Snellen in several languages. These contain not only letters, but dots and angular figures for the use of those unable to read. If vision is less than $\dfrac{1}{x\,x}$, it is usual to discard the letters, and test the power of counting fingers, and when they cannot be counted, it becomes not a question of vision, but of the quantitative or qualitative perception of light.

A very important point to be considered is the amount or intensity of light under which the examination of the acuity of vision is carried on. If daylight be used, it is not common to have the same degree of illumination upon different days, and hence comparative testing is not of much absolute value. It has seemed best to some experts, to use only artificial light for these examinations, and this light must of course come from a lamp in which the same kind of oil is always used under the same circumstances, in order to reduce to a minimum any possible source of error. At the best, we must regard these tests as but approximate.

In this test examination of the acuity of vision, it not infrequently happens that it would be advantageous to know the actual sensibility of the eye to light. Förster, of Breslau, has constructed an instrument for this purpose, a description of which will be found in "Graefe und Saemisch's Handbuch der Augenheilkunde," Bd. iii. p. 36. He claims that its use divides cases of impaired vision into two groups. In the first, where sensibility to light is but little diminished, are included those diseases in which the conducting portions of the optic nerve and retina are mainly affected. In the second class are those diseases in which the perceptive elements of the optic nerve and retina are involved. Förster gives a formula for the determination of L or the sensibility to light.—B.]

[Kuhnt's investigations upon colored-light induction are interesting. From experiments of various kinds, he deduces the general formula that each color possesses the power of inducing only its own color-quality. He then takes up the subject of successive colored-light induction, and from experiments deduces the general formula that for a fixation of forty-five seconds, the color of the after-image of a black velvet disk is always like or equal to the ground-color of the original. He next compares the color resulting from successive induction with an objective color, and concludes that the color resulting from successive induction appears almost the same as the disk of comparison, only a little darker and less saturated ("Archiv für Ophthalmologie," xxvii. 3).—B.]

Besides examining the acuteness of vision, it is often of much importance to ascertain with accuracy and care the condition of the field of vision, which may be readily done in the following manner: The patient, being placed straight before us at a distance of from fifteen to eighteen inches, is directed to look with the eye under examination (closing the other with his hand) into one of our eyes, his right eye being fixed upon our left, and *vice versa*. In this way any movement of the eye may be at once detected and checked. Whilst he still keeps his eye steadily fixed upon ours, we next move one of our hands in different directions throughout the whole extent of the field of vision (upwards, downwards, and laterally), and ascertain how far from the optic axis it is still visible; we then approach the hand nearer to the optic axis, and examine up to how far from it he is able to count fingers in different directions. The number of the extended fingers is to be constantly changed, and the examination to be repeated several times, so that we may ascertain whether the patient can count them with certainty, or whether he hesitates in his answers, or only guesses at their number. We may thus readily discover whether the field of vision is of normal extent, or whether it is defective or altogether wanting in certain directions.

We may term that part of the field in which the patient can still distinguish an object (a hand, a piece of chalk, etc.) the *quantitative* field of vision, in contradistinction to that small portion in which he is able to count fingers, and which may be designated the *qualitative* field.

The following method of examining the field is still more accurate, and I should advise its adoption in all cases where it is of importance to have an exact map of the extent of the field, as in glaucoma, detachment of the retina, etc., so that a record may be kept of the condition of the field during the progress of the disease, or that we may be able to compare its extent before and after an operation. The patient, being placed before a large black-board, at a distance of from twelve to sixteen inches, is directed to close one eye and to keep the other steadily fixed upon a chalk dot, marked in the centre of the board and on a level with his eye. A piece of chalk, fixed in a dark handle, is then gradually advanced from the periphery of the board towards the centre, and the spot where the chalk first becomes visible is then marked upon the board. This proceeding is to be repeated throughout the whole extent of the field; the different points at which the object first becomes visible are then to be united by a line, which indicates the outline of the *quantitative* field of vision. [Fig. 5.] The extent of the *qualitative* visual field is next to be examined, and it is to be ascertained how far from the central spot the patient can count fingers in different directions. The points thus found are also to be marked on the board, and the marks afterwards united with each other by a line, which should be of a different color or character to that indicating the extent of the quantitative field, so that the two may not be confounded. It need hardly be mentioned that care is to be taken that during the examination the patient's eye remains steadily fixed upon the central spot, that the other kept closed, and that his distance from the board is not altered. The of the field inwards will, naturally, vary according to the prominence of the patient's nose.

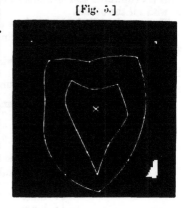

[Fig. 5.]

board is to be divided into four equal parts by a vertical and horizontal line (of about 4 feet in length), cutting each other at the central cross; each quadrant is then again to be divided into two equal parts by another line, so that the whole is divided into eight equal segments, as in the accompanying figure (Fig. 6), which represents the division of the field for the left eye.   For the right eye, the position of the letters must be reversed,

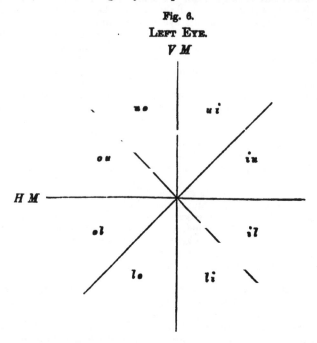

Fig. 6.

LEFT EYE.

V M

H M

thus *u i* (upwards and inwards) would be *u o* (upwards and outwards), and so with all the others.

The meaning of the letters is as follows:

V M—Vertical Meridian, dividing the field into two lateral halves (inner and outer).

H M—Horizontal Meridian, dividing the field into an upper and a lower half.

The upper half of the field is subdivided into four segments:

> *u o* upper and outer segment.
> *o u* outer "   upper   "
> *u i* upper "   inner   "
> *i u* inner "   upper   "

The lower half is also subdivided into four segments:

> *o l* outer and lower segment.
> *l o* lower "   outer   "
> *i l* inner "   lower   "
> *l i* lower "   inner   "

The method of examining the patient's field of vision is to be the same as that above described, when a plain board was used.   The object of the divisions is only to furnish a kind of framework for the map of the field, which enables us to sketch it with more ease and rapidity.   The boundary of the quantitative and qualitative fields is to be marked both upon and between each of the divisional lines, and the distance of each of these marks from the centre of the board is then to be measured, and its extent, in inches, is to be placed against each mark. A small fac-simile of the field of vision thus mapped out may then be drawn in the note-book, the field being here also divided into eight segments, the boundaries and measurements of the map being likewise copied; so that we may preserve, in a small and convenient form, an accurate record of the shape and extent of the visual field.

But the sight of the patient may be so much impaired that he can no longer count fingers, even in the optic axis, being only able to distinguish between light and dark, as in cases of mature cataract, severe cases of glaucoma, etc., and yet it may be of great importance to know whether or not the field of vision is of normal extent. This may be readily ascertained in the following manner: The patient is directed to look with the one eye (the other being closed) in the direction of his uplifted hand (held straight before him, on a level with his eye, and at a distance of from twelve to eighteen inches). A lighted candle is then held in different portions of the visual field, and the furthest point at which it is still visible in various directions is noted, the candle being alternately shaded and uncovered by our hand, so as to test the readiness and accuracy of the patient's answers. Care should also be taken to shade the candle when it is removed to another portion of the field. The light may likewise be thrown upon various portions of the eyeball by the mirror of the ophthalmoscope, and the patient questioned as to the direction from which the light appears to come.

Mr. Pridgin Teale has devised a modification of the above method, by subdividing the board (already divided by vertical, horizontal, and diagonal lines) by a series of concentric circles. There is, moreover, a travelling white disk of card-board, which can be moved from the outer edge of the board to the centre along the diagonal and other lines, thus forming a very convenient and easily recognizable object. There is also a rest to steady the patient's head, and maintain it at a certain distance. He marks the existence of good vision by a + sign, imperfect vision by —, and absence of vision by 0. Blank diagrams[1] are prepared, which are a copy of the markings on the board, on a scale of ¼ of an inch to 1 inch of the board.

Wecker employs the following mode of taking the field. He uses a large black-board, towards the centre of which can be moved, in a radiating direction, a number of small white ivory balls, thus marking the extent of the field; as soon as the ball reaches the limit of the field, it is turned round, and presents its black posterior surface to the patient. On the back portion of the board, the shape and extent of the field can be read off from the position of the white balls, which give its exact delineation.

Professor Förster's perimeter[2] is, however, by far the best instrument for measuring the extent of the field of vision. It consists of a semicircular band of brass, which is mounted on a stand. This band or arc is two inches wide, and curved at a radius of twelve inches; it revolves round a central axis, which permits of its being placed in different meridional positions. Each half of the arc is divided into 90°; 0° being situated in the middle, at the central axis, and the 90° at each extremity. The object for testing the field,

[1] These may be obtained at Messrs. Harrison's, 45 St. Martin's Lane.
[2] For a fuller description of this instrument, and the method of using it, I must refer the reader to Dr. Carl Möser's "Inaugural Dissertation on the Perimeter" (Breslau, 1866, published by H. Linder); also to the "Compte Rendu du Congrès D'Ophthalmologie," 1867, p. 125. The perimeter is made by Mr. Sitte, optician, 8 Alte Taschen-strasse, Breslau, and costs about £7.

a black movable knob, having a white centre
ma along to any point of the arc, by means of
m behind by a winch. At the back of the cent
a which a needle indicates the various meridia
a, and its inclination to the vertical meridia
to 180°, within these meridians. In order
in different directions, and to record the res
d circular maps, which are copies of the disk
le within each meridian. On these skeleton m
extent of the field in any given case. In ex
, he is not to have his visual line fixed on the
a little button placed 15° to the inner (nasal
ing the blind spot opposite the latter.[1]
Carter has recently devised an excellent mo
er, which is more simple in construction, less
ut of order. He gives the following descripti
Lancet," July 6, 1872:
a simple tripod, supporting a hollow stem (F
em (B) moves up and down, and can be fixed
e screw (C). At the top of the stem (B) is a
arrying the quadrant (E, E'), which turns in

unnecessary repetition, I must here explain the sig
e" and "blind spot." By visual line is understood t
yellow spot to the object point, and this line was forme
he optic axis, hence it is often said when a person is l
e axes are fixed upon it." This is, however, not stri
own that the visual line and optic axis are not identic

Fig. 7.

circle, and moves with just stiffness enough to remain wherever it is placed. On the quadrant is a travelling slide (F), with a white spot; and a second independent axis is inserted in the axis of the quadrant at G, and carries a short tube, in which may be placed a stem to support the fixing-point. The second or inner axis makes a complete revolution without affecting the position of the quadrant, and without being affected by it. At its attached extremity the quadrant terminates in a circular disk (E′), which is graduated

Fig. 8.

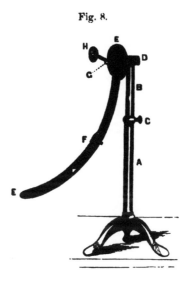

into degrees at the back, and a fixed index allows the exact position of the quadrant to be read off. The quadrant is also graduated from ten degrees to ninety, on its concave face, so as to show the exact position of the slide. The fixing-point may be either an ivory knob at the end of a wire, or, what is for most purposes better, a small disk with a central perforation, as shown at H, *through* which the patient looks at an object on the other side of the room, and obtains fixation without exercise of the accommodation and consequent fatigue to the eye. The travelling slide (F) may be made to carry a spot of any color or size that is desired, and it is furnished with a ring at the back, by which it may be moved by means of a hook set in a handle, so that its position may not be indicated by that of the hand of the operator. For the purpose of taking exact measurements of the blind spot, the quadrant is graduated at the back from eight degrees to twenty-five, in degrees and sixths of a degree; and a white spot is placed on the centre of the axis (G), to serve as a fixing-point for this particular purpose."

[Landolt's perimeter has a double arm, like Förster's, and is open to some of the same objections.

Scherk's perimeter consists actually of a hollow hemisphere, with a radius of one foot, attached tangentially to a vertical rod at its pole, blackened inside, and divided into meridians and concentric circles. The hemisphere is divided in the vertical meridian, and the two quadrants can be pushed aside from each other, to admit of more light. The method of examination is practically the same.

macula lutea, the chart is then spaced off—1st, by concentric circles, each 10° or 10 mm. apart (and the actual distance from the macula of a defect or lesion in the eye when it gives a break in the field of vision may, in some cases, be calculated); and 2d, by radii drawn at every 30° of the visual circle, intersecting the above concentric circles and numbered to correspond with the radii on the reverse side of the arc. The blind spot is noted at about 15° external to the centre of the chart. The clear space on the chart is an approximation only to the normal visual field; the variations at the periphery being so dependent upon individual conformations of face, prominence of eye, etc., that a standard scheme would, of course, be useless. This has been constructed as an average, from the observations of Förster, Aubert, Schoen, Hirschberg, etc., and it was thought desirable to indicate nearly the

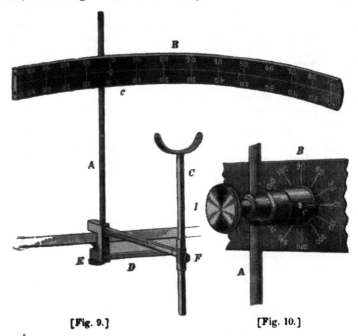

[Fig. 9.]   [Fig. 10.]

usual field, so that a striking variation would be detected at a glance. I have had it printed upon thin paper, for insertion in the book of histories which every one keeps.

The object of fixation (as stated, the proximal extremity of the axis) is an unpolished disk of nickel-plated brass, 15 mm. in diameter. I use, for the second or movable object, squares of thick card-board, capable of being inserted in a little spring clasp at the end of a stick serving as a handle. This handle is 35.5 cm. long, and may be used to determine with sufficient accuracy the position of the patient's head, or rather eye, at the centre of the curve of the arc, by measuring the length of the handle from two points (say zero and 90°) on the arc; where these intersect on the horizontal plane is the centre of the circle, and there the eye should be placed. The chin then resting upon the crutch is steady enough for practical purposes.

It is very often necessary to test the sense of color, and this is best done by testing the power of distinguishing between various colors without naming them. The best test-objects are dyed pieces of silk, or, better still, skeins of colored worsted, such as are recommended by Holmgren, of Upsala. A person who is color-blind will place together, as similar, certain colors which to a normal eye are very different. In the color-blindness which is the result of atrophy of the optic nerve and retina, the defect will be detected by asking the patient to name the colors; but in congenital color-blindness it is best to examine the patient without the colors being named.

Various instruments have, from time to time, been invented for determining and measuring the color-sense. One of the latest is that of Oliver, which consists of a blackened perforated disk, in which is inserted a movable graduated slide; the disk is then bolted to two circular cards, upon which are placed known colors. By the rotation of these color-bearing cards, and the movement of the slide, we can accurately determine the exposed area, the amount being registered by the graduated strip on the face of the slide. This strip has upon it an artificial division of the diagonal of the entire color-square into nine equal parts, each divided into ten equal parts. Each of the sides of the color-square is equal to ninety millimetres, and as the strip measures the diagonal, there is given by this measure an absolute answer for the actual increase of the side of the square in millimetres. The three primary colors and blue are placed on the first card. The second card has been added, in order to have a series of confusion colors in cases of color-blindness. ("Archives of Ophthal.," x. 4.)—B.]

Double images (*diplopia*).—An object only appears single when both visual lines are fixed upon it; any pathological deviation of either visual line must necessarily cause diplopia, as the rays from the object do not then fall upon identical portions of the retina. The slightest degree of diplopia is that in which the double images are not distinctly defined, but seem to lie slightly over each other, so that the object appears to have a halo round it.

We meet with two kinds of double images.

1. *Homonymous* (or *direct*) diplopia, in which the image to the right of the patient belongs to his right eye, the left image to the left eye.

2. *Crossed* double images, in which case the image to the right of the patient belongs to his left eye, that on his left to his right eye.

Homonymous diplopia is always produced (except in incongruence of the retinæ) in convergent squint, for if the eye deviates inwards from the object, the rays coming from the latter will fall upon the inner portion of the retina, and the image will (in accordance with the laws of projection) be projected outwards, as in Fig. 11.

Let I. be the right eye, whose visual line is fixed upon the object (b): II. The left eye, whose visual line (c d) deviates inwards from the object; the rays from b therefore fall upon e, a portion of the retina internal to the yellow spot (d), and the image is consequently projected outwards to f; b and f are, therefore, homonymous double images, the image b, which is to the right of the patient, belonging to his right eye, the image f to his left eye.

Crossed double images arise in divergent squint, for as the one eye deviates outwards from the object, the rays from the latter fall upon a portion of the retina external to the macula lutea, the image is projected inwards, and crosses that of the other eye, as in Fig. 12.

I. The right eye, whose visual line is fixed upon the object (b). II. The left eye, whose visual line (c d) deviates outwards from the object; the rays from the latter therefore fall upon e, a portion of the retina external to the macula lutea (d), and the image is projected to f, crossing the image b; the image f, which would lie on the patient's right hand, would, therefore, belong to his left eye, the image b, which would lie on his left side, to the right eye.

If one eye squints upwards, the rays will fall upon the upper portion of the retina, and the image be projected *beneath* that of the healthy eye. The reverse will be the case if the eye squints downwards, for then the rays will

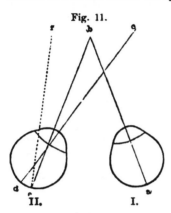

Fig. 11.

II.   I.

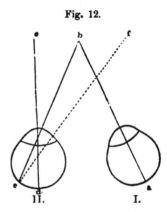

Fig. 12.

II.   I.

fall upon the lower portion of the retina, and the image will be projected *above* that of the healthy eye.

We should never forget to ascertain whether the diplopia be monocular or binocular; in the latter case, it will of course disappear upon the closure of either eye.[1] [If the diplopia is monocular, the lens and retina should be examined carefully, and the presence or absence of nervous symptoms should be looked into.—B.]

Let us now glance at the action of prisms. When a ray of light falls upon a prism, it is refracted towards its base. If, for instance, whilst we look at an object (*e. g.*, a lighted candle) at eight feet distance, with both eyes, a prism, with its base towards the nose, is placed before the right eye, the rays from the candle will be deflected towards the base of the prism, and fall upon a portion of the retina internal to the yellow spot, and be consequently projected outwards, giving rise to homonymous diplopia. As

Fig. 13.

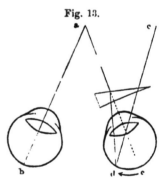

we are, however, very susceptible of double images, the eye will endeavor to unite them by an outward movement (its external rectus becoming contracted), which will again bring the rays upon the yellow spot, but at the same time of course cause a divergent squint. Fig. 13 will explain this.

---

[1] In examining the double images of a patient, it is convenient to place a slip of red glass before the sound eye, for we thus enable him readily to distinguish the two images by their color, and we also weaken the intensity of the image of the sound eye, and approximate it more to that of the affected one, whose image, owing to the rays from the object falling upon an eccentric portion of the retina, will be less intense in proportion to the distance of the spot, upon which the rays fall, from the macula lutea.

[This difference in the distinctness of the images is not always noticed by the patient, and, when they are very wide apart, the false image may not be noticed at all.—B.]

Let a b be the visual line of the left eye fixed (with the other) upon a candle eight feet off. Now, if a prism (with its base towards the nose) be placed before the right eye, the rays are refracted towards the base of the prism, and do not, as in the other eye, fall upon the yellow spot, but upon a portion of the retina (d) internal to the latter, and the image is projected outwards to e; homonymous diplopia therefore arises, and, to avoid this, the external rectus muscle contracts and moves the eye outwards, so as to bring the macula lutea (c) to that spot (d) to which the rays are deflected by the prism. As the rays from the object will now fall in both eyes upon the macula lutea, single vision will result, accompanied, of course, by a divergent squint of the right eye.

The reverse will occur if we turn the prism with its base to the temple, for then the rays will be deflected to a portion of the retina to the outer side of the macula lutea, and the image will be projected inwards across that of the left eye, and crossed diplopia will be the result. In order to remedy this, the internal rectus will contract and move the eye inwards, so as to bring the macula lutea to that spot to which the rays are deflected. [Prisms are occasionally useful in examining feigning patients; for the correction of diplopia from slight strabismus; for estimating the strength of the internal and external recti, and other purposes. The internal rectus can overcome a much stronger prism (base outwards) than the external (base inwards), whilst the superior and inferior recti are still less able to cause compensatory movements (base downwards or upwards); and, in endeavoring to cause diplopia in an examination for malingering, it is best to use a rather weak prism (about 6° or 8°) with its base up or down (Nettleship).—B.]

The Compress Bandage.—The form of bandage to be employed, as well as its mode of application to the eye, is of much practical importance, and it should vary according to the effect which we desire to produce. If the bandage is applied only for the purpose of keeping the dressing upon the

[Fig. 14.]

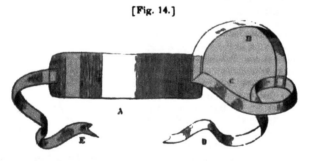

eye, of preventing the movement of the latter and of the eyelids, or of guarding the eye against the effect of light or cold, it need but be of a very simple kind, and I think Liebreich's bandage answers these purposes best. But Von Graefe has shown that the compress and bandage may often be made of great therapeutical value, especially in arresting and limiting suppurative inflammation of the cornea, such as is apt to occur in old and decrepit persons after injuries to the cornea, or an operation (e. g., extraction of cataract). In such cases Liebreich's bandage does not suffice, and we must employ the pressure-bandage of Von Graefe.

Liebreich's bandage [Fig. 14] consists of a knitted cotton band [A] about *hes* long and 2½ inches wide. At the one end are two tapes, the one

[C] going round the back of the head, the other [B] forming a cross-bar with the first, and passing over the top of the head. The other end of the bandage also carries a tape [E] which is to be tied at the side of the head, opposite the affected eye, to the one [CD] coming round from the back. [Fig. 15 represents the bandage applied.—H.] The principal advantages offered by this bandage are—that it perfectly retains its position without slipping, and that it can be undone and the dressings changed without the patient's head having to be raised from the pillow. If the thick knitted band proves heavy and hot, I substitute for it a band of fine muslin or of elastic web. The bandage is to be applied over the following dressing: The patient being directed gently to close his eyes, a piece of soft linen is laid over the lids so as to soak up any discharge; small oval pledgets of charpie' or carded cotton-wool are then placed over this, more especially in the hollows at the inside of the eyeball and beneath the upper edge of the orbit, so as to fill these out, and bring the padding nearly to the same level as in the centre. The pressure of this cushion should be quite uniform, and not greater upon one portion of the eye than another, more especially upon the centre of the eyeball, otherwise it will produce pain and discomfort. The succession of the pledgets of charpie should be applied in such a manner that the upper lid is gently

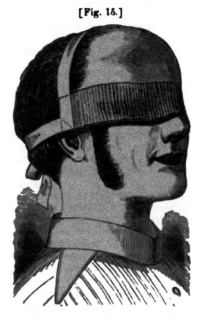

[Fig. 15.]

stretched across the eyeball in a lateral direction, and the lids thus kept immovable. The two principal points of pressure should be at the inner and outer canthus, so that the eyeball is only pressed by the upper lid being stretched gently across it.

Von Graefe' makes use of three different forms of compressive bandages —1, the temporary; 2, the regular compress; 3, the pressure compress.

1. The *temporary bandage* simply consists of a knitted cotton band about fifteen inches in length and one and three-quarters inch in width, which is to be placed over the eye and fastened by a couple of tapes. For this purpose, I think Liebreich's bandage is to be greatly preferred, but with the next two forms of bandage it is different, for here we can regulate the degree and mode of pressure desired with a nicety and accuracy not to be obtained with Liebreich's.

2. The *Regular Compress.*—This bandage is about one and three-quarters yard long and one and one-half inch wide. Its outer two-thirds consist of fine

---

' Charpie consists of threads of very fine linen; the linen should be cut into small squares of about three or four inches in diameter, and the individual threads are then to be pulled out, thus forming the charpie, which should be folded into small pledgets. This is much cooler and more comfortable than cotton-wool.

' "A. f. O.," liv 2; *vide* also an abridgment of this paper, by the author, in "R. L. O. H. Rep.," v. 2

and very elastic flannel, its central third of knitted cotton. The eye having been padded with charpie or cotton-wool, as above directed, the bandage is to be thus adjusted: One end is to be applied to the forehead just above the affected eye, and is then to be passed to the opposite side of the forehead and above the ear to the back of the head; the knitted portion is next carried on below the ear and brought upwards over the compress, the bandage being then again passed across the forehead and its end firmly pinned. The opposite eye may be closed with a strip of plaster, or, should it also require a compress, a separate bandage is to be applied.

3. The *pressure bandage* is made of fine and very elastic flannel, and should be about three and one-half yards long and one and one-quarter inch wide. It is intended to produce complete immobility of the eye, and to exert a considerable degree of graduated pressure. The one end of the bandage is to be placed upon the cheek, at a point about midway between the angle of the jaw and the ear of the affected side, and the bandage brought up over the compress (but not applied too tightly), and carried across the forehead to the back of the head; and then, passing beneath the ear, a second turn is to ascend (somewhat more vertically) over the compress, pressing firmly upon the latter. The bandage is then again carried across the forehead to the back of the head, and finally brought once more over the compress, but this time it is not to be pulled tight.

Baron Heurteloup's Artificial Leech.—This instrument is of the greatest service in the abstraction of blood in deep-seated intra-ocular diseases, as, for instance, in inflammations of the choroid, retina, and optic nerve. For, in order to relieve the intra-ocular circulation, it is necessary that the depletion should be rapid, and we find that in the inflammations of the deeper tunics of the eye, depletion by leeches is almost useless, whereas the effect of the artificial leech is very considerable. The instrument consists of a small sharp cylindrical drill, and of a glass exhausting tube, with an air-tight piston. The drill can be set so as to make the incision of the desired depth, and is worked by a string, on pulling which, a rapid revolution of the drill is caused, and the skin consequently deeply incised. The instrument is to be applied to the temple, and the hair should be previously shaved off at this spot, otherwise it will get between the skin and the edge of the exhausting tube, and thus cause the admission of air. The incision should be made tolerably deep (the depth varying of course with the thickness of the skin), in order that the blood may flow freely and rapidly. The air-tight piston is then to be applied over the incision, and a few rapid turns given, so that the skin may be somewhat sucked up into the tube. The blood will now flow very rapidly, and the screw in the piston must be moved in accordance with the flow of blood, so that no vacuum exists between the plug and the column of blood, nor should the screw be moved roughly and too quickly, otherwise it may produce great pain. The glass cylinder (which holds about one ounce of blood) should be filled in from three to four minutes. The plug of the cylinder should be soaked in hot water, previous to the operation, so that it may swell up and fit very tightly into the tube, and the edge of the latter, which is applied to the skin, should be greased or soaped, in order that it may fit closely to the skin, and prevent the entrance of air. With a little practice, the operation may be gently yet effectually performed without giving much pain to the patient. Hot fomentations should be applied afterwards, so that there may be free after-bleeding. As the abstraction of blood near the eye always causes considerable increase in the flow of blood to the part and its vicinity, the patient should be kept in a darkened room for the first twenty-four hours, until the period of reaction is passed. At first, the sight will be a little dim and indistinct, but after thirty or thirty-six hours have elapsed, the beneficial effects of the depletion will generally be marked. [There are some objections to Heurteloup's leech, the chief of which is that a permanent scar often results from the irregular incision made by the drill, which is worked by a lateral motion. A modification of this apparatus has been made by Dr. F. B. Loring, of Washington, in which the lateral motion has been changed to a vertical one, by putting the drill in a cylinder, and working it by two lateral pistons, joined at the extremities to a disk of the same diameter as the inclosing cylinder. A full description of the instrument may be found in the "Archives of Ophthalmology," vol. viii. No. 4.—B.]

The Eye-douche.—The best and cheapest form of this instrument consists of a piece of India-rubber tubing about four and one-half feet in length, carrying a rose at one end, and at the other a curved piece of metallic pipe, which is to be suspended in a jug of water placed on a high shelf. The fine jet of water thrown up through the rose will be about twelve or fifteen inches in height, and the force with which it plays upon the eye may be regulated by approximating or removing the latter from the rose. This form of eye-douche is to be preferred to that which is applied by means of a cup to the eye itself, as the jet is in this case far too strong, and often increases instead of alleviating the irritation. It is to be employed night and morning, or oftener if the eyes feel hot and tired, for two or three minutes at a time. The eyelids are to be closed, and the stream of water is to play gently upon them.

Mathieu's (Paris) water atomizer, or the instrument used for Dr. Richardson's ether spray, will also be found very useful and agreeable.

[Various forms of atomizers have at different times been recommended, and in some cases they are extremely useful adjuncts in the treatment of conjunctival and corneal affections, though ophthalmic surgeons are divided in opinion as to their practical value over the ordinary way of employing moist cold and warmth to the eye.—B.]

CHAPTER I.

DISEASES OF THE LACHRYMAL APPARATUS.

1.—DISEASES OF THE LACHRYMAL GLAND.

[*Functional anomalies* in the lachrymal gland consist in abnormally diminished or increased secretion. The former is especially noticeable in xerophthalmia, and is not due to a closure of the excreting ducts of the gland, but to a spread of the disease from the conjunctiva to the gland, and an actual lessening of the secretion with eventual atrophy of the gland.

An increased secretion is met with in almost all inflammatory affections of the eye, especially when blepharospasm is present; also in cases of neuralgia of the trigeminus, when the first and second branches are involved. When there is an obstruction to the passage of the tears, the latter become neutral, and act as an irritant in the conjunctival sac, and cause a new overflow of tears. This lachrymation is the earliest symptom of the complications that may arise from alteration of function in the lachrymal passages, and is followed by a sense of the presence of some foreign body beneath the lids. This is succeeded by a conjunctivitis, which in its turn brings a marginal blepharitis, and in many instances an obstinate blepharospasm. If the patient is of advanced years, ectropium of the lower lid is frequently observed, with more or less extensive superficial keratitis. Finally appear the symptoms of dacryo-cystitis and stricture of the nasal duct. A second class of complications consists solely of subjective symptoms, such as photopsia and phosphenes, photophobia and uniocular diplopia, due to the prismatic effect of the layer of tears in the cul-de-sac and reaching over the cornea. (See "Recueil d'Ophthalmologie," March, 1880.)—B.]

Inflammation of the lachrymal gland (Dacryo-adenitis) is generally chronic in character, and gives rise to a more or less considerable, firm, nodulated, immovable swelling at the upper and outer margin of the orbit. The upper portion of the tumor disappears beneath the edge of the orbit, but can be readily followed if the tip of the little finger is inserted beneath the upper and outer orbital ridge. The skin is movable over the tumor, and the upper eyelid is somewhat reddened and puffy, sometimes, indeed, the redness and swelling may be very considerable, so that the upper eyelid hangs down in a thick, massive fold over the lower. The conjunctiva is somewhat injected and swollen, especially at the retro-tarsal fold, and there may also be considerable chemosis. As a rule, the swelling is but slightly painful, either spontaneously, or to the touch; but if the inflammation is very acute, the pain may be severe, and extend to the corresponding side of the face and head. If the swelling acquires any considerable size, the eyeball will be displaced downwards and inwards, and its movements be impaired in the opposite direction. The inflammation generally runs a very chronic and protracted course, the swelling either gradually undergoing absorption, or chronic suppuration occurring; but if the tumor is so large as to displace the eyeball, or impair its mobility, it will be necessary to remove it. Sometimes both lachrymal glands[1] become simultaneously inflamed, giving rise to a symmetrical swelling at the upper and outer edge of each orbit. In rarer instances, the inflammation assumes an acute and sthenic character, there being great heat, redness, and swelling of the part, with perhaps a rapid formation of pus, so that the disease assumes all the appearances of an acute abscess. The latter points, the skin gives way, and there is an escape of pus, which may continue to ooze out for some length of time; subsequently the opening closes, the inflammatory products become absorbed, and the swelling gradually disappears. Sometimes, however, the aperture remains patent, and a minute fistulous opening is established, through which the tears ooze forth. The fistula may also occur in chronic suppuration of the gland, being situated either on the external skin or on the conjunctival surface. Such fistulæ prove extremely obstinate and intractable in the treatment, and if the aperture should become accidentally stopped up, severe inflammatory symptoms may supervene.

Inflammation of the lachrymal gland may be due to cold, or to a traumatic origin. It may also supervene upon chronic inflammation of the conjunctiva or cornea. Von Graefe mentions cases in which chronic swelling and congestion of the gland were produced by the protracted use of a compress bandage, the retention of the tears in the gland probably exciting irritation.

In chronic dacryo-adenitis, we may endeavor to produce absorption of the inflammatory products by the local application of ointments containing iodide of potassium, iodine, or mercury; or by painting tincture of iodine over the part. In the acute form, hot cataplasms and leeches should be applied, and if suppuration threatens, a free incision should be made into the swelling. The same is to be done if pus is formed in chronic cases. [When chemosis is present, the conjunctiva should be scarified.—B.]

Simple hypertrophy of the lachrymal gland is a rare affection, and may occasionally be somewhat difficult to diagnose with certainty. It may ensue upon repeated inflammatory attacks, or occur spontaneously, and is most frequently met with in children; indeed it may even be congenital. This condition is particularly characterized by the extreme slowness with which the swelling increases in size, and the absence of all redness, pain, or other inflammatory symptoms. The tumor is circumscribed, more or less firm, elastic, and nodulated, and may, in time, acquire so considerable a size as to displace the eyeball and curtail its movements. Attempts should be made to disperse it by the application of iodine, mercurial ointment, etc.; but these generally prove unavailing, and recourse must be had to operative interference.

Cysts of the lachrymal gland[2] (Dacryops) are of very rare occurrence, and present the appearance of a little tumor, varying in size from a small bean to a hazel-nut, in the upper and outer portion of the upper eyelid, and extending back beneath the edge of the orbit. If at all considerable in size, it becomes observable to the eye, and readily so to the touch. On everting

---

[1] Vide Haynes Walton, "Med. Times and Gazette," 1854, p. 817; and Horner, "Kl. Monatsbl.," 1866, p. 257.

[2] Vide a very interesting paper on this subject by Mr. Hulke, "R. L. O. H. Rep.,"

the lid there is noticed, close beneath the conjunctiva, a bluish-pink, semi-transparent, elastic, and somewhat fluctuating swelling, consisting, perhaps, of several nodulated segments of varying size. It springs still more into view, if the lid is retracted and pressed in a downward direction. The swelling, moreover, increases suddenly and markedly in size if the patient cries, or the secretion of tears is stimulated by the application of some irritant to the conjunctiva.

The cyst is generally due to the stoppage of one or more of the excretory ducts of the gland, so that the tears are retained, and distend the portion of the duct and gland above the point at which the obstruction is situated. The duct is sometimes, however, patent, so that the tears may slowly ooze out, and the cyst be emptied by pressure.[1] According to Schmidt,[2] the disease is sometimes congenital. The best mode of treatment is to establish an artificial opening on the inside of the conjunctiva, so that a free exit may be afforded for the escape of the tears. For if an attempt is made to remove the cyst entire, we shall generally fail, as its wall is very delicate, and the tumor is very apt to recur. Moreover, there is much fear of leaving a small, fistulous opening, which may prove extremely obstinate and intractable in the treatment. De Wecker has, however, lately recorded a successful case of removal of a dacryops.[3] An artificial opening of sufficient size may be gained by simply making a linear incision of from one and a half lines to two lines in extent, and keeping it patent by passing a probe every day along its edges, until the latter have become cicatrized. Or again, von Graefe's[4] plan may be adopted, of passing a fine, threaded, curved needle through the aperture of the duct (if this is patent) and carrying it along the anterior wall of the cyst to a distance of about two lines, at which point it is again to be brought out, so that a bridge of the anterior cyst wall of about two lines in extent is included within the thread, which is to be tied in a loose loop. The intermediate bridge may either be allowed to slough through, or may be divided at the end of a few days, and thus an artificial opening will be established, through which the lachrymal secretion can flow off.

Fistula of the lachrymal gland is occasionally observed, and may ensue upon dacryops or an acute or chronic abscess, or be due to a traumatic origin, supervening upon some injury of the gland or some operation, as for instance the opening or removal of a cyst. The fistulous opening is generally extremely minute, only admitting, perhaps, the point of a very fine bristle. Through this little aperture the tears ooze slowly forth, and their quantity increases with the augmentation of the secretion of the lachrymal gland during any mental excitement, or irritation of the eye from dust or wind, astringent applications, etc. The affection often proves somewhat obstinate and intractable. The edge of the fistulous opening may be touched with a fine point of nitrate of silver, after the edges have perhaps been first pared; or the obliteration may be attempted by the galvano-caustic apparatus. Again, we may succeed in occluding it by freshening the edges of the aperture, and then closing it with a fine suture. Sometimes, however, severe inflammatory symptoms, followed by the formation of pus, ensue upon the healing or blocking up of the fistulous opening, recurring again and again with great severity. Alfred Graefe[5] narrates a case of this kind, in which he was finally obliged to excise the lachrymal gland, in order to cure the disease and relieve the patient of this constant suffering and annoyance. Mr. Bowman[6] succeeded in

[1] *Vide* Von Graefe, "A. f. O.," vii. 2, 1.
[2] " Lehre von den Augenkrankheiten," 1817.
[3] " Kl. Monatsbl.," 1867, p. 34.
[4] "A. f. O.," vii. 2, 2.
[5] "A. f. O.," viii. 1, 279.
[6] "R. L. O. H. Rep.," 1, 288.

curing an obstinate and long-established external fistula of the lachrymal gland, by establishing an artificial opening on the conjunctival surface by a small seton, and then closing the external aperture.

[Hulke's method also seems to give good results. The two ends of a silk ligature, each armed with a needle, are passed through the external fistulous opening in such a manner that one needle penetrates the conjunctiva of the upper lid above the other. Both ends of the ligature are thus brought out in the conjunctival cul-de-sac, and, being drawn tight, inclose a triangular piece of the upper lid in their grasp, the apex of which is at the fistula, and the base in the conjunctiva. The ends are then cut off, and the fistula soon heals.—B.]

Various kinds of tumor are met with in the lachrymal gland, but by far the most frequent are those of a sarcomatous nature. Cancer is of very rare occurrence, and is probably always secondary, extending from the neighboring tissues to the gland. Knapp,[1] however, reports a case of hypertrophy of the lachrymal gland with carcinoma.

[New growths in the lachrymal gland are rare occurrences. Many different kinds of neoplasms have been described by various authors as met with here, such as simple hypertrophy, adenoma, adenoid, colloid, sarcoma, myxoma, fungus medullaris, encephaloid cancer, scirrhus, etc. Becker's investigations have, however, rendered it probable that these all probably represent different stages of development of the same growth. (See "Bericht ueber die Augenklinik der Wiener Universität," 1863–65.) A case of mixed enchondroma and hypertropy of the lachrymal gland has been reported by Busch. Schirmer is inclined, with Becker, to classify all the various growths under the common name of *adenoid*. Chloroma has been described as a greenish, homogeneous, hard mass, always malignant, and causing death by attacking the dura mater. Isolated cases have also been reported of angioma, hydatid cysts, and dermoid growths. (See "Graefe und Saemisch's Handb.," vii. p. 10.) The symptoms are the same for all these growths, one of the first being exophthalmus, with more or less pain in the orbit and upper lid. A careful examination will always lead to a recognition of the trouble, and the operative removal of the tumor and glands should be done as early as possible, in order, if possible, to prevent permanent damage to the eye and optic nerve.

Mollière and Chandelux report a case of intra-acinous colloid epithelioma(?) in a boy, æt. 15. Its growth was of unknown duration, and had been accompanied by orbital pains. There was moderate exophthalmus; the tumor was ovoid, its long diameter being transverse, and was not adherent to the skin of the upper lid. It was hard, somewhat painful, lobulated, and adherent to the upper and outer wall of the orbit. It was enucleated with facility. It proved to be an epithelioma, developed within the acini of the gland, and had undergone colloid degeneration. Five months after the operation the tumor reappeared, and a second operation was done nine months after the first. This time, the growth had involved more of the orbital tissue. It again recurred, and ten months later had filled the entire orbit, and there were nodules beneath the skin all around the orbital region, and the bones of the face were deeply involved. ("Lyon Méd.," November 1881.)—B.]

Sometimes the secretions of the gland may undergo chalky degeneration and dacryoliths be formed. [This tendency to concretion is known as lithiasis, and is exceedingly rare. The concretions should be removed from the conjunctival surface, as they occasion conjunctivitis, episcleritis, and pannus. ("Centralblatt für prakt. Augenheilk.," December, 1880.)—B.]

---

[1] "Kl. Monatsbl.," 1865, 378.

Extirpation of the lachrymal gland may have to be performed for hypertrophy or chronic inflammation of this organ, if it produces much disfigurement or displacement of the eyeball. It has, however, been lately strongly recommended as a cure for very obstinate and severe cases of lachrymal disease. This operation has been particularly practised by Mr. Zachariah Laurence for the latter class of diseases, and a full description of the mode of operating will be found in his paper upon the subject.[1] The patient having been placed under the influence of chloroform, the surgeon is to divide with a scalpel the skin, muscle, and fascia over the upper and outer third of the orbit to the extent of about an inch, so as freely to enter the orbit at the situation of the lachrymal gland. The latter may easily be felt with the tip of the little finger as a small, hard body. If there is any difficulty in finding the gland, Mr. Laurence recommends that the external commissure of the lids should be at once divided by a horizontal incision, which should meet the inner extremity of the first. Thus a triangular flap will be formed with its apex inwards and the gland can be more readily reached. The latter is then to be firmly seized with a sharp hook, drawn forth, and carefully excised. Tolerably free hæmorrhage generally ensues, but this can be readily arrested by the application of a stream of cold water. The wound is to be closed with fine silver wire sutures; this should not, however, be done until all bleeding has ceased, otherwise, there may be extensive extravasation of blood into the cellular tissue of the upper lid.

2.—IMPEDIMENT TO THE FLOW OF TEARS—☞ STILLICIDIUM LACHRYMARUM.

Although the term epiphora is generally applied to every kind of "watery eye," this is, strictly speaking, erroneous and hence it should only be used in those cases in which there is an undue secretion of tears and of the mucus secreted by the conjunctiva, so that the canaliculi cannot carry the tears off, but they flow over the lids and cheek. The epiphora may be due to some irritation conveyed to the lachrymal nerves from the conjunctiva or cornea. Thus if a foreign body is lodged in the conjunctiva or cornea, a considerable degree of lachrymation at once takes place. The same occurs in many of the inflammations of the eye, more especially in some of the forms of keratitis and also in some of the morbid changes of the deeper tissues of the eyeball. Mental emotion will also produce it. The degree of lachrymation will, of course, vary with the nature and intensity of the morbid process and also according to individual circumstances. From this condition, we must distinguish that in which there is no oversecretion of tears but the lachrymation is due to an impediment or obstruction to their efflux through the lachrymal passages. This is termed "stillicidium lachrymarum." In such cases the tears collect at the corner of the eye, causing the patient frequently to wipe the eyes, or else they slowly flow over the edge of the lower lid which gradually becomes sore, red, and swollen, from constant moistening. This constant wiping of the lids then tends still more to increase the lachrymation, and to alter the position and the structure of the punctum and canaliculi. The eyes often become very irritable, the patients complaining much of a constant smarting, heat, and itching in them, which is much aggravated by reading, sewing, writing, and by exposure to bright light, wind, or dust. In the later stages of this irritability of the eye and of the lachrymation is increased, very obstinate and intractable inflammation of the edge of the lid and of the conjunctiva may ensue, which sets defiance to every form of collyrium or topical application, but readily yields if the impediment in the lachrymal apparatus is removed, and the stillicidium cured. The obstruction to the efflux of the tears may be situated at any point of the lachrymal canal, in the puncta, the canaliculi, the sac, or the nasal duct.

We sometimes notice in elderly persons, or after a severe illness, that the orbicularis palpebrarum is so much relaxed, that the tears are no longer propelled by it into the puncta, but that they collect in the central portion of the lower lid, which is sunk down and somewhat everted, in the form of a little pouch or hollow. In such cases, the fluid does not readily pass into the puncta, even although these may be patent. This *relaxation of the orbicularis is, in elderly persons, often due to atrophy of the orbital cellular tissue, and perhaps of the orbicularis muscle.

[*The edge of the lids* may be *abnormally situated*, being turned too far in towards the eye from cicatricial contraction of the conjunctiva, or too far out by contraction of the skin. In either case, there will be an overflow of tears. The same occurs from *abnormal size* or *position* of the *caruncle*, and here the latter must be removed.—B.]

The *puncta lacrymalia* may undergo certain *changes of position* and *form, or even become obliterated*. In their normal position, they are turned directly inwards towards the eyeball, so that the tears which collect in the lacus lacrymarum near the caruncle may be readily guided into the puncta and canaliculi, thence to make their way through the lachrymal sac and nasal duct. Now, when the position of the punctum is changed, so that instead of being just sufficiently inverted, it stands erect or is everted, the tears can no longer enter it, but must collect in the corner of the eye and overflow the lid, and a very slight, perhaps almost imperceptible, displacement will suffice for this. It has already been stated that this constant moistening of the lids soon makes them very irritable, swollen, and inflamed, which will tend still more to evert the punctum. The malposition of the punctum is most frequently met with after diseases which cause a shrinking of the external skin of the eyelid, as, for instance, eczema, or inflammation of the edge of the lid, erysipelas, &c. Also, if the conjunctiva or caruncle is much swollen or hypertrophied, so that the edge of the lid is somewhat pushed away from the eye. Small tumors or cysts, situated close to the punctum, may also produce it. On the other hand, the malposition of the punctum may not consist in its being everted, but in the edge of the lid and punctum being turned in, which may occur when the eye is much sunken in the orbit. This faulty position of the punctum is very frequently overlooked. The punctum, and a portion of the canaliculus, may also be dilated and have lost its contractility, appearing in the form of a prominent nipple, so that the entrance of the tears is rendered difficult. Or again, the punctum may be greatly contracted in size, or even quite obliterated, having become covered by a layer of epithelium. This is apt to be the case in very chronic inflammation of the conjunctiva and edge of the eyelid, in which the secretions are altered and diminished, and a thin layer of desiccated epithelium is formed over the free edge of the lid and the punctum.

The best mode of treating malposition of the punctum—whether it be erect, everted, or turned in—is by Mr. Bowman's operation of slitting up the punctum and the canaliculus, and thus changing the closed into an open channel, into which the tears can gain ready entrance. This little operation may be performed in various ways, and although it appears simple and easy enough, yet it sometimes requires a certain degree of nicety and care to perform it quickly and with success, more especially if the patient is timid and restless. Let us suppose that the lower punctum of the right eye is to be divided. The patient should be seated with his head supported against the back of an arm-chair, or the chest of the surgeon. The latter should then, standing behind the patient, introduce a very fine sharp-pointed grooved director (Fig. 16) vertically into the punctum, and then, turning it horizontally, he should run it (with the groove upwards) along the canaliculus as far as the inner edge of the lachrymal sac. Whilst the director is passing along the canaliculus, the skin of the lower eyelid should be put tightly on the stretch, by being drawn outwards and somewhat downwards with the forefinger of the left hand. Otherwise, if the lining membrane of the canaliculus is swollen or lax, it may become tucked up in front of the director, and thus somewhat impede its progress. When the point of the director has reached the further end of the canaliculus, the instrument is to be taken into the left hand, between the forefinger and thumb, the lower lid being at the same time put upon the stretch by the ring finger of the same hand. The patient being then directed to look upwards, the point of a cataract knife (held between the forefinger and thumb of the right hand, the ring finger of which is at the same time to raise the upper lid) is inserted into the punctum, and its edge run along the groove of the director to the inner wall of the sac, so that the lower canaliculus may be slit up to its whole extent. If the patient is very timid and restless, and nips his eyelids very firmly together, the aid of an assistant is generally required. To obviate this, some surgeons employ a very fine pair of straight, blunt-pointed scissors, the one blade of which is to be inserted into the punctum and run along to the extremity of the canaliculus, which should be at the same time put upon the stretch and then divided at one sharp cut. I myself prefer Bowman's narrow probe-pointed canaliculus knife to any other instrument. It should, however, be made very narrow, and its probe-point be very small, otherwise it may be difficult to enter it if the punctum is very minute. In such a case, the latter should first be somewhat dilated with the point of the director, and this will generally suffice for the ready admission of the point of the knife, which should then be run along, with its sharp edge upwards, quite up to the extremity of the canaliculus, and the latter be divided along its whole course, by lifting the knife somewhat from heel to point. Care should be taken that the canaliculus is divided to its full extent. For slitting the upper punctum and canaliculus, this knife, or the grooved director and cataract knife, may also be employed, although I generally prefer Weber's beak-pointed knife for this purpose. In selecting this instrument, we must be particular that the nodular point, as well as the cutting portion of the blade, is not made too large, else a difficulty will be experienced in inserting it into the upper punctum, and passing it along the canaliculus. The beak point should be passed well down into the sac, so that the upper canaliculus may be divided to its whole extent. The bleeding which follows the slitting up of the canaliculus is generally but very slight, and when it has ceased, the film of blood-coagulum should be removed with a small pair of forceps, from the whole length of the wound, and a little olive oil be applied to the latter, so as to prevent its closing. Moreover, it is advisable to pass a director along the incision every day for a few days, so as to keep this patent.

Fig. 16.

But the canaliculi may also be contracted, or partially or wholly obliterated, their passage being narrowed by a swollen and inflamed condition of the lining membrane, or from cicatricial changes which the latter has undergone, in consequence, perhaps, of preceding inflammation. Such cicatrices are most frequently met with after a granular condition of the lining membrane, for the granular inflammation may extend from the conjunctiva into the canal, and even into the lachrymal sac. The cicatrices may, however, be of traumatic origin, having been perhaps produced by wounds or burns, or by the bruising and tearing of the canal caused by a clumsy and rude passage of the probes. The swollen and turgid condition of the canaliculus is due either to an inflammation extending to it from the conjunctival or the lachrymal sac, or may be caused by the presence of some foreign body within it, such as an eyelash, a dacryolith, or a small fungus. Although the stricture may exist at any point of the canaliculi, it is most frequently situated at the spot where the latter open into the sac. [Small tumors like hordeola may compress the canaliculus and obliterate its calibre, or the canal may be blocked by concretions of lime. Polypi have also been found in the canal. The presence of all these obstructions is easily recognized by a fine probe, and the treatment is to slit up the canaliculus and remove them at once.—B.]

Should the lower punctum be obliterated (atresia) and quite invisible on the most careful search (aided by a magnifying lens), an ingenious operation of Mr. Streatfeild[1] may be performed; viz., after the upper punctum and canaliculus have been divided, a fine director (suitably bent) is to be passed by this aperture into the inferior canaliculus, and, if possible, through the lower punctum; if not, the lower canaliculus can easily be laid open upon it. This operation will also be found very serviceable in those cases in which the lower punctum and a portion of the lower canal are obliterated. The converse may also be done, the director may be introduced by the lower punctum, and brought out by the upper. These operations, however, often require considerable dexterity and patience.

If the canaliculus is only narrowed, it should be well laid open in the manner above directed. If the stricture exists at the neck of the sac, and is firm and contracted, it should be freely divided with a canula knife, which is to be introduced sheathed, and then, when it has arrived opposite the point of stricture, the sheath is drawn back, and the blade uncovered. This instrument is best introduced by the upper canaliculus, which should have been previously divided; or the stricture may be incised by Weber's knife. After the division, the stricture must be treated by the use of probes. I shall return to this subject, and to these instruments, in treating of stricture of the lachrymal passages. If the lower canaliculus (owing to a swollen and thickened condition of the lid) remains everted, even after having been divided, Mr. Critchett[2] advises that a portion of the posterior wall of the canal should be seized and snipped out with scissors, "thus effecting the treble objects of drawing the canal more inwards towards the caruncle, of forming a reservoir into which the tears may run, and of preventing any reunion of the parts." [When there is any eversion of the lid, it is better to incise the canaliculus in a direction backwards towards the eyeball, and not directly upwards, as is usually done. If this does not succeed in curing the overflow, then Critchett's method can be resorted to.—B.] If the whole or the greater portion of the lower canaliculus is obliterated, it will be different. In such cases, if the patient is troubled with epiphora, the upper canaliculus should

[1] " R. L. O. H. Rep.," iii. 4.
[2] Lectures on the Diseases of the Lachrymal Apparatus, " Lancet," 1868, vol. ii. p. 697.

be freely slit open along its whole extent, so that the tears may gain an easy entrance; but if this should not suffice, and the lower canal be only partially obliterated, we should endeavor to pass back a very fine grooved director from the opening in the upper canaliculus into the lower one, and lay this open upon the director.

3.—[PHLEGMONOUS] INFLAMMATION OF THE LACHRYMAL SAC. DACRYOCYSTITIS [PURULENTA-BLENNORRHŒA.—B.].

This disease is frequently very acute in character, and is then accompanied by intense pain, which extends to the corresponding side of the head and face, and there is, moreover, often marked constitutional disturbance or feverishness. The skin over the region of the lachrymal sac and its vicinity becomes swollen, red, and glistening, and an oval swelling of varying size appears at this spot. The inflammatory swelling often also extends to the eyelids and face. The former become very puffy, and œdematous, so that they are only opened with difficulty, and then it is perhaps noticed that the conjunctiva is injected and swollen, and that there is a certain degree of chemosis. From this great swelling of the lids and face, the case assumes somewhat the appearance of erysipelas of the face, for which it might indeed be mistaken by a superficial observer. The swelling is often very sensitive, the patient involuntarily shrinking back from any attempt to touch it. If the inflammatory symptoms are but moderate, the sensitiveness is much less marked, and on exerting a certain degree of pressure, we may be able to press out a small quantity of pus through the puncta, or it may pass down the nasal duct. The swelling and thickening of the lining membrane of the passages may, however, be so considerable, as to prevent the exit of any discharge. Moreover, the opening into the sac may have become somewhat displaced, on account of the swelling of the lining membrane and the enlargement of the cavity of the sac, and thus offer another obstacle to the escape of the contents.

But when the inflammatory swelling has somewhat subsided, and the size of the ducts is thus increased, the discharge may often be very freely squeezed out of the puncta, welling up at the inner angle of the eye and flowing over the lid. Together with the pain, the patient experiences a feeling of dryness and weight in that side of the nose; and if the disease has been preceded by blennorrhœa of the sac, or a stricture in the lachrymal passages, there is always a distinct history of the pre-existence of a more or less considerable and obstinate epiphora. In the acute inflammation of the sac, the onset of the disease is generally very rapid and intense, reaching its acme in the course of a few days. It may, however, be more protracted and chronic in its course, and all the inflammatory symptoms be less marked and severe. If the disease is left to itself, we find that the swelling gains in size, the skin over it becomes thinner and thinner, a distinct feeling of fluctuation is experienced, and finally the abscess makes a spontaneous opening through the skin, and a considerable amount of pus escapes. The perforation is rapidly followed by a great diminution in the intensity of the inflammatory symptoms. For some time, matter will continue to ooze out through the opening, but, finally, the latter may close and cicatrize firmly, and the disease become cured; or there may remain a chronic inflammation of the sac, which often proves very obstinate and intractable. Fresh inflammatory exacerbations supervene, pus be again collected, and thus a relapse take place. In ⸱ instan the inflammation is so severe as to destroy the lining membrane of the sac, and the latter may thus become obliterated. Or again, the aperture in the skin may scab over, pus become again collected in the sac, and force its way once more through the opening; this, perhaps, occurring again and again, until finally a fistulous opening is left, through which a thin muco-purulent discharge and the tears constantly ooze. In yet other cases, the sac may undergo ulceration at one point, and the matter escape into the neighboring cellular tissue, thus giving rise to a secondary sac or pouch, perforation may finally take place, and a fistulous opening be established, leading (perhaps by a long track) into this diverticulum. In some instances, there are several such pouches burrowing beneath the skin in different directions. They are, however, generally, only met with in the chronic form of dacryocystitis.

Inflammation of the lachrymal sac is often due to an extension of the inflammation of the mucous lining of the nostril to the nasal duct and the sac, or downwards from the conjunctiva and canaliculus. Hence, it may supervene upon nasal catarrh, or conjunctivitis (more especially the granular form). [This is a much more frequent cause than is generally supposed. It is the editor's opinion that the majority of cases both of catarrhal and purulent dacryocystitis are caused by a primary inflammation in the lining of the nose, be it catarrhal or syphilitic. Periostitis of the duct and nose is a very common complication.—B.] It may also follow blennorrhœa of the sac. Periostitis and caries of the nasal bones, more especially in persons of a scrofulous or syphilitic diathesis, may likewise produce it. It sometimes occurs as a primary affection, being then generally due to exposure to cold and wet. It is often stated that erysipelas is a frequent cause, but it would rather appear that the latter disease is the effect, and not the cause.

Our chief effort in treating these cases must be directed towards the establishment of a free and ready exit for the discharge. This is best done by dividing the punctum and canaliculus quite into the sac. If the opening into the latter is somewhat contracted, I am in the habit of dividing the upper canaliculus with Weber's knife, and then passing the latter into the sac, and freely incising its neck. In this way, a very free opening is obtained, through which the contents of the sac can be readily emptied, for a slight pressure upon the latter will suffice to cause the escape of the pus. A probe may then be passed, so as to dilate the neck of the sac and the nasal duct. Agnew[1] sometimes opens the sac between the commissure of the lids and the lower punctum; this is easily done, as the swollen lachrymal sac forms a prominence here. If the mucous lining is much inflamed and swollen, it is wise to abstain from too much meddling and probing, as this only tends to irritate, and excite fresh inflammation. A free exit having been obtained for the discharge, the pain and inflammatory symptoms soon subside, and, moreover, all danger of perforation is prevented. Indeed, by at once employing this mode of treatment, we may often avert this danger, even when the skin over the swelling has already become very thin. To aid in allaying the inflammation, warm poppy fomentations, or a leech or two, may be applied; but if the disease has advanced so far that perforation is imminent, the sac should be freely laid open with a scalpel, and the pus evacuated. The incision should run in a downward and outward direction, and be sufficiently large to permit of the ready escape of the discharge. A narrow strip of lint should be inserted into the sac, so as to keep the wound open for a few days, and allow of the draining off of the matter. A warm poultice is to be applied after the operation, and frequently changed for the first day or

[1] "Medical Record," Oct. 15, 1870.

two. When the inflammation has considerably abated, the canaliculus should be divided and a probe passed into the nasal duct, so that a free passage may be made for the discharge and the tears. The opening into the sac will then soon close firmly, leaving but a very slight cicatrix behind. To hasten the cicatrization, the edge of the opening may be lightly touched with sulphate of copper. If perforation has already taken place before the surgeon is consulted, the canaliculus and neck of the sac should be divided, and a probe passed. In such cases, the edges of the perforation are often very ragged and granular: indeed, there may even be an ulcerated opening of a considerable size. This should be touched with sulphate of copper, a probe be passed daily through the duct, and then the fistulous opening will soon be found rapidly to heal. If any fistulous openings exist in connection with diverticula, they should be laid open, and caused to heal from the bottom.

Should a condition of chronic inflammation of the sac, accompanied by a muco-purulent discharge, persist for some time after the perforation is closed, and the more acute inflammatory symptoms have disappeared, the sac should be syringed out with an astringent lotion. Before employing this, it is well to inject the sac with water so as to dash out all the discharge, and then a weak astringent injection, zinc. sulph. gr. ij–iv, or alum gr. ij. aq. dest. f $\bar{3}$j) should be employed. This will diminish the inflammatory swelling and secretion of the lachrymal passages. This injection should be used every day, or every other day, according to circumstances, and will generally soon produce very considerable improvement. Its strength should gradually be increased. Various kinds of syringes have been devised for this purpose, but the best is a small graduated glass syringe holding about half an ounce. I am in the habit of employing one made for me by Messrs. Weiss, which differs somewhat from that in ordinary use. The instrument consists of two separate parts, the canula and the syringe.

The silver canula is of the size of Bowman's No. 6 probe, and is about three inches in length. At the top is a cross-bar, by which it can be easily bent and directed, and beyond this bar is a portion of India-rubber tubing about one and a quarter inch in length, ending in a silver mount into which the nozzle of the syringe fits firmly. The advantage of the India-rubber tubing is, that when the canula is passed quite down into the nasal duct, the patient can lean forward with his face over a basin, and the surgeon, standing in front of the patient, can bend the India-rubber tube forward to the necessary extent, and readily insert the nozzle of the syringe, and thus inject the fluid without any difficulty: whereas, with the ordinary silver canula, it is often difficult to do so, on account of the prominence of the brow. The fitting of the nozzle into the canula by a plain mount is much better than by a screw, because, if the screw sticks a little, or the patient is restless, the lining membrane of the lachrymal passages may easily be injured in the endeavor to screw the nozzle on. The instrument is to be used in the following manner. The canula is to be passed down, by the upper or lower canaliculus, through the sac into the nasal duct, and allowed to remain there for five or ten minutes, so as to dilate the passage. The patient being then directed to lean his face well forward over a basin, the nozzle of the syringe is gently inserted into the canula, and the fluid slowly injected, which will flow out through the nostril into the basin. Whilst injecting, the surgeon should, with his left hand, seize the canula by the cross-bar, and steady it carefully, so that the fluid may come in contact with every part of the duct and sac. The first injection should consist of water, in order to wash away the discharge; the canula should then be re-introduced, and the astringent injection be used. Mr. Bowman employs a small India-rubber ball syringe, but the stream from this is often too weak to force its way through, if the lining membrane of the sac and duct is greatly swollen, or the stricture very firm. If the case proves very obstinate, and the patient cannot possibly submit to a lengthened course of treatment, and is yet anxiously desirous to be relieved of the complaint, it may be necessary to destroy the sac, but such a course should only be followed in very rare and exceptional instances. I shall, however, return to this subject when treating of blennorrhœa, and of obstinate strictures of the duct and sac.

4.—[CATARRHAL INFLAMMATION] OF THE SAC (MUCOCELE).

This disease is often developed very slowly and insidiously, coming on almost without the patient being aware that there is anything the matter, except perhaps a little epiphora, and a slight and occasional swelling in the region of the lachrymal sac, accompanied, if the latter is pressed, by a little oozing out of turbid, viscid discharge, which, passing over the cornea, dims the sight. The swelling of the sac varies considerably in size and hardness. It is generally elastic and firm, and the skin somewhat red; on squeezing out the discharge, the tip of the finger sinks a little into the skin. The distention of the sac undergoes considerable alterations, varying with the changes in the temperature, and the exposure to which the patient subjects himself. As long as the weather is warm and dry, the patient may be quite free from any trouble, but as soon as he exposes himself to a cold bleak wind or a damp atmosphere, the sac becomes inflamed and swollen, the eye is watery, and on pressure upon the sac, a copious discharge wells up through the puncta. The frequent recurrence or long existence of this condition leads to a thickened and villous state of the lining membrane of the sac and ducts, and the secretion becomes more thick and muco-purulent in character. If it constantly regurgitates through the puncta, these and the canaliculi may become somewhat dilated. Stricture of some part of the nasal duct, or of the canaliculus near its opening into the sac, if it has not already occurred, will generally soon supervene.

In some cases, the sac, instead of being thickened and hypertrophied, becomes thinned and greatly distended; being filled with a thin, glairy, viscid fluid which flows down the nasal duct, or oozes up through the puncta.

[Catarrh] of the lachrymal sac is almost always met with as a secondary affection, being often consecutive upon an inflammation of the Schneiderian membrane, which, ascending along the nasal duct, has reached the sac. Hence nasal catarrh, and periostitis or caries of the nasal bones, are not unfrequent causes of the disease. Or it may supervene upon inflammation of the conjunctiva (more especially granular ophthalmia), or of the edge of the lid. Malposition or contraction of the puncta, or a narrowing or stricture of the lachrymal canal, also often produce it. Indeed, obstructions in the lachrymal passages, either above or below the sac, are very fruitful sources of blennorrhœa. This disease is, therefore, often met with in cases in which there is a narrowing, obliteration, or eversion of the puncta; or a contraction or stricture of the canaliculus or of the nasal duct, which may be due to inflammatory swelling of the lining membrane, or to the presence of cicatrices. Polypi or other growths, which by compression narrow or obstruct the duct, may also give rise to it. Persons in whom the root of the nose is very flat and broad, and the eyes far apart, are very subject to diseases of the lachrymal apparatus, on account of the diminution of the antero-posterior diameter of the duct; but the same thing may occur, as Arlt and de Wecker point out, if the nose is very prominent and narrow, so that the passage is much narrowed laterally. Blennorrhœa of the sac often supervenes upon acute inflammation of the latter, which, after having perhaps caused repeated perforation and escape of the discharge, passes over into a state of chronic inflammation, accompanied by a thin muco-purulent discharge. Acute inflammatory exacerbations recur every now and then, and a more or less extensive and firm stricture of the lachrymal or nasal duct is almost always present.

Only in very rare instances do we find that the disease, if left to itself, undergoes any considerable or permanent improvement, much less a cure. For even in spite of the best and most patient treatment, it often proves very obstinate and intractable. The lining membrane of the sac and duct becomes hypertrophied and swollen, and often undergoes extensive cicatricial changes, being transformed into a fibro-tendinous tissue, and the discharge becoming thin, glairy, and viscid, or in some cases of a thick gluey character (Stellwag). [In mucocele of the sac with simple lachrymation, Landolt probes the canals with the conical sound, without incising them, and then injects a solution of sodium borate (1–200). If it does not pass, he incises the upper canal, and injects a solution of sodium sulphate (1–150).—B.]

Strictures of the lachrymal passages vary very considerably in extent, firmness, and situation. Their most frequent seat is the point where the canaliculi open into the sac, or where the latter passes into the nasal duct;

[Fig. 17.] but they may also be situated at a lower part of the duct, and hence the necessity of always passing the probe through the whole length of the latter, in order that we may ascertain whether any stricture exists at its lower portion. If the stricture be due to a thickened swollen condition of the lining membrane, and if it be considerable in extent, it will oppose a certain degree of obstruction to the passage of the probe, and will embrace the latter firmly and closely, but will yield to the gentle yet steady pressure of the instrument. The dense cicatricial stricture affords a more obstinate resistance, and it may be difficult to pass even a very small probe, without employing a considerable degree of force. The symptoms to which a stricture gives rise are epiphora, blennorrhœa or inflammation of the sac, and a glairy, viscid, or muco-purulent discharge.

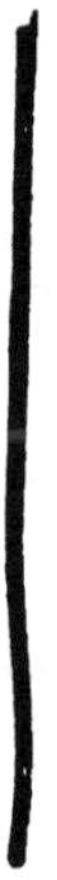

The first and fundamental principle in the treatment of blennorrhœa of the sac and stricture of the lachrymal passages is, to divide one or both puncta and canaliculi, and to pass a probe down through the nasal duct. The mode of dividing the puncta and the canaliculi has been already described. The probes which are best adapted for catheterization, are those of Mr. Bowman,[1] which are made of silver, and of six different sizes. No. 1 is very small, like a fine hair probe; No. 6 is about one-twentieth of an inch in diameter [and is represented of its actual size in Fig. 17.—H.]. Mr. Pridgin Teale, of Leeds, recommends a bullet probe, which is also preferred by Mr. Critchett,[2] who thinks that it passes more readily, and is less apt to lacerate the mucous lining, or to make a false passage. [Dr. Williams,[3] of Boston, advocates the use of flexible probes with bulbous extremities, of the size of Bowman's series, but slender for one-third of the distance from the bulb to

[1] "R. L. O. H. Rep." i 10.   [2] "Lancet." 1864. vol. i. 147.
[3] "Transactions of the Ophthalmological Society." 1869.—H.]

the flat disk in the middle. They are of alloyed silver, and have an elastic flexibility without being able to bend upon themselves in encountering obstructions. Dr. Williams has found in practice, that these probes adapt themselves to the sinuosities of the passages, and can be introduced with more facility and less pain, and are less likely to take a wrong passage than Bowman's probes, which, if not bent so as precisely to correspond with the direction of the duct in each particular individual, often lacerate the mucous lining of the passages, giving rise to pain and hemorrhage, and retarding cure by causing local inflammation.—H.] I, as a rule, use Mr. Bowman's probes, but frequently employ a considerably larger size than No. 6. The instrument is to be introduced in the following manner: The end of the probe having been slightly bent, so that it may pass more readily forward into the nasal duct, its point should be inserted vertically into the lower punctum, the skin being at the same time put on the stretch, and then passed horizontally along the opened canaliculus until its extremity reaches the inner wall of the sac, which is easily recognized by its presenting a hard, bony obstruction to the probe. The latter is then to be turned vertically, the convexity of the bend looking backwards, and slowly and gently passed into the sac; when the latter is gained, the direction of the instrument must be slightly altered, the point being directed somewhat outwards and forwards, so that it may readily pass into the nasal duct, through which it is to be pushed until it reaches the floor of the nose. When the lining membrane of the sac and of the duct is much swollen and hyper-trophied, it is sometimes rather difficult to find this entrance, as it may be somewhat displaced or contracted, or more or less covered by a small fold of the mucous membrane, which thus forms a little valve over it. If, after some careful searching, we do not succeed in finding the opening into the nasal duct, it is better to withdraw the probe, and to wait for a day or two until the inflammatory swelling has subsided, than to attempt to force the passage of the probe; for this may not only produce severe laceration of the membrane, but lead to the formation of a false passage, or the probe should be withdrawn, its curvature somewhat altered, and then be again inserted, in the hopes of finding the aperture. The first probe that is passed should only be of medium size (No. 3 or 4 of Bowman), but if the stricture is very considerable, No. 2, or even No. 1, may have to be tried before it can be passed. The instrument should be allowed to remain in the duct for five or ten minutes, and be then gently withdrawn, and this catheterization should be repeated every day or every other day, according to the exigencies of the case. The size of the probe should be increased until we arrive at No. 6, or it may be necessary to go even beyond this. [It is better to increase the size of the probes rapidly up to No. 10, and allow them to remain in the duct for from twenty minutes to half an hour.—B.] If the probe is arrested at the point where the canaliculi join the sac, the skin near the tendo-oculi will be moved with the movement of the probe, and an elastic obstruction be felt; whereas, when the instrument has entered the sac, the skin does not wrinkle or move.

If from the displacement of the puncta or stricture of the canaliculi, the sac has been emptied for a long period, it may become considerably diminished in size and its walls much thinned. We then find great difficulty in intro-ducing the probe into the sac, as it repeatedly slips out again. In many cases, it suffices to open the lower canaliculus and to pass the probe through it; in others, it may be necessary also to divide the upper one. This is more especially the case if we desire to get a very free opening into the sac, to pass an extra sized probe, or if there exists any stricture at the

5

The probes are passed through the entire length of the lachrymal passages from the punctum lacrymale to the floor of the nostril. The probe is preferably introduced into the lower punctum, and in the following manner:

The lower lid is drawn tense with the thumb of the left hand; the patient is directed to look upwards, and the probe, held vertically with the convexity of the bend looking backwards, is introduced into the punctum; its direction is then almost immediately changed to the horizontal, and by a gentle pressure is pushed inwards, until it reaches the inner wall of the lachrymal sac, which is recognized by the bony obstruction to its progress. The direction of the probe is then again changed to the vertical, and with moderate pressure is gently pushed onwards until the stricture is passed, and the point of the instrument rests upon the floor of the nostril. Folds of mucous membrane sometimes interfere with its passage, and to avoid tearing them requires perseverance and delicacy of manipulation. On no account should violence be used, for injury would then undoubtedly result. By the aid of continued moderate pressure, a passage can often be effected through a stricture which at first was impermeable.

Fig. 20.

The probe should be allowed to remain in the passage about ten minutes, and its introduction should be repeated every few days, as soon as the irritation caused by the previous operation has subsided. The size of the probe used should be gradually increased until the tube is fully dilated. Should these means prove unsuccessful, the canaliculus may be slit up, as recommended by Mr. Bowman.—H.] [It is not advisable to introduce a probe into the sac without first slitting up the canaliculus.—B.]

For some years past, bougies of laminaria digitata have been used by several surgeons of eminence. They were first introduced for this purpose by Mr. Couper, and have been extensively employed by him and Mr. Crimpett. I have also often used them with marked success in cases of very obstinate stricture. Their peculiar advantage consists in their imbibing the fluid in the lachrymal passages, and swelling up to double and treble their original size. But there is the danger that they may swell up to such an extent beyond the point of stricture, that the dilated bulbous part can only be drawn back through the stricture at the expense of much contusion or even laceration of the lining membrane at this point, or, what is still worse, that in the great effort to extract the probe it may break short, and have to be pushed. The best mode of obviating these difficulties, and yet at the same time to produce a slow and gradual dilatation, is to draw back the probe a very little at intervals of a minute or two, in order that it may not have time to swell up considerably below the stricture. By this gradual extraction, the latter will, moreover, be gently dilated by the enlarging probe. By pursuing this method, and by always being extremely careful to use these bougies with delicacy and gentleness, I have found great benefit from their employment. Their use, however, requires so much supervision, that it is somewhat difficult to find sufficient time in hospital practice, where the patients are so numerous, that one may easily forget to withdraw the probe a little at short intervals, and let it swell up too much. In order to limit the dilatation to the point of stricture, the rest of the bougie may be covered with copal varnish.

If the blennorrhœa proves obstinate, and the discharge as well as the swelling of the sac and duct continue, great benefit is found from the systematic use of astringent injections, of sulphate of zinc, alum, or acetate of lead. Their strength must vary according to the amount and nature of the discharge, and the degree of swelling of the lining membrane. Before their use, the sac must be washed out with an injection of water. The patient should also be directed frequently to press out the discharge, for if it is allowed to accumulate in the sac, and to become decomposed, it proves a source of considerable irritation, and may even set up an acute inflammation of the sac.

Dr. Stilling, of Cassel, has devised a cure for strictures of the lachrymal passages by internal incision.[1] The punctum having been divided, he passes down a probe and finds the exact seat of the stricture, then withdraws the probe and passes down his knife[2] (Fig. 21) to the stricture, and divides it in three or four directions. This having been done, he withdraws the knife, re-introduces the probe, and if another stricture is found further down, also divides this. Dr. Warlomont, in an article in the "Annales d'Oculistique,"[3] speaks in the warmest terms of his great and immediate success with this operation, and narrates several cases. He operates in the following manner: The upper punctum having been divided with Weber's knife, he next passes Weber's biconical sound down into the nasal duct, and leaves it there for a few minutes. On its removal, he immediately passes Stilling's knife completely down into the nasal duct, so that its whole blade disappears, and then incises the duct in three or four directions, until the knife can be turned quite freely in all directions. No dilator or probe is introduced after the operation; and according to Stilling and Warlomont, even severe and obstinate cases are thus immediately and permanently cured. The favorable action of this operation appears to be chiefly due to its affording a very free exit to the contents of the sac. As the operation is very painful, chloroform or the nitrous oxide gas should be given. I have tried the operation in numerous instances, with varying success. In only a few cases did I obtain a complete and permanent cure; in most of the others considerable benefit was derived, but the operation had subsequently to be supplemented by the occasional use of probes or Weber's sound, and of injections, which subsequently led to favorable results. In a few instances, I have found that, after a time, the nasal duct was greatly contracted, almost as if the periosteum had become swollen, so that the probe was very firmly grasped, and could only be passed with difficulty at first. On the whole, I have found most benefit from Stilling's operation in cases of obstinate chronic blennorrhœa of the sac, accompanied by a copious secretion of muco-purulent discharge, and but a slight stricture. In such, its favorable action appears to be principal due to its affording a permanent and very free exit for the contents of thely

Fig. 21.

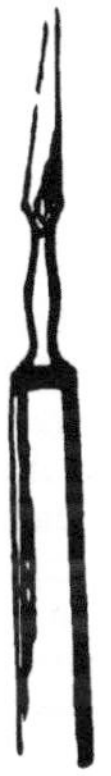

Vide Dr. Stilling's brochure, "Ueber die Heilung der Verengerungen der Thräwege-mittelst der Innern Incision." Cassel, 1868. A somewhat similar proceeding been recommended by Jaesche in "A. f. O.," x. 2, 166.

The blade of this knife is thirteen millimetres long, three millimetres broad nearest handle, and gradually diminishes to three-quarters of a millimetre at the point, which is somewhat rounded but cutting. The blade passes over into a flat stem, which is about the size of Bowman's largest probe, and is attached to the handle. The back of the blade should be made strong and rather wedge-shaped, and it should not be too highly tempered, otherwise, it may easily break, or a portion of it chip off, in forcing it through, or in incising the stricture. The knife may be obtained of Messrs. Weiss.

[3] "Annales d'Oculistique," Oct. 1868.

Dr. Hermenstein proposes the forcible dilatation of the stricture, on the principle of Mr. Barnard Holt's dilatation of stricture of the urethra. [Dr. Theobald has recently advised the treatment of strictures of the nasal duct by the introduction of very large probes, the canaliculus having first been slit up. He employs a series of sixteen probes, made of silver, No. 1 measuring one-quarter of a millimetre, and No. 16 measuring four millimetres. The pain caused by the large probes is not especially severe, nor has he seen any ill consequences result from the great distention of the divided canaliculus. The ends of these probes are olive-shaped. (See "Archives of Ophthal.," vi., and "Trans. Amer. Ophthal. Soc.," 1879.)—B.]

We sometimes find that the alterations in the lining membrane of the sac are so great, that they persist even after the passage of the tears is unobstructed; and then it may be necessary to have recourse to some direct treatment of the sac. Thus, if the latter is not only much dilated, but also thickened and secreting much muco-purulent discharge, Mr. Bowman has dissected out the anterior half of the thickened sac. Mr. Critchett has treated such cases successfully, by laying open the sac, and destroying a portion of the interior with potassa cum calce. As this condition of the lining membrane of the sac, as well as the considerable dilatation of the latter, are to a great extent maintained and increased by the constant flow of the tears into the sac, Weber[1] has remedied this by producing an eversion of the punctum, so that the tears cannot flow into the canaliculus; thus causing them to collect in the little reservoir formed by the lower lid being slightly turned away from the eyeball. He gains this end, by passing a needle, armed with a stout thread, through the skin and muscle close to the punctum, and bringing it out again a little further inwards, so as to embrace the punctum and a small fold of the skin within the suture, which is to be tightly knotted. This will readily produce a slight ectropium, and the beneficial effect of preventing the entrance of the tears into the lachrymal sac will generally be already evident within twenty-four hours afterwards. I have sometimes gained great benefit, in such cases, from the application of a firm compress bandage over the sac, which prevents the entrance of the tears. This mode of treatment is also of great use in those cases in which the sac is much thinned and dilated, and secretes a large quantity of thin dairy discharge. Mr. Critchett[2] has devised an ingenious little truss, so as to keep up a gentle and continuous pressure.

If the stricture is very firm and dense, and there is much tendency to close after the removal of the probe, a style may be passed into the duct by the slit canaliculus, and left in for a few days. The upper portion is to be very thin and bent at a very acute angle, so as to be bent over the lower lid, thus keeping the portion in situ. The bent portion may also be made so thin and small, that it will lie along the opening made in the lower punctum, and thus be invisible. Mr. Bowman first introduced this mode of treatment, and it is often attended with success, but in some cases the style sets up a considerable degree of irritation, and may even give rise to ulceration if it is left in too long. The size of the style should be gradually increased as the stricture yields, until it has attained dimensions considerably larger than Bowman's probe No. 6. Dr. Green[3] recommends leaden styles for this purpose, as they readily adapt themselves to any irregularities in the direction of the curves of the nasal duct. The smaller sizes are made tubular, and contain

[1] "Kl. Monatsbl.," 1865, 106.
[2] "Lectures on Diseases of Lachrymal Apparatus," "Lancet," 1864, 1, 148.
[3] "Transactions of American Ophthalmological Society," second Annual Meeting, 1869, p. 15.

a steel-wire stilet, which renders them sufficiently rigid for introduction. Jaesche has likewise employed leaden styles for several years.[1] The old-fashioned style, which used to be inserted into the nasal duct through an external opening in the sac, has fallen into well-merited and almost entire disuse. [Attempts have frequently been made to treat the stricture from below, by the introduction of curved hollow sounds through the nasal opening of the duct, and after dilating the stricture, to inject various caustic and astringent fluids: these methods have, however, all been given up as impracticable. Sometimes, however, where there is a tight stricture at the nasal opening of the duct, it is possible to dilate this through the nasal meatus, and thus aid in making the duct patent.

It has long been recognized that women are more subject to diseases of the lachrymal apparatus than men, but why this is so has never been discovered. This is especially true of stricture of the duct. It has also been noticed that the left nasal duct is more frequently diseased than the right.

The prognosis of these cases is good so far as a marked improvement is concerned; but the physician should remember and the patient should be told that the course of treatment required is a long one, and must be systematically persevered in to the end.—B.]

In very severe and obstinate cases of chronic inflammation of the sac, accompanied perhaps by ulceration and periostitis, and a severe stricture or even closure of the duct, cases which resist every mode of treatment and prove a great and constant source of annoyance and trouble to the patient, it may be necessary to obliterate the sac. This is also indicated, if the patient cannot remain under medical care for a sufficient length of time to lead to any reasonable hope of benefit by the usual mode of treatment, and is yet very anxious to be relieved from this very troublesome affection. But this operation should, I think, be only adopted in very exceptional cases, which have resisted every other means of treatment. For it is surprising what a degree of improvement may often be attained by treating these cases with patience and care, although it must be confessed that a very long time is but too frequently required before much improvement takes place. Obliteration of the sac is, moreover, only indicated if the natural secretion of the tears is not considerable, so that they are nearly entirely carried off by evaporation, otherwise, great and annoying epiphora remains after the operation.

Various methods of destroying the sac have been devised and recommended. At one time, the actual cautery was extensively employed for this purpose, but lately the galvano-caustic apparatus has been largely substituted for it. The sac is to be opened by a free incision, which is to extend likewise through the tendo-oculi into the upper portion of the sac, which forms a cul-de-sac above the tendon, and thoroughly cleansed. When the hemorrhage has ceased, the lips of the wound are to be kept apart by Manfredi's speculum [Fig. 22], which is, moreover, provided with side plates to prevent the cheek from being burnt, and the actual cautery, or the galvano-caustic apparatus, can be applied. Instead of these, various caustics are often employed, e. g., nitrate of silver, butter of antimony, potassa c. calce, perchloride of iron, etc. I myself prefer the nitrate of silver, which I first saw employed for this purpose with great success by Von Graefe. It is easily manageable, very safe, and leaves the smoothest and least unsightly cicatrix of any caustic. Before attempting to destroy the sac, the puncta and canaliculi must always be first obliterated, so as to stop the entrance of tears to the sac, otherwise their admission will prevent, or at least greatly retard, the adhesive inflam-

[1] "Kl. Monatsbl.," Aug. 1869, p. 294.

mation and obliteration of the sac. The best method of closing the puncta and canaliculi is to pass into them a very fine probe, coated with nitrate of silver or a thin hot wire, which will set up adhesive inflammation, thus obliterating the puncta, and closing the canaliculi. When this end has been obtained, the sac must be laid open to its whole extent by a free incision, thoroughly cleansed out, and when the bleeding has entirely ceased, the walls of the sac should be touched with nitrate of silver. Cold compresses should be applied to diminish the inflammatory symptoms. The

[Fig. 22.]

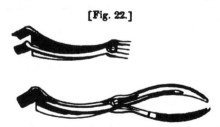

nitrate of silver should be used several times, at intervals of about two days, before the epithelium is formed; or, at the end of forty-eight hours, the thick eschar should be completely removed, and a small firm compress be applied to the sac, so as to bring its raw surfaces together, a firm bandage being placed over the compress, in order to keep it *in situ*.

[A better plan is to open the outer wall of the lachrymal sac through the conjunctival cul-de-sac, by a vertical incision either in front of or behind the caruncle, first incising both canaliculi. Then pull the lips of the wound apart by a sharp hook, and apply either nitric acid on a cotton probe, or the galvano-cautery directly to the wall of the sac. This effectually destroys the sac, and at the same time leaves no external scar. This operation was first suggested and practised by Dr. C. R. Agnew, of New York.—B.]

Dr. Pagenstecher strongly recommends the chloride of zinc paste (one part zinc. chlorid. to three parts of starch), which he uses extensively for the obliteration of the sac. He divides both canaliculi (with a peculiar knife made for this purpose by Weiss), in such a manner that the incisions meet in front of the caruncle. When all bleeding has ceased, he inserts into the sac a small portion of the paste (about the size of a split pea, this varying, however, according to the dimensions of the sac) wrapped in a thin layer of charpie or cotton-wool; a thick layer of charpie being pushed in after it in order to prevent any escape of the escharotic on to the conjunctiva. The paste is to remain in for twenty-four hours. At the end of two or three weeks the sac will generally be found to be obliterated by adhesive inflammation. Dr. Pagenstecher has been latterly induced to perform obliteration of the sac more frequently than in former years, not only on account of the relapses which sometimes occur after the treatment by probing, but more especially by the fact that he considers that eyes affected with chronic blennorrhœa of the sac are exposed to the greatest dangers, being exceptionally prone to suppuration of the cornea if they should become perchance affected with keratitis profunda, suppurative corneitis with hypopyon, etc. He states that when the atmosphere is dry and very hot, the secretions of the lachrymal sac become very readily decomposed, and if an eye affected with chronic blennorrhœa of the sac should then meet with an injury, producing perhaps only a slight abrasion of the corneal epithelium, it is almost always followed by a very dangerous and deleterious form of corneitis.

At the Ophthalmological Congress, held at Heidelberg in 1868, Dr. Berlin narrated several cases of very obstinate and severe disease of the sac, in which he obtained a successful result by extirpation of the latter.

[Schreiber gives the following indications for extirpation of the lachrymal sac: 1st. In very obstinate purulent dacryocystitis with stenosis of the nasal duct, which admits of being probed, but has existed so long that a slight bulging of the region of the lachrymal sac has been produced, with thickening of its walls. 2d. In fistula of the lachrymal sac, especially in cases in which frequently recurring attacks of inflammation have caused cicatricial adhesion of the skin with the wall of the sac, and induration. 3d. In tedious catarrh of the lachrymal sac with complete patency of the nasal duct. An incision, two millimetres long and four millimetres from the inner canthus, is to be made vertically with its upper end inclined slightly forwards, only through the skin, so as to avoid wounding the sac wall. The edges of this incision are to be carefully dissected up, and the anterior wall of the sac laid bare. The edges of the wound are then to be held apart with forceps or hooks, and the sac is to be seized with forceps and carefully dissected up from its attachments, keeping close to the lachrymal bone, either with scalpel or blunt-pointed scissors. If free bleeding follows, this must be arrested before the operation can be continued. After the sac has been removed, the cavity is to be carefully scraped with a Volkmann's sharp spoon, and the mucous membrane of the nasal duct scraped out and destroyed as far as possible with a smaller spoon of the same kind. The wound is then to be washed out with a two per cent. solution of carbolic acid, and the cavity is then to be closed accurately with sutures. (See "Archiv für Ophthalmologie," xxvii. 2.)—B.]

In severe and intractable cases of epiphora, inflammation of the sac, etc., the extirpation of the lachrymal gland has been strongly urged by several surgeons, more especially by Mr. Zachariah Laurence,[1] who has practised it extensively; it has also been employed by Mr. Carter, Dr. Taylor, Mr. Windsor, and others.

5.—FISTULA OF THE LACHRYMAL SAC, ETC.

By term is understood a communication between the lachrymal sac or passages and the external integument. I have already mentioned, when speaking of the inflammation of the sac, that after spontaneous perforation of the latter, a more or less extensive fistulous opening may be left, which may prove very obstinate and intractable if there is a very firm or impassable stricture, or considerable disease of the bone. Caries and necrosis of the bony walls of the sac are a very frequent cause of fistula. The latter, on the other hand, is but rarely produced by direct injury, or a wound of the sac. The fistula may either open directly into the sac, or there may exist a fistulous track of varying length. The edges of the fistula may be at first swollen, irregular, and somewhat ulcerated, the ulceration perhaps extending to some distance from the aperture. But after a time it contracts in size, its margin becomes smoother, and finally only a very minute opening, which hardly admits the finest probe, may be left; this is sometimes termed capillary fistula. If the orifice is retracted, and its edges covered with healthy-looking skin, the minute aperture may be easily overlooked, but on pressing

[1] Vide Mr. Laurence's article, "On Removal of the Lachrymal Gland as a Radical Cure for Lachrymal Disease," "Ophthalmic Review," No. 12.

the sac, a small tear-drop will be seen to exude. [Congenital lachrymal fistula has been observed by Agnew. (See "Trans. Amer. Ophth. Soc.," 1874.)—B.]

The best treatment for lachrymal fistula is that of slitting up the puncta, dividing the internal palpebral ligament, and passing a probe down frequently. If the passage is free, this will generally cause the fistula to heal in the course of a few days. But if the passage is impermeable, or the disease of the bone extensive, it may be necessary to obliterate the sac, or to force the passage. The latter is to be done with one of Bowman's probes or Weber's dilator. But extreme care must be taken to do this with delicacy, for if rude force be used, much mischief is sure to accrue. In the capillary fistula, the edges of which are covered by smooth skin, it is sometimes advisable to pare the edges, so as to make them raw, and then to close the minute aperture with a suture, which will cause the opening to heal by first intention.

[Chiralt advises destruction of the sac for the cure of fistula, and against the use of Bowman's probes, except in a limited number of cases. He uses, as a cauterizing agent, the acid nitrate of mercury, and claims that it cures almost certainly within a period varying from twelve to twenty-four days, and that in most cases there is no subsequent lachrymation. (See "Rev. de Méd. y. Cirug. Pract.," October 7, 1880.)—B.]

Polypi of the sac are of rare occurrence. They closely resemble nasal polypi in structure, and may attain the size of a small nut. They give rise to a peculiar feeling of resilience and elasticity to the finger, and although on pressure a certain quantity of glairy or muco-purulent fluid may be evacuated, yet we cannot empty the sac completely. On incising it, some fluid escapes, and the polypus (like a gelatinous mass) springs into the wound.[1] If the sac is extensively diseased, or there is a very firm stricture of the nasal duct, it may be necessary to obliterate the sac after the removal of the polypus.

Cases of hemorrhage into the sac, producing thus an impermeability of the latter, are of rare occurrence. Two instances of this kind have been recorded by Von Graefe.[2] The presence of chalky concretions (dacryoliths) in the ducts or in the lachrymal sac is also but rarely observed.

In some rare instances a peculiar fungus (leptothrix) is met with in the lower canaliculus, resembling very closely the leptothrix buccalis, which has been observed by Leber and Rottenstein[3] in carious teeth. Several cases of leptothrix have been described by Von Graefe,[4] and one by Förster.[5] According to the former, the affection commences with a certain degree of epiphora, which is followed by redness of the caruncle and neighboring portion of the retro-tarsal fold, as well as of the conjunctiva and margin of the lid in the vicinity of the lower canaliculus. The patients, at the same time, complain of a sensation of heat and itching at the inner angle of the eye, at which also small crusts of discharge are noticed, especially in the morning on waking. On closer examination, we now find that the shape and appearance of the margin of the lid along the lower canaliculus are somewhat changed, having become thickened and rounded, so that the edge of the lid does not lie in apposition with the eyeball; thus producing a tendency to ectropium, which is especially noticeable when the patient looks up. But

---

[1] Vide a case of Von Graefe's, "A. f. O.," i. 283.
[2] "A. f. O.," iii. 2, 857.   [3] Berlin, 1867.
[4] "A. f. O.," i. ii. and xv. 1, 324; also "Berl. Med. Wochenschrift," 1868, p. 264.
[5] "A. f. O.," xv. 1, 318. [Also, "Kl. Mon. f. Aug.," viii. p. 78; ix. p. 248. Also "Archives of Ophth. and Otol.," iii. 1.—B.]

CHAPTER II.

DISEASES OF THE EYELIDS.

1.—ŒDEMA OF THE EYELIDS, ETC.

ŒDEMA *of the lids* very frequently accompanies (as we have seen) the severer forms of inflammation of the conjunctiva, cornea, and iris. It may, however, be also dependent upon some disturbance of the general health, more especially in feeble and delicate persons. It is often due to an affection of the heart or kidneys, and should, therefore, always arouse our suspicions, and lead us to examine as to the presence of general dropsy, and of albumen in the urine. The degree of œdematous swelling of the lids is subject to much variation. If it be due to constitutional causes, it is often but inconsiderable in degree, giving rise only to a little puffiness and fulness of the lids, which is generally greatest in the morning, and diminishes during the day. Sometimes, the puffiness is principally confined to the lower lid, forming a little pouch or sac, which is very unsightly if it be considerable in size and if the subcutaneous veins are dilated, as the swelling then assumes a dusky, bluish tint. The swelling produced by œdema is smooth, pale, soft, and semitransparent, and is easily pitted with the point of the finger, the mark remaining for a little time.

If the œdema is due to constitutional causes, the treatment must be chiefly directed to their alleviation, when the swelling of the lid will soon subside. Where the puffiness of the lids occurs spontaneously in persons of a feeble, delicate habit, tonics should be administered, and the general health attended to. A compress bandage should be applied, and I have also found benefit from the use of warm aromatic bags (containing chamomile flowers, camphor, etc.) tied firmly over the eye. If the œdema is very obstinate and unsightly, a small horizontal fold of skin may be excised. Where this condition is dependent upon some other disease of the eye, this must be treated, and when it is alleviated, the puffiness will soon disappear.

Emphysema *of the lids* is due to the admission of air into the areolar tissue, and is generally caused by a fracture of the nasal bones or of the frontal or ethmoidal cells, and rupture of the mucous membrane; though generally produced by severe blows or falls, it may arise after blowing the nose very harshly. The swelling of the lid is tense and elastic, and there is distinct crepitation on pressure; the color of the skin is, however, unchanged. The treatment consists in the application of a compress bandage, with the use of a mildly stimulating lotion.

In erythema (hyperæmia) *of the eyelids*, the skin is very much reddened, and presents a bright scarlet flush, which temporarily disappears upon pressure. There is, however, but very little, if any, swelling of the lid, and no pain, although the patient complains of a sensation of great heat. The redness generally extends somewhat on to the cheek, and the palpebral and ocular conjunctiva may likewise be injected. The veins of the skin are also sometimes dilated. This affection is not unfrequently due to prolonged exposure to very bright sunlight or intense heat, and is also met with in persons suffering from some irregularity of the general circulation. Compresses, soaked in cold water or in Goulard lotion, should be frequently applied; and a solution of nitrate of silver (gr. iv ad f$\mathfrak{Z}$j) may be painted over the outside of the lids. If there is much vascularity of the conjunctiva, and a slight muco-purulent discharge, a weak collyrium of sulphate of zinc or alum should be prescribed.

A peculiar bluish discoloration of the eyelids (more especially the lower one is occasionally observed in persons of feeble health, and of a very transparent and delicate complexion. This dark tint is especially conspicuous beneath the lower lid, producing a dark-blue, semicircular ring. This appearance is due to a dilatation of the subcutaneous veins, which are more conspicuous on account of the delicacy of the skin. It is often difficult to cure this discoloration, more especially if a certain degree of œdema of the lid coexists. I have found the most benefit from the use of a solution of tannin gr. iv-viii, to f$\mathfrak{Z}$j of water, which is to be painted frequently over the outside of the eyelids. When this has been employed for some little time, a solution of acetate of lead or of nitrate of silver should be substituted. Care must, however, be taken that the nitrate of silver does not discolor the skin, which is especially apt to happen at the points where the latter is a little wrinkled. The general health should, at the same time, be attended to, irregularities in the circulation or the digestive functions be rectified, and abstinence from every form of dissipation strictly enforced.

[Hemorrhages beneath the skin and in the tissues of the lid occur as the result of rupture of the palpebral vessels, or from the extension of an orbital or intra-cranial hemorrhage into the lids. Any blow or fall upon the eyelids may cause a hemorrhage, and likewise any operation. The palpebral vessels may also be ruptured by any undue stretching of their walls, as during violent vomiting, or sneezing, or coughing. Symptomatic hemorrhages by diapedesis, without any rupture of the vessels, also occur in scurvy and purpura.—B.]

2—INFLAMMATION OF THE EYELIDS, ETC.

In the acute phlegmonous inflammation (abscess) of the eyelids, there is great redness, heat, and swelling of the lids, which are also acutely sensitive to the touch. The skin is greatly reddened, and, as the disease advances, it assumes a darker and more dusky hue. The conjunctiva is also injected, and there is often a considerable degree of chemosis. The swelling is firm and hard, and not œdematous: it often extends over the eyebrow and cheek, and may become so considerable that the upper lid is swollen up to the size of a pigeon's egg, or even larger. This hardness is at first especially conspicuous at one point, which feels like a little, firm, circumscribed nodule; this increases more and more in size, then the hardness gradually yields, the swelling becomes softer, more doughy, and there is a distinct sense of fluctuation. The skin becomes thinned and yellow at one point, gives way, and a large quanity of thick creamy pus escapes. In rarer instances, the perforation occurs through the conjunctiva. When the abscess forms at the inner angle of the eye, near the lachrymal sac, it has been termed *anchylops*, and may then be mistaken for acute inflammation of the sac. If it perforates at the inner canthus, it is called *ægilops*. It generally, however, occurs in the upper lid, which, on account of the swelling, hangs immovably down, so that the palpebral aperture is quite closed. The pain is mostly very great, and of a violently throbbing character, extending over the corresponding side of the head and face. There is often also much constitutional disturbance and feverishness. The course of the disease may, however, be more chronic, and all the inflammatory symptoms be subacute in character. Abscess of the eyelid is almost always of traumatic origin, being produced by wounds or blows upon the eye. It may, however, occur spontaneously, or supervene upon severe inflammation of the conjunctiva, or erysipelas of the eyelids. [Parinaud believes that alteration of the temporary or permanent teeth may provoke suppuration in the lower lid on a level with the orbital margin, or in the region of the lachrymal sac, where it simulates tumor or fistula of the sac. The course followed by the pus arising from an alveolo-dental periostitis is intra-osseous, and hence difficult to discover. Parinaud holds that there is a variety of suppuration around the eye, of dental origin, peculiar to children, due to the arrangement of the alveoles of the first and second dentition. In the adult, a suppurative process of dental origin is occasionally met with in front of the lachrymal sac. In these cases, the pus developed in the alveole may first penetrate into the maxillary sinus, where it provokes inflammation, and secondarily leads to the formation of a cutaneous fistula at the internal canthus; in another series of cases the lachrymal passages are free, the maxillary sinus is not involved, and the connection between the abscess or fistula at the internal canthus and the dental process cannot be discovered. The vascular canals which open constantly by one or two orifices upon the ascending ramus of the maxilla, in front of the lachrymal groove, and which communicate also with the foramina of the alveoles, explain the occurrence of these suppurative processes, which in so many instances are accompanied by necrosis of the orbital margin. (See "Archives générales de Médecine," June, 1880.)—B.]

If the disease is seen at the very outset, we should endeavor to produce the resolution of the inflammatory swelling by the application of cold (iced) compresses, leeches, etc.; but if we cannot succeed in this, hot poultices or sedative fomentations should be applied, in order to accelerate the formation of pus, and as soon as fluctuation is felt, a free incision should be made into the swelling parallel to the edge of the lid, so as to give ready exit to the discharge; for, if this is not done, but the abscess is allowed to perforate spontaneously, the sufferings of the patient are not only greatly aggravated and prolonged, but the opening will be ragged and insufficient, and by the contraction of the cavity of the abscess, will tend to produce ectropium. If perforation has already occurred, the opening should be enlarged if it is insufficient for the free discharge of matter; and if several apertures exist close together, they should be laid open into one large wound. After the escape of the pus, warm poultices should be applied, and subsequently warm-water dressing and a compress bandage, so as to keep the lid in position and the walls of the abscess in contact, and thus hasten the union. A generous diet and tonics should be prescribed. Any eversion or malposition of the eyelid or puncta must be treated at a subsequent period.

In erysipelas of the lids the swelling is not firm, hard, and of a dusky-red hue, but œdematous, softer, and of a more rosy, semitransparent hue, the color disappearing on pressure. The cuticle is frequently elevated in the form of small blisters by an effusion of serum. The swelling of the lid is often very considerable, and extends over the eyebrow and down the cheek; the conjunctiva is injected, and there is more or less chemosis. There is generally much constitutional disturbance; the patient is feverish, his tongue is much loaded, and he is often extremely weak and feeble. The pain is generally not very great, nor of a throbbing or pulsating character. If pus is formed, the swelling assumes greater firmness, the skin becomes more tense and of a livid, dusky-red tint, and the pain, heat, and throbbing increase in severity. The swelling becomes softer, there is a distinct feeling of fluctuation, and then, if left to itself, the abscess points and perforates. The matter may extend freely into the connective tissue, and give rise to extensive sloughs. But erysipelas may produce much more serious complications, for the inflammation may extend to the cellular tissue of the orbit, giving rise to abscess within the latter and great exophthalmus, followed perhaps by sloughing of the cornea or suppurative irido-choroiditis; or the inflammation may extend backwards from the orbit, along the optic nerve to the brain, and set up meningitis; or, again, the erysipelatous inflammation may also become diffuse, and extend to the face. The sight may likewise be much impaired or lost by the inflammation extending to the neurilemma of the optic nerve and setting up optic neuritis, which may terminate in atrophy of the nerve. Or the latter may be produced by the great pressure upon, or stretching of, the optic nerve. The purulent matter, as Mackenzie points out, may likewise make its way into the lachrymal sac, which becomes filled with pus from without; in the production of which, its lining membrane has no share.

Erysipelas of the eyelids may be spontaneous in origin, being caused by exposure to cold and wet, more especially if the patient is already in feeble and delicate health from want or dissipation. It is often, however, of traumatic origin, being due to injuries, wounds, etc., of the lids. Our first object in the treatment must be to strengthen the patient. If the stomach is much deranged, the tongue loaded, the breath fetid, a brisk purgative or an emetic should be at once administered. Then tonics should be given, more especially the tincture of steel, or preparations of steel and quinine. The diet must be generous, and stimulants, particularly port wine and brandy, should be freely administered. Warm poppy or laudanum fomentations should be applied to the lids, or they may be painted with collodion. If pus is forming, a free incision must be made at once, in order to permit of its ready escape. If the chemosis is very considerable and firm, so that it presses upon the vessels which supply the cornea, and thus endangers the nutrition of the latter, the chemotic swelling should be incised at different points; but if the pressure of the swollen lids is threatening this danger, the outer canthus should be divided. When the erysipelatous inflammation has extended to the orbital cellular tissue, and the eye is protruded from a collection of pus or an effusion into the orbit, a free and deep incision should be made so as to evacuate it.

Cases of anthrax (carbuncle) of the lids generally occur in elderly persons of feeble health. The inflammatory swelling is of a dusky, livid red, and firm and circumscribed, and there is a great tendency to sloughing. Vesicles form on the lid and burst, discharging sanious matter; the skin and areolar tissue become black and gangrenous, and, sloughing out, leave a more or less deep cavity, which then granulates and cicatrizes. A crucial incision should be made into the swelling at an early stage, so as to allow the escape of matter and facilitate the separation of the slough, and warm poultices should then be applied. The patient's strength must be sustained by a liberal administration of brandy, wine, tonics, and a good diet. If the pain is great, opium must be given, either internally or by the subcutaneous injection.

Malignant pustule of the lids is said to be somewhat common in certain parts of France and of the continent, but I have never heard of its having been met with in England in its true type. According to Mackenzie, it is characterised by the formation of a vesicle filled with bloody serum, which is accompanied by great and firm swelling of the lids, the skin of which is dusky and red. The base of the pustule is hard and nodular, and soon sloughs, the gangrene spreading with great rapidity. There is severe constitutional disturbance, much fever, and intense pain. The disease is almost always produced by contact with decomposing carcasses of cattle, or with animals suffering from farcy; hence it is most frequently met with amongst tanners, butchers, drovers, etc. It is so extremely dangerous that it may prove fatal within twenty-four hours of the outset, the inflammation extending to the head and neck, and the eye being either destroyed at the time, or subsequently from exposure. Mackenzie states that the best treatment is a deep crucial incision of the swelling, followed by the immediate application of the actual cautery. Tonics and stimulants should be very freely administered.

8.—SYPHILITIC AND EXANTHEMATOUS AFFECTIONS OF THE EYELIDS.

[Syphilitic lesions of the lids are of three kinds: 1st. Chancre or the initial sclerosis; 2d. Exanthemata; 3d. Gummata. The exanthematous variety is merely a local symptom of the constitutional disease, and the gumma is a late manifestation of the disease.

The exanthematous lesions of the lids are usually of the papular or tubercular variety. The result is frequently an ulcer, the centre of a papule or tubercle breaking down and sloughing on the surface. It may be confined to the skin or involve the entire thickness of the lid. The tubercular syphilide presents the same characteristics as the gumma, and microscopically they are one. The tubercle may be cutaneous or subcutaneous, and the latter is apt to be very painful. The papular syphilide, though generally of rapid growth and often extending over the entire lid, does not extend very deeply into the tissues, and the destructive process is consequently superficial.—B.]

Syphilitic ulceration of the eyelid generally commences at its free edge, along which it rapidly spreads, more especially towards the skin, showing a greater tendency to extend in this direction than inwards towards the conjunctiva. The eyelid is much inflamed and swollen in the vicinity of the ulcer, and of a dusky, livid hue. The swelling is firm and hard, and feels indurated. The ulcer has a hard, cartilaginous base, its edges are irregular, and its bottom presents a peculiar dirty and lardaceous appearance. The whole surface of the lid is often swollen and indurated, and of a dusky-red tint, the inflammation extending generally to the conjunctiva, and being accompanied by a muco-purulent discharge. If the disease is not recognized and properly treated, the ulcer will rapidly spread, become deeply notched, and perhaps soon eat its way through the whole substance of the lid, destroying skin, cartilage, and conjunctiva. Indeed its ravages may be so great, that the whole of the eyelid may become destroyed, and the disease even extend to the other lid. In rarer instances, the ulcer may occupy the internal surface of the eyelid, and spread over a considerable portion of the palpebral conjunctiva without appearing externally. If the ulcer is situated in the inner canthus, or the inner edge of the lower lid in the vicinity of the lachrymal sac, it may be mistaken for a fistula of the latter; indeed it may penetrate into the sac. It is often somewhat difficult to determine with certainty the true nature of the disease, or to make the differential diagnosis between the syphilitic ulcer and the different forms of lupus and epithelioma.

The syphilitic character of the ulceration must, however, be suspected, if it proves very obstinate, and instead of yielding to the usual remedies, gets worse and spreads more and more. We must then carefully and searchingly inquire into the history of the case, and ascertain whether any other symptoms of syphilis are present, such as eruptions of the skin, ulceration of the throat, etc., or whether there has been any chance of direct contagion; for, although these ulcers are almost always secondary, a primary hard chancre of the lid may be met with. [The chancre may occur on the edge of the lid, and the induration extends upward some distance upon the tarsus. It is usually very slow in its course, and resists treatment obstinately. The induration occurs very rapidly in the margin of the lid. Both macroscopically and microscopically the chancre bears a close resemblance to the gummy induration which has undergone ulceration.—B.] The softer variety appears, however, to be of rare occurrence. The ulceration may also extend to the eyelids from the neighboring parts, such as the nose, etc. [The condition of the glands nearest the lesion should always be ascertained. It may happen that induration of the sore is absent or but slightly marked, but it very rarely if ever, happens that glandular induration and induration of the ... are both absent. Out of sixteen hundred and forty-six cases of induration ... tabulated by Sturgis, the ... was situated on the eyelid in ... —H.] The gumma of the lid may be circumscribed or diffuse. The ... appears as a nodule near the ciliary margin. The latter may ... the whole lid, and is then known as Tarsitis syphilitica. The circumscribed gumma which is situated is a tubercular syphilide; it may be acute or ... Circumscribed induration of the entire lid is rare, though a number of cases have been recently reported. In these cases the skin is ... involved. The isolated gumma sometimes follows hard after the initial sclerosis, though ... as a ... and as syphilitic ... See a paper on Syphilis ... in ... N. Y. Med ... March 1878, and one on Tarsus Syphilitica in Trans. Amer ... Soc., 1878, by the Editor.—B.] The treatment must consist of ... the patient as rapidly as possible ... of ... mercurial baths; and ... be kept ... for some time, otherwise a relapse may occur ... The latter should be freely touched with ... red precipitate ... and the ... resists the action of ... Allmann's ... skin ... If this ... same purpose.

In adults he ... heals itself ... the ... the ... baths and should be ... important ... danger of ... and ... should be ... the red precipitate ... should be ...

The ... affections ... a ... in ... consequently ...

upon the eyelids. Psoriasis, pityriasis, and urticaria are also occasionally found upon the lids.—B.] Eczema of the lids occurs very frequently in conjunction with eczema of the face. It is also due to severe and protracted inflammation of the conjunctiva or cornea, more especially phlyctenular ophthalmia, and is caused by the irritation of the constant discharge, and of the hot scalding tears flowing over the edge of the lid and down the cheek. The proper mode of treatment is described in Chapter IV.

Herpes zoster frontalis seu ophthalmicus is not infrequently accompanied by inflammation of the eye, and is hence of peculiar interest to the ophthalmologist. Mr. Hutchinson has called special attention to this fact, and has also shown that it is of far more common occurrence than is generally supposed, being but too often mistaken for erysipelas. To him and to Mr. Bowman,[1] we are chiefly indebted for some admirable papers upon this disease. The affection is generally ushered in by more or less severe pain and tenderness in the brow and head, which last for several days, then the skin becomes red and swollen, and numerous small herpetic vesicles make their appearance, being arranged in groups (generally of an oval shape). The individual vesicles become confluent, their contents dry up into scabs, which afterwards drop off, and leave deep and characteristic scars, which are very diagnostic of the pre-existence of zoster. The eruption extends only along that portion of the skin which is supplied by the ophthalmic division of the fifth nerve, and is therefore confined to the forehead, the anterior portion of the scalp, the upper eyelid, and the side of the nose; the neck and lower lid are often swollen, but are quite free from vesicles. It may, however, affect only certain branches of the ophthalmic, e. g., the frontal, the trochlear and nasal branch escaping; but sometimes the middle division of the fifth may also be affected, as well as the first (Hebra), and then the eruption appears likewise on the cheek. The disease is probably mostly due to cold, which causes an inflammation of the superficial portion of the trunk of these nerves and their cutaneous ramifications, which is succeeded by the eruption of vesicles.

According to Hutchinson[2] the eye hardly ever suffers much in herpes frontalis, unless the oculo-nasal branch is affected, and the vesicles appear on the side of the nose, and its tip, the severity of eruption being usually in direct relation with the severity of the ocular inflammation. The eye does not inflame till the eruption is at its height, or beginning to decline; it is most commonly observed in old persons, in whom indeed herpes zoster frontalis is also most apt to occur. The parts of the eye affected are chiefly the cornea, upon which small, frequently marginal, ulcers form, and the iris, which may become inflamed. The iritis is generally only slight in character, but if the corneal ulcer is large and perforates, and the iritis is severe, serious complications may ensue, and the sight be even lost. There is often great swelling of the lids, together with a varying degree of photophobia, lachrymation, and conjunctival redness. The temperature of the affected part is markedly increased, but its sensibility is diminished. According to Horner[3] the earliest symptom observed in the eye is the appearance of transparent vesicles on the cornea; they are generally situated at or near the margin and arranged in groups, or they may appear in single file like the beads of a rosary. They are accompanied by slight cloudiness of the epithelium. These

[1] "R. L. O. H. Reports," v. and vi.; *vide* also a case of Steffan's in "Kl. Monatsbl.,"
1873, 360.

[2] "R. L. O. H. Reports," vi. 3, 182.   [3] "Kl. Monatsbl.," 1871, 321.

and lotions have been recommended for this disease, and in very chronic and obstinate cases it is advisable occasionally to change the remedy.

In the milder forms, the application night and morning, of the weak nitrate of mercury, or the red or white precipitate ointment will suffice. [An ointment of yellow or red precipitate of mercury, from three to ten grains to the drachm of vaseline, is an excellent preparation.—B.]

If the edge of the lid is much excoriated, a solution of nitrate of silver (gr. v–x ad f℥j) should be lightly painted over it every day; or pledgets of lint, dipped in a weaker solution of nitrate of silver or of sulphate of zinc, should be periodically applied. If small pustules or ulcers have formed, these should be touched with a finely pointed crayon of sulphate of copper or the mitigated nitrate of silver. I have also found very great benefit from the use of Hebra's ointment, which consists of equal parts of Oleum Lini and Emplastrum Plu ... th ... le Balsam of Peru. This is spread on a pledget of lint and ... bed-time, being kept on all night. On its removal in ... to be well sponged with warm water. Dr. McCal ... the use of a solution of potassa fusa (usu ... little of which is to be painted ... h by the surgeon himself ... di-
ness to stop the
or two of a col
or three times
and cold win
treatment, g
he is of a
quinine sh
digestible
Indeed,
these p
stinate
arseni

A
sm
fo
s

... s
... for

ther-
... ne of
tion of
red; so
l in the
ize and

No. ...
Date: ... 188
Prepare for ...
℞
A. M. Gardner, M. D.
...ISTOGA, CAL.

junctivitis or corneitis, more especially if the latter are accompanied by a great discharge of hot scalding tears, which constantly moisten and excoriate the edges of the lids. But it occurs also as a primary disease, and is then generally due to prolonged exposure to wind, cold, bright glare, or to an impure smoky atmosphere. Its intensity is much aggravated by dirt and want, and it is, therefore, most frequently met with amongst the poorer classes, and especially amongst those nationalities in which habits of cleanliness do not prevail. It occurs most frequently amongst children, but it is also met with in adults, and is especially prone to attack persons of a delicate, feeble, and scrofulous constitution, or who suffer from impairment of the digestion; in such, it proves especially obstinate and apt to recur. Dr. McCall Anderson considers t at this disease ¸ neither more nor less than a pustular eczema (impetigo) attacking the edges of the lids.[1] [In a considerable proportion of the patients affected, the disease is associated with some error of refraction or muscular defect, which renders the ordinary treatment of little or no value. Therefore, it is well always to test the refractive and muscular conditions of such eyes, and where any error is discovered, correct it by the necessary glasses before using local remedies. Often the disease will disappear without any local treatment when the refractive or muscular error has been corrected.—B.]

In the *treatment* of this disease, the greatest attention must be paid to the most scrupulous cleanliness. In mild cases, the eye should be frequently washed with tepid water, or warm milk and water, so as to remove the crusts from the lashes, and when this has been done, a little of the weak nitrate of mercury ointment should be applied to the roots of the lashes with a fine camel's-hair brush. [A better application is a solution of sodic bicarbonate in the proportion of grs. xv–xx to the ounce of hot water, to soften the crusts.—B.] If this prove too irritating, we should diminish the strength of this ointment by an admixture of one or two parts of lard. If the crusts are thick and firm, and the edges of the lids very swollen and red, mere ablution with warm water will not suffice, but compresses, steeped in hot water, should be applied for ten or twenty minutes, and frequently changed during this period. This should be repeated three or four times a day, or hot bread and water or linseed-meal poultices may be applied instead of the compresses. This will greatly alleviate the inflammation, and the crusts will be so thoroughly soaked and softened, that they will either become detached spontaneously, or can be removed without difficulty or injury to the lid. The hot compresses or poultices will be found especially useful in the morning, when the crusts are thick, and the lids firmly glued together by the nocturnal discharge. After the removal of the crusts, the lids may be bathed with tepid water, and then some astringent ointment or lotion should be applied. Before doing so, any diseased or stunted eyelashes should be extracted with the cilia forceps, as this favors the growth of the new ones, and renders the application of the topical remedy more easy. Indeed, if the disease is severe, and implicates the greater portion of the lid, it will be well to remove the greater part of the lashes, or, as suggested by Mr. Streatfield, to cut them down quite close to the margin. Malposition, or a faulty shedding of the lashes, is a not unfrequent cause of a very obstinate, though perhaps mild, form of blepharitis. In such cases, we find that on passing the lashes lightly through our finger and thumb, many of them come out at once, their root being often black. Great benefit is derived from careful and repeated epilation of the affected lashes. A great number of ointments

---

[1] "A Practical Treatise upon Eczema," by Dr. McCall Anderson, p. 197.

and lotions have been recommended for this disease, and in very chronic and obstinate cases it is advisable occasionally to change the remedy.

In the milder forms, the application night and morning, of the weak nitrate of mercury, or the red or white precipitate ointment will suffice. [An ointment of yellow or red precipitate of mercury, from three to ten grains to the drachm of vaseline, is an excellent preparation.—B.]

If the edge of the lid is much excoriated, a solution of nitrate of silver (gr. v–x ad f$\mathfrak{z}$j) should be lightly painted over it every day; or pledgets of lint, dipped in a weaker solution of nitrate of silver or of sulphate of zinc, should be periodically applied. If small pustules or ulcers have formed, these should be touched with a finely pointed crayon of sulphate of copper or the mitigated nitrate of silver. I have also found very great benefit from the use of Hebra's ointment, which consists of equal parts of Oleum Lini and Emplastrum Plumbi, with a little Balsam of Peru. This is spread on a pledget of lint and applied to the lids at bed-time, being kept on all night. On its removal in the morning, the eyes are to be well sponged with warm water. Dr. McCall Anderson strongly recommends the use of a solution of potassa fusa (usually ten grains to an ounce of water), a very little of which is to be painted every day on the edges of the lids with a fine brush by the surgeon himself. A large brush, soaked in cold water, should be in readiness to stop the action when desired. If any conjunctivitis coexists, a drop or two of a collyrium of sulphate of zinc or of alum should be applied two or three times a day. The eyes should also be protected against bright light and cold winds by a pair of blue eye-protectors. Together with this local treatment, great attention must be paid to the patient's general health. If he is of a scrofulous habit, or in delicate health, cod-liver oil with steel or quinine should be administered. His diet should be nutritious, but easily digestible, and all excess, more especially in drinking, should be avoided. Indeed, even the moderate use of stimulants cannot be borne by some of these patients, causing an aggravation or a relapse of the disease. In obstinate cases, I have also derived much benefit from the prolonged use of arsenic.

Acne ciliaris is not unfrequently met with; we then notice one or more small nodules, which are due to an inflammation of the sebaceous or hair-follicles, and situated close to the edge of the lid, which is more or less swollen, red, and inflamed; indeed, if the attack is severe, the whole lid may be very œdematous. These nodules are situated in the subcutaneous cellular tissue, and are somewhat movable, and several cilia may sprout out from the apex of the pustules. The latter gradually increase in size, and, after having attained a certain volume, may undergo resolution; but they generally suppurate, the pus escaping either through the duct of the follicle, or making its way through the external skin. In other cases, the nodule becomes hardened and indurated (*acne indurata*), and may thus exist unchanged for a very long time.

This disease is mostly met with in youthful individuals, who may be otherwise in very good health, excepting that they show a disposition to acne of the face. It may, however, occur independently of this, if the secretion of the sebaceous follicles of the eyelids is from any cause morbidly altered; so that, either from its excess in quantity or hardness, it becomes confined in the gland, and then sets up inflammation. On account of the larger size and number of the sebaceous follicles in the upper lid, acne occurs more frequently in this than in the lower. The causes of acne ciliaris resemble those of acne in general, and, like the latter, this disease generally runs a protracted course, and is very apt to recur. Amongst the principal causes, I may mention irregularities in diet, free indulgence in wine, spirits, or other excesses; and, in females, derangement of the uterine functions. Exposure to dust, dirt, cold winds, bright glare, etc., increases the severity and obstinacy of the disease, and favors the tendency to relapses. If the affection has lasted for some time, and is accompanied by a good deal of inflammation, it may become complicated with blepharitis marginalis.

[Kummerfeld's lotion is highly recommended as a preventive of recurring attacks. It consists of gum. camphoræ, 0.4; lac sulphur. 4.0; calcis aquæ et aq. rosæ, ãã 40.0; gum. Arab. 0.8: and should be painted over the edges of the lids at night.—B.]

Great attention should be paid to the cleanliness of the lids, which should be frequently washed, so that any discharge which clogs the lashes, or has become encrusted on the lids, may be removed. The loose or affected eyelashes should be frequently plucked out. If the nodule and the neighboring portion of the lid are red, inflamed, and painful, cold compresses should be applied, but if signs of suppuration appear, hot poultices or fomentations should be substituted, and the pustule be punctured, in order that the discharge may find a ready exit. In the indurated form, an ointment containing mercury or iodide of potassium should be applied. The diet and habits of the patient should be carefully regulated, and if he is feeble and delicate in health, tonics should be administered.

The presence of lice[1] on the eyelashes (phthiriasis ciliarum) might be mistaken for tinea, but the crusts present a more circumscribed and beaded form. The citrine or red precipitate ointment should be applied twice daily, which will generally kill the pediculi in a few days. If they are numerous, it may be necessary to clip the lashes very close.

5.—EPHIDROSIS AND CHROMHYDROSIS.

An excessive secretion of the sudoriferous glands of the lids, more especially the upper, is occasionally met with. The perspiration exudes so freely that the surface of the lid is covered by a thin layer or film of fluid, reaching perhaps nearly up to the edge of the orbit. This condition is termed Ephidrosis [or Hyperidrosis.—B.]. On wiping the skin dry with a fine dossil of linen, we can easily notice (with the aid of a magnifying-glass) that the moisture exudes from innumerable little pores, flows together into large drops, and finally covers the lid with a thin layer of fluid (Von Graefe).[2] Soon the conjunctiva becomes somewhat injected and inflamed, the edges of the lids become sore and excoriated (more especially at the angles of the eye) from the constant irritation of the moisture, and an obstinate blepharitis marginalis, with a slight degree of conjunctivitis, is set up. The patient at the same time complains of a peculiar itching and biting sensation on the outer surface of the lid. The affection is very obstinate and protracted, for although astringent lotions and collyria benefit the inflammation of the conjunctiva and the edge of the lid, they exert but little, if any, influence upon the secretion of fluid. Wecker recommends "Hebra's ointment" (p. 85). The general health, and especially the action of the skin and kidneys, should be attended to.

Chromhydrosis (stearrhœa nigricans of Erasmus Wilson). Under this title has been described a very peculiar pigmented condition of the eyelids, which is characterized by the appearance of a dark-brown or brownish-black discoloration of the lids, more especially the lower, which is chiefly noticeable in the folds of the skin, and does not reach up to the lashes. It can be readily removed with oil or glycerine, but, apparently, not with water. It has been chiefly met with in females, more especially those of a nervous, hysterical temperament, and there can be but little doubt that it is artificial, being due to some pigment painted on by the patient in order to deceive her medical attendant, and to awaken interest or compassion. [Both Rothmund and Michel are not willing to admit this in all cases.—B.] For a very full account of this condition, I would refer the reader to the French translation of Mackenzie, iii. 44, and to a paper read by Dr. Warlomont, before the Heidelberg Ophthalmological Congress, 1864, *vide* "Kl. Monatsbl.," 1864, 381.

Xanthelasma palpebrarum [Xanthoma, Vitiligoidea, Fibroma lipomatodes.—B.] is the name given by Mr. Erasmus Wilson to peculiar yellow spots or patches, which are sometimes met with on the eyelids of middle-aged persons, generally near the inner or outer canthus. They vary in size from a small speck, like a pin's head, to an oval or crescentic patch, perhaps one-third of an inch in magnitude. The spots or patches are yellowish in tint, flat, somewhat elevated above the level of the skin, and their centre is generally marked by a black point. Mr. Hutchinson[1] has lately called special attention to this affection, and since then numerous cases have been recorded. Virchow[2] narrates an extraordinary one, in which there were small yellow nodules on the cornea, and a number of yellowish tumors all over the body (xanthelasma multiplex).

[Mr. Hutchinson[3] thinks that it is not impossible that these patches result from derangement in the nutrition of the skin of the eyelids which frequently occurs in association with hepatic and ovarian disturbances. The patches of true xanthelasma are always persistent, and usually tend slowly, but steadily, to increase.—H.]

[The patches are sometimes nodular, and grow quite large, and not infrequently occur all over the body and extremities. Icterus is very often present in these cases. A very early symptom of the development of xanthoma is a twitching and pricking in the lid. Anatomically, the change consists, says Waldeyer, in a hyperplasia of the connective-tissue cells and their consecutive fatty metamorphosis, especially between the hair-bulbs and sebaceous glands. Another view, is that the disease is a hyperplasia of the cells of the sebaceous glands, with obstruction and dilatation of the glands. The treatment consists in excising the discolored skin and subcutaneous tissue, and should only be done for cosmetic purposes.—B.]

6.—HORDEOLUM (STYE).

This disease is not, as is sometimes supposed, an inflammatory affection of the Meibomian glands, but is a furuncular inflammation of the connective tissue of the lids, having its seat generally in the vicinity of the hair-follicles, and near the margin of the lid. In most cases there is only one boil, in others there are several. At the outset of the disease, we notice a small circumscribed nodule or button near the edge of the lid, the skin being freely movable over it. If the development is very acute, the lid is often much inflamed, very red, and œdematous; and although these symptoms are generally confined to the portion of the lid in the vicinity of the stye, they may extend to the whole eyelid, and the ocular conjunctiva may also become

---

[1] "R. L. O. H. Rep.," vi. 4, 1869. [2] Virchow's "Archiv," lii. 504.
[3 "Med.-Chir. Trans.," vol. liv. 1871.]

œdematous. If the upper lid is the one affected, it may hang down in a massive fold, and quite close the palpebral aperture, there being at the same time, perhaps, a good deal of photophobia and lachrymation. The patient generally complains of very considerable pain, and the swelling in the vicinity of the nodule is exquisitely tender to the touch; sometimes there is also a good deal of feverishness and constitutional disturbance, the sufferings of the patient being quite out of proportion to the extent of the disease. The latter may, however, run a more subacute or chronic course. The prominence produced by the nodule is generally at once evident to the eye, assuming the appearance of a little circumscribed tumor, about the size of a pea, the skin of the lid in its vicinity being of a dusky, angry red. Sometimes several lashes project from its apex, if it is situated at the margin of the lid. If it be not visible, its presence may be easily detected by lightly passing the tip of the finger over the surface of the eyelid. On eversion of the latter, the conjunctiva will generally appear smooth and unaltered, but if the nodulum points inwards, the circumscribed nodule will appear on the inner surface of the lid, the conjunctiva over and around it being reddened and swollen. If suppuration has set in, and the matter "points," the apex of the little button presents a grayish-yellow tint. If the disease is allowed to run its course, it may sometimes undergo resolution, but, as a rule, suppuration sets in, and perforation takes place, more or less thick purulent matter being discharged, together with which there is often mixed some grayish-white gelatinous substance, consisting of ill-developed or broken-down connective tissue. This is discharged in little lumps. The disease shows a very great tendency to recur again and again, so that its existence may be prolonged for very many months, and this has led some authorities to consider it dependent upon some peculiar diathesis. It is most frequently met with in youthful individuals, more especially in those of rather delicate health, who are often subject to acne, or who are addicted to free living or dissipation. If the course of the disease is protracted, and more especially if there are frequent relapses, it is not unfrequently followed by chalazion, being due to inflammatory changes in the Meibomian glands, and followed by fatty or chalky degeneration of their contents.

At the very onset of the disease, more especially if there are severe inflammatory symptoms, cold compresses should be applied; but, as a rule, I prefer the use of hot poultices which should be changed very frequently; for this will greatly accelerate the formation of pus, and expedite the progress of the case. When suppuration has set in, and the skin has become thinned and yellow at one point, a small incision should be made to permit of the ready escape of the pus, with which will generally be mixed some of the gray gelatinous connective tissue. The pain is immediately and greatly relieved by the incision. When cicatrization has taken place, I have found much benefit in preventing a recurrence of the disease, from the use of a weak ointment (ointment of nitrate of silver, gr. ij–iv ad ℥j). If the patient is feeble in health, tonics must be given, and the digestive functions thoroughly regulated.

TUMORS OF THE EYELIDS.

Tarsal Tumor. Tarsal cyst is a tumor due to inflammatory changes in the Meibomian glands and ducts, giving rise to an alteration and obstruction of the secretions. Any disturbance in the nutrition of a Meibomian gland gives rise to a chronic thickening of the connective tissue around the gland, which thickens and infiltration of the latter with small cells. By a coalescence of several groups of cells there results a nodule, which consists of granulation tissue with giant cells. The result is softening, perforation outwards, and healing by a scar in the tarsus. (See a paper by Fuchs, "Ueber das Chalazion," "Archiv f. Ophth.," xxiv. 2).—B.] If the inflammation has been acute, or if an acute inflammatory exacerbation has occurred, suppuration may take place and pus be formed. In other cases, the contents of the cyst, instead of being purulent or muco-purulent, are fluid, and gelatinous, fatty, or sebaceous and clotted. The tumor is generally about the size of a little pea, but may increase to that of a small bean; it is situated at some distance from the free margin of the lid, and is generally most manifest on its inner surface, lying close beneath the conjunctiva (which is often considerably thinned), and forming here a small, circumscribed, bluish or yellowish-white tumor, which springs prominently into view when the lid is well everted and the conjunctiva put upon the stretch [Fig. 23]. In other and rarer cases, the tumor points outwards, and lies close beneath the skin, which is frequently somewhat reddened and thinned over and around it.' It occurs far more frequently in the upper than in the lower lid. Sometimes it may exist in both eyelids, or in both eyes.

[Fig. 23

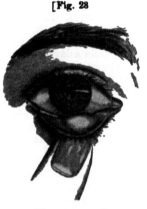

After Mackenzie.]

If the tumor is small and hard, and its formation has been extremely slow, we may endeavor to favor its absorption by the use of red precipitate or iodide of potassium ointment, but, as a rule, this proves quite ineffectual, and we must generally have recourse to operative interference. If the tumor presents upon the conjunctival surface, the lid should be thoroughly everted, and the conjunctiva put upon the stretch, so as to render the little nodule prominent and tense. A free crucial incision should then be made into it with a cataract knife or small scalpel, so that it may be laid well open. If the contents are fluid or muco-purulent, they will at once escape; if this is, however, not the case, and they are somewhat coherently gelatinous, a small curette should be introduced, and gently turned round, so as to break down and scoop out the contents. Should small portions of the latter adhere to the wall of the cyst, they should be snipped off with a pair of scissors curved on the flat. After making a free crucial incision, we may often succeed in more completely and readily emptying the contents of the cyst, by nipping it firmly between the thumb and nails, than by the use of the curette. If the tumor is deeply seated and near the outer surface, the incisions must be proportionately deep, and extend through the tarsus, as it is generally better to open the tumor, if possible, from within, for we thus avoid the formation of a cicatrix in the skin. Special attention must be paid to this if the chalazion is situated near the margin of the lid, and particularly near the punctum, for then the cicatrix would be very prone to produce a certain degree of eversion of the edge of the lid, and displacement of the punctum; but if the tumor is situated at some distance from the edge of the lid, and in its central or outer portion, lying close beneath the skin, and if the latter is lax, the incision may be made from the outside; for the wrinkles of the loose skin will hide the cicatrix, and prevent the danger of eversion. The removal of the contents is generally accompanied by considerable bleeding, and the tumor may, hence, appear to be hardly reduced in size. But in the course of a few days, the adhesive inflammation supervening on the operation will cause a contraction of the cyst, and it, together with the thickening of the structures in its vicinity, will rapidly disappear. This adhesive inflammation may be augmented by lightly touching the interior of the cyst with a finely pointed crayon of nitrate of silver. [It is better in all cases where the tumor is not too large or too far removed from the ciliary margin, to open the lid with a narrow knife along the ciliary margin, carrying the point of the knife well into the tumor. Then the contents can be squeezed out between the thumb and finger, or a small spoon can be introduced through the wound and the contents evacuated. This avoids leaving a scar either on the external or internal surface of the lid.—B.]

If the tumor is hard and firm, I generally direct the patient to apply hot poultices for a day or two before the incision, as this accelerates any tendency to suppuration, and softens the contents, so that they are less tenacious and more easily removed. As patients affected with chalazion often suffer from irregularities of the digestive functions, these should be carefully attended to.

The Meibomian follicles sometimes become obstructed, without there being any swelling or dilatation of the glands. These obstructions are due to an accumulation of the secretion in the ducts, giving rise to small yellowish-white concretions, either studded irregularly about the smooth conjunctival surface, or arranged, perhaps, in single file, like little pins' heads, along the course of the duct. If these are very small, few in number, and unattended with any inconvenience or irritation, we need not interfere; but if they are numerous, large in size, and productive of irritation, they should be pricked with the point of a knife, and the hardened contents squeezed out, or their removal may be facilitated by using a grooved spud.

Milium is a minute white tumor, about the size of a millet-seed, hence its name, which is mostly situated at or near the free edge of the lid. It generally occurs isolated, although perhaps in considerable numbers, or the tumors may be arranged in clusters. The cilia sprout forth from the centre of, and between, these little nodules. The latter should be pricked, and their soft, suet-like contents squeezed out.

Molluscum, or albuminoid tumor, is of the same nature as milium, but attains a much more considerable size, and is generally situated at some little distance from the edge of the lid, and is quite painless. The skin over it is, as a rule, somewhat thinned, so that its yellowish-white color and nodulated surface are very evident. In its centre is sometimes noticed a minute opening, through which a little white fluid exudes, and drying, forms a little brittle crust upon it. In recent cases, this matter is contagious. If the tumor exists for a very long time, its attachment to the skin may be stretched and elongated, so that it has a more or less distinct neck or pedicle, which renders it pendulous. Molluscum is generally not confined to the lids, but occurs at the same time upon the face and other parts of the body. The crust upon its apex should be detached with a pair of forceps, the nodule pricked or slightly incised, and the contents squeezed out between the thumb-nails. If it is not emptied at once, the pressure should be repeated. When several mollusca exist on the eyelids and face, it is better to operate upon them all at one sitting. Ebert[1] narrates an extraordinary case of a girl aged four, whose eyelids were so covered with mollusca some reaching the size of a hazel and walnut' that she could not open her eyes.

Michel describes two varieties of molluscum: the M. contagiosum or sebaceum, and the M. fibrosum, the first of which is described above. Their contagiousness is both affirmed and denied, and is said by those who affirm it, to be due to the so-called molluscous bodies, which resemble fat, though no true fat globules are present. It occurs in both sexes and at all ages, and no special cause can be assigned to it. When the tumors are of large size, it is better either to ligate them or to remove them with the scissors.

The fibroma molluscum is more apt to be pedunculated and to attain a larger size. The molluscous bodies are wanting, and they consist of a soft, finely fibrillated connective tissue with few cells.—B.]

Sebaceous tumors occur most frequently in children, and resemble mollusca in their nature, but attain a still more considerable size, reaching perhaps that of a large filbert or even a small walnut. They occur most frequently at the outer and upper margin of the orbit, close to the eyebrow. The skin over the tumor generally retains its normal appearance, or may become somewhat reddened. The contents are inclosed in a cyst-wall, the posterior portion of which is somewhat thickened and hypertrophied, and are suet-like and sebaceous, consisting of broken-down epithelial cells, fat molecules, and hairs. In other cases, the tumor is softer, and its contents are more oily. If it is very small, and its appearance does not annoy the patient, it may be left untouched, but otherwise it should be removed at an early stage. As, in order to prevent its return, it is necessary to remove it whole, it is better not to puncture it and squeeze out its contents, but to dissect it out, if possible, without tearing or pricking the cyst-wall. Hence, a free incision should be made through the skin, with a cataract knife or small scalpel, and parallel to the edge of the orbit. When the tumor is of considerable size, a crucial incision may be made so as to facilitate the dissection, but generally one long incision will suffice. The tumor should then be slowly and carefully dissected away, the adhesions between the cyst-wall and the surrounding cellular tissue being delicately severed with the point of the knife, or detached by gentle traction, assisted, perhaps, with the end of the handle of the knife.

An assistant should be ready with a sponge to wipe away the blood, so that the operator may constantly have a good view of the outline of the tumor and its adhesions, otherwise the cyst-wall may easily be pricked, and its white pultaceous contents begin to escape, which greatly increases the difficulty of completely removing the tumor. If the cyst-wall has not been removed entire, the remaining portions may be lightly touched with nitrate of silver. In order to accelerate the union, the edges of the wound should be brought together with fine sutures, and cold-water dressing be applied.

[Under the general head of sebaceous tumors, occur the atheromatous cysts and dermoid tumors. All these tumors may be congenital or acquired. They are more apt to occur in the upper lid and eyebrow, and may reach an enormous size. They belong to the class of retention tumors, and their contents may undergo marked alteration. Serous and colloid cysts are also met with in this region. True dermoid cysts are always congenital, and where they have existed for a long time, they have been known to produce absorption and even perforation of the underlying bone by their steady, long-continued pressure. They occasionally undergo calcareous degeneration. (See a paper on "Encysted Tumors of Eyelids and Vicinity," by the Editor, "Amer. Journ. Med. Sciences," April, 1879.)—B.]

Fibroma is met with in the eyelids in the form of a small, hard, circumscribed tumor, being sometimes congenital, and occasionally exquisitely painful to the touch. These tumors sometimes assume a cartilaginous character, and spring prominently into view when the eyelid is everted, looking like a second tarsal cartilage (Wecker). Von Graefe[1] reports a tumor of

---

[1] " Kl. Monatsbl.," 1863, p. 23.

this kind, occurring at the outer angle of the eye, and which had attained the size of half a hazel-nut. It was situated in the submucous connective tissue, and, on removal, was found to consist of true bone tissue.

Fibromas increase but very slowly in size, and this forms the chief distinguishing feature between them and sarcomatous tumors, for they cannot be distinguished with certainty from the latter, except with the microscope.

Under the term *cylindroma*, Von Graefe describes a peculiar tumor[1] which is sarcomatous in its nature, and is met with in close vicinity to the eye, e. g., the eyelids, orbit, etc., or the head. It is particularly distinguished by the fact that, together with its sarcomatous structure, it shows peculiarly club-shaped outgrowths from the capillaries and veins (Recklinghausen[2]). The tumor is very painful if firmly pressed, but spontaneous pain only occurs periodically. It shows a tendency to recur after removal, as it is very difficult to extirpate it completely.

Warts occasionally form on or near the edges of the eyelids, and should be snipped off with a pair of scissors, or touched with caustic or acetic acid. If the base is narrow, a silk or fine horse-hair ligature should be applied, so as to strangulate it, which will cause the wart to drop off in the course of a few days.

[*Papillomata*, in which the papillæ are isolated from the beginning, are also met with on the margins of the lid.

Ichthyosis has also been seen here by Arnold, in a case of general congenital ichthyosis.—B.]

Fatty tumors are not of frequent occurrence in the eyelids; they may generally be readily recognized by their smooth, circumscribed, somewhat lobulated form, and are firm and elastic to the touch. Their progress is, as a rule, extremely slow, and they can be readily removed.

In rare instances, *cutaneous horns* are observed growing from the lid. The only case of the kind which I have seen, occurred in a patient of Mr. Bowman at Moorfields, whose history (for which, as well as the drawing, I am indebted to Mr. Fairlie Clarke) was as follows: J. H., aged 76, farm laborer, applied at Moorfields on May 18, 1869, on account of a horn growing from the lower lid of the left eye. It began about ten months ago as a small wart, and it gradually increased in size until it has now reached a length of about an inch, and is the thickness of a crow-quill. It is situated at the centre of the ciliary border of the right lower lid, and hangs down in a pendulous manner (side Fig. 24). It is of a dark color, hard and horny, except just at its base, where it is continuous with the skin. By its weight it has drawn the eyelid slightly down and everted it a little. On May

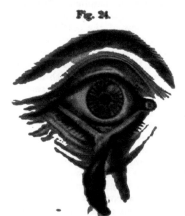

Fig. 24.

the Mr. Bowman excised the "horn," including the base within the limits of a V-shaped. The edges of the wound were brought together with a pin, and secured with a figure-of-eight ligature. On May 28th the pin and ligature were removed, and the patient was discharged from the hospital; cured.

[1] "A. f. O.," x. 1, 184.   [2] "A. f. O.," x. 1, 190.

Another remarkable case is reported by Dr. Henry Shaw,[1] of the Massachusetts Eye and Ear Infirmary. The man was fifty-six years of age, and the horn, which was situated on the right lower lid, attained a length of one and three-fourths inch, its circumference at its base being one and seven-eighths inch; it was curved, and looked like the beak of a bird. Dr. Shaw excised it with success.

Epithelial cancer is almost the only malignant tumor which occurs primarily in the eyelids, for the other forms, such as scirrhus, medullary cancer, etc., are generally only secondarily met with in this situation.

Epithelial cancer shows itself most frequently in the lower eyelid, and near the outer canthus. [It is of three kinds: the superficial, the deep, and the papillomatous; and it is said that these are all different stages of the same disease.—B.] It occurs generally in persons above the age of forty, or even in those much more aged, being rarely met with in youthful individuals. At the outset, the disease assumes the appearance of a small, circumscribed, slightly elevated induration, situated at, or close to, the edge of the lid, and looking like a wart or a small thickened crust. It is covered by healthy-looking, uninflamed skin, and a few varicose vessels are perhaps seen to pass over or near it. The surface of the little nodule often looks rough and scaly, as if the cuticle were thickened. It may remain in this condition for a very long period, and years may elapse before it increases materially in size, or becomes ulcerated. On this account, and from its being quite painless, it is often entirely disregarded by the patient, who supposes it to be simply a wart. When the disease occurs in the skin over the lachrymal sac, it has been mistaken for dacryocystitis. Thus Mackenzie mentions one instance, in which the patient called to have a style introduced, and another, in which one had actually been worn. But, sooner or later, it gradually and almost imperceptibly increases somewhat in size, creeping along the edge of the lid and assuming a lengthened, ovoid shape. Its surface becomes broken and excoriated, and a thin grayish-yellow discharge exudes from it, which hardens upon it in the form of dark rough crusts. Then ulceration sets in, and the tumor slowly spreads in circumference and depth, the edges of the ulcer being somewhat elevated, and studded, perhaps, with a few palish-red tubercles, which rapidly form again if abscised. The skin around the tumor is but little thickened, swollen, or discolored, and this distinguishes the disease from lupus, and also from a syphilitic ulcer. Moreover, the slowness of its growth and the history of the case, would prevent its being mistaken for the latter. When the ulceration sets in, the pain increases, but seldom to any considerable degree, nor is it of a very acute, lancinating character; but if any nerves are exposed by the ulceration, the patient's suffering will, of course, be much augmented. The discharge is of a yellowish color, healthy in nature, and free from fetor.[2] Sometimes, the ulcer may become temporarily cicatrized, either completely or in part, and then remain apparently healed for a certain time; but soon a breach of surface again occurs, and fresh ulceration sets in. In time, the ulcer invades the lid more and more, spreading along its surface and extending deeply into its structure, until it may eat its way completely through its whole thickness, and appear on the conjunctival surface; thence, perhaps, extending to the orbit. If the lids are destroyed, the eyeball will be exposed, and suppuration of the cornea may ensue, accompanied perhaps by loss of the lens and a considerable portion of the vitreous humor, and followed by atrophy of the globe. Mac-

[1] "Boston Med. and Surg. Journal," 1860, Feb. 11.
[2] Vide Dr. Jacob's able paper on this disease, "Dublin Hospital Reports," vol. iv., 1827.

kenzie[1] has witnessed the most excruciating pain ensuing upon implication of the eyeball, or when the ulceration affected the infra-orbital and supra-orbital nerves. The disease may also extend to the face, finally opening into the mouth. The veins which pass over the ulcer often give way and cause very considerable hemorrhage.

The cause of the disease is frequently dubious, but sometimes we are able distinctly to trace its origin to some injury or blow, or the existence of some prolonged course of irritation.

If the disease is moderate in extent and circumscribed, so that there is hope of entirely removing it, the treatment by extirpation is, I think, as a rule, the best; care being taken to carry the incisions through the healthy integuments, for fear of leaving any of the morbid tissue behind. This incision is generally made of a V-shape, and sufficiently large to include all the diseased portion within it. The edges of the wound should be brought together with fine sutures; or if the loss of substance is considerable, a plastic operation should be performed, and the skin brought from the temple or cheek. Mackenzie, however, prefers to make a semilunar incision, and to allow the wound to heal by granulation. It must be admitted, however, that even when the operation has been followed by a firm cicatrix, and the disease has appeared to have been cured, after a time a relapse has taken place, and hence the treatment by escharotics and other agents has been strongly recommended. Potassa fusa and the chloride of zinc paste have been especially used as caustics. Mackenzie[2] strongly recommends the sulphate of zinc for this purpose. The water of crystallization of the sulphate of zinc having been driven off by heat, and the residuum reduced to a fine powder, he mixed it with a little glycerine, so as to form a thick tenacious paste, and on the point of a bit of stick, applied it over the scab and the hard edges of the ulcer; the part being then covered with a bit of dry lint. This treatment was repeated two or three times, and produced a firm, healthy cicatrix, and apparently an excellent cure.

Dr. Broadbent's treatment by injection of acetic acid (one part of strong acid to about four of water) may also be tried, and has proved very successful in the hands of several distinguished surgeons, amongst others, Mr. Power,[3] De Weeker,[4] etc. Dr. Althaus' treatment by electrolysis may likewise be tried, being quite free from any pain or discomfort. Mr. Bergeron[5] recommends the internal and local use of chlorate of potash.

[Better results are obtained from sliding flaps than by the methods of transplantation of flaps ordinarily in use. The epithelioma or diseased tissue is to be removed by a four-cornered or rectangular excision. Then if the sliding flap is to come from the nose, horizontal incisions are to be made through the skin over the nose, inclosing a flap of skin broad enough to cover the defect in the lower lid. This is to be dissected up and made to slide forward until it meets skin on the other side of the defect, to which it is to be united. If the flap is to slide from the temple, the incisions are to be made towards the region, the upper one being a prolongation of the external canthus, and the lower one diverging from it somewhat downward. Sometimes both flaps are made to slide towards each other. This mode of operating has been practised quite extensively in this country by Knapp, Noyes, and others. (See "Arch. für Ophthal.," xiii.; "Arch. of Ophth. and Otol.," i. 1 and 2. A modification of this operation has been practised by

[1] Diseases of the Eye, 4th edit., 187.　　[2] R. L. O. H. Rep.," ii. 5.
[3] Mr. Power, Diseases of the Eye, p 108.
[4] De Weeker, Maladies des Yeux, 2d edition, p 659.
[5] H. p 659.

Noyes, of New York, for the purpose of remedying defects about the inner portion of the lower lid, and which succeeds very well in some cases of epithelioma. It consists in sliding the whole cheek, together with the remaining portion of the shortened lid, inward and upward. Its advantage over the other operation by sliding flaps, is that the necessary incisions are not so conspicuous. The flap does not slough; it lies in perfect coaptation and is fully adequate to cover any defect. One of the incisions runs perpendicularly downward in the furrow alongside of the nose, as far as the ala nasi, and the other one is made horizontally outward across the temple towards the ear, a varying distance in different cases. It is, in short, a bucco-temporal flap instead of a naso-buccal flap. (See "Trans. Amer. Ophth. Soc.," 1879.)—B.]

Sarcoma and carcinoma of the eyelids are extremely rare affections. Hirschberg[1] describes a case of small-cell sarcoma involving the lower lid, in which the tumor reached the size of an apple, and was removed by him together with the eyeball. [Sarcomatous tumors which originate in the orbit, however, frequently involve the lids in their progress. Primary sarcoma of the lids mainly occurs in childhood or youth, and begins as an œdematous swelling beneath the movable skin. It is elastic, grows rapidly, and soon infiltrates the interstitial tissue of the orbicular muscle. A case of inelastic sarcoma of the lid has been reported by Gibson ("Phil. Lancet," No. 2, 1851); and a case of cysto-sarcoma by Daucher ("Allg. Wien. Med. Zeit.," 1859). During the last few years several cases have been reported, among them two by Samelsohn and Schirmer. Prout has reported an interesting case of sarcoma of the tarsus and conjunctiva, in a young girl, which involved the lower lid. The growth was removed without difficulty from the conjunctival surface of the lid, and on examination proved to be a round-cell sarcoma of the tarsus and conjunctiva with admixture of club-shaped or cylindroid cells. Portions of the growth had undergone extensive amyloid degeneration. In places the epithelium of the conjunctiva was very much thickened. (See "Arch. of Ophthalmology," viii. 1, pp. 73–78.)—B.]

Rodent cancer of the eyelids generally commences by a small mole or pimple, which has existed perhaps for many years, beginning to itch and becoming somewhat tender to the touch, and then a breach of surface occurs, which becomes covered with a scab. Gradually, the solid pimple increases in size and involves the healthy structures, and the central crack assumes the appearance of an ulcer. The margin of the latter is indurated and broad, but is quite free from tubercles, and there is but very little inflammatory congestion. The solid growth slowly spreads to the adjacent structures, advancing in depth as well as in circumference, and without any regard to difference in the tissues; although there is a considerable difference in the rate of progress in the various tissues, the skin always yielding most rapidly. The disease, as a rule, only after the age of fifty, produces no cachexia, and but little pain, and is never followed by enlarged glands or deposits in the viscera. With regard to the *prognosis*, it is favorable if the disease is seen at an early stage, while complete removal by the knife or escharotics is possible. Its progress is the more rapid, and the tendency to return the more marked, the younger the patient. When the disease occurs in the eyelids it is best to excise it, and to fill up the gap by transplantation of the skin, for in this region the use of a very powerful escharotic, such as the chloride of zinc paste, is generally not advisable. If excision is not practised, it is therefore better to employ some other caustic, such as nitrate

---

[1] "Knapp's Archiv," 2, 1, 229.

of silver, nitric acid, or acid nitrate of mercury. To relieve the pain of the application of the latter, the part should be painted immediately afterwards with collodion[1] (Nayler).

[A few cases of *adenoma* of the lids have been reported. They grew near the edge of the lid, ulcerated and developed fistulous tracts. The surrounding infiltration was extensive. A microscopical examination showed a neoplastic growth of epithelial tubes with sparse anastomotic connections. In a case reported by Nettleship ("R. L. O. Hosp. Rep.," vii. 2) the tumor was as large as a raspberry, projected both from the outer and inner surfaces of the lid, was solid throughout, and its cut surface did not bleed. Sections showed it to be composed of numerous gland-follicles with secondary pouches, and an overgrowth of the connective-tissue elements of gland structures.

Neuroma-fibrillare of the lid is mentioned by Billroth as congenital. He removed a tumor from the upper lid of a boy six years old, which extended upon the temp , and was very sensitive to the touch. It was removed with difficulty, and showed on examination nodular branched cylinders, in the axis of which were the remains of small nerve branches. Bruns has described three such cases. ("Graefe u. Saemisch, Handb.," iv. p. 428.)

Amyloid degeneration of the tarsus has only been recognized of late years. One of the first to call attention to it was Vogel, who observed it in a case of enormous infiltration of the lid with great thickening of the walls of the vessels. The application of iodine and sulphuric acid proved the existence of amyloid disease. The symptoms are very characteristic: enormous thickening and elongation of the lids, which are very hard and cannot be everted; the absence of all signs of inflammation in the external skin, which usually remains freely movable; entire absence of pain, and steady growth of the disease. Bull has reported an interesting case of amyloid infiltration of the lid, in which the disease began in the orbit, and eventually spread to the brain and caused death. Both lids were involved to an extreme degree, and a piece being excised and examined proved the case to be one of amyloid degeneration. ("Trans. Amer. Ophthal. Soc.," 1878.) Von Hippel has an interesting article upon the subject, based upon the careful examination of one case (see "Archiv für Ophthal.," xxv. 2), and Mandelstamm has also reported some observations upon the subject, based upon cases ("Archiv für Ophthal.," xxv. 1). In Prout's case of sarcoma, which had undergone amyloid degeneration, the latter was most extensive in the interior of the tarsus, finally crowding out entirely the sarcoma cells. In this region of pure amyloid infiltration, the vessels were more numerous, and the walls of the smaller arteries and capillaries showed well-marked signs of infiltration, the internal one being the first affected. The connective tissue in the vicinity was also involved. ("Archives of Ophthal.," viii. 1.)

Lupus has been met with in the eyelids as a secondary growth from the neighboring parts of the face. It sometimes extends with great rapidity along the edge of the lid, which leads to marked shrinking and cicatrization of the lid, with sometimes anchyloblepharon, and sometimes ectropium.

Lepra, or *Elephantiasis Græcorum* of the eyelids, has been frequently observed as the first symptom of the disease. Bull and Hansen have observed a large number of cases of lepra, and among the first symptoms noted a loss of the eyebrows, and the formation of nodules in the lids, with loss of the lashes. These nodules may reach the size of a hazel-nut, are brown in color, and lie in the skin, or just beneath it. The cellular infiltration belongs

---

[1] For admirable descriptions of this disease, *vide* Mr. Moore's work, "On Rodent Cancer," and Mr. Hutchinson's "Clinical Report on Rodent Ulcer," "Med. Times and Gazette," 1860, vol. ii.

alone to the vessels, and may obliterate them. The nodules ulcerate on the surface or break down in the centre, but there is rarely any suppuration. Ectropium is the final result. These nodules may be extirpated early in the disease, but when ulceration has once begun, it is useless. ("The Leprous Diseases of the Eye," 1873.)

Cysticerci have been found in the cellular tissue of the upper and lower lid, and even between the bundles of fibres of the orbicular muscle. The skin is freely movable over the tumor, and there are no signs of inflammatory irritation. They are to be removed by excision. ("Graefe und Saemisch, Handb.," iv. p. 433).—B.]

8.—[ANGIOMA.—B.]—NÆVUS MATERNUS (TELANGIECTASIS).

[*Angiomata* occurring in the eyelids include cavernous tumors, as well as telangiectasiæ. The former are rare, not congenital, but appear in childhood or youth, and may involve the entire lid, which is markedly swollen, bluish-red, and drooping.—B.]

The telangiectatic tumor is more frequently met with on the eyelids, and may vary considerably in size and appearance. Its surface may be smooth and even, or granulated, and perhaps divisible into two or three distinct portions. The color also varies from a light scarlet to a dark bluish-red or purple. Nævi may be quite superficial and confined to the skin, or extend deeper and implicate the subcutaneous tissue, perhaps to a considerable extent. They have also been divided into an arterial or active, and a venous or passive form. The former are firm and distinctly pulsatile to the touch, and cannot be emptied, except the vessels which supply them are compressed (Mackenzie). The venous are softer and more elastic, and can be easily emptied by pressure. On the patient's stooping down, the nævus rapidly swells up, and becomes dark and very tense.

The nævus is almost always congenital, and may gradually increase up to a certain point, and then remain almost stationary, or else it may spontaneously diminish in size, and slowly disappear, without leaving a trace behind.

Various modes of treatment have been recommended for this disease. Of these the best are, I think, the application of threads soaked in perchloride of iron, the various forms of ligature, and electrolysis. Injection of the perchloride of iron is excessively dangerous, and several cases of instantaneous death have been recorded. Hence it is far wiser to traverse the tumor in different directions with threads dipped in perchloride of iron, and to allow them to remain in for a few days. The subcutaneous ligature, either in a figure-of-eight, or circular, also proves very successful. If the tumor is considerable in size, and divisible into several portions, one of these may be taken at a time, and the operation repeated several times. De Wecker[1] transfixes the base of the little tumor by two needles crossed at right angles (+), and then firmly strangulates the base with a thread passed beneath the needles.

The application of electrolysis to these nævi, appears to me to be very serviceable. Dr. Althaus,[2] to whom we are indebted for the introduction of this mode of treatment, has found it very successful, and narrates a case in which a nævus of the eyelid (in a patient of Mr. White Cooper) was rapidly cured without leaving any trace behind. The great advantages of electrol-

---

[1] De Wecker, " Maladies des Yeux," 2d edition, i 653.
[2] *Vide* Dr. Althaus' interesting work on " Electrolysis."

ysis are, that it is free from all pain and danger, and that it does not leave any scar or disfigurement.

Galvano-puncture has also been recommended. [This method may be employed where the angioma is not very large, as it reduces the cicatrization to a minimum. But many of these nævi, and even the larger angiomata, can be extirpated by the knife, care being taken to use Desmarres' lid-clamp or other contrivance for controlling the blood-supply. Generally speaking, less deformity results from the use of the knife than from caustics or the galvano-cautery. Knapp's lid-forceps are better than Desmarres', for they give more space for operating. After the tumor has been excised and the cavity washed out, a careful application of pins and twisted sutures will almost always arrest the hemorrhage, and, if not, it can always be controlled by the lid-clamp. See a paper by Knapp in "Arch. of Ophthal.," iii. 3 and 4. See also a paper by the Editor in the "Trans. Amer. Ophth. Soc.," 1880, and "New York Med. Journ.," September, 1880.—B.]

6.—[PARALYSIS OF THE LEVATOR PALPEBRÆ SUPERIORIS.—B.]
—PTOSIS.

In this affection the upper eyelid droops down, so that the palpebral aperture is greatly narrowed, and the cornea more or less covered, the patient being unable by a voluntary effort to raise the lid. In the chapter upon the Paralytic Affections of the Muscles of the Eye, it will be mentioned that ptosis is a frequent symptom in paralysis of the third nerve, on account of the *levator palpebræ superioris* being supplied by this nerve. In complete paralysis of the third nerve we find, besides the ptosis, that on lifting the eyelid, the eye is immovable in all directions except outwards, and slightly downwards and outwards, that the pupil is dilated, and the accommodation paralyzed. The ptosis may be partial or complete; in the former case, the upper lid can still be somewhat lifted, and does not droop to the full extent; in the latter, it hangs down immovably, and has to be lifted up by the assistance of the finger. The palpebral aperture may, however, be somewhat widened, and the upper lid slightly elevated by the relaxation of the orbicularis and the contraction of the frontalis muscle. The causes of paralysis of the third nerve will be mentioned further on, and I need not here consider them. It must be stated, however, that in some rare instances the branch to the levator palpebræ may be alone implicated, owing to its direct compression by an exostosis, tumor, etc., the other branches of the third nerve being unaffected. Or, again, some traumatic lesion, implicating the nerve or the muscle itself, may be the cause. Ptosis may also occur independently of any paralytic affection, being due to some want of development or congenital insufficiency of the levator palpebræ, which coexists sometimes with epicanthus. Or it may remain after the great swelling of the lid and hypertrophy of the conjunctiva accompanying purulent or granular ophthalmia, the levator not being sufficiently strong to overcome the weight. A certain degree of ptosis is also sometimes observed in aged people, if there is a great superabundance of flaccid skin, and the levator palpebræ is at the same time somewhat weak.

An interesting form of partial and slowly developed ptosis is occasionally observed in adults; it is accompanied by myosis of the same eye, and there is an entire absence of paralysis of any of the other muscles supplied by the third nerve. Horner records an interesting instance of this kind, in which there was also, during any excitement, marked increase in the temperature and redness of the corresponding half of the face, which stopped exactly in the median line; this side of the face being also quite free from any perspiration. The eye-tension was slightly diminished. He considers that this form of ptosis is evidently due to paralysis of the plain muscular fibres of the upper lid, which are supplied by the sympathetic, thus forming the opposite condition to the retraction of the upper lid, which is met with in exophthalmic goitre, and which is due to irritation of these fibres.

The *treatment* must be varied according to the cause of the affection. If it be due to paralysis, the general line of treatment laid down in the chapter upon the Paralytic Affections of the Muscles of the Eye must be followed. Electricity often proves of considerable benefit. But if the disease resists all these remedies, recourse must be had to operative interference. In those cases in which the ptosis is simply due to an over-abundance of hypertrophy of the skin, a horizontal fold of the latter, parallel to the edge of the lid, should be pinched up with a pair of forceps and excised, the edges of the wound being united by fine sutures.

The attempt has, moreover, been made by Bowman and Von Graefe to bring forward the insertion of the levator palpebræ, and thus augment its power, on the same principle upon which the insertion of some of the ocular muscles is sometimes brought forward. But the results were not favorable. Von Graefe[1] has more lately devised the following operation: A transverse incision is made through the skin of the upper lid about two and a half lines from its free margin, and extending the whole length of the lid, the incision being made to gape by a vertical traction upon its edges, and by separating the subcutaneous cellular tissue with a knife. When a sufficient breadth of the orbicularis has been thus exposed, it is to be seized with the forceps, and a portion of about four or five lines in width is to be excised, care being taken not to injure the subjacent fascia. The incision is then to be united by sutures, which are to be carried through the skin and the cut edges of the orbicularis. The effect of this operation is to cause a subcutaneous shortening of the upper lid, to weaken the action of the orbicularis, and thus to assist that of the levator. If the length of the lid is increased, Von Graefe, after having finished the transverse incision, makes a second, having its convexity upwards, so that a shortening of the skin may be combined with the subcutaneous shortening of the lid.

10.—PARALYSIS OF THE ORBICULARIS PALPEBRARUM.

In this affection we find that the eyelids cannot be completely closed, on account of the inefficient elevation of the lower lid, so that a chink of varying size exists between the two lids. By a strong effort of the will, the patient may succeed (more easily if the other eye is closed) in almost shutting the lids by the relaxation of the levator palpebræ. The wide gaping of the eyelids gives a peculiarly staring appearance to the patient, and is termed *lagophthalmos*. The paralytic lagophthalmos is present even during sleep, and resists the action of reflex irritants applied to the conjunctiva. Paralysis of the orbicularis is soon followed by other symptoms. There is marked epiphora, and the constant flowing of tears over the cheek soon causes irritation and excoriation of the edges of the lids, upon which thickening and eversion supervene. The exposure of the eye to external irritants (such as

[1] "A. f. O.," ix. 2, 57.

particles of dust, etc.) soon produces conjunctivitis and superficial keratitis, ending, perhaps, in pannus and xerophthalmia.

The affection of the orbicularis is due to paralysis of the facial nerve. The orbicularis may be alone affected, or the paralysis may extend to several, or all the branches of the facial nerve. It is only very rarely met together with hemiplegia. The causes of the disease may be peripheral or central. Amongst the former, exposure to cold air, damp, etc., is the most frequent. It may also be caused by direct pressure (as from a tumor) upon any part of the nerve, or by injuries which implicate the latter. Amongst the cerebral causes need only be mentioned the presence of tumors, syphilitic exudations, hemorrhagic or purulent effusions, etc., and different lesions situated at the base of the brain. [Diseases of the ear, the lymphatic glands and parotid gland, may all produce lesions of the facial nerve. According to Eulenburg, facial paralysis originating from lesion of the pons involves the orbicularis; while if it proceed from the cerebral peduncles, or from the central ganglia, or from progressive paralysis of cranial nerves, or from affections of the spinal cord, the orbicularis is likely to escape. (See "A Treatise on Diseases of the Eye," by Henry D. Noyes, 1881.)—B.] If the disease is due to paralysis, the treatment laid down in the article upon "The Paralytic Affections of the Muscles of the Eye" should be pursued. In order to guard the eyeball against the effect of external irritants, we may pare to a slight extent two corresponding points of the tarsal margins of the upper and lower lid, and then unite them by two or three stitches; the eyeball being thus protected until the orbicularis has regained its power.

11.—BLEPHAROSPASM.

This affection varies much in intensity. In the slighter forms, there may only exist a moderate degree of temporary twitching and contraction of the lids, which soon passes off again. If the affection is more severe, the spasm of the orbicularis may be so great, that the eyelids are firmly pressed together, and that it is quite impossible for the patient or the surgeon to open them even to a slight degree. The endeavor forcibly to open the eye is intensely painful, and may even almost throw the patient into epileptiform convulsions. At the outset, the disease is generally but moderate, but if the cause persists, or efficient treatment is not adopted, it gradually increases in severity, and the spasm, which was before perhaps only periodical, becomes permanent, so that the patient cannot open his eye at all. Then the other eye may become affected in a similar manner, and the muscles of the face, and even of the extremities, may undergo spasmodic contractions.[b]

Blepharospasm is often met with in the course of inflammatory affections of the cornea and conjunctiva, or if a foreign body has become lodged within the folds of the latter. In such cases, it is evidently due to a reflex neurosis produced by irritation of some of the branches of the fifth nerve. This likewise occurs in severe cases of hyperæsthesia of the retina. It is also seen in connection with neuralgia of the supra-orbital nerve, or of the fifth; the exact seat of these affections being perhaps a certain spot is found where firm pressure will at once ... It must be mentioned, however, that in some instances ... upon the facial nerve at its exit) through the stylo-mastoid ... the blepharospasm (Romberg).

b "A. f. O.," i. 1, 440.

The treatment of the disease must vary with the cause and duration. Thus the severe blepharospasm often noticed in the course of corneal affections disappears with them; or, if it persists, it frequently yields to tonics, immersion of the head in cold water, sea bathing, and the subcutaneous injection of morphia. Indeed, the latter remedy is often found of great benefit in the treatment of these spasmodic affections. From one-sixth to one-third of a grain of morphia should be injected at the point where pressure will stop the spasm, and be occasionally repeated. If, however, these remedies fail to cure the blepharospasm, and if pressure upon the supra-orbital nerve stops it, and enables the patient momentarily to open his eye, this nerve must be divided. This operation was first performed by Von Graefe, at Romberg's suggestion, in a case of intense blepharospasm which had supervened upon the lodgement of a foreign body in the folds of the conjunctiva. It was evidently a case of hyperæsthesia of the orbicularis from contusion, and was considered by Romberg to be a reflex spasm due to a pathological irritation of the sensory nerves. He, therefore, advised the division of the supra-orbital nerve, from which recurrent (sensory) branches are probably distributed to the orbicularis. The operation proved perfectly successful, and has since then been often repeated with much benefit by Von Graefe and other surgeons. The supra-orbital nerve should be divided close to its exit from the supra-orbital foramen, and, in order to facilitate this, the eyebrow should be drawn well upwards, so as to make the skin tense. If the nerve is not completely divided, the effect will only be slight or temporary, and the operation should be repeated. As this non-success may sometimes be due to a reunion of the divided ends of the nerve, some surgeons have cut out a piece of the latter. After the operation, there should be a certain degree of anæsthesia just above the divided portion of the nerve, and in the upper lid. The operation should be performed under chloroform, more especially in children. Prior to its performance, the surgeon should, of course, try whether the firm compression of the supra-orbital nerve alleviates the blepharospasm, for only in such cases can we expect a favorable result. [Subcutaneous division of the orbicular muscle was recommended and practised by Dieffenbach, but without much success.

Dr. Mathewson, of Brooklyn, has proposed a method of treating blepharospasm, which has been sometimes employed for the relief of ptosis. A slender band of rubber, a out one line broad, half a line thick, and an inch long, is to be attached byb one end to the surface of the upper lid near its lower edge, at the middle of its horizontal length; a strip of isinglass plaster, notched so as to adapt itself accurately, is applied across the band, and the whole is covered with collodion and allowed to dry till firmly adherent. The band is then to be stretched upward to an inch and a half, so as to elevate the lid moderately, and fastened to the forehead in the same way, and to be kept in place until the blepharospasm is overcome. The size, length, and tension of the band may be varied to suit circumstances. ("Trans. Amer. Ophth. Soc.," 1874.)

Among the remedies for internal administration which have been recommended in the treatment of this disease, the most important is conium, a very powerful and somewhat dangerous drug. Its effects must be very closely watched, and the first dose should never be more than ten drops of Squibb's fluid extract, repeated from three to six times daily. The physiological symptoms will be vertigo, incoördination of muscles, thickness of speech. The administration of the drug must then be stopped, and at this stage the eyelids will open. Another remedy, recommended by Dr. Oppenheimer, and suited to children with strumous inflammation, is the dropping of iced water upon the exposed eye every fifteen minutes or half hour. (See Noyes, loc. cit., p. 146.)—B.]

Nictitation, or involuntary convulsive twitching of the eyelids, is o sionally met with in a varying degree, and is generally owing to a re neurosis producing a spasmodic contraction of the orbicularis; these twi lugs following each other in rapid succession. The affection may be lim to one eye, or involve both, the upper lid being more frequently implicated than the lower. It is always markedly increased by any nervousness or agitation of mind, and is frequently met with in persons in a weak, nervous, or hysterical condition. It may also be due to some local irritation, as an inverted lash, slight inflammation of the conjunctiva, etc. It is sometimes observed in cases of hypermetropia in which glasses are not worn, and will then disappear with the removal of the cause. In nervous and delicate persons, the general health should be attended to, an aromatic and slightly stimulating lotion applied to the lids, and the eye-douche be used. In hypermetropia, the proper glasses should be ordered, and then the twitching will soon disappear.

12.—TRICHIASIS AND DISTICHIASIS.

These conditions are characterized by an irregularity in the growth and direction of the eyelashes, which are more or less inverted. In trichiasis,

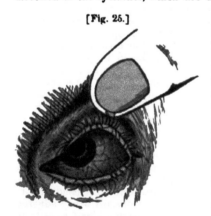

[Fig. 25.]

the lashes are irregular, some perhaps having a natural position and appearance, whilst others are incurved, thin, pale, straggling, and stunted [Fig. 25]. In distichiasis, there are two distinct rows of lashes, the outer being in the usual position, the inner being situated further back and turned inwards. The double arrangement is, however, often only apparent, being due to a thickening and stretching of the edge of the lid, and a consequent alteration in the direction of the hairbulbs and the cilia. Both trichiasis and distichiasis may affect the whole length of the lid, or be limited to a certain portion or portions of it; and if the malposition only involves a very few, colorless, thin cilia, it may readily be overlooked, and maintain a prolonged and very annoying irritation of the eye and lids.

This faulty position of the cilia is generally accompanied, or soon followed by a certain degree of inversion of the eyelid (entropium), and perhaps by a shortening and incurvation of the tarsus. But in the simple and true trichiasis or distichiasis this is not the case, and the position of the lid and the condition of the tarsus are perfectly normal.

The most frequent causes of these conditions are long-continued and severe inflammations of the conjunctiva (purulent and granular ophthalmia, etc.), and of the edge of the lid; in which the hair-follicles have undergone inflammatory and suppurative changes, so that they are either destroyed, or their functions so much impaired that the growth of the lashes is injured, and they become weak, stunted, and distorted. Ulcers and small abscesses at the roots of the cilia, or injuries (burns, cuts, etc.) of the edge of the lid, may also produce these affections.

The irregular growth and inversion of the lashes, even although only a few may be involved, set up considerable irritation of the eye, which becomes watery, red, and irritable, the patient complaining of a constant pricking and itching in it, as if a minute foreign body, or a little sand or grit, were lodged beneath the lid. If the affection is allowed to continue, the symptoms of irritation increase in severity, and there may be considerable lachrymation and photophobia. The constant spasmodic contraction of the eyelids causes an inversion of the edge of the latter, which may, in time, become permanent, so that an entropium is superadded to the trichiasis. After a time, the constant friction of the inverted or stunted lashes against the cornea sets up a superficial corneitis, and a more or less severe degree of pannus will supervene.

[Fig. 26.]

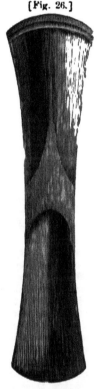

The treatment of distichiasis and trichiasis must vary with the extent and severity of the disease. If only a few, straggling cilia are misplaced, their repeated evulsion may eventually cure the affection. By frequently extracting the lashes, we may, in time, succeed in causing an atrophy of the hair-bulbs, and thus arrest the growth of the cilia. Indeed, many patients learn to do this very well for themselves, or are satisfied to have the lashes extracted every few weeks by their medical attendant. If the trichiasis is confined to a very few and scattered lashes, this treatment may suffice; but the oft-repeated evulsion occasionally leads, after a time, to a certain degree of irritability of the eye, and may thus become a source of annoyance to the patient. Sometimes, the destruction of the hair-follicles by the application of liquor potassæ also proves successful, where only a few cilia are implicated. A horn spatula [Fig. 26] having been inserted beneath the eyelid, and the edge of the latter put on the stretch and somewhat everted, so that the row of lashes is brought well into view, the point of a needle (dipped into liquor potassæ) should be run up to the roots of the distorted lashes, so as to reach their follicles; or liquefied potassa fusa may be employed for this purpose, and in the same manner, as has been proposed by Dr. Williams.[1] This will generally soon cause their destruction. Some surgeons also produce the latter by means of the application of a strong caustic solution (e. g., the sulph-hydrate of calcium). In order that it may not extend to the conjunctiva or the cheek, and set up considerable inflammation, the surrounding parts should be smeared with oil, the edge of the lids be well everted, and the solution very carefully applied. The calcium is to be washed away with a sponge after four or five minutes. But if a considerable extent of the lid is treated in this manner, a very unsightly baldness (madarosis) will ensue. And hence it is always wiser to endeavor, where a considerable length of the edge of the lid is involved, to perform some operation which shall prove a cure, and yet pre-

---

[1] "R. L. O. H. Rep.," lii. 219.

serve the eyelashes.   Very numerous operations have been proposed for the
cure of trichiasis, more especially when combined, as is generally the case,
with entropium.   Some of these consist in the complete excision of some or
all of the eyelashes, others in giving the latter a different direction, but not
destroying them.

When only a limited number of lashes is misplaced, the following is the
best mode of excising them.

If the upper lid is the seat of the disease, Snellen's modification of Desmarres' clamp, Fig. 27, should be used.   The lower blade should be inserted

Fig. 27.

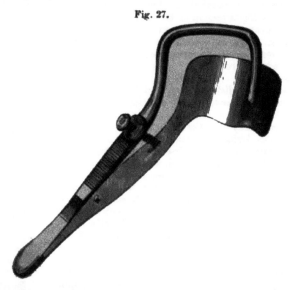

beneath the upper eyelid, and the two blades then screwed down, so as to
compress the eyelid firmly between them and control the bleeding [Fig. 28].
[Mr. Laurence has slightly modified Snellen's forceps (Fig. 29), and adapted
the same principle to the lower lid.—H.]   In the operations for slight partial
trichiasis, it is not so necessary to use this instrument, as for those which are
performed when a considerable portion of the lid is implicated.   An incision
is then to be made with a small scalpel (or with a broad iridectomy knife)
at the edge of the lid, just between the Meibomian ducts, so that the cilia
are included in the anterior portion of the incision.   The latter is to extend
upwards to about three lines, and its length should include all the distorted
lashes.   Two incisions are then to be made through the edge of the lid and
the skin, these incisions meeting at the centre, so as to form two sides of a
triangle, the base of which is formed by the lower incision along the margin
of the lid.   This triangle, which includes the bulbs of the misplaced lashes,
should then be removed.   The lateral incisions may also be made with a
pair of curved scissors, one point of which is to be inserted at the angles of
the longitudinal wound.   The lateral edges of the incision are to be brought
together with fine sutures.

Herzenstein has devised the following operation for trichiasis, which
appears to be especially applicable to the partial forms, where only a few
lashes are implicated.   It consists in the insertion of a thread, which sets up

considerable irritation, and the accompanying suppuration causes the destruction of the follicles of the displaced cilia. Dr. Herzenstein performs the operation in the following manner: He enters a needle (*N*, Fig. 30),

[Fig. 28. Fig. 29.]

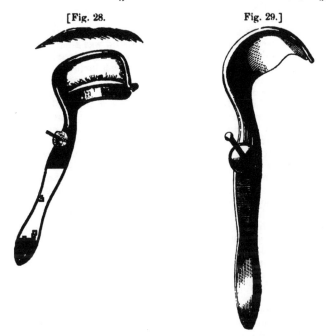

carrying a fine silken thread, at the edge of the lid between the cilia and the openings of the Meibomian ducts, at *a* (Fig. 30), passes it along subcutaneously in a vertical direction, and brings it out at *b*, slightly above the margin

Fig. 30.

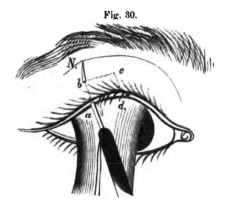

of the lid. The one thread is here drawn through, and the needle again inserted at the same opening, *b*, and passed along subcutaneously and parallel to the margin of the lid, to the extent of the distorted lashes (to *c*). The thread is here again drawn through, and the needle reinserted at the same orifice, *c*, and passed down vertically to make its way out at a point (*d*) between the borders of the margin of the lid. The two ends of the thread are then firmly tied, and permitted to cut their way out. Cold compresses should be applied. If numerous little yellow spots of suppuration appear, the thread should be at once removed. He has also operated successfully in cases where a very considerable extent of the lid was affected.[1]

When a considerable number of the lashes are misplaced, we must remove a long narrow strip of the edge of the lid, which includes these faulty cilia, or even "scalp" the whole lid. Snellen's clamp having been applied, an incision is to be made with a scalpel or cataract knife along the free edge of the lid between the eyelashes and the opening of the Meibomian glands, so as to split the tarsus into two, and sufficiently deep to pass beyond the roots of the lashes. A second incision is then to be made on the external surface of the lid, and carried along, and parallel to, its edge, just behind the row of lashes, so that the two incisions meet, and the strip of skin and integument, containing all the faulty lashes and their roots, is then to be excised. This operation may be partial or extend nearly to the whole length of the lid, according to the extent of the faulty lashes. On completing the excision, the part should be sponged and the tarsus be closely examined, to discover if any of the hair-bulbs (which appear like minute black spots) have escaped, in which case they should be excised, otherwise the cilia will, of course, grow again. Sutures need not be employed, but a cold wet compress should be applied.

The above operation is certainly efficacious in curing the trichiasis, but it is unsightly, more especially in the upper lid, and the entire absence of the eyelashes and their protective influence may give rise to a good deal of inflammation, from exposure of the eye to external irritants, such as dust, etc. However, in persons who are careless as to their personal appearance, and are anxious to be quickly and effectually cured of the disease, this operation will be found a very suitable one. But in those cases in which it is of importance to preserve the eyelashes, and simply to give them a different and better position, so that in place of being turned in, they are well everted, the operation of transplantation is to be much preferred. Indeed, I almost invariably perform it in preference to that of scalping, even although the personal appearance may be of no particular importance. The two following are, I think, the best operations for transplantation.

1. Arlt's modification of Jaesche's operation. As this is a tedious and painful proceeding, the patient should be put under the influence of an anæsthetic. Snellen's clamp having been applied, an incision is to be carried along the free edge of the eyelid, between the cilia and the openings of the Meibomian ducts, and reaching to a depth of about two lines, care being taken to avoid the punctum. In this way, the free edge of the lid will be split into two portions, the anterior containing the integuments, eyelashes, and their bulbs, etc., and the posterior the cartilage and the efferent ducts of the Meibomian glands. When this incision is completed, a second is to be carried along the outer surface of the lid, about one and a half or two lines above the eyelashes, and parallel to them. This incision is to extend through the skin and the orbicularis down to the cartilage, and be of sufficient length to pass at each extremity somewhat beyond the first incision. In the next place, a third, semicircular incision is to be made from one extremity of the

second incision to the other (as in Fig. 31), so that a semicircular portion of skin is included within it. This portion of skin is then to be very carefully dissected away, without any injury to the orbicularis. The size of the flap must vary with the amount of eversion which we desire; in simple cases of

Fig. 31.

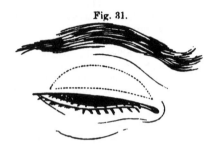

trichiasis, without any entropium, it need be but small. When this has been done, the edges of the incisions should be brought together by fine sutures. The effect of this shortening of the skin of the eyelid will be to roll out the edge of the lid and the eyelashes, which can be the more effectually done as the edge of the lid has been split into two, and the external portion is thus greatly liberated.

I have found this operation generally very successful, but it must be confessed that it does occasionally fail in two ways. 1st. The change in the position of the faulty cilia which are situated near the extremities of the incision may not be sufficient. 2d. The nutrition of the narrow bridge containing the eyelashes may be here and there impaired, leading to a partial slough and loss of the lashes at this point. To obviate these ill-results, and yet to preserve all the advantages of this method of operating, Von Graefe has devised the following modification:[1]

Fig. 32.

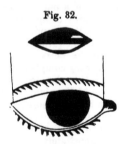

2. Von Graefe's operation (vide Fig. 33). He makes two vertical incisions four lines in length, which pass upwards from the anterior edge of the lid through the skin and orbicularis, and from the lateral margins of the portion of the lid which is to be transplanted. Hence, if the trichiasis is complete, and extends the whole length of the eyelid, the external vertical incision will be at the outer commissure, the inner at the upper lachrymal punctum (which should be preserved intact). In the next place, an incision is to be carried along the free edge of the lid between the cilia and Meibomian ducts, just as in Arlt's operation. The lashes can now be well everted, and in order to assist still further in maintaining this position, an oval portion of skin may be excised (vide Fig. 32), or this may be effected by the application of two or three vertical sutures, without excision.

In cases of partial trichiasis of the upper lid, the following operation of Anagnostakis' will be found very successful. He includes the cilia which are to be excised between two vertical incisions (Fig. 33), which diverge somewhat above. The cilia having been excised, he resects a portion of the

[1] "A. f. O.," x. 2, 226.
[2] Vide "Annales d'Oculistique," 1857, and French translation of Mackenzie, vol. ii. p. 80.

flap of skin (Fig. 34) lying between the incisions, draws it down until it reaches about half a line beyond the margin of the lid, and then attaches it by a suture at each corner (Fig. 35). The suture is removed about twenty-four hours afterwards. By this proceeding is avoided all shortening of the external lip of the margin of the lid. Where the trichiasis or entropium affects the greater portion of the lid, he makes a long incision through the skin, parallel to the edge of the lid, and about three millimetres distant from it, and if the skin is very abundant, he removes a horizontal fold. He next excises some of the fibres of the orbicularis which cover the upper segment of the tarsus, and then unites the incision by sutures.

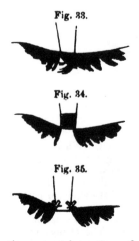

Fig. 33.

Fig. 34.

Fig. 35.

In those cases in which a few cilia only have a faulty position, the following operation of Snellen is indicated: The two free ends of a silken thread are to be drawn through the eye of a curved needle so that a sling is formed on the other side. The point of the needle is to be inserted at the free margin of the lid, as close as possible to the misplaced eyelash, and the needle is then to be brought out, in a line with the normal cilia, at the external portion of the lid, about one line from its margin. With the aid of a pair of forceps the faulty eyelash is laid into the sling, and the two drawn completely through, so that the lash is laid into the tract of the needle wound, and its point should issue from the external opening of the latter. [Nicati has described a case of what he calls true distichiasis, in which the hairs grew from the ducts of the Meibomian glands. The case was a very complete one, the rows of hairs extending from one end of all four lids to the other, and emerging regularly from the orifices of the ducts of the Meibomian glands. From a pathogenetic standpoint, the presence of these hairs is another proof that these glands partake of the nature of sebaceous follicles. Nicati recommends the following operation: he makes a vertical incision with a cataract knife throughout the whole length of the lid, immediately behind the faulty cilia, and parallel to the conjunctiva, so as to detach the tarsus from the conjunctiva, which incision should be two millimetres deep. Parallel to this, but immediately in front of the cilia, he makes a second incision of the same length and depth. Then with scissors he extirpates this circumscribed portion with the hairs. (See "Archives d'Ophthalmologie," Jan.–Feb. 1881).

When the faulty position is limited to a few hairs, especially if these are isolated, and not grouped together, the hair-bulbs may be destroyed and a cure effected by the galvano-cautery. The needle is introduced into each hair-bulb separately, and thus the follicle is most surely and effectively cauterized. No bad results follow this method of treatment. (See a paper on this subject by Dr. G. H. Fox, entitled "The Permanent Removal of Hair by Electrolysis," in the "New York Medical Record" for March 11, 1882.)

Another simple way of treating slight cases of trichiasis, which is sometimes effective, is to pass three or four ligatures vertically through the lid; entering them along the ciliary margin of the lid, passing them beneath or behind the orbicular muscle, and bringing them through the skin just beyond the curved border of the tarsus. They are then to be tied tightly and the ends cut off. They may be removed on the fifth or sixth day, or allowed to slough out.—B.]

In severe cases of trichiasis and entropium, Dr. Pope,[1] of New Orleans, recommends the extirpation of the tarsus. Having first performed all the steps of Arlt's operation, and removed a portion of the orbicularis, he next extirpates the tarsus, beginning by an incision in the posterior flap, along its free margin, between the tarsus and conjunctiva. The tarsus is best removed piecemeal, until nothing remains but its upper rim, to which the levator palpebræ superioris is attached; this rim is to be bevelled off. The wound in the outer flap is then to be united by sutures.

18.—ENTROPIUM.

In this condition, the free edge of the eyelid is more or less inverted, so that the eyelashes are turned in and sweep against the eyeball. The entropium may be either partial or complete, and be limited to one eyelid, or affect both. We must distinguish two principal forms of the disease: 1. The spasmodic or acute entropium; and 2, the chronic entropium, which is caused by inflammatory changes in the conjunctiva and cartilage.

The spasmodic entropium is acute in character, and occurs chiefly in elderly persons (hence it is often also termed senile entropium), the skin of whose eyelids is very lax, and who have perhaps had their eyes bandaged up for some length of time; thus, it is often observed if a firm bandage or pad has been worn, either on account of some operation on the eye, or for some inflammatory affection. Indeed, the photophobia and long-continued spasm of the lid attendant upon the latter, may give rise to entropium by the spasmodic contraction of the orbicularis, which causes the edge of the lid to roll in, more especially if the skin of the lid is very abundant and lax [Fig. 36]. In this form of spasmodic entropium we observe that the lashes have become tucked in towards the eyeball, and are quite hidden from view, the margin of the lid being rolled in upon itself, and presenting its smooth, rounded edge upwards. On gently drawing back the eyelid into its normal position, we notice that it looks, perhaps, quite healthy, or only slightly swollen and red; but its edge is not sore or notched, and the eyelashes are perfectly regular and well developed, being neither distorted nor dwarfed. The lid can be temporarily retained in its natural position, but very soon it rolls in again, especially if the patient should wink. This form of entropium is particularly met with in the lower eyelid, but may also affect the upper. In the chronic entropium the appearances are very different, for on everting the edge of the lid, we generally find it inflamed, excoriated, contracted, and notched. The eyelashes are sparse and irregular in their growth, showing the characters of distichiasis or trichiasis, and being dwarfed and stunted. Instead of the eyelid presenting folds of superabundant lax skin, it often looks rather shortened and tightly stretched, the cartilage being contracted and incurved; and on version of the eyelid (which is frequently performed with difficulty), the conjunctiva shows the remains of inflammatory, and often deeply marked cicatricial changes. The length of the palpebral opening (from angle to angle) is frequently considerably

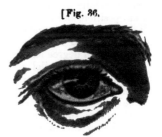

[Fig. 36.

After Mackenzie.]

[1] "Arch. of Ophth. and Otol.," vol. i. p. 10.

diminished in size, so that the eye looks smaller and sunken. The induration and contraction of the cartilage are often very marked, and it may be
shortened horizontally or transversely. These changes in the cartilage are
especially observed as a consequence of severe and long-standing granular
ophthalmia. This form of entropium is generally caused by various inflammations of the conjunctiva and the edge of the lid, more especially if there
is much photophobia, and, in consequence of this, severe blepharospasm.
Long persistent distichiasis or trichiasis may also, as has been already stated,
give rise to a certain degree of entropium. The latter may likewise occur
when the eyeball is atrophied and shrunken, so that it no longer fills out the
orbit and sustains the lids, which consequently show a tendency to become
rolled in. Entropium may also be of traumatic origin. Thus burns, scalds,
injuries from lime, or wounds of the inner surface of the eyelid, may produce
it, by causing a destruction and cicatricial contraction of the conjunctival
and subconjunctival tissue. In such cases, symblepharon often coexists.

The presence of entropium generally soon sets up great irritation of
the eye, producing photophobia, lachrymation, and blepharospasm. Subsequently, superficial keratitis supervenes, and a more or less dense pannus
may be formed, leading to still graver complications if the inversion of the
lids is not cured. In some instances, however, even a tolerably severe degree
of entropium may exist for some time without setting up much irritation.

The treatment of entropium must vary according to the nature and extent
of the disease. In the slight and recent cases of spasmodic or senile entropium (especially of the lower lid), it may suffice to replace the lid in its
normal position, and then to paint its external surface with collodion.[1] This
will dry at once, and prevent the lid from again inverting. The collodion
must be renewed every two or three days. But if the entropium is too
considerable in degree for this mode of treatment, a narrow horizontal fold
of skin, running parallel and close to the edge of the lid, and a portion of
orbicularis should be removed. A fold of skin of the requisite size, having
been caught up between the branches of the entropium forceps [Figs. 37, 38],
is to be excised by a few rapid snips of the scissors, and then a portion of
the orbicularis should, if necessary, be also removed. Before beginning
the excision of the skin, we should see what effect the pinching up of the
fold between the forceps has upon the position of the lid. If it does not
evert the latter sufficiently, a larger fold must be seized; if its effect is too
great, the size of the fold must be diminished. As a rule, no sutures will
be required, but a light pad and bandage should be applied, when the
bleeding has ceased. It has been also recommended to excise one or more
small portions of integument in a vertical direction, the edges being united
by fine sutures. The removal of a horizontal fold of skin is, however, in
my experience, to be preferred.

As the palpebral aperture is frequently considerably shortened in chronic
cases of entropium, so that the eye looks very small, much benefit is often
derived from slitting up the outer canthus (canthoplasty). The canthus
may be divided with a bistoury or with a pair of strong scissors. If the
latter be employed, one blade should be passed behind the outer canthus,
the other in front, and the commissure be divided with one sharp cut. An
assistant is then to stretch the incision in a vertical direction, so as to cause
it to gape. The conjunctival surface of the incision is to be united at one
or more points to the skin by a fine suture, in order to prevent union taking
place. One suture should be applied at the upper angle, another at the

1 Vide Mr. Bowman's paper. "Braithwaite's Retrospect," 1851.

lower, and, if advisable, a third may be inserted at the outer extremity of the wound. Dr. Noyes pushes a narrow knife between the conjunctiva and skin at the outer canthus, making a vertical incision (one and one-half line long), next a horizontal cut (three-eighths to one-half of an inch long), through the skin and orbicularis. The cut edge of the conjunctiva is seized with forceps, slight cuts are made into it with scissors above and below, so as to form a small flap. The bands of connective tissue which hold down the outer canthus to the edge of the orbit must also be cut across. Sutures are then to be applied to the edge of the conjunctiva and skin.

[Fig. 37.   Fig. 38.]

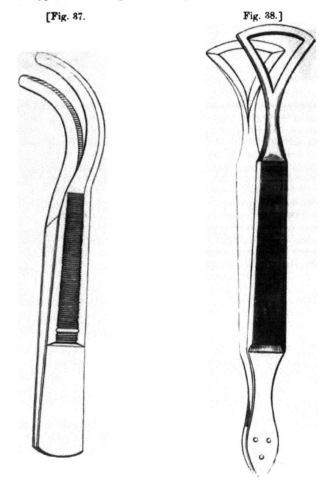

Von Graefe[1] strongly recommends the following operation for spasmodic entropium. He makes a horizontal incision (Fig. 39) through the skin, parallel to the edge of the lower lid and about one and one-half line from its

[1] "A. f. O.," x. 2, 222.

anterior margin, the extremities of the incision runing up to within one or two lines of a vertical line passing through each commissure. He then removes a triangular portion of skin (*A*), the two lateral flaps *B* and *C* are

Fig. 39.   Fig. 40.   Fig. 41.

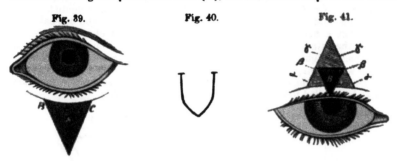

somewhat dissected up and united by two or three fine horizontal sutures. The horizontal wound is left to cicatrize. He varies the height and breadth of the triangle, according to the degree of relaxation of this portion of the lid. The height is of little consequence, but the breadth may have to vary from three to five lines. If we desire to gain a still more considerable effect, the vertical incisions may be made of the shape represented in Fig. 40.

If, together with a spasmodic entropium of the upper lid, the cartilage is contracted, Von Graefe, after having made the horizontal incision and removed a triangular portion of skin (Fig. 41), carries a horizontal incision through the fibres of the orbicularis muscle close to the edge of the lid, and pushes them up so as to expose the external surface of the tarsus. A triangular portion of the latter (*B*) is then to be removed, the position of the triangle being the reverse of that in the skin, so that the base of the triangle (varying in extent from two and a half to three lines) reaches close to the upper edge of the tarsus, and its apex lies close to the margin of the lid. The whole thickness of the tarsus should be removed, so that only the conjunctiva remains. The middle suture (*ββ*) should pass through the edges of the incision in the tarsus. It is generally necessary to combine canthoplasty with this operation, as it may otherwise diminish the size of the palpebral aperture too much.

In those cases of entropium in which the tarsus is unaffected and has retained its normal curvature, the operation of transplantation of Arlt or Von Graefe (pp. 106, 107) will be found very serviceable. But if the entropium is considerable, a larger portion of the skin should be removed (together with some of the fibres of the orbicularis) than in the case of simple trichiasis.

The following operation of Pagenstecher[1] will also be found an exceedingly good one. He commences by dividing the external commissure of the lids to such an extent that the wound in the conjunctiva equals from two lines to three lines, and that in the skin from three to four lines. By moderately stretching the edges of the incision downwards, the horizontal wound is changed into a vertical one, and the opposed surfaces of skin and conjunctiva are then to be united by sutures. By this proceeding the palpebral aperture is enlarged, a slight ectropium is produced, and the action of the

[1] "Klinische Beobachtungen," 1861; also "Compte-Rendu du Congrès d'Ophthalmologie," 1862, p. 241.

orbicularis is diminished by the interposition of the conjunctiva between its fibres. The lid being everted, he next inserts several ligatures, more especially at those points where the cilia have a faulty position. For this purpose, the lax skin of the lid and the fibres of the orbicularis are to be lifted up into a horizontal fold with a pair of forceps, and a curved needle (armed with a strong, waxed thread) passed through the base of the fold, quite close to the external surface of the tarsus. The point of the needle is then to be brought out at the edge of the lid, slightly to the outer side of the apertures of the Meibomian ducts. The ligature is to be firmly tied and allowed to suppurate out, which generally occurs in from six to ten days. As a rule, two or three ligatures will suffice to produce a considerable eversion of the margin of the lid. The effect of each suture can be calculated according to the width of the fold of skin which is lifted up. The advantages which Pagenstecher claims for this operation are: 1. That the pressure which the lid exercises upon the eyeball is diminished by the widening of the palpebral aperture; 2, the prevention of the cilia coming into contact with the cornea; 3, the eyelashes are preserved and their normal growth promoted. The little scars left by the sutures very soon disappear, without leaving any trace behind them. Cold-water dressing should be employed in order to alleviate the inflammation, which is sometimes severe, and a bandage should be applied so as to keep the parts quiet. In some cases the sutures may be removed before they slough out.

Snellen[1] recommends a ligature to be inserted in the following manner: The lid being very much everted, he passes two needles (attached to each end of a silken thread) from within outward through the whole thickness of the lid, so that the one needle pierces the upper margin of the tarsus, and the other passes a little above this edge. The needles are then reintroduced at the points of exit, passed down to the interior surface of the tarsus and along it, beneath the orbicularis, towards the edge of the eyelid, being brought out just in front of the lashes, close to each other, at about a distance of two millimetres. The upper edge of the tarsus is thus inclosed in a sling, and in tying the threads near the ciliary border, we evert the edge of the lid and draw it upwards. The thread may be removed about the third day, care being taken that no portion of it remains behind, otherwise sloughing may occur. It must be admitted, however, that ligatures alone often prove but of slight or only temporary benefit.

When the entropium is paired with contraction and incurvation of the tarsus, operations which simply act upon the position of the lid by the removal of a portion of skin, and perhaps some of the fibres of the orbicularis, no longer suffice; but we must then also remove a portion of the tarsus, so that the cicatrization may cause a contraction of the outer portion of the tarsus, and thus counteract the incurvation.

For this purpose Mr. Streatfeild[2] devised his operation of "grooving the tarsus," which answers very well when the latter is simply incurved without being contracted. He performs the operation thus: "The lid is held with Desmarres' forceps [Fig. 42], the flat blade passed under the lid, and the ring fixed upon the skin, so as to make it tense and expose the edge of the lid. An incision with a scalpel is made of the desired length, just through the skin, along the palpebral margin, at a distance of a line or less, so as to expose but not to divide the roots of the lashes; and then just beyond them the incision is continued down to the tarsus (the extremities of this wound are inclined towards the edge of the lid); a second incision, farther from the

<hr>

[1] "Compte-Rendu du Congrès d'Ophthalmologie," 1862, p. 236.
[2] "R. L. O. H. Rep.," i. 121.

8

palpebral margin, is made at once down to the tarsus in a similar direction to the first; and at a distance of a line or more, and joining it at both extremities; these two incisions are then continued deeply into the tarsus in an oblique direction towards each other. With a pair of forceps the strip to be excised is seized and detached with the scalpel."

[Fig. 42.]

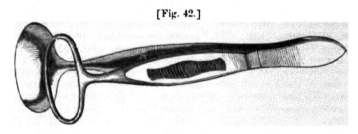

I have succeeded in curing severe cases of entropium of the upper lid with marked contraction and incurvation of the tarsus by a combination of Arlt's and Streatfeild's method. The first steps of the operation are identical with those of Arlt's (p. 106); but after the removal of the oval portion of skin, I make a longitudinal incision through the fibres of the orbicularis down to the tarsus. The latter being well exposed, I make two longitudinal incisions (inclining towards each other) in it, nearly down to its inner surface. The incisions should slope so much that they meet near the posterior surface of the tarsus, and thus include a wedge-shaped strip of the latter, the base of the wedge being turned towards the skin, and the apex towards the conjunctiva. This strip of tarsus is then to be excised with the scalpel. The size of this strip will depend upon the degree and extent of the incurvation and contraction of the tarsus. The edges of the incision in the skin should be neatly brought together by sutures, which are to be passed somewhat deeply, so as to include a portion of the orbicularis, but need not be passed through the tarsus.

Snellen[1] performs a somewhat similar operation. He makes an incision through the skin of the upper lid about three millimetres from the margin, parallel to it and extending along its whole length. A corresponding portion (about two millimetres in width) of the orbicularis is excised, and next a triangular wedge-shaped piece of the tarsus along the whole length of the lid. Three sutures are then inserted in the following manner: A suture armed at each end with a needle is to be passed through the upper edge of the incision in the tarsus, and both needles are then to be carried through the lower margin of this groove and brought out through the skin just above the line of lashes, the points of exit lying four millimetres apart. The two other sutures are to be inserted in the same way, care being taken that the points of exit are about four millimetres from each other. A bead is then passed over each end of the sutures (to prevent their cutting the skin), and the latter carefully tied, so that the two opposite sides of the incision in the tarsus are accurately approximated. The upper edge of the skin wound is left open.

Dr. Berlin[2] recommends that a portion of the tarsus, inclusive of the conjunctiva, should be excised. An incision is made about five millimetres above the margin of the upper lid, extending along its whole length if neces-

[1] "Relève Statistique de la Clinique du Dr. D. Weeker," 1873.
[2] "A. f. O.," xvii. 2. 91.

sary, and including skin, muscle, tarsus, and conjunctiva, then a corresponding portion of tarsus about two to three millimetres in width is excised, together with the conjunctiva. The wound is then, as a rule, closed with sutures.

[Schneller's operation ("Arch. für Ophthal.," xix. 2) for trichiasis and entropium consists in making two incisions through the skin, parallel to the edge of the lid, and uniting them at their ends so as to include an elliptical portion of skin, which is left in position. The skin above and below is then dissected up, and the two free margins are united throughout their whole extent by sutures *over* the circumscribed portion, which is thus buried. He claims that the buried elliptical piece aids in stiffening the lid, and thus opposes the tendency to inversion. After a time it seems to fuse with the skin covering it.

A modification of Von Ammon's tarsotomia horizontalis has been proposed by Von Burow. The lid is everted and the point of the knife is pushed through the tarsus near its outer end a line or more from the cilia, and carried along between tarsus and muscle from the outer to the inner end. If the tarsus is very much thickened, a wedge-shaped piece should be cut from the upper side of the incision. A narrow strip of skin is then excised from the length of the lid, and then from three to five sutures are inserted in the skin and the external wound closed. The incision through the tarsus may be made with a pair of scissors. This operation has been done by Green, of Saint Louis, with good results. Von Burow claimed success in more than one thousand cases. (See "Berl. Kl. Woch.," 1873, No. 24, and "Trans. Fifth Internat. Ophth. Congress," N. Y., 1876.)

In entropium of the lower lid, Noyes, of New York, has employed a method of operating which is of the nature of blepharoplasty. A horizontal incision is made outward a varying distance, usually about three lines, beginning at the outer canthus, and the canthal ligaments of both lids carefully severed; the conjunctiva is also loosened from its attachments. A narrow tongue of skin is then formed by making incisions upwards towards the temple, just beyond the end of the eyebrow, constructing a small flap, which has its base below and its apex above. This being loosened, is turned downwards and inserted between the edges of the wound, room being made at the palpebral angle by nicking the margins of the lids above and below. In closing the wounds, the first step is to draw together the edges of skin where the flap was removed. The apex of the flap is next attached in its new position to the conjunctiva, and then quite a large number of sutures must be introduced to make a close adaptation of the parts. The effect is, however, satisfactory. ("Trans. Fifth Internat. Congress of Ophth.," 1876.)

Another operation for entropium has recently been recommended by Hotz, who discards both the lid-clamp and the horn spatula. While an assistant fixes the skin of the eyebrow firmly against the supra-orbital margin, he seizes the centre of the ciliary margin of the lid and draws it tightly downward. He then makes a horizontal incision through the skin and orbicularis across the entire length of the lid, two millimetres above the level of the canthi. He then excises a strip of muscular fibres three millimetres wide from end to end of the lid. Four sutures are then introduced through the skin of the lid two millimetres below the border of the incision, are passed through the aponeurosis upon the upper third of the tarsus, a little above the junction with the fascia tarso-orbitalis, and finally through the upper cutaneous border. The sutures are then tied with a firm, deep knot. Cold-water dressings are then to be applied for twenty-four hours, and the sutures may be removed on the third day. ("Arch. of Ophthal.," viii. 2.)

In all the various operations proposed for the severer forms of entropium, especially where there is an incurvation of the tarsus, it is generally necessary to perform some little operation at the same time at the external canthus. This latter operation, hitherto known as canthoplasty, was first proposed by Von Ammon for the widening or lengthening of the interpalpebral aperture. The operation, as generally performed, is not, strictly speaking, a plastic operation. The external canthus is prolonged outward by a horizontal incision, which is sometimes extended as far as the bony margin of the orbit. A pair of scissors or a scalpel is then used to dissect up the conjunctiva, and the canthal ligament is then divided, either of the upper lid alone, or of both. The skin and conjunctiva are then stitched together. (See a valuable paper by H. Althof in "Trans. Amer. Ophth. Soc.," 1874.)—B.]

14.—ECTROPIUM.

In this condition, the eyelid is more or less everted and its conjunctival surface exposed. The degree of ectropium varies greatly, being in some cases so slight that the edge of the lid is but a very little turned out and drooping, whereas in others, the whole eyelid is everted and its lining membrane apparent [Figs. 43, 44].

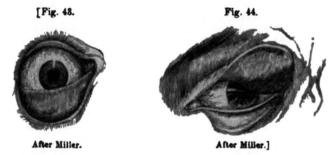

[Fig. 43.   Fig. 44.

After Miller.   After Miller.]

Slight degrees of ectropium are often seen in elderly people, more especially if they are affected with a chronic inflammation and thickening of the conjunctiva and edge of the lids. This, together with a certain degree of atrophy and relaxation of the orbicularis, causes the edge of the lid (especially the lower) to become somewhat everted and drooping, so that its margin is no longer applied to the eyeball, but sinks away from it. In consequence of this slight eversion, the punctum lacrymale is no longer turned in towards the eyeball, but is erect or everted. The tears, instead of being carried off through the canaliculus, collect at the inner corner of the eye, so that the eye appears to be always moist and swimming in tears; the latter flow over the edge of the lid, and thus maintain and increase any existing excoriation or inflammation of its margin. Severe inflammations of the conjunctiva (especially purulent and granular ophthalmia) are frequently the cause of ectropium, particularly if they are accompanied by great swelling and hypertrophy of the conjunctiva, and by such considerable chemosis, that the latter protrudes perhaps between the lids; for if the œdematous infiltration and swelling of the lid subside, but those of the conjunctiva continue, the lid is apt to become everted by the action of the orbicularis; being assisted in this by the hypertrophy of the conjunctiva, to which the external portion of the lid can offer no counterpoise, and also by the great degree of chemosis.

If such an eversion occurs, and is not at once replaced, the compression of the cartilage and of the upper portion of the lid soon produces great strangulation and a serous and hemorrhagic infiltration of the lid, which greatly increase the swelling. Hence the tumor, as Mackenzie remarks, is occasioned in a great measure by strangulation, like the swelling of paraphimosis. We not unfrequently observe such cases of ectropium in children suffering from purulent ophthalmia, in whom the lid has become accidentally everted during the application of local remedies, etc.; and instead of having been at once replaced, some time, perhaps several days, has elapsed before medical aid was sought. The strangulation is greatly increased in children by their violent fits of crying and struggling. In chronic cases of purulent and granular ophthalmia, the conjunctiva is not only swollen and hypertrophied, but the cartilage becomes relaxed and stretched, so that it no longer maintains the proper curvature and position of the lid, but assists materially in the production of the ectropium. The lid becomes at the same time elongated; indeed, ectropium seldom exists for any length of time without causing a certain, often considerable, increase in the length of the lid.

Paralysis of the facial also causes ectropium (especially of the lower lid) and lagophthalmos. Intra-orbital tumors, abscess of the orbit, etc., often produce eversion of the lid, on account of the exophthalmos to which they give rise.

But the most frequent cause of ectropium is found in the presence of cicatrices, excoriations, etc., in the vicinity of the edges of the lids, for by their contraction, during cicatrization, the margin of the lid becomes more or less everted [Fig. 45]. Thus, in long-continued excoriation or eczematous inflammation of the edge of the lid and its vicinity, we find that a contraction of the skin takes place, and the lid becomes somewhat everted. This can often be observed in cases of inflammation of the conjunctiva and cornea, accompanied by severe lachrymation. The edge of the lid becomes swollen and inflamed, its margin rounded, the eyelashes stretched and displaced, and the punctum everted and perhaps obliterated. Various injuries to the external surface of the lids of the integuments in their vicinity, such as burns, scalds, wounds, etc., which produce loss of substance, may give rise by their cicatrization to more or less considerable ectropium.

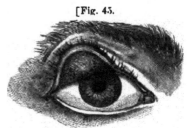

[Fig. 45.

After Lawson.]

Caries of the orbit, more especially at its outer and lower margin, is a fruitful source of very severe and obstinate forms of ectropium; for the caries is frequently accompanied by the destruction of a considerable portion of the substance of the lid, which may be implicated in the cicatrix and adherent to the bone. Thus we sometimes find the smooth surface of the lid drawn at one point into a small funnel-shaped aperture, which extends deeply down as far as the bone, to which its apex is adherent. Abscess of the frontal sinus, which perforates by a small opening through the upper portion of the lid, may be followed by an adhesion of the lid to the aperture in the bone, and a considerable degree of ectropium. In cases of ectropium of the upper lid, due to caries, we may often notice (as Mackenzie points out) the vicarious action of the lower lid, which becomes somewhat raised, so as to accommodate itself to the deficiency of the upper.

Ectropium generally soon produces a chronic inflammation of the conjunctiva and cornea, on account of the exposure of the eye to the irritating influences of the atmosphere, and of foreign substances, such as dust, etc. After a time, the conjunctiva becomes thickened, swollen, and desiccated, its epithelial layer hypertrophied and roughened, and at length xerophthalmia may be produced, the conjunctiva and tarsus undergoing atrophic changes. The cornea becomes inflamed, pannus supervenes, or deep ulcers are formed, which may lead to extensive perforation and all its dangerous consequences, such as staphyloma, or even atrophy of the eyeball. We often find, however, that the effect of the ectropium upon the eye is but inconsiderable, and is not followed by any marked inflammation of the conjunctiva or cornea. This is due to the fact, that the eyeball is rolled upwards, and is thus protected by the upper lid (the wrinkling and contraction of the brow often assisting in this), which thus guards it against external irritants. Hence, we sometimes find that patients apply to us for treatment of the ectropium far less on account of the inflammatory or other affections, than for the sake of having their personal appearance improved, which is rendered extremely unsightly from the exposure of the red, fleshy conjunctiva. In consequence of the ectropium and the malposition of the puncta, the tears cannot enter the latter, but flow over the cheek, and from the lachrymal sac being in a constant state of emptiness and non-use, it may in time shrink and become permanently diminished in size (Weber),[1] its walls being thinned and atrophied.

In the eversion consequent upon inflammation and hypertrophy of the conjunctiva, the lid should be *at once* replaced, if we see the case sufficiently early, and should be retained in its proper position by a compress bandage. Directions should also be given to the attendants in cases of purulent ophthalmia, etc., more especially in children, immediately to replace the lid if it becomes everted during the application of topical remedies. If this treatment does not suffice, and there is great hypertrophy and proliferation of the conjunctiva, the surface of the latter should be touched with mitigated nitrate of silver, the effect of which is, however, to be at once neutralized with salt and water. The conjunctiva is then to be freely scarified, which will generally cause a considerable diminution in the size of the lid. In some cases it is, however, necessary to excise a more or less considerable portion of the swollen and hypertrophied conjunctiva. If these remedies fail, we must have recourse to operative interference; but I may mention that the operations proposed and practised at different times are far too numerous to be entered upon here, and I shall consequently confine myself to a description of those which have been found to be the most useful and successful. I must state, however, that no very definite or precise rules can be laid down as to the exact method of operating, for we constantly meet with cases of ectropium so variable in degree and extent, that we are obliged to modify and alter the mode of operating, in order to adapt it to the exigencies of each individual case.

In the above form of ectropium, as well as in the senile, the best treatment is the diminution of the palpebral aperture by the operation of tarsoraphia, more especially if there is a certain degree of lengthening of the eyelid. Before proceeding to operate, the surgeon should take the outer edges of the lids between his forefinger and thumb, and draw them somewhat out towards the external canthus, and then approximate them towards each other at this point, in order that he may be able accurately to estimate the extent to

---

[1] "A. f. O.," viii. 1, 95.

which the palpebral aperture should be narrowed. The effect which this narrowing has upon the edge of the everted lid should likewise be noted, as also the fact whether the lid has to be a little raised or depressed, in order to bring it into a proper position. If the puncta are erect or everted, they should be slit up, so as to facilitate the entrance of the tears into the sac.

Tarsoraphia, which was first devised by Walther, is to be performed as follows: The operator, having inserted a horn or ivory spatula between the lids at the outer canthus, makes an incision through the skin and connective tissue parallel to the edge of the upper lid, and about three-quarters of a line from its margin. This incision is to be commenced at the outer canthus, and carried along the edge of the lid to a distance of from one and a half lines to three lines; it is then to be carried vertically down to, and through the anterior edge of the lid. This portion of the lid, including its cilia, is then to be completely excised from this point to the outer canthus, care being taken that the hair-follicles are not divided obliquely, but entirely removed, otherwise they will grow again. The same proceeding is then to be repeated in the lower lid, so that the two raw surfaces of the edges of the lids can be accurately applied to each other, and united by two or three sutures. In order still more to facilitate the union, and to give the lashes a more perfect and favorable inclination, Von Graefe[1] has modified the operation in the following manner: He carries on horizontally the inner portion of the vertical incision (which has been made perpendicularly through the edge of the lid) to the extent of about one line or one and one-half line toward the nose, along the posterior border of the margin of the lip, and pares the latter by removing a small slip of conjunctiva. This is to be done in each lid, the cilia being of course left at the outer portion of this part of the lid. In those cases in which there is a considerable elongation of the edge of the lower lid, as well as of its cartilage, an unsightly pucker or fold is apt to be produced by the sutures at the outer canthus. To obviate this, a triangular portion of the substance of the lower lid should be excised near the outer commissure, the base of the triangle being turned toward the edge of the lid. The operation of tarsoraphia will also be found very useful in lagophthalmos due to paralysis of the portio dura, as well as in that which is sometimes noticed after the old squint operation.

For the senile or spastic forms of ectropium, tarsoraphia will be found greatly preferable to the operation of Adams, which consists in the removal of a triangular, V-shaped piece from the whole thickness of the lid, the base of the triangle being turned toward the margin of the latter, and the apex toward the cheek. [Fig. 46.] The edges of the wound are then to be brought accurately together by sutures, one of which should be inserted close to the margin of the tarsus, so that the lips of the wound may be brought very closely together at this point. [Fig. 47.] The chief disadvantage of this operation is that, when it is done near the central part of the lid, it shortens the edge of the latter without elevating it at the outer canthus, hence it is closely pressed against the eyeball, which may, moreover, be somewhat irritated by the pucker or fold to which the cicatrix gives rise. If this operation is adopted, it should, therefore, be performed close to the outer canthus, as this tends to elevate the edge of the lid at this point.

We have now to turn our attention to those cases in which a partial or complete ectropium is due to a cicatrix, which is situated at a short distance from the edge of the lid, and causes eversion of the latter by traction.

[1] "A. f. O.," iv. 2, 201.

Very numerous operations have been devised to remedy this defect, of which I shall only mention those of Wharton Jones (sometimes also termed Sanson's operation), Dieffenbach, and Von Graefe, for they are, I think, the most generally useful and successful.

[Fig. 46.   Fig. 47.]

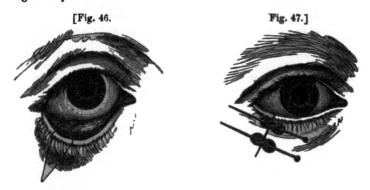

Mr. Wharton Jones' operation is to be performed in the following manner:[1] "The eyelid is set free by incisions made in such a way that when the eyelid is brought back into its natural position, the gap which is left may be closed by bringing its edges together by sutures, and thus obtaining immediate union. Unlike the Celsian operation, the narrower the cicatrice the more secure the result. The flap of skin embraced by the incisions is not separated

Fig. 48.   Fig. 49.

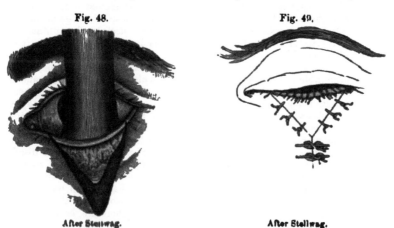

After Stellwag.   After Stellwag.

from the subjacent parts; but advantage being taken of the looseness of the subcutaneous cellular tissue, the flap is pressed downwards,[2] and thus the eyelid is set free. The success of this operation depends very much on

[1] Vide Mr. Wharton Jones, "Treatise on Ophthalmic Medicine and Surgery," p. 625.
[2] Mr. Jones is here describing the method in which the operation is to be performed on the upper lid; in the lower lid, of course, the flap would be pressed upwards, and the natural position of the edge of the lid would be thus regained.

the looseness of the cellular tissue. For some days before the operation, therefore, the skin should be moved up and down, in order to render the cellular tissue more yielding."

In Figs. 48 and 49 the method of performing this operation upon the lower eyelid is illustrated. A horn spatula having been inserted beneath the lower lid, so as to render this tense, two straight incisions are to be made from the edge of the lid, in such a manner that they converge toward each other, and meet at such a distance below the lid, that the cicatrix is completely included within the triangular flap thus formed. The flap is then to be pressed upwards, so as to bring the edge of the lid into its normal position, and all the opposing bridles of cellular tissue are to be divided, without, however, dissecting off the flap from the subjacent parts, except, perhaps, very slightly at the periphery. The edges of the wound existing below the apex of the flap are next to be closely united by two common or twisted sutures (Fig. 49), and then the two edges of the flap are to be accurately united by sutures at each side to the opposite margin of the wound. If it be necessary somewhat to shorten the edge of the lid, tarsoraphia may be united with this operation. The above method of operating is especially indicated in those cases of ectropium in which the shape and form of the lid are but little changed, its margin being chiefly elongated.

Dieffenbach devised the following operation for eversion of the lower lid, due to a cicatrix situated at a short distance from it. The cicatrix is to be included within a triangular flap, the base of which [Fig. 50, c c] is to

[Fig. 50.   Fig. 51.]

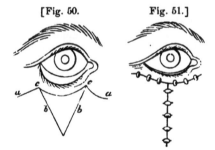

be turned towards the margin of the lid, the apex to the cheek. This triangular portion is then to be removed, and the incision, which represents the base of the triangle, is to be prolonged horizontally on each side to a short distance [a], in order to facilitate the approximation of the lateral edges [b b] of the triangle, which should be raised from the subjacent parts by a few incisions with the scalpel. The two lateral incisions of the triangle are to be united by fine sutures, and then the horizontal incision, on each side of the base of the triangle, is also to be brought together by sutures [as is represented in Fig. 51].

Von Graefe has lately introduced the following method of operating for the severer cases of ectropium of the lower lid, more especially those which are the result of chronic blepharo-adenitis. He makes a horizontal incision just behind the edge of the lid, in the intermarginal space, from the lower punctum to the outer canthus. From the extremities of this line (Fig. 52), two incisions are then to descend vertically down the cheek, for a distance of from eight lines to ten lines. The square flap A is next to be dissected up, and, if necessary, somewhat raised subcutaneously beyond the lower extremities of the vertical incisions. The flap is then to be seized at its upper edge by two pairs of broad forceps, and forcibly stretched upwards, and maintained in this position by sutures, which are to be applied first at the vertical incisions, commencing at their lower extremity. The two upper angles, which now project considerably above the upper margin of the opposite edge of the wound, should next be sufficiently bevelled off, and this is best done by making a somewhat bent incision ($B B$) whose acute angle C is then to be drawn up and united to D. The effect of this bent incision ($B B$) is twofold, viz., it shortens the edge of the lid, and elevates the flap. The closer to the edge of the lid the point C is brought, the less does it elevate the flap, but the more does it shorten the edge of the lid;

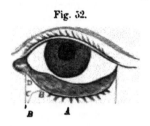

Fig. 52.

whereas, the closer the point C lies to the vertical incision, the more is the flap elevated, and the less is the edge of the lid shortened. The more exact measurements as to the size of the incisions, etc., can only be determined during the performance of the operation, more especially the adaptation of the flap in its new position, as we must shape and modify them according to circumstances. Indeed this holds good in all plastic operations. Finally, the horizontal wound is to be closed with sutures, and in such a manner that the latter include broad portions of skin, but only narrow ones of conjunctiva; as this is more favorable for the subsequent fastening of the flap, for the different threads of the sutures are to be tolerably tightly fixed to the forehead. A firm compress bandage is to be applied during the first twenty-four hours. Von Graefe has found this operation much more successful than that of Dieffenbach.[1] [For a further consideration of the various modifications of tarsoraphy that have been proposed, see the following references: "Giornale Internaz. delle Sci. Med.," ii. 3; "Progres Medical," Sept. 18, 1880; "Bull. et mem. de la Soc. de Chirurgie," August and September, 1881; "Trans. Amer. Ophthal. Soc.," 1880.—B.]

In those instances of ectropium in which extensive cicatrices involve a considerable portion, or even the whole thickness of the lid, as often occurs in caries or necrosis of the bone, or in cases of cancer, etc., it may be necessary completely to excise the affected portion, and to fill up the wound by transplanting a flap taken from the adjacent integuments. This operation of making a new eyelid is termed blepharoplasty, and very numerous modifications of it have been from time to time devised: Dieffenbach and Fricke having been amongst the first to practise it. The flap is sometimes taken from the temple and forehead, in other cases, from the cheek or side of the nose, according to the size and position of the cicatrix or growth which is to be excised. The flap has even been formed from the back of the hand.[1] I shall, however, only describe a few of the more important and most generally successful modes of operating, which will suffice to illustrate the principles that are to guide us, but the details of which must be modified and altered according to the exigencies of special cases. There are, however, a few points which apply to all these cases of blepharoplasty, and attention to which greatly increases the chance of a favorable result. Thus, the size of

[1] A. f. O. v. 9, 255.
[1] The Wharton Jones, "Ophth. Med. and Surg."

the flap should always be larger than the wound into which it is to be fitted, in order that this may be completely filled up, and its edges and those of the flap be readily united without any undue stretching; a certain degree of latitude being also allowed for a little shrinking or contraction of the flap. Care must likewise be taken that the surrounding skin is not too much stretched when the flap is fastened in its new position; hence, if any undue tension exists, a few superficial incisions should be made in the skin near the base of the flap so as somewhat to liberate it. The base of the flap should always be made sufficiently broad to maintain the vitality of the transplanted portion, which is otherwise prone to slough. This vitality may, however, be also impaired by the unhealthy condition of the skin from which the flap is taken; by it being too firmly pressed against the bone by a very tight compress bandage; or, on the other hand, by its not being kept in sufficiently

Fig. 53.

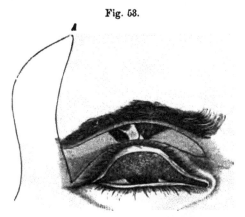

After Stellwag.

close contact. The prospect of the success of the operation is always best when the integuments from which the flap is taken are quite healthy, and are free from all cicatricial or inflammatory changes.

In Fig. 53 is illustrated the method of excising a large cicatrix of the upper lid, which has produced extensive ectropium. The cicatrix is to be included within two horizontal incisions, which converge towards each other at the inner (nasal) side, but diverge and descend somewhat at the temple. The diseased portion of the lid is then to be carefully dissected away from the subjacent tissue, so as thoroughly to liberate the lid, which is then to be drawn into its normal position. The extent and shape of the wound which is thus made, are to be estimated with as much accuracy as possible, and a corresponding flap (A, Fig. 53) is then to be dissected from the skin of the temple. For reasons stated above, the size of this flap should, however, be somewhat larger than the wound into which it is to be fitted. When the flap has been carefully dissected off, so that only its base remains standing, it is to be twisted somewhat upon itself, fitted into the wound, and carefully fastened there by numerous fine sutures; the incisions in the temple being closed in the same way.

In Fig. 54 is shown the method of fastening a flap which has been dissected out from the temple into a wound in the lower eyelid.

Dieffenbach made three incisions, which formed an equilateral triangle, and included the cicatrix; the one incision being carried parallel to, and somewhat below, the margin of the lower lid, Fig. 55. He then excised the portion included within the triangle, and next dissected an oblong flap of

Fig. 54.

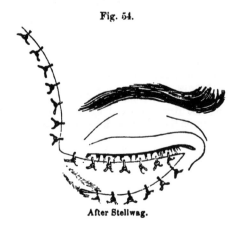

After Stellwag.

skin (Fig. 55, A) from the parts immediately adjacent to the wound, and shifted it laterally into the latter, retaining it in its position by sutures (Fig. 56).

Fig. 55.   Fig. 56.

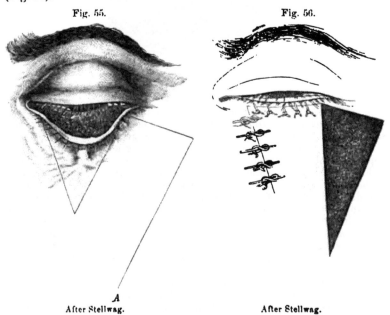

A

After Stellwag.   After Stellwag.

If the margin of the lid is implicated in the disease, it must also be included in the part which is excised; and the upper, horizontal incision of the new flap should then be made somewhat longer, so that this portion of the flap may form the edge of the lid.

Knapp has described[1] an ingenious modification of blepharoplasty, performed by him in a case in which a cancerous tumor occupied the inner two-thirds of the lower lid (including its edge), extending somewhat beyond the inner angle of the eye, and involving the skin of the nose to an extent of from two lines to three lines. As the flap is apt to contract when it is made with its base downwards, and may thus give rise to ectropium, Dr. Knapp, at the suggestion of Dr. Fritz Pagenstecher, operated in the following manner: He included the tumor between straight incisions (which were carried well into the healthy tissue). After the morbid growth had been thoroughly removed, he prolonged the internal horizontal incisions towards the nose, and thus prepared a square, horizontal flap at this point. He then made (in the prolongation of the palpebral aperture) an incision from the outer canthus slightly upwards into the skin of the temple; and next a second incision, which was at first a straight prolongation of the lower edge of the wound, but was then somewhat arched downwards on to the cheek, the concavity looking downwards. The long flap thus formed, and which increased considerably in width towards its base, was then dissected off from the subjacent tissue, drawn forwards, and its inner angles united by twisted sutures to the vertical edge of the nasal flap. Both flaps, though tightly stretched, entirely covered the wound, and formed a very successful artificial lid. The external fourth of the latter, which had remained standing, now formed the most internal portion. The edges of the wound were then carefully united by very numerous sutures, and a compress bandage applied for forty-eight hours. Perfect union resulted, and the patient was discharged fourteen days afterwards, completely cured. The palpebral aperture was slightly (about two lines) diminished in length, but could be easily and perfectly opened and closed by the action of the upper lid. The lower lid was closely applied to the globe, and Knapp states that this was one of the most successful cases of blepharoplasty with which he has met. [Knapp[2] has since operated by the same method upon similar cases, and the result left nothing to be desired. But, although this method produces very excellent results, it is limited in its efficiency, and Knapp has not ventured by its means to repair the loss of more than three-quarters of the lower lid.—H.] In cases in which we unite the opposite edges of two flaps, care must always be taken to allow a sufficient amount of skin, so as to permit a certain degree of contraction and gaping of the edges of the flaps, in case they should not unite by first intention, which is not unlikely to occur.

In those cases in which cicatrices or cancerous growths implicate the inner or outer canthus, and to a small extent the opposite edges of the two lips, the flap which is to cover the wound may be taken from the skin of the nose or the temple, according to the situation of the disease. In such instances, the following operation, devised by Hasner, will be found useful: If the morbid growth be situated at the outer canthus, and implicates to a certain extent the edges of the upper and lower lid, the tumor is to be included above and below between elliptical incisions, which should be laid well in the healthy integument. The line of junction of these two incisions should then be slightly prolonged outwards, and a sufficiently large flap be excised from the temple. The upper extremity of this flap is to be bifurcated, so as to fit easily into the wound made in the edges of the lid at the outer canthus. If the disease is situated at the inner canthus, the flap should be taken from the side of the nose.

[1] "A. f. O.," xiii. 1, 183.   [2 "Archiv of Ophthal. and Otol.," vol. ii. p 209.]

If the cicatricial adhesions are narrow and not very firm, it may suffice to divide them subcutaneously, and thus to liberate the lid, and allow it to assume its normal position. [Landolt has described a new method of blepharoplasty, which is quite ingenious. He considers the lid as formed of two leaves or laminæ; an external leaf, comprising skin and orbicular muscle with the cilia, and an internal leaf comprising the submuscular connective tissue, tarsus, and conjunctiva. In cases of loss of the lower lid it is generally merely the external leaf that is lost, while the conjunctiva is usually preserved. In such a case the conjunctiva of the lower lid is freshened, and detached as far as possible from the subjacent tissue, as far as the cul-de-sac. The upper lid is then divided into its external and internal leaves, and the conjunctiva of the lower lid is inserted between them, and carefully united by sutures passing from within outward through the external leaf of the upper lid. The latter may easily be extended and elongated, and thus there is a solid occlusion of the eyeball. At the end of several months the upper lid has regained its suppleness, and the interpalpebral aperture may be reëstablished through the upper lid. Of course, there will be no cilia in the new-formed upper lid. Landolt claims success in every case in which it has been tried. (See "Archives d'Ophthalmologie," Nov.–Dec. 1880.)

Certain observations of the Editor upon the natural course of development and transformation in scars of the face, involving the lids directly or indirectly, have led him to think that the natural process of change may be assisted and perhaps hastened by a combination of massage and traction, and thus the parts made more movable and put into a better condition for the performance of any blepharoplastic operation, the chances of the success of which are thereby enhanced. We know that in time the tissue of a scar assimilates more and more to the structure of a part, and its deep attachments become more movable. The scar, which at first is thin, bluish, and shining, and composed of undeveloped fibrous tissue, becomes white and depressed, and its structure comes very slowly to resemble that of the part where it is situated, though of course it never becomes true skin. The loosening of such scars from their deep attachments is due to a slow absorption of certain tissue-elements and the formation of a loose network of connective tissue, more or less elastic and pliable, at the base of the scar. Great changes occur in this regard in course of time; but, as D. Hayes Agnew says, external agents, such as rubbing and kneading the parts, or massage, and even soaking and steaming the parts, are useful in hastening the process of interstitial absorption. We can readily see that the act of massage, by pressure on plastic deposits, causes an absorption of a certain amount of intercellular material, and thus the texture at the base becomes more open. Persistent rubbing and kneading of scars of the face, both those due to burns and those resulting from bone-caries, as preparatory to blepharoplasty, have, in a number of instances in the Editor's experience, yielded most excellent results. Adhesions of scars, slight or extensive, to the subjacent parts, have been slowly, cautiously, and painlessly detached, and a gradual absorption of the firm material in the dense part of the scar has been brought about. So considerable has been the result obtained in some cases that the Editor has come to regard this gradual extension and loosening as an important part of the treatment in these cases. It is astonishing how soft and pliable the seams in these scars become under this treatment, and this pliability and elongation of the cicatrix is probably permanent. The depressed scars due to bone disease, in which, after the casting off of the sequestrum, the fistulous sinus has closed and the scar has become depressed and firmly adherent to the bone or periosteum, generally prove intractable to this method of treatment by massage. In these cases it will be necessary to divide the adhesions subcutaneously, and then keep up motion in the parts by rubbing, until all danger of re-adhesion of the old attachments has passed. This operation has been advocated by Mr. Wm. Adams, of England, who has practised it in a number of cases with success. (See "British Med. Journal," April 29, 1876). He describes it as an operation for the obliteration of depressed scars after glandular abscesses or exfoliation of bone. The operation consists, first, in subcutaneously dividing all the deep adhesions of the cicatrix by a tenotomy knife, introduced in healthy tissue, a little beyond the margin of the cicatrix, and carried down to its base. Then the depressed cicatrix is carefully and thoroughly elevated, lifting it up as it were, so that the cicatricial tissue remains prominently raised, and the cicatrix maintained in its elevated position for several days by passing two hare-lip pins or needles through the base at right angles to each other. The needles or pins are generally removed on the fourth day, and the cicatricial tissue, somewhat swollen and infiltrated, is allowed gradually to subside to the proper level of the surrounding skin. Adams thought that after subcutaneously dividing all the deep adhesions of the cicatrix, elevating the cicatricial tissue, and retaining it so raised for a few days, the depression would become filled up by inflammatory infiltration, so that the scar could not again sink below the level of the surrounding skin; the depression would thus become obliterated, and all the adhesions of the cicatrix would be effectually removed. The doubtful point is whether, in the course of time, absorption and recontraction of the inflammatory lymph would take place, so that the depression would return.

After the operation the cicatricial tissue always loses its shiny, membranous character, and becomes looser and of an opaque white color.

So far, this method of treatment of depressed, adherent scars from bone-caries has been employed by the Editor in but three cases, but in all with satisfactory success. One was for complete eversion of the lower lid by a broad, depressed cicatrix, firmly adherent to the superior maxilla below the orbital margin. The original trouble was probably extensive caries of the bone from scrofulous disease. After the loosening of the scar had been done, and subsequent massage treatment had been carried on for four weeks, the lid was inverted, and the space opened by the incision was filled in the ordinary way by transplantation of a flap of skin with pedicle from the temple.

The second case was also complete eversion of the lower lid from the same cause, the original injury having been a pistol-shot wound. The adhesions here were not so broad as in the first case. The subsequent method of treatment was the same.

The third case was one of almost complete eversion of the upper lid, produced by a long and somewhat broad scar on the forehead, just above the eyebrow, the cicatrix being markedly depressed and firmly adherent, throughout its whole length, to the bone. There had been quite extensive destruction of bone from a severe blow received many years before. In this case also the same steps were carried out, and the resulting gap filled by transplantation of a flap from high up on the forehead. As before stated, the ultimate result was excellent in all the cases. (See "Trans. Amer. Ophthal. Soc.," 1881, and "Amer. Journ. Med. Sci.," October, 1881.)

In the repair of lesions about the inner halves of the lids, or in cases where there is no skin available for flaps either upon the forehead or temple or outer portion of the cheek, Noyes, of New York, makes use of a naso-

buccal flap, in which the incisions are made down the side of the nose and
cheek, as far as the upper lip; the free end being below, and the attached
end or base above. The incisions are so made as to include vessels which
come from the supra-orbital, ethmoidal, and nasal branches of the orbital
arteries; and also some branches from the other side of the median line, by
laying the incision obliquely across the nose. When this flap is twisted
upon its base upwards and laid in position, there is left a large gap in the
face, which is filled by sliding the cheek in towards the median line, and
uniting the edges by pins and figure-of-eight sutures. The deformity resulting is sometimes, however, very considerable. ("Trans. Fifth Inter.
Ophth. Congress," 1876.)—B.]

Skin-grafting has lately been much advocated as a substitute for the various
blepharoplastic operations in cases of ectropium, injury of the eyelids from
burns, etc. Some operators follow Reverdin's original method of inserting
a few small isolated portions of skin on the granulating surface, to act as
centres of new dermic cell-formation. De Wecker,[1] who has had great experience in the employment of skin-grafting in diseases of the eyelids, however, recommends that the *whole* granulating wound should be covered with
small pieces of skin measuring six or eight millimetres, just like mosaic
work. Transparent isinglass plaster, or gummed gold-beater skin, is to be
placed over it, so that the condition of the little portion of skin may be
watched, this being covered by a pledget of cotton-wool and a bandage, as
it is of much importance to maintain the temperature of the part. If it is
found that some of the pieces have not taken, fresh ones must be substituted
for them. De Wecker considers skin-grafting especially indicated in the
following cases:

1. It should always be employed in burns of the eyelids or neighboring
parts, which give rise to suppurating wounds, the faulty cicatrization of
which threatens deformity or displacement (eversion) of the eyelids.

2. In partial or complete ectropium, due to neighboring cicatrices (from
burns, caries, etc.).[1] In such cases the lid is to be so thoroughly freed by
dissection from its cicatricial adhesions that it can be with ease drawn into
its normal position. In order to maintain it there, two opposite points of the
margins of the lids are to be pared, and united by sutures. This causes the
wound to be kept open and level, and after good fleshy granulations have
sprung up (i. e., after six or eight days) they are to be completely covered
by a mosaic of little portions of skin.

3. Skin-grafting may advantageously replace many of the methods of
blepharoplasty in cases of destruction of the eyelids. In a case of complete
destruction of the eyelids, De Wecker freshens the parts next to the edge of
the orbit; he then dissects off a strip of skin (from one and a half to two
centimetres in width) on the forehead and cheek by curved incisions, which
meet near the temple. These strips should be sufficiently freely dissected
off to permit of their sliding easily into the proper position, and of a very
exact coaptation of their freshened borders. They are to be fastened by
a series of deep and superficial sutures, which are to be kept in for three or
four days.

4. In all cases in which the eyelids have suffered, either through accident
or operation, a considerable loss of substance, leaving a suppurating surface,
as for instance after the removal of cancerous growths.

---

[1] " Annales d'Oculistique," Juillet–Août, 1872, p. 64; *vide* also "Relevé Statistique
· la Clinique Ophthalmologique," du Dr. de Wecker, 1873.
Vide also cases by Mr. Lawson, "Clinical Society's Transactions," 1871, p. 49.

[Lawson, Sattler, and Horner have all had good results from this method of filling in defects by the "greffe dermique."

More recently Mr. Wolfe, of Glasgow, has devised a new method of skin-grafting by transplanting a large piece of skin, without pedicle, upon the surface of a fresh wound. Wolfe began his operations in cases of loss of conjunctival substance, by shifting portions of conjunctiva from one spot to another, without keeping a pedicle. He then carried the principle further, and supplied conjunctival deficiencies by transplanting portions of conjunctiva from the rabbit to the human subject. In applying this principle to the filling up of cutaneous deficiencies, he came to the conclusion that if it is desired to make a skin-flap adhere to a new surface by first intention or by agglutination, it must be carefully and completely cleared of all areolar tissue, and properly fixed in its new place. He reports two cases of destruction of the lower lid, in which the skin-graft, two inches long by one inch wide, was taken from the forearm. He does not cut away any cicatricial tissue in the skin, but makes a horizontal incision through the skin parallel to the ciliary region, and two lines from it, and dissects up the cicatricial skin all round. He then pares away the cicatricial subcutaneous tissue till a clean surface is made. Then the two lids are fastened together at their ciliary margins by sutures. Next a flap of skin is removed from the forearm, or chest, or from any point where the skin is thin, carefully prepared free of all areolar tissue, and placed accurately in the space that is to be filled, so that the cicatricial skin-tissue surrounds it like a frame. No sutures are to be used, but the graft and surrounding skin are covered by a fine gutta-percha tissue or gold-beaters' skin, next by a layer of collodion, and finally by a lint compress and a bandage. ("Med. Times and Gazette," June 3, 1876.)

Wadsworth, of Boston, has reported a most successful result from Wolfe's method. The case was complete ectropium of the lower lid from a burn. The flap was removed from the inner side of the forearm. The case did well from the beginning, and the patient was discharged eighteen days after the operation with complete union, and the ectropium completely relieved. ("Trans. Fifth Internat. Ophthal. Congress," 1876.)

Aub, of Cincinnati, has also reported two successful cases, operated on by this method. It is of great importance to make the transplanted graft sufficiently large to compensate for great shrinking, and to clean the graft thoroughly of all subcutaneous tissue. ("Arch. of Ophthal.," viii. 1.) Noyes, of New York, has also operated successfully by this method in two cases, restoring the entire lid. In a recent paper on the same subject, Wolfe defines carefully his method of operating. The dressing consists of dry lint, though he thinks Martin's recommendation of hot dressing a decided improvement; and he has also become gradually reconciled to the use of very fine sutures. He does not employ antiseptic dressing, because he considers it desirable to keep the cuticle from peeling off, and thinks the carbolized applications have a tendency to lead to its detachment. (See "Brit. Med. Journ.," March 19, 1881.) Mathewson has recently reported two cases of ectropium treated successfully by Wolfe's method of transplantation of skin flaps without pedicle. In the first case the transported skin flap was taken from the left side, over the seventh rib, was elliptical in shape, and measured three inches in length by one and a half in breadth. In the second case the flap was removed from the inner surface of the upper arm, and measured two and six-tenths inches in length by one and seven-tenths in breadth. (See "Trans. Amer. Ophthal. Soc.," 1880.) Howe, of Buffalo, also reports a successful case in a young woman, who had complete eversion

9

of the right upper lid, and dense cicatrization of the skin of the forehead, from a burn in childhood. The piece of skin was taken from the inner aspect of the right forearm, and measured three and one-eighth inches in length by one and three-eighths in breadth. Three months after the operation the effect was excellent. (See "Trans. Amer. Ophthal. Soc.," 1880. See also articles on "Blepharoplasty," in the "Lancet," April 17, 1880; "Bull. et mém. de la Soc. de Chirurgie," April 5, 1880.)—B.]

15.—INJURIES, WOUNDS, ETC., OF THE EYELIDS.

Ecchymosis of the eyelids is of frequent occurrence, being chiefly the consequence of a severe blow or fall upon the eye, and is hence often met with in pugilistic encounters. It is due to a sanguineous effusion into the areolar tissue of the eyelids, which gives rise to a dark, livid discoloration, commonly termed "black-eye." As a rule, it occurs within a few hours after the accident; it may, however, come on at once, the discoloration extending from the eyelids to the neighboring parts. These facts distinguish this form of ecchymosis from that which is due to a counter-fracture of the orbit, for then the reverse obtains, the discoloration shows itself after a much longer interval, and gradually extends to the eyelids. Together with the effusion of blood into the areolar tissue of the lids, there is often much serous infiltration and swelling of the latter and of the surrounding parts, the lids being perhaps so swollen that the eye is firmly closed. The discoloration is at first dark and livid, but gradually undergoes various changes of tint, turning bluish-red, green, yellow, etc. A black-eye generally disappears in two or three weeks' time, but the absorption of blood may be accelerated by various local remedies. Directly after the injury, compresses of lint dipped in ice-cold water should be applied, and very frequently changed, being retained in position by a firm bandage. This application of a cold compress tends greatly to limit the effusion of blood. The absorption of the latter is subsequently much hastened by the continuous application of a firm bandage, together with which an evaporating lotion should be employed. Of the two, the bandage will, however, be found to render the greater service in accelerating the absorption. The tincture of arnica has long enjoyed a great and special reputation for curing black-eyes. It should be employed as a lotion (tr. arnicæ mont. f 3ij, ad aq. dest., or mist. camphor. f 3iv). A compress of lint is to be soaked in this, and applied to the lids by a firm bandage. The following formula, recommended by Mr. Lawson, is also a very good one: R. Tr. arnic. mont. f 3iv; Liq. ammon. acet. f 3j; Sp. rosmarini f 3iv; Mist. camph. ad f 3viij.—M. f. lotio. A poultice of black bryony-root is likewise much in vogue amongst the public. The swollen parts should never be pricked or punctured, as this tends to produce suppuration and erysipelas.

Wounds of the eyelids vary in danger according to their situation and extent, and according to the fact whether they are simply incised, or are punctured, and accompanied perhaps by considerable bruising and contusion of the parts. If the incision is superficial and horizontal, and has only divided the skin and a few of the fibres of the orbicularis, it will soon heal by first intention, if the edges of the wound are brought together by sutures and strips of plaster, and little, if any, mark will be left behind. But when the wound is extensive, and has penetrated deeply into the upper lid, implicating perhaps the tarsus, and dividing the fibres of the levator palpebræ, its consequences are much more serious. For not only may it produce a considerable degree of ptosis, but, on account of the suppuration which may supervene, contraction and shrinking of the integuments may ensue, and give rise to a severe and obstinate ectropium. If the cut is vertical, it may divide the tarsal edge of the lid, slitting it up and laying it open to a more or less considerable extent, thus giving rise to an unsightly gap or coloboma. If the rent is situated near the inner angle of the eye, it may divide the canaliculus, and tear it away from the punctum lacrymale. In a small punctured wound, the danger is but slight, if it is confined to the eyelid and has not extended into the orbit or injured the eyeball, otherwise it may produce more or less orbital cellulitis; or, if the globe has been injured, serious consequences may arise, and the eye be perhaps completely lost. If the wound or tear in the eyelid has been accompanied by severe contusion of the parts, there is always much danger of suppuration or even of sloughing setting in. Wounds of the eyelids implicating the infra-orbital nerve have been noticed to produce amaurosis, which was termed sympathetic. The cases of this kind which have been narrated, occurred, however, before the discovery of the ophthalmoscope, and hence the true condition of the fundus oculi was not known.

Wounds of the skin of the eyelids should be brought accurately together with fine sutures and strips of plaster, the part being kept cool and at rest by the application of a moist compress and a bandage. Even where the wound extends deeply into the tissue of the eyelid, and is accompanied by much bruising, it is better to unite its edges by sutures than to leave it to heal by granulation, as this will produce a more or less considerable loss of substance, contraction of the integuments, and very probably ectropium. If the tarsal edge has been divided by a vertical cut [Fig. 57], the edges of the

[Fig. 57.

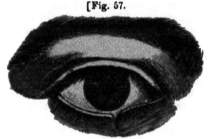

After Lawson.]

gap should be very carefully brought together, and maintained in accurate apposition by the insertion of one or more twisted sutures. One suture should always be applied as closely as possible to the edge of the lid, so that the margin of the latter may become accurately united. The edges of the gap may, if necessary, be pared; the needle should be a very fine one, and should be inserted through the tarsus. If the canaliculus has been divided, its opening should be searched for, and a director (Fig. 16, p. 58) should be inserted, and the canaliculus be slit open into the sac, with a cataract knife. [When the edge of the lid is divided, thus forming a traumatic coloboma, the first step is to remove carefully all cicatricial tissue. If the coloboma is extensive, the adjacent skin must be dissected up so as to relieve the resulting tension, and sometimes Knapp's method of lateral or sliding flaps becomes necessary. It is advisable after operating on such a case to close both eyes, thus keeping the parts in absolute apposition. If there has been a good deal of gaping of the edges of the laceration owing to contraction of the fibres of the orbicularis, vertical incisions may be made through skin and muscle on one or both sides of the wound, which aid in relaxing the parts. (See a paper by Knapp in "Arch. of Ophth. and Otol.," v. 1.)—E.]

The eyelids are often also injured by burns or scalds from hot seething fluid, the flame of a candle, etc., the explosion of gunpowder, or the action of strong caustic fluids. If the edges of the lids are severely injured, these may become adherent, and a more or less extensive anchyloblepharon be produced, or symblepharon may ensue, if the conjunctiva has been implicated in the injury. Moreover, a very severe and obstinate form of ectropium often follows burns of the lids, on account of the shrinking and contraction of the skin which accompany and supervene upon the cicatrisation. This is especially observed in the lower lid. If the injury is so extensive that little is left of the eyelids except the tarsus and the conjunctiva, the ectropium and consequent lagophthalmos are so great, that severe inflammation of the cornea and other structures of the eye supervenes, and the latter is generally soon destroyed. In slight cases of scalds or burns of the eyelids in which the cutis is not destroyed, cold-water dressing should be applied and constantly renewed for the first twenty-four or thirty-six hours. If a blister forms, this should be pricked and the serum allowed to escape, the water dressing being then re-applied. If the injury has been so severe that the skin is destroyed, simple cerate dressing should be applied and great care be taken that the lid is kept upon the stretch during the period of cicatrization, in order that new skin may be formed, and ectropium be thus avoided. A bandage should, therefore, be so applied as to keep the lid upon the stretch, and the patient should not be allowed to use his eyes until complete cicatrization has taken place.

The eyelids often become greatly inflamed and swollen from the stings of insects, such as bees, gnats, etc. The sting should be removed as soon as possible, and cool-water dressing or evaporating lotions be prescribed.

Amongst the congenital malformations of the eye, we sometimes meet with epicanthus and coloboma of the eyelid.

Epicanthus consists in the presence of a crescentic fold of skin, which passes from the nose to the eyebrow, and overlaps and hides, to a greater or less extent, the inner canthus. If it is considerably developed it is very unsightly, and it may be necessary to cure it by operative interference; but we should wait with an operation until the child gets older, for it is often found that the deformity gradually disappears as the bones of the nose become more developed, and the latter more prominent. If this should not, however, occur, an elliptical fold of skin (the size of which must vary with the amount of effect we desire to produce) is to be excised from the upper portion of the nose [Fig. 58]. The edges of the wound should be somewhat dissected up, so that they may be the more readily approximated, and the lips of the wound closed with sutures.

Coloboma or fissure of the eyelids is a congenital deformity, which is but of rare occurrence. It is sometimes associated with cleft palate, harelip, coloboma of the iris and choroid, dermoid tumor on the cornea, and other arrests of development. The fissure may be confined to one eyelid, or be present in both; or, again, a double cleft may exist, the two fissures being, perhaps, close to each other, and connected by a small intervening bridge. It occurs most frequently in the upper lid. Manz[1] has recorded a case in

[1] "A. f. O.," xiv. 2, 145.

which there was coloboma of both upper lids, with cutaneous fræna arising from the cornea, and running through the fissure into the skin of the forehead. To cure this condition, the edges of the coloboma should be pared, and then accurately brought together by fine twisted sutures, which should pass through the tarsus, the one suture being quite closely applied to the

[Fig. 58.]

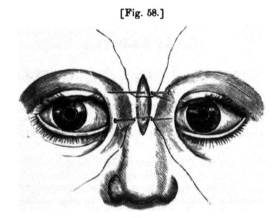

free edge of the lid, so that the lips of the cleft may here be very evenly and accurately united.

[In rare cases the lids are wanting, either entirely or in part, and this may occur alone without corresponding defect in the eyeballs, though the latter and even the orbits may be entirely wanting, the skin of the forehead and cheek being continuous. ("Graefe u. Saemisch, Handb.," ii. p. 103.—B.]

CHAPTER III.

DISEASES OF THE CONJUNCTIVA.

1.—HYPERÆMIA OF THE CONJUNCTIVA.

WE not unfrequently meet with a hyperæmic condition of the conjunctiva, and it is of practical importance to distinguish this from a mild form of conjunctivitis. In the former condition we find, on everting the eyelids, that their lining membrane is abnormally red, and perhaps a little swollen, and traversed by well-marked meshes of bloodvessels, which render the Meibomian glands somewhat indistinct. This increased redness may extend to the retro-tarsal fold, caruncle, semilunar fold, and even to the ocular conjunctiva, so that the white of the eye appears flushed and injected. The papillæ of the conjunctiva may also be slightly swollen and turgid, which gives a somewhat rough and velvety appearance to the inside of the lids. The patient is generally troubled by a feeling of smarting and itching in the eye, and a heaviness and weight in the eyelids, so that he experiences some difficulty in keeping them open. These sensations become worse in the evening, more especially in bright artificial light. Sometimes there is a slight tendency to lachrymation when the eyes are exposed to wind or a smoky atmosphere, but there is no trace of any mucous discharge.

This hyperæmic condition may be produced by long-continued work at small objects, such as reading, engraving, microscopizing, more especially by strong artificial light. It is also not unfrequently a reflex symptom of hyperæmia of the choroid and retina. Thus, in very short-sighted persons affected with sclerotico-choroiditis posterior, we often notice that the conjunctiva becomes flushed if they persist long in reading, sewing, etc. Again, we frequently meet with the same thing in persons suffering from hypermetropia, who either do not use spectacles at all, or of insufficient power, so that their accommodation is strained and fatigued. [The presence of myopic astigmatism, one of the most annoying of all errors of refraction, is not an uncommon cause of chronic conjunctival hyperæmia, which may end in marginal blepharitis if uncorrected.—B.]

It may also be caused by an irritating condition of the atmosphere, e. g., cold wind, dust, etc. Or it may be due to mechanical irritants, such as a foreign body lodged under the eyelids or in the cornea, to inversion of the lashes, or an obstruction of the lachrymal passages.

The treatment of hyperæmia of the conjunctiva is very simple, and should chiefly directed to the removal of the cause. If it be brought on by ~work, cessation from this must be enforced, and if the patient suffers 1 hypermetropia, this must be treated by the proper use of spectacles.

The eye-douche or the atomizer must be frequently used, and the eyelids should be bathed with an evaporating lotion, which greatly relieves the
1. R. Sp. æther. nit. f3j; Acet. aromat. gtt. vj; Aq. destill. f3vj. To be feeling of heaviness in the lids. The following lotions will be found very useful for this purpose:
sponged over the closed eyelids and around the eyes three or four times daily, and allowed to evaporate.
2. R. Ætheris f3ij–f3iv; Spir. rosmar. f3iv. To be used the same way as the above, but in smaller quantities, especially if the skin be very delicate and susceptible. The best astringent lotions are those composed of two to four grains of sulphate of zinc or acetate of lead, in four to six fluidounces of water. A piece of folded lint saturated with this lotion is to be laid over the eyelids for fifteen or twenty minutes, several times a day, and a few drops may be allowed to enter the eye. [A solution of one drachm of powdered borax in four fluidounces of camphor water is a very useful and soothing lotion in these cases.—B.]
But if the hyperæmia has become chronic, these applications will not suffice, and it will then be necessary to apply a drop or two of a weak collyrium (gr. j–ij to f3j of water) of sulphate of zinc or copper, or even of the nitrate of silver, to the conjunctiva;[1] or the sulphate of copper or the lapis divinus[2] may be lightly applied in substance. The eye-douche or cold compresses should be used after these applications. I must here call attention to a very prevalent popular error, namely, that it strengthens the eyes to dip the face into cold water with the eyelids open. This habit is, however, to be condemned, as it often produces much irritation and hyperæmia of the conjunctiva.
[Bernett has recently called attention to a circumcorneal hypertrophy of the conjunctiva, which is characterized by the presence of a yellowish-gray elevation at the limbus corneæ, and encroaching more or less on the surface of the cornea itself. It has a soft, succulent appearance, but no indication of pus-formation or ulceration. The conjunctiva itself appears thickened and dull. Associated with these changes, there are alterations in the palpebral conjunctiva in the shape of papillary excrescences, and the conjunctival surface looks as if covered by a thin layer of milk. The disease is aggravated during the hot months of the year. In the negro race there is a brownish discoloration of the conjunctival tissue, most intense at the scleral base of the mass, and gradually fading away towards the equator. The subjective symptoms are identical with those of the worst cases of hyperæmia of the conjunctiva. It seems to be a disease mainly of childhood. It may disappear without leaving any trace, or the corneal limbus may become prominently thickened, or it may result in genuine corneal opacity. No treatment is of much avail. (See "Archives of Ophthalmology," x. 4.)—B.]

[1] Collyria are best applied with a camel's-hair brush or the hollow part of a quill pen, which is not to be cut pointed (as for writing), but rounded off, a small hole being cut in the upper part, so that the air may enter and force out the liquid. The surgeon should stand in front of the patient, and, directing him to look upwards, raise the upper lid with the forefinger of his left hand, and depress (and slightly evert) the lower lid with the thumb, in this way a little pouch is formed between the lower lid and the eyeball, into which the drop is to be poured. The patient should then rub the lids well together, so that the collyrium may come in contact with the whole of the conjunctival surface. Instead of the quill or brush, the stopper of a drop-bottle, as sold by most chemists, may be used.
[2] Lapis divinus is composed of equal parts of sulphate of copper, nitrate of potassium, and alum, which ingredients are to be moulded into sticks.

2.—CATARRHAL OPHTHALMIA[1] [CONJUNCTIVITIS.—B.].

The term 'simple conjunctivitis" should, I think, be altogether discarded. It is, in fact, only the mildest form of catarrhal ophthalmia, and hence there is no reason to make it a distinct disease.

On everting the eyelids in a case of catarrhal ophthalmia, we notice that the conjunctiva is red, vascular, and swollen, so that the Meibomian glands

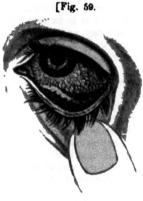

[Fig. 59.

After T. W. Jones.]

are nearly or entirely hidden. The hyperæmia commences at the tarsal portion of the conjunctiva, to which it may indeed remain confined in very mild cases. Generally, however, it soon extends to the retro-tarsal fold, caruncle, semilunar fold, and ocular conjunctiva, reaching perhaps quite up to the edge of the cornea. As the disease subsides, the vascularity retraces its steps in the reverse direction. It is important to distinguish the vascularity of the ocular conjunctiva from that of the subconjunctival tissue.[2] The former is characterized by a superficial network of vessels of a brick-red or scarlet color, which run up to the edge of the cornea, and are freely movable upon the sclerotic. [Fig. 59.] The meshes of this network are coarse and large, more especially towards the region of the retro-tarsal fold. On and between them are often noticed coarse red patches of extravasated blood, particularly near the cornea. But these effusions are also seen on the palpebral conjunctiva and retro-tarsal fold. If the ocular conjunctiva is alone implicated, the white sclerotic can be seen shining through the vascular meshes. But it is different if the subconjunctival tissue is also injected, for we then notice fine parallel vessels of a rosy tint, radiating towards the cornea, around which they form a pink zone. These vessels are not movable upon the sclerotic.

The eyelids are generally somewhat swollen and red, and their temperature is perhaps slightly increased; but none of these symptoms are so marked as in purulent ophthalmia. Occasionally, the œdema of the eyelids is so considerable that the upper lid hangs down in a massive fold, and overlaps the lower. The edges of the lids are usually somewhat red and swollen, and at a later stage they often become sore and excoriated from the discharge

---

[1 The term "ophthalmia" being of wide significance, it is a mistake to use it when speaking of conjunctival diseases, and, though frequently so employed, it seems better to use the term "conjunctivitis," and confine the word "ophthalmia" to the general inflammations of the eyeball, especially that form which has its seat in the uveal tract, and which is known as "sympathetic."—B.]

2 We may distinguish three kinds of vascularity on the eyeball: 1. The conjunctival vessels, which are brick-red, large-meshed, and freely movable. They consist both of veins and arteries. 2. The subconjunctival vessels, which are of a pink, rosy tint, their meshes being smaller, and the vessels radiating in a parallel direction towards the edge of the cornea, around which they form a rosy zone; these vessels are chiefly venous. 3. The sclerotic vessels, which do not appear in the form of distinct individual vessels, but as small ill-defined red patches, which lend a bluish-red blush to the surface of the sclerotic. For information as to the bloodvessels of the eye, I must refer the reader to Leber's important researches, "A. f. O.," xi. 1, 1; and also to those of Donders, "Klin. Monatsblät.," 1864.

and the altered secretion of the Meibomian glands. Indeed, this irritation may in time give rise to marginal blepharitis.

The degree of swelling of the lids does not, however, necessarily correspond to the intensity of the disease, or the redness of the conjunctiva. Thus, in feeble subjects, we sometimes find that there is great œdema of the lids, leading us to suspect a severe form of the disease, and yet, on opening the eye, we are surprised to find but slight injection of the palpebral and ocular conjunctiva, and but little, if any, discharge. In such cases we should examine as to the existence of an hordeolum, or whether the patient has been stung on the lid by an insect.

In the severer cases of catarrhal ophthalmia, we find that the conjunctiva becomes very swollen, more especially in the region of the retro-tarsal fold, so that, on considerable eversion of the eyelids, it springs into view in the form of one or more thick red girdles encircling the eyeball. The caruncle and semilunar fold are also swollen, and assume a dark red and fleshy appearance. At an early stage of the affection, the swelling of the conjunctiva is firm, and lends a peculiar lustrous and glistening appearance to the inner surface of the lids; but later it becomes more flaccid and soft, and falls more readily into folds. The papillæ of the conjunctiva generally become swollen and turgid, often to a considerable degree, so that they give a rough, velvety, and so-called "granular" appearance to the conjunctiva.[1] In severe cases, especially in old decrepit persons, and after the long-continued use of cold applications, the ocular conjunctiva may also become swollen (chemosis), which is due to a serous, or perhaps even plastic, infiltration of the conjunctiva and subconjunctival tissue. In the majority of cases, however, the chemosis is but very slight.

The discharge varies in quantity and quality, according to the stage and intensity of the affection. In the early stages, there is generally only an increased secretion of tears, but the discharge soon becomes more opaque and stringy, and of a yellowish-red tinge, consisting chiefly of albumen and broken-down epithelial cells. As the disease advances, and the inflammatory symptoms increase in severity, the discharge becomes more copious and of a muco-purulent character, the pus cells being suspended in the mucus. It then also assumes a light yellow color, and a thicker and more creamy consistence. In very mild cases it is often so slight in quantity that it might easily escape detection. Perhaps it is only on very considerable eversion of the lids, that a thin yellow string of matter is observed to be embedded and almost hidden in the folds of the conjunctiva, or collected in the form of a small yellow bead at the angle of the eye. The lashes are generally found to be somewhat glued together in the morning by the discharge, and the altered and increased secretion of the Meibomian glands.

There is generally very little pain in catarrhal ophthalmia. The patient only complains of a feeling of heat and itching in the lids, which causes him to rub them frequently. These sensations increase towards night, and manifest themselves especially during reading or writing by artificial light, or in a crowded and smoky room. The eyelids feel stiff and heavy, so that it is difficult to open them; this is especially the case if the lids are rather tight

---

[1] In using the term "granular" for this appearance of the conjunctiva, I must strongly insist upon the great necessity of not confounding this condition with that of true granular lids, which is but too often done, and which has led to very great confusion, not only in the diagnosis, but also in the treatment recommended for these affections. In the former case, the granular appearance is simply due to the infiltrated and turgid condition of the papillæ, whereas the true granulations are a new formation of a perfectly different character.

and press upon the globe. One of the most characteristic symptoms is the sensation as if a foreign body, such as sand, grit, or finely powdered glass, were lodged under the lids. This is evidently due, as was pointed out by Mackenzie, to the friction of the swollen papillæ [or more likely of the enlarged bloodvessels—B.] against the ocular conjunctiva. This sensation should, however, remind us of the fact that the symptoms of catarrhal ophthalmia, viz., conjunctival and subconjunctival injection, lachrymation, pain, etc., may be produced by a foreign body, and the inner surface of both lids, as well as the cornea, should therefore be carefully examined, in order that we may ascertain whether a foreign body be present or not.

There is generally only a slight degree of photophobia. If it is severe, and accompanied by much lachrymation, subconjunctival injection and considerable pain in and around the eye, more particularly over the brow and down the side of the nose (ciliary neuralgia), it is a sign that there is much irritation of the ciliary nerves.

Vision is only in so far affected, that objects may appear somewhat hazy and indistinct, as if seen through ground glass, which is due to the presence of a little of the discharge upon the cornea. The patients also notice muscæ volitantes in the shape of strings of fine beads floating through the field of vision, these are produced by mucus and little flakes of epithelium being washed over the cornea by the movements of the eyelids. For the same reason, the flame of a candle often appears to be surrounded by a colored ring, which, however, also disappears when the lids are rubbed. I need hardly point out that this should not be confounded with the luminous ring round a flame, which is one of the premonitory symptoms of glaucoma.

Catarrhal ophthalmia may be caused by sudden changes in the atmosphere, by exposure to cold, draught, and wet, or to great heat and glare, as, for instance, from a blacksmith's forge, or a large cooking fire. [It is a very common disorder among cigarmakers, who are constantly exposed to an atmosphere loaded with fine particles of tobacco-dust, and whose fingers, furthermore, being constantly coated with this same dust, keep up the irritation in the eyes whenever they are brought in contact with them.—B.] Long confinement in hot, smoky, crowded, and ill-ventilated rooms may likewise produce it, as also excessive use of the eyes, especially by artificial light. Or it may show itself in conjunction with, and be a part symptom of, the affections of the mucous membrane of the nose or respiratory organs. As a continuation of the common integument, the conjunctiva may, moreover, become affected in the acute exanthemata, as in smallpox, scarlatina, and measles, also in erysipelas, herpes zoster, and eczema of the face. It may suffer consecutively in affections of the eyelids, as for instance in ectropion or distichiasis, or in those of the lachrymal apparatus. Indeed epiphora, dependent upon some impediment to the free efflux of the tears, is a not unfrequent cause of obstinate and chronic inflammation of the conjunctiva, which readily disappears as soon as the lachrymal affection is cured. Undetected foreign bodies, or injuries from mechanical or chemical irritants, may also give rise to conjunctivitis.

Finally, it may be produced by contagion, more especially if the disease is at all severe, if the swelling extends to the retro-tarsal fold of the upper lid, and the discharge is of a muco-purulent character. It almost always reproduces catarrhal ophthalmia, and only in rare cases gives rise to the purulent or diphtheritic form.

The *prognosis* of catarrhal ophthalmia is favorable, for the affection is amenable to treatment. The milder forms generally run their course few days, the more severe in two or three weeks. The cornea becomes but seldom implicated, and even if ulcers should form upon it, they are generally quite superficial and peripheral, so that at the worst they only give rise to a slight opacity. Only in very severe cases and under very injudicious treatment do the cornea and iris participate to any dangerous extent.

If the affection is neglected, it may become chronic, and prove very obstinate and intractable, more especially in old persons. The conjunctiva becomes flaccid and rough, and this may give rise to superficial [keratitis.—B.] or ectropion, particularly of the lower lid.

The *treatment* must vary according to the stage and the severity of the disease. If the eye is very irritable, and there is much photophobia, lachrymation, and ciliary neuralgia, accompanied by conjunctival and marked subconjunctival injection, astringent lotions should be carefully avoided, as they would increase the irritability, or might even set up inflammation of the cornea or iris. In such cases, the lids should be well everted, and a careful examination made as to the presence of a foreign body beneath them, or upon the cornea. If none is detected, the condition of the palpebral and ocular conjunctiva and of the cornea and iris should next be ascertained, as these symptoms of irritation may be due to phlyctenular ophthalmia, or to a commencing inflammation of the cornea or iris. In this condition of the eye, it is often impossible to decide whether it is simply a case of commencing catarrhal ophthalmia accompanied by unusually severe symptoms of ciliary irritation, or whether it is a case of incipient corneitis or iritis. It is, therefore, always the wisest plan to leave the question of diagnosis open, until the real character of the affection becomes more pronounced, and to endeavor to alleviate the symptoms of irritation by soothing applications (such as atropine and warm fomentations). By so doing, we guard ourselves against committing, perhaps, a serious error in treatment; for if it should turn out to be a case of catarrhal ophthalmia, astringents may be employed as soon as the symptoms of irritation have somewhat subsided, and the discharge has assumed a muco-purulent character; if, on the other hand, it should prove to be a case of keratitis or iritis, the treatment has been most appropriate and judicious, whereas the use of astringents, more especially the more powerful ones, would have been very injurious.

The patient should be warned to guard his eyes against exposure to wet or cold; and to abstain from all reading, etc., more especially by artificial light.

In order to relieve the ciliary neuralgia, hot poppy fomentations should be applied to the eye; but if the patient should be of a rheumatic habit, the moisture may produce considerable œdema of the lids, and hot dry flannels are therefore to be preferred.

A solution of atropine (gr. ij to f ℥j of water) should be dropped into the eye two or three times a day [Atropine is unnecessary except when the pain is severe, and should not be used in these cases generally, because of its effect on the vision, which is sometimes depressing to the patient.—B.], and the following compound belladonna ointment should be rubbed over the forehead: — ℞. Extract. belladonnæ gr. x; Hydrarg. ammon. chlorid. gr. v; Adip. ℥j. ℞.—A portion of this is to be rubbed over the forehead three or four times daily, and should be covered by a piece of thin tissue-paper, so as to prevent its drying and becoming hard. It should not be washed off until it is time for its re-application. In the course of two or three days a slight papular eruption will appear, when the ointment is to be discontinued. [Relief in severe cases is sometimes obtained by painting the external surface of the eyelids and the skin of the forehead and temple with balsam of copaiba.—B.]

When the acute symptoms of irritation have subsided, and those of catarrhal ophthalmia—more especially a muco-purulent discharge—begin to show themselves, astringents must be applied. In the milder cases, in which there is not much conjunctival redness, and the discharge is chiefly of a mucous character, lodging in the form of thin, yellowish, stringy flakes in the retrotarsal fold, or the angles of the eye, a solution of sulphate of zinc or copper (one or two grains to the fluidounce of distilled water) should be dropped into the eye two or three times daily. [Solutions of zinc or copper are painful, and therefore often objectionable. A solution of alum, grs. v–x to the ounce of water, is the most useful application in most cases for the patient to apply.—B.] If the bloodvessels are much dilated, and the conjunctiva relaxed and flaccid, a solution of tannin (gr. iv–viij to f ℥j of water) is to be preferred. I have also found much benefit from the chloride of zinc (gr. ss–j to f ℥j), which is strongly recommended by Mr. Critchett.

But if the inflammation is severe, if the discharge is copious, thick, and creamy, these remedies will no longer suffice, and we must have recourse to nitrate of silver, the strength of the solution varying according to the amount and thickness of the discharge. For general purposes a solution of two or three grains to the ounce will be found the best. A large drop of this should be applied with a camel's-hair brush or a quill to the inside of the lower eyelid three or four times a day. The lids should then be rubbed with the finger, so that the solution may come in contact with the whole of the conjunctiva. The feeling of grit and sand in the eye as well as the lachrymation are much relieved, and will disappear for five or six hours. On their appearance, the collyrium should be again applied. It may, however, be necessary to apply a still stronger solution (gr. iv–vj to f ℥j) if the discharge is very copious and thick, and if the affection has lasted for some time, or the mitigated nitrate of silver should be applied in substance. Before the collyrium is applied, the discharge must be removed by the injection of lukewarm water beneath the lids. This renders the action of the collyrium far more efficacious. After each instillation of the astringent collyria,[1] cold-water compresses should be applied to the lids for the space of from a quarter to half an hour, being changed as soon as they become at all warm. This will give great relief to the patient, and subdue the pain and irritation produced by the lotion.

Lukewarm water should be injected between the lids every two or three hours, so as to wash away the discharge. Or the following lotion, recommended by Mackenzie, may be employed with advantage for this purpose: ℞ Hydrarg. bichlorid. gr. j ; Ammoniæ muriat. gr. vj ; Aq. destill. f ℥vj. Misce. A tablespoonful of this lotion is to mixed with a tablespoonful of hot water. In mild cases the eyes should be fomented with it three or four times daily, a little being permitted to enter the eye. In severer cases it should be injected over the whole conjunctiva.

A little simple cerate or unscented cold cream is to be applied to the edges of the lids to prevent their sticking. [Vaseline is a very useful application for this purpose.—B.] If crusts have formed upon the lashes, they are to be soaked with warm water, and then carefully removed so as not to produce any excoriation. If the edges or angles of the lids are sore and excoriated, the red precipitate ointment (gr. j–ij to the drachm of lard) is to be applied
' and morning, or the weak nitrate of mercury ointment may be used.
' attendants must be warned that the discharge in catarrhal ophthalmia
'gious, and that the sponges, towels, etc., used for the patient must be

ollyria of nitrate of silver are more properly caustic than astringent.—B.]

carefully kept apart, and not employed for any other purpose. Some authors have expressed a doubt as to the contagiousness of catarrhal ophthalmia, but in out-patient practice, we have very frequent opportunities of seeing several members of the same family affected consecutively with the disease. Constitutional treatment will hardly be required; the bowels should be kept freely open, and, if the patient is feeble and out of health, tonics should be administered.

8.—PURULENT OPHTHALMIA.

(Syn. Egyptian ophthalmia, contagious ophthalmia, military ophthalmia.) [The disease represented by these three terms is far oftener a granular conjunctivitis than a suppurative process. Purulent conjunctivitis would be a better synonym. Conjunctival blennorrhœa.—B.]

We cannot draw a sharp line of demarcation between acute catarrhal and purulent ophthalmia. The latter may indeed be regarded as a more severe form of catarrhal ophthalmia, in which all the symptoms of this affection are intensified in degree. The lids are more œdematous, hot, and red, the palpebral and ocular conjunctiva more injected and swollen, and the papillæ more turgid and prominent. The chemosis is also more considerable, and the discharge is thicker, more copious, and more contagious. The inflammation is, moreover, not confined to the conjunctiva, but extends deeper, and involves also the subconjunctival tissue; so that there is not only a secretion of muco-purulent discharge upon the free surface of the conjunctiva, but also an infiltration of sero-plastic lymph into the substance of this membrane. The cornea is, moreover, far more frequently and more seriously implicated than in catarrhal ophthalmia.

At the commencement, the patient experiences a sensation of heat and itching in the eye, as if a foreign body, more especially sand or grit, were lodged beneath the eyelids. The edges of the latter become slightly glued together, and small beads of matter collect and harden on the lashes and at the corners of the eye. On eversion of the lids, their lining membrane is found to be very vascular, swollen, and of a uniform redness, so that the Meibomian glands can no longer be distinguished. The retro-tarsal fold, the caruncle, semilunar fold, and ocular conjunctiva are also abnormally red and swollen. The eyelids are red, glistening, and perhaps somewhat puffy. At first, there is only considerable lachrymation, but the discharge soon assumes a muco-purulent character, having yellow flakes of pus and broken-down epithelial cells suspended in it.

Up to this point, all these symptoms are only those of catarrhal ophthalmia; but, as the disease advances, they soon become more severe in character. The patient often experiences great pain in and around the eye, which may even extend to the corresponding half of the head, especially if the inflammation be of a sthenic character, in which case marked febrile symptoms may also present themselves. Generally, the pain diminishes as soon as the discharge becomes purulent. It may, however, again increase in severity if the cornea becomes affected, and especially if the iris or other tissues of the globe should become involved in the inflammation. In general inflammation of the eyeball (panophthalmitis) the pain is often excruciating.

The lachrymation and photophobia increase, the lids become very swollen, so that the upper hangs down in a thick heavy fold, and they can only be opened or everted with difficulty. [Fig. 60.] They are red, glistening, and œdematous, and, if deeply pressed, somewhat tender. [The tenderness and pain on pressure of the swollen lids is a very constant sign in this disease.—B.] Their temperature, though markedly increased, never reaches a very high degree, and this, together with the absence of tenderness, is of importance in the

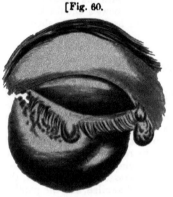

[Fig. 60.

After Dalrymple.]

differential diagnosis between purulent and diphtheritic ophthalmia. The conjunctiva becomes vascular and swollen, and patches of effused blood are noticed both on its palpebral and ocular portion. The papillæ are very turgid and prominent, giving a rough and villous appearance to the inside of the lids. As they increase in size they become flattened at the sides, from being pressed against each other, and they appear arranged in rows without a distinct base. The prominence may be so considerable that they assume the appearance of cauliflower excrescences. They often bleed freely on the slightest touch, as their epithelial covering is very thin and easily shed. The retro-tarsal fold is much swollen, and, on eversion of the lids, springs into view in the form of thick, red, fleshy girdles, which encircle the eyeball. The ocular conjunctiva becomes very vascular, and a serous

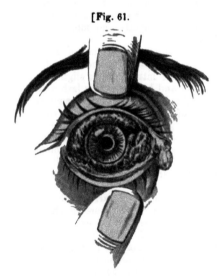

[Fig. 61.

Shows the swollen and chemotic condition of the conjunctiva of an eye in which the disease has existed four or five days. After Dalrymple.]

or even plastic effusion takes place into it, and the subconjunctival tissue. [Fig. 61.] This chemosis is far more marked than in catarrhal ophthalmia, and may be so considerable as to rise like a high, red, semi-transparent mound round the cornea, overlapping its edges more or less considerably, and even perhaps protruding between the lids. The chemosis is most prominent at the outer and inner side of the cornea, at the triangular spaces opposite the palpebral aperture; for the pressure of the lids keeps down the chemotic swelling above and below. On account of the great swelling and weight of the eyelids, and the great chemosis, the vessels supplying the cornea become much compressed, and its nutrition proportionately impaired; and this explains the great tendency to ulceration and suppuration of the cornea in severe purulent ophthalmia. For the idea that the irritating and noxious character of the discharge produces the affection of the cornea is erroneous.

As the disease advances, the discharge increases in quantity, becomes more opaque, thick, and creamy, and, on account of its admixture with blood, frequently assumes a reddish-yellow tint. It is often so considerable in quantity that it wells out from between the eyelids when these are opened, and flows down over the cheek; the lashes become clogged with it, and glued together into little bundles. It collects in the retro-tarsal fold and on the surface of the cornea in the hollow formed by the chemosis, and this appearance may easily be mistaken by a superficial observer for suppuration of the cornea. The discharge should, therefore, always be wiped away from the cornea before any opinion is formed as to the condition of the latter. On cleansing away the matter from the surface of the palpebral conjunctiva, we notice that the latter looks red, glistening, villous, and succulent, which enables us at a glance to distinguish the disease from diphtheritic conjunctivitis. Sometimes, however, the discharge is more tenacious, and clings to the surface of the conjunctiva like a thin membrane, so that it cannot be easily wiped away, but requires to be stripped off, when it comes off in the form of thin flakes. But, on its removal, we find that the membrane was quite superficial, and that the appearance of the conjunctiva beneath is the same as that described above. Hence it is erroneous to call this "diphtheritic conjunctivitis," simply because the discharge is more tenacious and comes off in flakes, for the symptoms of true diphtheritic ophthalmia are not only very different, but demand a very different course of treatment; but there can be no objection to terming it "membranous ophthalmia." We sometimes, however, meet with mixed forms of purulent and diphtheritic ophthalmia. [See the section on Membranous Conjunctivitis.—B.]

The chief danger in purulent ophthalmia is the implication of the cornea. Any cloudiness of the latter must, therefore, be always regarded as an untoward symptom, more especially if it already shows itself at an early stage of the disease, and if there is any tendency to a diphtheritic character in the ophthalmia. At a later period it is less to be feared. The appearance of the cornea must be carefully watched from day to day, and in severe cases its condition should be examined, if possible, at the interval of a few hours. Implication of the cornea is especially likely to occur if the inflammation is very severe, the temperature of the lids much increased, the chemosis considerable and firm, and accompanied by great photophobia, lachrymation, and ciliary neuralgia. The pain is generally intermittent, and often very severe, especially towards night; it may extend deep into the orbit and over the corresponding side of the head and face. On examining the condition of the cornea, we may then perhaps discover small phlyctenulæ or infiltrations at its edge or upon its surface, which soon pass over into ulcers. Sometimes there is a serous infiltration (œdema) into the cornea, which may remain confined to the periphery, giving it a slightly steamy or clouded appearance. If this opacity is considerable, and extends over the centre of the cornea, the sight may be greatly impaired, or a circumscribed light-gray infiltration may show itself at one portion of the cornea and disappear again as the ophthalmia subsides, or it may become more dense and assume a yellow tinge. Generally, the infiltration soon changes into an ulcer, which may, in favorable cases, remain superficial, and ultimately leave only a very slight, or even no opacity of the cornea; but if the infiltration or ulcer is of considerable size and rather deep, a dense opacity may remain behind, and greatly impair the sight, if it be situated in the centre of the cornea. The ulcer, instead of remaining superficial, may, however, rapidly increase in circumference and depth, and soon lead to extensive perforation of the cornea, accompanied by prolapse of the iris, escape of the lens, and perhaps a certain quantity of vitreous humor, and be followed probably by the formation of a considerable staphyloma.

When the cornea gives way, the patient experiences a sudden remission of the violent pain, accompanied by a gush of fluid over the cheek. If the ulcer is large, the cornea, on account of being thinned and softened at this point, may become somewhat bulged forward before perforation occurs. The dangerous character of the ulcer, of course, increases with its extent, as the perforation will be proportionate in size.

Sometimes several infiltrations are formed near to each other, and then coalesce, thus giving rise to one large ulcer. In many cases the perforation, if it be but of limited extent, is the best thing that can occur, for the ulcer, instead of increasing in circumference, then begins at once to heal.

Perforation of the cornea may give rise to the following complications: 1. Prolapse of the iris; 2. Anterior synechia; 3. Central capsular cataract; 4. Displacement or obliteration of the pupil; 5. Anterior staphyloma. For further information upon this subject, I must refer the reader to the chapter on ulcers of the cornea.

If the perforation of the cornea is small, a little portion of the iris will fall against it; when the aqueous humor escapes, lymph will be effused at the bottom of the ulcer, and the iris will become adherent at this point to the cornea, giving rise to an anterior synechia. The pupil will be dragged towards the adhesion and more or less displaced; or it may be partially or wholly implicated in it. If the perforation was extremely small (such as would be produced by a fine needle), the reaccumulation of the aqueous humor may tear through any little adhesion that has taken place between the iris and cornea, and no anterior synechia will be left. When the perforation occurs at the centre of the cornea, the lens will come in contact with the bottom of the ulcer, and a central anterior cataract may be formed. If the cornea gives way to a greater extent, a knuckle of iris may be pushed into the ulcer and cause a prolapse of the iris, which may increase to a very considerable size from the aqueous humor collecting within it and swelling it out. A small protrusion of this kind has been termed a myocephalon. Or the lens may escape together with some of the vitreous humor, if the rupture of the cornea is large, and then the eyeball may become atrophied. Or the iris falls into the gap, becomes adherent to the cornea, and covered with lymph, which assumes a cicatricial character, and yielding gradually to the intra-ocular pressure, becomes more and more prominent, and a partial or total staphyloma results.

A very dangerous kind of ulcer is that which makes its appearance in the form of a small crescentic ulcer near the edge of the cornea (generally the lower), looking as if it had been scratched by a finger-nail. Its edges soon become infiltrated, and assume a yellow tint. It increases in depth, and rapidly extends further and further round the cornea, until it may give rise to a very considerable perforation or slough of the latter. On account of its being situated so closely to the edge of the cornea, this form of ulcer is often hidden by the chemosis, and thus easily overlooked at the outset.

In very severe cases of purulent ophthalmia, with intense inflammatory symptoms, sloughing of a great portion or even of the whole of the cornea may take place within a few hours. The cornea loses its transparency, becomes of a grayish-white color, which soon passes into a yellow tint, and looks shrivelled and quite opaque. It soon yields to the intra-ocular pressure, gives way, and the eyeball becomes atrophied.

Iritis may supervene when the ulceration has extended to the deeper layers of the cornea, or when perforation has occurred. If severe, it generally gives rise to great ciliary neuralgia, photophobia, and lachrymation. If a portion of the cornea remains sufficiently clear to permit of our seeing the iris, we find the latter discolored, and the pupil contracted, irregular, and perhaps blocked up with lymph, or there may be pus in the anterior chamber. The inflammation may extend from the iris to the other tissues of the eye, and general inflammation of the eyeball (panophthalmitis) set in, accompanied by excruciating pain. Pannus occurs but seldom in acute purulent ophthalmia, and only in cases where the papillæ have been much swollen from the very commencement of the disease, and from their rubbing against the cornea have induced a superficial vascular keratitis. It is more frequently met with in chronic ophthalmia. It is an interesting circumstance, that if the cornea has been suffering from pannus before the attack of purulent ophthalmia, there is far less danger of its ulcerating or suppurating than if it is quite transparent. This important fact has been utilized in the treatment by inoculation of pannus dependent upon granular lids.

Purulent ophthalmia generally runs its course in three or four weeks. It may, however, become chronic, and last for many months or even years, and prove very obstinate. This is especially the case if the papillæ remain swollen and prominent, for by their constant friction against the cornea, pannus is but too often produced. The relaxed condition of the conjunctiva may also give rise to ectropion, or this may be produced by the lids having become everted during the progress of the disease, and not having been properly replaced.

Causes.—[Purulent ophthalmia is generally due to contagion from the same disease, or from an acute or chronic discharge from the urethra or vagina, whether gonorrhœal or not. (Nettleship.)—B.] It may become developed from an acute catarrhal ophthalmia, by the symptoms of the latter increasing in severity, either through a continuation of the original acute, through neglect, or through a mistaken course of treatment. The same causes which may give rise to catarrhal ophthalmia, viz., exposure to cold or draught, great glare, etc., may also produce the purulent form. We sometimes find that it occurs epidemically, and that mild irritants, which would at other times only have caused a simple catarrhal conjunctivitis, now produce purulent ophthalmia. An unhealthy locality, a vitiated atmosphere, crowded and badly ventilated rooms, exposure to great heat or cold, dust, and glare, intensify the character of the epidemic. Some of these causes are frequently met with in places where many persons are collected together, as in work-houses, foundling hospitals, and large barracks. If purulent or even catarrhal ophthalmia once breaks out in such establishments, it is often very difficult to arrest it before it has spread widely amongst the inmates and committed great ravages. If soldiers on their march or in camp are exposed to great heat and glare, and to hot winds carrying before them clouds of sand and dust, as occurs in India or Egypt, ophthalmia will soon show itself amongst them. Hence the terms military and Egyptian ophthalmia. These names should, however, be abandoned, for this affection shows no special characteristics warranting its being classed as a disease *sui generis*. The ophthalmia is in such cases generally one of purulent ophthalmia, but sometimes it may assume the character of severe catarrhal or granular conjunctivitis. Or these affections may pass one into the other, or exist side by side in the same army. This being so, we can easily understand how such various, and often conflicting and confused accounts have been given of the character, the severity, and the contagiousness of the so-called military ophthalmia.

Contagion is the most frequent cause, as the contagious power of the discharge is often very great. This varies, however, according to the severity and stage of the disease. Piringer,[1] who made a great number of valuable and interesting experiments to test the contagious power of the discharge, found that during the earliest stage, and also in chronic cases, in which the discharge is thin, watery, and transparent, it is hardly, if at all, contagious; but it becomes slightly so when, though still watery, it assumes a somewhat mueo-purulent character, and then it generally reproduces a mild form of the disease. The contagiousness increases in proportion to the intensity of the affection, and the purulent nature of the discharge. According to the same authority, the discharge of a severe purulent ophthalmia, if applied to a healthy conjunctiva, may reproduce the disease in from six to twelve hours; that from a moderately severe form in from twelve to thirty-six; the mild, in sixty to seventy; and that from chronic ophthalmia in seventy-two to ninety-six hours. It is of the greatest practical importance to remember that the discharge from purulent ophthalmia does not always reproduce the purulent form, but may give rise to catarrhal, granular, or even diphtheritic conjunctivitis—just as the discharge from catarrhal, diphtheritic, and acute granular ophthalmia may produce purulent ophthalmia. [That purulent conjunctivitis ever causes diphtheritic conjunctivitis is doubtful. Most modern authorities hold that they are two distinct diseases, differing in their pathology and pathogenesis.—B.] The special form of conjunctivitis which may arise will depend upon atmospherical, local, and constitutional causes, and also upon the age of the patient. Thus Von Graefe states[2] that in Berlin the matter from ophthalmia neonatorum, when applied to the eyes of children of two or three years of age, generally produces diphtheritic conjunctivitis, whereas when applied to adults it mostly gives rise to purulent or sometimes to granular ophthalmia.

Healthy eyes are more rapidly and severely affected by the inoculation of contagious matter than those suffering from vascular forms of keratitis, more especially pannus. Repeated inoculation diminishes the contagious power of the discharge. This is also diminished by diluting the latter with water, it being altogether lost when it is diluted with about one hundred parts of water. Gonorrhœal and vaginal discharges may also produce purulent ophthalmia. It appears certain that the air is often a carrier of the contagion, especially if many persons suffering from severe purulent ophthalmia are crowded together in one room, and this is perhaps small and ill-ventilated. Von Graefe thinks that in such cases the propagation is partly caused by the suspension of the constituents of the discharge in the atmosphere, and partly by the air expired from the lungs, from the discharge passing down the lachrymal passages into the nose—just the same, in fact, as what occurs in common nasal catarrh, the contagious nature of which depends chiefly upon the expired air.

The *prognosis* which may be given in a case of purulent ophthalmia will depend upon the stage and severity of the disease, and also upon the prevailing character of the epidemic, should such exist. It may be favorable, if the affection is of a mild muco-purulent character and is due to spontaneous causes; or, having been produced by contagion, if the inoculating matter was mild and chiefly mucous in character; also, if the redness and swelling of the eyelids and conjunctiva are but slight; if the inflammation is chiefly confined to the palpebral conjunctiva; or, should it extend to the ocular, if the chemosis is serous and soft, not plastic and hard; if the discharge is thin and scant, the cornea unaffected, the character of the epidemic

[1] Piringer "Die Blennorhoe im Menschenauge," Gratz, 1841.
[2] "Deutsche Klinik," 1864, p. 79.

mild, without any tendency to the diphtheritic form of conjunctivitis. We must, on the other hand, be extremely guarded in our prognosis, or even form an unfavorable one, if the inflammation is very intense, the chemosis hard and lardaceous, and so considerable as completely to surround the cornea and overlap it; if there is any ulceration of the cornea, especially if this be considerable in extent, and occurs early in the disease; if the inflammation shows a diphtheritic character.

Treatment.—If the attack is severe, the patient should be confined to a darkened room, or even to his bed. The room must, however, be well ventilated, and plenty of fresh air be admitted, particularly if it is occupied by several patients. Those who have the disease in a severe form should, if possible, be separated from the milder cases. I need hardly point out that in barracks, unions, schools, etc., the healthy inmates should be strictly kept apart from those who are suffering from ophthalmia. Their eyes should, moreover, be examined every day, in order that the first symptoms of the disease may be detected. The patients and attendants should be made aware of the contagious character of the disease, which continues as long as the discharge remains opaque and mucous. Special care must be taken that the sponges, towels, water, etc., which are employed for the patients are not used by others. To guard them against the risk of contagion, the medical attendants and nurses should wear the curved blue eye-protectors, more especially whilst applying the collyria or syringing out the eyes, as a little of the matter may otherwise be easily splashed into their eyes. If by accident, any of the discharge should have got into a healthy eye, lukewarm water should be at once injected under the lid so as to wash it away, and then a drop of a weak solution (two grains to the fluidounce of water) of the nitrate of silver or sulphate of zinc should be applied to the conjunctiva. If only one eye is affected with purulent ophthalmia, the other must be at once, without loss of time, hermetically closed. The common compress bandage will not suffice for this purpose, for the discharge might soak through, especially during the night, when it may run over the bridge of the nose from the affected to the healthy eye. The best protection is the following compress, recommended by Von Graefe. A pad of charpie or cotton-wool should be applied to the eyelids and covered by diachylon plaster, which is to be fastened down by collodion, so as to completely exclude the air. This compress should be removed twice daily, and the eye cleansed and carefully examined. [Another protective method is that recommended by Dr. Buller, of Montreal, which consists of a piece of mackintosh about four and a half inches square, with a watch glass fastened to a hole in the centre, through which the patient can see; this is fixed by broad pieces of strapping to the nose, forehead, and cheek, its lower and outer angle being left open for ventilation. (Nettleship.)—B.] If there is any redness or swelling of the conjunctiva, or any discharge, the pad should be discontinued, although in some cases the continuance of the firm pressure appears to cut short the attack. A drop of a weak solution of nitrate of silver or sulphate of zinc should be at once applied. Ice compresses may also be applied to the eyelids, as they, according to Piringer, will often cut short the attack.

There is generally not much constitutional disturbance, except the disease is severe, in which case, more especially in gonorrhœal ophthalmia, it is often accompanied by marked febrile symptoms. If the tongue is foul and loaded, a brisk purgative should be administered, and the bowels be kept well opened. If the patient is plethoric and feverish, cooling salines must be prescribed, and the diet be kept low. Formerly, the depletory plan of treatment was carried to great excess, and venesection employed to such an extent that we read of cases in which the patient was bled "as long as the blood could be got from the arm." (Wardrop.) Now, however, this course of treatment has fortunately almost completely exploded, and venesection is hardly ever employed. Indeed, we not unfrequently find that patients suffering from purulent ophthalmia are of a weakly and cachectic habit, in whom such a line of treatment would be most injudicious and injurious. In all such cases tonics, especially quinine and steel with perhaps some ammonia, should be freely administered, the patients being at the same time put upon a good, nourishing, and easily digestible diet, with meat once or twice a day, and if necessary, they may even be allowed a moderate quantity of stimulants. In this we must, however, be guided by individual considerations. If the patient is restless and sleepless, a narcotic should be given at night, as it is a great relief if he can obtain a good night's rest.

The greatest attention must be paid to the local treatment. The eye should be frequently cleansed of the discharge. The eyelids being opened, a small stream of lukewarm water [or a warm saturated solution of boracic acid in water—B.] should be allowed to play gently upon them, until all the discharge is washed away. Still better is it to employ for this purpose a small syringe, the nozzle of which is to be gently inserted between the eyelids. The syringe should be very carefully and delicately handled, otherwise it will bruise and irritate the eye, or even perhaps rub against the cornea. [A fountain syringe may be applied more advantageously for this purpose, the force of the current being regulated by the height at which the reservoir is placed.—B.] The nurse must also be very careful that no drop of the returning fluid is thrown into her eye. In severe cases the eye should be thus cleansed every hour or two, in milder cases three or four times daily will suffice. The crusts which form upon the eyelashes should be well soaked with warm water and then gently removed, so as not to excoriate the lids. A little simple cerate should be applied to the edges of the latter, night and morning, to prevent their sticking, or if they are getting sore the citrine ointment may be substituted. If the temperature of the lids is but moderately increased, it is only necessary to employ cold compresses for an hour or two after the application of caustics, for we thus assist the astringent action of the caustic upon the bloodvessels, and also moderate the reaction produced by it; but if the attack is very severe, and the eyelids very red, swollen, and hot, a temporary use of cold water will not suffice, and we must have recourse to a constant application of iced compresses. They should be applied in the following manner: slightly moistened pledgets of lint, of a sufficient size to cover both eyelids, should be laid upon a lump of ice until they are quite cold, when they are to be applied to the eyelids and changed as soon as they get the least warm. Several of such pledgets should be kept lying upon the ice, so that one is always ready for use. If the temperature of the lids is very high, the lint may require to be changed every one or two minutes. It is, therefore, absolutely necessary to have a nurse for each patient, or at least for every two. Instead of the lint, small caoutchouc ice-bags may be employed. If great attention cannot be paid to the application of the iced compresses, it is better to abstain altogether from their use, as they may otherwise do more harm than good. We must then rest satisfied with the cold-water dressing or Goulard lotion. When the eyelids become cooler and less red, the patient begins to find the extreme cold disagreeable, and then cold-water dressing should be substituted for the iced compress, or it may even be necessary to pass over to the use of warm fomentations. A constant small stream of cold water may also be allowed to play upon the eyelids by means of a small siphon connected with a little reservoir placed at the bed-head. [Dor recommends the benzoate of sodium, because of its supposed energetic disinfectant qualities. He uses it as a disinfectant solely in solutions of one to twenty, as often as is deemed necessary. (See the "Lyon Médical" for March 7, 1880.)—B.]

Local depletion is often of great benefit. If there is much ciliary neuralgia, accompanied by great swelling, heat, and redness of the eyelids, and if these symptoms do not readily yield to cold compresses, leeches should be at once applied. The best place for their application is on the temple, about an inch from the outer canthus; for, if they are put close to the eyelids, they often produce great œdema of the lids which may even extend to the cheek. Their number should vary from four to eight, according to the requirements of the case. They should be applied two at a time, so that the effect may be prolonged, and free after-bleeding is to be encouraged by warm fomentations.

If the eyelids are much swollen, very tense, and press greatly upon the eyeball, and especially if the cornea is beginning to become affected, the outer commissure of the lids should be divided. This will not only mitigate the injurious pressure of the lids upon the eyeball and cornea, but it will also give rise to free bleeding from the vessels which are divided, and thus greatly relieve the circulation of the external portions of the eye. The incision is to be carried through the skin and fibres of the orbicularis, but not through the mucous membrane, otherwise an ectropion might be produced. [This operation of canthotomy is extremely necessary in all cases where there is much swelling of the lids, and should be done at once.—B.]

We have now to consider the most important part of the treatment, namely, the topical application of caustics and astringents. At the commencement of the disease, whilst the discharge is still but moderate in quantity, we must be careful not to employ too strong a caustic, more especially if the eyelids are hard and the conjunctiva and papillæ not much swollen, for fear that there should be a tendency to diphtheritic conjunctivitis, which would be greatly aggravated by free cauterization. As soon as the discharge has become copious, and the symptoms of true purulent ophthalmia are well pronounced, astringents must be employed more energetically. The choice of the astringent and the mode of its application will depend upon circumstances. If we have to treat the person as an out-door hospital patient, and shall perhaps only see him every second or third day, it will be necessary to give him a remedy which can be readily and efficiently applied by some attendant. Under these circumstances I have found the injection of zinc and alum, as employed at the Royal London Ophthalmic Hospital, Moorfields, by far the best. Its strength, and the frequency of its application, must vary according to the severity of the disease. I generally employ a solution of two grains of sulphate of zinc and four or six grains of alum to the half ounce of distilled water. This is to be injected between the eyelids with a small glass syringe every fifteen or thirty minutes during the day, and every two hours at night. As the condition of the eye improves, it is to be applied less frequently. Before its application, the discharge should be thoroughly washed away by an injection of lukewarm water, in order that the collyrium may come everywhere in contact with the surface of the conjunctiva. Every second or third day, the surgeon should apply a drop or two of a strong solution of nitrate of silver (gr. x to f℥j of water) to the inside of the lids, or it should be brushed over the conjunctiva with a camel's-hair brush; the patient in the interval continuing with the injection.

Much benefit may also be derived from a solution of nitrate of silver (gr. x

to f ʒj of water if the case is severe), which should be dropped into the eye
every five or six hours, with a quill or camel's-hair brush. But it is more
difficult to apply these drops properly and efficiently than the injection, and
it is therefore always better that the surgeon should, if possible, do this
himself. My friend, Mr. Moss, has very successfully treated, at the Moorfields Hospital, out-patients suffering from very severe purulent or gonorrhœal ophthalmia, in the following manner, which was, I believe, suggested
to him by Professor Donders: The lids being well everted, he applies with
a camel's-hair brush a very strong solution of nitrate of silver (gr. xxx–xl
to the f ʒj) to the conjunctiva once a day. In the intervals, the patient uses
an injection of alum every half-hour or hour. Quinine or steel is, at the
same time, given internally.

But if the patient is in the hospital, or can be frequently seen by the
surgeon, I greatly prefer to apply the nitrate of silver in substance. It has
this great advantage, that we can regulate and limit its effect, and prevent
its coming in contact with the cornea and the ocular conjunctiva, which is
quite impossible with the solution. Moreover, the latter is easily decomposed
if the discharge is copious, and its effect is thus impaired. It is, however,
absolutely necessary that the surgeon or a skilful assistant should apply it,
as it cannot be entrusted to a nurse. We are indebted to Von Graefe[1] for
the scientific explanation of the action of the nitrate of silver in purulent
ophthalmia, and for very exact and comprehensive directions as to its use.
During a prolonged stay in Berlin, I saw it employed most successfully in
this way by Von Graefe in many cases of purulent ophthalmia.

Pure nitrate of silver is too strong to apply in substance to the conjunctiva, as its escharotic action is too severe. It produces a thick eschar which
is thrown off with difficulty, hence the superficial portion of the conjunctiva
is very liable to become destroyed, and deep cicatrices may be produced.
Its strength should, therefore, be diluted by mixing it with one-half or two-
thirds of nitrate of potassium.

The application is to be made in the following manner: The eyelids having been thoroughly everted, so as to bring the retro-tarsal fold well into
view, the folds of the conjunctiva of the upper and lower lid should be
allowed to cover the cornea, and thus protect it from the action of the caustic.
The crayon of mitigated nitrate of silver should then be lightly passed over
every part of the surface of the palpebral conjunctiva, especially in the
retro-tarsal region. A solution of salt and water should then be freely
applied with a large camel's-hair brush, in order to neutralize the nitrate of
silver. The caseous shreds of chloride of silver, which are thus formed,
should be washed away with clean cold water, before the lids are replaced.
We can very easily regulate the action of the caustic. When but a slight
effect is required, the crayon should be passed but once or twice very lightly
over the conjunctiva. If a stronger action is desired, it may be used with
more freedom. The neutralization with the salt and water should not take
place immediately after the application of the caustic, except where the effect
of the latter is to be but very slight. It should not, however, be postponed
longer than from ten to fifteen seconds.

The caustic should not, as a rule, be applied to the ocular conjunctiva, for,
... but secondarily affected, its swelling and inflammation will gener-
as the condition of the palpebral conjunctiva improves. It may,
ecessary to do so, if the chemosis is so considerable as to pro-
the lids, and does not yield to free incisions. But it should

only be touched here and there, and the salt and water should be immediately applied.

If the swelling of the conjunctiva is very considerable, it should be freely scarified with a scalpel or Desmarres' scarifier, directly after the neutralization of the caustic; and the bleeding should be encouraged by the application of hot sponges, and by slightly kneading the lids between the fingers. The incisions in the papillæ should be very superficial, otherwise deep cicatrices will be left. The lids should on no account be scarified before the application of the nitrate of silver, for the latter would act too severely upon the incised conjunctiva. If the chemosis is great, incisions radiating towards the cornea should be made in it, either with a pair of scissors or a scalpel: or a small fold of conjunctiva may be snipped out with the scissors near the outer edge of the cornea. Ice compresses are to be applied directly after the cauterization, for they diminish the inflammatory reaction, and assist in the contraction of the bloodvessels.

If we watch the condition of the eye, we shall find that it becomes very hot and painful directly after the cauterization, and that this is accompanied by increased lachrymation and a mucous discharge. The eschars which are formed upon the palpebral conjunctiva are shed in from thirty to sixty minutes, in the form of little yellowish-white, rolled-up flakes. Those on the ocular conjunctiva remain somewhat longer. The inflammatory symptoms soon subside, the conjunctiva becomes less turgid, the lachrymation and purulent discharge diminish, and the stage of remission sets in, during which the epithelium is regenerated. When this has taken place, the original condition, as it existed before the application of the caustic, begins to reappear. The conjunctiva becomes more red and swollen, the discharge increases in quantity, and the inflammatory symptoms in severity. It is of consequence to endeavor, by renewed cauterization, to cut short this third period at the outset, before it has regained its original intensity. We shall thus be able, by degrees, to extend the duration of the stage of remission, and to diminish the intensity of the inflammatory stage. Generally, it will suffice to apply the caustic once in twenty-four hours; in very severe cases it may be necessary to do so more frequently, but it should never be applied until the purulent discharge has again set in.

Von Graefe has shown that the effect of the nitrate of silver (although it momentarily increases the congestion) is to contract the bloodvessels, and to accelerate the circulation, which is retarded in purulent ophthalmia, the conjunctiva being at the same time very vascular and congested, and its vessels dilated; moreover, the serous infiltration of the conjunctiva is greatly relieved by the copious serous effusion which follows the cauterization. This is the period of remission, during which the epithelial layer of the conjunctiva is regenerated.

If the cornea becomes cloudy, a solution of atropine (gr. ij to f℥j of distilled water) is to be dropped into the eye three or four times daily. Where the caustic is employed, the atropine should not be used until the period of remission has set in. If the nitrate of silver drops are used, the atropine should be applied during the intervals, and about two hours after the former. It is better to use atropine in all cases of purulent conjunctivitis from the beginning, as a possible aid in preventing serious corneal disease. In cases in which the cornea becomes infiltrated very soon in the course of the disease, it has been recommended to employ eserine in place of atropine, and much benefit has been recorded in its favor. It was formerly supposed that it exerted a specific antiseptic effect upon the purulent infiltration, but this is now generally discredited. It was also supposed that, owing to its diminishing the intra-ocular tension, it assisted in the furtherance of the osmotic processes by counteracting the interference in the nutrition of the cornea produced by the disease. More extended experience has not substantiated the former evidence in its favor. The strength of the solution used has been from two to four grains of the sulphate to the fluidounce of distilled water.—B.]

If there is a deep ulcer of the cornea, which threatens to perforate the latter, we should at once perform paracentesis by pricking the bottom of the ulcer, and letting the aqueous humor flow off very gently. The opening in the cornea will thus be extremely small; a little portion of iris will fall against it, lymph will be effused, and the intra-ocular pressure being now taken off, the ulcer will begin to heal at the bottom. The re-accumulation of the aqueous humor will generally suffice to detach the portion of iris from the cornea. If, however, a small anterior synechia should persist, atropine drops should be applied, in order, if possible, to tear it through. It may be necessary to repeat the paracentesis several times, if we see that the bottom of the ulcer is being bulged forwards by the aqueous humor. By such a timely paracentesis we often limit the ulcer to a small extent, and finally little or no opacity of the cornea may remain. But if we permit the ulcer to perforate of its own accord, the opening will be much larger, for the bottom of the ulcer becomes attenuated and extended in size before the cornea gives way. The aqueous humor will then escape with considerable force, and carry the iris, or even, perhaps, the lens, if the perforation be large, into the opening in the cornea, and thus a considerable anterior synechia or prolapse of the iris may occur. If the latter is considerable it should be pricked with a fine needle, and the aqueous humor distending it be allowed to flow off, which will cause the prolapse to collapse. This may be repeated several times, until it shrinks and dwindles away. If this does not occur, the prolapse should be stripped off with a pair of scissors, after having been pricked. Should the lens have fallen into the opening and be presenting through, it should be at once removed, together, perhaps, with a little of the vitreous humor. An incision should be made through the central portion of the perforated cornea, with Von Graefe's narrow cataract knife. If a piece of iris protrudes, this should be somewhat drawn out and snipped off. The capsule should be freely lacerated with the pricker, and the lens will then readily escape if a little pressure is made upon the eye. A little vitreous humor will generally exude, and the lips of the incision fall into close apposition. A firm compress bandage should be carefully applied, so as to keep the eye immovable and the vitreous pressed back. Should the latter show a tendency to protrude through the incision, and thus interfere with its firm cicatrization, it should be pricked, and a little be allowed to escape, the bandage being then re-applied. We may thus be able to save a sufficient portion of clear cornea to permit of the subsequent restoration of some useful degree of sight, by the formation of an artificial pupil.

If the disease has become chronic, the nitrate of silver must be less frequently applied, or it should be exchanged for, or alternated with, the use of sulphate of copper in substance. A crayon of this should be passed lightly over the palpebral conjunctiva, more particularly in the retro-tarsal region, once every day. Or, a solution of sulphate of copper (gr. ij ad f℥j) should be dropped into the eye once or twice daily. The astringent must be occasionally changed, as the conjunctiva after a time becomes accustomed to it, and it loses its effect. Thus, we may alternate the sulphate of copper with a collyrium of the sulphate, acetate, or chloride of zinc, alum, acetate of lead, or vinum opii, or the red or white precipitate ointment may be applied to the conjunctiva. If the papillæ are much swollen and very prominent, like cauliflower excrescences, it may be necessary to snip them off with a pair of scissors.

4.—GONORRHŒAL OPHTHALMIA.

[Syn. Gonorrhœal conjunctivitis.—B.]

Gonorrhœal ophthalmia is one of the most dangerous and virulent diseases of the eye. In the majority of cases it presents the symptoms of a very severe purulent ophthalmia, accompanied sometimes by marked constitutional disturbance.

Shortly after the infection, the patient experiences a feeling of tingling and smarting in the eye, as if a little grit or sand had become lodged beneath the lids. The eye becomes red, watery, and irritable, and the edges of the eyelids somewhat glued together by a slight grayish-white discharge. These symptoms rapidly increase in severity, and the disease quickly assumes the character of purulent ophthalmia of an aggravated type. The eyelids become greatly swollen, hot, red, and œdematous [Fig. 62], the conjunctiva

[Fig. 62.   Fig. 63.

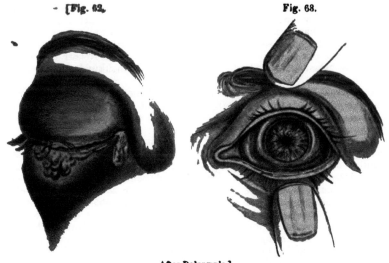

After Dalrymple.]

very vascular, swollen, and villous; the chemosis is also very considerable [Fig. 63], enveloping and overlapping the cornea, and protruding between the lids. The discharge is thick and creamy, and perhaps so profuse that it oozes out between the lids, and when they are opened streams over the cheek. There is always great danger of the cornea becoming affected with deep and extensive ulceration, which frequently quickly leads to perforation. The constitutional symptoms are often severe; the patients being generally in a feeble and weakly condition, their general health having, perhaps, suffered from the existence of the gonorrhœa.

Sometimes, the disease shows from the outset a marked tendency to assume the character of diphtheritic conjunctivitis, and this proves especially dan-

gerous to the eye. In such cases, we notice that the conjunctiva, instead of
presenting the usual red, vascular, succulent appearance common to purulent
ophthalmia, becomes pale, smooth, and infiltrated with a fibrinous exudation.
The discharge is also quite different, being thin, gray, and watery. The
cases of gonorrhœal ophthalmia which prove so virulent as to destroy the
cornea in the course of a few hours, are probably mostly of this diphtheritic,
or, at all events, of a mixed character. In England, however, this form is
very rare, and, amongst the numerous cases of gonorrhœal ophthalmia which
have come under my care and observation, I have only met with the purulent disease.

Gonorrhœal ophthalmia is always due to contagion, and the doctrine of
metastasis (which was formerly much in vogue) is quite untenable. It may
be produced during any stage of the urethral disease, but about the third
week of the existence of the latter is the most dangerous period, the discharge being then very copious, thick, and noxious. I have, however, seen
the discharge from a gleet give rise to severe and even destructive gonorrhœal ophthalmia. Medical men unfortunately sometimes altogether neglect
to warn their patients of the danger of contagion from the urethral discharge.
I have met with several instances of severe and destructive gonorrhœal
ophthalmia, in which the patients had never been informed by their medical
men of the very contagious character of the discharge from the urethra, and
had accidentally inoculated one of their eyes. [The secretion of gonorrhœal
conjunctivitis has been found to contain micrococci, as well as pus cells and
epithelial cells; the masses of micrococci being partly free, and partly enclosed in the pus and epithelial cells. This corroborates Neisser's discovery.
(See the "Centralblatt für die praktische Augenheilkunde," September,
1881.)—B.]

Gonorrhœal ophthalmia is far more frequent amongst men than women,
and the right eye is the one usually attacked, the corresponding hand being
most used for the purpose of ablution, etc., and, consequently, most prone to
be the carrier of the virus to the eye.

If we see the patient very shortly after the inoculation, the eye should be
thoroughly syringed out with lukewarm water, and a drop or two of a weak
solution of nitrate of silver (gr. ij ad f℥j) be at once applied, and repeated
at the intervals of a few hours. [Stronger solutions, of the strength of x-xx
grains to the fluidounce, are more useful in cutting short the disease.—B.]
Iced compresses must also be employed. The other eye should be at once protected by the hermetical bandage (vide p. 147) against the danger of contagion. The treatment must be the same as that for purulent ophthalmia,
the patient's health being sustained by tonics and a generous diet. [Where
there is much swelling of the lids, the pressure upon the eyeball should be
lessened by the operation of canthotomy, as in purulent conjunctivitis.
Fuchs recommends splitting the external commissure with the scissors, and
then deepening it with the knife until the lids are entirely relaxed. He
then everts the lower lid by a long deep suture in the cheek; this is removed
five days later. (See "Centralblatt für die praktische Augenheilkunde,"
July, 1881.) Critchett divided the upper lid vertically from ciliary margin
to eyebrow in a case of gonorrhœal conjunctivitis in a child; he then separated the two angles of the divided tarsus, and fixed them with fine sutures
to the skin of the eyebrow. The immediate effect was to diminish the redness and swelling of the lid and conjunctiva. At the end of six weeks, the
edges of the divided lid were freshened and brought together with sutures.
Union occurred with very little deformity and the functions of the lid were
well performed. (See "Lancet," April 3, 1880.)—B.]

1.—OPHTHALMIA NEONATORUM. [PURULENT CONJUNCTIVITIS OF NEW-BORN INFANTS.—B.]

[True purulent conjunctivitis of infants begins, probably in the majority of cases, as a catarrhal inflammation, with mucoid or muco-purulent secretion; but the latter rapidly becomes thicker, more cloudy, yellow, and really purulent. Sometimes the change from catarrhal to purulent inflammation is so rapid that the former stage escapes observation. The disease begins on the second or third day after birth, though it may appear on the first day, or may be postponed to the fifth. If it does not appear until after the fifth day, the suspicion is aroused that the contagion has occurred since birth, and from some other cause than inoculation with the vaginal discharge of the mother during parturition, as the irritation of bright light, or cold wind, or contagion from some other case.

The symptoms of a well-marked case are: swelling of the tissue of the eyelids; redness of the cutaneous surface, sometimes amounting to lividness; more or less sticking of the lid-margins together; the appearance of a purulent discharge when the lids are opened; marked injection of the ocular conjunctiva, accompanied generally by some chemosis; sometimes the lids are so swollen as to prevent their eversion; but where they can be turned out, the retro-tarsal fold is found enormously swollen, as is also the papillary portion of the tarsal conjunctiva, and covered by a yellowish exudation, which may be more or less flocculent, or even stringy. There is

[Fig. 64.

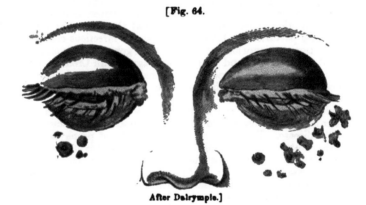

After Dalrymple.]

great heat of skin in the immediate vicinity, and sometimes a slight rise in the general temperature. This condition lasts usually from four to six days, and then the acute inflammatory symptoms begin to subside, though the purulent discharge may be very profuse for a much longer period. Both eyes are almost always affected, though usually one before the other. In some instances the ropy, fibrinous exudation which is noticed in the beginning continues to the end, and is accompanied by patches of coagulation upon the conjunctiva itself. In other, not very rare cases, the flocculent fibrinous material is deposited continuously over the whole tarsal surface of the conjunctiva, and very closely resembles a membrane. It is, however, friable and easily removed by the forceps, coming away in small bits or shreds, and leaving a raw, bleeding surface, and the hemorrhage is sometimes quite profuse. This may not form again, though it usually does. With this pseudo-membranous formation there is also an abundant purulent discharge, which lasts long after the pseudo-membrane has ceased to be formed. These cases resemble closely the cases described by some of the German authors as croupous conjunctivitis, though the membrane in the latter is usually coextensive with the palpebral conjunctiva and moderately thick. They seem to be cases of the disease in which the products of inflammation are of a more highly organized type. Though comparatively rare in the higher classes, the disease is of very frequent occurrence among the lower orders, and is especially rife in hospitals for the confinement of women. (See "Annales de Gynécologie," March, 1881; "Archiv für Gynækologie,'" xvii. 1, 1881; "Centralblatt für Gynækologie," Jan. 22, 1881.) As regards the causation of the disease, all recent authors agree that the disease is, in the great majority of cases, due to inoculation during parturition with the discharge from the vagina of the mother. Cases of purulent conjunctivitis now and then occur, however, where the mothers have had no discharge from the vagina. This vaginal secretion need not be purulent, for an ordinary vaginal catarrh or the lochial discharge has been known to cause many cases of purulent conjunctivitis in infants. The disease may be, and often is, communicated by carelessness and uncleanliness on the part of nurses, mothers, and other attendants, often in the washing of the children after birth, or in handling them subsequently, by carrying the vaginal discharge upon the fingers or upon the bedding or clothing. Credé states that in his experience the cases of purulent conjunctivitis in new-born children have been, almost without an exception, caused by direct contact of the vaginal secretion with the eyes during parturition. He believes that the infectious character of a vaginal secretion continues long after the specific gonorrhœal symptoms have disappeared. Galezowski and Abegg both agree with Credé in the belief that the disease is *always* caused by the introduction of the leucorrhœal or gonorrhœal vaginal secretion between the eyelids of the infant during parturition.

Recognizing this fact in the etiology of the purulent conjunctivitis of infants, our main endeavors should be directed towards preventing the occurrence of the disease. The practical question is one of prophylaxis, and to this end, the care of the disease must be placed in the hands of the obstetrician and nurse, and on them must rest the responsibility of the result. As a precautionary measure, the vagina of the mother should be kept thoroughly cleansed for some days before confinement, though the uncertainty of the occurrence of the latter renders the duration of the former equally uncertain. The methods of disinfection of the mother's vagina and the child's eyes consist in the application of solutions of carbolic acid, salicylic acid, boracic acid, and nitrate of silver, of varying strength. The prophylactic measures recommended by the Editor are as follows: In all cases of vaginal discharge in parturient women, whether specific or not, the vagina should be carefully cleansed and disinfected repeatedly, before parturition begins, with a two per cent. solution of carbolic acid. As soon as the child is born, the external surface and edges of the lids should be carefully cleansed with a one or two per cent. solution of carbolic acid, and then the conjunctival cul-de-sac washed out with some of the same solution, or with a saturated solution of boracic acid. This must be done by the attending physician, or by a skilled nurse under his supervision. The eyes of all new-born children should be carefully watched for the first week or ten days, and whenever any signs of an ordinary catarrhal conjunctivitis appear, the conjunctiva should be thoroughly brushed over with a solution of silver nitrate, from two to five grains to the fluidounce of water. If the conjunctivitis has become purulent, the child should, if possible, be isolated from all healthy infants, and have its own bath-tub. If this is not possible, the diseased infant should be bathed last, and no sponges used, but only cloths, which can afterwards be destroyed. If one eye only is affected, do not apply the hermetically sealed bandage to the sound eye, but envelop the arms and hands of the baby so as to prevent the secretion from being carried to the fellow-eye, and lay the child upon the side corresponding to the diseased eye. The most important feature in the treatment is enforced cleanliness. This requires constant attention and the frequent use of some soft cloths and plenty of water. The use of cloths, dipped in ice-water, or laid on blocks of ice and then placed on the lids, must be regulated by the amount of swelling of the lids and heat of the parts. As soon as the lids can be everted, the proper treatment is a thorough application of nitrate of silver to the conjunctiva of the lid and retro-tarsal fold, daily and sometimes twice a day. If this is thoroughly done, a five-grain solution will, in most cases, suffice; but where there are profuse secretion and considerable swelling of the conjunctiva, a ten-grain solution becomes necessary. When, owing to marked hyper-trophy of the papillary structure of the conjunctiva, a stronger caustic becomes necessary, it is better to discard solutions and employ the lapis mitigatus (one part of nitrate of silver to two parts of nitrate of potassium), and neutralise its effect by a subsequent washing with a solution of chloride of sodium.

It is well to employ a one-grain solution of sulphate of atropia in a saturated solution of boracic acid in every case of purulent conjunctivitis, as the great danger in this disease is purulent infiltration and perforation of the cornea. Should this infiltration occur at the centre of the cornea, the atropia should be instilled frequently, for if perforation occurs, the dilatation of the pupil will prevent a large prolapse of the iris through the perforation. If the infiltration of the cornea, on the contrary, be at or near the margin, it is better to employ a two-grain solution of the sulphate of eserine, as thus an extensive prolapse of the iris may be prevented if the ulcer perforate. In all cases, the cleansing and washing of the lids and conjunctiva should be done with a saturated solution of boracic acid, and the atropine and eserine should be dissolved in the same. The prognosis will depend upon the severity of the attack and the condition of the cornea. It is by no means uncommon for the cornea to become infiltrated early in the disease, and end in perfora-tion and prolapse of the iris in spite of the most careful and methodical treatment. The frequency of large leucomata with adhesions of the iris to the cornea, proves that this is no uncommon result. An interesting point in the pathology of this disease is the discovery of micrococci in the discharge of purulent conjunctivitis in every case, and sometimes the bacillar bacteria also. (See "Centralblatt für die praktische Augenheilkunde," Sept. 1881.)

In cases of perforation of the cornea and prolapse of the iris, resulting in the formation of an adherent leucoma, the vision can be improved by the formation of an artificial pupil, by means either of an iridectomy or an iridotomy. But this should not be done until the child is at least several months old.—B.]

6.—DIPHTHERITIC CONJUNCTIVITIS.

[The rarest form of conjunctival inflammation, as it is the most dangerous to the eye in its destructive tendencies, is the diphtheritic. This disease, though not uncommon in Berlin and some portions of northeastern Germany, is relatively rare in other parts of the Continent of Europe, and absolutely rare in Great Britain and the United States. Isolated cases are met with here, but the disease never assumes the *quasi* epidemic character that it does in some of the German cities.

Diphtheritic conjunctivitis is characterized by a rapid and very marked swelling of the lids, due to a more or less *extensive infiltration*, not only of the *entire conjunctiva*, but also of the *other tissues of the lid*, sometimes even including the *integument*, by an inflammatory product of marked coagulability. This infiltration is *into the tissue* of the conjunctiva, and not an exudation *upon its surface.* The local heat of the parts is very pronounced. The infiltration into the lids is so great that they become almost like a board, look and feel like brawn, and cannot be everted. This dense infiltration often drives all the blood out of the eyelids, and instead of presenting a livid appearance, as in the purulent form of conjunctivitis, they appear dusky yellow, and even blanched. As a consequence of this extensive and rapidly occurring infiltration, the nutrition of the parts is interfered with or entirely cut off, and the conjunctiva changed into a necrotic mass and cast off as a slough. This necrosis sometimes extends deeper than the conjunctiva, and an extensive loss of substance in the lid tissue occurs. When the strangulation is not so extensive in the lid, and the skin looks angry and reddened, the dense, hard, brawn-like condition of the lids is sufficient to distinguish the case as one of diphtheritic conjunctivitis. Such a case cannot be mistaken for purulent conjunctivitis. Where it is possible to evert the lid in part, the inner surface is seen to be of a green or grayish-yellow color, usually bloodless, which appearance is due to an infiltration of the entire thickness of the conjunctiva, and not to the formation of a membrane on its epithelial surface.

During this first stage of the disease the exudation from the conjunctiva is usually slight, and consists of a thin, dirty, very hot, ichorous fluid, containing yellowish shreds and some cells.—B.]

Even deep scarification of the conjunctiva fails to produce a copious sanguineous discharge, for the latter is either thin, scanty, and of a reddish-yellow tint, or the incisions remain almost dry.

The discharge on the surface of the conjunctiva often assumes the form of thin, yellowish, reticulated patches, of varying size. In some cases, thick opaque membranes are formed, which are so coherent that they can be stripped off in large pieces, forming casts of the lids and the surface of the eyeball. Their forcible removal may cause considerable bleeding, but we do not find, as is the case in purulent ophthalmia, that the denuded conjunctiva presents a red, succulent, villous surface, but we come down upon another layer of yellowish-gray fibrinous infiltration. In fact, the latter is not confined to the surface of the conjunctiva, but extends more or less deeply into its stroma.

[In the second stage the exudation changes in character, and becomes puriform and finally purulent. The disease is rapid in its progress, and reaches its height usually within a few days. The ocular conjunctiva becomes densely infiltrated, and surrounds the cornea like a hard, unyielding wall. There are usually but few bloodvessels to be seen, but numerous petate hemorrhages are not infrequent. After the disease has lasted from : to eight days, the hard, board-like condition of the lids diminishes, small rhs begin to appear in the conjunctiva, the latter becomes loose, red, and ng, and assumes the appearance of a suppurating or granulating surface. lar conjunctiva takes on the same change; the lids can be everted, n becomes purulent, and the second stage has begun. This stage ng time, differing in no respect from an ordinary purulent conjunctivitis, and terminates in the third or cicatricial stage. This last stage is deeper and more extensive; dependent in direct ratio upon the amount of destruction by necrosis following the infiltration.—B.]

Diphtheritic conjunctivitis is a far more dangerous disease than purulent ophthalmia, on account of the frequency and severity of corneal complications. Extensive ulceration or suppuration of the cornea is but too frequent. The dense, hard, infiltrated conjunctiva presses upon the cornea and upon the bloodvessels which supply it, hence the nutrition of the cornea is greatly impaired, and its suppuration may rapidly ensue. If the cornea is about to be implicated, we notice that its lustre is slightly diminished, its surface faintly clouded, and its epithelial layer somewhat abraded. A yellow infiltration appears, which rapidly passes over into an ulcer, the latter extending quickly in circumference and depth, until a very considerable portion of the cornea may be involved. In some cases, when the ulcer has extended nearly as far as the membrane of Descemet, its floor becomes somewhat more transparent, and bulged forward by the aqueous humor. The patient's sight is temporarily much improved, and he is buoyed up by the vain hope that his eye is safe; but perforation generally rapidly ensues. If the disease is very severe, and the cornea has become affected at a very early stage, the whole cornea may suppurate, give way, and a considerable amount of the contents of the globe escape. The perforation is soon blocked up by a glutinous exudation, which also glues down the edges of the prolapsed portion of iris to the cornea. The earlier the cornea becomes affected, the greater is the danger, for the ulcers which occur at a later period of the disease spread less rapidly, and show a greater tendency to limitation. We also find, as in purulent ophthalmia, that those eyes are safest in which there exist either vascular ulcers of the cornea or a vascular pannus, for then the nutrition of the cornea is carried on by the bloodvessels upon its surface, and there is far less danger of its undergoing suppuration.

[This description of the disease in its various stages we owe originally to Von Graefe, who first differentiated it as a distinct affection. Usually the general condition of the patient affected with diphtheritic conjunctivitis is bad. The eye may be the only organ affected by the disease, though often the nose, the throat, and the eyes are all involved in the process. The local manifestation of the diphtheritic poison may appear first in the conjunctiva, or it may spread from the nose or throat to the eye. In North Germany, diphtheritic conjunctivitis is a not infrequent complication of malignant scarlatina. It occurs more often in children than in adults, thus resembling the croupous form of inflammation. The diphtheritic process in the conjunctiva is probably caused by the presence of lower organisms, and the chief part in the infiltration is taken by cellular elements, which are so numerous and so densely packed together as to obliterate the vessels and cut off the circulation. Micrococci have been found in the secretion, mixed with pus-cell and epithelial cells.

From this rapid survey of the symptoms and course of a diphtheritic conjunctivitis, it will be seen that there are always necrosis of tissue, loss of substance, and cicatrization in the lid, none of which evils occur in the purulent or membranous forms of conjunctivitis. In all three stages of the purulent and membranous conjunctivitis, the great danger is ulceration and necrosis of the cornea; and the more the ocular conjunctiva is involved, the greater is the danger. The nutrition of the cornea may be so greatly interfered with that it may become entirely opaque within forty-eight hours; and when this occurs, it may slough out entire, like a watch-glass from its frame. When the cornea is not entirely surrounded by the brawny conjunctiva, part of it can generally be saved, even in its transparency, though this is rare.

In making a prognosis, we must be chiefly guided by the severity of the inflammatory symptoms, the amount of the fibrinous exudation, the swelling and hardness of the lids, the chemosis, and especially by the condition of the cornea. The prognosis is almost always bad, owing to the very rapid strangulation of the tissues. Not uncommonly the lower lid becomes excoriated upon its skin surface by the acridity of the discharge in 'the first stage, and becomes covered by a diphtheritic membrane. Fortunately the disease is rare among new-born children; it occurs more frequently between the ages of two and seven. It is extremely contagious, and this is now the explanation of the occurrence of epidemics, the disease being propagated by infection with the secretion.

One point in the pathology of the disease has given rise to an almost endless discussion, which in some quarters has not yet been satisfactorily settled, viz.: whether the disease is ever produced by infection with the purulent secretion from a non-diphtheritic case. There seems no good reason for doubting that diphtheritic conjunctivitis has been produced by infection with the purulent secretion of a gonorrhœal conjunctivitis, for it was frequently seen at Von Graefe's clinic in Berlin and elsewhere. Yet Von Graefe himself defined the affection as a general constitutional disease, and clearly differentiated it from purulent conjunctivitis. In view of the authenticity of the cases above referred to, we must agree with the modified statement of Von Graefe that, while in many cases diphtheritic conjunctivitis is a symptom of a general disease, yet there are cases in which it is a local disorder, caused by infection with the secretion from a purulent conjunctivitis. The reverse of the case has also been stated to be true on the authority of Horner, who asserts that though the discharge from a case of diphtheritic conjunctivitis, when applied to a healthy conjunctiva, usually reproduces diphtheritic conjunctivitis, it does not always; for purulent conjunctivitis has been known to result from such infection. This would look as if purulent and diphtheritic conjunctivitis were intimately connected, and leaves the pathogenesis of the latter still in an unsettled state. The infection may be carried by the atmosphere, and not be due to direct contagion from sponges, towels, etc.

The disease is not always binocular, and great care must therefore be taken of the unaffected eye. If the case be seen early enough, some impermeable or hermetically sealed bandage should be applied, the best being that of Dr. Buller, of Montreal, through the glass centre of which the eye may be constantly watched. Yet this is not always a protection, for when there is a constitutional blood disorder at the bottom of the disease, of course no external protective bandage would be of any avail.—B.]

With regard to the *treatment*, it must be confessed that we have, unfortunately, but little control over the disease during the first period.

Our first care must be to remove the patient from all noxious influences that may keep up and intensify the disease, and every effort must be made to prevent its spreading.

We must endeavor to diminish the inflammatory symptoms, more particularly if they assume a sthenic type. If the eyelids are greatly swollen, and very red, hot, stiff, and painful, iced compresses must be employed almost without intermission, being changed as soon as they become at all warm. They must be less frequently employed when the second period (that of vascularization) is setting in, and when this has become fully established, they must be only used after the cauterization. The effect of the cold is to counteract the stasis by causing contraction of the vessels, and it also acts as a sedative, giving great relief to the intense pain. But if there is extensive ulceration of the cornea, the cold compresses should be replaced by warm fomentations, so that we produce an acceleration in the vascularity of the conjunctiva. Indeed, lately some surgeons, especially Berlin[1] and Mooren[2] have recommended the substitution of warm fomentations for the iced compresses, on the ground that they bring about the second period more rapidly. Thus they may prove of advantage when ulceration of the cornea occurs during the first period, and the ulcer shows no tendency to become limited or vascularized, for the tendency to necrosis is markedly aggravated by the application of cold or of caustics. Mooren formerly always employed iced compresses, but in later years he has substituted the use of warm poultices, together with derivatives internally. But then he himself admits, that the disease never appears in Düsseldorf with the extreme intensity which it so often assumes in Berlin.

Local depletion also proves of much service. Unfortunately, the disease occurs so frequently in anæmic and cachectic individuals, that we generally cannot make a full use of this. In adults, more particularly if the disease is due to contagion, and the patient robust and strong, leeches should be applied in large quantities to the temples, or at the upper angle of the nose. Three or four leeches should be applied at a time, and as soon as these drop off they are to be replaced by others. But care must be taken not to push this remedy too far, especially in feeble persons, for by greatly weakening the patient we increase the danger of sloughing of the cornea. In very severe cases as many as thirty to forty leeches (Wecker) or even a greater quantity (Graefe) may have to be applied before any impression is made upon the disease.

[The division of the external canthus by the operation of canthotomy is not as a rule advisable in these cases, even where the lid-tension is marked, for a diphtheritic membrane is almost certain to form upon the incised surfaces and complicate the case. Hence it is better to apply leeches to the temple, where depletion is desired.

No caustics should ever be employed in the first stage, as they would do positive harm. When the second or purulent stage has fairly begun, then the application of caustics is indicated under the same rules as apply to true purulent conjunctivitis. The same rules also apply to the use of atropine or eserine in the diphtheritic as in the purulent form. As soon as the stage of cicatrisation has begun, it is better to stop the use of caustics, as they do no good and may do harm. Cleanliness in all three stages is very important, and the best means thereto is a one per cent. solution of carbolic acid, applied with a brush or injected gently under the lids. Tweedy recommends the local application of sulphate of quinine. He uses a lotion of four grains of the drug to the fluidounce of water and a minimum of dilute sulphuric acid, using it constantly in the eye, and keeping compresses soaked in it upon the closed lids. He believes the quinine to be a specific in the diphtheritic exudation, checking and controlling the inflammatory process, and limiting the inflammatory neoplasm. He does not believe that the bacteria or the micrococci destroy the cornea. Vossius recommends a four per cent. solution of salicylic acid in glycerine, brushed over the conjunctiva every half hour. In almost all cases a strongly tonic general treatment is indicated from the beginning, quinine and iron being especially valuable.—B.]

---

[1] "Kl. Monatsbl.," 1864, p. 259.
[2] "Ophthalmiatrische Beobachtungen," p. 70.

[7.—MEMBRANOUS OR CROUPOUS CONJUNCTIVITIS.

Though most German authorities, and some others, regard croupous or
membranous conjunctivitis as a distinct disease, differentiating it from purulent and from diphtheritic conjunctivitis, the Editor regards this as extremely
doubtful as far as the purulent form of inflammation is concerned. Saemisch
defines croupous conjunctivitis as that variety of inflammation which is characterized by the formation of a more or less extensive membrane upon the
surface of the palpebral conjunctiva. The intensity of the inflammatory
process varies in different cases: in some the membrane is a very thin, perfectly transparent, thread-like gelatinous layer, while in others it is denser,
thicker, opaque, and yellowish-white in color; and this may sometimes be
removed in one entire membrane from the *surface* of the conjunctiva. When
the membrane is of the latter character, it adheres with tolerable firmness to
the conjunctiva, and cannot be easily wiped off, but must be removed with
the forceps, and always leaves a bleeding surface beneath it. The gelatinous
layer of exudation, on the other hand, is easily removed with a small brush
or bit of muslin, and if this is done carefully, does not leave a bleeding surface beneath it. The lids are reddened and swollen, as in the purulent form
of the disease, and there is, moreover, a more or less abundant flocculent
secretion, which may be purulent from the beginning. The pathological
process here consists mainly in the deposit of an albuminous exudation,
probably fibrine, *upon the surface* of the inflamed conjunctiva, which deposit
rapidly coagulates on exposure to the air, and thus assumes the form of a
membrane. This deposit contains cells which have made their exit from
their mucous membrane, and upon the number of these cells depend more
or less the firmness and density of this membrane, as may be shown by a
microscopic examination. When this membrane is removed, either as a
slough by the processes of nature, or by the forceps in the hand of the surgeon, the mucous membrane lies bare, deprived of its epithelium throughout
a varying extent; but there is no loss of substance of the conjunctiva, and
but very little infiltration of its tissue. When the membrane has been removed, it may form again, or the exudation may assume the purulent form.
It is highly probable that those cases of conjunctivitis in which the formation of a pseudo-membrane is the characteristic feature, are cases in which
the conjunctival inflammation is of the same nature as the purulent form,
but in which the exudation is for a time of a higher organization. Even
those authors who insist most strenuously that membranous conjunctivitis
should be regarded as a distinct disease, admit that in very many cases of
purulent conjunctivitis the exudation at first coagulates very rapidly on exposure to the air, and thus forms a pseudo-membrane over the surface of the
conjunctiva. The tendency to this coagulation of the exudation is very
often seen in cases of catarrhal conjunctivitis, though a continuous pseudo-
membrane, covering the entire surface, is never formed. The *treatment*
of these cases of membranous formation does not differ from that of the
ordinary form of purulent conjunctivitis. It must be locally, strictly antiphlogistic and disinfectant, by the application of iced cloths and the use
of a saturated solution of boracic acid or of a one per cent. solution of carbolic acid for cleansing purposes. As fast as the discharge appears it must
be removed, either with a small brush or with a piece of soft muslin. If the
pseudo-membrane be of the thin gelatinous variety, it may easily be removed; but if it be dense and firm, no attempt at removal should be made,
as it is better to wait until it is cast off as a slough. During the early stage

no caustics should be employed, but when the purulent secretion has become established, the same remedies are indicated as in the purulent form of the disease. The indications for the use of atropine or eserine are the same as before mentioned. Attempts have been made to cut short the tendency to the pseudo-membranous formation by the insufflation of powdered sulphate of quinine, but hitherto without much effect, and the application is often quite painful. Micrococci have sometimes been found in the secretion of croupous conjunctivitis, but not always.—B.]

8.—GRANULAR CONJUNCTIVITIS—TRACHOMA.

It has been already mentioned that in catarrhal and purulent ophthalmia, the papillæ of the conjunctiva are often much swollen and hypertrophied, forming more or less prominent elevations on the palpebral conjunctiva. [Fig. 65.] They appear in the form of bright or bluish-red, velvety, succulent elevations, which have no distinct pedicle, but seem to pass over into the tissue of the conjunctiva. They are ranged in rows, and are, of course, confined to that portion of the conjunctiva which contains papillæ. Commencing at about a line from the free margin of the lid, they extend slightly beyond its tarsal border; their sides are generally flattened, on account of the papillæ being pressed against each other. They are often very conspicuous at the angles of the eye, and assume also a considerable size near the retro-tarsal fold, looking perhaps like large warty excrescences. The name of granular lids is but too often given to this hypertrophied condition of the papillæ, instead of being limited to the true granulations, which are neoplastic formations, and not swollen papillæ. On account of this error, the greatest confusion still reigns upon this subject, a confusion which not only materially affects the diagnosis, but also the treatment of the disease. What has tended still more to foster this misconception of the real nature of granular ophthalmia, is the fact that true granulations are generally accompanied, in the course of their development, by a more or less swollen and hypertrophied condition of the papillæ. If the latter gain a considerable prominence, the granulations may even be hidden by them. Stellwag von Carion[1] applies the term of "*papillary trachoma or granulations*" to these hypertrophied papillæ, and I see no objections to retaining this name, if it be only remembered that these differ altogether in their nature and mode of development from the true granulations.

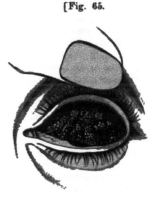

[Fig. 65.

After T. W. Jones.]

Before proceeding to the consideration of granular ophthalmia, I must call special attention to a peculiar vesicular condition of the conjunctiva, which is frequently premonitory of that affection. It is a matter of surprise that this condition, which has been so carefully and elaborately described by several eminent continental writers, more especially Stromeyer, Bendz, and

[1] "Praktische Augenheilkunde," 3d edition, p. 404. 1867.

Warlomont, should have apparently altogether escaped the attention of many English ophthalmic surgeons; indeed, we are principally indebted to two distinguished English military surgeons[1] for giving this subject due prominence in our medical literature, and calling the attention of the profession, and more especially of army medical men, to a condition of the eye which is very important to all who have the charge of large bodies of men, e. g., soldiers, paupers, convicts, etc.

This vesicular condition of the conjunctiva is distinguished by the following symptoms: On everting the lower eyelid, we notice upon it small, round, transparent bodies like little sago grains or herpetic vesicles, which are situated· directly beneath the epithelium. They mostly make their appearance first on the lower eyelid, and may, indeed, remain confined to it, but they generally extend to the upper eyelid, and I have seen a few rare instances in which they encroached considerably upon the ocular conjunctiva. The vesicles are sometimes isolated, and but few in number, being sparsely scattered about the conjunctiva, especially near the outer angle of the eye. In other cases, they are studded thickly over the palpebral conjunctiva and retro-tarsal fold. They cannot be emptied of their contents by pricking, and differ in this form from the sudamina of herpes, and the serous elevation of the epithelium of the conjunctiva, which is occasionally met with in catarrhal ophthalmia; moreover, in the latter condition the vesicles are much larger. The vesicles consist of a stroma of connective tissue containing nucleated cells like lymph corpuscles, with a little fluid. They are surrounded by a delicate layer of condensed connective tissue, which has no proper enveloping membrane, but passes over into the neighboring less condensed tissue. With a fine needle we may often succeed in removing them entire. They seem to be identical in structure with the closed follicles of the intestines, etc. Sometimes these vesicles appear without any change in the conjunctiva. Generally, however, there is an increased vascularity of this membrane with some swelling, more especially at the retro-tarsal fold. The vessels of the conjunctiva are very apparent, and often of a dusky bluish-red color, sending small branches towards the vesicles, which may appear arranged in rows like little transparent beads. But this hyperæmic condition may sometimes mask the presence of the vesicles, especially if they are small and not very numerous, so that they might readily be overlooked by a superficial observer. If the conjunctiva is, however, examined through a magnifying glass, they will be easily distinguished.[2]

If the hyperæmia of the conjunctiva is but slight, these vesicles may exist for a very long time, for months or years, without producing any sensible discomfort or symptoms of inflammation. The patient may either be quite unaware that there is anything the matter with his eyes, or he may only notice a slight sensation of pricking of itching in the eye, the lashes being perhaps somewhat glued together in the morning. There may also be a

<hr>

[1] I refer here to the excellent and very interesting articles on "Military Ophthalmia," by Dr. Frank, late of the Army Medical Department, and by Dr. Marston. Both deserve the careful study of all surgeons. The first appeared in the "Army Medical Blue Book," of 1862; the second in Beale's "Archives of Medicine," No. xi., 1862.

[2] In a recent article on trachoma, in Graefe's Archiv (xv. 1, 129), Dr. Blumberg states that his researches have led him to consider the trachoma granulations as circumscribed hyperplasia of the lymphoid cells, which pre-exist in the normal conjunctiva, and are scattered about in its reticulated connective tissue. In the further progress of the disease, the trachoma follicles undergo fatty and caseous (tubercular) degeneration, and finally cicatricial changes, which lead to a contraction of the surrounding conjunctival tissue. In this last stage, such complications as entropion, trichiasis, pannus, etc., begin to manifest themselves.

tendency to irritability of the eyes during reading or writing, more especially by artificial light. Sometimes, however, even these symptoms are entirely absent.

This vesicular condition of the conjunctiva is due to an enlargement of the closed lymphatic follicles of Krause, which are situated directly beneath the epithelium, and which are not apparent in a normal state of the conjunctiva, but become swollen and enlarged when this membrane is in an irritable condition. Stromeyer[1] called special attention to these vesicular granulations, but supposed that they were pathological products, and did not exist in a healthy conjunctiva. The researches of Krause and Dr. Schmidt, of Berlin, have, however, distinctly proved that they are physiological [structures.—B.], which are not apparent to the naked eye whilst the conjunctiva is in a normal condition, but are apt to become enlarged into these sago-grain vesicles from a proliferation of their contents, more especially of their connective-tissue elements, when there is any chronic irritation of the conjunctiva.

Now it is a very important question, and one which has not at present received a decided and satisfactory answer, whether the true granulations are developed from these vesicular bodies, or rather the follicles of Krause, or whether they are a distinct neoplastic formation, due to a proliferation of the contents of the connective-tissue cells of the conjunctiva. The former view is maintained by several observers of eminence, more especially Bendz and Stromeyer. But one weighty argument against this view is furnished by the fact that true granulations sometimes occur in situations where these follicles are more or less completely wanting, as for instance on the ocular conjunctiva. Wecker strongly advocates the view that the true granulations are neoplastic formations, akin to tubercle, and are due to a proliferation of the contents of the connective-tissue cells, and that they consist of a mass of closely packed nuclei with little or no connective tissue between them. At a later stage, the connective tissue becomes increased in quantity, and forms a semitransparent, gelatinous, grumous mass containing a small quantity of fat. The nuclei diminish in number, and are finally only sparsely scattered amongst the connective tissue. It is an important fact that this gelatinous mass becomes transformed at a later stage into a dense fibrillar tissue, and that the latter shows a great tendency to contraction, thus causing more or less destruction of the true conjunctival tissue. A firm cicatricial tissue is formed, which gives a streaky, tendinous appearance to the inner surface of the lids; the latter gradually become shortened, the retro-tarsal fold almost obliterated, the tarsal cartilages incurved, thus giving rise to trichiasis and entropion.

I have never had the opportunity of distinctly tracing the transformation of the vesicles into true granulations, as they are far less frequently met with in civil than in military practice. Moreover, we cannot watch the patients so constantly and closely. They attend perhaps for some length of time with vesicular granulations, and are then lost sight of. The same difficulty exists with regard to the determination as to whether a given case of acute or chronic granulations has been preceded by a vesicular condition of the lids, for it has been already stated that the latter may exist for a long time without the knowledge of the patient. The definite settlement of these questions will, I think, depend very much upon the observations by our military *confrères*, who enjoy every opportunity of constantly watching the development of the disease from its earliest (vesicular) stage to the latest,

[1] Stromeyer, "Maximen der Kriegsheilkunst." 1861.

and their experience upon these points is, therefore, of the greatest importance.

[According to most recent investigations, granular conjunctivitis is regarded as distinct from the follicular form of inflammation. The granulations consist of elevations, over which the epithelium passes, due to infiltration into the conjunctival stroma, which extends to the papillæ and submucous tissue, thus producing more or less organized new tissue. This infiltration is afterwards partly absorbed and partly changed into dense cicatricial tissue, which in passing through the shrinking stage occasions much trouble. Briefly, the granulation of the conjunctiva is a neoplasm. Nettleship makes a good point in stating that "it should be remembered that these prominences into the conjunctiva are not *granulations* in the pathological sense. Though these vesicular granulations, if neglected, tend to the development of true granular conjunctivitis, the latter is very often developed in cases where the vesicular formation was not present.

Sattler's investigations into the *nature* of *trachoma* are of considerable pathological interest. He regards the trachoma granules as a characteristic and specific product of the trachomatous process. In his opinion, lymph-follicles do not exist in the normal conjunctiva. He has examined the secretion from the different phases of the trachomatous process, and has never found but one form of schizomycetes, the circular micrococcus, which is of somewhat smaller size than the microcaccus of blennorrhœa, but in other respects exactly like the latter. Isolated micrococci occurred but rarely. The division of the micrococci occurred very rapidly, so that sometimes it was impossible to note it. The isolated micrococci never touched each other, and when they occurred in groups, they seemed to be surrounded by a clear sac or envelope. This peculiar arrangement is characteristic of the trachomatous secretion, as it is of the secretion in ophthalmia neonatorum. If trachoma be a localized infecting disease, and these schizomycetes the bearers as well as the producers of the infection, we must not look for the origin and place of development of these organisms in the secretion of the mucous membrane, or even in the epithelium, but in the tissue of the conjunctiva itself. The same micrococci which are met with in the secretion, occur also in the trachoma granules; not only upon the nuclei, but also in the intervening spaces, both isolated and in groups. In the tissue surrounding the trachoma granules are to be seen small groups of nuclei, some filled with, others covered by, micrococci. Another noticeable appearance in many cases of trachoma is a more or less extensive infarction of the lymphatics with elements resembling those of infiltrated connective tissue. In old cases of trachoma, there is often seen a considerable and irregular thickening of the adventitia of the vessels; and in many, an obliteration of their calibre and conversion of the vessel into a solid cord. In very many cases the process eventually is a gradual disappearance of the trachoma granules, ending in atrophy of the conjunctiva. Sattler thinks that it is not improbable that the exciting cause of trachoma is originally from some genital secretion, and this latter from a micrococcus. The reason why in these cases a distant infection occurs so rarely, is that the schizomycetes of conjunctival blennorrhœa soon lose, in a dried condition, their specific properties, or at least the latter become so modified that in the struggle for existence with other schizomycetes and cells, they die. (See the "Klinische Monatsblätter für Augenheilkunde," Beiträge for 1881.)—B.]

But whether we accept or not the theory that vesicular granulations are the first symptoms of granular ophthalmia, and may become developed into true granulations, there cannot be the slightest doubt that they must be regarded as a strongly predisposing cause of the latter. It is, therefore, of great importance that their existence should be detected as early as possible, more especially where a large number of persons are collected together, as in barracks, workhouses, and schools. For this vesicular state of the conjunctiva must be watched with care and anxiety, as it chiefly occurs in individuals living in a confined and vitiated atmosphere, and under faulty sanitary arrangements. Proper hygienic measures should, therefore, be at once adopted, and the patients, if necessary, submitted to treatment; for if these vesicular granulations be allowed to exist unchecked, and such eyes are exposed to the usual irritating influences met with in marches and encampments, as for instance exposure to wind, dust, draughts of cold air, or bright glaring sunlight, an epidemic of granular ophthalmia is but too likely to break out, the ravages and extent of which cannot be foretold. It is an interesting fact that Stromeyer[1] also met with these vesicular granulations amongst many of the domestic animals, more especially pigs, and that they existed in proportion to the dirty condition in which these animals were kept. These observations, moreover, entirely agree with those made amongst human beings, for he found that vesicular granulations occur especially amongst persons inhabiting crowded, close, dirty, and ill-ventilated dwellings.

Dr. Marston, who has enjoyed great opportunities of studying the phenomena of granular ophthalmia, holds similar views. He found[2] vesicular granulations very prevalent amongst the poorer classes in Gozo, especially where there was a large family, who live in wretchedly confined cabins, often with their domestic animals. With regard to the importance of vesicular granulations, as being indicative of a vitiated state of the atmosphere, he says, "So certain do I feel that the prevalence of vesicular disease of the lids is in direct ratio to the amount and degree of defective sanitary arrangements, that I conceive the palpebral conjunctiva offers a delicate test and evidence as to the hygienic conditions of a regiment."[3]

It is, therefore, of much importance to discover the presence of vesicular granulations as early as possible, in order that the hygienic conditions of the ward or sleeping apartment of the patient may be thoroughly examined. Such patients should be placed in large, airy, well-ventilated rooms, which are not exposed to the bright sunlight. Strict orders should also be given that the same sponges, towels, or water are not used for others. Indeed, it is advisable that even healthy persons should always wash in perfectly clean water which has not been already used by others. It is better to separate those affected with vesicular granulations from the healthy, for I think that there can be little doubt that vesicular granulations are contagious, more especially when they are accompanied by conjunctival swelling, and a little muco-purulent discharge. The patients should be in the open air as much as possible, care being taken, however, that they are not exposed to dust, wind, and bright sunlight. Their diet should be nutritious and easily digestible. If they are weak or scrofulous, quinine, steel, cod-liver oil, etc., should be administered. If there is slight conjunctivitis, with a little discharge, or small yellow shreds are formed on the conjunctiva, a weak astringent collyrium (Zinc. sulph. or Plumb. acetat., gr. 1–4 ad f$\mathrecal{z}$j Aq. destill., or Boracis gr. iv–vj ad f$\mathrecal{z}$j) should be used, or the lids may be very

[1] Stromeyer, "Maximen der Kriegsheilkunst," p. 49.
[2] Idem, p. 201.
[3] To the military surgeon I would especially recommend the admirable article on "L'Ophthalmie Militaire en Belgique," by Drs. Warlomont and Testelin, in their French translation of Mackenzie. Also the valuable paper by Dr. Hairion, published in the "Archives Belges de Médecine Militaire," 1848.

lightly touched with a crayon of sulphate of copper, or, still better, of the lapis divinus. Pricking the vesicles with a needle does little or no good. The eye-douche or the atomizer is found to be very beneficial and agreeable to the patient. I have occasionally met with this vesicular condition of the eyelids amongst wealthy persons, in whom the conjunctiva was in a state of irritation from exposure to cold, bright light, etc., and where no faulty hygienic arrangements could be discovered. The affection readily yielded to mild astringents, the eye-douche, and careful guarding the eyes against exposure and too much reading, etc. Vesicular granulation may also be produced by the long-continued use of atropine. I have lately met with some striking examples of this. The disuse of the atropine and the employment of a weak astringent collyrium, soon caused the granulations to disappear; but, on the reapplication of atropine, a fresh crop rapidly sprung up.

[The use of atropine sometimes gives rise to a peculiar irritation and inflammation of the conjunctiva and skin of the lids—*atropine irritation.* The conjunctiva is reddened, and on the lids it becomes thickened, and even granular. The skin is reddened, somewhat shining, though lax, and whilst not losing its wrinkles, it becomes glazed and slightly excoriated. This effect of atropine is commonest in old people. Some persons are very susceptible, and cannot bear even a drop or two without suffering in some degree. Daturine is to be used instead of atropine, unless it be safe to disuse all mydriatics for a few days. An ointment containing some lead and zinc should be applied to the lids, and an astringent zinc lotion to the conjunctiva; in other cases glycerine to the skin is better than anything, and sometimes a bread poultice gives most relief.—*Nettleship.*

The new mydriatic Duboisin has been recommended in these cases, but its use has not yet been extensive enough to enable us to judge whether it is free from the same objection.—B.]

We must now pass on to the consideration of "Granular Ophthalmia." In practice we find that we may distinguish two special forms under which the disease shows itself, viz., the *acute*, which is often accompanied by severe inflammatory symptoms, and the *chronic*, in which these are sometimes but moderate, and occasionally almost entirely absent. Of course, we meet with numerous cases which cannot be properly placed in either category, but show a mixed character. Practically, it is, however, of much consequence to distinguish between the acute and chronic forms, for a great and serious mischief may accrue from a mistaken diagnosis and treatment of a case of severe acute granular ophthalmia.]

ACUTE GRANULAR CONJUNCTIVITIS.

If the attack is severe, there are generally marked inflammatory symptoms; the eyelids are red, swollen, and œdematous, and on opening the eye, we see that there is a good deal of conjunctival and subconjunctival injection. The degree of conjunctival swelling varies; sometimes it is considerable, more especially in the retro-tarsal region, and there may also be marked serous chemosis. The photophobia and lachrymation are often very great, so that the patient is quite unable to open the eye, and directly it is attempted, hot, scalding tears flow over the cheek. There is often severe throbbing pain in and around the eye, and perhaps over the corresponding half of the head. On eversion of the lids, we find that the conjunctiva is vascular and swollen, and that the papillæ are prominent, red, and succulent. On closer inspection (with or without a magnifying glass) we notice, scattered between the papillæ, and perhaps almost hidden by them, numerous small, round, white bodies, like sago grains, which are not, however, confined to the palpebral conjunctiva, but extend to the retro-tarsal fold. If we examine the cornea in such a case by the oblique illumination, and through a magnifying glass, we find that the opacity is composed of a quantity of small elevated gray dots, with the epithelium raised over them. Numerous blood-vessels run over from the conjunctiva to these spots, giving a more or less red tint to the opacity of the cornea. This vascular opacity may involve a considerable portion of the cornea, and is not chiefly confined to the upper half, as is the case in the pannus produced by the friction of granulations or inverted eyelashes of the upper lid upon the surface of the cornea. Sometimes small ulcers appear at the edge of the cornea. When the acute stage has lasted for a few days, the symptoms of irritation begin to diminish. The severe pain, photophobia, and lachrymation decrease, the papillæ at the same time becoming more turgid, vascular, and prominent, thus hiding the granulations; whilst the discharge, which has hitherto been chiefly watery, with perhaps only a few yellow flakes suspended in it, becomes thicker and muco-purulent in character. The intensity of the conjunctival inflammation varies greatly; sometimes it reaches only the catarrhal form, at others it assumes a severe purulent type. The stage of purulent ophthalmia generally lasts for several weeks, and then the symptoms gradually subside; the papillæ diminish in size, and the white sago-grain granulations are then perhaps found to have disappeared, they having in fact been absorbed during the inflammatory state of the conjunctiva. But so favorable a result is not always obtained, for on the decrease of the inflammatory symptoms, and the diminution in the size of the papillæ, the white, and now more prominent, spots may reappear between them, the inflammation having been insufficient for their absorption. If the patient is exposed to any fresh exciting cause, a relapse may occur, and a renewed attack of more or less severe acute ophthalmia may take place. This is, however, far less common than in the chronic form.

Contagion is a very frequent cause, for the discharge from an eye affected with acute granulations is very contagious, more especially during the muco-purulent stage. It does not necessarily reproduce the same affection, but, like purulent or even diphtheritic ophthalmia, may give rise to catarrhal, purulent, or diphtheritic conjunctivitis. [This cannot but be regarded as a questionable statement, so far as diphtheritic conjunctivitis is concerned. If the latter could be produced by contact with the discharge of acute granulations, we must necessarily regard it as a purely local disease, and in no sense connected with any constitutional symptoms of the severity that we are apt to see in that form of conjunctivitis.—B.] This will depend upon local and individual circumstances, and upon the character of any epidemic of conjunctivitis that may be prevailing at the time. Another very fruitful source of acute granulations is defective hygiene; the long-continued use of atropine may also produce them.

The *prognosis* in acute granular conjunctivitis is generally favorable, if the true nature of the affection is recognized at the outset, and a proper course of treatment is adopted. But if the disease is mistaken for a case of purulent ophthalmia, and freely treated by strong caustics, the intensity of the irritation will be greatly increased, and the inflammation may even assume a diphtheritic character. At the best, the salutary inflammation of the conjunctiva will be suppressed, and the absorption of the granulations checked.

The *treatment* must vary with the nature and stage of the affection. We must especially remember that, when the acute symptoms of irritation have subsided, our chief object is to obtain, if possible, the absorption of the granulations by keeping up a certain amount of inflammation of the conjunctiva. The degree of the latter should just suffice to promote this absorption, but should never be allowed to become so considerable as to arrest or retard it.

If there is much photophobia, lachrymation, and ciliary irritation, the greatest care must be taken to avoid all stimulating applications. Atropine drops (gr. ij ad f℥j) should be applied three or four times daily. If they are, however, found to keep up or increase the irritability, they should be at once exchanged for a belladonna collyrium (Ext. bellad. ℨss ad aq. destill. f℥j), which should be applied somewhat more frequently, and in larger quantity. [Solutions of the other mydriatics, such as duboisia, hyoscyamia, and hydrobromate of homatropine, will sometimes be found useful, where atropine increases the irritability.—B.] At the same time, the compound belladonna ointment should be rubbed into the forehead every four or six hours, until a slight papular eruption is produced. If the pain in and around the eye is very severe, of a pulsating, throbbing character, and increases much toward night, a few leeches should be applied to the temple. Cold compresses are also of much benefit in subduing the irritation and relieving the pain. They must, however, be applied with circumspection, and their effect watched. If the cold is disagreeable to the patient, warm poppy or belladonna fomentations should be substituted. If the conjunctiva is much swollen, more especially in the retro-tarsal region, it may be lightly scarified, care being taken to make the incisions very superficial, so that no cicatrices may be left. Much benefit and comfort are often experienced from the application of a bandage, for this keeps the eye quiet, and prevents the irritation caused by the constant movements of the lids.

When the symptoms of irritability subside, and the disease assumes the character of purulent ophthalmia, it must be treated on the same principles as that affection. The same rules as to the choice and mode of application of caustics apply as in the latter disease ; the only difference being, that the cauterization must not be repeated so frequently, as we must remember that it is desirable to maintain a certain degree of inflammation in order to favor the absorption of the granulations. But care must be taken not to commence the use of caustics too early, whilst there is still considerable irritability of the eye, otherwise this will be greatly increased, and infiltrations, or even ulcers, of the cornea may be produced. In those cases in which we are in doubt as to whether the irritability of the eye is not still too great for the application of the nitrate of silver or sulphate of copper, it is always wiser to feel our way with some milder application. For this purpose we may try a weak solution (gr. vi–x ad f℥j) of [alum—B.], a little of which should be painted over the granulations with a brush, and at once washed off with warm water ; and if this is well borne, and causes a subsidence of the inflammatory symptoms, we may, in the course of a day or two, pass over to the use of the stronger caustics. Von Graefe[1] strongly recommends chlorine water for the purpose of paving the way for the use of stronger caustics in acute granulations.

When the crayon of nitrate of silver and potash is applied, it should be at once neutralized by the application of salt and water. As a rule, the cauterization should not be repeated more frequently than every forty-eight hours. Great care must be taken if any ulcers of the cornea exist, for they may be easily aggravated by too free a use of the nitrate of silver. If there is a great deal of irritation, I often apply atropine drops in the interval of the cauterization. When the swelling of the conjunctiva has considerably subsided, and the purulent discharge diminished, the sulphate of copper in substance, or a collyrium of [sulphate of zinc (gr. v–x ad f℥j)—B.] may be employed with advantage. If it is found that, together with the diminution of the inflammation and the size of the papillæ, the granulations assume a more prominent character and increase in size and number, this tendency to a neoplastic formation must be checked at once, and their absorption hastened, by exciting a more considerable amount of inflammation by means of a freer use of some caustic, especially the sulphate of copper, which possesses the great advantage of increasing the inflammation without giving rise to thick firm eschars.

CHRONIC GRANULATIONS.

[Syn. Granular lids, Trachoma, Chronic granular conjunctivitis.—B.]
Instead of the very pronounced symptoms of irritation and inflammation which are met with in acute granular conjunctivitis, the inflammation accompanying the chronic form is often very slight, and may, indeed, be almost absent at the commencement of the affection; so that, in fact, persons may be suffering from chronic granulations without being aware that there is anything particular the matter with their eyes; the eyelids being only a little glued together in the morning, or there being perhaps a slight feeling of roughness under the eyelids. At the same time, the upper lid may hang down somewhat, its natural folds being more or less obliterated, and the palpebral aperture consequently narrowed. During all this time the conjunctival inflammation may be almost absent; indeed, it is never very prominent, or in proportion to the amount of the granulations. On eversion of the lids, we at once notice the presence of the granulations in the form of small grayish-white bodies, like tapioca grains, more especially at the retro-tarsal fold, and in the vicinity of the angles of the eye. They may also appear on the palpebral conjunctiva, which is somewhat injected and swollen. In this situation, however, their size and number are less than at the retro-tarsal fold. These may be termed "simple granulations," or, according to Stellwag, "granular trachoma." [These have been called frog-spawn granulations, from their resemblance to the spawn of frogs.—B.] Generally, however, this condition is soon followed by inflammatory symptoms. The conjunctiva becomes vascular, thickened, and swollen, and the papillæ hypertrophied and prominent, having the granulations scattered between them. Here, therefore, we have true granulations existing side by side with the swollen papillæ, and hence Stellwag calls this form "mixed granulations." The lids are more or less pulpy, the conjunctiva red and swollen, especially in the retro-tarsal region, and there is, perhaps, some chemosis round the cornea. The discharge, which was at first thin and watery, with only a few yellow flakes suspended in it, becomes thicker, more copious, and of a muco-purulent character. The eyes are very irritable, and the patient experiences a sensation as of grit or sand in them, especially under the upper lid, and is unable to expose them to wind, bright glare, dust, or to long-continued work, without their becoming very red, watery, and inflamed.

But all these symptoms vary considerably in intensity, according to the degree of the accompanying conjunctival inflammation. Sometimes this assumes a mild catarrhal form; in other cases it is more severe and of a purulent type. The course of the disease is often extremely protracted, extending over many months, or even years. A source of danger, as well as of annoyance and discomfort, is the tendency to relapses, the intensity of which also varies. Thus a mild attack of chronic mixed granulations may be nearly cured when, from an exposure to some irritating cause, a relapse occurs, accompanied, perhaps, by a more severe form of conjunctivitis than the original one, and a fresh crop of granulations appears before the former ones have been absorbed. These inflammatory symptoms are, however, rather due to a renewed swelling of the papillæ than to a new formation of granulations. Sometimes these relapses are accompanied by considerable infiltrations of the cornea. Such relapses may occur again and again, leaving the eye in a worse condition each time, and gradually giving rise to various serious complications, such as pannus, trichiasis, entropion, etc.

If the attack is severe, and the crop of granulations very considerable, the infiltration but too often extends from the surface to the substance of the conjunctiva. The granulations then become more velvety, red, prominent, and diffused in appearance (hence the "diffuse trachoma" of Stellwag), and are often divided by deep chinks. They are, therefore, less distinguishable from the papillæ, especially as the latter often assume a brownish-red color, and their epithelial layer becomes somewhat thickened.

If the development of the granulations cannot be checked, and they extend deeply into the stroma of the conjunctiva, the latter often contracts, atrophies, and becomes gradually changed into a fibrous cicatricial tissue. These changes may even extend to the tarsus, and the cicatrices lend a peculiar glistening or tendinous appearance to the surface of the conjunctiva. We then see the latter occupied by narrow tendinous streaks, the longest and most marked generally running parallel to, and about one line from, the edge of the lid. Other tendinous streaks extend in a reticulated manner towards the retro-tarsal fold. But if the atrophy of the conjunctiva and tarsus is very considerable, the bloodvessels gradually become obliterated, and the surface of the conjunctiva then assumes a pale, waxy, uniformly tendinous apppearance; the papillæ, follicles, and finally the Meibomian glands becoming destroyed. It is important to remember that too free a use of caustics (especially the nitrate of silver in substance or in strong solution) will destroy the delicate structure of the conjunctiva, and produce more or less extensive cicatrices.

These changes often extend to the retro-tarsal fold, which becomes contracted and tendinous, so that its free border is shortened and rounded. It no longer springs into folds at the point where it is reflected from the lid on to the eyeball, but, on account of this shortening, it passes almost straight on, so that the fold or cul-de-sac which should exist at this point is obliterated. This condition has been termed symblepharon posterius. If it is very considerable, the lids cannot be completely closed, and thus a certain degree of lagophthalmos may be produced.

These changes in the conjunctiva are of course accompanied by an alteration and diminution in its normal secretions, so that its surface becomes dry, rough, and scaly. This dryness (xerophthalmia) is often increased by the narrowing or even obliteration of the ducts of the lachrymal gland by the inflammation of this portion of the conjunctiva.

On account of the atrophy and contraction of the conjunctiva and tarsus,[1] latter becomes shortened and incurved. If this be but slight, it may ice an inversion of the eyelashes (trichiasis), which now sweep and t the surface of the cornea. This inversion may be confined to of the lashes, or extend to the whole row. If the contraction of

---

reliable investigations having shown that there are no cartilage cells in the ⁴l it, but that the latter consist mainly of a very dense connective-tissue rm tarsal cartilage is a misnomer.—B.]

the tarsus is considerable, not only the eyelashes, but the free edge of the lid will be rolled in, and thus an entropion will be produced. The constant friction of the lashes and the edge of the eyelid against the cornea irritates the latter, and soon gives rise to superficial vascular keratitis (pannus). This pannus may be termed "traumatic" (Arlt), being produced by the friction of the inverted lashes, or of prominent granulations or papillæ, etc., in contradistinction to the pannus which is due to an extension of the granulations on to the cornea. [The term "mechanical" would be better than "traumatic," as pointing more surely to the cause.—B.] The differential diagnosis between these two forms is generally not difficult. In the latter, we can trace the extension of the disease from the ocular conjunctiva on to the cornea. Small, round, elevated, gray infiltrations are formed on its surface just beneath the epithelium, and extend over a considerable portion or even the whole of the cornea. Between these little nodules, bloodvessels appear in more or less considerable number. These infiltrations often leave behind them depressions or small ulcers on the surface of the cornea. The traumatic pannus almost always commences at the upper portion of the cornea, extending from the periphery. This is due to the fact, that the granulations are generally more prominent, and trichiasis is more frequent in the upper lid than in the lower. The pannus frequently remains confined to the upper portion of the cornea, the lower continuing transparent. Besides the incurvation of the edges of the lids and consequent entropion, we often find that the palpebral aperture becomes much shortened (blepharophimosis) in chronic granulations. The pressure thus exerted on the eyeball increases any existing pannus, and greatly retards the cure of the granulations.

Chronic granulations occur most frequently in adults, and are but seldom met with in children or the very aged. Both eyes generally become affected either at the outset or after a time. It has been maintained by some ophthalmic surgeons of eminence (more especially Arlt), that the disease is often due to constitutional causes, particularly scrofula. This does not, however, appear to be the case, although it must be conceded, that it is frequently met with in weakly, cachectic, and scrofulous individuals. But ill-health is, I think, rather the effect than the cause, for the very protracted course of the disease is sure to tell more or less severely upon the health and spirits of the patient.

Defective hygiene and contagion are also the chief causes of chronic granulations. The muco-purulent discharge is very contagious, and may produce a similar affection, or it may cause catarrhal, purulent, or even diphtheritic conjunctivitis,[1] just as, conversely, these diseases may produce granular lids.

It is probable that, as in purulent conjunctivitis, the disease may also be propagated by the air, more especially if it is accompanied by severe purulent discharge, and the cases are crowded together in small, close, ill-ventilated rooms. The disease may occur epidemically and endemically. It spreads rapidly amongst the inhabitants of closely crowded dwellings, such as barracks and workhouses. It is very prevalent amongst certain nationalities, where the people are crowded together for a length of time in small dirty cabins, filled, perhaps, with smoke and ammoniacal exhalations. Thus it is very common amongst the poorer Irish, and also amongst the Russian peasants (Weeker). [The prevalence of this disease among certain races is very marked. Thus, in addition to the Irish and Russian peasants, it is

[1 This statement has been questioned in a previous paragraph.—B.]

very common among the Jews and certain Oriental races. On the contrary,
it is exceedingly rare among the negroes of the United States.—B.]

The *prognosis* of chronic granular conjunctivitis may be favorable, if the
granulations have been but limited in number, and the patient has been
treated from the outset. It must, however, be always remembered that the
course of the disease, even in the most favorable cases, is apt to be very protracted. This will be more especially the case, if the granulations have
appeared in considerable quantity; if they have invaded the stroma of the
conjunctiva, and if there is a tendency to relapses. For then serious complications, such as trichiasis, entropion, and pannus, are likely to occur, and
will not only aggravate the symptoms, but greatly retard the cure.

In the *treatment* of this disease, our first care must be to place the patients
under the most favorable sanitary conditions. They should take a good deal
of out-door exercise, their eyes being protected against wind, dust, and bright
light by blue glasses. They should be warned not to expose themselves to
any irritating causes, as, for instance, tobacco smoke. I have often known
the disease aggravated and kept up by the patient spending much time in a
room filled with tobacco smoke. For this reason no smoking should be
allowed, except in the open air, and then only to a limited extent. The
general health must also be attended to. Not only may the patient be
naturally weak and feeble, but the severity and protracted course of the disease are but too likely to affect the health, and at the same time to exert a
most depressing influence upon the mind. The diet should be nutritious,
and easily digestible, and malt liquor and wine will generally be very beneficial. If the patient is scrofulous, or weak and feeble, cod-liver oil, steel,
and quinine should be freely given, and every care taken to invigorate the
constitution as much as possible by open air exercise, sea-bathing, or even a
voyage.

In our local treatment we must be chiefly influenced by the fact, that
the maintenance of a certain degree of inflammation of the conjunctiva is
necessary and desirable, in order to produce and hasten the absorption of the
granulations. Our chief efforts must, therefore, be directed to maintain the
requisite degree of inflammation, and so to balance it that it shall not on
the one hand be too considerable, nor on the other too slight for promoting
the absorption.

The greatest stress must be laid upon the fact, as Arlt and Stromeyer
remind us, that the purpose of the cauterization is *not* that of chemically
destroying the granulations, for this would lead to great and lasting injury
of the conjunctiva from the destruction of its secreting organs, and the formation of dense cicatrices; but its object is to maintain a certain degree of
hyperæmia and inflammation of the conjunctiva, in order to hasten the
absorption of the granulations. The nature and strength of the caustic
must vary with the effect we desire to produce. If there is much swelling of
the conjunctiva and papillæ, together with a thick, copious, muco-purulent
discharge, the crayon of nitrate of silver and potash should be applied, its
effect being at once neutralized by the solution of salt and water. The
cauterization may be repeated every forty-eight hours. If the patient cannot
be seen sufficiently frequently for this, he should use a collyrium of nitrate
of silver (gr. ij–iv ad f 3j), or of sulphate of copper of the same strength, two
or three times daily. In these cases we may also first try the effect of a
collyrium of acetate of lead, gr. ij–iv ad f 3j, or the chlorine water, in order
to see if the conjunctiva will bear the nitrate of silver. The use of very
strong solutions of nitrate of silver (gr. x–xx ad f 3j) are not judicious, as
they are but too likely to destroy the granulations, and with them the normal

structure of the conjunctiva, instead of simply favoring their absorption. I think the crayon of nitrate of silver or sulphate of copper is always to be preferred to the use of collyria, as we can regulate and limit the effect of the cauterization according to our wish, confining it, if necessary, chiefly or entirely to certain portions of the conjunctiva. If there is considerable swelling of the conjunctiva, especially at the retro-tarsal fold, superficial scarification may be employed with much advantage. After the cauterization, cold compresses should always be applied to the eyelids, in order to diminish the inflammatory reaction; or the cold douche or atomizer may be employed. If the conjunctivitis is so slight as not to produce the absorption of the granulations, but rather to encourage their development, it will be necessary to increase the hyperæmia and inflammatory swelling of the conjunctiva. The repeated application of sulphate of copper in substance is very effectual for this purpose. The same effect may also be produced by the application of warm compresses over the eyelids. Von Graefe[1] has found this treatment very successful, especially in those cases in which the granulations tend to extend deeply into the conjunctiva, and in which there is not a sufficient degree of hyperæmia and swelling of this membrane. These warm compresses should, however, only be applied for a limited period, otherwise they may produce too considerable an inflammation and too great an irritability of the eye. [A useful application in allaying irritation and photophobia may sometimes be found in the balsam of copaiba, applied to the external surface of the lids and forehead.—B.]

In treating chronic granulations, it will be necessary occasionally to change the caustic, as it loses its effect after a time, from the conjunctiva becoming accustomed to it. Thus alum, acetate of lead, or tannin, may be substituted with advantage for the nitrate of silver and sulphate of copper. Some patients are more benefited when the astringent or caustic is applied in the form of an ointment than of a collyrium. If it is, therefore, found in obstinate cases of chronic granulations or chronic ophthalmia that the various collyria are doing but little good, an ointment must be substituted for them, containing sulphate of copper, nitrate of silver, or acetate of lead. The strength of the ointment must vary with the severity of the case, but as a rule it is best to employ it rather weak at first, for fear of setting up too much irritation. The following proportions will be found most generally useful: 1. Cupri sulph. gr. j–iv ad Axung. ℥j. 2. Argent. nitrat. gr. ss–iij ad ℥j. 3. Plumb. acet. gr. iv–xij ad ℥j. The glycerine plasma may be substituted for the lard. A small portion (about the size of a split pea) of the ointment should be placed with a probe or the end of a quill on the inner side of the lower lid; the eye is then to be closed and the lids rubbed over the globe, so that the ointment may come in contact with the whole conjunctival surface. [An application which is sometimes found useful is an ointment made of ten grains of the red precipitate of mercury to the drachm of vaseline. Care should be taken that the mercury is thoroughly rubbed up before incorporation with the vaseline.—B.] Great care must be taken never to order any preparation of the salts of lead if there is any abrasion of the epithelium of the cornea or any ulcer of the latter, as it will produce an indelible lead stain. Hairion[2] strongly recommends the use of tannin in cases of chronic ophthalmia, etc. etc. He employs it in two forms, as a collyrium, and as a mucilage. The former contains about twelve grains of tannin to f℥j of distilled water, and is chiefly indicated in cases of catarrhal ophthalmia. The mucilage is much stronger, and is employed in chronic granulations, chronic

[1] "A. f. O.," vi. 2, 147.   [2] French Translation of Mackenzie, i. p. 753.

ophthalmia, pannus, etc. It is to be prepared in the following manner:
One part of tannin is to be dissolved in four parts of water, and this solution
strained through fine muslin; then two parts of gum arabic are added,
and the whole carefully mixed and worked up into mucilage. A small
quantity is to be applied with a fine camel's-hair brush to the conjunctiva
of the lower lid. In chronic granulations, etc., and chronic ophthalmia,
much benefit is often derived from the application of astringents and caustics
to the external surface of the lids. Thus a solution of nitrate of silver (gr.
iv–viij ad f $\mathfrak{z}$j) may be painted over the external surface of the upper lid, or
a compress of lint dipped in it and laid over the closed lids. Care must,
however, be taken that the solution is not too strong, or repeated too often,
otherwise it may easily stain the skin. Compresses soaked in either of the
following lotions and laid over the closed lids will also be found very bene-
ficial: 1. Liq. plumb. diacet. f $\mathfrak{z}$j; aq. dest. f $\mathfrak{z}$iv. 2. Liq. plumb. diacet. f $\mathfrak{z}$j;
boracis, $\mathfrak{Z}$ij; aq. amygdal. amar. (Prussian Pharmacopœia) f $\mathfrak{z}$ss; aq. dest. f $\mathfrak{z}$vj.
These compresses are to be changed every three or four minutes, and con-
tinued for twenty to thirty minutes, this being repeated two or three times
daily. In some cases the acetate of lead should be rubbed in (finely powdered) between the granulations. This treatment, which was first adopted
by Buys,[1] has been practised with great success, especially in Belgium. I
have employed it with much benefit in those cases in which, together with
but a slight secretion and lachrymation, the granulations are prominent
and fleshy, being arranged in rows, with deep furrows or chinks between
them. Finely powdered acetate of lead should be freely rubbed into these
furrows until they are quite filled up. The effect of this is, so to speak, to
choke the granulations, their vitality is impaired, and they gradually dwindle
down in size and disappear. After the application, the conjunctiva looks
marbled or tatooed of a red and white color, the chinks are filled up, and it
soon becomes smooth and even. An important fact in connection with this
treatment is, that the discharge is now no longer contagious; at least in
Belgium it is always considered, when the acetate of lead has been rubbed
in, that the patients may go with impunity amongst healthy persons; so that
soldiers affected with granular lids need no longer be confined and separated
from the others, but may, if they are able, resume their duties without
danger of spreading the disease. The acetate of lead is best applied in the
following manner: The eyelids having been thoroughly everted and the
retro-tarsal fold brought well into view, a small portion of very finely powdered acetate of lead is then taken up in a small curette and dusted over
the granulations, being well rubbed into the chinks, so as to fill them up.
The watery discharge from the conjunctiva changes the powder into a thin
plasma, which runs through and fills up the furrows between the granulations. When it has been applied to every portion of the granular conjunctiva, a small stream of cold water, either from a sponge or an India-rubber
ball syringe, should be made to play upon the conjunctiva, in order to wash
away any superfluous quantity of the powder, which comes away in small
white flakes. Both eyelids may be everted at the same time, so as to fold
over and protect the cornea, the powder being rubbed over both eyelids,
and the stream of water applied before they are replaced. But if the simultaneous eversion of both lids is difficult, or the patient very restless and
unruly, it is better to evert one lid at a time. It is best to commence with
the lower lid, for if the lead be applied first to the upper, the lower becomes
reddened and bathed in tears, so that it will not only be difficult to see the

[1] French Translation of Mackenzie's Treatise, i. 748.

chinks, but the powder will be readily washed away by the tears; whereas the conjunctiva of the upper lid, from its greater expanse, can be more readily dried, and the tears are hence of less inconvenience.

Directly after the application, there is an increased flow of tears, the ocular conjunctiva becomes injected, and this is accompanied perhaps by considerable irritation, heat, and smarting in the eye, but these symptoms will soon yield to the application of cold compresses. In about half an hour, the lid should be everted and the conjunctiva again washed by a stream of water, in order that any remains of the lead may be removed. The conjunctiva will now be more smooth and even, the chinks between the granulations being filled up and obliterated by the powder. If the application has been insufficient or too superficial, the granulations will reappear after a time, and increase in size and prominence, rendering a fresh application of the remedy necessary. If the acetate of lead is carefully applied and the surplus well washed away, I cannot say that I have ever seen any disadvantage arise from its employment, nor have I found that it roughens the lids and thus irritates the surface of the cornea. The best mode of applying the solution of the acetate of lead is to evert the lids, and after drying the conjunctiva with a piece of linen, to apply it with a small brush to the granulations, this being neutralised after a few seconds with tepid water. The strength of the solution should vary from six to ten or twenty grains to the fluidounce, according to the condition of the conjunctiva, and it should be applied every day or every other day.

I must strongly object to the application of undiluted liquor potassæ to the granulations, as this not only more or less destroys the stroma of the conjunctiva, but gives rise to very considerable cicatrices, leading to entropion, etc.

Should any ulcers of the cornea exist, the treatment of the conjunctivitis by caustics must be continued, but atropine should be applied in the intervals. The application of a firm compress bandage often acts very advantageously in checking the growth of the granulations, and hastening their absorption; but other local remedies must be at the same time applied. It has even been suggested to keep up a considerable degree of compression by ivory plates adjusted to the lids.[1]

[Mr. Bader speaks highly of the application of sulphate of quinine to the conjunctiva in cases of granular lids accompanied by pannus. About as much as would go on the point of a penknife is to be applied twice daily, with a camel's-hair brush, to the inside of the lower lid.[2] Nagel[3] has also found collyria of quinine beneficial in chronic conjunctivitis and suppurative keratitis. This is probably due to the influence which quinine exerts in checking the amœboid movements and migrations of the white-blood corpuscles, and in restraining the dilatation of the bloodvessels, as shown by Binz.—B.]

The treatment of the pannus must vary according to its cause, its degree, and length of existence. If it be dependent upon the friction of inverted lashes, prominent granulations or papillæ, or upon entropion, these affections must be treated, and when they are cured, the pannus will soon disappear; but if the granular lids and the pannus have become very chronic, they may set an obstinate defiance to the most varied treatment. Caustics and stimulant applications of every kind may be tried, and yet the disease prove intractable. In some cases, in which the pannus was not too dense and vas-

[1] *Vide* Dr. Stokes' paper on this subject. "Dub. Quart. Journal Med. Sci.," xli. 88. [2 "Lancet," Oct. 28, 1871.—B.] [3 "Kl. Monatsbl.," 1869, p. 480.—B.]

cular, I have found considerable benefit from a collyrium composed of one part of oil of turpentine to two or four parts of olive oil. A drop of it should be applied once or twice daily to the inside of the lid. This collyrium was, I believe, first recommended by Donders. If, on the disappearance of the pannus, we find the curvature of the cornea considerably altered, or a central opacity remaining, it may be necessary to make an artificial pupil either by an iridectomy or an iridodesis. If the palpebral aperture is much shortened, and the eyelids thus press on the eyeball, the outer canthus should be divided with a pair of scissors, so as to widen the opening of the lids and relieve the pressure. (Vide operation of Canthoplasty.)

Von Graefe[1] has found great benefit from chlorine water in cases of even severe complete pannus. He especially mentions two cases in which the pannus was so advanced that the patients could only distinguish light from dark, and were quite unable to count fingers. In both, not only had various caustics, such as nitrate of silver, sulphate of copper, acetate of lead, been applied for many months without avail, but syndectomy had been performed, and in one, inoculation, without any beneficial result. After using the chlorine water for six or eight weeks, they were both so much improved as to be able to find their way about tolerably well. In other, less severe, cases of pannus, he has also experienced much benefit from its use. The chlorine water is either to be used as a collyrium and dropped into the eye once or twice daily, or it is to be lightly brushed over the everted conjunctiva.

For very inveterate cases of pannus, more especially if it only involves a portion of the cornea, syndectomy may be tried. This operation, which was first introduced by Dr. Furnari,[2] proves useful in cases of inveterate pannus, in which a portion of the cornea is clear, so that it would not be safe to perform inoculation, or, if the latter is for some reason inapplicable, in cases of complete pannus. The object of the operation is to cut off the supply of blood from the cornea by a division and partial removal, not only of the conjunctival, but also of the subconjunctival vessels. It is a less dangerous and troublesome proceeding than inoculation. It must, however, be also admitted that it is not always successful, the cases improving perhaps somewhat at first, and then a relapse takes place.

[Scarification of the large superficial vessels of the cornea, frequently repeated, has been advised in obstinate cases of pannus, and in some instances has proved efficacious. It acts probably in the same way as peritomy.—B.]

Syndectomy is to be performed in the following manner: The patient should be placed thoroughly under the influence of an anæsthetic, as the operation is very painful and protracted, and the eyelids should be kept apart by the stop speculum. The operator then seizes with a pair of forceps a portion of the conjunctiva and subconjunctival tissue, near the cornea, so as to fix the eye steadily. He next with a pair of curved scissors makes a circular incision through the conjunctiva, all round the cornea, and about an eighth of an inch from the edge of the latter, and parallel to it. This circular band is then dissected off, and excised close to the edge of the cornea, so that a wide circle of conjunctiva may be removed all round the cornea. For the purpose of more easily rotating the eye, two small portions of conjunctiva should be left standing near the cornea until the operation is completely finished, when they are to be snipped off. A circular portion of the subcon-

[1] "A. f. O.," x. 2, 198.

[2] "Gazette Médicale," 1862, No. 4, etc.; vide also an article upon the subject by Mr. Bader, "Roy. Lond. Ophth. Hosp. Reports," iv. 22. This operation has received various names; at one time it was termed Circumcision of the Cornea. It is now generally called either Syndectomy or Peritomy.

junctival tissue, corresponding to the wound in the conjunctiva, is next to be removed, quite close to the sclerotic, so as to bare the latter completely; if small portions of subconjunctival tissue remain adhering to it, they may be scraped off with the edge of a cataract or iridectomy knife. Some of the larger vessels upon the cornea may also be divided near its edge. Dr. Furnari advises that the exposed sclerotic should be cauterized with nitrate of silver. This is, however, a most dangerous proceeding, as it is but too likely to produce inflammation and sloughing of the sclerotic and cornea. Cold compresses should be applied until the symptoms of inflammatory reaction have subsided. These are, as a rule, but moderate, and the photophobia, pain, and lachrymation generally disappear in about forty-eight or sixty hours. It is wise to keep the patients in the hospital for a few days, so that, if severe inflammatory symptoms should supervene, they may be treated at once.

In those cases of inveterate pannus in which the latter is thick, very vascular, and covers the whole of the cornea, and in which, on account of the cicatricial changes in the conjunctiva, it is impossible to excite sufficient hyperæmia and swelling of the conjunctiva for the absorption of the granulations, it may be necessary to produce a purulent inflammation of the conjunctiva by the inoculation of pus, in order that the granulations may, if possible, be absorbed and the cornea cleared during the progress of the inflammation. This proceeding, which was first advocated by Piringer, has long been extensively and successfully practised in Belgium, where granulations are very common amongst the soldiers. In England it has also been very largely and successfully employed at the Royal London Ophthalmic Hospital, Moorfields, where Mr. Bader first introduced it. I have seen many admirable cures produced by it, and patients restored to the enjoyment of excellent sight (some being able to read No. 1 of Jaeger) who had been suffering from so dense a pannus that they were unable even to count fingers. In many of these cases most other remedies had been tried without avail. The chief danger is, of course, that the purulent inflammation which is induced should be so severe as to produce suppuration of the cornea and loss of the eye. But it is surprising what a degree of inflammation a very vascular and completely opaque cornea will bear with impunity, and be, perhaps, finally restored to almost normal transparency. It may be laid down as a rule, that the more vascular the cornea, the less danger is there of its sloughing, for the numerous bloodvessels on its surface will maintain its vitality during the purulent inflammation. Inoculation is, therefore, much less safe where the vascularity of the cornea is but moderate, and is inadmissible if a portion of it remains transparent. Another danger of inoculation is, that the matter, instead of setting up purulent ophthalmia, may give rise to diphtheritic conjunctivitis. Happily this danger is but very slight in England, but we have seen that in certain parts of the continent, more especially in Berlin, this affection is but of too common occurrence, and that the mild forms of conjunctivitis often produce the most virulent form of diphtheritic conjunctivitis. For this reason, it is there hardly safe to inoculate a case of pannus with even the mildest purulent matter, for we have no ... t it may not give rise to diphtheritis. Von Graefe has called ... ion to this fact, and has been obliged, in consideration of so great a risk, to abandon almost entirely the employment of inoculation in the treatment of pannus. In England, the occurrence of diphtheritis is ex- ... and I have not seen a single case of inoculation in which it

Many surgeons are still very much afraid of inoculation, but, I think, when we consider how utterly hopeless most cases of severe chronic pannus are, that we are justified in strongly recommending the patient to run some slight degree of risk for the chance of obtaining a useful amount of sight. I do not, therefore, hesitate to employ it in cases of inveterate, complete, vascular pannus, in which the other remedies have been tried without avail, for in such we must admit that it is our last resource, and that no other chance of restoring the sight remains.

Care must, however, be taken in the choice of the purulent matter, and in regulating its strength according to the exigencies of the case. The more dense and vascular the pannus, the stronger may the matter be. The best and safest is that obtained from the eyes of an infant suffering from purulent ophthalmia, more especially if the disease is in its decline, and no affection of the cornea, or only a very slight one, exists. Yellow pus is more active and powerful than the whitish discharge, as is also that taken from the eye during the acute stage of the disease.

The matter from an eye suffering from inoculation is stronger than that from an infant, as its activity appears to be increased by the inoculation. Gonorrhœal matter is far too strong and dangerous. Even in the worst cases, I prefer the whitish discharge from an infant. Mr. Lawson, who has had very great experience in this subject of inoculation, has also very justly pointed out[1] that, in using gonorrhœal matter, there is the risk of its being tainted by the syphilitic virus through a chancre perhaps existing in the urethra.

The mode of inoculation is as follows: A drop of pus from the eye of an infant affected with purulent conjunctivitis is to be placed with the tip of the finger (or a camel's-hair brush) on the inside of the lower eyelid, and left there. Within twenty-four hours of the inoculation, the eyelids generally begin to swell and become œdematous, often to a very considerable degree; this is accompanied by more or less irritability of the eye, photophobia, and lachrymation. In the course of three or four days, all the symptoms of an acute purulent conjunctivitis set in, together with a copious, thick, creamy discharge. The disease mostly runs its course in from three to four weeks, by the end of which time the cornea is generally much more clear, and the granulations diminished. This improvement, however, continues to increase for many weeks, or even months. No treatment is to be adopted for checking the course of the inflammation. After the second or third day, the patient may be permitted to wipe away the discharge with a sponge or a bit of linen, so as to cleanse the eye. But, however severe the inflammation may be, it must be allowed to run its course unchecked by the use of astringent or caustic lotions.

One eye should be inoculated at a time, the other being carefully closed by the hermetic collodion compress. This must be more especially done if this eye is sound. Indeed, in such a case, it may be a question whether the diseased eye should be inoculated at all, for fear that, through any mischance or carelessness, the healthy eye should become affected. In deciding this point, we must be chiefly guided by individual considerations. The compress should be removed every day, in order that the eye may be washed and cleansed, during which process, of course, the greatest care must be taken that no pus gets into it.

A very interesting and important fact has been pointed out by Mr. Lawson,[2] viz., that a preliminary syndectomy appears to render the inoculation a safer proceeding, for, the conjunctiva and subconjunctival tissue having

---

[1] "Roy. Lond. Ophth. Hosp. Reports," iv. p. 188.   [2] Ibid., p. 186.

been removed from around the cornea, the intensity of the inflammation at this point is greatly diminished, and the cornea less apt to suffer. In cases, therefore, in which the pannus is not very vascular, or does not involve the whole of the cornea, and where, therefore, inoculation might prove dangerous, it would be advisable to precede it by a syndectomy, and then, when the eye has quite recovered from this, to employ inoculation.

[Mention should here be made of those cases of obstinate pannus in which iritis has supervened. This is usually of the serous form, and exerts an influence upon the continuance of the pannus. A small iridectomy in these cases will sometimes exert a curative effect upon both diseases where other means have failed.—B.]

9.—PHLYCTENULAR [CONJUNCTIVITIS. HERPES CONJUNCTIVÆ. PUSTULAR CONJUNCTIVITIS.—B.]

The disease is generally ushered in by a feeling of heat and itching in the eyelids, and a watery and irritable condition of the eye. These symptoms of irritation increase until there may be a very considerable amount of photophobia, lachrymation, and pain in and around the eye (ciliary neuralgia). The latter, however, is never so severe when the phlyctenulæ are confined to the conjunctiva, as when they also invade the cornea. There is also more or less conjunctival and subconjunctival injection, the degree and extent of which vary with the intensity and extent of the disease. Sometimes the injection is only partial and confined to a certain portion of the ocular conjunctiva. We then notice a triangular, fan-like bundle of conjunctival vessels, extending from the retro-tarsal region towards the edge of the cornea. The base of the triangle is turned towards the palpebræ, and the apex is at the cornea. Beneath the conjunctival injection is observed a corresponding rosy zone of subconjunctival vessels. At this spot there is also generally a slight œdematous swelling of the conjunctiva (serous chemosis). At the apex of the triangle of vessels, one or more small herpetic vesicles or pustules make their appearance, which are semitransparent, or of a yellowish-white color, and about the size of a small millet-seed. They are especially apt to occur at the outer side of the cornea, and are often symmetrical, being formed at the outer side of each eye. The epithelium which covers the phlyctenula is soon shed, leaving a small excoriation or ulcer, which generally dwindles down and becomes completely absorbed. In other cases, the ulcer increases somewhat in size and depth, and its contents become yellow and opaque; but after a time it is covered again by epithelium, and its contents then gradually undergo absorption. With the appearance of the phlyctenula, the symptoms of irritation generally diminish, especially when the epithelium is shed and the contents of the vesicle escape. As the latter is being absorbed the vascularity decreases, but at the same time the conjunctiva may become somewhat swollen, especially in the retro-tarsal region, and this is accompanied by a muco-purulent discharge; so that we have in fact a combination of catarrhal and phlyctenular conjunctivitis. The affection may, however, have this mixed character from the outset.

If the phlyctenulæ are not confined to one portion of the ocular conjunctiva, but are scattered about on various parts of it, in perhaps considerable numbers, the vascularity is diffuse and well marked. The symptoms of irritation are more pronounced, and the ciliary neuralgia, lachrymation, and photophobia greater. The latter, indeed, is sometimes excessive in phlyctenular conjunctivitis, more especially in scrofulous children, and is

en quite disproportionate to the amount of the vesicles. The p
quently form at the edge of the cornea, surrounding it like a ro
they occur at the limbus conjunctivæ, lying partly on the cornea
the conjunctiva. Very often the affection appears simultaneo
junctiva and the cornea. The pustules sometimes increase c
size and depth, the inflammation extending to the subconjunc
iscleritis), and even perhaps to the superficial layers of th
e corresponding portion of the conjunctiva and subconjunctiva
n often very vascular, and considerably thickened and swollen,
stules appear situated upon a prominent base. The vascularity
the subconjunctival tissue) is of a peculiar dusky, bluish-red ti
very easily recognized. This form is extremely protracted and
relapses, so that many months may pass before it is cured.
stules are very numerous, it has been termed *pannus herpeticus.*
The *prognosis* of phlyctenular conjunctivitis is generally very
ecially if the case is seen early; if the phlyctenulæ are few
l limited to one portion of the conjunctiva; if the cornea is no
l there is no episcleritis. In favorable cases, the disease gene
course in from ten to fifteen days, and disappears without le
ce behind it. ·Very mild cases, in which only one or two sma
he form near the edge of the cornea without much irritability
lty of the eye, may even be cured in five or six days, simply
nffilations of calomel, without any other treatment whatever.
rce of trouble and annoyance is the great tendency to relapses.
t as the disease seems to be all but cured, fresh symptoms of
ervene, and a new crop of phlyctenulæ appears. If the dis
omes complicated with episcleritis, its course may be very obsti
tructed.
Phlyctenular conjunctivitis occurs by far most frequently amongst
ecially those of a feeble, scrofulous habit, and of a highly ner
ble temperament. Stellwag is of opinion that local irritants acti
ciliary nerves may give rise to it; as, for instance, the prema
essive use of strong astringent collyria in some cases of conju
list the iritability of the eye is still very great. The irritation
propagated from other branches of the fifth to the ciliary nerv
as of eczema, impetigo of the cheek, the mucous membrane of the n
lnrd, he thinks that the disease is of an herpetic nature, and henc
herpes conjunctivæ." Some of its varieties do not, however, be
mblance to herpes in their course.
The *treatment* must be especially directed to the following poi
inish the irritability of the eye, to prevent any graver complicati
ten the absorption of the phlyctenulæ, to prevent if possible the occu
relapse, and to improve and strengthen the patient's general heal
The eye should be washed with lukewarm water, and the crusts rem
n the edges of the lids. If the latter are excoriated, a little simple
weak oxide of mercury ointment should be applied to them. The
eailes are to be applied to the nostrils if they are excoriated, or a
ill of lint soaked in olive oil should be inserted into them. If the
ah thick discharge from the nose, the inside of the nostril should
ntly touched with a finely pointed crayon of nitrate of silver. Liebre
nsly recommends the "Eau de Labarraque" (a solution of soda imp
sl with chlorine gas) for this purpose. If the lower lid and cheek

---

[1] "Klin. Monatsbl.," 1864, p. 393.

stecher for the more accurate indications as to its use, and for showing the advantage of employing it in considerably stronger doses than was formerly done. He has more lately substituted the yellow amorphous oxide of mercury for the red oxide, which is in the finest possible state of division, and, being entirely free from any crystalline form, does not adhere by any fine points to the conjunctiva.[1] He uses an ointment of very considerable strength, viz., half a drachm or one drachm of the yellow oxide of mercury to an ounce of lard.[2] I have generally found that a much weaker ointment (gr. x–xxiv to the ounce) was equally beneficial, and caused less irritation. [For most cases an ointment of the strength of two or three grains of the yellow oxide to the drachm of vaseline, is strong enough.—B.] It should be applied once a day with a small brush to the inside of the eyelids, which, on being closed, will sweep off the ointment from the brush. After a few minutes it should be wiped off from the lids (between which it becomes exuded) with a piece of fine linen. The ointment is especially indicated when the symptoms of severe irritation have subsided, but it may even be applied with advantage in the acute stage, if care be taken to remove it completely from the conjunctival sac. It is also of great benefit in checking the tendency to relapses

In cases in which the phlyctenular ophthalmia is accompanied by much swelling of the conjunctiva and symptoms of catarrhal conjunctivitis, Von Graefe has found much benefit from chlorine water, as it diminishes the catarrhal symptoms, especially the swelling, without setting up too considerable a degree of irritation, which is the chief danger in employing the nitrate of silver or any strong astringents in these cases. It is also indicated in the prominent ulcers, accompanied by episcleritis, as it considerably hastens the formation of the epithelial covering over the ulcer. Some touch the latter with the point of a crayon of nitrate of silver, but this is not always free from risk, especially when the ulcer is situated near the cornea, and the chlorine water appears to act more beneficially. [With a finely pointed crayon of nitrate of silver, this may be carefully done, and sometimes renders great service in cutting short the disease.—B.]

It is not advisable to apply blisters to the temple, as the skin is often extremely irritable, and there is frequently a great tendency to eczema. Great attention should be paid to the constitutional treatment of the patient. He should be placed upon a nutritious and wholesome diet, and be allowed as much exercise in the open air as possible. Cleanliness should be strictly attended to, and cold bathing insisted upon if the patient is not too weak. Nothing is so injurious as to confine him in the dark on account of the photophobia, for in this way the eye will become so sensitive that no light will be borne. Children are especially prone to seek the dark, burying their heads in their mother's lap, or in a sofa or bed in the corner of the room, and only the strictest injunctions will make them face the light. They should be gradually accustomed to it, their eyes being perhaps protected by a shade, or a pair of blue glasses. [The local application of pilocarpine, in the form of a solution of the hydrochlorate, has been recommended in these cases, but its success has not been especially gratifying.—B.]

The bowels should be kept regulated, and an occasional purge of rhubarb and jalap, or calomel and jalap, should be given, particularly in children. If the children are very irritable, and there is much pain, sedatives should be prescribed, e. g., small doses of hyoscyamus, conium, or morphia.

---

[1] "Nassauer Corresp. Bl.," No. 10, 1858.
[2] An interesting and valuable paper, by Dr. Pagenstecher, on the use of this ointment, will be found in the "Ophthalmic Review," vol. ii. 115 [and in the "Amer. Journ. of Med. Sci.," Oct. 1865, pp. 507 and 550].

Tonics, more especially quinine, are of great benefit. These may be given in combination with steel, or also with cod-liver oil. In infants and young children, the liquor cinchonæ or the vinum ferri should be administered. [The systematic and prolonged use of cod-liver oil in these cases is perhaps the most important part of the treatment. These cases are so very frequently of stramous origin that it is well also to combine with the oil either the syrup of the iodide of iron, or the syrup of the hypophosphites of lime and magnesia. In many cases of puny, marasmic children, a daily inunction of one or two ounces of cod-liver oil is a great aid in building up a satisfactory state of health.—B.]

The photophobia often proves very obstinate and intractable, but as a rule less so than when the cornea is also implicated. This spasm of the lids (blepharospasm) is a reflex neurosis, due to an irritation of the nerves of the conjunctiva and cornea, which produces hyperæsthesia of the orbicularis muscle (vide blepharospasm). The photophobia dependent upon exposure of the denuded nerve fibres of the cornea, should, as has been recommended above, be treated by the application of a compress. As the health of the patient improves, and he becomes more and more accustomed to the light, the photophobia will generally disappear. In children, it may be very advantageous to employ a remedy which I first saw very successful in Von Graefe's hands, viz., the dipping their heads under water, as this breaks the circuit of reflex action by the intense fright of the child. This should, if necessary, be repeated several times, even at one sitting, until the child opens its eyes properly. I have often seen surprising results from this treatment, when all other remedies had failed. The head must, however, be well dipped under water, so that mouth, nose, and eyes are immersed, the child being kept in this position for a few seconds, which will effectually frighten it.

In adults I have also obtained much benefit in severe blepharospasm from the subcutaneous injection of morphia in the region of the supra-orbital nerve. The division of this nerve will not be necessary in the photophobia accompanying phlyctenular ophthalmia.

10.—EXANTHEMATOUS [AFFECTIONS OF THE CONJUNCTIVA.—B.]

The eyes often become affected in measles and scarlatina. In the milder cases the conjunctiva becomes hyperæmic, and perhaps symptoms of catarrhal conjunctivitis supervene. Exceptionally, however, the inflammation may assume a more severe muco-purulent character, leading perhaps to perforating ulcers of the cornea, prolapse of the iris, and anterior staphyloma; this is more especially liable to occur in children of a weakly, scrofulous diathesis. Not unfrequently the conjunctivitis presents the phlyctenular form, being accompanied by much photophobia, lachrymation, and general irritability of the eye. Extensive ulcers of the cornea, or iritis, are only of rare occurrence. In the majority of cases the treatment need only be very simple. The eye should be guarded against the light, be frequently washed, so that any discharge may be cleansed away, and if there is much hyperæmia or any inflammation of the conjunctiva, a mild astringent collyrium of sulphate of zinc, acetate of lead, or alum should be prescribed. If there is much photophobia and lachrymation, together with phlyctenulæ on the conjunctiva or cornea, atropine or belladonna drops should be applied to the eye, and the compound belladonna ointment be rubbed in over the forehead. The general health should at the same time be attended to.

In smallpox, the eyes are apt to suffer in a far more dangerous manner, for the inflammation is not only more severe, but the variolous pustules may form on the lids, the conjunctiva, and even on the cornea, leading to grave, and often very dangerous complications. Happily, since the introduction of vaccination, the variolous ophthalmia is far less dangerous than formerly, when it led but too frequently to destruction of the sight.

If a considerable number of pustules form on the eyelids, the swelling of the latter is often so great that it is impossible to open the eye. They are also apt to form at the very edge of the lid between the eyelashes, and often destroy the hair-bulbs, thus producing perhaps permanent loss of the eyelashes (madarosis). If they are situated on the palpebral conjunctiva near the edge of the eyelid, they may obliterate the openings of the Meibomian glands, and cause a stoppage and alteration in their secretions; or the growth and arrangement of the lashes may become affected, and distichiasis or trichiasis be produced. If the pustules form on the limbus conjunctivæ, they are chiefly dangerous inasmuch as they may extend to the cornea. The very prevalent opinion that variolous pustules often form on the conjunctiva and the cornea, during the eruptive stage, has been distinctly denied by Drs. Gregory and Marson. The latter especially maintains most strongly that no pustules form on the eye. The conjunctival inflammation met with in smallpox may assume the catarrhal, muco-purulent, or phlyctenular character. The latter is perhaps the most common. The eyelids and lachrymal apparatus are often affected, and this frequently gives rise to very obstinate and troublesome complications. But the eye may become implicated at a later stage of the disease, when the scales have fallen off from the pustules. Hence this has been termed by some writers, "secondary variolous ophthalmia." Mackenzie mentions that he has often seen both central abscess of the cornea and onyx at its lower edge produced, after the general eruption has completely gone. Although this mostly occurs about the twelfth day, he states that it may even take place five or six weeks after the patient has recovered from the primary disease. At first an infiltration of the cornea occurs, which generally soon passes over into an ulcer, and this, increasing in circumference and depth, may perforate the cornea, producing prolapse of the iris or partial staphyloma. If several such infiltrations should coalesce, a large ulcer or abscess will be formed, giving rise to an extensive leucoma, even if the cornea does not perforate. Should the whole cornea be destroyed by suppuration, a complete staphyloma will be the result. Again, the inflammation may attack the other structures of the eye, and the latter be lost from panophthalmitis.

The *treatment* should be much the same as that recommended for the conjunctivitis of measles and scarlatina. In order to prevent the formation of pustules on the eyelids, glycerine, olive oil, or unscented cold cream should be freely rubbed over them three or four times daily. Mackenzie recommends that two or three leeches should be applied to the temples, or behind the ears. The general health should be kept up by tonics, and the bowels properly attended to. If pustules form on the lids or conjunctiva, they should be pricked and emptied of their contents. If the cornea becomes implicated, and perforation is threatened, this must be treated according to the rules laid down in the treatment of ulcers of the cornea.

[In eczema of the scalp and face, especially in the bad cases which are so frequent among the infants and young children of the poor, a very severe conjunctivitis of the phlyctenular and catarrhal type is a very common accompaniment of the skin disease. The eyes are tightly closed by dried crusts, and when these are washed away, and the lids opened, a quantity of muco-pus exudes. When this has been removed, we often find pustules in the conjunctiva and not infrequently on the cornea. Cleanliness and atropine are the main reliance as local means of cure, while the eczema is to be carefully looked after. Though these cases are usually cured without any worse result than a macula on the cornea, yet the corneal infiltration may lead to perforation and prolapse of the iris with its consequences.—B.]

In erysipelas of the face, the conjunctiva is often affected, and this is accompanied by very great swelling of the eyelids. The cornea becomes but seldom implicated.

11.—XEROPHTHALMIA.

[Syn. Xerosis conjunctivæ, Xeroma.—B.]

In this condition, the conjunctiva is thickened, dry, and of a dusky-red color, its epithelial surface being rough and scaly. If the affection exists to a considerable extent, both the palpebral and ocular conjunctiva assume a dirty, grayish-white appearance, and become rough, dry, and cuticular. This condition is due to atrophy of the conjunctiva, subconjunctival tissue, and even of the tarsus, all of which undergo cicatricial changes, the nature of which has been already mentioned under the head of granular ophthalmia. The secreting apparatus of the conjunctiva is more or less destroyed, and this membrane assumes more the character of the cutis. On account of this disturbance in the secretions of the eye, the latter appears dry, and the patient experiences a most annoying sensation of heat, dryness, and stiffness in the eyes, and the puncta are generally much contracted, or even obliterated. The semilunar fold is hardly apparent. There is, moreover, always more or less posterior symblepharon, so that the hollow in the retro-tarsal region is obliterated, and the palpebral conjunctiva passes abruptly on to the eyeball. Sometimes small frena exist between the lid and the globe. During the movements of the eye, the ocular conjunctiva is thrown into small concentric folds round the cornea. The latter is generally opaque, often very considerably so; the opacity assuming perhaps the character of pannus, and extending over the greater portion, or even the whole, of the cornea. The surface of the cornea is generally rough and uneven, and its sensibility, as well as that of the conjunctiva, is greatly impaired, so that mechanical irritants, dust, dirt, foreign bodies, etc., are hardly felt, and excite little or no irritation.

Xerophthalmia is generally caused by long-continued and severe inflammation of the conjunctiva, more especially by the chronic diffuse granular ophthalmia, which is so apt to give rise to extensive atrophy and cicatrices of the conjunctiva and tarsus. It may also arise after diphtheritic conjunctivitis, or be produced by injuries to the conjunctiva, from strong acids, lime, etc., and the excessive and long-continued use of strong caustics, more especially the nitrate of silver. In the latter case, we find not only that the palpebral and ocular conjunctiva have become dry and cuticular, but that they are very markedly discolored, being of a dirty, olive-green tint, which is extremely unsightly.

Unhappily, no treatment is of much avail. We can only endeavor to remedy the dryness of the eye, due to the absence of its normal secretions, by the frequent use of some bland fluid employed as a collyrium. I have found milk answer far better than any other, which has been also strongly recommended by Von Graefe. Benefit is also sometimes experienced from the use of glycerine, which was first proposed by Mr. Taylor. The effect of these applications is to soften and wash away the hardened epithelial scales, and sometimes perceptibly to clear the opacity of the cornea.

[Clinically, it is possible to recognize two forms of xerosis, the epithelial and the parenchymatous, though the latter is by far the more common. The former is the more amenable to treatment, and Saemisch affirms that a complete restoration to the normal condition of the conjunctiva results. This condition is probably what existed in the cases of cholera patients described by Von Graefe. The parenchymatous form is almost certainly destructive of vision, owing to the cornea being involved. Perhaps the best results in the way of treatment, in addition to the bland collyria, have been obtained from the long-continued use of moist heat and the protective bandage. Recently, attempts have been made to replace the atrophied conjunctiva by transplantation of healthy mucous membrane taken from the conjunctiva of a rabbit. Wolff was the first to propose this, and a full account of his method may be found in the "Annales d'Oculistique," lxix. and lxx. Since then a number of others have attempted the same procedure, among them De Wecker, who is somewhat enthusiastic upon the subject. (See Masselon's "Relevé Statistique," Paris, 1874.) The results, when viewed fairly, have not been very satisfactory.—B.]

12.—PTERYGIUM

This affection is due to hypertrophy of the conjunctival and subconjunctival tissue, showing here and there tendinous or fibrillar expansions. The elevated portion of the conjunctiva is traversed by numerous bloodvessels, which run a horizontal course. If the vascularity is but slight, and the hypertrophy of the tissue but inconsiderable, it is termed *pterygium tenue* [Fig. 66]; whereas, if the thickening is excessive and the development of bloodvessels great, so that it looks like a well-marked red elevation—somewhat resembling a muscle—it is called *pterygium crassum* [Fig. 67]. It is

[Fig. 66.   Fig. 67.

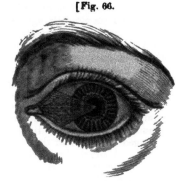

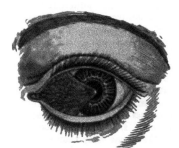

After Guthrie.   After Guthrie.]

always triangular or fan-like in shape, having its base, which is often very wide, turned towards the semilunar or retro-tarsal fold, and its apex towards the cornea. It sometimes passes close up to the edge of the latter and stops short just at the limbus conjunctivæ; in other cases it passes beyond this, and extends more or less on to the cornea, even reaching, perhaps, to the centre, but very seldom extending beyond the latter. Its apex is generally not very acute or pointed, but rather rounded off or indented. The portion situated on the cornea looks tendinous rather than vascular, or is made up of loose connective tissue like that on the sclerotic. It may be so superficial as to be readily shaved off, or it may extend deeper into the substance of the cornea, so that, when it is removed, an irregular hollow or furrow is left behind. The pterygium is mostly but loosely connected with the sclerotic and cornea, and with a pair of forceps it can readily be lifted up in a fold. But if the tendinous bands in its conjunctival portion are considerable and dense, this laxity is a good deal impaired and the elevation is rather tense and stretched, thus impeding the movements of the eyeball to a certain extent, which gives rise to a sensation of tightness or dragging when the eye is moved. The pterygium is most frequently met with at the inner angle of the eye, corresponding to the situation of the internal rectus muscle. It is occasionally symmetrical in the two eyes. It is less frequently seen at the outer angle, and still less upwards or downwards. In some rare cases, two or even more have formed on the same eye. It occurs in adults, but is most frequently seen in persons beyond middle age, and very rarely in children.

The *causes* of pterygium are often somewhat obscure and uncertain, as its formation is generally very slow and gradual. There can be no doubt that long and constant exposure to heat, glare, wind, dust, and chemical irritants may produce it, by setting up a state of chronic irritation of the conjunctiva, which gradually leads to a thickening and hypertrophy of this membrane and of the subconjunctival tissue. This occurs particularly in situations which are specially exposed to these influences, namely, at the inner and outer angle of the cornea, which lie in the palpebral aperture, and are unprotected by the lids. I have frequently met with this affection in persons who have long resided in hot climates, especially in several natives of the West Indies, and this agrees with the experience of other observers. Pterygium may also be produced by phlyctenular and even catarrhal ophthalmia.

Arlt[1] has, I think, offered by far the most reasonable and probable explanation of the formation of pterygium in many cases. He thinks that it is frequently produced in the following manner: If a superficial ulcer or abrasion (due perhaps to some chemical or mechanical injury) exists at the very edge of the cornea, the conjunctiva near it, particularly if it be somewhat excoriated and relaxed, as is often the case in old people, falls against it, and becomes adherent to the ulcer, being at the same time dragged somewhat toward it. This is always accompanied by a certain degree of irritation and serous infiltration of the conjunctiva, which, on the serum becoming absorbed, causes a certain amount of contraction and dragging of the membrane. Should the external irritants continue to act upon the eye, we can easily understand how this condition is not only maintained but increased in extent, the conjunctiva being gradually more and more dragged upon and involved in the process. Hasner[2] has more lately pointed out that the connection between the conjunctiva and subconjunctival tissue at the limbus conjunctivæ is often relaxed, more especially in aged persons, and that this forms a frequent predisposing cause of pterygium. A simple hypertrophy of the tissue may then suffice to draw up the neighboring conjunctiva, but this will, of course, be much more likely to occur if an ulcer or excoriation is formed, for, during the cicatrization the conjunctiva will be more or less dragged upon. The pterygium is often but of slight extent, and may increase but very slowly, remaining indeed almost stationary for a length of time, and without perhaps encroaching upon the cornea. In other cases its

[1] " Die Krankheiten des Augues," 1855, 1, p. 160.
[2] " Clinical Observations," Prague, 1865.

course is more rapid, and it may extend quite to the centre of the cornea, thus more or less affecting the sight and impairing the movements of the eye. Even if the pterygium is in such cases removed, some opacity of the cornea will remain, so that it may be necessary to make an artificial pupil.

[There may be absolutely no signs of any ulcerative action in the cornea. Microscopical examination of some cases has proved, on the authority of Schweigger, that the apex of the pterygium which is upon the cornea is covered by epithelium, not only on its anterior, but also on its posterior or adhering surface. With this there is also a folding in of the tissue along the sides of the apex. Arlt has shown that the growth of the pterygium forward is *into* the substance of the cornea, beneath the epithelial layers, instead of over them. Poncet has advanced the singular theory that pterygium is a parasitic conjunctival sclerosis, but holds that the theory of a primitive ulcer is absolutely necessary for the *début* of the affection. According to his theory, beneath the conjunctival growth are the parasitic vibriones, which he describes as the sole cause of the slow, onward march of the pterygium. This onward progress he calls "microbiotic ulceration." Singularly enough, however, he states that in cases where the pterygium has recurred after removal, few or no microbia have been found.—B.]

If the pterygium is but small, and is chiefly confined to the sclerotic, benefit is often derived from the application of astringent collyria, such as the sulphate of copper or zinc, the vinum opii, or even the nitrate of silver, more especially if there is any catarrhal ophthalmia. The application of the powdered acetate of lead (as recommended in granular ophthalmia) has also been advocated (Decondé). But if the disease is considerable, so that it annoys the patient during the movements of the eye, or if from its position on the cornea the sight is affected, these remedies will not suffice, and we must have recourse to operative treatment. [As the tendency of the pterygium when once it has encroached upon the cornea, is to grow over the cornea toward the centre, it is better to remove it at once, before it has covered the space in front of the pupil, as it always leaves an opacity behind it.—B.] Unfortunately, this is not always so successful as we could desire, for, if the pterygium encroaches much on the cornea, an extensive opacity will be left; and, if the base of the pterygium is large, the loss of substance will be considerable, and the resulting cicatrix will be dense, tendinous, and more or less prominent, giving rise to what has been termed "secondary pterygium," which may even necessitate a further operation. This is especially apt to occur if excision has been performed, and the wound has been made triangular in shape.

Numerous modes of operating for pterygium have been advocated, but I shall confine myself to the description of the three following, viz.: 1. Excision; 2. Transplantation; 3. Ligature. Of these, I have found the transplantation the most successful.

1. Excision.—This operation is to be performed in the following manner: The patient having been placed under the influence of an anæsthetic and the eyelids kept apart by the spring speculum, the operator seizes the pterygium with a pair of finely toothed forceps, and, raising it up, carefully abscises the corneal portion either with a cataract-knife or a pair of curved scissors. When the pterygium has been removed from the cornea, its conjunctival portion is to be excised up to about one and a half or two lines from the edge of the cornea. The lines of incision should run along the upper and er edge of the pterygium for the desired extent, and should then be made onverge toward each other, so that the wound may not assume a triar but a rhomboidal shape. The hypertrophied tissue having been

thoroughly removed, the edges of the conjunctival wound are to be accurately brought together by two or three fine sutures. As the edges of the incision a   apt to be somewhat uneven and ragged from the irregular dragging of the conjunctiva into the pterygium, I have found it advantageous to pass the threads through the conjunctiva prior to the excision, so as to embrace the pterygium to the desired extent, and then to make the incisions within the lines of the sutures, which will be a guide to the operator and enable him to render them more straight and even. The suggestion of making the wound rhomboidal, instead of triangular, is due to Arlt. The chief advantage of this is, that its edges can thus be made to fit more neatly and closely together, that it yields a more even and straighter line of adhesion, and that the tendency to the formation of a thick, prominent cicatrix is thus greatly diminished; whereas, if the wound is made triangular, the angles of the base of the triangle become puckered and projecting when the edges are united by sutures, and the central portion of the base is apt to be drawn toward the cornea, thus increasing the tendency to a prominent cicatrix.

It is not necessary, nor indeed desirable, to remove the pterygium as far as the semilunar or retro-tarsal fold, for the extent mentioned above will generally suffice. Pagenstecher[1] does not excise the pterygium, but, having separated it from the cornea and the sclerotic to the required extent, he simply turns it back, and brings the edges of the wound together by sutures. The pterygium soon shrinks, dwindles down, and gradually disappears altogether.

2. Transplantation, which is chiefly applicable when the pterygium is very large, was first introduced by Desmarres.[2] He detaches the pterygium from the cornea and sclerotic quite up to the base, and then turns it back towards the nose. He next makes an incision in the conjunctiva near and parallel to the lower edge of the cornea, and sufficiently large to receive the pterygium; the latter is then inserted into the incision and retained in this position by a few sutures. The chief advantages of this proceeding are, that the conjunctiva is preserved, that the pterygium soon shrinks in its new situation, and that there is far less chance of recurrence than when excision is practised. To avoid the prominence produced by the transplantation of a large pterygium, Knapp[3] practises the following modification of Desmarres' operation: Having dissected off the corneal portion of the pterygium, he makes two curved incisions, running from the upper and lower borders of the base of the pterygium towards the corresponding retro-tarsal fold. He then excises the corneal part of the pterygium, and, with a pair of straight scissors, divides the remaining portion by a horizontal incision. Next, a small square flap of conjunctiva is to be dissected off from the subjacent tissue above and below the wound, so as to cover the latter. The contraction produced by this causes the curved incisions to gape sufficiently to receive the horizontal halves of the pterygium, which are to be fastened in these incisions by sutures. The line of junction of the conjunctival flaps is also to be united by a couple of sutures.

3. The ingenious operation by ligature was suggested by Szokalski.[4] A couple of small needles having been armed with the ends of a fine silk thread, the operator, lifting up the pterygium with a pair of forceps, inserts one needle at its upper edge, near the cornea, and passing it beneath the

[1] "Klinische Beobachtungen," 1861, 15.
[2] "Maladies des Yeux," 2, 169.   [3] "A. f. O.," 14, 1, 267.
[4] "Arch. f. Physiol.-Heilkunde," 1845, 2.

pterygium, brings it out at the lower edge. (Fig. 68.) The other needle is then passed in the same manner beneath the pterygium, near its base. The needles are next cut loose, and the ligature will consequently be divided into three portions, viz., an outer, an inner, and a central one. The ends of the inner thread are then to be firmly tied, so as to tightly embrace this portion of the pterygium, then the ends of the outer thread are to be united, and finally, the two ends of the central ligature, which lie at the lower edge of the pterygium, are to be firmly tied. The ends of the ligatures may be snipped off, or fastened to the cheeks by strips of adhesive plaster. At the end of four days, the strangulated portion of the pterygium may generally

Fig. 68.

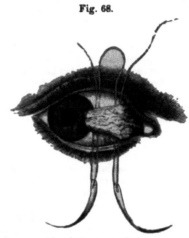

After Stellwag von Carion.

be easily removed with a pair of forceps. The affection is said never to recur after this operation.

[Galezowski advises operating on pterygium by the method of turning the growth upon its base. The apex of the growth is seized with the forceps, separated very carefully from its corneal adhesions, and then carefully dissected up to its base. When the pterygium is free throughout its entire length, he takes a thread, armed at each end with a curved needle, and pierces the apex with both needles, so as to include it in a small loop. Then turning the needles inward, he brings them out at the base of the growth, one near the upper and the other near the lower margin. The two ends are then tied in a tight knot, and thus the apex of the pterygium is turned inward towards the base, and the latter is strangulated by the knot. The pterygium, abandoned to itself, atrophies, and the ligature is left to ulcerate its way out. Lotions of a carbolic acid solution are employed several times a day, for the purpose of destroying any microbia that may be present.—B.]

We must not confound a little yellow spot near the cornea (pinguecula or pterygium pingue) with true pterygium. It often appears on the conjunctiva of elderly persons, near the edge of the cornea, in the form of a small yellow elevation. It is not of a fatty nature, but is due to hypertrophy of the subconjunctival tissue, accompanied by thickening of the epithelium. It but seldom causes any inconvenience; should it do so, it may be snipped off with a pair of scissors.

18.—SYMBLEPHARON.

In this affection there exists an adhesion between the conjunctiva of the eyelid and that of the eyeball. This fraenum may be extensive, and nearly the whole length of the palpebral conjunctiva (of one or both lids) be adherent to the opposite surface of the globe, producing a considerable limitation of the movements of the eyeball; or the adhesion may be very limited, so that only a narrow bridle exists. In the latter case, there may be simply a small bridge of conjunctiva passing from the lid to the eyeball, readily permitting the passage of a probe beneath it; or, the adhesion may include a portion of the retro-tarsal fold, in which case no passage would exist. In some cases, we have a combination of the two, the probe passing only part of the way. If the palpebral conjunctiva adheres to the cornea, it has been termed "symblepharon cum corneâ" [Fig. 69], and it then assumes somewhat the character and appearance of a pterygium. The most frequent causes of symblepharon are injuries from red-hot metal, molten lead, strong acids, or quicklime, or from gunpowder exploding near the eyes. These produce more or less extensive sloughing and excoriation of the conjunctiva of the lid and eyeball, granulations form, and the opposite excoriated surfaces become firmly united. If these adhesions are but of limited extent, the constant movements of the eyeball will gradually stretch them, until the fraena become perhaps considerably elongated. Wounds penetrating through the eyelids into the globe may also produce symblepharon. It is but seldom due to ulcerations or pustules accompanying non-traumatic inflammation of the conjunctiva.

[Fig. 69.

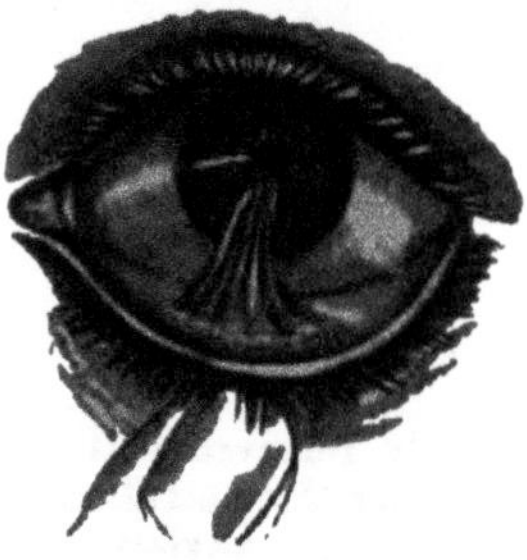

After Mackenzie.]

The effect which an operation will have in the cure of a symblepharon will depend chiefly upon the extent of the latter. If it is very considerable, embracing the retro-tarsal fold, and producing a close adhesion between the lid and the eyeball, but little good can generally be done by an operation. The most favorable cases are those in which a narrow band passes like a bridge from the palpebral to the ocular conjunctiva, so that a probe can be freely inserted beneath it. But even those cases in which the adhesion passes to the retro-tarsal fold may sometimes be much improved if the fraenum is but small. If one or two narrow membranous bands exist, they should be put on the stretch and divided close to the globe, and reunion should, if possible, be prevented by frequently passing a probe, dipped in a little oil or glycerine, between the raw surfaces; or, these may be touched lightly with a crayon of nitrate of silver, in order that an eschar may be formed, and adhesion prevented.

When the adhesion is more extensive, a simple division of the fraenum will not suffice, for the raw surfaces will be so considerable in size, that they are sure to reunite, for, as they contract during granulation, the opposing surfaces will be again drawn towards each other. Many of these cases appear to do very well at first, but, after a time, a relapse generally occurs, so that finally they are hardly, if at all, improved by the operation. In order to prevent this reunion of the raw surfaces, it has long been proposed to interpose a small shield of glass, horn, or ivory between the lid and eyeball. This has often been tried, but has almost always failed, except where the fræna are very narrow, for as the wound cicatrizes, the parts in its vicinity contract, and thus gradually push out the shield. Mr. Wordsworth[1] uses a glass mask, instead of a metal shield. It is a glass shell, like an artificial eye, having a central aperture for the cornea. He has found it very successful in the treatment of extensive fræna, and in cases of destruction of the epithelium of the conjunctiva, in which symblepharon was imminent.

In order to obviate this tendency to reunion, Arlt has introduced and practised with success the following operation.[2] The eyelid having been drawn away from the globe, so as to put the frænum well on the stretch, the operator passes a curved needle, armed with a fine silk thread, through the symblepharon, close to the cornea, the adhesion is then to be carefully dissected off from the cornea and sclerotic as far as the retro-tarsal fold. Two curved needles having been armed with the thread, the symblepharon is doubled down, so as to bring its conjunctival surface in contact with the raw surface of the globe, and the needles are then passed through the thickness of the lid, close to the orbital edge, and the sutures tied on the outside of the lid, so as to keep the symblepharon folded down in the required position. If the frænum is not very broad, the edges of the wound in the ocular conjunctiva should be brought together by two or three fine sutures. After the operation, cold compresses are to be applied. When the conjunctival wound is healed, the turned-down symblepharon, which will by this time have shrunk considerably, may be excised if it should prove irksome to the patient.

The operation which I have found most successful for the permanent cure of moderate cases of symblepharon, is that of transplantation, for which we are indebted to Mr. Teale.[3] He describes the mode of operating, as follows:

"Having first made an incision through the adherent lid, in a line corresponding to the margin of the concealed cornea (see A, Fig. 70), I dissected the lid from the eyeball, until the globe moved as freely as if there had been no unnatural adhesions. Thus, the apex of the symblepharon (A, Fig. 71), being part of the skin of the lid, was left adherent to the cornea.

<table>
<tr><td>Fig. 70.</td><td>Fig. 71.</td></tr>
</table>

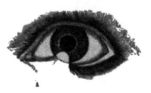
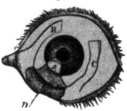

"In the next place, two flaps of conjunctiva were formed, one from the surface of the globe, near the inner extremity of the raw surface, the other from the surface of the globe, near the outer extremity. I first marked out, with a Beer's knife, a flap of conjunctiva (B, Fig. 71), nearly a quarter of an

[1] "R. L. O. H. Rep.," 3, 216.   [2] "Prager Vierteljahreschrift," xi. 161.
[3] "R. L. O. H. Rep.," 8, 263.

inch in breadth, and two-thirds of an inch in length, with its base at the
sound conjunctiva, bounding the inner extremity of the exposed raw surface,
and its apex passing towards the upper surface
of the eyeball. The flap was then carefully
dissected from the globe, until it was so far at
liberty as to stretch across the chasm without
great tension, care being taken to leave a sufficient thickness of tissue near its base. A second
flap was then made on the outside of the eyeball in the same manner. In making the flaps,
conjunctiva alone was taken, the subconjunctival tissue not being included. The two flaps
thus made were then adjusted in their new situa-
tion (see Fig. 72). The inner flap, B, was made to stretch across the raw
surface of the eyelid, being fixed by its apex to the healthy conjunctiva, at
the outer edge of the wound. The outer flap, C, was fixed across the raw
surface of the eyeball, its apex being stitched to the conjunctiva near the
base of the inner flap. Thus, the two flaps were dove-tailed into the wound.
The flaps having been adjusted in their new position, their vitality was
further provided for by incising the conjunctiva near their base, in any
direction in which there seemed to be undue tension, and by stitching
together the margins of the gap whence the transplanted conjunctiva had
been taken (e. g., D, E, Fig. 72). One or two other sutures were inserted,
with a view to prevent doubling in of the edges of the transplanted conjunctiva." The apex of skin left on the cornea soon atrophies and disappears.

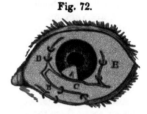

Fig. 72.

More lately Mr. Teale has devised the following very ingenious mode of
treating symblepharon by transplantation.[1] The operation is to be performed as follows: 1. The patient being under the influence of an anæsthetic,
the eyelid is to be first set perfectly free from the eyeball. The separation
of the lid is commenced at the margin of the cornea (A, Fig. 73), so as to

Fig. 73.

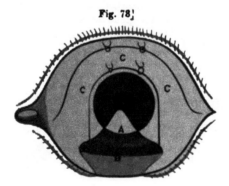

leave behind any skin or opaque material adherent to the cornea, and is
carried deeply into the fossa (B) between the lid and eyeball. 2. A nearly
circular band (ccc) is marked out in the sound conjunctiva about a quarter

[1] Mr. Teale first described this operation in a paper read before the International
Ophthalmological Congress, held in London, August, 1872, and showed some patients
on whom it had been successfully performed.

of an inch in breadth by a very sharp scalpel, the outer incision being made first. This band commences at one end of the gap resulting from the liberation of the lid, passes round the sound margin of the cornea, and terminates at the opposite end of the gap. 3. Four stitches are then inserted near the middle of the flap, two on each edge in order (a) to prevent the flap from curling up with the mucous surface downwards; (b) to facilitate the manipulation of the flap whilst it is being separated from the eyeball. These stitches are to be inserted as follows: A fine silk thread is passed twice through the eye of a small curved needle. The needle held in a holder is inserted at the edge of the flap and tied into a single knot of the thread, and allowed to hang down at one side, it being prevented from slipping off the thread by the double passage of the thread through the eye. The four stitches are thus attached each with its needle ready to complete the suture after the flap has been transferred to its new bed. 4. Separation of the flap is completed by small curved scissors, the flap being held and raised by the forementioned sutures. 5. The flap having been separated on its *under surface*, whilst its extremities are continuous with conjunctiva, is then brought over the front of the cornea, raw surface downwards, into the new bed provided by the liberation of the eyeball from the lid. 6. The sutures already inserted are now used for fixing the flap as deeply as possible into the fossa between the lid and globe. Other stitches are inserted so as to steady the flap without making it tense.

[Knapp has described a somewhat similar operation for the relief of a case of broad pterygium-like symblepharon with granulations growing from its apex, attaching the lower lid to the cornea. The details of the operation, however, differ somewhat from Teale's, and the conjunctival flaps have a slightly different direction. The description may be found in the "Archiv für Ophthalmologie," xiv. 1, 1868, p. 270.

The transplantation without pedicle, or better the grafting of small pieces of healthy conjunctiva, from the human eye or from some of the lower animals, into the raw space made by the detachment of a symblepharon, has been recommended as likely to prove successful, and, in the hands of several surgeons, has given excellent results. Mr. Wolfe, of Glasgow, who first brought this method to the notice of the profession, operates as follows:[1] The patient is anæsthetized, and the conjunctival adhesions are separated completely, so that the eyeball can move in every direction, and the space to be filled up carefully prepared. He next marks the boundary of the portion of a rabbit's conjunctiva, which he wishes to transplant, by inserting four black silk sutures, which he secures with a knot, leaving the needles attached. These also indicate the epithelial surface, which would be difficult to distinguish after separation. The portion of conjunctiva from the rabbit which he chooses is that which lines the inner angle, covers the membrana nictitans, and extends as far as the cornea, on account of its vascularity and looseness. The sutures being put on the stretch, he separates the conjunctiva with scissors, and transfers it quickly to replace the lost palpebral or ocular conjunctiva of the patient, securing it in its place by means of the same needles and sutures, and adding other stitches if necessary. Both eyes are then bandaged. For the first forty-eight hours the conjunctiva has a grayish look, but gradually becomes glistening, and finally assumes a red appearance. If any irritation set in, he uses warm fomentations. He considers quick transplantation, without previous handling of the conjunctival graft, very necessary to success.—B.]

[1 "Lancet," April 8, 1876.—B.]

14.—ANCHYLOBLEPHARON.

By this is meant a more or less extensive, thin, membranous or cicatricial adhesion of the edges of the eyelids to each other. It frequently coexists with symblepharon, the same injury having given rise to both these conditions. Sometimes the adhesion is confined to the inner angle of the eye, leaving perhaps a small opening through which the tears can escape and a probe may be passed. [Fig. 74.] Extensive membranous adhesions between

[Fig. 74.

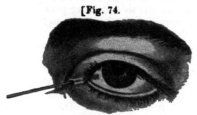

After Lawson.]

the edges of the lid are generally congenital. The most frequent causes of anchyloblepharon are chemical and mechanical injuries, such as burns or scalds from hot iron, molten lead, strong acids, etc. In these cases there is generally also symblepharon. Blepharitis, accompanied by ulcerations at the edge of the lids, may produce it, if the ulcers are situated opposite to each other on the two lids, and kept for a long time in contact by the eye being bandaged (Stellwag).

Before an operation is attempted for the cure of anchyloblepharon, the surgeon should ascertain whether or not symblepharon coexists, and if so, what is its extent, and whether it involves the cornea or not; for if the lid be widely adherent to the cornea, little or no benefit will accrue from an operation. If a small opening exists at the nasal side, or if the anchyloblepharon is but partial, a probe should be passed in underneath the lid, so as to ascertain whether any adhesions exist between it and the eyeball. If the adhesion between the eyelids is complete, the best way of determining this is to pinch the upper eyelid into a fold, so as to draw it away from the globe, and then to order the patient to move his eye in different directions, when we can easily estimate the freedom of the movements. We should also examine what perception of light the patient still enjoys, in order, if possible, to ascertain whether the cornea and retina are healthy or not.

If the adhesion between the eyelids is not very considerable, consisting perhaps of one or more small bands, it should be simply divided close to the edge of the lid. In order to prevent readhesion of the surfaces, these should be touched with collodion (Haynes Walton). If the anchyloblepharon is complete, but a small opening exists near the nasal portion; a grooved director should be passed in through this, and run behind the adhesion, which is to be divided upon it with a scalpel. If no opening exists, the operator should at one point lift up the lids from the eyeball in a vertical fold, and divide the adhesion here, then introduce a director through this incision, and finish the operation with its aid.

In any operative procedure for the relief of anchyloblepharon, it is necessary that at least one of the divided surfaces should be covered with epithelium, especially where the two surfaces come together, as at either canthus, otherwise it will be impossible to prevent readhesion of the parts.—B.]

15.—INJURIES OF THE CONJUNCTIVA.

These may be of a mechanical or chemical nature. The former may prove injurious by their contact with the conjunctiva, setting up irritation and inflammation, or from their wounding and lacerating this membrane. The foreign bodies most frequently met with on the conjunctiva are bits of steel, iron, glass, coal, straw, dust, etc., which may remain lodged on its surface, or become more or less deeply embedded in its structure. The presence of a foreign body in the eye generally sets up at once severe symptoms of ciliary irritation. The eyelids are spasmodically contracted, the ocular conjunctiva becomes injected, and a bright rosy zone appears round the cornea; there is also much photophobia, lachrymation, and a feeling as of sand and grit in the eye or under the upper lid. Sometimes, the pain and ciliary neuralgia are considerable, and the pupil is markedly contracted. If the foreign body is small, and simply lies on the conjunctiva, the movements of the eyelids, the rubbing of the eye by the patient, and the copious lachrymation will often suffice to extrude it. If the surgeon suspects the presence of a foreign body, he must carefully and closely examine the surface of the palpebral conjunctiva of both lids, as well as the ocular conjunctiva and the cornea. The lower eyelid is to be depressed by the fore and middle finger so as to bring its inner surface, and especially the retro-tarsal fold, well into view, the patient at the same time being directed to look upwards.

The upper lid is next to be well everted, and its lining membrane thoroughly scanned, more particularly the retro-tarsal region, within the folds of which the foreign body often lies hidden, and may easily escape detection. Cases are narrated in which an undiscovered foreign body has set up a severe and obstinate ophthalmia. When found, the foreign body

[Fig. 75. Fig. 76.] 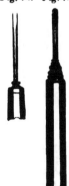 should be removed with the spud [Fig. 75], which should be inserted beneath it, and gently lift it out. If it has got somewhat embedded in the conjunctiva, Mr. Haynes Walton's gouge [Fig. 76] will be found very serviceable. If the foreign bodies, more especially shot or small splinters of glass or steel, etc., are buried in the conjunctiva, their exact situation should be ascertained by lightly passing the finger over the surface of the conjunctiva, and they should then be excised with perhaps a small portion of the latter. Sometimes, impalpable bits of dust or dirt get upon the conjunctiva, and set up a good deal of irritation. The lids being well everted, a blunt probe should be passed over their lining membrane and behind the retro-tarsal fold, which will sweep off any such portions. The surface of the conjunctiva should then be washed by a stream of lukewarm water, directed upon it from a sponge or a syringe. If sand or grit has got into the eye, it should also be washed away in this manner.

After the removal of a foreign body a little castor or olive oil should be dropped into the eye, and if there has been great irritation, cold compresses should be applied to the lids.

Chemical injuries may produce a more or less extensive abrasion of the epithelium, or excoriation of the surface of the conjunctiva, if the injury was severe or the chemical agent very strong, a deep slough of this membrane may occur, which, in cicatrizing, will cause a considerable contraction of the

boring tissues. Plastic lymph is effused, and the opposite raw surfaces
conjunctiva become closely adherent, hence these injuries so frequently
rise to symblepharon and anchyloblepharon. Sometimes, deep and
late ulcers are formed, the surfaces of which become covered with
ting granulations.

uries from lime are unfortunately of common occurrence, and are very
rous in their nature, for this agent is strongly irritant, producing not
destruction of the epithelium and the surface of the conjunctiva, but
or less deep and extensive sloughs of this membrane and of the cornea.
erefore, frequently destroys the sight, or in more favorable cases gives
an extensive symblepharon. If the patient is seen at once, a weak
on of vinegar and water (f3j to f3j of water), or of dilute acetic acid,
d be freely injected under the lids; this will produce an innocuous
te of lime. A few drops of olive or castor oil should be applied to the
ns to lubricate the surface of the conjunctiva; and then the surgeon,
ing both lids, should proceed to remove every particle of lime. This
g been done, the eye should be well washed by letting a stream of luke-
water from a sponge or syringe play upon the surface of the conjunc-
A few drops of olive oil should be applied three or four times a day.
schars which form on the conjunctiva must be removed with a pair of
s. If there is much conjunctivitis with a muco-purulent discharge,
astringent collyria of sulphate of zinc or nitrate of silver must be
yed, or the eye may be frequently washed with a glycerine lotion
erin. f3j ad Aq. dest. f3vij), a little being allowed to flow into the eye.
vhen the sloughs are detached, astringents should not be used, as they
xcite too much irritation. Nor should they be used if the eye is very
ble and painful, or the cornea is affected. In such cases soothing ap-
ions are indicated, such as the belladonna lotion, compound belladonna
ent rubbed on the forehead, poppy fomentations.

ong acids, such as the sulphuric or nitric, produce extensive sloughing
conjunctiva and cornea, accompanied by severe symptoms of irrita-
Generally, however, the eyelids suffer the most, and the deep sloughs
may be produced frequently give rise to entropion.
ter an injury from strong acids, the eye should be syringed out with a
solution of carbonate of soda or potassa (Đj to f3iv–vj Aq. destill.),
ter to neutralize the acid. Afterwards, olive oil is to be dropped in.

16.—TUMORS OF THE CONJUNCTIVA, ETC.

lypi are occasionally met with in the conjunctiva, especially at the
nnar fold or caruncle. They appear in the form of small pink lob-
d elevations or excrescences, and have a distinct pedicle. Although
are generally small, they may reach the size of a hazel-nut,[1] and pro-
between the aperture of the lids. They may be readily snipped off
a pair of curved scissors, or a scalpel, but are apt to bleed rather freely.
hemorrhage may, however, be easily arrested by a light touch with a
n of nitrate of silver, which will, moreover, check the tendency to a
rence of the disease.
ignicula [Syn. Interpalpebral blotch.—B.] might be mistaken by a
ficial observer for a slightly developed pterygium, as it is a small tri-
lar elevation, situated generally close to the edge of the cornea, toward
its base is turned. It occurs at the outer or inner edge of the cornea,

---

[1] Graefe, "A. f. O.," i. 1, 289.

and is due to hypertrophy of the conjunctival and subconjunctival tissue, as well as of the epithelial cells, but it does not contain any fat, as might have been suspected from its yellow tint. It is chiefly met with in old persons, and is due to a chronic irritation of the conjunctiva. It generally remains small and stationary, and produces no particular inconvenience or disfigurement. Should it, however, increase in size, or its appearance prove disagreeable to the patient, it may easily be excised.

Fatty tumors [Lipomata—B.] are of rare occurrence, and are most frequently observed on the ocular conjunctiva at some little distance from the cornea, and between the recti muscles, more especially on the superior and external rectus, in the vicinity of the lachrymal gland. They are often due to hypertrophy and extension of the adipose tissue of the orbit. They appear in the form of smooth, yellow, lobulated, elastic tumors, and may reach a considerable size. They are mostly congenital, and do not become very noticeable or increase greatly in size until a much later period. When they attain considerable proportions, they may push the eyeball aside, and by pressure impede the functions of the lachrymal gland.

If the tumor is inconsiderable in size, it may be easily removed, but care should be taken to preserve the conjunctiva as much as possible, and the incision should be closed by a fine suture.

Dermoid tumors are not of unfrequent occurrence. They are situated at the limbus conjunctivæ, partly on the cornea, and partly on the sclerotic

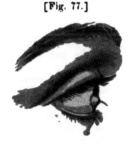

[Fig. 77.]

[Fig. 77], are of a pale, whitish-yellow color, about one or two lines in diameter, and somewhat raised above the level of the cornea. The surface of the tumor is generally smooth, but it may be lobulated, and from it one or two short hairs may protrude. Wardrop[1] mentions an extraordinary case in which twelve very long hairs grew from the middle of the tumor, passed through between the eyelids, and hung over the cheeks; these hairs had not appeared till the patient was sixteen years of age, at which time his beard also began to grow. The tumor is generally congenital, and almost completely stationary, increasing very slowly in size with the growth of the body. It may, however, become developed later in life, and augment considerably in size. The largest tumor of the kind that I have met with, I saw in Von Graefe's clinique, in 1860. It extended over the outer two-thirds of the cornea, was prominent, lobulated, and very disfiguring, almost hiding the cornea. From their close analogy to the structure of the skin, these tumors have been called "dermoid." They sometimes, however, appear to consist only of elastic fibrillar connective tissue, rudiments of true skin, fat, hairs, and sebaceous follicles. Marked increase in their size, or recurrence after removal, appear to be due to an increase in their fatty constituents. They may be readily excised, but care must be taken not to endeavor to remove them thoroughly from the cornea, as they sometimes extend deeply into its structure.[2]

[Dr. Taliaferro, of Kentucky, has recorded[3] an interesting case of a female, aged fifteen, who had a congenital dermoid tumor on each eye. Each tumor was of a delicate pink color at its base, becoming brownish at

[1] Wardrop's "Morbid Anatomy of the Human Eye," 1, 32.
[2] *Vide* Graefe's articles "On Dermoid Tumors," "A. f. O.," vii. 2, and xii. 2, 227.
[3] "American Journal of the Medical Sciences," 1841, N. S., ii. 88.

its apex. The tumor on the left eye, Fig. 79, at its base measured five lines in one diameter, by three and a half in the other, and rose in a conoidal form to about six lines in height. It almost covered the lower two-thirds of the pupil. From the apex grew some ten or twelve hairs, about sixteen lines in length, and a shade darker than the cilia. The tumor of the right

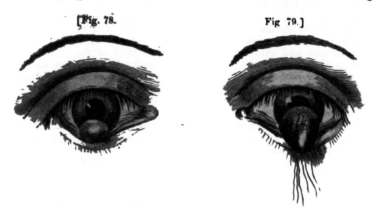

[Fig. 78.

Fig 79.]

eye, Fig. 78, was in shape and position similar to the one on the left, but of about half the size, and covering only the lower sixth of the pupil. The tumors were excised with excellent results.—H.]

[Dermoid growths are generally considered under the head of corneal tumors, as they are almost always situated upon the corneal margin.—B.]

Warts are occasionally seen on the conjunctiva, forming small, red, flesh-colored excrescences, being met with either singly, or in little clusters. They may occur on the palpebral or ocular conjunctiva, and also on the semilunar fold, and bear a strong resemblance to the warts upon the prepuce. They are generally accompanied by a certain degree of conjunctivitis, and a thin muco-purulent discharge. They should be at once snipped off with scissors before they attain any size, or have time to spread, and, if necessary, the cut portion should be lightly touched with nitrate of silver.

[Mackenzie relates a case in which the removal of a wart from the external surface of the lower lid was followed by the development of a number of warts upon the ocular conjunctiva.—B.]

Cysts of the conjunctiva may be readily distinguished by their circum-scribed round form, and their pink, translucent appearance, the transparency of their contents being easily recognized with the oblique illumination. They may occur in different portions of the conjunctiva, and vary in size from a small pea to that of a hazel-nut, or they may even exceed this. If they extend into the orbit, and attain a considerable size, they cause more or less protrusion of the eyeball. The walls of the smaller cysts are generally very thin, and only so slightly connected with the conjunctiva that they may be very readily removed.

[There are certain forms of cystic tumors, occurring beneath the conjunc-tiva, chiefly of the eyeball, but also of the eyelids, which occupy compara-tively little room in the cavity of the orbit, and hence may be separated from the larger and better known class of orbital cysts. There are two forms of these cysts: First, those in which the space filled by the fluid is a natural cavity; and, second, those in which the cavity is of new formation. They are always simple or barren; that is, they contain fluid or unorganized matter. They seem always to be formed by the enlargement and union of the spaces in areolar tissue. If the pressure of the contained fluid continues, the cavity eventually gains a perfect wall, which, under the microscope, is seen to consist of fine fibro-cellular tissue, sometimes lined by a single layer of squamous epithelium. This wall is, however, so thin that it is extremely difficult to remove the cyst entire. Their causation is still unsettled. They occur most often in children and young adults, and are met with at the internal and external angle of the lid. They are also found overlying or immediately in front of the lachrymal sac, but having no connection with it. Their contents here strongly resemble olive oil, and in this they resemble certain cysts of the thyroid body and ovary. There is one case reported of the development of a serous cyst in the lachrymal caruncle. A full account of these subconjunctival cysts will be found in the "American Journal of the Medical Sciences," January, 1878.—B.]

Cysticerci have been found several times beneath the ocular conjunctiva, and in one instance (Sichel) beneath the palpebral. There is seen at some part of the ocular conjunctiva, near the angle of the eye, a transparent, cyst-like elevation, which is round, sharply defined, and somewhat movable, and varies in size from a pea to a small bean. The conjunctiva over the cyst, and in its vicinity, is somewhat hyperæmic, but if it is sufficiently thin and transparent, we may be able to distinguish at the outer wall of the cyst a peculiar yellow or grayish-white spot, which is the head and neck of the entozoon, and Sichel[1] states that this appearance is quite characteristic.

CANCEROUS TUMORS are sometimes met with as primary affections, but far more frequently as secondary diseases, after cancer of the lids or of the eyeball.

Epithelial cancer [does occur] as a primary disease in the conjunctiva, though generally it extends from the eyelids. It appears as a small, smooth, or slightly nodulated excrescence or button, at the edge of the cornea, and often bears a very striking resemblance to a pustule or phlyctenula. It may, however, be distinguished from the latter by the absence of all inflammatory chemosis and irritation, and arterial injection, only a few dilated tortuous veins converging toward the little tumor; there is often also some serous infiltration. Subsequently the tumor increases in size, and assumes a redder tint, and its surface becomes more nodulated (cauliflower excrescences), being covered by dry, thickened epithelium; or there may be a breach of surface, and a thin, muco-purulent discharge exudes from the ulcer. The tumor may invade the cornea to a considerable extent, but is generally but slightly adherent to it, so that it may be nearly entirely removed. It may, however, produce a dense opacity of the cornea beyond the limits of the tumor, or lead to deep and extensive ulceration, or even perforation. If the tumor is stalked, it may be freely movable upon the surface of the cornea. Like all cancerous growths, it should be removed at the earliest possible period, and the edges of the conjunctival wound should be closed with fine sutures, in order that the sclerotic may not be exposed. It is, however, very apt quickly to recur, when the operation should be repeated without loss of time. But if the tumor has invaded the cornea to a considerable extent, is intimately connected with its tissue, and has greatly impaired the sight, it will be better to excise the eye; but even this does not always guard against recurrence, the new growth springing from the lids, or

[1] "Iconographie Ophthalmologique," p. 702.

from the bottom of the orbit. In such cases it is, therefore, always advisable to apply the chloride of zinc paste to the orbit, after the removal of the lids. [According to Alt, the beginning of epithelial tumors is an excessive cell-formation, a true hyperplasia of the epithelial layer of the conjunctiva or cornea. The next stage is when the underlying tissue becomes hyperæmic and shows a large and abnormal amount of round cells. He thinks that only in a few instances do the epithelial cells themselves show the conditions of proliferation, but he is positive that their condition mainly occurs in the round cells of the conjunctival stroma. The formation of round-cell cylinders and their partial transformation into epithelioid cells show that the connective tissue itself is also acting in the formation of epithelium. ("Transactions of Canada Medical Association," 1877.)

Melanotic epithelioma is excessively rare. An interesting case, in which the growth involved the cornea but began in the conjunctiva, and was successfully removed with preservation of perfect vision, has been reported by Dr. H. D. Noyes in the "Archives of Ophthalmology," viii. No. 2.—B.]

Melanotic [*sarcoma*] appears in the form of a small darkish-red or brownish-black spot or tumor in the subconjunctival tissue near the cornea, at the semilunar fold or caruncle. As it increases in size, it may implicate the lids, extending beneath them and giving rise to more or less considerable adhesions. The tumor may remain stationary for a long period and then rapidly increase, and it is very prone quickly to recur after removal. It must be remembered that many of the little black tumors which are often erroneously called melanotic cancer are only sarcomata.

[The development of *sarcomata* in the conjunctiva is not very uncommon. They usually start from the sclero-corneal margin and grow into the conjunctiva, though they may begin in the conjunctiva. The latter are generally pigmented, are usually of the small-cell variety and very vascular. When situated in the palpebral conjunctiva they usually have a pedicle. Cases have been reported by Müller, Graefe, Horner, Wecker, Estlander, Talko, and others. A case of sarcoma of the palpebral conjunctiva and tarsus which had undergone amyloid infiltration is reported by Dr. J. S. Prout, in the "Archives of Ophthalmology," viii. No. 1. The tumor developed from a trachomatous conjunctiva, and was removed entire, leaving the skin and muscle of the lid intact. Another case, reported by Dr. E. Dyer ("Trans. Amer. Ophthal. Society," 1879), began in the ocular conjunctiva, extended to the eyeball and orbit and brain, and the child died: this was a spindle-cell sarcoma.

Primary carcinoma of the conjunctiva is a very rare disease, as it almost always starts from the lids, eyeball, or orbit. Conjunctival carcinomata may be pigmented or unpigmented, and may occur as a mixed tumor with sarcomatous tissue. A very interesting paper, by Dr. H. D. Noyes, on a critical study of one hundred and twenty-seven cases of tumors growing from the front of the eyeball and eyelids ("Archives of Ophthalmology," vol. viii. No. 2), gives some points in regard to the frequency and locality of these growths.

Medullary cancer almost always extends to the conjunctiva from the lids or from the eyeball itself, the cornea or sclera giving way, and the tumor sprouting forth and very rapidly spreading thence into the neighboring tissues.

De Wecker has observed cases of growths in the ocular conjunctiva, resembling polypi, which grew very rapidly, and when removed soon returned. They were painless, but were accompanied by swelling of the tonsils. They spread with great rapidity.—B.]

Nævi sometimes extend from the external portion of the eyelid to the palpebral or even ocular conjunctiva, and may reach a very considerable size if they are not treated at an early period. They may, however, occur primarily on the conjunctiva or the semilunar fold, and should be removed as early as possible.

[*Papillary fibromata* are sometimes met with on the conjunctiva. Horner reports a case which extended from one canthus to the other and covered the upper part of the cornea, though it was not adherent to it. It was removed, but returned, and the patient died subsequently of carcinoma of the stomach. ("Graefe u. Saemisch's Handbuch," iv. p. 152.)

Subconjunctival osteomata have been observed in two cases. In all probability, however, these growths proceeded from the sclera. ("Graefe und Saemisch's Handbuch der Augenheilk.," iv. p. 151.)

Adeno-papilloma of the conjunctiva is a rare disease. Some cases have been described by Fontan, who examined them microscopically, and found the glandular hypertrophy the most marked feature present. The development of the papillæ was marked, but secondary in importance. The remaining fibrous and vascular elements were entirely accessory. They are benignant growths, but under rare circumstances may undergo transformation into epithelioma. (See " Recueil d'Ophthalmologie," December, 1881.)

Lymphangiectasia has occasionally been observed in the conjunctiva. Leber reports a case of hemorrhagic lymphangiectasia in a woman who, from childhood, had been subject to conjunctival hemorrhages. The enlarged vessels filled with blood were evidently lymphatics, for they lay deeper than the bloodvessels, and were much smaller in size and in their anastomotic meshwork, especially near the corneal margin. The production of this condition was due to the frequent hemorrhages into the conjunctiva, by which the lymphatics were kept constantly distended, and finally remained in a state of abnormal distention.

Lymphadenoma of the conjunctiva is a rare affection and presents nothing of special interest. (See " Recueil d'Ophthalmologie," April, 1880.)—B.]

Lithiasis is a term applied to a hardening or calcification of the secretion of the conjunctival glands, more especially the Meibomian glands. The affection appears in the form of white, round concretions of the size of a pin's head, which may, however, attain larger dimensions on the inner surface of the conjunctiva. They occur either singly, being scattered about over the surface of the lid, or they may appear arranged in single file along the tract of the ducts leading from the gland. The latter is, however, much more rare. On account of the roughness which they produce on the lid, considerable irritation and even a certain degree of conjunctivitis may be set up. The little calculi are easily removed by incising the conjunctiva over them, and lifting them out with the point of a cataract-needle, or a grooved spatula. Sometimes the concretion is soft and semitransparent, and appears at the opening of the duct, whence it may be readily pressed out.

The secretions of the caruncle also sometimes undergo cretefaction; and chalky deposits are likewise met with in the caruncle, often giving rise to irritation and swelling.

Pemphigus of the conjunctiva is a very rare affection, of which, I believe, only two cases have been recorded, viz., one by White Cooper,[1] the other by Wecker.[2] The symptoms are very characteristic, for one or more large vesicles form in the palpebral and perhaps also on the ocular conjunctiva; they contain a turbid serum and look exactly as if they had been caused by a burn or scald. There is generally a good deal of conjunctivitis, accom-

[1] " R. L. O. H. Rep.," 1, 165.   [2] " Kl. Monatsbl.," 1868, 282.

panied by lachrymation, photophobia, and perhaps some muco-purulent discharge. On bursting, the vesicle leaves a raw excoriated surface, which
secretes a thick muco-purulent discharge. If repeated crops of vesicles have
appeared, they may gradually give rise to symblepharon. The treatment
should consist of mild astringent collyria, and the frequent application of
glycerine to moisten the lids (Wecker). Internally, arsenic should be administered, for these patients always suffer from pemphigus of some other
part of the body.

Hemorrhage into the conjunctiva is generally produced by blows or falls
upon the eye or face, or by severe straining as in coughing, sneezing, etc.,
causing a rupture of some of the minute bloodvessels of the conjunctiva.
Such ecchymoses are also often met with in the course of inflammations of
the conjunctiva, or in persons suffering from scurvy. In other cases, they
occur spontaneously without any apparent cause; I have met with several
instances of this kind in which the ecchymosis had come on during the
night. But the effusion of blood may not be due to a rupture of any of the
conjunctival bloodvessels, but have gradually made its way forwards from
the orbit beneath the conjunctiva. Thus a blow upon the skull may, by a
contre-coup, produce a fracture of some portion of the walls of the orbit, this
is followed by more or less severe hemorrhage, and the effused blood may
make its way forwards beneath the conjunctiva. The ecchymosis does not,
however, in such cases appear directly after the accident, but only at an
interval of several hours.

The ecchymoses are generally situated on the ocular portion of the conjunctiva in the vicinity of the cornea, or in the retro-tarsal fold. The effusion
mostly gives rise to uniformly red patches, which vary in size and number,
but it may be so considerable that it extends round the whole cornea.

The treatment should consist chiefly in the application of stimulating
lotions, e. g., Tr. arnic. f3j, Aq. dest. f3iv, to be applied to the eye, or a
compress moistened with this lotion should be firmly tied over the eye; indeed a firm compress bandage accelerates the absorption of blood more than
any other remedy. A poultice of black bryony-root is also useful.

Œdema of the conjunctiva is met with very frequently in the course of
many inflammations of the conjunctiva and inner tunics of the eye, but it
may also occur spontaneously, more especially in elderly, feeble persons,
affected perhaps with disease of the kidney. The treatment should consist
in the application of a firm bandage, and the use of mild astringent collyria.
A few superficial incisions may be made in the chemosis with a pair of
curved scissors. The health of the patient should be at the same time attended to. Dr. Lawson Tait[1] has called attention to the important fact that
severe œdema of the conjunctiva is sometimes a symptom of surgical fever
(pyæmia), being dependent on a thrombus in the cavernous or ophthalmic
sinus.

[Œdema of the conjunctiva is a very marked symptom in orbital cellulitis,
and in bad cases of purulent conjunctivitis.—B.]

Subconjunctival emphysema is caused by fracture of the nasal parietes,
which admits the air into the subconjunctival tissue; or by a rupture in the
walls of the lachrymal sac, when the air is also admitted beneath the conjunctiva, if the nose is blown. The nature of the affection may be recognized
by the peculiar crackling which is heard when the swelling is pressed with
the finger; firm pressure causing it to disappear. A bandage should be
applied, and, if necessary, the swelling may be pricked with a needle and
the air allowed to escape.

<hr>

[1] "Edinburgh Med. Journal," No. 45, p. 798.

[17.—SYPHILIS OF THE CONJUNCTIVA.

Syphilitic lesions of the conjunctiva existing independently, and not connected with lesions of the eyelids on the one hand, or of the eyeball on the other, are not common.   In syphilitic patients, an obstinate catarrhal conjunctivitis is often met with, and this is especially noticeable in some cases of obstinate iritis.   The syphilitic lesions of the conjunctiva are eruptions, ulcerations, and infiltrations; and under the second head are to be included not only the chancre, but also secondary ulcers resulting from the breaking down of infiltrated masses.   The chancre is a rare lesion on the conjunctival surface alone, as in most of the reported cases the initial ulcer was on the margin of the lids, and involved both skin and mucous membrane; but it does occur as a conjunctival lesion alone, as in cases reported by Desmarres, Sturgis, Galezowski, Bumstead, Bull, and others.   The conjunctival chancre is apt to be a deep ulcer, with sharp edges and eroded walls, the bottom being covered by a gray pultaceous slough, and there is engorgement of the preauricular gland, and sometimes of the parotid, and even of the submaxillary glands.   This latter sign has come to be regarded by authorities as pathognomonic of syphilis.   There seems to be little doubt that either the ciliary margin of the lids or the cul-de-sac is the part most frequently the seat of the conjunctival chancre.   There are some cases reported where the lesion was in the ocular conjunctiva at the edge of the cornea, but they need confirmation.

The *secondary lesions* of the conjunctiva are much more frequent than the initial lesion.   They have been described by Lancereaux as small circumscribed spots, elevated, non-vascular, and of a reddish-gray or copper color. Galezowski affirms that syphilitic affections of the conjunctiva are either chancres or mucous patches, but in this he is mistaken; for papules and pustules are not rarely seen here, accompanying other signs of constitutional syphilis.   Certain specific sores with tawny surfaces are not very uncommon here, and are probably ulcerated mucous patches.   These ulcerate very easily, and it is not improbable that some of the reported cases of soft chancre of the conjunctiva are ulcerated mucous patches.   A secondary conjunctival ulcer is distinguished by its fatty-looking coating, irregularly eroded edges, and uneven base; if properly treated, they cicatrize rapidly.

A point of interest in these superficial ulcers on the conjunctiva is their isolated occurrence as a symptom of syphilis.   The patient may have been free from all symptoms of the disease for several years, when suddenly the conjunctival lesion makes its appearance, runs its course, is healed, and again the patient is free from all symptoms.

A third variety of conjunctival lesion in constitutional syphilis is the gummy infiltration, circumscribed, and diffuse, and this is probably the least common of all.   Late manifestations of syphilis, occurring in the tertiary period, are rarely limited to the conjunctiva; but usually beginning in other tissues, involve the mucous membrane by contiguity of tissue.   The term "conjunctivitis gummosa," used by Hirschberg, has no advantage over "gummy infiltration of the conjunctiva," and hence the latter term is retained.   This gummy infiltration may be in the form of small discrete tumors, or of a general thickening of the mucous membrane.   There is an infiltrated yellow base, a more or less marked swelling of the conjunctiva around the infiltration, and ulceration may set in rapidly.   Gummy infiltration of the ocular conjunctiva is very rare, but when it occurs may be entirely distinct from scleral infiltration.   (See "Amer. Journ. of the Med. Sciences," Oct.

1878, p. 413 et seq.) For a more detailed account of syphilis of the conjunctiva, the reader is referred to a paper on the subject by the Editor in the "American Journal of the Medical Sciences," October, 1878; and to the fourth edition of "Bumstead on Venereal Diseases," Chapter on "Diseases of the Eye," by Dr. Loring.

18.—RARE DISEASES OF THE CONJUNCTIVA. LUPUS, LEPRA, LARDACEOUS DISEASE, TUBERCULOSIS, PSORIASIS.

Lupus of the conjunctiva, as an independent disease, is but seldom met with. It appears first in the palpebral conjunctiva, and oftener in the lower lid than in the upper. The conjunctiva is injected, covered by small and large prominences, which are grouped together and resemble a granulating denuded surface. Later, the lupus nodules shrink and cicatrize, while new ones are developed elsewhere on the conjunctiva.

[Histologically, lupus is a granulation tumor, the substratum being distinguished by an abundant development of formative cells and giant cells. The products of lupus are histologically much more like ordinary inflammatory neoplasms than tubercles. The lupus nodule is often nothing more, in the early stage, than a circumscribed mass of granulation tissue, and is sometimes vascular, even when it contains giant cells. It may suppurate directly and then cicatrize. The usual stages of its metamorphosis, absorption, softening, and disintegration, are not distinguishable from the modes of involution of ordinary inflammation infiltration. (See an article by Baumgarten in the "Archiv für Patholog., Anat. und Phys.," lxxxii. 3.)—B.]

The final cicatricial degeneration may be very extensive and destructive. Generally the disease attacks the conjunctiva secondarily from the lids or vicinity of the face, though in very rare cases it may precede the development of the process in the skin. An interesting case of conjunctival lupus is reported by Dr. E. S. Peck in the "Archives of Medicine," June, 1880.

The disease occurs more often in one eye than in both. The treatment is, of course, to destroy the lupoid formation, and the best agent is probably the nitrate of silver in substance, though the growths may be removed more rapidly by the knife or scissors.

Lepra, though generally involving the cornea mainly, also affects the conjunctiva. It is met with in those cases in which the skin is red and swollen into folds, and appears as a slightly circumscribed, circular, whitish or pale yellow swelling, non-vascular, and looking like the rind of bacon, which either extends into the cornea or towards the cul-de-sac. Ole Bull and Hansen, however, think that the conjunctiva is not involved except in cases of rapid infiltration of the cornea and sclera.

Lardaceous, or Amyloid disease of the conjunctiva, is very rare, and has only very recently been recognized. During the last few years, cases have from time to time been reported, and Leber has published the results of a very careful investigation into its origin and mode of development in the conjunctiva as well as in other parts of the eye. ("Archiv für Ophthalmologie," Bd. xxv. 1, pp. 257–340.) In regard to the origin and development of the amyloid bodies, Leber believes that they are secreted by the cellular layer of the conjunctiva, and that lardaceous degeneration is a purely local lesion, and not the expression of a disease of the general organism. Clinically, the disease has by some authors been described as strongly resembling trachoma, and by others as perichondritis of the tarsus, but it differs markedly from both, though in some cases it may certainly be regarded as the result of trachoma. It may involve both ocular and palpebral conjunctiva, though it is usually confined to the latter. The lid is hard and swollen, the conjunctiva not much injected, of a faint yellow color, markedly thickened and infiltrated, and generally with a smooth surface. The whole lid may be everted, but without any special increase in the secretion. If the ocular conjunctiva is involved, it rises like a wall around the cornea. When the conjunctiva is seized with forceps, it seems almost cartilaginous or like brawn, but very brittle, as small pieces easily come away. If the infiltration does not involve the entire conjunctival lining of one lid, there may be sometimes seen a trachomatous condition of the conjunctiva not involved by the disease, and the lids of the other eye may be trachomatous. When incised, it feels like brawn, and there is no hemorrhage. An incised surface, when treated with solution of iodine and sulphuric acid, turns violet and then brown, thus answering to the test of lardaceous disease. Under the microscope, the amyloid infiltration is seen to extend mainly in the course of the vessels, the walls of which are also infiltrated, though detached masses of bodies which have coalesced are not uncommon.

The treatment consists in a careful and complete removal of the infiltrated tissues by the knife, either at one operation or gradually. The disease does not show any tendency to return.

[Rachlmann regards amyloid degeneration as entirely independent of conjunctival trachoma. He thinks that it is always preceded by a stage of hyaline degeneration, and that there may be a retrograde metamorphosis of the growth after partial extirpation. (See "Archiv für Augenheilkunde," x. 2.) Kubli considers four phases in the development of this growth: 1st. The phase of simple adenoid proliferation in the subconjunctival tissue. 2d. The phase of hyaline degeneration of adenoid structure. 3d. The phase of marked amyloid degeneration. 4th. The phase of calcification and ossification. The presence of few or many vessels gives to the neoplasm either a bright-yellowish, glassy color, and firm, elastic consistence, or a more reddish-yellow or reddish-brown color and soft, elastic consistence. In the third phase the tissue of the tumor is not elastic, but inelastic and brittle. Kubli regards the disease as unique, and having nothing in common with trachoma. He advises radical extirpation in every case where this can be done without causing very great loss of substance. In cases where this is not admissible, he recommends partial extirpation, in hopes of setting up spontaneous retrogressive metamorphosis of the growth. (See "Archiv für Augenheilkunde," x. 4, and final part.)—B.]

Cases have been reported by Kyber, Mandelstamm, Leber, Von Hippel, Prout, Shambach, and others (see "Archiv für Ophthalmologie," Bd. xxv. 1 and 2; "Archives of Ophthalmology," vol. viii. No. 1). In a case reported by Bull, the disease began in the orbit, and involved the lid and conjunctiva secondarily (see "Transactions of the American Ophthalmological Society," 1878).

Tuberculosis of the conjunctiva is also a disease of great rarity and comparatively recent recognition. Koester, in 1873, published a case of tubercle in the conjunctiva without tubercular disease of any other organ; hence a purely local disease. Sattler and Walb have both seen cases in which tubercles were found in the bottom of a conjunctival ulcer, and the former has described a case of miliary tuberculosis which involved conjunctiva, episclera, sclera, and cornea. Baumgarten's two cases are undoubted: in one, the tuberculous infiltration was found at the bottom of an ulcer; and in the other, small tumors formed in the conjunctiva, which were composed of small masses resembling in structure the giant-cell tubercle, and later underwent caseous degeneration. [Real tubercle is destitute of vessels, never undergoes direct suppuration or cicatrization, and its metamorphosis occurs through the medium of a tissue destruction totally different from that occurring in ordinary chronic inflammatory products; that is, by cheesy necrobiosis.—B.]   A microscopical examination of all the cases reported gives a picture of a specific character, and proves that not unfrequently we have to do not with a purely local process, but with the local expression of a general pathological condition.   The lymphatics of the eye are especially involved, as may be seen in the enlarged glands of the ear and lower jaw.   If the case is at all marked, one or both lids are very much thickened, and the patient cannot open the eye.   The lids are reddened and feel soft and elastic.   When the lid is everted, the conjunctiva bulges forward with luxuriant granulations, like the granulating surface of a wound.   The tarsal conjunctiva may be entirely free from granulations.   There is usually a purulent discharge, and some pannus.   The tubercular eruption may occur in the ocular conjunctiva.   T e proportion between tubercle and granulation tissue varies somewhat, but the microscopic pictures are all about alike.   [Manz reports an interesting case in a boy, two years and a half old, in whom both lids of the right eye were swollen, and under the skin of the lower lid was a small movable nodule.   The temporal half of the lower lid was destroyed, and the inner part was strewn with grayish-white nodules, which extended into the fornix.   On the conjunctival surface of the upper lid were two small, shallow ulcers, with infiltrated edges, and also several small nodules like those in the lower lid.   The child died at the end of three months, with all the signs of tubercular meningitis.   The tuberculous deposit seemed to be confined to the conjunctiva of the lids, fornix, and eyeball, as none was found in the choroid.   (See "Klinische Monatsblätter für Augenheilkunde," January, 1881.)—B.]

The treatment is first constitutional, and secondly local.   The granulations should be cut off before they have reached the period of caseous metamorphosis, and the raw surface should then be cauterized; and this may be done rather freely without fear of producing disagreeable cicatrization.   For a full account of the subject, see "Archiv für Ophthalmologie," xxv., abth. 4; articles by Hänsell, Haab, Leber, and Deutschmann, same journal, xxiv. 3; "Bericht der Ophthal. Gesellsch.," 1877; "Klin. Monatsbl. für Augenheilk.," xiii., xv.

Psoriasis of the conjunctiva has been described by some authors, among them Terrier ("Arch. gén. de médecine," 1876), accompanying psoriasis of the skin of the face and eyelids.   It is said to tend to a consecutive sclerosis.—B.]

limbus conjunctivæ, where it forms a bright rosy zone. If the vascularity is considerable, these parallel vessels are very numerous, and give a very red appearance to the edge of the cornea, which is often also somewhat swollen. When the cornea is extremely vascular and opaque, so that it assumes a very red or even fleshy appearance, the disease is termed *"pannus crassus;"* whereas if the bloodvessels are few and scattered, and the cloudiness inconsiderable, it is called *"pannus tenuis."*

In the acute form of the disease, there is often considerable photophobia, lachrymation, and ciliary neuralgia, accompanied by marked conjunctival and subconjunctival injection. But if the affection runs a very protracted and chronic course, the irritability of the eye is generally but slight, except if acute exacerbations occur. The surface of the cornea gradually becomes more opaque, rough, and irregular, and its epithelial layer hypertrophied and thickened, so that the cornea may finally assume almost a cuticular appearance. Or the epithelium may be shed at different points, giving rise to superficial facets and irregularities. But the loss of substance may extend much deeper, and extensive ulcers be formed, which may even lead to perforation of the cornea, and subsequently to anterior synechia, staphyloma, etc. After the pannus has existed for some time, the cornea is apt to become somewhat thinned, and, yielding gradually to the intra-ocular pressure, to lose its normal curvature and become bulged forward. This fact is of great practical importance, for even although the cornea should hereafter regain much of its transparency, this faultiness in its curvature will produce considerable deterioration of vision.

Amongst the causes which may produce pannus, granular conjunctivitis is by far the most frequent; in fact, in the vast majority of those cases in which the opacity is confined to the upper half of the cornea, it is due to granular lids. When speaking of granular conjunctivitis, I mentioned that pannus might be produced by the friction of the roughened surface of the lid on the cornea, or by a direct extension of the granulations on to the ocular conjunctiva, and from thence on to the cornea. In the latter case, small gray or yellow infiltrations appear near the margin of the cornea, and, if the attack be acute, may even extend over the whole of the cornea. Between these infiltrations bloodvessels are seen to be passing.

Phlyctenular or purulent conjunctivitis may also give rise to pannus. In the former case, the opacity and vascularity are not considerable in extent, and the affection is chiefly characterized by the appearance of scattered phlyctenulæ, or small infiltrations on the surface of the cornea.

The disease may likewise be produced by the constant friction and irritation of the cornea, caused by inverted eyelashes, with or without entropion, by suppuration of the Meibomian glands (chalazion), and by the desiccation and exposure of the cornea to external irritants, as in cases of lagophthalmos, etc. In such cases, the disease may be termed "traumatic pannus." In the chronic form, pannus may exist for many years without undergoing any particular change, except perhaps thinning and prominence of the cornea. Inflammatory exacerbations may, however, occur again and again, and each time leave the sight and the opacity of the cornea in a worse condition.

[In bad cases of "pannus crassus" it may be necessary to shave off the corneal granulations, and then carefully apply the mitigated stick of nitrate of silver to their base.—B.]

The *prognosis* is favorable in proportion as the pannus is inconsiderable and of recent origin, and the cause remediable. In very chronic cases, especially of the pannus crassus, the disease, even if eventually cured, generally leaves behind it extensive and dense opacities. If there is a central leucoma, or if iritis has occurred during the progress of the disease, and the pupil is closed, it will be necessary to perform iridectomy.

The *treatment* to be adopted must depend upon the cause, for if the latter can be cured, the pannus will also disappear. As I have already, in the article upon granular ophthalmia, entered very fully into the mode of treating pannus produced by that disease, I need not recur to this subject. In cases of traumatic pannus, our efforts must be at once directed to the removal of the cause, e. g., the entropion, inverted lashes, chalazion, etc. The opacity of the cornea which may remain after the disappearance of the original disease, must be treated by mild local irritants, amongst which may be especially recommended insufflation of calomel, the application of the red or yellow precipitate ointment, vinum opii, oil of turpentine, sulphate of copper, etc. These applications hasten the absorption of the morbid products, by producing a temporary inflammatory congestion of the blood-vessels.

[Critchett recommends, in every case of chronic pannus, that the treatment be begun by a peritomy, which consists in dissecting up from the corneal margin a bridge of conjunctiva of varying thickness, and its removal. He has found that when sufficient time has been allowed, usually from four to six months, for the resulting cicatrix to become dense, white and atrophied, thus cutting off the vascular supply to the pannus, the cornea gradually becomes transparent, and the granulations either disappear or become more amenable to treatment.—B.]

2.—PHLYCTENULAR KERATITIS (HERPES CORNEÆ).

[Syn. Pustular ophthalmia.
The term "corneitis," as applied to inflammation of the cornea, is used almost solely in England, while in the United States and on the Continent of Europe the term "keratitis" is employed, which is etymologically more correct.—B.]

This disease often accompanies phlyctenular conjunctivitis. In fact, the two affections are alike in character, and demand a very similar mode of treatment.

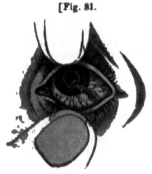

[Fig. 81.

After T. W. Jones.]

As in phlyctenular conjunctivitis, the appearance of the vesicles on the cornea is generally preceded by a sensation of heat and itching in the eyelids, which is soon followed by conjunctival and subconjunctival injection, photophobia, lachrymation, and ciliary neuralgia. The latter, which is often but slight when the affection is confined to the conjunctiva, is frequently very severe in herpes corneæ. The same is the case with the photophobia, which is often most intense and persistent. The characteristic little phlyctenulæ soon make their appearance on the surface of the cornea. [Fig. 81.] Their number and mode of distribution vary greatly. Sometimes, there are but one or two near the margin of the cornea, in other cases they are more numerous, and are either scattered freely over the surface of the cornea, or are chiefly confined to one part. Or again, they may be ranged along its edge in single file, surrounding a more or less considerable portion of the cornea, like a string of beads. If the phlyctenulæ are numerous, and extend over a considerable expanse of the cornea (pannus scrofulosus), the vascularity is general, and the cornea is surrounded by a bright, rosy zone of vessels; whereas, if the pustules are confined to one portion of the cornea, the injection is generally also partial. Sometimes, the phlyctenulæ are very superficial, and appear in the form of small, transparent vesicles or blisters, whose epithelial covering is soon shed, leaving a small excoriation, which may easily escape detection, and lead to an erroneous diagnosis and mode of treatment. Generally, however, the phlyctenula is more apparent, and is embedded in the cornea, its summit rising slightly above the surface. It appears in the form of a small, circumscribed, gray infiltration, surrounded by a zone of slightly opaque and swollen cornea, the latter being especially the case if several phlyctenulæ are situated close together. At its apex a little transparent vesicle often forms, which bursts and leaves an excoriated surface, the bottom of which is opaque, and of a gray or grayish-yellow color. This excoriation may gradually extend somewhat in circumference and depth, and assume the character of a small ulcer, which is especially apt to occur if the phlyctenula is situated near the centre of the cornea, and the affection has been injudiciously treated by strong astringents. If no transparent vesicle forms at the apex of the phlyctenula, this becomes somewhat more opaque and infiltrated, and then, losing its epithelial covering, is changed into a superficial, yellowish-gray ulcer. These ulcers generally run a very favorable course if they are judiciously treated, and show little or no tendency to extend much, either in circumference or depth. The ulcer becomes covered by a layer of epithelium, and gradually fills up, and the cornea regains more or less of its transparency. But if the infiltrations are situated very close to each other, two or three may coalesce, and thus give rise to one extensive ulcer, which may increase in depth, and even lead to perforation. This may also occur if the infiltrations are situated somewhat deeply in the cornea, and if strong local irritants (nitrate of silver, sulphate of copper, etc.) are employed. In the majority of cases there is no fear of this complication, for under judicious treatment the excoriations or little ulcers soon fill up, the corneal substance is regenerated, and perhaps no opacity is finally left. In other cases, the result is not so favorable, for a more or less dense opacity may remain behind.

There is great tendency to relapse. Just as the symptoms of irritation and vascularity are subsiding, the phlyctenulæ disappearing, and the disease seems to be almost cured, all the acute symptoms of irritation return, a fresh crop of pustules makes its appearance, and a severe relapse takes place. This may occur again and again, and the affection gradually assume a chronic character; vessels are developed upon the cornea, which run towards the infiltration, and this condition might be mistaken by a superficial observer for that of fascicular keratitis. On closer examination it will, however, be seen that the bloodvessels are few in number, and more scattered, not rising prominently above the surface of the cornea, and not pushing along the infiltration before them, but rather stopping short of it. When numerous phlyctenulæ are crowded together on the cornea, and interspersed with bloodvessels, it is often termed "herpetic or scrofulous" pannus, more especially if they are situated in the upper half of the

The causes which may produce this affection are the same as those which give rise to phlyctenular conjunctivitis, and it also occurs most frequently amongst children and young persons of a weakly, scrofulous constitution, and nervous, excitable temperament.

Sometimes, as has been especially pointed out by Prof. Horner,[1] we meet
with herpetic vesicles in the cornea in the course of catarrhal affections of
the respiratory organs, also in pneumonia, and they generally follow shortly
upon, or occur simultaneously with, herpes of the lips or nose.   This form is
characterized by the formation of numerous transparent vesicles on the
cornea, mostly arranged in groups; they are generally situated near the
margin, but may also occur at the centre.   The vesicles soon burst, and
leave behind them small excoriations deprived of epithelium, followed perhaps by infiltrations and suppurative keratitis.   The affection is very painful
and obstinate, and closely resembles the form met with in herpes zoster frontalis, excepting, as Horner shows, that in the latter there is diminution of
the intra-ocular tension and extensive anæsthesia of the cornea.

In the *treatment* of herpes corneæ accompanying catarrh of the respiratory organs, the insufflation of calomel generally greatly relieves the pain
by causing rupture of the minute vesicles.   Atropine and a bandage should
also be applied.   In the form accompanying herpes zoster, injections of morphia and electricity are often very serviceable in alleviating the sufferings
of the patient.

The *treatment* should also be similar to that which was recommended for
phlyctenular conjunctivitis.   I must here lay the greatest stress upon the
necessity of avoiding the use of caustics, more especially the nitrate of silver,
for this greatly increases the irritability of the eye, aggravates the character
of the disease, and augments any tendency to necrosis and breaking down of
the corneal tissue.   It may also cause the inflammation to extend to the iris
and ciliary body.   Indeed it may be laid down as a rule, that in all affections of the cornea, except those of a very chronic character, the use of
caustics should be most strictly avoided.   In phlyctenular keratitis our chief
endeavor must be to diminish the great irritability of the eye, to prevent the
extension of the phlyctenulæ or ulcers, and to facilitate and assist the regeneration of the corneal tissue.   The agent which we shall find of the greatest
service for these purposes is atropine.   Indeed, this remedy is invaluable in
the treatment of affections of the cornea and iris.   It exerts a beneficial influence upon the cornea by acting as a local anæsthetic during its passage
through the cornea into the aqueous humor, thus greatly diminishing the
irritability of the cornea and of the ciliary nerves.   This is often witnessed
when a drop of atropine is applied to an eye affected with acute keratitis,
accompanied by intense symptoms of irritation; for if such an eye is examined half an hour after the application of the atropine, we find a very
marked diminution in all these symptoms; the patient expressing himself
greatly relieved.   The atropine also acts by decreasing the intra-ocular tension, and thus relieving the cornea of a certain degree of pressure;[2] hence its
nutrition and the regeneration of its substance are greatly facilitated.   This
diminution in the intra-ocular tension is of special advantage in deep ulcers
of the cornea, as will be readily understood when we remember that the
thinnest portion of the cornea (the bottom of the ulcer) has to sustain the
same degree of intra-ocular pressure as the healthy part.[3]   The solution of

---

[1] "Kl. Monatsbl.," 1871, 321.

[2] This statement needs modification.   According to the most reliable and recent
tonometrical investigations, atropine diminishes the intra-vascular tension by paralyzing
the muscular coat of the vessels, but the general intra-ocular tension in the vitreous is
increased by its use.—B.]

[3] I must, however, strongly insist upon the absolute necessity of the solution of atropine being quite pure, and perfectly free from any admixture of strong acid or spirits of
wine.   A few drops of strong sulphuric acid are sometimes added by chemists when the
sulphate of atropine is not quite neutral, and therefore imperfectly soluble.   I have met

atropine (gr. ij ad f℥j of water) should be applied to the eye three or four times a day. If it should, after a time, be found rather to increase than alleviate the irritation, a collyrium of belladonna must be substituted. If it has already produced considerable irritation of the conjunctiva and a crop of vesicular granulations, an astringent collyrium of alum, borax, or nitrate of silver (gr. j ad f℥j) should be employed. The belladonna ointment is to be rubbed on the forehead three or four times daily, until a slight papular eruption is produced. If there is much pain in and around the eye, and more especially if the latter is very painful to the touch, much relief is often experienced from the application of two or three leeches to the temples, or a blister should be applied behind the ear. If, together with the photophobia and lachrymation, the temperature of the lids is much increased, I have often found very marked benefit from the periodical application of cold compresses. [If the case is marked by obstinate photophobia, the forcible opening of the lids and dropping iced water directly upon the cornea, as recommended by Dr. Oppenheimer, will very often prove beneficial.—B.] These are to be applied three or four times a day, for a space of twenty to thirty minutes, and are to be changed every two or three minutes, as soon as they get the least warm. The photophobia is often, however, very obstinate and intractable. When it is chiefly due to an abrasion of the epithelium and exposure of the corneal nerves, a compress bandage should be applied. But sometimes it resists all remedies, and a severe spasm of the lids (blepharospasm) remains even after the affection of the cornea is cured. In such cases, the different remedies which I have mentioned in the articles on phlyctenular conjunctivitis, should be tried, viz., subcutaneous injection of morphia, immersion of the face in cold water, and if all these fail, and the spasm is arrested by pressure upon the supra-orbital nerve, we must have recourse to a division of this nerve. I have often found that a prolonged stay at the seaside, together with sea-bathing, tonics, a generous diet, and plenty of out-of-door exercise will cure cases of photophobia which have obstinately resisted all other remedies.

[Solutions of daturine and duboisine, in the form of sulphate, have been used in place of atropine where the latter has caused irritation, but there seems to be no special advantage in either. Both irritate the conjunctiva when used for a length of time, and often give rise to vesicular granulations, just as the atropine does. Duboisine has only recently been made

with several instances in which a pure solution of atropine proved of the greatest benefit in allaying the irritability of the eye and in alleviating the inflammation, and in which a fresh supply of atropine (made up after the same prescription, but obtained from a different chemist) has at once set up severe irritation of the eye, accompanied by considerable pain, redness, lachrymation, etc., but these symptoms soon disappeared again on the use of a pure solution of atropine. On examination, the impure solution was found to contain a small quantity of strong sulphuric acid. Such cases as this completely disprove the theory that a small quantity of strong acid or of alcohol can have any prejudicial effect upon the eye, even although there may be much ciliary irritation and a severe inflammation of the cornea or iris. I must state, however, that we occasionally meet with exceptional cases in which there exists a peculiar idiosyncrasy which renders the patient most intolerant of the use of even a weak and imperfectly pure solution of atropine. I have seen instances in which a drop of a weak and quite pure solution of atropine has produced great irritation and pain, or even an erysipelatous condition of the eyelids and cheek, accompanied by redness and chemotic swelling of the conjunctiva. This is, however, a very exceptional occurrence, and bears not the slightest analogy to those cases in which the irritation is caused by the impurity of the atropine; for in such, a pure solution is not only well borne, but greatly alleviates the ciliary irritation and inflammatory symptoms. Mr. Lawson also mentions some interesting instances of this peculiar idiosyncrasy, in a paper in the "R. L. O. H. Reports," known to ophthalmic surgeons, but it contains many of the constituents of atropine. It has not, however, been sufficiently long in use to admit of definitely settling its place in ophthalmic therapeutics.—B.]

Arsenic has been strongly recommended in this form of keratitis, on the supposition of its similarity to eczema. This remedy often proves very serviceable, especially if the keratitis is accompanied by an eczematous eruption of the forehead and face. In the latter case, the lotion of acetate of lead and glycerine (p. 183) should be applied to the face; or the following lotion may be used for the same purpose: R. Boracis ʒij, Glycer. fʒss, Aq. sambuci fʒij, Aq. dest. ad fʒviij. A powder containing oxide of zinc may be dusted over the face. The patient's general health should be attended to, and, if he is of a weakly and scrofulous habit, tonics, cod-liver oil, and a nutritious and generous diet, together with the use of ale and wine, should be prescribed. The bowels should be kept well regulated, and special attention should be paid to the free action of the skin, as this exerts a marked influence upon the symptoms of ciliary irritation, especially the photophobia. When the acute symptoms have subsided, we must have recourse to the insufflation of calomel, and, if this is well borne, the yellow oxide of mercury ointment (gr. j–ij ad ʒj) should be applied; this will not only hasten the absorption of any remaining opacity, but check the tendency to relapses. In chronic and very obstinate cases, especially if they are accompanied by much vascularity of the cornea, great benefit is often experienced from a seton.

[Within the last few years a great deal has been said and written upon the use of eserine and pilocarpine in conjunctival and corneal affections. Dr. H. W. Williams, of Boston, was the first to make any extended experiments in this country, and he reports very favorably on both drugs as valuable in conjunctival and corneal diseases, especially ulcers ("Boston Medical and Surgical Journal," March 14, 1878; "Trans. of Amer. Ophthal. Soc.," 1878). In those forms of disease met with so frequently in strumous children, the photophobia and blepharospasm are very often relieved by eserine sulphate (gr. ij ad fʒj). In the ordinary form of conjunctival herpes, eserine does not seem to do any good, but where the vesicles are large and coalesce, with zones of infiltration, eserine acts like a charm. In ulcers of cornea, eserine sometimes does good, especially in the serpiginous form, but, in the long run, better results will be obtained from atropine. The hydrochlorate of pilocarpine, in solutions of two or four grains to the fluidounce, seems to be of much more limited application than eserine, and, though in the hands of Dr. Williams and some other observers it has proved very useful, it has not answered the expectations of ophthalmic surgeons. An ointment of iodoform has been recommended in these herpetic affections of the cornea and conjunctiva, and seems in some cases to do good in allaying photophobia and irritation. The chief objection to its use is its disagreeable odor (Iodoform gr. v–x ad Vaseline ʒj).—B.]

In rare instances, we meet with a peculiar formation of transparent vesicles upon the surface of the cornea, which are produced by slight elevations of the epithelial layer and the anterior elastic lamina from the surface of the cornea proper. The appearance presented by these little blisters is very characteristic, and is generally accompanied by very severe symptoms of irritation, especially photophobia and lachrymation. These symptoms subside when the vesicles burst, but a fresh crop of the latter is generally formed every three or four days. In a case mentioned by Mooren, the disease assumed the character of a regular tertian type, and was cured by the energetic use of quinine; indeed this remedy, combined perhaps with steel, should be given in all cases, atropine and a compress bandage being applied to the eye.

3.—FASCICULAR KERATITIS.

This peculiar form of keratitis, which is very common in Germany, is extremely rare in England, for whilst I saw many instances of it in Berlin, I only remember having met with four pure cases in England during the last eight years.

The symptoms of this affection are very characteristic, and easily recognised. The attack is generally ushered in by considerable photophobia, lachrymation, and ciliary neuralgia. On examining the eye, the ocular conjunctiva is found to be injected, and there is also seen a bright rosy zone of subconjunctival vessels round the cornea. Near the edge of the latter may perhaps be noticed at one spot a few small phlyctenulæ, and the limbus conjunctivæ is at this point also somewhat swollen. The parallel subconjunctival vessels are seen at this spot to pass on to the cornea and extend more or less on to its surface, forming a narrow bundle or leash of vessels (hence the term "fascicular" keratitis), which lies in a somewhat swollen and elevated portion of the cornea. This fasciculus of vessels consists both of veins and arteries; at its apex, and rising somewhat above the level of the vessels, is noticed a small, crescentic, yellowish-gray infiltration, surrounded by a somewhat opaque and swollen portion of cornea. As the disease progresses, the infiltration is gradually pushed further and further on to the cornea in front of the vessels; its epithelial covering is shed, it assumes a yellowish tint, and becomes changed into a small superficial ulcer. In some instances the original leash of vessels may bifurcate, so that it assumes a Y-shape, having a separate infiltration at each apex. The disease may extend far on to the cornea, and prove dangerous from its leaving a dense opacity in the centre of the cornea just over the pupil; but the ulcer generally remains superficial, and does not extend very deeply into the cornea or lead to perforation. During the progressive stage, the symptoms of irritation are very marked and obstinate. When the disease has reached its acme, it generally remains stationary for some little time (perhaps even several weeks) and then gradually diminishes in intensity and slowly retrogrades, the symptoms of irritation rapidly disappearing. The time which elapses during these several stages will depend upon the size of the fasciculus of vessels and of the infiltration. The vascularity gradually diminishes, the ulcer is again covered by a layer of epithelium, and begins to fill up from the periphery towards the centre; the corneal tissue is more or less regenerated, and after a time but little opacity may be left.

This disease is generally due to the same causes as phlyctenular conjunctivitis, and is most frequently met with in weakly and scrofulous persons, and in them it is very apt to run a most protracted course.

If the symptoms of irritation are very acute, only soothing remedies should be applied. Atropine should be dropped into the eye, the compound belladonna ointment should be rubbed in over the forehead, a blister should be applied behind the ear, and a leech or two to the temple if the eye is very painful to the touch. If the vascularity is very marked and the case severe, benefit is often derived from dividing the bundle of vessels close to the cornea, either with a small scalpel or a pair of curved scissors; for after this has been done, the bloodvessels on the cornea and the infiltration are generally shrink and diminish in size. When the acute symptoms of irritation have considerably subsided, the insufflation of calomel should be at once commenced, or the yellow oxide of mercury ointment (gr. ij–viij ad ʒj) should be applied. Both these remedies, but more especially the yellow oxide, are almost specifics for this disease. The ointment may be applied from the very commencement, if the symptoms of irritation are not very marked; it must, however, be used with care, and its effect should be closely watched. If we find the next day that it has excited considerable redness and irritation, its use should be temporarily abstained from, and calomel should be substituted. It is also of much use in checking the tendency to relapses, in cutting these short, and in hastening the absorption of the corneal opacity. Frequently, we must alternate between the ointment and the calomel, as after a time they temporarily lose some of their effect.

A seton at the temple sometimes also proves of much benefit in this affection, not only in shortening the course of the disease, but also in preventing the occurrence of relapses.

4.—SUPPURATIVE KERATITIS..

[Syn. Abscess of the cornea.—B.]

Practically, it is of importance to distinguish two principal forms of suppurative keratitis. The one is accompanied by more or less marked inflammatory symptoms, whilst in the other these are entirely absent, and the chief danger of the disease is found in their absence, as the suppuration spreads very rapidly, and an extensive abscess or slough of the cornea speedily ensues. These two forms also demand a totally opposite plan of treatment. In the inflammatory, we must endeavor to check and subdue the symptoms of irritation and inflammation by local antiphlogistics; whereas in the torpid, non-inflammatory form, we must most carefully eschew such treatment, and at once attempt to produce a certain degree of inflammation, in order to check the tendency to necrosis and purulent infiltration.

Whilst drawing special attention to these two opposite types of the disease, I must state that in practice we constantly meet with mixed forms, showing some of the symptoms of each type. Indeed, the surgeon will chiefly display his skill and judgment by distinguishing whether any of the symptoms have attained an undue prominence and require to be checked, in order that a just balance may be maintained between the necessary degree of inflammation and the suppurative condition of the cornea; so that whilst on the one hand the inflammatory symptoms are not allowed to become excessive, they are, on the other, not too much suppressed.

The inflammatory suppurative keratitis is often accompanied by great photophobia, lachrymation, and intense ciliary neuralgia; there is also much conjunctival and subconjunctival injection, the cornea being surrounded by a bright rosy zone, accompanied perhaps by some chemosis. On account of the irritation of the ciliary nerves, the pupil is often greatly contracted. On examining the cornea, we notice a small circumscribed infiltration, which is generally situated near the centre, but sometimes at the periphery of the cornea. Its position varies, sometimes it is situated in the superficial layers of the cornea, and then the latter may become somewhat raised above the level at this point, or it may lie in the central or deeper portion of the cornea, in which case the surface remains unaltered. The infiltration soon increases in density, and assumes a creamy, yellowish-gray color, being surrounded by a well-marked line of demarcation in the form of a light-gray zone, which gradually shades off into the transparent cornea; the latter also shows a certain degree of inflammatory swelling at the point occupied by this zone. The epithelium may be shed, and a portion of the contents of the infiltration break down and be thrown off, so that a more or less deep ulcer is formed. Although the subconjunctival vessels may pass slightly on to the cornea, they never reach the ulcer, even when this is situated near the periphery. When it is in the centre of the cornea, the latter appears quite free from bloodvessels, except a few which may just pass over its margin. The retrogressive stage generally soon sets in, the infiltration changes its yellow hue for a light-gray tint, and becomes gradually absorbed, leaving perhaps hardly any opacity behind. The disease as a rule shows a tendency to remain localized, and not to extend superficially, but rather in depth. Relapses are apt to occur, and the affection may thus assume a chronic character.

But the disease does not always run so favorable a course. Thus, several superficial infiltrations may be formed close to each other, and, gradually extending in circumference and depth, may coalesce, and thus give rise to a considerable abscess of the cornea. Their contents undergo suppurative and fatty degeneration, the cells and nuclei break down, the infiltration assumes a yellow color, being surrounded, however, by a grayish-white zone of demarcation. If this occurs near the centre of the cornea, it may prove dangerous from its leaving a dense opacity just over the pupil, or from its perhaps leading to an extensive slough of the cornea. Again, if the infiltration is situated deeply in the cornea, it may lead to perforation of the latter, or give rise to onyx, hypopyon, and iritis. The pus may sink down between the lamellæ of the cornea to its lower margin, and thus produce a peculiar opacity, termed onyx or unguis, on account of its supposed resemblance to the white lunula of the finger-nail. If the onyx is but small, and confined to the very edge of the cornea, it may easily be overlooked, more especially if it be somewhat covered by the swollen limbus conjunctivæ. If it is more considerable, so that it reaches nearly up to one-third of the cornea, or even higher, it may be mistaken for an hypopyon; but on careful examination (more especially with the oblique illumination) it will not be difficult to distinguish it from the latter, for it will be seen to lie on the corneal side of the anterior chamber, a portion of transparent cornea perhaps dividing it from the latter; and it is situated at some distance from the iris. But the differential diagnosis is of course more difficult if, as is sometimes the case, an hypopyon coexists with the onyx.

The hypopyon which not unfrequently accompanies suppurative keratitis (more especially the non-inflammatory form) may be produced either from the iris or from the cornea in the following ways:

1. An inflammation of the iris may supervene upon the keratitis, lymph be effused into the aqueous humor, and, falling to the bottom of the anterior chamber, thus produce an hypopyon.

2. The abscess may perforate the cornea, and its purulent contents be carried into the aqueous humor and be precipitated at the bottom of the anterior chamber. Sometimes such a mode of production of hypopyon is completely overlooked, from the fact that the communication between the anterior chamber and the abscess in the cornea is not large and direct, but is brought about by a small sloping canal, through which the contents of the abscess have made their way into the anterior chamber. Special attention has been called to this fact by Weber,[1] who has, moreover, frequently passed a minute probe from the ulcer through the canal into the anterior chamber, and thus verified the communication. With the oblique illumination, this little canal appears like a white streak, running from the abscess to the anterior chamber.

[1] "A. f. O.," viii. 1, 322.

3. When the abscess is situated deeply in the cornea, near the membrane of Descemet, inflammatory proliferation and fatty degeneration of the epithelial cells lining the posterior portion of the cornea may occur. They are thrown off, and, mixing with the aqueous humor, render this turbid, and if these deposits are considerable in quantity, they may fall down to the bottom of the anterior chamber, and thus produce an hypopyon. It has been also supposed that the latter is often due to a transudation of some of the contents of the deep-seated abscess into the aqueous humor.[1] Weber, however, asserts that he has never met with an instance in which the communication between the abscess and the anterior chamber could not be distinctly proved by means of probing. I have, however, met with cases of abscess in the middle portion of the cornea which have been accompanied by an infiltration situated at the membrane of Descemet, and an hypopyon evidently produced by the latter (for there was no iritis), and in which I have failed, on the most careful examination by the oblique illumination, to trace any communication between the abscess and the posterior infiltration.

Inflammatory suppurative keratitis is met with in severe and aggravated cases of phlyctenular keratitis, and also in severe cases of purulent, granular, and diphtheritic conjunctivitis. It is very frequently caused by mechanical and chemical injuries, such as the lodgement of chips of steel, a bit of wheat-ear, etc., in the substance of the cornea, which perhaps remain there undiscovered. This is especially the case in old or very feeble persons. It may also follow operations upon the eye, more particularly those for cataract.

In the milder cases of inflammatory suppurative keratitis, atropine should be applied three or four times daily, and the compress bandage employed. If there is much irritability and ciliary neuralgia, and if the eye is very painful to the touch, two or three leeches should be applied to the temple. Subcutaneous injections of morphia may also be employed with great advantage. If the abscess resists all treatment, great benefit is often derived from slightly opening it with the point of an extraction knife. But if it is deep-seated, and threatens to perforate the cornea, paracentesis should be performed by passing a fine needle into the anterior chamber through the bottom of the abscess. If a considerable hypopyon exists, paracentesis should also be performed, but with a broad needle, the object of the operation being not so much to remove the lymph from the anterior chamber as to diminish the intra-ocular pressure, and thus to arrest the progress of the disease, to hasten the absorption of the infiltration, and facilitate the regeneration of the corneal tissue. This operation may have to be repeated several times (vide treatment of ulcers of the cornea by paracentesis). In order to diminish the intra-ocular pressure still more completely, and more effectually to subdue the inflammation, it may be very advisable to perform iridectomy in cases in which suppurative keratitis is extensive, threatens perforation, and is accompanied by hypopyon. This is more especially the case if the abscess is deep, and situated in the centre of the cornea, for even if it should not perforate, it will leave a dense leucoma, which will subsequently necessitate the formation of an artificial pupil. It is, therefore, much wiser to make an iridectomy at once, as this will exert a beneficial influence upon the course of the disease, and leave an artificial pupil opposite a clear portion of the cornea.

In the non-inflammatory suppurative keratitis there is generally a very marked absence of all the usual symptoms of irritation and inflammation. There is no photophobia, lachrymation, or pain, and the eye appears, in fact,

[1] Roser, "A. f. O.," ii. 2, 151.

abnormally insensible to external irritation (bright light, etc.). It may, however, supervene upon a circumscribed infiltration of the cornea, accompanied by severe symptoms of irritation and intense ciliary neuralgia. These symptoms suddenly yield, and the abscess shows a tendency to necrosis, extending quickly in circumference and depth. There is formed very rapidly, often in the course of a few hours, in the centre of the cornea, a small yellow spot, which is sharply defined against the clear and transparent cornea, and is not surrounded by an opaque gray zone, as is the case with the inflammatory infiltration. Indeed, the adjoining portion of the cornea may even appear abnormally lustrous, which is probably due to serous infiltration. The yellow color is also more deep and pronounced than in the inflammatory form. The disease rapidly extends in circumference, and consecutive yellow layers are formed around the original infiltration. The tissue of the cornea becomes quickly broken down, undergoes fatty degeneration, and pus-cells are formed in large quantity, and the abscess soon gains a considerable extent, both on the surface and in depth, reaching, perhaps, nearly to the membrane of Descemet. When the suppuration has attained a certain depth, the epithelial cells lining the membrane of Descemet undergo inflammatory proliferation, and, being thrown off, mix with the aqueous humor, rendering this turbid, and perhaps sinking down in the anterior chamber in the form of a hypopyon. The iris becomes swollen, hyperæmic, and of a yellowish-red color, due probably in part to the hyperæmia, and in part to a purulent infiltration of its tissue. There are generally no firm adhesions between the edge of the pupil and the capsule of the lens. The tendency of this non-inflammatory form of suppurative keratitis is to extend rather in circumference than in depth, so that it leads to very considerable opacity or even extensive suppuration of the cornea, with all its dangerous consequences.

[In abscess of the cornea, iritis with adhesions is a very common complication.—B.]

When the process of reparation sets in, we find that the yellow and sharply defined infiltration becomes surrounded by a grayish zone, and that there is at the same time an increase in the vascularity of the eye. Much of the danger is now past, for the disease assumes more of the character of inflammatory suppurative keratitis and shows a tendency to become limited, and there is, consequently, much less fear of purulent necrosis and sloughing of the cornea. Gradually the yellow color is changed to a whitish gray, the purulent infiltration breaks down and is absorbed, and the corneal tissue is regenerated. It may, after a time, even regain its normal transparency, especially in children, and if the infiltration was but small and superficial. Otherwise, a more or less dense opacity is left behind, which, if it be situated in the centre, may cause great impairment of vision. But if a sufficient portion of the margin of the cornea is transparent and of normal curvature, excellent sight may often be restored by the formation of an artificial pupil. But, unfortunately, so favorable a result is not always obtained in severe and extensive suppurative keratitis. Perforation of the cornea but too frequently takes place, followed by anterior synechia or staphyloma, or the inflammation extends to the other tissues of the eyeball, and panophthalmitis occurs, ending in atrophy of the globe.

Non-inflammatory suppurative keratitis occurs frequently in very aged and feeble persons, more especially after operations involving the cornea (such as those for cataract, particularly the flap extraction), or after injuries to the cornea from foreign bodies striking it or becoming lodged on its surface or in its substance. Thus, it is not unfrequently met with amongst aged country people, if a bit of wheat-ear, or perhaps the wing of an insect, becomes embedded in the cornea and is not removed at once. I have seen it produced in some instances by a simple concussion from a blow against the eye by a bit of wood, the bough of a tree, etc., without any wound of the cornea. Von Graefe ("A. f. O.," xii. 2, 250) has also described cases of suppuration of the cornea occurring in infants suffering from encephalitis.[1] It may likewise supervene upon severe constitutional diseases, which have greatly weakened the general health, such as typhus fever, cholera, encephalitis, diabetes, etc.

It may also follow paralysis of the fifth nerve, and is then termed neuroparalytic keratitis. The affection of the cornea is generally chronic, and occurs some time after the paralysis. If the latter is partial, the cornea is but rarely affected, and then only partially, and not to a severe extent. The eye loses its sensibility, so that when irritants (e. g., astringent collyria) are applied to it, they excite redness, but no feeling of pain or discomfort; indeed their presence is unfelt. The cornea then becomes opaque, ulcers may form, and suppuration may take place, leading perhaps to perforation, hypopyon, etc., and the inflammation may even extend to the iris. The epithelium of the cornea and conjunctiva becomes rough and desiccated, so that a certain degree of xerophthalmia is produced. One very interesting fact is, that paralysis of the fifth nerve always produces a diminution of the intraocular tension, and this is a point of the utmost importance with regard to the whole question of glaucoma and increased intra-ocular tension.

[Haase thinks that the Gasserian ganglion is not the seat of the centre of nutrition for certain definite nerve-fibres, but that this centre is situated at the origin of the nerves; and that disturbances of innervation in the eye occur also from pathological changes above the ganglion of Gasser, the nervous structure of the ganglion itself being found unaltered. (See "Archiv für Ophthalmologie," xxvii. 1.)—B.]

The affection of the cornea which may ensue upon paralysis of the fifth nerve is apparently not due to malnutrition of the part, but simply to mechanical injuries, caused by the action of external irritants (dust, sand, etc.) to which the eye is exposed, and whose presence, on account of its insensibility, it does not resent or feel. That this is so, has been uncontrovertibly proved by the experiments of Snellen[2] and others. Snellen divided the fifth nerve in rabbits, and sewed their ears over their eyes, so as to protect the latter from all external irritants, and he found that when this was done the cornea did not become affected, whereas it began to become opaque the very day after the eye was left uncovered. More lately he has reported[3] a very interesting case, which fully bears out this view. A man, thirty-six years of age, was affected with complete paralysis of the left fifth nerve, together with paralysis of the sixth nerve of the same side. In consequence of the latter, there existed a convergent squint of the left eye, and on the outer side of the cornea there was a superficial ulcer, surrounded by a tolerably broad gray zone. The eye was quite insensible, and the acuteness of vision diminished to $\frac{11}{cc}$, and its tension was much decreased. In order to ascertain with certainty whether the affection of the cornea was due to malnutrition of the eye, or to its exposure to external irritants, Snellen fastened, by means of strips of plaster, a stenopaic shell over the eye, in order to protect it. A small central aperture was left for the patient to see through, so that he might ascertain whether the shell retained its proper position, for

[1] Vide also Hirschberg's article, "Berl. klin. Wochenschrift," 1868, No. 31.
[2] "Virchow's Archiv," vol. xiii., 1868.   [3] "Jaarlijksch Verslag," etc., 1868.

from the want of sensibility of the eye, he could not determine it otherwise. The shell was removed twice a day, in order that the eye might be washed and cleansed. The improvement in the condition of the cornea and the sight was very marked, for within two days the vision $= \dfrac{20}{LXX}$, and the cornea cleared so rapidly, that in eight days after the application of the shell the acuteness of vision was normal, viz., $= \dfrac{20}{XX}$. Only a small opacity remained at the outer side of the cornea, but the loss of sensibility and the diminished tension continued. The application of turpentine and nitrate of silver produced the same symptoms of congestion as in a normal eye, without, however, being felt by the patient. The stenopaic cup was left off, and the eye exposed; within two days the eye became again more inflamed, and the vision became diminished to $\dfrac{20}{C}$. It shortly regained its normal standard after the reapplication of the shell.

Meissner[1] is, however, of opinion that this tendency to inflammation of the cornea is not altogether due to the loss of sensibility, for he has observed three cases[2] in which no keratitis ensued after division of the ophthalmic branch of the fifth nerve, although the eye was quite insensible, and not guarded against external irritants. On examination, it was found that in all these instances the innermost portion of the nerve had escaped division. He, therefore, considers it probable that the fibres of this portion of the nerve render the eye more able to resist the effect of external irritants, etc. This supposition is strengthened by another case, in which Meissner incompletely divided the fifth nerve in a rabbit, and, although the sensibility of the eye was not impaired, the inflammation of the cornea ensued in the customary manner. On examination, it was found that only the median (innermost) portion of the nerve had been divided. Schiff[3] has repeated these experiments, with exactly the same results.

The very dangerous character of non-inflammatory suppurative keratitis is chiefly due to the rapidity with which the infiltration extends, more especially in circumference, and to the great tendency to purulent necrosis of the corneal tissue, which leads but too frequently to very extensive suppuration of the cornea, or even to purulent disorganization of the eyeball. This disease proves especially disastrous if it be treated by the ordinary antiphlogistics, e. g., cold compresses, leeches, etc., more particularly in severe cases. Thus Von Graefe found, that, when he pursued this mode of treatment, he lost about three-fourths of the severer cases; whereas his success was very marked as soon as he substituted warm fomentations and the compress bandage. The object of the warm fomentations is to excite a certain degree of inflammatory reaction and swelling in the conjunctiva and cornea; for in the total absence of these is to be sought the chief danger of the disease. They also hasten the limitation of the suppuration, expedite the absorption of the infiltration, and favor the process of reparation. After their application the eye becomes more injected, and this is accompanied by inflammatory swelling of the conjunctiva. The vascularity also extends more or less on to the cornea. The infiltration is no longer sharply defined against the transparent cornea, but a gray halo appears around it, and this portion of the cornea is somewhat swollen, and the line of demarcation soon becomes well

[1] Henle and Pfeuffer's "Zeitschrift" (3), xxix. 96.
[2] These experiments were made on rabbits.
[3] Henle and Pfeuffer's "Zeitschrift" (3), xxxix. p. 217.

marked. If an hypopyon exists, and is not very considerable in extent, we often find that it becomes rapidly absorbed after the use of warm fomentations. Von Graefe[1] generally uses warm chamomile fomentations, varying in temperature from about 90° to 104° of Fahrenheit, according to the condition of the eye. The less the symptoms of inflammatory irritation, the higher should the temperature be. They should be changed every five minutes, and their use suspended for one-quarter in every hour. The temperature should be lowered and the fomentations changed less frequently, or a longer interval be allowed to elapse between their application, as soon as the zone of demarcation and the inflammatory swelling make their appearance, and the necrosed portions of cornea begin to be thrown off. If these points are not attended to, we may set up too great an inflammatory reaction, so that it may even become necessary to check it by antiphlogistic applications (cold compresses, leeches, etc.). Saemisch,[2] who has extensively studied the effect of warm fomentations, advocates their continuation for a somewhat longer period in certain cases, in order to promote the exfoliation of the necrosed portions, and to expedite the absorption of the morbid products. Their effect must then, however, be closely watched, in order that too much inflammation is not set up. Indeed, the employment of warm fomentations requires great circumspection and attention, and cannot be entrusted to a stupid or careless nurse, for if they are applied too hot, changed too frequently, or continued too long, they may produce an excess of inflammation; or if, on the other hand, they are permitted to get cold, they are even still more injurious, by diminishing the vitality of the part, and thus increasing the tendency to necrosis. Where I cannot rely upon the care and attention of the nurse, I am in the habit of ordering the occasional use of warm poppy or chamomile fomentations at stated periods; for instance, three or four times a day for the period of half an hour; the fomentations being changed every five minutes during that time. In this way, considerable benefit may be derived from their use, without incurring any risk.

Warm fomentations are indicated in all forms of non-inflammatory suppurative keratitis, whether of spontaneous origin, or caused by injuries to the eye or operations (especially those for the removal of cataract). They may also be necessary in cases of inflammatory suppurative keratitis if the symptoms of inflammation have sunk below a certain point.

Great advantage is also experienced from the use of a firm compress or the "pressure bandage" (vide p. 48), for this is of much service in limiting the extent of the suppuration and hastening the formation of the zone of demarcation. Its application should alternate with the warm fomentations.[3] Even a certain degree of iritis does not contraindicate its use. According to Von Graefe, it is not, however, applicable in those cases in which the purulent necrosis occurs rapidly, after the sudden cessation of severe symptoms of irritation and ciliary neuralgia, with which the disease was ushered in. After the pain had been alleviated by a subcutaneous injection of morphia, and warm fomentations had been applied, Von Graefe found much benefit from the use of chlorine wate.[4] [Solutions of salicylic acid and of borax (the latter in the proportion of 3j to the Oj) have been recommended in these cases when the chlorine water proves too irritating.—B.] If there is any iritis and the aqueous humor is turbid, with or without the presence of hypopyon, it is most advisable to perform iridectomy without delay. This

---

[1] "A. f. O.," vi. 2, 133. Vide also the author's abstract of this paper in "Roy. Lond. Ophth. Hosp. Reports," vol. iii. 128.
[2] "Klinische Beobachtungen von Pagenstecher und Saemisch," ii. 102; 1862.
[3] "A. f. O.," vol. ix. 2, 151.   [4] Ibid., vol. x. 2, 205.

will generally at once cut short the progress of the disease and stop the extension of the suppuration. But if it is found that this improvement is but temporary, and lasts but for a few days, Von Graefe advises that the chlorine water should be again applied. He has done this even within thirty hours after the operation, if fresh crescentic infiltrations showed themselves around the original abscess, and he found that there extension was decidedly and markedly checked by this remedy.

In the neuro-paralytic form of keratitis, a light bandage should be applied over the eye, so as to protect it against all external irritants. It should be removed two or three times daily, and the eye washed and cleansed. If the case be seen sufficiently early and before any considerable mischief has been done, this remedy will generally suffice rapidly to cure the affection of the cornea. [Good results have occasionally been obtained from the use of the constant galvanic current, applied daily for from fifteen minutes to half an hour, one pole over the closed lids and the other behind the ear, and the direction of the current reversed during the sitting.—B.]

Atropine drops should always be applied, as they not only act as an anodyne, but also diminish the intra-ocular tension. They are of especial importance if there is any iritis. Dr. Warlomont speaks very highly of the use of Van Roosbroeck's ointment in cases of indolent, necrotic corneal ulcers. Its composition is as follows: Hydrar. subsulph. gr. 4, 6, or 8, Bals. Peruv. ℥ 10–15, Axung. ℥ss.

If perforation of the cornea appears imminent, and the ulcer is not of considerable size, a paracentesis should be made with a fine needle through the bottom of the ulcer, so as to allow the aqueous humor to flow off very slowly. This will diminish the intra-ocular tension and facilitate the absorption of the infiltration, and the filling up of the ulcer. But if the infiltration or ulcer is deep seated, of considerable extent, and shows a tendency to increase still more, or to perforate the cornea, paracentesis should be at once performed. It is also indicated if a certain degree of hypopyon is present, with or without iritis. It has been already stated, that our object in tapping the anterior chamber is less to remove the lymph than to diminish the intra-ocular pressure, and thus to stop the progress of the disease, hasten the absorption of the morbid products, and facilitate the regeneration of the corneal tissue. The incision is to be made with a broad needle in the cornea near its lower edge, and the aqueous humor should be allowed to flow off very slowly indeed. It may be necessary to repeat the operation several times, or, in order that its effect may be more lasting, the little wound may be kept patent by the occasional insertion of a small probe once or twice a day.

But if the hypopyon is considerable in size, occupying perhaps one-third or one-half of the anterior chamber, if there is much iritis, or if the abscess in the cornea extends very deeply, and threatens to cause an extensive perforation, it is of great importance that an iridectomy should be made without loss of time; for the intra-ocular tension will be thus more completely diminished, and for a longer period, than by the paracentesis. We generally find that the iridectomy exerts a most beneficial influence upon the suppuration of the cornea, and also as an antiphlogistic upon the inflammation of the iris. The progress of the suppuration, both in circumference and depth, is arrested, the deeper layers of the cornea do not become necrosed, and the absorption of morbid products and the process of repair are hastened. Indeed, I think that an iridectomy should generally be preferred to a paracentesis, if the disease be at all severe and threatening perforation, more especially if the abscess or ulcer be of considerable size

15

... for them it will leave a dense
... the formation of an artificial

... follow an iridectomy in these cases.
... the pupil becomes blocked by a
... the corneal process. Opening the
... ...sion of any portion of iris, is a
...—B.]
... iridectomy should be made down-
... that the lymph may escape with
... ...cision. If it does not escape readily,
... ...rior chamber than to pull and drag
... this may set up great irritation. I
... ...king the iridectomy upwards and
... by a pair of forceps, for this will
... and may produce much irritation

... paracentesis should be made with a
... abscess, so that it may be split across;
... the incision will carry with it more or
... and thus cleanse it and favor its filling
... performed (vide p. 232).
... recommended by Fuchs and others, as a
... I: should be heated to a faint red heat.
... and the subsequent reaction is very slight.
... ...ently opaque.—B.]
... ...tive keratitis it is of great importance to
... ...th. As this affection is most prone to
... and is old and feeble individuals, tonics
... freely administered, and the patient be
... wine or malt liquor. I have been occa-
... ...is kind as hospital out-patients, and have
... ...very successful results, even although the
... and accompanied by some hypopyon and
... applied atropine, warm poppy fomenta-
... and a compress bandage, and performed
... when the hypopyon had reached to more
... ...mber. I have at the same time prescribed
... ...mbined perhaps with ammonia or mixed
... stimulants.
... ...ate of uterine in all asthenic corneal ulcers;
... ...ss of scrofulous and cachectic subjects; in
... ...uro-paralytic keratitis. (See "Annali di

... ...ld induce us to treat such cases as out-
... gravest nature, and demands the frequent
... constant care of a good nurse.

OF THE CORNEA.

... in importance and danger according to
... in some cases their course is acute and
... protracted, obstinately defying almost
... less important and dangerous than the

deep-seated ulcers. In the former, we should not include mere abrasions of the epithelium such as may occur after slight injuries from foreign bodies, or from the bursting of the vesicle in phlyctenular corneitis. The term ulcer should, I think, be confined to cases in which there is a breaking down and elimination of the affected corneal tissue, so that there is a distinct loss of substance.

When speaking of phlyctenulæ and the inflammatory infiltrations of the cornea, it was mentioned that their contents often break down, soften, and are thrown off, giving rise to an ulcer, which may either remain superficial or extend somewhat deeply into the corneal tissue. But the tendency to ulceration may also show itself from the outset. Then there is noticed, near the centre of the margin of the cornea, a small opacity, the edges of which are somewhat irregular, swollen, and of a gray color, which shades off to a lighter tint towards the centre, so that the latter may even seem quite transparent. The ulcer, whose epithelial covering is lost, is surrounded by a zone of gray and somewhat swollen cornea; it gradually assumes a more yellow tint, and extends in depth and circumference, its contents breaking down and being cast off, so that it may reach a considerable extent before its progress can be stopped. It is often accompanied by severe symptoms of irritation, great photophobia, lachrymation, and ciliary neuralgia. When the process of reparation sets in, we notice that the epithelial layer is gradually formed, this reparation commencing from the periphery. Then the ulcer assumes a grayer tint and is gradually filled up by new tissue, which may resemble very greatly the normal corneal tissue, although the intercellular substance is apt to be not quite transparent, thus giving rise to a certain amount of opacity. Sometimes the process of repair is extremely slow, and many months elapse before the ulcer is healed. As soon as the layer of epithelium is regenerated, the symptoms of irritation, more especially the pain and photophobia, rapidly subside. Bloodvessels (both venous and arterial) appear upon the cornea [Fig. 82] and run towards the ulcer, hastening the process of reparation and absorption, and dwindling down and disappearing when their task is done. Sometimes the reparative process is incomplete, and a more or less deep, opaque depression or facet, of a somewhat cicatricial appearance, remains behind.

[Fig. 82.]

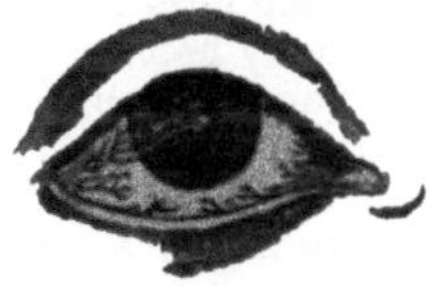

We sometimes meet with a peculiar form of funnel-shaped ulcer, which shows a very marked tendency to extend in depth and perforate the cornea, obstinately and persistently resisting all and every kind of treatment until perforation has taken place, when it at once begins to heal.

Another and very dangerous form is the crescentic ulcer, which commences near the edge of the cornea, and looks as if a little portion had been chipped out with the finger-nail. It shows a great tendency to extend more and more round the edge of the cornea like a trench (in which the cornea is much thinned), until it may even encircle the whole cornea. The vitality of the central portion is generally greatly impaired, and it becomes more and more opaque, and shrivels up until it may look like a yellow, dry, friable, or cheesy substance, portions of the surface of which may be thrown off, or it may give way and a very extensive rupture of the cornea take place. This crescentic ulcer is extremely dangerous and intractable, resisting often most obstinately every form of treatment. In some cases great advantage has been derived from syndectomy, either partial, if the ulcer was but of slight extent; or complete, if a considerable portion of the cornea had become involved. In other cases I have, however, seen it do but very little good. Iridectomy has also been sometimes found of benefit, and should be preferred to paracentesis. The patient should be placed upon a very nutritious and generous diet, and tonics, together perhaps with mixed acids, should be administered.

Whilst these different forms of corneal ulcer are always accompanied by more or less irritation and inflammation, there are some forms in which the inflammatory symptoms are almost entirely absent; they, indeed, in their character and course may closely resemble the non-inflammatory suppurative keratitis. We notice that the ulcer is white in color, and clearly defined against the transparent cornea, and not surrounded by a gray, swollen zone of demarcation. It is accompanied by very little, if indeed any, photophobia, lachrymation, redness, or pain; there is also more tendency to necrosis, and extension in circumference than in the other forms.

One peculiar and very dangerous kind of non-inflammatory or indolent ulcer is that which is often met with in very aged and decrepit individuals, and is generally accompanied by hypopyon. In character it closely resembles the non-inflammatory suppurative keratitis; in fact, the latter very frequently passes over into this form of ulcer, more especially when it has been produced by an accident, such as a foreign body. Like it, it commences with a grayish-white infiltration, perhaps in the centre of the cornea, which soon passes over into an ulcer and extends very rapidly in circumference and depth, the affected tissue breaking down and being cast off until a large sloughing ulcer is the result. When it has reached a certain depth it very frequently becomes complicated with hypopyon, which may be due to iritis, to inflammation of the posterior layers of the cornea and proliferation of the epithelial cells, or to perforation of the ulcer and a discharge of its contents into the anterior chamber. One portion of the margin of the ulcer is swollen and of a grayish-white tint, this opacity assuming sometimes a semilunar or crescentic form, and from it small striated opacities run deeply into the corneal tissue. The cornea in the vicinity of the ulcer is generally clear and transparent, or only faintly clouded. From the dangerous character of the disease, and its tendency to spread, Prof. Saemisch proposes to call it "ulcus serpens corneæ."[1] There is a marked absence of all inflammatory symptoms, and in this consists its chief danger, as it leads to rapid and extensive sloughing of the cornea. In other cases there are great ciliary irritation and neuralgia, and in these there is generally no hypopyon (Saemisch).

Sometimes we may observe a peculiar transparent ulcer of the cornea, in which both the margins and the bottom of the ulcer are quite translucent, and free from any opaque halo; there is also an absence of vascularity. These ulcers are very intractable, and may persist for a long time. They may, however, heal rapidly if a sufficient degree of vascularity can be established.

The complications to which ulcers of the cornea may give rise are often very serious, and may even prove destructive to the eye. If the ulcer is superficial, of but slight extent, and occurs in a young healthy subject, it may heal perfectly, and finally leave very little, if any opacity behind; the cornea in time regaining its normal transparency. Indeed, even small perforating ulcers which have given rise to anterior capsular cataract, may gradually disappear without leaving almost any trace behind them.

[1] Vide a very interesting brochure, by Prof. Saemisch, "Das Ulcus Corneæ Serpens, seine Therapie." Bonn. Max Cohen, 1870.

I have not unfrequently met with cases of central capsular cataract in old persons whose corneæ were apparently clear, and it was not until the cornea was examined by a strong light or with the oblique illumination, that a small opacity could be detected just opposite the centre of the lens; then, on inquiry, it was perhaps ascertained that the patient had as a child suffered from inflammation of the eye.

When the ulcer has extended very deeply into the cornea, nearly as far as the posterior elastic lamina (membrane of Descemet), the latter may yield before the intra-ocular pressure and bulge forward, looking like a small transparent vesicle at the bottom of the ulcer. This condition has been termed hernia of the cornea, or "keratocele." If the membrane of Descemet be very tough and elastic, it may protrude even beyond the level of the cornea, and thus produce a transparent, prominent vesicle, like a tear-drop. This generally soon bursts, and gives rise to an ulcer, or a fistulous opening may remain, and prove very intractable; but it may exist for weeks or even months, when it gradually becomes thicker, flatter, more opaque, and changed into a kind of cicatricial tissue. It was generally supposed that the walls of this vesicle consist only of the membrane of Descemet pushed forward by the aqueous humor, but Stellwag states that they also always include some of the deepest layers of the cornea, traces of which may even be found at the sides of the vesicles, and sometimes also at the apex.

The chief danger of the ulcers, apart from the dense opacities which they may leave behind, is to be found in their perforating the cornea, and the degree of this danger varies with the extent and situation of the perforation.

If the perforation is but small, the iris will fall against it when the aqueous humor flows off, without protruding through it; plastic lymph will be effused at the bottom of the ulcer and this may at once commence to heal, the iris becoming slightly glued against the cornea. The aqueous humor reaccumulates, and if the adhesion between the iris and cornea is but very slight, it will yield before the pressure of the aqueous, and the iris be liberated and fall back to its normal plane. The muscular action of the sphincter and dilator of the pupil during the action of the pupil, will also assist in breaking through the adhesion, but if the latter is at all considerable and firm, the iris will remain adherent to the cornea, and a more or less extensive anterior synechia be formed. If the perforation is large, as it must be if the iris falls into it and protrudes through it [Fig. 83], this protrusion may gain a considerable size by the collection of aqueous humor behind it, which causes it gradually to distend and bulge more and more. The color of the prolapse is soon changed from black to a dirty, dusky-gray tint, and its base is surrounded by a zone of opaque cornea. The portion of protruding iris which lies against the edges of the ulcer, generally becomes united to the latter by an effusion of plastic lymph, the aqueous humor is again retained, and the anterior chamber re-established, with the exception of the portion in the vicinity of the prolapse, for here the iris is lifted away from the anterior surface of the lens, and a more or less considerable posterior chamber is formed. The pupil is distorted and dragged towards the perforation, and the extent of this distortion varies with the size and situation of the prolapse. If a portion of the pupil is included in the prolapse, it will be irregularly displaced and dragged towards the latter, and diminished in size correspondingly to the amount of the pupil which is

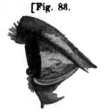

[Fig. 83.

After Miller.]

involved. When the whole pupil is included, the iris will be tensely stretched towards the perforation; if the latter is considerable in size, and the aqueous humor has gushed forth with much force, the lens, and even some of the vitreous humor, may be lost. If the prolapse is small and seen shortly after it has taken place, it may often be replaced under judicious treatment, and the ulcer perhaps heal without even an anterior synechia remaining behind; but if it is considerable in size, the result will be much less favorable, for the protruding portion of iris, exposed to the action of external irritants, e. g., the air, movements of the lids, etc., becomes inflamed and covered by a thin grayish-white layer of exudation, which gradually becomes thicker and more organized, and assumes a cicatricial texture. Now, if this cicatricial covering and the adhesions of the iris to the edges of the ulcer are not sufficiently strong to withstand the intra-ocular pressure, the prolapse will gradually increase in size, and the surrounding portions of the cornea will also bulge more and more, until an extensive staphyloma may be produced. If the cornea is perforated at several points, through which small portions of the iris protrude, it is termed "Staphyloma racemosum."

If the perforation is very small, and situated at or near the centre of the cornea, capsular cataract may be produced in the manner already described. Again, the sudden escape of the aqueous humor, and falling forward of the lens, may cause a rupture of the capsule, and thus give rise to lenticular cataract.

With regard to the treatment of ulcers of the cornea, we must be chiefly guided by the amount of inflammation which is present. Whilst we endeavor to check an undue degree of inflammation, we must be on our guard not to subdue it too much, as this would favor the tendency to necrosis, and protract the process of reparation. In the progressive stage of an acute inflammatory ulcer, the patient should be kept in a somewhat darkened, but well-ventilated room, and be guarded against the effects of bright light, cold wind, and other external irritants. It may be necessary to administer a brisk purgative and saline diuretics, together with a light, non-stimulating diet, if there are marked inflammatory symptoms and the patient is of a strong, plethoric habit. But we must be upon our guard not to prescribe this kind of treatment in all cases, for very frequently ulcers of the cornea occur in persons of delicate, feeble health, and then it would prove injudicious and injurious, for it would increase the tendency to necrosis, and retard the filling up of the ulcer. In such cases, the patient should be placed on tonics, and a very nutritious diet. When the process of repair has set in, he should be permitted to get into the open air, indeed this is especially indicated if the disease shows a tendency to become indolent and chronic. Much benefit is then experienced from out-of-door exercise, and a residence in the country or at the sea-side.

The object of our local treatment must be to endeavor to diminish marked symptoms of inflammatory irritation, to stop the progress of the ulcer, and to hasten its repair and the absorption of the morbid products. If there are much injection, photophobia, lachrymation, and ciliary neuralgia, atropine should be dropped into the eye, the compound belladonna ointment should be rubbed over the forehead, and perhaps a blister applied behind the ear. If the pain in and around the eye is very great, and especially if the latter is very tender to the touch, two or three leeches should be applied to the temple. Much relief will also be experienced from the subcutaneous injection of morphia. A great amount of mischief is but too often caused by the use of strong caustic or astringent lotions, during the acute, progressive stage of the ulceration. Not only do they greatly augment the irritation, but they increase the tendency to necrosis and extension of the ulcer. It is only in the chronic, torpid ulcer which has already become covered by epithelium, that caustics are at all applicable, and even then they must be used with great caution and circumspection. In the chronic, indolent, non-inflammatory ulcer we must apply atropine, a compress bandage, and above all, warm fomentations, in order to excite a certain degree of inflammatory swelling; or the yellow oxide of mercury ointment may be employed, for this remedy hastens the process of absorption and tends to prevent relapses. The patient's health must be invigorated by tonics, a generous diet, and stimulants; indeed, the same line of local and general treatment must be adopted as in non-inflammatory suppurative keratitis. We must never forget to apply a compress bandage over the eye, in order not only to guard it against external irritants, but to support the thinned ulcerated portion of the cornea against the intra-ocular pressure, and to prevent the constant movements of the eyelids, which greatly impede the formation of an epithelial covering over the ulcer; which, as we have seen, forms the commencement of the retrogressive and reparative stage. If the photophobia is very intense and obstinate, and the firm pressure of the lids prevents the process of reparation in the ulcer, much benefit is experienced from the division of the outer canthus, as recommended by Mr. Carter,[1] which speedily relieves the photophobia and greatly accelerates the healing of the ulcer.

In all ulcers of the cornea, but more especially in those which extend deeply into its substance, the process of repair is greatly retarded by the high amount of intra-ocular pressure which the thinned portion of the cornea at the bottom of the ulcer has to bear. In consequence of this, the latter is very apt either to give way completely, and to perforate; or else it yields somewhat before the intra-ocular pressure, bulges forwards, sloughs, and is partly thrown off, and thus the process of repair is much impeded. Now we possess three principal means of diminishing the intra-ocular pressure, viz., atropine, paracentesis, and iridectomy. The beneficial action of atropine, both as a direct sedative and in reducing the intra-ocular tension, has been already explained.

In very obstinate and chronic ulceration of the cornea in which the corneal vascularization is either absent or very deficient, and in which there is much lax swelling of the conjunctiva, especially at the retro-tarsal fold, Dr. Hosch strongly advises the application of pure nitrate of silver to the retro-tarsal fold. It must, however, be only applied to a narrow rim of the latter by means of a finely-pointed crayon of nitrate of silver, and at once neutralized by salt and water. It should not be re-applied until the eschar is entirely removed.[2]

If the ulcer has extended so deeply into the substance of the cornea as to threaten perforation, no time should be lost in performing paracentesis at the bottom of the ulcer; by so doing, we shall be able to limit the perforation to a very small extent; for if we permit the spontaneous perforation of the ulcer, we find that, before this occurs, the bottom of the ulcer extends somewhat in circumference, and thus a considerable ragged opening may result, and the latter will certainly be much larger than if it had simply been made with a fine needle. Moreover, the escape of the aqueous humor will, in the former case, be more sudden and forcible, which is apt to produce considerable hyperæmia *ex vacuo* of the deeper tunics of the eyeball; prolapse of the

---

[1] "The Practitioner," January, 1869.
[2] "Kl. Monatsbl.," 1872, p. 321; also Graefe, "A. f. O.," vi. 2, 165.

iris, which may lead to suppurative iritis or irido-choroiditis; or rupture of the capsule, and consequent cataract; or, again, the suspensory ligament of the lens may be torn, and the lens partially dislocated. The paracentesis should not be postponed until the deepest layers of the cornea are implicated, for we then run the risk of a large spontaneous perforation occurring before we have time to interfere. The puncture should be made with a fine needle at the deepest portion of the ulcer, and the aqueous humor allowed to flow off as gently as possible. The iris will gradually move forward, and come in contact with the back of the cornea; a thin layer of lymph will be effused at the bottom of the ulcer, under which the regeneration of the corneal tissue will take place, the iris being generally more or less glued to the perforation by the effusion of lymph. As soon as the opening is stopped by this plug of lymph, the aqueous humor will re-accumulate, and, if the adhesion between the iris and cornea is but slight, it will readily yield to, and be torn away by, the force of the aqueous humor and the action of the muscles of the iris. But, if the layer of lymph at the bottom of the ulcer is thin and weak, the force of the intra-ocular pressure may rupture it, or may cause it to bulge forward, and thus necessitate a repetition of the paracentesis. The latter should also be repeated, perhaps even several times, if we notice that the process of repair becomes arrested, and that the ulcer again shows a tendency to increase in depth. After the operation, a compress bandage should be applied. If the ulcer is extensive, and if hypopyon or iritis coexist, the puncture should be made with a broad needle at the edge of the cornea [Fig. 84], or an iridectomy should be substituted. The indications which

[Fig. 84.

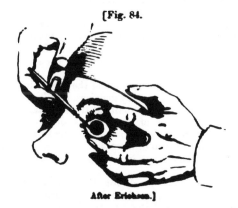

After Erichsen.]

should guide us in selecting between these two operations have already been considered in the article upon suppurative corneitis.

In the indolent hypopyon ulcer (ulcus serpens of Saemisch), described at p. 228, a vast number of remedies have been tried, of which the most successful have been warm fomentations, paracentesis, and iridectomy, together with tonics and a generous diet. It must, however, be confessed that such success has been but limited, more especially when the ulcer was extensive, rapidly spreading, and accompanied by a considerable hypopyon. Saemisch has lately devised the following operation for the purpose of dividing the base of the ulcer, and maintaining a diminution of the intra-ocular tension for some length of time, so that the progress of the disease may be arrested, and the process of repair accelerated. His results have been very favorable, for out of thirty-five cases in which the operation was performed, the progress of the affection was at once arrested in thirty-four. The amount of sight which was saved varied, of course, according to the circumstances of the case. The eyelids being kept apart with the stop-speculum, and the eyeball fixed with a pair of forceps, a puncture is made with Von Graefe's narrow cataract-knife at the temporal side of the ulcer in the healthy portion of the cornea, about one millimetre from the margin of the ulcer. The point of the knife having entered the anterior chamber, the blade is to be carried through the chamber behind the bottom of the ulcer (towards the bottom of which the edge is to be turned), and the counter-puncture made at a point corresponding to the puncture, and likewise situated in the healthy cornea, slightly beyond the margin of the ulcer. The fixing forceps are now laid aside, and then, with a slight sawing movement, the knife is to cut its way out through the ulcer, the blade being several times turned a little on its axis, so that the aqueous humor may flow off very gently beside the blade. The last portion of the cornea should be divided as slowly and gent y as possible. If there is any hypopyon, it generally escapes through the incision. A light compress is to be applied, and within an hour or two the wound is generally already closed, and then atropine should be used. The wound is to be opened twice daily for the first few days with a probe, or, still better, with Weber's beak-pointed canaliculus knife, the blunt point of which is to be inserted between the lips of the incision; but care must be taken that this is delicately done, so that the aqueous humor flows off very gently. The wound must be reopened every day until the process of repair has become thoroughly established, which is known by the fact that the opaque and swollen margin becomes narrower and narrower, breaks up into punctated or faintly striated opacities, until it finally disappears altogether, and then the incision may be allowed to close. This generally occurs at about the second or third week. When the symptoms of irritation have subsided, the red precipitate ointment may be applied, to accelerate the healing of the ulcer and the absorption of the opacity. [Continued experience with Saemisch's method of treating the serpiginous corneal ulcer has not been very satisfactory, at least among ophthalmic surgeons in the United States. Though the operation is very generally practised, yet more reliance is placed on the local application of heat, and the strong tonic and stimulating general treatment.—B.]

In cases of obstinate ulceration of the cornea, confined chiefly or entirely to one portion of the latter, much benefit is sometimes derived from syndectomy of the corresponding segment of the sclerotic; so that the blood supply of the affected portion of the cornea may be more or less cut off. In obstinate, chronic, vascular ulcers of the cornea, which have long resisted every form of treatment, and show a great tendency to recur, the insertion of a seton at the temple often renders the most marked and striking benefit, the disease being rapidly cured, and the relapses prevented, if the seton is worn for some time after the corneal ulcer is healed.

[Fuchs advises the use of the actual cautery, heated to a faint red beat, in "hypopyum keratitis," in "ulcus corneæ serpens," in the "ulcus rodens" of the cornea, and in all torpid or rapidly destructive ulcers of the cornea. Martin employs the actual cautery for all corneal ulcers. He thinks the iron at a red heat diminishes the intra-ocular tension, and in this lies its value as a therapeutic agent. He makes one or two applications, according to the size of the ulcer, and does not hesitate to perforate if there is any tendency to necrosis.—B.]

Indolent Hypopyon Ulcer.—Operative interference is, however, only indicated in the more advanced and graver cases, when the ulcer is considerable in extent, its bottom and edges infiltrated with pus, and the hypopyon large. In such cases either a large iridectomy, or Saemisch's operation should be performed; on the whole, I have found the former the more successful proceeding of the two, although this may to some extent be due to the fact that I was not always able to insure the incision being kept properly open for a sufficient length of time. In the milder cases, and during the earlier stages, when the ulcer is of a grayish-white tint, not considerable in depth or breadth, accompanied by but a small hypopyon, a compress bandage, atropine, and warm fomentations will suffice. The patients are generally in feeble health, and should therefore mostly be put upon a good diet, with stimulants, and tonics should be prescribed. Occasionally I have been obliged to treat persons suffering even severe forms of the disease as out-patients, and I have been surprised to see sometimes very unfavorable cases recover under the above treatment, and without an operation. A very interesting and valuable account of the pathology and the treatment adopted in Professor Horner's practice will be found in Mad. Bokowa's brochure on "Hypopyon Keratitis."[1] Out of two hundred and twenty-four cases, one hundred and eighteen were cured without operation. She has also found iridectomy more successful than Saemisch's operation; she, however, does not operate in the milder cases, whereas Saemish operates even in such, which would probably do well without any operation at all.

We are especially indebted to Mr. Critchett for introducing this mode of treatment[2] in certain cases of chronic vascular ulcers of the cornea, which are particularly characterized by their protracted course, their great tendency to recur, and the obstinacy with which they resist all ordinary methods of treatment. Mr. Critchett has favored me with the following description of the manner in which the seton is to be applied:

"I generally use rather stout silk or fine twine, such as a large suture needle will carry. I select a spot near the temporal region under the hair, so as to avoid as far as possible a visible scar. Care is required not to wound the temporal artery; this may generally be avoided by drawing the skin well away from the temporal fascia, holding it firmly by the hair. The needle is thus passed through at a level, anterior to the artery; about an inch is usually included, and a loose loop is formed, which may be placed behind the ear: it requires to be dressed and moved daily; it usually continues to discharge for

---

[1] Alfred Graefe recommends that in Saemisch's operation the incision should not be made through the ulcer itself, but close to its margin in the healthy cornea, so as to cut off the sound from the diseased portion. "Kl. Monatsbl.," 1872, p. 173.

[2] Professor Horner believes that pus cannot sink down between the lamellae of the cornea, and that this can only occur between the cornea proper and the membrane of Descemet. He is, moreover, of opinion that the purulent deposit in cases of hypopyon keratitis, which, when observed in profile, appears at the first glance to be between the lamellae of the cornea, is mostly really situated in the anterior chamber. From its being tough and tenacious it adheres firmly to the membrane of Descemet: and if it be inconsiderable in quantity, a space is left between it and the iris, thus causing it to closely resemble an onyx; this little interspace is only filled up when the purulent deposit becomes more considerable, and then produces a well-marked hypopyon. *Vide* "Hypopyon Keratitis," by Mad. Marie Bokowa. Zürich, 1871, Zürcher and Furrer.
Horner is of opinion that the hypopyon is often due to a direct migration of cells from the bottom of the ulcer into the anterior chamber; the epithelial layer of the membrane of Descemet (Endothel) playing then only a passive part. This idea has been substantiated by experiments on rabbits, etc. (loc. cit.).

[3] Mr. Spencer Watson has also published some able papers upon this subject in the "B. L. O. H. Rep.," and in the "Medical Mirror."

two or three months, and then either cuts its way through, or dries up. In severe and obstinate cases, where it is necessary, it may be renewed, selecting a spot near to the previous scar. I have sometimes found it desirable to continue the influence of a seton for twelve months. There are certain inconveniences that occasionally arise to which I may briefly allude. It will sometimes happen that in spite of every care and precaution a branch of the temporal artery is pricked by the point of the needle as it traverses the skin; this accident is at once recognized by the rapid outflow of arterial blood from one or both openings, through which the silk passes. In the event of such an accident, it is better at once to remove the silk, and then moderate pressure checks the bleeding, and in a few days a neighboring spot may be selected for the reintroduction of the silk; but if this precaution be not taken, and if an effort be made to retain the seton in spite of the hemorrhage, there is a great liability to secondary bleeding, to extravasation of blood beneath the scalp, burrowing abscesses, and other untoward casualties, and in one instance I observed the formation of a small traumatic aneurism. In certain exceptional cases, the introduction of the seton is followed by considerable swelling of the surrounding parts, with a tendency to erysipelas, and suppurative inflammation cannot be established. As soon as these symptoms show themselves the silk should be removed."

If an ulcer is situated at or near the centre of the cornea, and perforation appears inevitable, the pupil must be kept widely dilated with atropine, in order that, when the cornea gives way and the aqueous humor escapes, the edge of the pupil may not be involved in the perforation. On the other hand, if the ulcer is situated near the margin of the cornea, the reverse is indicated, and the pupil should be allowed to remain undilated, or even stimulated to extreme contraction, by the application of the extract of the Calabar bean [or, better, a solution of Eserinæ sulph. gr. ij ad Aq. dest. f℥j.—B.], in order to remove the edge of the pupil as far as possible from the situation of the threatening perforation. Either of these remedies is also indicated when a slight adhesion exists between the cornea and iris (anterior synechia), for, by the strong action of the muscles of the iris which they produce, the adhesion may be forcibly torn through. Mr. Pridgin Teale informs me that he has often derived much benefit from dividing anterior synechiæ. This is done both with the view of causing a diminution of the corneal opacity, at the site of adhesion, and of releasing the iris from its drag.

[This is a very useful procedure in many cases, and changes a "leucoma adhærens" into a simple leucoma. It can be done in almost all cases of slight anterior synechiæ, by a simple application of the various steps employed in Passavant's operation for the division of posterior synechiæ. A small linear incision is made in the cornea, near the margin, and then the adhesion of the iris to the cornea divided by the cutting hook of Passavant, or torn away from its attachment by a pair of delicate iris forceps. The division of these adhesions in a case of opacity of the cornea, often renders a subsequent iridotomy or iridectomy much simpler. Galezowski's operation of synechotomy for adherent leucoma is a very similar method. He uses a needle with a cutting edge, shaped like a pruning-knife, or of a short synechotome made for the purpose. He punctures the cornea at the side opposite to the synechia, and a little above the horizontal diameter of the leucoma, directing the point of the instrument between the iris and the cornea, with the edge toward the synechia. Then, by repeated saw-like movements, the iris is cut loose from the cornea.—B.]

If a slight prolapse has occurred, we must at once attempt to replace it by pressing it gently back with a spatula or probe, or we may endeavor to cause it to recede by widely dilating the pupil by atropine. A firm compress should be applied in all cases of prolapse, for it will favor the consolidation of the wound by the formation of a layer of lymph over the prolapse, and will prevent the latter from yielding to the intra-ocular pressure and increasing in size. The protruding portion of iris should also be pricked with a fine needle, and the aqueous humor be allowed to escape; for this will cause the prolapse to shrink and gradually dwindle down. This operation may be repeated several times, and generally with the best results; but if the prolapse is large and prominent, it should be first pricked with the needle, and then, when the escape of the aqueous humor has caused it to collapse, it should be seized with the iridectomy forceps, and snipped off with a pair of curved scissors quite close to the cornea, a firm compress being at once applied. The same treatment is to be pursued in staphyloma iridis.

Some surgeons recommend that the prolapse should be touched with a point of nitrate of silver, or with a little vinum opii; but this is apt to set up great irritation, and may even produce severe iritis. If it be done at all, a weak solution of nitrate of silver should be lightly applied to the apex of the prolapse, with a fine camel's-hair brush. In a considerable and obstinate prolapse, much benefit is generally derived from making a large iridectomy in an opposite direction, for this will often cause the prolapse to recede and flatten. This operation is likewise indicated when the pupil is partly or wholly implicated in the prolapse or anterior synechia; also, when there is a partial staphyloma, and, above all, when this is accompanied by an increase in the intra-ocular tension. For, as has been pointed out by Von Graefe, in cases of partial or complete staphyloma, or of leucoma prominens, the degree of blindness is frequently quite disproportionate to the optical condition. In such cases, there is often contraction of the visual field, eccentric fixation, increase in the intra-ocular tension, and excavation of the optic nerve. When glaucomatous symptoms supervene upon partial staphyloma or leucoma prominens, we find the cornea becomes at this point markedly prominent, even after it has already become thickened and consolidated.

Fistula of the cornea often proves very obstinate and intractable, and even dangerous to the eye, leading perhaps finally to irido-choroiditis and atrophy of the eyeball. A fistulous opening of the cornea may result in consequence of a small perforating ulcer, or from a wound of the cornea, with or without injury to the lens. The fistulous opening may become temporarily closed, so that the aqueous humor re-accumulates, but after a short interval it again gives way, the aqueous flows off, and the anterior chamber is obliterated. This may occur over and over again. When fistula of the cornea exists, the eye remains irritable and injected, the intra-ocular tension is greatly diminished, the anterior chamber obliterated, and a small drop of fluid may be noticed exuding through the aperture in the cornea. Various modes of treatment have been advocated. At the outset, a firm compress bandage should be applied, as well as a strong solution of atropine, and if this fails to heal the fistula, the latter may be touched with the point of a fine camel's-hair brush dipped in a weak solution of nitrate of silver, this being repeated several times, at an interval of a day or two. The disadvantage of this mode of treatment is, however, that it often produces an indelible cicatrix. An iridectomy frequently proves of more service. Wecker[1] considers that the fistula is due to an eversion of the membrane of Descemet at this point, and has therefore devised the following treatment. He introduces into the opening a very fine, smooth-pointed, straight pair of forceps, and, seizing the wall of the fistulous track, bruises its lining, and thus denudes the corneal tissue. This having been done at several points, atropine and a compress bandage must be applied. Great care and delicacy are required not to rupture the capsule with the point of the forceps. He has thus cured a case of fistula of the cornea, which had resisted, for ten months, different modes of treatment. Zehender[1] has found the prolonged use of the extract of Calabar bean of great service in curing a corneal fistula.

6.—DIFFUSE KERATITIS (PARENCHYMATOUS, INTERSTITIAL, SYPHILITIC).

In this disease we may also distinguish two principal forms. The one is accompanied by marked symptoms of inflammation, and is hence called "diffuse vascular keratitis." In the other, or "non-vascular" form, these symptoms are entirely absent.

1. In the *vascular diffuse keratitis*, we notice, together with a certain varying degree of conjunctival and subconjunctival injection, a zone of vessels passing from the margin of the cornea more or less towards the centre, where they terminate in a sharply defined line. They are not situated on the surface of the cornea, as those in pannus, but enter deeply into its substance. They consist in part of vessels derived from the junction of the conjunctival and subconjunctival vessels near the margin of the cornea, and in part also of branches coming from the bloodvessels of the ciliary body. Sometimes the vascularity at the edge of the cornea is so great, that it looks like a bright red zone of extravasated blood. Soon there is noticed at one or more points, a slight opacity of the cornea, which generally commences at the margin where its density is greatest, and gradually shades off towards the centre into transparent cornea. Sometimes, however, the opacity begins at the centre, whence it slowly extends towards the periphery. The cloudiness gradually increases in extent and thickness, until the whole surface of the cornea may become diffusely opaque. The density and color of the opacity vary a good deal. Thus, it may be but thin, and of a grayish-white color, having very much the appearance of frosted glass, or it may be thicker and of a yellowish creamy tint, more especially in the centre of the cornea. Indeed, at this point we not unfrequently see a large circular patch of a pale yellow color, which is evidently deeply seated in the substance of the cornea. This central patch may gain a considerable size, even of two or three lines in diameter. Sometimes several such denser patches may be noticed at different points. The epithelial layer at first retains its normal smoothness, but after a time it becomes somewhat rough and thickened, as if it had been lightly pricked by a pin, or a fine powder had been strewn over it. The disease shows very little tendency to ulceration or to purulent necrosis, unless it has been very injudiciously treated by caustics or strong astringent collyria. But the whole surface of the cornea may be swollen and become somewhat prominent, yielding here and there to the intra-ocular pressure and bulging forward. Generally these prominences disappear with infiltration, but if they have been considerable, they may leave behind some impairment of the true curvature of the cornea. The amount of inflammation and ciliary irritation vary very much. Sometimes, there is very considerable and obstinately persistent photophobia, together with lachrymation and a certain degree of ciliary neuralgia. In other cases, these symptoms never assume

any particular prominence. The sight is always greatly impaire
the patient can hardly see a hand moving, which is due to the dif
acter of the opacity, for it is as if he were looking through a piece
glass. If both eyes become affected, which is generally the case, th
this total loss of sight is most depressing, and demands the greatest c
in the surgeon to prevent the patient from seeking other and perl
dicious advice. For the disease runs a most slow and protracte
months and months elapse before any, even slight improvement
show itself, and during all this time no treatment appears of an
service. We can but let the disease run its course, and endeavor t
in its progress. It may take from six to eight weeks until it has re
acme ; the cornea being then, perhaps, almost covered with closely
bloodvessels, which reach nearly up to its very centre, where is see
yellow infiltration. The red appearance of the cornea is often incl
small extravasations of blood, caused by the giving way of som
The disease may now remain stationary for a few weeks, and then
cess of reparation sets in. The vascularity diminishes ; the vessel
closely arranged at the edge of the cornea, and show more or less
able gaps between them ; and the infiltration becomes thinner and
color, gradually disappearing more and more from the periphery
the centre, which is the last to clear up.

The *prognosis* of the disease is, on the whole, favorable, for, all
runs a most protracted course, which may extend over many mo
although the opacity of the cornea may be so dense as to prevent th
from even counting fingers, there is no tendency to ulceration of th
and the opacity gradually disappears until there is finally perhaj
slight cloudiness left. Both eyes are generally affected, and this re
disease of course the more harassing and alarming to the patient,
thus remain for many weeks almost totally blind. Iritis is a free
companiment of the inflammation of the cornea, and may be qui
pected during the progress of the case, as the iris is hidden from vie
opacity of the cornea ; and it is only when the latter becomes cle
the iris is found somewhat discolored, and the pupil irregular and
But a still graver and more dangerous complication is inflammatic
ciliary body, which is especially apt to occur if the case has bee
ciously treated, and caustic or strong astringent collyria have been
We must suspect this complication, if the symptoms of inflammato
tion are greatly increased in intensity, if the vascularity, photophobi
mation, and ciliary neuralgia are severe, if the sight is rapidly di
and the field of vision markedly contracted, and if the eye at the
the ciliary body is extremely sensitive to the touch.

Diffuse keratitis is especially apt to occur between the ages of
twenty, but it may be met with up to thirty-five or forty. It
occurs in persons in a feeble, delicate state of health, which may l
numerous causes, such as want and privation, very hard and fatigui
more especially in a confined and vitiated atmosphere ; and it is o
with in persons affected with a scrofulous diathesis, or with inherited
I cannot at all agree with the view that diffuse keratitis is always d
herited syphilis, for although I have often seen it associated with tl
yet in many cases not the slightest trace of a syphilitic taint could
tained, and there was a marked and complete absence of the
syphilitic features and the notched teeth. Indeed, I think that we
too apt hastily to jump to the conclusion that hereditary syphilis exi
on a more careful and searching examination into some of these hi

would be found that the miscarriages, early deaths of children, etc., were due
ŏctly natural causes, and quite independent of any syphilitic taint. I
f course, be met with the constantly recurring argument that it is im-
o to get at the truth of the history, but I think that we are justified
ng the patient and his parents the benefit of the doubt, if no reliable
proof of the presence of inherited syphilis can be made out. For this reason,
I must completely disagree with those authors who term this disease "syphilitic
keratitis;" for, as I have already stated, it is frequently met with in persons
in whom not the slightest trace of a syphilitic taint can be detected. Whilst
combating some of these views, I must, however, seize this opportunity to
express my admiration for the very important and interesting researches of
Mr. Jonathan Hutchinson,[1] into the frequent connection between inherited
syphilis and many of the diseases of the eye, a discovery which has proved
of great importance and use in the treatment of these affections.

[If the keratitis occur in connection with hereditary syphilis, the existence
of the latter may generally be diagnosticated, as pointed out by Mr. Hutchinson, by certain peculiarities presented by the *permanent teeth*, especially by
the upper central incisors, which are the most reliable for purposes of diagnosis.
The characteristic malformation of the upper central incisors consists chiefly
in a dwarfing of the tooth, which is usually both narrow and short, and in
the atrophy of its middle lobe. This atrophy leaves a single broad notch
(vertical) in the edge of the tooth. This notching is usually symmetrical,
as shown in Fig. 85. It may vary much in degree in different cases. Sometimes the teeth diverge, and at others they slant towards each other. The
ended woodcut, Fig. 86, affords a good illustration of the deformity. In
ority of cases the condition of the teeth is sufficient only to excite

Fig. 85.   Fig. 86.

 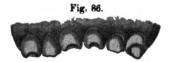

suspicion, and not to decide the question, although in a marked case of malformation, Mr. Hutchinson states that he would feel "no hesitation in pronouncing the possessor of the teeth to be the subject of inherited syphilis,
even in the absence of other testimony."[1] In a considerable number of cases
of hereditary syphilis, the teeth show no deviation whatever from the normal
standard, and in such the diagnosis must be guided by other and well-known
symptoms.—H.]

[The interstitial keratitis, which is one of the symptoms of congenital
syphilis in association with the notched incisor teeth, is almost always symmetrical, and usually occurs between the ages of six and fifteen, sometimes
as early as two or three years, and very rarely as late as twenty-five or
thirty.—B.]

Mr. Brudenell Carter points out that the absence of syphilis in the parents
does not necessarily preclude its existence in children, as the taint may have
been introduced by vaccination."[2]

In the treatment of this disease, we must be chiefly contented with guarding
the eye against all noxious influences, such as bright light, wind, draughts, etc.,
and must endeavor to prevent the inflammatory symptoms from gaining an
undue prominence. Unfortunately, we do not at present know of any means

[1] *Vide* Mr. Hutchinson's admirable work, "Syphilitic Diseases of the Eye and Ear."
[2] Reynolds' "System of Medicine," vol. i. page 317.   [3] "Lancet," 1868; 1, 765.

of checking the progress and development of the disease, or of curtailing its protracted course. The use of caustics or astringent collyria must be most carefully avoided, as they only tend to increase the inflammatory irritation and to produce complications, such as ulcers of the cornea, or inflammation of the iris or ciliary body. At the outset, atropine should always be applied, although when the cornea becomes diffusely clouded, it is but of little use, as it is not absorbed, and it is apt to increase the inflammation if it be too long continued. But when the cornea begins to clear, atropine or the belladonna collyrium should be again applied. Local depletion and very antiphlogistic treatment are not well borne, on account of the weakly and feeble health of the patient. Moreover, they tend to impede the formation of bloodvessels on the cornea, and to protract the course of the disease. But if symptoms of cyclitis make their appearance, leeches should be applied to the temple, and paracentesis should be performed; and if the sight deteriorates greatly, the field becomes contracted, and especially if the intra-ocular tension increases, an iridectomy should be made at once. When the cornea is beginning to clear up, the absorption of the morbid products may be hastened by applying slight irritants. The best to commence with is the insufflation of calomel, which should be employed once daily. If the eye bears this well, without becoming too much irritated, the yellow precipitate ointment should be substituted for it. At first, I generally employ it of about the strength of two grains to the drachm, and use but a very small quantity. If it excites much irritation, I apply a still weaker ointment, or postpone its use for a few days. I have found it by far the best remedy for accelerating the absorption of opacities of the cornea. A collyrium of iodide of potassium (gr. ij ad f ʒj) is also serviceable for this purpose. In very obstinate cases of diffuse keratitis, I have also occasionally found much benefit from the application of a seton to the temple. Hasner has practised paracentesis.

[Massage of the eye is a remedial measure worth trying in this form of keratitis. It is an easy procedure, the motion is rapid and painless, and is useful in all varieties of chronic corneal affections. It is sometimes well to associate with the massage the use of the ointment of the yellow oxide of mercury.—B.]

In some cases, iridectomy proves beneficial not only in accelerating the cure, but also in the early stage sometimes arresting the progress of the disease. Mr. Pridgin Teale informs me that he has practised it with success in cases in which the progress of the disease was rapid and unchecked by other remedies, and in which there had been a diminution of the eye tension before the operation.

It is of great importance to attend to the general health of the patients, as they are as a rule of a feeble, cachectic habit. Tonics, especially the syrup of the iodide of iron, quinine, or the citrate of quinine and steel, should be administered. Cod-liver oil, with or without quinine or steel, is also of much benefit. If a syphilitic taint is suspected, the iodide and bromide of potassium in combination with the bichloride of mercury and cinchona, may be given with much advantage. [These cases of congenital syphilis are very apt in children to be complicated with struma, and hence all preparations of mercury must be administered with extreme caution.—B.] The diet should be nutritious and easily digestible. Meat may be allowed two or three times daily, and wine and malt liquor may be freely administered. In fact, everything should be done to strengthen the patient. In hospital practice, I have often been obliged to take such patients into the house for many months, in order that they might have more attention, and a more generous diet than they would have obtained at home. When the acute stage is past, and the cornea is beginning to clear, the patient should, if possible, be sent into the country, or, still better, to the seaside, and enjoy a great deal of out-of-door exercise. The obstinate photophobia and chrouic irritability of the eye, which often prove so troublesome, yield sometimes most rapidly to change of air.

[Hot fomentations frequently repeated and kept up for a long time, with the interrupted use of atropine, are two extremely useful agents in treating this disease.—B.]

2. In the non-vascular diffuse keratitis, we notice that a small cloud appears in the centre of the cornea, unaccompanied by any but the slightest symptoms of irritation, and there is only a very faint rosy injection around the cornea, but not extending on to it. In the course of ten or fourteen days, the opacity extends over the whole surface of the cornea, giving it the appearance of ground glass, or of a mirror that has been lightly breathed upon. The symptoms of irritation, especially the photophobia, may now increase somewhat, but the vascularity remains slight. The vessels never become very numerous or closely crowded together, as is the case in the vascular form; but individual vessels struggle on towards the infiltration, and do not terminate uniformly in a defined line. The opacity gradually becomes somewhat more dense and yellow towards the centre, and then, after a time, clears up at the periphery, and the infiltration slowly disappears in a centripetal direction. The course of this form is also extremely protracted, and many months may elapse before the cornea regains its transparency. The prognosis is still more favorable than in the vascular form, for there is far less tendency to complications with inflammation of the iris and ciliary body, or to ulceration of the cornea; although the latter may be produced if strong caustics or astringents be employed.

The causes are the same as in the vascular form. If there is any marked irritability of the eye, this should be treated by atropine, cold compresses, blisters, etc. In the majority of the cases the progress of the affection languishes and becomes torpid, and there is a complete absence of all symptoms of inflammatory irritation. In such, it is advisable to apply a slight irritant, more especially the yellow oxide of mercury ointment, every day for a few days. This will excite a little irritation, the central portion of the infiltration will become somewhat more thick and yellow, and the progress of the disease will be accelerated. It has often been noticed that a certain amount of conjunctivitis is very favorable. Thus, if the patient suffering from this form of keratitis, by accident, contracts catarrhal conjunctivitis, the progress of the affection of the cornea will be greatly hastened, and an infiltration disappear in a few weeks, which would otherwise have taken many months before it had become absorbed. This fact led Von Graefe to employ warm fomentations in these cases, in order to excite a certain degree of inflammatory swelling of the conjunctiva. They are indicated if the vascularity and irritation are but very slight, and the progress of the disease extremely protracted and sluggish. They must be employed with care and circumspection, so that they may not excite too much inflammation of the conjunctiva, which would retard instead of hastening the absorption of the infiltration, and perhaps leave it incomplete.

[There is a peculiar variety of keratitis known as "band-shaped" keratitis, which occupies the region of the centre of the cornea, the rest of the cornea being perfectly transparent. The opacity begins on the nasal and temporal sides, and slowly advances towards the centre. The opacity is dull, and its surface has a stippled appearance. The pericorneal injection may be very

slight, and the progress of the disease very slow. After a varying length of
time other symptoms of a deeper trouble are developed, mainly of a glaucomatous nature. The treatment consists in doing an iridectomy as early as
possible in the progress of the inflammation. Galezowski describes a calcareous degeneration of the corneal epithelium, as developing very slowly,
and states that the patient does not completely recover his vision until after
five, six, and even eight years have elapsed. It is generally idiopathic and
presents no complications in other parts of the eye. When these opaque
epithelial pellicles are removed and examined microscopically, they are found
filled with small granules pressed closely together, so as to hide the outline
of the cells. They are hard, and resist compression; spherical, yellow, and
highly refracting. They are insoluble in ether and chloroform, but are dissolved by hydrochloric acid. The deep layer of epithelium is almost always
unaltered. Galezowski regards the disease as a calcareous keratitis, the result
of a particular diathetic influence. He employs dilute hydrochloric acid
in the treatment of the affection, and says that when this opaque epithelium has once been removed, there is no reproduction of it. (See "Recueil
d'ophthalmologie," June, 1881.)

Hocquard speaks of two varieties of epithelial patches upon the cornea,
which he calls hyperplastic and emulsioned. In both there is found beneath
the white substance, removed by scratching, a slight, superficial ulceration,
scarcely more than an erosion, toward which are seen converging some conjunctival vessels. Two conditions must exist, supplementing each other, before
these epithelial patches can be developed: 1st, a modification of the anterior
layers of the cornea; 2d, a slight irritation long continued, acting upon the
surface of the transparent membrane thus transformed. He recommends
daily scraping of the patch, followed by brushing the ulcerated corneal surface with a brush soaked in ether. (See "Archives d'Ophthalmologie,"
Sept.–Oct. 1881.)—B.]

7.—OPACITIES OF THE CORNEA

These vary much in situation, extent, and thickness. If they are quite
superficial and thin, looking like a faint, grayish-blue cloud, they are termed
nebulæ. If the opacity is of a denser, white, pearly, tendinous character,
and situated more deeply in the substance of the cornea, it is called an
albugo or leucoma.

A temporary diffuse opacity of the cornea may be produced by sudden
increase of the intra-ocular pressure, as in certain forms of glaucoma, etc.
This opacity is probably due in part to a displacement of some of the corneal
elements, and also, perhaps, to a disturbance of the nutrition of the cornea
from the compression of the nerves.

We meet with a very superficial opacity of the cornea, which is due to
changes in the epithelial layer. Here and there the epithelial cells become
thickened, aggregated together, and opaque, their contents having perhaps
undergone fatty degeneration. These opacities are of a faint gray, or bluish-
gray color, with an irregular margin. In their centre, the reflection of an
object, for instance the bars of a window, will be found indistinct, or more
or less distorted. Generally, the opacities are easily observable. They may,
however, be so slight as to escape detection, except with the oblique illumination, when they become very evident. They are chiefly met with as the
result of the superficial forms of keratitis, especially pannus due to distichiasis or granular lids, and also of the superficial ulcers of the cornea.

The deeper opacities, which are situated in the substance of the cornea itself, may be confined to a certain portion of it (partial leucoma) [Fig. 87], or extend over its whole surface (total leucoma). The cloudiness may either be of a uniform grayish-blue, or grayish-white color, or may be made up of several opaque, white patches or spots of varying extent and shape. The outline of these opacities is irregular and not sharply defined, being shaded gradually off into the normally transparent cornea. Their thickness and color also vary much, from a grayish-blue to a yellowish-white and densely opaque tint. The epithelial layer is often irregular and punctated, as if a fine powder had been dusted over it, and this causes a distortion of the reflected image. Or, again, the opacities may look like little opaque, chalky nodules strewn about on different portions of the cornea (generally near its surface), and are the remains of phlyctenulæ.

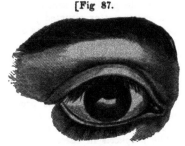

[Fig 87.

After Dalrymple.]

Fine punctate opacities are also met with on the posterior surface of the cornea. They are generally arranged in the form of a pyramid, with its base downwards, and are chiefly due to a precipitation of lymph on the posterior wall of the cornea, but also perhaps to inflammatory changes in the posterior epithelial layer. These peculiar opacities are observed in serous iritis (sometimes termed aquo-capsulitis, keratitis punctata, etc.), and also in inflammations of the deeper tunics of the eyeball, and in sympathetic ophthalmia. In the latter cases, similar punctate opacities may also occur on the anterior surface of the cornea. The different opacities which we have mentioned are chiefly due to inflammatory changes in the corneal and epithelial cells, and are capable of undergoing almost complete absorption, so that they may hardly leave a trace behind them. It is necessary to distinguish from them another form of opacity, which is dependent upon permanent change, often of a tendinous or cicatricial nature, and hence does not undergo absorption, but remains indelible. These opacities are more regular and sharply defined in their outline, and have a more uniform, tendinous, glistening-white or chalky appearance, having, perhaps, a deposit of fatty or earthy matter in the centre. The epithelial layer is smooth and not irregular. These cicatrices vary in extent and shape, in accordance with the size and depth of the original ulcer; they do not, however, correspond exactly to it, because a portion of the latter is very frequently filled up by transparent corneal tissue. These cicatricial opacities occur very frequently in combination with those due to inflammatory changes, so that we have the two forms existing together. The cicatrix, instead of being sharply defined, is then surrounded by a more or less wide, opaque areola of inflammatory infiltration. The latter may in time become completely absorbed and transparent, and leave only the cicatricial opacity, which will, of course, be now considerably less in size than the original leucoma.

In cases of perforating ulcers of the cornea, accompanied with anterior synechia, the cicatrix to which the iris remains attached is termed *leucoma adhærens*. If it be situated near the centre of the cornea, a portion of the pupil will be included in it, leaving, perhaps, the other part of the pupil free, and opposite a transparent portion of the cornea.

A peculiar superficial opacity of the cornea is sometimes met with, which is due to calcareous deposits (consisting of phosphate and carbonate of lime) in the anterior elastic lamina. These opacities are of a mottled brownish hue, with an indistinct margin, which shades off, more or less abruptly, into the healthy cornea. Their course is very protracted, and they are apt simultaneously to affect both eyes. Two very interesting cases of this peculiar opacity, which occurred about the same time, have been described by Mr. Dixon[1] and Mr. Bowman.[2] In each of these cases, a portion of the opacity opposite the pupil was scraped off with a scalpel, and was found to consist of hard gritty matter, situated just beneath the epithelium. The result of the operation upon the sight was excellent. Sometimes earthy or metallic incrustations are formed upon the cornea, and give rise to peculiar opaque or chalky-looking specks. This occasionally occurs from the contact of quicklime or the deposits formed from lead lotion in cases of ulcers or abrasions of the cornea. Here I must again warn the reader against the use of collyria containing lead in cases of ulcer of the cornea or even abrasion of the corneal epithelium, for the precipitation of the lead gives rise to a very marked white stain, which produces great impairment of sight if it be situated in the centre of the cornea.

The *prognosis* in cases of opacity of the cornea will depend very much upon the age and constitution of the patient, and upon the duration, extent, situation, and nature of the opacity. Thus, in children and young persons in good health, opacities, the result even of extensive keratitis or deep ulcers, may in time disappear almost completely, without leaving, perhaps, any trace behind. I have already stated that this may even occur in small perforating ulcers, which have given rise to central capsular cataract. With regard to the opacities due to inflammatory changes in the corneal tissue, it may be laid down as a general rule that the more recent, superficial, and limited such opacities are, the more rapidly and completely do they disappear. By the application of irritants to the eye, we may greatly assist in removing the cloudiness due to inflammatory changes in the corneal and epithelial cells. We thus excite hyperæmia of the parts, increase the interchange of material, and accelerate and stimulate the process of absorption. When the opacities are due to permanent cicatricial changes, these applications are of no avail, and we must then have recourse to other remedies if the opacity causes any impairment of vision. If the opacity is dense and situated in or very near the centre of the cornea, the sight may be very considerably affected, as it will more or less cover the pupil. But even slighter opacities may somewhat impair and confuse the vision, by the diffusion and irregular refraction of the rays of light which they produce. But, apart from this effect upon the sight, these opacities may give rise to other complications. Thus, on account of the indistinctness of the retinal region produced by the cloudy state of the cornea, the patient will bring small objects (as in reading, sewing, etc.) very close to the eye, in order to gain a larger and more distinct image. But this constant accommodation for a very near point, after a time causes the lens to forfeit some of its elasticity, so that it cannot resume its original form, and the accommodation cannot relax itself completely when the eye is looking at distant objects. The lens remains too convex, and the eye has become myopic. The myopia may be also in part due to a change in the shape of the eyeball, produced by constant and long-continued accommodation for near objects (*vide* article "Myopia"). Opacities of the cornea may also give rise to oscillation of the eyeballs, and to strabismus.

[1] " Diseases of the Eye," 3d edition, p. 114.
[2] " Lectures on the Parts concerned in the Operations on the Eye," etc., pp. 38, 117.

Innumerable local remedies have been recommended for the dispersion of opacities of the cornea. From amongst these we may select the following as the most trustworthy and efficacious: The insufflation of calomel, the use of the red or yellow oxide of mercury ointment, collyria of iodide of potassium, vinum opii, nitrate of silver, sulphate of copper, and the sulphate of soda. A small quantity of the latter may be dusted into the eye, or it may be used as a collyrium, about one or two grains to a fluidounce of water. Together with the use of any of these agents, atropine should be applied, as it diminishes the intra-vascular pressure, and thus facilitates the interchange of material and the process of absorption. I have generally found it best, first to dust in calomel for a few days in order to see how the eye bears this, and then, if it does not excite too much irritation, to employ a stronger irritant, especially the red or yellow oxide of mercury ointment. At first its strength should not, I think, exceed one or two grains to the drachm of lard. A little portion, about the size of a couple of pins' heads, should be placed on the inside of the lower eyelid, by means of a probe, and the lids should then be rubbed over the cornea, so that the ointment may come well in contact with it. If the yellow precipitate ointment be used of greater strength than that mentioned above, it should be removed after a few minutes, otherwise it will produce too much irritation. If it is found that the ointment excites a great deal of irritation, redness, and pain, a smaller quantity, or a weaker preparation should be used, or the calomel should again be substituted for a few days. Generally, it is better if the surgeon can himself apply these remedies, as he is then able to watch their action upon the eye; but if the proper mode of using the calomel or the ointment be explained and shown to the patient, I have found no difficulty in getting these remedies applied by the patient himself, or his friends. But if I do not apply the ointment myself, I never prescribe it stronger than gr. j–ij and even the stronger preparation requires to be removed from the conjunctiva after two or three minutes. I have also found advantage from the application of iodide of potassium, either in a collyrium or mixed with the yellow precipitate, in the following proportion: Potass. iodid. gr. j, Hydrar. ox. flav. gr. ij, Adipis ʒj–ʒij. The instillation of a little vinum opii also proves very useful. Nitrate of silver or sulphate of copper is only indicated when there is any inflammatory swelling of the conjunctiva, accompanied by muco-purulent discharge. After any of these remedies have been used for a length of time, they should be exchanged for some other agent, as the eye becomes accustomed to them, and they appear temporarily to lose their effect. Inoculation was formerly in vogue for the cure of opacities of the cornea. It has, however, fallen into disuse.

Von Hasner,[1] of Munich, has strongly recommended the subconjunctival injection of tepid salt and water in cases of dense non-vascular opacities, such as remain after diffuse keratitis. The strength of his solution varies from a scruple to a drachm of salt to a fluidounce of water.

De Wecker[2] has recently advocated the method of tattooing for the removal of the cosmetic defect produced by dense leucomata. The operation, as a rule, causes very little pain or irritation, is best performed with a number of the finest needles firmly bound, with the points on a level, in a handle, such as a penholder. The substance which De Wecker recommends for tinting is India ink; Mr. Taylor has also employed[3] with

[1] "Klinische Monatsblätter f. Augenheilkunde," 1866, p. 161.
[2] "Archives of Ophthalmology and Otology," vol. ii., No. 2, p. 224.
[3] "American Journal of the Medical Sciences," October, 1872, p. 561.—H.]

advantage sepia, ultramarine, and other colors, and, when an immediate and deeply colored effect has been desired, a combination of lampblack with India ink, and a solution of nitrate of silver. The needles are dipped into the pigment solution, which should be made as thick as possible, and, the eye being steadied, the superficial layers of the cicatrix are rapidly punctured in an oblique direction, and layers of the solution applied just as in the ordinary tattooing.—H.]

[A better method is to use a single grooved needle, rub up the India ink to a thick solution, and cover the leucomatous spot thickly with it; then fill the groove in the needle with the pigment, and puncture the cornea obliquely in various directions. This takes more time than the other method, but the work is better done. The puncture of any bloodvessel is of course a great disadvantage, as the blood washes away the pigment. A number of sittings is necessary for the completion of the operation, and, after a varying length of time, ranging from a year to eighteen months, the operation must be repeated, as the pigment stain wears away.—B.]

The chalky incrustations, or deposits of lead upon the cornea, should be carefully scraped off with a cataract or sickle-shaped knife [Fig. 88]. If they are extensive, the whole need not be removed, but only a portion sufficiently large to uncover the pupil. As this operation is sometimes very painful, it had better be done under an anæsthetic, especially in children. Afterwards, a little olive oil or atropine should be applied to the eye.

[Fig. 88.]

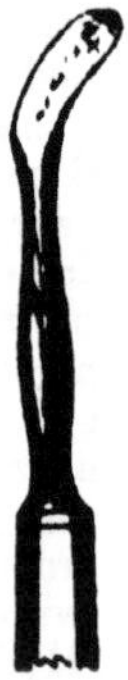

But if the opacity resists all these remedies, and materially impairs the sight, we must endeavor to improve vision, either perhaps by some optical arrangement, or by the formation of an artificial pupil opposite a clear portion of the cornea. For the purpose of diminishing the effect of the diffusion and irregular refraction of the rays produced by the cloudiness, the stenopæic spectacles will often be found of great use (Donders).[1] They consist of an oval metal plate, having a small central aperture. The effect of this is to permit only the central rays, which fall in the optic axis, to pass, whereas all the peripheral, diffused light is excluded. If necessary, convex or concave lenses may be applied behind the apparatus. Although these stenopæic spectacles often answer admirably for any employment at near objects, e. g., reading, sewing, engraving, etc., they cannot be used for walking about, as they produce too great a contraction of the field of vision.

An artificial pupil may be made either by means of an iridectomy, an iridodesis, or iridencleisis. If the opacity is confined to the centre of the cornea, it will be best to perform iridodesis or iridencleisis, for, by so doing, we can draw the iris somewhat forward opposite the opacity, and thus diminish the diffusion of light produced by the latter; moreover, the apex of the artificial pupil will be opposite the edge of the lens, and will thus prevent the irregular refraction which would be caused if the periphery of the lens were widely exposed by an iridectomy. But if the opacity is more considerable, and does not leave a wide margin of clear cornea, the artificial pupil thus made will be insufficient, more especially with regard to the amount of light admitted into the eye; and in such cases it is better to make an iridectomy, which should, however, be but small. If the margin of transparent

[1] "A. f. O." t. 1, 251; vide also Donder's "Anomalies of Accommodation and Refraction of the Eye," p. 128. New Syden. Society.

cornea is very narrow, there is always the danger that the wound made in the performance of iridectomy may produce a certain degree of fresh opacity of the small portion of clear cornea near it, and thus militate against the benefit derived from the operation. In order to obviate this danger, we may make the artificial pupil by coredialysis, which would, of course, produce no cloudiness of the cornea opposite to the new pupil, the incision being made at another portion of the cornea. An artificial pupil should always be made opposite that portion of the cornea which is the most clear, and has the truest curvature. The direction inwards, or slightly downwards and inwards, is by far the best for optical purposes, for not only does the artificial pupil then correspond to the visual line, but it also assists better in the binocular vision (Gemeinschaftlicher Sehact) with the other eye. If any anterior syne-chia exists, and its extent is but small, it may be divided with the point of the broad needle or iridectomy knife, in the performance of iridodesis or iridectomy. If it is of recent formation (as after an incised or punctured wound of the cornea), the adhesion is often so slight that it may easily be detached with a blunt hook or a small spud.

[Aehmrleth has proposed, in cases of total opacity of the cornea, to admit light through an opening in the sclera; but no practical results have ever been obtained from this method.—B.]

[A mode of treatment of dense leucomata has recently been devised by Mr. Henry Power,[1] of London, and practised on the human subject with "promising results." It consists in removing a portion of the opaque cornea of the patient with a sharp punch specially devised for the purpose, and obtaining, by the same means, an exactly corresponding portion of a healthy rabbit's cornea, and transferring it to the space in the human eye. The lids are then to be fixed together, and, in a week, Mr. Power has found union to be complete. Whether the portion transplanted will become perfectly clear is as yet, from want of experience, say.—H.]

[The operation of "corneal transplantation" has been perfected by Mr. Wolfe of Glasgow, who has had some excellent results. His instruments are a lance-knife with a stop, a broad-grooved director, and a double-bladed knife which fits into the grooves of the director. A flap, broad at the base and converging towards the cornea, is taken from the ocular conjunctiva on each side, and dissected up to the transition fold. These are turned over on the cornea and removed in the usual way. The lance is then introduced in the limbus so as not to injure the conjunctival flap, and pushed in as far as the stop will allow. The director is then passed through one of the openings and pushed in front of the iris and lens out through the opposite side. The knife is then placed in the grooves, and the corneal flap separated and put in tepid water. A similar conjunctival and corneal flap is then removed from the other patient; but here the lance must be used so as not to interfere with the pillars of the iris, and it must be rapidly withdrawn, so as to prevent as much as possible the escape of the aqueous humor, and consequent falling forward of the iris. The transparent graft is then placed in position, and secured by stitches in the corners of the conjunctival flaps. Wolfe thinks the success depends upon the graft being taken from a freshly enucleated human eye, the smoothness of the corneal incisions, and the exactness of the measurements of the graft. Moreover, no damage must be done to the subjacent structures, and hence the whole cornea must not be removed. Sellerbeck has also reported cases operated upon in this way (see "Medical Times and Gazette," Nov. 22, 1879; "Archiv für Ophthalmologie," xxiv. 4).—B.]

[[1] "Med. Times and Gaz.," Aug. 10, 1872.]

[The subject of corneal transplantation has been the subject of investigations by Neelsen and Angelucci, whose observations have been made upon quite a number of experiments upon animals. They draw the following conclusions from their own experience: In the majority of cases the transplanted portion of cornea partially sloughs, while what is left becomes inclosed in opaque cicatricial tissue. A permanent adhesion, with maintenance of the transplanted piece, is possible only when the latter is nourished not only from its margin, but also from its inner surface by old or newly formed subjacent tissue. Thus, in a successful case of transplantation, there lies upon the inner or under surface of the transplanted portion an opaque layer, which eventually so diminishes the transparency of the graft itself, that the final result is practically a failure. It would also appear from these experiments that an artificial, flat or shallow corneal wound may, without the transplantation of a flap, be filled by transparent tissue, which probably comes from the conjunctiva. (See "Klinische Monatsblätter für Augenheilkunde," August, 1880. Also an article by Zehender in the same journal for May, 1880.)—B.]

I need hardly say that the experiments made by Nussbaum and others, to cut a hole in the opaque cornea and insert a piece of glass, have completely failed.

8.—ARCUS SENILIS.

[Syn. Gerontoxon.—B.]
This peculiar marginal opacity of the cornea is due to fatty degeneration of the corneal tissue, which generally commences first in the upper portion of the cornea. It then shows itself in the lower, and the extremities of the two arcs increase more and more, until at last they meet and encircle the whole cornea. We are chiefly indebted to Mr. Canton[1] for an exact and extensive knowledge of this condition; he has found that it generally occurs about the age of fifty, but that it may appear at a much earlier age, especially in families in which it appears to be hereditary. He also considers that the arcus senilis affords us the best indication of the proneness of other tissues to fatty degeneration.

The opacity is at first of a light gray color, appearing like a narrow silvery rim near the edge of the cornea, but not reaching quite up to the latter, being always divided from it by a transparent portion of cornea. At a later period, the opacity assumes a denser and more creamy tint, and increases in depth and width, being generally broader above and below than at the sides. It might be supposed that the fatty degeneration of the corneal tissue would impede or prevent the union of an incision lying in this part of the cornea. This is, however, not the case, for we find that a section carried through the arcus senilis heals perfectly, as may be often observed in cases of extraction of cataract.

9.—CONICAL CORNEA. [KERATOCONUS.—B.]

When this affection is but slight, a cursory observer may easily overlook it, and mistake it, perhaps, for a case of myopia, complicated with weakness of sight (amblyopia); but a marked case cannot well be overlooked. On regarding such an eye from the front, we notice that the centre of the cornea

---

[1] Vide Mr. Edwin Canton's work, "On the Arcus Senilis," London, 1863.

appears unusually glistening and bright, as if a tear-drop were suspended from it. If we then look at it in profile, the size and shape of the conicity will become at once apparent. [Fig. 89.] Sometimes the conicity is not in the centre, but nearer the margin of the cornea. But by means of the ophthalmoscope, even the slightest cases of conical cornea may be diagnosed with cer-
tainty, as was first pointed out by Mr. Bowman.[1] For this purpose the mirror alone is to be used, without the convex lens in front. On throwing the light upon the cornea, we receive a bright red reflection through the centre of the cornea, which gradually shades off and becomes darker

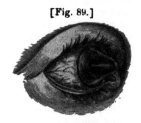

[Fig. 89.]

towards the base, so that the central bright red spot is surrounded by a dark zone, which in its turn is again encircled by a red ring. If we throw the light upon the centre of the cornea at different angles, the side of the cone opposite to the light is darkened. The central red zone (in which we obtain a reverse image of the disk, etc.) is due to the reflection of the fundus through the central conical portion of the cornea, and the outer red ring to the reflection through the normal peripheral portion of the cornea. The dark zone between the two is, according to Knapp,[2] due to the diffusion and complete reflection of the rays of light at the base of the cone, where it passes over into the normal curvature of the cornea.

On the ophthalmoscopic examination of the fundus of an eye affected with conical cornea, we notice a considerable parallax on moving the convex lens in front of the patient's eye.[3] In this way we can produce a distortion and displacement of a certain portion of the disk and retinal vessels, whilst the other part of the disk remains immovable, just as occurs in glaucomatous excavation of the optic nerve.

Even in slight cases of conical cornea, the patients always complain of considerable, and often great impairment of sight. On account of the conicity of the central portion of the cornea, the antero-posterior axis is increased in length, and hence the eye has become more or less myopic, and the patient consequently holds small objects (as in reading, etc.) very close to the eye. But the impairment of sight is chiefly due to the astigmatism caused by the irregular curvature of the cornea, which gives rise to great distortion and confusion of the retinal images. [The astigmatism may be simple myopic, or mixed, or even simple hypermetropic astigmatism.—B.] Concave spherical lenses, therefore, generally produce but slight improvement, but some benefit is occasionally derived from cylindrical glasses, although the astigmatism is, as a rule, too irregular to admit of much correc-
tion. More improvement is found from the use of a circular or slit-shaped stenopæic apparatus, fitted, perhaps, with a suitable concave lens, as this diminishes the circles of diffusion upon the retina by cutting off the periph-
eral rays of light. We often notice that the patients endeavor to accomplish this for themselves by nipping their eyelids together, so as to change the palpebral aperture into a narrow slit. After the disease has existed a certain time, and reached a high degree of development, the apex of the cone often becomes opaque, and thus the sight is still more deteriorated.

The bulging forward of the cornea is not due to an increase in the intra-
ocular tension (which is indeed rather slackened), but to a diminution in

[1] " R. L. O. H. Rep.," ii. 154.   [2] " Kl. Monatsbl.," 1864, 318.
[3] Donders, " A. f. O.," 7, 199; also Donders, op. cit., 551.

the power of resistance of the cornea, and as this bulging increases, the portion of cornea embraced in it becomes thinner and thinner. It is an interesting fact, that, however attenuated the apex may become, it never gives way, except through an accidental injury. Mr. Bowman thinks that the reason of this is, that, "as the cornea becomes thinner, the escape of the aqueous humor by exosmose is facilitated, and thus the internal pressure is reduced, so as to be no longer in excess of the diminished resisting power of the cornea. A balance is established like that of health, only that there is a more than ordinary outflow of the aqueous humor by transudation through the cornea. This accords with my previous observation, as to such eyes being rather unduly soft."

The progress of the disease is generally very slow. It may become stationary at any point, stopping short when the conicity is still but slight, or going on until it is very considerable and the apex has become clouded. It generally sooner or later attacks both eyes. It occurs frequently, but not always, in persons of a delicate constitution, and commences chiefly between the ages of fifteen and thirty. Mr. Bowman has observed a very few cases in which it occurred in more than one member of the same family. Any considerable and protracted use or straining of the eye in reading, sewing, etc., will tend to increase its development and produce local irritation and congestion.

Innumerable remedies have been suggested and tried for the relief and cure of conical cornea, but almost all of them without success. If the patient is in delicate health, tonics and a nutritious diet with plenty of fresh air and exercise should be prescribed, and the use of the eyes for reading, etc., should be forbidden if both are affected. In order to neutralize the myopia produced by the conicity of the cornea, Sir W. Adams removed the lens. Mr. Wardrop recommended frequent tapping of the anterior chamber. Mr. Tyrrell was the first to make an artificial pupil in this disease, and this is the treatment which has hitherto proved most successful. The purpose we have in view in making an artificial pupil is twofold: 1st. To improve vision by making a pupil opposite a portion of the cornea which has retained its normal curvature; 2d. To arrest the progress of the disease, and, if possible, to cause it to retrograde somewhat by diminishing the intra-ocular pressure.

The artificial pupil may be made either by an iridectomy or an iridodesis. By the former operation, we certainly bring the pupil opposite a marginal portion of the cornea, but there is this disadvantage, that the original pupil remains opposite the conicity, and therefore the rays which pass through it are diffused and irregularly refracted, and thus confuse the retinal image and diminish its distinctness; whereas, by means of an iridodesis we can draw the iris well forward towards the incision, and thus displace the pupil towards a portion of the cornea which is less irregularly curved, and bring the iris opposite the cone. The incision should be made slightly in the sclerotic, so that the plane of the iris may not be moved away from the lens. The best direction for the iridodesis is slightly downwards and inwards. In order to obtain the advantages which are derived from a slit-shaped stenopaic apparatus, Mr. Bowman has made a double iridodesis, so that an oblong slit-shaped pupil is obtained. This may be made either vertical or horizontal. In the former case, we have the advantage that a considerable portion of the angles of the slit is covered by the lids, which renders it much less unsightly, more especially if the irides are light in color, than the horizontal slit, which gives the appearance of a cat's eye. The operation should not be performed in opposite directions at the same sitting, as the point first tied is apt to yield and be drawn into the anterior chamber again, when the iris is drawn towards the opposite incision. It is best to make the second iridodesis about eight or ten days after the first. The incision should be made in the sclerotic, so as to retain the normal plane of the iris.

Not only does this operation produce a beneficial effect in an optical point of view, but it also sometimes causes a considerable diminution in the bulge of the cornea and the progress of the disease. At present it is very difficult to decide upon the point as to which operation is really the best, as the results have varied considerably. For instance, in some cases benefit has been produced in the sight by the second iridodesis, whereas in others again this has not been the case. The improvement is, however, never so conspicuous as after the first operation. My own experience rather tends to the opinion that, on the whole, the progress of the disease is most arrested and the bulging of the cornea most diminished by an iridectomy. Care must, however, be taken to make it only moderate in size, and perhaps slightly upwards and inwards, so that a part of the base of the artificial pupil may be covered by the upper lid. In slight cases, in which the conicity is either almost stationary or but very slowly progressive, I think iridodesis is indicated; whereas if it is considerably and markedly progressive, an iridectomy is to be preferred.

Von Graefe has lately published a very interesting case of conical cornea, in which he produces ulceration of the apex of the cone, and subsequent contraction and flattening of the cicatrix.[1] The fact that the cicatricial contraction which follows extensive ulcers or infiltrations of the cornea always produces a certain degree of diminution or flattening of the curvature of the cornea, led Von Graefe to the idea that a similar effect might be brought about in severe cases of conical cornea, by the artificial production of a little ulcer. The operation is to be performed in the following manner: The point of a very small knife, made of the shape of Von Graefe's narrow cataract-knife, but smaller in size, is to be passed into the middle layers of the cornea, just at the apex of the cone, to the extent of about a line, and then brought out again; so that a very small superficial flap may be formed, which is then to be seized with a very fine pair of forceps and snipped off at its base with a pair of curved scissors, thus leaving a superficial gap at this point. Great care must be taken that the knife does not penetrate the cornea, of which there is the greatest risk, on account of the extreme tenuity of the cornea at the apex of the cone. Should, however, perforation occur, the operation should be postponed for a few days, until the aperture is closed. The day after the operation, the floor of the gap is to be lightly touched, at two or three points, with a finely pointed crayon of mitigated nitrate of silver (nitrate of silver one part, nitrate of potassium two parts), the effect of the cauterization being at once neutralized by the application of salt and water. The application of the caustic is to be repeated at intervals of from three to six days, until a slight, faintly yellowish infiltration is formed, with but a moderate degree of pericorneal injection, when we may consider the effect as sufficient, and simply apply atropine to the eye and guard it against exposure. The cauterization generally produces but very little irritation. Should the infiltration show a tendency to assume the character of a perforating ulcer, the compress bandage must be employed alternately with warm aromatic fomentations, and it may even be necessary to perform paracentesis. The improvement of the sight will not be at once apparent, indeed at first it may even be deteriorated, but at the end of five or six weeks, when

---

[1] "A. f. O.," 12, 2, 215. More recently Von Graefe has published an elaborate and interesting paper upon this subject in the "Berliner klinische Wochenschrift," 1868,

the infiltration begins to contract, it rapidly increases, the little cicatricial opacity gradually diminishes in size and density, and leaves the sight greatly improved. Von Graefe has performed this operation with great success in several cases of severe conical cornea, and has gained much better results than from the formation of an artificial pupil. Mr. Critchett has lately likewise obtained a most successful result by this proceeding in a case of double conical cornea.

Mr. Bader[1] has obtained very favorable results from excising an elliptical piece of the apex of the cone. The operation is best done by transfixing the apex of the cone with Graefe's cataract-knife, and then cutting out from within outwards; in this way a small flap is made, which is then to be seized with iris forceps and excised with a pair of scissors. Originally he transfixed the apex of the cone with a small curved needle, carrying a suture, prior to making the incision with the knife, so that the flaps could afterwards be united by suture. It has been found, however, that the wound heals very readily without a suture. A bandage should be kept over the eye until all redness and watering have disappeared; if a suture has been applied, it may remain in for four or five days, but must be removed if there is any chemosis or swelling of the lids. The chief disadvantage of this operation is, that it often leaves a very extensive adhesion of the iris to the cicatrix, which may not only impair the acuity of vision, but prove of subsequent danger to the eye, in the same way as ordinary anterior synechia. As it is often difficult in this way to get both sides of the opening of equal size and shape, Mr. Critchett has invented the following ingenious knife. It consists of two Sichel's blades (the backs of which touch, and the point of one being a little longer than the other), which are set upon one handle. They are hinged together, so that they can be set at any required angle, and be fixed there by a screw. The operation is to be performed as follows: "The blades being firmly fixed at the desired angle, the points are to pierce the cornea at the point of the cone to which the excision is to reach, passed steadily on through the anterior chamber, brought out at the opposite point of the cone, and pushed on until they have cut their way out. Thus a small elliptical piece (both sides of which are exactly equal and sharply defined) of the cornea will be excised. Should one side of this piece remain slightly adherent, it is to be snipped off with scissors.

Mr. Bowman has lately employed a drill for excising a portion of the cone, and has favored me with the following description of this operation:

"In 1869 I had some small cutting trephines,[2] made by Messrs. Weiss, adapted, among other uses, to excise a defined circular portion of the apex

---

[1] "Lancet," January 20, 1873.

[2] De Wecker has also lately devised a trephine, which is constructed on the same principles as Heurteloup's artificial leech. The cutting cylindrical blade is inclosed in a solid tube, from which it does not protrude, except upon pressure of a spring. At present he only thinks the instrument indicated—1. In cases of complete cicatrix of the cornea, more especially if the lens has escaped during the suppuration, a small circular portion of the centre of the cicatrix is to be pinched out, so as to leave a permanent fistula. By this proceeding the patients may gain a fair qualitative perception of light, sufficient perhaps to enable them to find their way about, or even to decipher large letters. 2. In cases of absolute glaucoma, in which a satisfactory iridectomy cannot be made on account of the advanced atrophy of the iris, and a simple sclerotomy would not suffice. Here the chief objects of the operation are to relieve the patient of the severe pain, and to avoid the necessity for enucleation of the eyeball. A circular portion of one or one and one-half millimetre in diameter is to be removed at the edge of the cornea, care being taken to avoid all risk of injury to the lens, or of approaching too closely to the ciliary body. Thus a large filtrating cicatrix is established. *Vide* "Annales d'oculistique," October, 1872.

of a conical cornea. The instruments vary in diameter, so as to remove portions of different sizes, as required. They are also provided with a movable 'stop,' to regulate the depth of penetration. They are rotated by the finger and thumb.

"Having found the application of caustic to the abraded surface, according to Graefe's method, to be followed by prolonged irritation, I soon abandoned its use, and employed the trephines to remove at once a circular piece of cornea in its whole thickness, the portion included in the instrument being seized by small forceps and excised by scissors as soon as the escape of aqueous humor showed that the chamber was penetrated at any part of the circle. A satisfactory modification of the curvature was thus obtained, but with the occasional disadvantage which is apt to attend the complete removal of an elliptical or other shaped portion by any other method, viz., that during the healing of the gap, the pupillary region of the iris, always contracted while the aqueous leaks, is liable to become engaged in the wound, and an anterior synechia result. To prevent this, I practised iridectomy simultaneously in some cases, but I have recently operated in another way. Instead of carrying the trephine quite through the cornea, I withdraw it when it has nearly reached the membrane of Descemet, and then, seizing the place with fine forceps, dissect it off with a broad needle. The floor thus left immediately bulges like a hernia, and is then either punctured at its centre, or a small central portion of it is excised, the object being to allow temporary drainage of the aqueous, and thus promote the contraction of the cornea, without the risk of anterior synechia; for the small orifice made ought to correspond with the centre of the pupil, and, to insure accuracy in this respect, I would suggest the use of Calabar bean immediately before operating, so that the site of the contracted pupil may be a guide to the surgeon. If during the ensuing two or three weeks the aqueous is found to have reaccumulated, the central point is again opened at intervals of a few days, no pain or irritation being thereby occasioned. Indeed, it is remarkable how little inconvenience attends the whole proceeding, provided ordinary prudence be observed.

"The improvement of the curvature goes on during several weeks after the final closure of the orifice, and should any conicity be found remaining afterwards, a repetition of the operation on a smaller scale will furnish the means of correcting it.

"The opacity resulting from this mode of operating seems to be unexpectedly slight, but, if required, it may be concealed by the tattooing process.

"My experience thus far induces me to recommend this operation in even the earlier stages and slighter degrees of conical cornea, as a smaller extent of cornea need then to be involved, and there must be a much better prospect of recovering a quite normal curvature than if the operation be delayed until the bulge grows greater. A considerable advantage, therefore, of this method would seem to be that, by its harmlessness, it will admit of being applied to a number of slight and incipient cases, which the surgeon has hitherto been very timid in meddling with, notwithstanding that they are attended with great defects of vision, which no optical contrivance will correct."

At present, it must be admitted that all these modern methods of treatment of conical cornea are still upon their trial, and nothing decisive can as yet be said as to their relative advantages or disadvantages. The simplest and easiest is, without doubt, the formation of a central ulcer (Graefe's method), especially if the denudation be made as I have suggested, by simply scraping off the epithelium and superficial layer of cornea. It certainly requires a longer time than excision or drilling out of a piece, but it is also much easier. Should a central leucoma be left, an iridectomy would improve the sight, and tattooing the opacity would improve the appearance.[1]

[Del Toro describes a method which he has employed for some time for the cure of conical cornea. He first does an iridectomy, and waits twelve or fifteen days for the wound to heal. Then, with a very fine knife heated to a white heat, he destroys the vertex of the conical cornea, which can be done immediately and with scarcely any pain. He then applies a compressive bandage for two weeks, and at the end of that period a cure is obtained, leaving a slight opacity. This cauterization also seems to exercise a beneficial influence on the existing kerato-malacia, while the early iridectomy diminishes the intra-ocular tension. The only precaution necessary is to carefully avoid opening the anterior chamber with the hot knife. (See "La Crónica oftalmológica," May 12, 1881.)—B.]

10.—KERATO-GLOBUS (HYDROPHTHALMIA ANTERIOR. HYDROPS OF THE ANTERIOR CHAMBER).

This disease is characterized by a uniform spherical bulging of the whole cornea, so that it is increased in size in all its diameters. [Fig. 90.] Gener-

[Fig. 90.

After T. W. Jones.]

ally, however, this increase in size is not confined to the cornea, but extends to the neighboring portion of the sclerotic. The augmentation in the size of the anterior half of the eyeball is often so considerable, that the eye protrudes between the palpebral aperture, and prevents the easy closure of the eyelids. On account of the peculiar staring appearance which this gives to the eye, the disease has also been termed "buphthalmos." True hydrophthalmos or buphthalmos is always congenital. For an important and very interesting account of this disease, I would refer the reader to a dissertation on "Hydropthalmus Congenitus," by Dr. Wilhelm v. Muralt, of Zurich,[2] based on cases which occurred in Professor Horner's clinique.

The cornea may either remain transparent or become slightly opaque near the periphery; in other cases the cloudiness may be more considerable, and extend over the greater portion of the surface of the cornea. The anterior portion of the sclerotic is much thinned and of a blue tint, which is due to a shining through of the choroid. The size of the anterior chamber is much increased, both in depth and circumference. The aqueous humor is generally clear. The iris is also enlarged, and the fibres near its ciliary margin are stretched and opened up; the pupil is generally somewhat dilated and sluggish, and perhaps here and there adherent to the capsule. The iris is often somewhat cupped back, which increases still more the depth of the anterior chamber, and it may also be tremulous, which may be either due to dislocation of the lens, caused by a stretching and giving way of its suspensory ligament, or to the iris being no longer in contact with the anterior surface of the lens, but divided from it by a collection of fluid in the posterior chamber. Sometimes, however, the iris is bulged forwards.

[1] "Annales d'Oculistique," lxviii. p. 187; "Clinique Ophthalmologique," Paris, [2] "Trans. of the Internat. Ophthal. Congress," p. 72.—B.]
       [2] Zürich, published by Zürcher and Furrer, 1869.

But as the disease advances, the optic disk becomes excavated from the permanent increase in the intra-ocular tension, the lens becomes opaque, the vitreous humor fluid, the retina perhaps detached, and atrophy of the eyeball may close the scene. On account of the great attenuation of the anterior portion of the coat of the eye, even a slight blow may suffice to rupture the globe. But whether this may occur spontaneously is doubtful. The state of the sight varies considerably. In some cases the patient can still decipher moderate-sized print; in others it is greatly impaired, which may be due to the opacity of the cornea, or to inflammation of the deeper tunics of the eye. As a rule, the disease terminates sooner or later in blindness.

The affection does not appear to be due to an increased secretion of the aqueous humor, but to a thinning and diminution in the power of resistance of the cornea, following generally upon severe and extensive inflammation of the cornea, as, for instance, vascular keratitis or pannus. The opacity may afterwards disappear, but the bulging remains, and even gradually augments. Treatment, unfortunately, is but too often of little avail. The most is to be expected from a large iridectomy. The patient's general health should be strengthened, and the eyes be but moderately employed. If the protrusion is very considerable, the cornea opaque, and the sight almost entirely gone, an operation for staphyloma may be indicated, not only for the sake of appearance of the eye, but also to alleviate the inconvenience and constant irritation kept up by the incomplete closure of the eyelids.

11.—STAPHYLOMA OF THE CORNEA AND IRIS.

We have already seen that when an ulcer of the cornea causes perforation of the latter, the aqueous humor flows off, the iris falls forward, and may become adherent to the cornea. If the perforation is of but slight extent, an

Fig. 91.   Fig. 92.

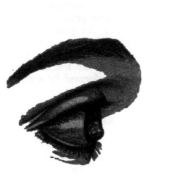
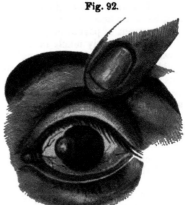

Side view. After Mackenzie.   Front view. After Dalrymple.]

anterior synechia will be produced, without perhaps any bulging of the cornea at this point. But if the opening is large, a considerable portion of iris will fall against or into the gap, and perhaps protrude through it, giving rise to a more or less extensive prolapse. This is soon covered with a layer of lymph, which becomes organized, gradually assumes a cicatricial character, and replaces the cornea at this point, to which it may indeed bear a certain outward resemblance.   It is, however, much weaker and less elastic, so that it readily yields to the intra-ocular pressure, gradually bulges forward, and gives rise to a partial staphyloma.   [Figs. 91, 92.]   If the latter is situated at the margin of the cornea, the pupil may remain partially or entirely free, and a certain amount of sight be preserved ; but if the prolapse occurs in the centre, the whole pupil will be involved.   A partial staphyloma may gradually increase, until it implicates the surrounding cornea to a considerable extent, and if the perforation was originally of large size, it may, finally, even involve the whole cornea, and become changed into a total staphyloma. When the projection has become at all considerable, so as to protrude somewhat between the lids, its exposure to the action of external irritants is apt to produce occasional inflammatory exacerbations, which tend to cause a still greater increase in the size of the staphyloma.

The most frequent causes of partial staphyloma are sloughs and ulcers of the cornea, wounds and injuries, and also certain operations upon the eye, as, for instance, flap extraction, which may be followed by a considerable prolapse of the iris and the formation of a partial staphyloma.

No time should be allowed to elapse before the tendency to staphyloma is checked.   Thus if a prolapse of the iris has occurred, it should be treated at once by the proper remedies.   The best treatment for partial staphyloma is undoubtedly by iridectomy, as this, by diminishing the intra-ocular pressure, not only prevents the increase of the bulging, but generally also causes it to decrease in size.   The artificial pupil should be made opposite to the most transparent portion of the cornea.   I must here again mention the very important fact that cases of partial or complete staphyloma are sometimes accompanied by marked increase of tension, so that the eye is in a glaucomatous condition, and the degree of impairment of vision quite disproportionate to the amount of staphyloma and opacity of the cornea.   In such cases there will be increase of tension, accompanied perhaps by contraction of the field, eccentric fixation, and excavation of the optic nerve. In all cases of staphyloma the degree of tension, the state of the sight and of the field of vision must therefore be carefully watched, and an iridectomy must be on no account delayed if symptoms of glaucoma supervene.   I think this treatment of partial staphyloma by iridectomy greatly preferable to that which was formerly much in vogue, viz., the touching the protrusion with nitrate of silver, and thus changing it into an ulcer, which, on cicatrizing, would produce a flattening and shrinking of the staphylomatous tissue. This is apt to set up considerable irritation, and proves far less efficacious than an iridectomy.   Partial abscission may also be performed by a modification of Critchett's operation.

12.—TOTAL STAPHYLOMA OF THE CORNEA AND IRIS.

This only occurs in cases in which there has been an almost total destruction of the cornea by sloughing or ulceration.   Its shape is generally spherical [Fig. 93], although occasionally it may be conical.   The neighboring portion of the sclerotic mostly becomes implicated in the process, and the staphyloma may, in time, involve the anterior half of the eyeball.   The lens may either have escaped at the time of the perforation, or have remained behind, in which case it often becomes opaque.   Its position within the eye varies; it generally lies in close contact with the iris and the cicatricial tissue, to which it becomes adherent; it may, however, be separated from the iris by a considerable amount of aqueous humor, which forms a large posterior chamber; or, again, it may have become detached from the suspensory ligament, and have sunk down into the vitreous humor.

The presence or absence of the lens after an extensive perforation of the cornea exerts great influence upon the formation of a staphyloma. If the lens escaped at the giving way of the cornea, a firm cicatrix is formed, which will generally resist the intra-ocular pressure, and not bulge forward; but will often become consolidated, contract, and lead, perhaps, to a certain degree of shrinking of the globe. It is different, however, if the lens has remained within the eye, for it then bulges forward, and presses upon the newly formed cicatricial tissue, which gradually yields and becomes staphylomatous. If, therefore, a case of extensive perforation of the cornea, with a tendency to staphyloma, is seen at an early stage, and the lens is found pressing against the cicatrix, it is best to remove it at once, so as to allow the cicatrix to become firm and consolidated. The lens

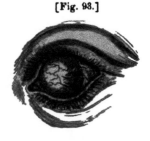

[Fig. 93.]

may be removed by making an incision into the staphyloma with Graefe's cataract-knife, dividing the capsule, and allowing the lens to escape. Or, it may be done according to the following proceeding of Mr. Bowman, which I have seen answer remarkably well in several cases. He passes a broad needle through the staphyloma into the lens, and breaks this freely up. The needle having been withdrawn, a curette is passed through the same opening, and the soft lens-matter allowed to escape. The breaking up of the lens may be repeated at intervals of a few days. The staphylomatous protrusion will gradually subside, the cicatrix will become firm and consolidated, and the eye perhaps shrink somewhat. When all symptoms of irritation have subsided, an artificial eye may often be worn without the necessity of any further operation.

As we cannot restore any sight in cases of total staphyloma, the object of our treatment must be to remove the protrusion, so as to free the patient from the pain and inconvenience which generally attend this disease, and also to improve the personal appearance and permit of the adaptation of an artificial eye. There are numerous modes of operating for staphyloma, of which the following only require mention: 1. Excision. 2. Mr. Critchett's operation of abscission. 3. Graefe's seton operation. 4. Borelli's operation. [Total and even partial abscission of the staphyloma is dangerous, when there are signs of increased intra-ocular tension and consequent amaurosis; in other words, secondary glaucoma. In these cases, enucleation is the only permissible operation.—H.]

1. *Excision.*—This is best performed in the following manner: The point of a cataract-knife (the edge of which is turned downwards, as in Fig. 94) is to be passed into the sclerotic, near the edge of the staphyloma, and somewhat above its horizontal diameter, so that about two-thirds of the staphyloma may be included in the incision. The blade of the knife is to be carried on parallel to the base of the tumor, until its point makes its exit at the opposite side, at a spot corresponding to the puncture. The knife should then be pushed slowly on, until it has cut its way out and divided the lower two-thirds of the staphyloma, by a large flap-shaped incision. The remaining portion is next to be divided by the aid of a pair of scissors. A bandage is then to be applied, either together with water dressing or a simple pledget

of lint.   Lymph will be effused from the edges of the incision
or less firm cicatrix result; the eyeball will shrink somewhat,
haps a tolerably good stump for the application of an artific
result of the operation is not, however, always so favorable.   A
gush of vitreous humor may follow upon the excision of the an

Fig. 94.

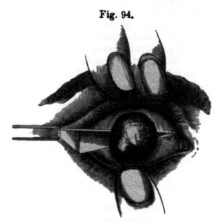

After Stellwag.

of the eye, and intra-ocular hemorrhage ensue.   Or, again, suppura
the eye may take place, accompanied, perhaps, by very violent pa
inflammation.   The eyeball then shrinks and dwindles down, leaving
very small and inefficient stump, with a slight degree of movement,
application of an artificial eye.   To obviate these disadvantage
Critchett has employed the following ingenious and valuable opera
abscission, which leaves an excellent, large, movable stump.

Fig. 95.

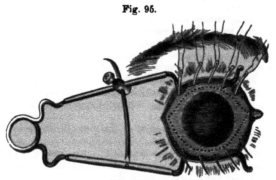

After Lawson.

2. Mr. Critchett's[1] operation of abscission is to be performed thus:
patient being placed under the influence of chloroform, the staphyl
freely exposed by means of a wire speculum; a series of four or five

1 "Roy. Lond. Ophth. Hosp. Reports," iv. 1.

small needles, with a semicircular curve, are passed through the mass, about equidistant from each other, and at such points as the lines of incision are intended to traverse (Fig. 95). These needles are left in this position, with both extremities protruding to an equal extent from the staphyloma. The advantages gained by this part of the proceeding are: 1. That a small quantity of the fluid parts of the distended globe escapes, thus diminishing pressure, and preventing a sudden gush of the contents, when the anterior part is removed. 2. That the points of emergence indicate the lines of incision. 3. That the presence of the needles prevents, or rather restrains, to some extent, the escape of the lens and vitreous humor, after the anterior part of the staphyloma has been removed. The next stage of the proceeding is to remove the anterior part of the staphyloma. This requires some judgment and modification in size and form, in accordance with the extent of the enlargement, so as to leave a convenient globe. My usual plan is to make an opening in the sclerotic, about two lines in extent, just anterior to the tendinous insertion of the external rectus, made with a Beer's knife [Fig. 96]. Into this opening I insert a pair of small probe-pointed scissors, and cut out an elliptical piece, just within the points where the needles have entered and emerged. The needles, armed with fine black silk, are then drawn through each in its turn, and the sutures

[Fig. 96.]

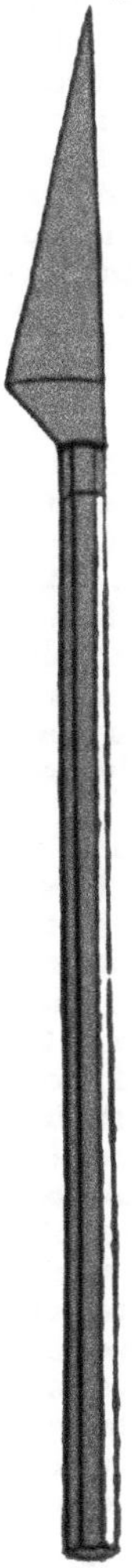

Fig. 97.

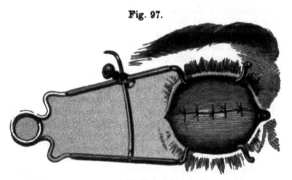

After Lawson.

are carefully tied, so as to approximate as closely as possible the divided edges of the sclerotic and conjunctiva (Fig. 97). The operation is now finished; the speculum may be removed so as to allow the lids to close, and wet lint may be applied to keep the parts cool. In a large majority of cases, union of the divided edges takes place by the first intention." . . . . "I generally leave the sutures in for some weeks. Sometimes they come away spontaneously, and when this is not the case, they may readily be removed after all irritation has passed away, and after firm union has taken place. If the case be examined three or four months after the operation, a movable globe is seen with a flattened anterior surface, traversed by a white line of cicatrix, and having rather a prominent external angle. Upon this an artificial eye can be readily adapted, which moves to a greater extent than I have observed previous to adoption of my present method."

Care must be taken in making the incision, so to slope and bevel off the angles, that the lips of the wound here fit very accurately and neatly, otherwise an awkward pucker may be left at those points, which will interfere materially with the comfort of wearing an artificial eye. It is always best, except perhaps in young children, or where the staphyloma is small, to employ five sutures, in order that too great an interval may not be left between them, for if this be the case, beads of vitreous will protrude, become covered with granulations, and suppurate somewhat. My experience of Mr. Critchett's operation has certainly been most favorable, and I can entirely endorse his statement, that we gain by it a better and more perfectly movable stump for an artificial eye, than by any other operation. I do not, however, think it indicated in those cases in which the disease is not confined to the anterior portion of the eyeball, but the inflammation has extended to the retina and choroid. For in such cases, the operation is not only often followed by perhaps immediate and severe intra-ocular hemorrhage leading to suppuration of the globe, but we leave behind a part of the diseased structure, which may not only become again inflamed, but, what is still more to be dreaded, be the cause of sympathetic inflammation in the other eye. In all such cases, it is therefore undoubtedly by far the safest plan to remove the whole eyeball, as this frees us from all fear of sympathetic ophthalmia. If the patient is in good circumstances, and is so situated that he can at once apply to a surgeon, if the stump becomes inflamed, or symptoms of sympathetic irritation show themselves, and if he is extremely anxious about his personal appearance, abscission may be performed, otherwise it is safest to remove the staphylomatous eye altogether. I must here state, that in the "Dublin Quarterly Journal of Medical Science" for 1847, vol. iii. p. 242, Mr. (now Sir William) Wilde drew attention to a new operation which he had devised for the removal of staphyloma. This consisted in the introduction of a curved needle through the base of the staphyloma, then removing the conical projection with a cataract-knife and scissors, drawing the needle through, and tying the ligature. Sir William Wilde subsequently sometimes employed several ligatures.

In order to avoid, if possible, any risk of sympathetic irritation of the other eye, which might be awakened by the passage of the needles through the ciliary region, or the presence of the threads at this point for eight to fourteen days, Knapp[1] has devised the following modification of Critchett's operation: Instead of passing the needles and sutures through the ciliary region or cornea, he passes them through the conjunctiva by means of two needles. This proceeding is illustrated in Fig. 98. A fine, threaded needle is inserted in the conjunctiva, about four or five millimetres above the base of the staphyloma, and somewhat to the inner side of the vertical meridian (Fig. 98, a), it is passed beneath the conjunctiva and subconjunctival tissue towards the nose, and brought out at the inner edge of the base of the staphyloma (b). Thence the same needle and thread are passed over the staphyloma to its lower margin c, and there again inserted in the conjunctiva and passed beneath it to d. The same proceeding is repeated on the outer portion of the staphyloma at e, f, g, h. The threads are then well laid back out of the way of the lines of the incision, and the staphyloma excised as in Critchett's operation. The two ends of the thread, l l' and m m', are then firmly tied, so that the lips of the incision are brought into close contact. The threads are to be removed at the end of three or four days.

3. Von Graefe's[2] operation by seton consists in passing a double thread parallel to the cornea, through the coats of the eyeball (but not where they

[1] "A. f. O.," xiv. 2, 275.   [2] "Archiv f. Ophthalmologie," ix. 2, 106.

are thinned) and the vitreous humor, so as to include them within a suture to an extent of four or five lines. The threads are not to be tied tightly, but left in a loose loop, and their ends are to be snipped off close to the knot. A light compress is to be applied to the lids. Within from fifteen to thirty-two hours, acute symptoms of suppurative choroiditis generally supervene, accompanied by subconjunctival chemosis, slight immobility of the lateral movements of the eye, and perhaps a certain degree of protrusion of the globe. The threads are then to be removed, and warm chamomile or poppy

Fig. 98.

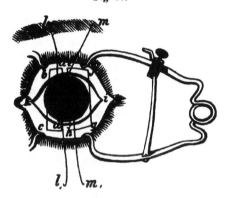

fomentations should be applied to alleviate the pain. The eyeball after a time becomes shrunk and atrophied. I have seen one case successfully treated by Mr. Bowman in a somewhat similar manner. The threads were, however, left in for some time and occasionally moved. There were no severe symptoms of inflammation, and the eye gradually diminished to about half its original size, and an artificial eye is now worn with comfort. The great advantage of this proceeding is, that there is no tendency to sympathetic inflammation, which appears never to ensue upon suppurative choroiditis.

4. Dr. Borelli transfixes the staphyloma by two needles, which are passed through the base of the protrusion, so as to cross each other at right angles. The one is entered at the temporal side, midway between the vertical and horizontal meridian of the cornea, passed beneath the tumor, and brought out at a corresponding point at the opposite side. This pin may be entered either above or below the horizontal meridian, as appears most convenient to the operator. The second pin is then to be introduced at right angles to the first, so that they form a cross (×). A thread is then passed round the staphyloma behind the pins, and tightly tied; the ends may be twisted and fastened to the cheek. Simple cerate dressing and a compress bandage should be applied. At the end of the third day the protrusion, together with the pins and thread, is generally found to be detached, and on the eighth or ninth day the wound is firmly cicatrized. If the staphyloma is very large, as little as possible should be included between the pins, and the tumor should not be drawn too tight, lest the strangulated portion should give way, or severe ophthalmitis be set up. In partial staphyloma more of the base should be included, and the threads tied close and tight within the remaining cornea. I have had no personal experience of this operation,

but it has been strongly recommended by several eminent surgeons, more especially for partial staphyloma, as it leaves a good portion of clear cornea, behind which to make an artificial pupil. The operation is almost free from danger, and leaves, at the worst, a firm movable stump for an artificial eye.[1]

De Wecker has lately devised the following operation, and has favored me with the subjoined description of his mode of operating: The patient having been anæsthetized, the lids are to be kept apart by Desmarres' lid holders (as they separate them very widely and thus afford more room for the operation). The conjunctiva is then to be carefully divided with scissors all round the cornea, and near the edge of the latter, the scissors being passed freely between the conjunctiva and sclerotic so as to detach the former as much as possible up to the equator of the eyeball. Four sutures are then to be inserted. A needle should be passed from without inwards through the conjunctiva near the lower edge of the cornea; the same needle should then be made to perforate the conjunctiva about the upper margin of the cornea at an equal distance from the corner of the flap; this perforation must be from within outwards, so that the needle issues about two or three millimetres from the edge of the flap. Four loops are to be made in this way (as is shown in Fig. 99, *a a*, *b b*, *c c*, *d d*), two of which should be turned over towards the temple, the other two towards the nose, before we proceed

Fig. 99.

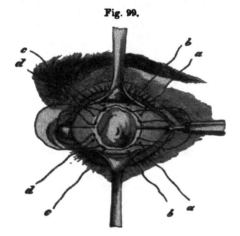

to excise the staphyloma. The latter is to be done by transfixing the base of the tumor with Graefe's knife, and then cutting straight out, the two halves being then carefully excised with scissors by two semicircular incisions near the edge of the cornea. If the lens is not spontaneously expelled, the capsule should be opened with the cystitome, and after the exit of the lens the sutures should be brought together. In order to avoid any mistake being made between them, we may employ fine silk of different colors. On account of the conjunctiva gliding very readily over the sclerotic, we can obtain a most accurate coaptation of the edges of the wound, and if the patient has been thoroughly under the influence of chloroform there will probably be no escape of vitreous humor. Should the vitreous show a tendency to bulge

[1] Vide an excellent description of this operation in the French Translation of Mackenzie's "Diseases of the Eye," vol. III., 1867.

between two of the sutures, another should be inserted at this point, so as to compress it and keep it back.

[In young subjects, as infants or children, all palliative measures should be tried in preference to enucleation. In cases of very marked staphyloma, total evulsion of the iris has been performed by Dr. H. D. Noyes, with excellent results.—B.]

18.—INJURIES AND WOUNDS OF THE CORNEA.

Foreign bodies are frequently met with on the cornea, and amongst the most common are chips or splinters of iron, steel, wood, glass, etc., which have become lodged or impacted on the surface, or more or less deeply in the substance of the cornea. The presence of a foreign body on the cornea generally at once excites considerable reaction. The eye becomes flushed and painful, and this is accompanied by photophobia and lachrymation. There is a well-marked rosy zone around the cornea, and, on account of the ciliary irritation, the pupil is contracted. There is generally no difficulty in detecting the presence of a foreign body in the cornea, more especially if the former is dark (e. g., a chip of steel or iron), and if the eye is turned sideways to the light. But if any doubt exists as to the presence and exact situation of a foreign body, atropine should be applied, and the eye examined with the oblique illumination, and, if necessary, with the aid of a magnifying glass. The advantage of employing atropine is, that the dark background afforded by the widely dilated pupil throws the cornea into strong relief, and thus facilitates the detection of a foreign body, particularly if this be light colored, as, for instance, a splinter of glass.

If the foreign body is situated superficially, and is early removed, no trace of its presence may remain. If, however, it has escaped detection, or the patient has not sought relief, and the foreign body is allowed to remain in the cornea, it may set up very considerable keratitis, and even iritis, accompanied, perhaps, with hypopyon. The cornea around the foreign body becomes infiltrated, and even a more or less extensive ulcer may be formed, or suppurative keratitis may supervene, with hypopyon, iritis, and sloughing of the cornea. This is often observed in aged and decrepit individuals, when a foreign body (e. g., a portion of wheat-ear, a splinter of glass) has become impacted in the substance of the cornea. In other and rarer instances, a layer of lymph surrounds and encloses the foreign body, which remains innocuous in the very substance of the cornea. Sometimes a splinter of steel or iron passes partly through the cornea, and projects somewhat into the anterior chamber, lying half in the latter, and half in the cornea.

There is generally no difficulty in removing chips of steel, iron, or glass lodged upon the the anterior surface of the cornea, close beneath the epithelial layer. As a rule, I always prefer to keep the eyelids apart with the stop-speculum, and to fix the eye with a pair of forceps. By so doing, we avoid all risk from any sudden movement or start of the patient, and can accomplish the removal of the foreign body very quickly and efficiently. The application of the speculum and forceps undoubtedly causes some degree of pain, but this is more than counterbalanced by the advantage of having the eye completely under our control. I have but too often seen that, after numerous ineffectual and painful attempts to remove the foreign body, they had, after all, to be employed. The patient should sit on a chair, either directly facing the light, or, if the foreign body can be better seen, with the face turned sideways towards it, and his head should lean back against the breast of the operator, who should stand behind him. Having applied the speculum, the surgeon steadies the eyeball with a pair of forceps held in his left hand, and endeavors to remove the foreign body with the spud, by passing the instrument behind it, and thus lifting it out. If the foreign body is impacted deeply in the substance of the cornea, there arises the danger that in our efforts to remove it we should push it further in, or cause it to perforate and fall into the anterior chamber. A broad needle should in such a case be carefully passed behind the foreign body, and thus be lifted out. If it lies very near the posterior wall of the cornea, the needle may be passed into the anterior chamber, and the broad part of its blade pressed against that portion of the posterior wall of the cornea which is opposite the foreign body, so as to steady this, and then it may be removed with another needle, or a very fine pair of forceps. A similar proceeding is to be adopted if the foreign body protrudes partly into the anterior chamber, for then an iridectomy knife or a broad needle should be passed into the latter and pushed behind the foreign body, gently pressing this back into the cornea; its anterior end should be seized with a pair of forceps, and in this way it may be readily extracted. [A better way is to transfix the cornea with either a broad Graefe's cataract-knife, or even a Beer's cataract-knife, making the points of entrance and exit on either side of the foreign body. Then press the flat side of the knife against the posterior surface of the cornea, or against the foreign body, if it reaches into the anterior chamber, thus holding it in place, and preventing it falling to the bottom of the chamber. Then enlarge the wound in the cornea made by the foreign body, and remove the latter either by forceps or scoop.—B.] If a bit of steel is situated on the surface of the cornea, it may also be removed with a magnet. After the removal of a foreign body from the cornea, a drop or two of castor oil should be applied to the eye, to lubricate the parts. Afterwards atropine should be applied, in order to allay the irritation. If the latter is considerable, and accompanied by severe ciliary neuralgia, cold compresses and leeches are indicated, followed by warm poppy fomentations. The use of the eyes must be forbidden until all symptoms of irritation have subsided.

The effects which burns, injuries from quicklime, molten lead, and chemical agents may have upon the cornea, have already been described in the section on injuries to the conjunctiva (p. 198), and the same course of treatment is to be pursued as was advocated before.

Wounds of the Cornea.—The danger to be feared from these varies according to their extent, situation, and nature. It occasionally happens that a very superficial cut with a sharp instrument does not perforate the cornea, but simply penetrates into its substance, and forms a small flap, which may heal readily, by the first intention, without leaving any trace. Thus a small, clean cut or puncture of the cornea frequently heals without leaving any mark behind, as is daily evidenced by operations upon the cornea, as, for instance, those for cataract, either performed with a knife or by the needle. The chief danger of penetrating wounds of the cornea is that they may cause considerable prolapse of the iris, or that they should implicate the iris and lens, and thus set up severe iritis or traumatic cataract. In such cases, the condition not only of the cornea, but also of the iris and lens, must be carefully watched, for any implication of the structures of course greatly enhances the danger of the accident. Bruises of the cornea by blunt instruments also often prove very dangerous, as, on account of the contusion of the injured part and its vicinity, severe inflammation, perhaps of a suppurative character, is set up, which may even lead to suppuration of the cornea.

In the treatment of injuries or wounds of the cornea the first indication is to subdue the symptoms of irritation and inflammation. If there is great pain, cold compresses should be sedulously employed, or a few leeches should be applied to the temple, followed by hot poppy fomentations, so that free after-bleeding may be encouraged. A strong solution of atropine should be prescribed, the compound belladonna ointment be rubbed over the forehead, and a light, though firm compress bandage be applied, in order that the parts may be kept perfectly at rest. If the symptoms of inflammation do not readily yield to such treatment, the eye should be again most carefully examined, in order that it may be ascertained whether a little foreign body has not remained undetected in the cornea, anterior chamber, or iris. The various complications, such as prolapse of the iris, iritis, traumatic cataract, etc., must be treated according to the general rules laid down in the sections in which these affections are described. If an incised wound is situated partly in the cornea and partly in the sclerotic, it occurs sometimes that the portion in the latter situation does not heal readily, and that a little fistulous opening may remain. In such cases, the treatment is to unite the wound in the sclerotic by means of one or two fine sutures, according to its extent. This will keep the lips of the incision in contact, plastic lymph will be effused, and a firm union will soon be effected. The thread should carry a needle at each end, so that we may be able to insert the suture into the sclerotic from *within outwards*, otherwise a sudden start of the patient might cause the point of the needle to penetrate the eye.

[14.—TUMORS OF THE CORNEA.

Tumors of the cornea are very rarely found originating in the tissue of the cornea itself, but begin in the conjunctiva either at the limbus or elsewhere, and involve the cornea through the medium of its epithelium. They may be benign or malignant.

The *dermoid* tumor is of the most frequent occurrence, and has been already described in detail in the article upon tumors of the conjunctiva (p. 200). In its pure form it is a congenital growth, but a mixed growth of dermoid and lipomatous tissue is sometimes met with after birth, and even in adult life.

Pure *Melanoma* must be regarded as a benign growth, though it may become malignant. It is a rare tumor in the cornea, and generally develops from the small pigment patches met with on the conjunctiva near the cornea, either spontaneously or as the result of injury.

Sarcoma of the cornea is almost always of the pigmented or melanotic variety. It proceeds from the limbus, passes over to the cornea, has sometimes a smooth, sometimes a lobulated surface, and is very vascular. It is of a brown or black color, and of varying consistency. Though it may involve the corneal parenchyma, it usually does not, but pushes in between the epithelium and the corneal tissue proper. The epithelial covering is usually enormously hypertrophied, and the sarcoma is almost always of the small round cell variety. It may involve the sclera quite extensively.

Epithelioma of the cornea begins generally as a small nodule on the limbus, resembling a phlyctenule, and may remain for a long time quiet, until it suddenly begins to grow very rapidly. It may be very painful. The tumor is grayish-white or reddish, and may in very rare cases be black. It has an irregular, fissured surface, and is usually soft. These tumors are generally removed with ease, and the corneal parenchyma is but very little changed. The growth pushes in over the cornea beneath the epithelium, and the ocular conjunctiva is usually extensively infiltrated. When removed, they generally return.

The *Melano-carcinoma* begins also at the limbus, and may grow to an enormous size, so that the eyelids cannot be closed. These tumors are always black or brown, soft, fungoid, and so vascular that they bleed on the slightest touch. Though usually growing over the cornea under the epithelium, they may involve the parenchyma very extensively, the membrana limitans externa being destroyed.

As regards treatment, operative removal is the only method of any use. If the growth is seen early enough, it can generally be removed without any difficulty, and with very little damage to the cornea. Even if the tumor is of some size, its removal, leaving the eye in place, should always be attempted, and will generally succeed, though it will probably return. Where we have, however, to deal with a fungoid mass of melano-carcinoma, its removal will be of no use on account of its rapid reappearance, and the eyeball should be enucleated together with most of the ocular conjunctiva, in order to prevent if possible its return in the orbital tissue.—B.]

In general leprosy the cornea in rare instances may also show a leprous condition. Professor Sylvester, of Bombay, has kindly furnished me with some particulars of leprous tubercle of the cornea, with a very few cases of which he has met. In one patient thirty-five years of age, and a confirmed leper, "The tubercle on the sclero-corneal junction of the left eye is about the size of a large split pea, smooth on the surface, and precisely resembles those on the skin, except that, wanting the brown pigment of the dermal covering, it is of a paler flesh color, and is covered with conjunctiva in which two stray, tortuous vessels ramify. It has a hard feel when taken between the blades of the forceps, and when pressed gives little or no pain; it is but slightly vascular and firmly incorporated with the cornea proper; it is, moreover, surrounded by a zone of decided opacity which extends completely through to the membrane of Descemet; the opaque zone slightly overlaps the pupillary aperture, which is dilated; the iris is as yet unaffected, and the fibres of its stroma distinct." In another case the whole cornea was involved, causing it to resemble an ordinary staphyloma. Professor Sylvester believes that the disease commences in the conjunctiva and extends thence to the cornea, and that the eye may be lost by the extension of the tubercle, the base of which presses on and involves the iris, which becomes inflamed, and subsequently the deeper tunics become implicated. He has never seen the eye implicated in the anæsthetic form of lepra; Chisolm, however, has recorded such a case.[1] Dr. Pedraglia has published a very interesting paper[2] on diseases of the eye in lepers, giving the history of fourteen cases which he observed in Bahia and Rio de Janeiro. He found the following the principal changes which take place in the eye: 1. The *eyelids* lose their lashes, and become thickened and red; 2. The *conjunctiva* also is thickened and red, which he believes to be less of a tuberculous character than due to a proliferation of the connective tissue, but this only occurs in those cases in which the skin is hypertrophied, for when the latter is pale and anæmic both the eyelids and conjunctiva remain normal: 3. The *cornea* may be affected with superficial keratitis, or with opacities due to the extension of thickened conjunctiva, tubercles (?), or else it may become stretched and assume a greater conicity; 4. In nearly all cases in which there is opacity of the cornea, there was also a chronic affection of the uveal tract, *e. g.*, atrophy of

[1] "R. L. O. H. Rep.," vi. 2, 126. [2] "Kl. Monatsbl.," 1872, p. 65.

iris tissue, anterior synechiæ, closed pupil, and in some even opacity of the lens. Mr. Hutchinson has observed one case of leprous tubercle of the cornea, a portrait of which is given in the New Sydenham Society's "Atlas of Skin Diseases" (Pl. 29).

DISEASES OF THE SCLEROTIC.

1.—EPISCLERITIS AND SCLERITIS.

[Though episcleritis may exist alone, yet, if it is at all chronic, the superficial layers of the sclera are always involved, and hence the process may be termed scleritis. The injected vessels are of three kinds: First, the long tortuous conjunctival vessels; secondly, the episcleral or subconjunctival vessels, which are shorter; and, thirdly, the deep ciliary vessels, short and straight, and only appearing when iris or cornea is involved.—B.]

Though not a dangerous affection, episcleritis often proves extremely troublesome on account of the protracted and obstinate course which it runs, and also on account of the tendency to frequent recurrence which it often manifests. It is distinguished by the appearance of a small dusky-red, or reddish-yellow elevation on the sclerotic, in close proximity to the insertion of one of the recti muscles, and at a short distance from the edge of the cornea. It occurs most frequently at the temporal portion of the sclerotic, near the insertion of the external rectus muscle. The appearance of the little nodule is generally preceded and accompanied by more or less conjunctival and subconjunctival redness, more especially of that segment of the eyeball upon which the elevation is situated, to which, indeed, the vascularity is often confined. The subconjunctival tissue is at this point markedly thickened and swollen, and of a peculiar rusty, dark, purplish hue, its bloodvessels (as well, perhaps, as those of the conjunctiva) being here somewhat dilated, tortuous, and of a dusky tint. Frequently the conjunctiva is hardly at all affected, the vascularity and swelling being confined to the subconjunctival tissue and the superficial layers of the sclerotic. There is sometimes considerable photophobia, lachrymation, and a certain degree of ciliary neuralgia, but in many cases these symptoms are almost entirely absent, and the patient experiences only slight discomfort, or a feeling of dull, heavy pain in and around the eye. The affected point of the sclerotic may also be more or less sensitive to the touch. At the outset, this affection might be mistaken for phlyctenular or pustular conjunctivitis, but the little nodule soon increases in size, and assumes a dusky, reddish-brown appearance, having a broad base, and showing no tendency to ulcerate or suppurate. Gradually it becomes more pale, diminishes in size, and slowly disappears, after it has existed perhaps for many months. Or it may recur again and again, either at the same spot, or at some other point of the eyeball, so that the disease may travel round the cornea from point to point.

There is an acute form which must be distinguished from the chronic, though it tends to run into the latter, and is very rare.

The consequences of a chronic scleritis are important, and sometimes disastrous; the corneal complication almost always existing in the form of an infiltration, and very rarely tending to the development of ulceration, is by no means a constant result. It begins at the margin and advances towards the centre, and leaves behind it deep and permanent opacities. Inflammation of the uveal tract, especially of the iris, according to Saemisch, occurs in all cases of corneal complication. Functional disturbances in scleritis may be very pronounced or scarcely perceptible. The disease may disappear without leaving any trace, but this is not common unless it is of syphilitic origin. As rare complications may be mentioned: 1st, the ulceration of the inflamed scleral tissues; and 2d, the development of scleral ectasia. This latter results from a thinning of the membrane, is very rare, and must be distinguished from that form of ectasia known as ciliary staphyloma, and due to other causes.

Scleritis is a rare disease, as a rule does not attack both eyes, and occurs oftenest in middle life.—B.]

The disease is not only very protracted and obstinate in its course, but also very little influenced either by general or local treatment. It occurs most frequently in females of an adult age, and does not appear to be due to any appreciable cause, except that it is perhaps more often met with in persons of a rheumatic or gouty tendency than in others. In some cases it would also appear to be due to a syphilitic taint, and is then apt to prove extremely obstinate, except it is treated by anti-syphilitic remedies. The cornea sometimes becomes implicated, more especially the part nearest the elevation, the superficial portions of the cornea becoming cloudy, and this opacity assuming somewhat the appearance of a partial arcus senilis. If there are much ciliary irritation and pain, atropine drops should be employed, and warm poppy fomentations be applied to the eye. The insufflation of calomel or the use of the red-precipitate ointment have proved of little benefit in my hands; indeed, I think them contra-indicated if there is any ciliary irritation, still more so is this the case with caustic collyria. I have, however, in some cases found marked and striking benefit from the use of a collyrium of chloride of zinc. I employ at first a very weak solution (gr. ss to f ℥j of water), and if this is well borne and does not augment the redness or produce much irritation, I increase the strength to gr. i–ij to f ℥j. The patient should be placed upon a generous diet, and tonics should be freely administered. Where there is a distinct gouty or rheumatic tendency, preparations of guaiacum, or colchicum together with tincture of aconite, should be given. If there are evidences of syphilis, iodide of potassium should be prescribed, and perhaps even mercurial inunction. [The hypodermic injection of the hydrochlorate of pilocarpine, in doses of one-fourth to one-half of a grain daily, is sometimes beneficial in cutting short the disease.

Massage has been highly recommended in scleritis and episcleritis by Pedraglia and others. In the former's hands it proved successful in several cases, no other treatment being employed (see "Centralblatt für prakt. Augenheilk.," April, 1881).

The following operative procedure has been recommended by Wickerkiewiez in cases of scleritis which have resisted the ordinary methods of treatment. The conjunctiva is divided freely over the scleral inflammation, so as completely to expose the diseased part. It is better to make this conjunctival incision parallel to the corneal margin. Then with a small, sharp spoon, made for the purpose, the operator scratches and scoops out the soft, spongy, very vascular, infiltrated tissue of the sclera, until healthy scleral tissue is reached. A crater-like excavation is thus formed. Iced compresses are then applied for an hour, and then an antiseptic bandage is put on. This bandage is reapplied daily, and if any purulent secretion appears, some astringent wash is used. In this way the duration of the disease is much shortened. (See "Centralblatt für prakt. Augenheilk.," October, 1880.)

yphilitica, or gummy infiltration of the sclera, is not an uncom-
in constitutional syphilis. This may be a circumscribed gummy
a diffuse infiltration. When circumscribed, it usually may be
e temporal side, either in the course of the external rectus muscle,
it and the superior rectus. Though somewhat chronic, it yields
y to proper anti-syphilitic treatment than the other varieties of
f, however, the gumma start from the ciliary body and spread
sclera, its termination is not so favorable.—B.]

IOR SCLEROTIC STAPHYLOMA. [CILIARY STAPHYLOMA, EQUATORIAL STAPHYLOMA.—B.]

matous bulging of the sclerotic may be chiefly or entirely con-
part of the anterior portion of the sclerotic, or it may involve,
s, the whole of the eyeball. The partial anterior staphyloma is
ear the ciliary region, or further back, near the equator of the
ty occur at any point from the edge of the cornea to the equa-
n of the eyeball, and frequently shows itself between the inser-
of the recti muscles, as there is less resistance offered at such a
protrusion of the sclerotic.
eat majority of cases, staphyloma of the sclerotic is due to irido-
accompanied by an increase in the intra-ocular tension, which
tention and bulging of the sclerotic at one or more points, the
f the sclerotic having moreover been perhaps also weakened by
atory thinning of its structure. The prominence of the inflam-
ptoms varies very greatly, according to the rapidity and acute-
hich the staphyloma is formed. If the course of the disease is
we find that there are marked symptoms of irido-choroiditis.
njunctival and subconjunctival injection, accompanied perhaps
a degree of chemosis, more especially over and around that part
otic which is beginning to bulge. The ciliary neuralgia is often
, and the ciliary region acutely sensitive to the touch. The edge
ea may be somewhat opaque, the aqueous humor hazy, the iris
ind inflamed, and its pupillary edge tied down by exudations of

pil is sufficiently clear to admit of an ophthalmoscopic examina-
treous humor is often found diffusely clouded, with large, dark
ing about in it. The tension of the eye is generally considerably
nd the sight and field of vision greatly impaired. The increase
ension is not, however, absolutely necessary to the production of
ua. For, on account of an inflammatory thinning of a certain
he sclerotic, the latter may not be sufficiently firm and strong at
resist the presence of even a normal degree of intra-ocular ten-
onsequently yields before it. In such a case there would, of
no augmentation of the eye-tension, no hardness of the globe.
are, however, rare in comparison to the others, in which the in-
he tension is the chief cause of the protrusion. Besides the
, the patient often complains of bright flashes of light (photop-
there is noticed at one point of the sclerotic a slight prominence
the outline of which may be circumscribed and clearly defined,
ular and pass gradually and insensibly over into the healthy
As the bulge increases, the sclerotic becomes more and more
rtly perhaps from inflammation and partly from distention) and

discolored, assuming at this point a dusky, dirty, bluish-gray hue, which is
due to the shining through of the choroid. Thus the staphyloma may attain
a considerable size, even in the course of a few weeks. [Fig. 100.] Together
with the increase in size of the staphyloma, the proximate portion of the
ciliary region, and even of the cornea, may become involved in it, and be
considerably changed in curvature, the corresponding plane of the iris and
the zonula of Zinn being stretched, and the attachment of the lens consequently relaxed and loosened.

[Fig. 100.

Fig. 101.

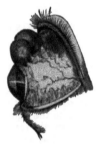

After Miller.

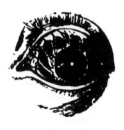

After Miller.]

As a rule, however, the progress of the staphyloma is very slow and gradual.
After a more or less acute and severe inflammation of the iris and choroid
has existed for some length of time, and its progress has been perhaps apparently arrested, it is noticed that the curvature of one portion of the
sclerotic is somewhat altered and more promi-
nent, and its surface traversed by dark, dilated
vessels. Gradually and slowly the protrusion
increases, the sclerotic becomes more thinned,
and exchanges its bright lustrous white color
for a dusky bluish tint. Sometimes the staphylomatous bulging is traversed by tendinous
glistening trabeculæ, forming a kind of framework, through the interstices of which the
darker portions bulge out, giving to the whole
a faint likeness to a mulberry. [Fig. 101.]
The staphyloma may now remain stationary
for a time, and the inflammatory symptoms
disappear. Then an inflammatory exacerbation supervenes, the eye becomes painful, irritable, flushed, and an increase in the size of the
staphyloma is noticed. But these symptoms
again disappear, and the progress of the disease

[Fig. 102.

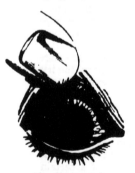

After Mackenzie.]

is temporarily arrested. Such exacerbations may be of frequent occurrence,
and lead, finally, to a considerable and very prominent staphyloma. Sometimes the staphylomatous bulgings are not chiefly confined to one portion of
the sclerotic, but occupy the whole of the ciliary region around the cornea,
and then the disease is termed "annular staphyloma." [Fig. 102.]
This distention and bulging are not limited to the sclerotic, but extend to
the choroid, which is generally adherent to the former, and consequently
stretched and bulged with it, undergoing in time perhaps almost complete

atrophy. The retina may either be adherent to the choroid, and therefore also stretched and altered in structure, or it may be separated from it at this point, and pass straight across the base of the staphylomatous bulge, the cavity of the latter being occupied by serous fluid. The vitreous humor is also more or less clouded and fluid. Sometimes it is, however, quite transparent, and we can then distinctly see (if the other refractive media are clear) the details of the fundus, and perhaps detect a deep excavation of the optic nerve. Generally, however, we are unable to see the fundus on account of exudations in the pupil, or the opacity of the lens and vitreous humor.

In complete sclerotic staphyloma, the anterior portion of the sclerotic and the cornea are greatly altered in curvature, being either distended into a conical, or sub-ovoid protrusion. The iris and zonula of Zinn are also much distended. The plane of the iris is greatly increased in size, and its surface is of a dirty slate tint, which is partly owing to inflammatory changes, and partly to the stretching and atrophy of its fibrillæ. It is, moreover, often tremulous, on account of the partial or complete dislocation of the lens, or on account of the latter being separated from its posterior surface by a considerable amount of fluid. From the distention and stretching of the zonula of Zinn, the attachments of the lens are relaxed and weakened, and the latter may be partially or completely dislocated into the vitreous humor. The depth and size of the anterior chamber are often greatly increased. Indeed the whole eye is much enlarged, and on this account as well as the protrusion of the eye from the orbit, this condition is often termed "buphthalmos." The sclerotic is traversed by dilated tortuous vessels, and is of a dusky, dark-blue tint, which is either diffuse and uniform in character, or chiefly confined to certain points, giving to the whole a dark, patchy appearance. The pupil is often occupied by lymph, the capsule of the lens opaque, and covered by masses of exudation, the lens itself being also frequently cataractous. If the staphyloma has formed after an extensive perforation of the cornea, there will be no anterior chamber, the iris and capsule of the lens are intimately connected with and adherent to the corneal cicatrix, the lens is cataractous, perhaps shrivelled and chalky, or altogether absent, having escaped through the corneal perforation.

Both the partial and complete staphyloma may after a time become arrested, the inflammatory exacerbations becoming less and less frequent, and finally ceasing. In other cases, severe suppurative irido-choroiditis supervenes, and gradually leads to atrophy of the eye. Or again, the bulging portion in a partial staphyloma may give way, either spontaneously or in consequence of a blow upon the eye, or a sudden and severe strain or exertion. A great portion of the contents of the eyeball escapes, this being often accompanied by profuse intra-ocular hemorrhage ; severe inflammation supervenes, and the globe shrinks and atrophies.

With regard to the treatment, I need only say that at the very outset of the disease, when the symptoms are only those of irido-choroiditis, the usual remedies—atropine, leeches, paracentesis, etc.—should be employed, but when the tension of the eye is markedly increased, and if the sclerotic shows at one point a tendency to bulge, these remedies no longer suffice, and a large iridectomy should be made at once. If this should not check the inflammation and the bulging of the sclerotic, repeated paracentesis may be tried, or a second iridectomy may be made opposite to the first, so as to divide the iris into two separate halves. But if the staphyloma is considerable and has existed for some time, the iridectomy no longer suffices to cause it to shrink, and we may then have to abscise it. This should be done with a cataract-knife, as in the case of staphyloma of the cornea (page 257). After the operation a firm compress bandage is to be applied. In cases of partial staphyloma, more especially if the base is small, I should prefer Borelli's operation (page 261) to abscission. In those cases in which the sight is greatly and hopelessly lost, and the eye is a source of constant irritation and discomfort, abscission by Critchett's method should be performed. [Critchett's method of abscission is by no means a safe operation in this region, as the resulting cicatrix comes to lie in the vicinity of the ciliary nerves, and may excite sympathetic irritation.—B.] But if the disease reaches far back, or involves the whole eyeball, it will be much wiser to excise the eye, for by abscising the anterior part, a portion of the diseased structures will be left behind, and the stump be prone to inflammatory complications, and thus prevent perhaps the possibility of wearing an artificial eye with comfort, and even endanger the safety of the other eye.

[Another method, which has found favor with some operators, consists in excising the anterior portion of the eyeball, and then completely eviscerating the contents, leaving nothing behind but the sclerotic, and the wound is then left to granulate.—B.]

8.—WOUNDS AND INJURIES OF THE SCLEROTIC.

Incised wounds of the sclerotic chiefly prove dangerous in so far that, if they are extensive, a considerable portion of the contents of the eyeball escapes, which is perhaps followed by profuse intra-ocular hemorrhage, suppurative choroiditis, and finally, atrophy of the eyeball. Or again, if the wound is smaller, its cicatrization may, by involving a portion of the retina, lead to a detachment of the latter, which, though limited at first, may gradually extend and threaten the safety of the eye. Again, the instrument producing the injury may wound the lens and cause traumatic cataract, accompanied perhaps by severe inflammatory complications leading to the destruction of the sight. Still greater is the danger if the point of the instrument is broken off and lodged in the interior of the eye, the same being the case if foreign bodies have perforated the sclerotic and entered the globe. If the wound is situated at the anterior portion of the sclerotic near the cornea, the iris generally protrudes, and the lens may be dislocated under the conjunctiva; this is especially the case after severe blows from blunt instruments, producing a rupture of the sclerotic. Indeed, ruptures of the sclerotic are generally far more dangerous than incised wounds, on account of the great force of the blow which was necessary to cause the sclerotic to give way. If the incised wound is not considerable in size, its edges should be carefully brought together by a fine suture or two. Any portion of protruding iris or vitreous humor being abscised, cold compresses should then be applied to allay the inflammatory reaction. In small punctured wounds a little head of vitreous may protrude through the aperture, and if the application of a firm compress does not accelerate union, this object may be obtained by lightly touching the wound with a crayon of nitrate of silver and potash every second or third day. When the wound is very extensive and a large portion of the contents of the globe has escaped, and there is no hope of restoring any sight, it is better to excise the eyeball at once, more especially if it is to the patient a matter of great moment (as amongst the poorer classes) to be cured as soon as possible, and to be free from further inflammatory attacks.

[A not uncommon occurrence after powder explosions is to find a number of grains of powder embedded in the sclera. These rarely give any trouble, and, as any attempt to extract them involves laceration of the conjunctiva, they had better be left undisturbed. Occasionally foreign bodies, as bits of stone or iron, have been found embedded in the sclera, though this is rare; for usually such particles impinge upon the sclera with such force as to perforate it and enter the eyeball. Incised wounds of the sclera are best treated by sutures, if they are not too large to call for enucleation of the globe.

Contusions of the sclera are of no special moment in themselves, except so far as they are to be regarded as contusion of the whole eye, with more or less severe injury to the contents of the globe, such as dislocation of the lens, rupture of iris and choroid, and intra-ocular hemorrhages.—B.]

A portion of the sclerotic may slough after injuries from burns, hot metal, etc. The injured part becomes covered with a whitish-gray eschar, which is thrown off together with portions of the sclerotic, until the vitreous humor becomes visible. The injury may be accompanied by inflammation of the cornea and iris, and opacity of the lens.

[4.—TUMORS OF THE SCLERA.

Tumors beginning in the sclera are rare. Those which, starting from some other source, whether intra-ocular or extra-ocular, involve the sclera secondarily, find that the latter offers considerable resistance to their progress. These usually begin in or near the ciliary and sclero-corneal regions, may be both benign and malignant, and may be classed as *dermoid, melanomata, sarcomata,* and *carcinomata;* and among the very rare forms occur fibromata, osteomata, and cysts.

The extra-ocular tumors which may involve the sclera are the dermoid and the melanomata, but by far the larger number of scleral tumors are of intra-ocular origin.

There is a case of *osteoma,* which originated in the sclera, reported by Watson; but many of the cases of scleral osteomata are merely *calcification* of the sclera, which is not so very uncommon.

Gummy tumors of the sclera have been considered under the head of scleritis syphilitica.

Tubercle of the sclera has been observed, but only as a secondary growth from some portion of the uveal tract.—B.]

CHAPTER V.

DISEASES OF THE IBIS AND CILIARY BODY.

1.—HYPERÆMIA OF THE IRIS.

HYPERÆMIA of the iris is of far more frequent occurrence than is generally supposed. Nor can we be surprised at this, when we remember the close connection which exists between the iris and cornea on the one hand, and the iris, ciliary body, and choroid on the other. Indeed, we may regard the iris as the anterior termination of the ciliary body and choroid, the whole forming, in reality, one tissue, the uveal tract. Hence the frequency with which inflammation of the iris extends to the ciliary body and choroid, and *vice versa.* In a hyperæmic condition of the iris, we find that there is more or less marked subconjunctival injection; that the pupil is somewhat contracted and sluggish, not reacting freely on the application of atropine; and that the iris is discolored, which is due to the increased vascularity imparting a reddish tint to the natural color of the iris. Thus a blue iris will become somewhat green, and a brown iris assume a slight admixture of red.

All causes which produce congestion of the deeper tunics of the eye may excite hyperæmia of the iris. Of these, the most frequent are over-exertion of the eyes in reading, engraving, etc., and inflammatory affections of the choroid, ciliary body, and cornea. But this condition may even be produced in acute granular conjunctivitis if this is injudiciously treated by caustics and strong astringent collyria.

The treatment must be chiefly directed towards a removal of the cause, and an alleviation of the irritation; hence, strict and prolonged rest of the eyes should be enforced, and they should also be guarded against exposure to strong light, cold, etc. Atropine should be applied to diminish the irritability of the eye.

2.—INFLAMMATION OF THE IRIS.

In iritis there are superadded to the symptoms of hyperæmia of the iris, those of an effusion of plastic lymph at the edge of the pupil, or on the surface and into the stroma of the iris.

Formerly, the inflammations of the iris were classified according to the dyscrasiæ of which they were supposed to be pathognomonic, and a formidable array of different forms of iritis was in this way established. By chiefly basing our classification on pathological anatomy, we can, however, greatly simplify the subject, and so embrace all shades of iritis within the following four groups: 1. Simple idiopathic iritis. 2. Serous iritis (Descemetitis, etc.). 3. Parenchymatous iritis. 4. Syphilitic iritis.

In order to avoid unnecessary repetition, I shall first describe the various symptoms which more or less accompany all inflammations of the iris, and then call attention to those which characterize the special forms.

Amongst the earliest symptoms of iritis are conjunctival, and especially subconjunctival injection, ciliary neuralgia, contraction and sluggishness of the pupil, and a discolored, dull, lack-lustre appearance of the iris.

There is generally some injection of the conjunctiva, which may be chiefly confined to the palpebral portion, or extend also to the ocular conjunctiva in the vicinity of the cornea. But a far more constant symptom is the subconjunctival vascularity, giving rise to a more or less broad, rosy zone of parallel vessels, closely ranged round the cornea. [Fig. 103.] This zone is generally of a bright rose color, and consists chiefly of small arterial twigs. It may, however, assume a somewhat blue or brownish tint, and the latter was formerly erroneously supposed to be symptomatic of syphilitic iritis. Although marked subconjunctival injection is present in the great majority of cases of iritis, we occasionally meet with severe cases in which it is not very conspicuous, as in typhus fever,

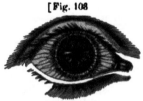

[Fig. 103

After Pirrie.]

pyæmia, etc. There is also more or less chemosis, and this may be so considerable that the conjunctiva is raised like a red or bluish-red mound round the cornea. The eyelids are often also swollen and puffy. In the milder cases they may retain their normal appearance, but if the attack is severe, the upper lid generally becomes red, glistening, and very œdematous and swollen. This is more especially the case in suppurative iritis or irido-cyelitis.

The intensity of the pain is very variable, for although it is generally severe, and often extremely so, it may in some cases be nearly entirely absent. The patient may at first only experience a feeling of itching and burning in the eye, but soon the pain becomes more severe, and assumes a sharp, cutting, lancinating character. It may be chiefly situated deeply in the eyeball, or extend to the forehead, temple, and corresponding side of the nose (ciliary neuralgia). Sometimes there is very intense neuralgia of the branches of the fifth nerve, extending over the corresponding side of the face and head, even as far as the occiput. The pain always increases in intensity towards evening, remaining very severe during the night, and diminishing towards morning. Although the patient may experience very acute pain in iritis, it is important to remember that the eye is not painful to the touch in a case of simple uncomplicated iritis. If sharp pain is caused when the ciliary region is pressed by the finger, it is indicative of the coexistence of inflammation of the ciliary body (cyclitis). Very frequently this tenderness is partial, and confined to the upper portion of the ciliary region.

The severity of the pain may give rise to some constitutional disturbance, and the exacerbations be accompanied by feverishness, a loaded tongue, impairment of appetite, and a tendency to retching and vomiting, which not unfrequently causes the disease to be mistaken for a severe bilious attack.

Although considerable photophobia and lachrymation may accompany iritis, they are seldom so severe and marked as in certain forms of keratitis.

We now come to the symptoms presented by the iris itself. Amongst the earliest are discoloration and dulness of the iris, and contraction of the pupil. The discoloration of the iris is partly due to hyperæmia and partly to an effusion into its structure. In order to estimate rightly the changes in color, we must always compare the affected with the other eye (if this be sound), otherwise an error may easily occur. We must also be upon our guard not to mistake the dulness and change in the tint of the iris, which may be produced by cloudiness of the cornea and of the aqueous humor, as being resident in the iris itself. Besides the discoloration, the iris presents a peculiar dull, lack-lustre appearance, its surface having lost its natural bright, glistening aspect, and appearing hazy and dull, as if covered by a fine veil. Its fibrillæ are also not sharply defined, but indistinct and blurred. This depends in a great measure upon the hypertrophy of the connective tissue elements of the iris, and upon the effusion of lymph into the stroma and upon the surface of the iris.

The pupil is sluggish and more or less contracted. This generally occurs in all but the very slightest cases of iritis, or in those in which there is a tendency to increase in the intra-ocular tension. This immobility of the pupil is partly caused by the hyperæmia of the vessels, but chiefly by the serous or plastic effusion which has taken place into the stroma of the iris, and impedes the action of the circular fibres of the iris. If the inflammation is but partial, the immobility of the pupil may be the same. In testing the mobility of the pupil, the patient should be placed so that the light falls sideways upon the eye. The other must be firmly closed with our hand, or by a handkerchief. The affected eye is to be shaded with the palm of our hand, which is then to be rapidly removed so as to admit the light, and the behavior of the pupil accurately watched, so that its size, mobility, and the extent of its contractions may be ascertained. It must be remembered that contraction and impaired mobility of the pupil may exist without any iritis; for they may be seen in keratitis, hyperæmia of the iris, or if a foreign body is lodged on the cornea, and are in these cases due to irritation of the ciliary nerves.

The edge of the pupil generally soon loses its circular form and becomes somewhat irregular [Fig. 104], and we may notice along it small exudations or beads of plastic lymph, which tie it down to the anterior capsule. These

[Fig. 104.   Fig. 105.

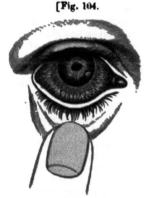

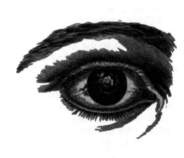

After T. W. Jones.   After Lawrence.]

may, however, be so minute as to escape detection, until the pupil is examined with the oblique illumination, or atropine is applied. The individual exudations often increase in size and coalesce, and, more lymph being effused, the whole circumference of the pupil may become fringed with them, and be tied down to the capsule of the lens, the centre of the pupil perhaps remaining clear and thus still permitting of good vision. This condition is termed "*circular*" or "*annular*" synechia, or "*exclusion of the pupil.*" We must distinguish this from the condition in which the effusion invades the area of the pupil, so that a more or less considerable portion of it is covered by a film of lymph, or even the whole of it occluded by a thick nodule of exudation, the sight being of course proportionately deteriorated; this is called "*occlusion*" of the pupil. [Fig. 105.] The exudation of lymph between the iris and the capsule of the lens is not always limited to the edge of the pupil, but may extend further back along the posterior surface of the iris, and thus produce broad and very firm adhesions. We shall see, hereafter, that this fact is of great importance in the performance of iridectomy for chronic iritis or irido-choroiditis. The partial adhesions between the pupil and capsule vary greatly in thickness, extent, and number, and become very apparent when atropine is applied, as they then give rise to various irregularities in the shape of the pupil.

[When the pupil is "excluded" or "occluded," the remainder of the iris being free, fluid is apt to collect in the posterior chamber, and by bulging the iris forwards, and diminishing the depth of the anterior chamber, excepting at its centre, to give the pupil a funnel shape. If such bulging be partial, or be divided by bands of tough membrane, a cystic appearance is given. *Secondary glaucoma* is likely to follow, and the tension of the globe should, therefore, be carefully noted whenever this bulging is present. "Total posterior synechia" always shows a severe iritis, though often one of chronic course; it often signifies deep-seated disease, and may be complicated by secondary opacity of the lens (cataract). Relapses of iritis are believed to be induced by the presence of synechiæ, even when there is no protrusion of the iris by fluid; but their influence in this way has probably been much overrated. (Nettleship.)—B.]

The surface of the iris may become covered with a film of exudation, or the lymph may mix with the aqueous humor, and render this turbid and clouded; or it may be precipitated against the posterior wall of the cornea in the form of small whitish opacities; or again, it may sink to the bottom of the anterior chamber, where it collects, in the form of an hypopyon. The amount of this yellowish deposit varies; it may be so slight as easily to escape detection, appearing like a small yellow fringe along the lower edge of the anterior chamber; or it may attain such a size that it fills half or even more of the anterior chamber.

In simple iritis the cornea is generally quite transparent, or shows but the faintest amount of cloudiness. Small portions of lymph may, however, be deposited from the aqueous humor upon the posterior wall of the cornea, giving rise to a punctate appearance. This occurs especially in the serous form of iritis. But the cornea may, also, become implicated in the inflammatory process.

Vision is often considerably impaired. This may be partly due to the cloudiness of the aqueous humor and of the area of the pupil. If the sight is much affected, and the pupil not occluded, we must suspect the coexistence of cyclitis, which is often accompanied by diffuse opacity of the vitreous humor. The power of accommodation is then, moreover, also affected. It is, therefore, very necessary accurately to test the degree of vision at the commencement of an iritis, in order that we may at once detect any marked deterioration, and ascertain to what cause this is due. The tension of the eyeball is normal in a case of common iritis, and the field of vision, although it may be somewhat contracted on account of the smallness of the pupil, or the presence of synechiæ, does not show the contraction peculiar to a glaucomatous condition of the eye.

We must now consider the symptoms by which the special forms of iritis are characterised.

1. *The Simple [Plastic] Iritis* is sometimes very slight in degree, and accompanied by only a very moderate amount of subconjunctival injection, photophobia, pain, or discoloration of the iris; indeed, its existence may remain quite unsuspected until atropine is applied, when the pupil is found to be irregular, and shows here and there a slender adhesion to the capsule. [Fig. 106.] This mild form of iritis is often met with after operations upon the eye (*e. g.*, cataract operations), or after injuries. The affection may, however, be more severe, and there is much pain, swelling of the lids, injection of the conjunctiva and subconjunctival tissue, chemosis, photophobia, and lachrymation. The iris is discolored, the pupil contracted and inactive, having deposits of lymph at its edge, and perhaps also in its area. A film of exudation covers the surface of the iris, rendering it dull and hazy, the aqueous humor is somewhat turbid, and the posterior surface of the cornea perhaps mottled with small deposits of lymph.

[Fig. 106.]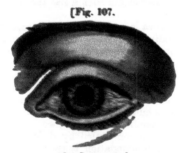

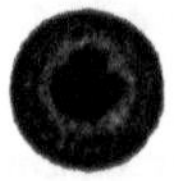

[In plastic iritis, the exudation occurs upon the anterior and posterior surfaces of the iris, on pupillary margin and anterior capsule of the lens. This form of iritis occurs idiopathically, or in constitutional syphilis, or as one of the signs of a rheumatic or gouty taint.—B.]

2. *Serous Iritis* (syn. Descemetitis, aquo-capsulitis, keratitis punctata, etc.) is chiefly distinguished by the absence of plastic exudation, and by the great tendency to hypersecretion of the aqueous humor. The symptoms of acute iritis are generally not very pronounced. The aqueous humor is secreted in greater quantity, and is somewhat clouded and turbid, and on closer observation we can often notice small particles of lymph floating about in it, before becoming deposited on the posterior surface of the cornea, or at the bottom of the anterior chamber. The latter is often markedly deepened, and the cornea appears somewhat bulged forward. The cloudiness of the aqueous humor often varies considerably and rapidly within the course of a few hours. The cornea may at first appear abnormally brilliant, but it soon

[Fig. 107.

After Dalrymple.]

loses its lustre and becomes slightly clouded, and small punctate opacities make their appearance upon its posterior surface. [Fig. 107.] These may be situated opposite the pupil, being perhaps grouped in a small circle; but they are generally arranged in the form of a pyramid, the base of which is turned towards the periphery of the cornea, and its apex towards the centre; the smaller opacities being situated at the apex, and the larger and coarser ones at the base. This proves that the opacities are composed of small masses of lymph, deposited from the aqueous humor upon the posterior wall of the cornea, and that they arrange themselves according to their size and weight, the larger and heavier ones gravitating downwards. The truth of this assertion has moreover been proved experimentally by Arlt.[1] He placed the head of the patient in different directions, sometimes keeping it for a e turned to the right side, sometimes to the left, and he found length of base of the pyramid always corresponded to the side of the eye this it had been maintained in the lowest position. But some of the opacities met with at the posterior portion of the cornea, are not due to these deposits from the aqueous humor, but are caused by inflammatory changes in the epithelial layer, or even in the posterior portion of the cornea proper. [This precipitate upon the posterior surface of the cornea, if extensive, may cause serious disease of the cornea, which may actually be of the parenchymatous variety, and lead to sclerosis of the cornea. This sclerosis, by its localization in the lower part of the cornea, and by its triangular shape, with base directed upwards, often proves the previous existence of a serous iritis.—B.]

The iris is but slightly discolored, and the pupil, instead of being contracted, as is generally the case in iritis, is somewhat dilated, often markedly so. This is due to an increase in the intra-ocular tension, which is often present in this disease, and the manifestation of which must be watched with the greatest care, for this serous form of inflammation shows a great tendency to extend to the ciliary body and choroid, which is accompanied by hypersecretion of the vitreous humor, marked increase in the intra-ocular tension, and a glaucomatous condition of the eye. The degree of eye-tension, the state of the sight and of the field of vision must, therefore, be frequently and carefully examined during the course of the disease, in order that the earliest symptoms of a glaucomatous complication may be detected and at once arrested. Adhesions between the edge of the pupil and the capsule are not of frequent occurrence in this form.

Serous iritis occasionally accompanies deep-seated inflammations of the eye, more especially chronic irido-choroiditis, and choroido-retinitis. Moreover, sympathetic ophthalmia sometimes appears in the form of serous iritis. It has also been supposed to be due to constitutional or hereditary syphilis.

3. *Parenchymatous and Purulent Iritis.*—In this affection the inflammation attacks the tissue of the iris, and its fibrillæ become much swollen and thickened. The plastic exudation is poured out into the parenchyma of the iris, along the edge and into the area of the pupil, and also on the posterior surface of the iris, giving rise to thick, broad adhesions between it and the capsule of the lens. On account of the exudation into the stroma of the iris, and the swollen and thickened condition of its fibrillæ, the circulation is generally considerably impeded, and large tortuous veins make their appearance on its surface. Along the edge of the contracted pupil are noticed a number of thick, firm nodules of exudation, of a creamy or reddish-brown color, tying down the edge of the pupil to the capsule; or they may even extend around the whole edge of the pupil, and thus give rise to a circular synechia (exclusion of the pupil). The effusion generally also invades the area of the pupil, indeed the latter may be completely blocked up by a thick yellow nodule of purulent exudation. The surface of the iris appears indistinct and hazy, its fibrillæ are swollen, and its anterior surface is covered by a layer of exudation, which varies considerably in appearance. In some cases it looks simply like a thin gray veil covering different portions or even the whole of the iris; in others it assumes a thick, creamy, purulent appearance, with small extravasations of blood scattered about here and there. Little yellow nodules (which are not to be confounded with the syphilitic nodules) may also appear strewn about on the surface of the iris. On

[1] "Augenheilkunde," II. 45.

account of the detachment of some of these nodules, and the effusion of lymph and purulent exudation into the aqueous humor, the latter becomes turbid and discolored. Flakes of purulent lymph and globules of pus are seen floating about in it, and, sinking down, give rise to an hypopyon, which may be so small as to appear only like a narrow yellow belt along the lower edge of the anterior chamber, or may be so considerable as to occupy one-half or more of the anterior chamber, reaching perhaps above the upper edge of the pupil. This parenchymatous or suppurative iritis may be accompanied by a similar form of inflammation of the ciliary body and choroid.

[The inflammatory products consist of lymphoid cells, large masses of free nuclei, and marked hypertrophy of the connective-tissue stroma. The latter occurs mainly in the vicinity of the pupil, and almost always gives rise to a membrane in the pupil which may become organized, vascular, and form part and parcel of the iris. This is the most destructive form of inflammation to the iris itself.—B.]

4. *Syphilitic Iritis* generally assumes the parenchymatous form. It is, however, especially characterized by the formation of peculiar nodules (gummy tubercles, Virchow). These are scattered about singly over a certain portion, or even the whole, of the surface of the iris, in the form of yellowish-red condylomatous nodules. They appear at first deeply embedded in the parenchyma of the iris (originating in the deeper portion of its connective tissue), and, as they increase in size, they push aside the fibrillæ of the iris, and protrude between them into the anterior chamber. They may attain a very considerable magnitude, their apex even touching the posterior wall of the cornea. They (according to Colbert) exactly resemble in structure the gummy tubercles (gummata) of Virchow. On account of the presence of pigment cells, and the great vascularity, the nodules frequently assume a dark reddish-brown sarcomatous appearance. They often undergo fatty and purulent degeneration, breaking down into a yellow, grumous, purulent mass, which becomes mixed with the aqueous humor. They may, however, undergo rapid absorption. These nodules, or condylomata as they are sometimes called, frequently remain confined to one portion of the iris, in which the inflammatory changes are moreover also more pronounced, so that the disease assumes a somewhat partial character, which is peculiar to the syphilitic form. We find, in such cases, that, although the whole cornea may be surrounded by a pink zone of vessels, this is most conspicuous at one point, and that the corresponding segment of iris is the most thickened and swollen, and that the nodules are chiefly or entirely confined to this portion. [These gummata are generally situated on the pupillary margin or in the peripherical zone of the iris. They sometimes spring from the posterior surface of the iris in the pupillary zone and push forward into the anterior chamber. In rare cases these nodules have been known to occur in such numbers and of such a size as to fill the anterior chamber and press against the cornea; and the rapidity of such development might lead to perforation of the cornea and destruction of the eye.—B.]

It must be distinctly remembered that, although the name of syphilitic iritis is given to the form of inflammation above described, the iritis which may occur in the course of, and be entirely due to, syphilis, does not necessarily always assume this type. For it may appear as a simple idiopathic iritis, or in a more or less severe parenchymatous form, so that the absence of the peculiar gummy nodule does not exclude the presence of syphilis in the system, or its being the cause of the iritis. But, on the other hand, the existence of these nodules may, in the vast majority of cases, be taken as a certain indication of the syphilitic nature of the inflammation. I can only remember having seen one case (a patient of Mr. Critchett's) in which there were well-marked nodules without the slightest evidence of syphilis. Some authors have stated that, in syphilitic iritis, the circumcorneal zone of injection is of a brownish tint, and that the pupil is displaced upwards and inwards. This is, however, not the case, for both these appearances may be met with apart from syphilis.

[*Gelatinous or Spongy Iritis* presents some clinical features different from any other variety, though it may be due to common constitutional causes. The exudation is peculiar, often occurs suddenly, may begin in the pupillary space or at the bottom of the anterior chamber, usually occurs very rapidly, and frequently entirely fills the chamber. This exudation has a gelatinous or spongy appearance, and sometimes seems to lie loosely like flocculi in the anterior chamber. This exudation has been examined by Knapp, Alt, and others, and found to be fibrous, consisting of a network of delicate fibrillæ, inclosing white and red blood-corpuscles and a finely granular substance. Alt thinks the presence of the fibrin is due to hemorrhages in the iris, the fluid parts of which percolate into the anterior chamber and coagulate there. But this latter may occur through the walls of inflamed bloodvessels without there being any hemorrhage, as Burnett very properly states. The exudation is usually completely absorbed, and sometimes with great rapidity. The absorption generally begins at the periphery, and the duration of the process varies between two and three weeks, though occasionally the inflammatory signs disappear in a few days. The treatment is the same as for plastic iritis. (See "Archives of Ophthalmology," vols. vi. and vii.; "Amer. Journ. of Med. Sciences," January, 1880.)—B.]

Amongst the *causes* of iritis, a very frequent one is exposure to sudden changes of temperature, cold draughts of air, rain, wind, etc. The disease is, in such cases, often termed rheumatic iritis. It may also accompany rheumatism in other parts of the body, being evidently produced by the same cause. It is erroneous, however, to speak of rheumatic iritis as a special form of the disease, for it has, in truth, no characteristic symptoms; it generally assumes the form of simple plastic iritis, and may vary greatly in severity, but is not, as a rule, accompanied by extensive exudative changes in the parenchyma of the iris, or by considerable hypopyon. The pain is frequently extremely severe, and may extend over the corresponding side of the head and face. The disease often runs a chronic and very protracted course, and relapses may take place on a recurrence of the rheumatic attack.

[*Rheumatism* is perhaps the most frequent cause of monocular relapsing iritis, and the relapses may occur in rapid succession or at intervals of months. *Gout* is another undoubted cause of iritis, and is of an insidious nature. The children of rheumatic and gouty parents are sometimes the victims of a very insidious chronic iritis, for which no treatment seems to be of any use.—B.]

Mr. Hutchinson[1] has observed a peculiar form of iritis occurring in children of gouty parents. It is chiefly characterized by occurring at an early age, and by being insidious and persistent; posterior synechiæ gradually form, leading to occlusion of the pupil, etc., and there are also probably opacities in the vitreous. The inflammation begins in one eye and generally almost entirely destroys the sight before it advances to the other.

Iritis is also often of *traumatic origin*, being caused by mechanical or chemical injuries, which either affect the iris directly or secondarily. Thus

[1] "Lancet," January 4, 1878.

foreign bodies may remain lodged for some time in the conjunctiva, cornea, anterior chamber, or in the deeper tunics of the eye, and then set up iritis. Clean incised wounds of the iris are not prone to give rise to it, as is proved by the operation of iridectomy, nor does strangulation or compression generally do so, as is evidenced by iridodesis. Wounds which bruise and lacerate the iris are the most apt to set up iritis. Injury of the lens, followed by traumatic cataract, very often produces it, more especially if the iris has been implicated in the injury, or the lens swells up very considerably and presses upon the iris. It also often supervenes secondarily upon other inflammations of the eye. Thus keratitis, especially the diffuse and suppurative forms, and deep or perforating ulcers of the cornea, are frequently accompanied by iritis; this is still more the case in inflammation of the choroid and ciliary body. [Iritis may also be secondary to intra-ocular tumors.—B.]

[Iritis may follow a punctured wound of the cornea and lens capsule, without any wounding of the iris. It is also often caused by the operation of extracting a cataract, and is often attended by chemosis, congestion, and the formation of tough membraniform exudations behind the iris.—B.]

Syphilis is a very frequent cause. When primary iritis occurs in infants or young children, it is almost always due to syphilis, and in such cases we generally meet with other symptoms pathognomonic of the syphilitic taint, such as condylomata about the anus, specific eruptions, etc. In adults it but seldom occurs together with the primary symptoms, but generally during the secondary or tertiary stage, being often the precursor of those symptoms, when the primary have disappeared. The iritis frequently occurs simultaneously with the syphilitic eruptions of the skin.

Some authors have asserted that gonorrhœa is sometimes the cause of iritis. Thus, Mackenzie[1] describes a special form, under the name of "gonorrhœal iritis." Mr. Wordsworth[2] has also narrated three cases in which iritis occurred together with gonorrhœa. It must, however, be stated that all three were complicated with rheumatism. I have myself never met with a case of iritis associated with gonorrhœa alone; but have only observed it in cases in which gonorrhœa coexisted with syphilis or with rheumatism, either of which diseases, as I have already stated, is a frequent cause of iritis. Nor does the so-called "gonorrhœal iritis" present any special or pathognomonic features. [The occurrence of a special form of iritis, a mixture of the plastic and serous forms, due to gonorrhœa, is still doubted by many ophthalmologists, especially in the United States. The iritis occurring in the course of or following rheumatic arthritis, has already been considered, and this may occur in the course of a gonorrhœa, but it is not yet proven that its occurrence at this time is more than coincidental.—B.]

Sympathetic inflammation of the iris is apt to occur after injuries to the eye, or to the lodgement of a foreign body within it, etc. The sympathetic iritis may assume the serous character, but generally appears in the form of suppurative irido-chroiditis. (*Vide* article on "Sympathetic Ophthalmia.") [The form of iritis occurring in sympathetic ophthalmia is almost always plastic, and but rarely suppurative.—B.]

Chronic Iritis is especially distinguished by the fact that the inflammatory symptoms are generally but slightly marked, or are almost so entirely absent that the patient is not aware that there is anything the matter with his eye, except a slight weakness or "cold" in it, as he frequently expresses it. The ocular conjunctiva and subconjunctival tissue are but slightly injected; there

---

[1] Mackenzie on "Diseases of the Eye," 652.   [2] "R. L. O. H. Rep.," iii. 301.

is only a faint pink blush around the cornea; there is but little photophobia, lachrymation, or ciliary neuralgia. The pupil is somewhat contracted and sluggish, and, at certain points, perhaps immovable. On examining it with the oblique illumination, we may frequently notice small adhesions between the edge and the capsule, which, as well as the irregularity of the pupil, become very evident upon the application of atropine. The color of the iris becomes gradually more changed, and this alteration in its tint is permanent, whereas in acute iritis it passes off again with the subsidence of the disease, without, perhaps, eventually leaving any trace behind. The normal brightness and lustre of the iris become faded and dulled, its fibrillæ indistinct and obliterated, and in the later stages of the disease it presents a yellowish-gray, dirty-brown, or slate-colored appearance, its tissue being thinned and atrophied, and traversed, perhaps, by enlarged and somewhat tortuous bloodvessels. The presence of such dilated vessels always indicates a state of congestion and stasis of the circulation in the iris and ciliary body. At this advanced stage, the iritis is generally, however, no longer simple in character, but has become complicated with inflammation of the ciliary body and choroid. (*Vide* the article on "Irido-choroiditis.")

Chronic iritis may supervene upon a more acute form of iritis, or the disease may manifest this chronic and insidious character from the very outset. It also frequently accompanies inflammations of the cornea, more especially the diffuse keratitis. Relapses are very apt to occur in chronic iritis; these recurrent inflammatory exacerbations being often produced by very slight causes, such as undue use of the eyes, particularly by artificial light, exposure to cold, wet, etc. This tendency to recurrence is especially marked in those cases in which numerous or extensive posterior synechiæ exist; for their presence is a constant source of irritation and teasing, as they prove a check to the free, spontaneous movements of the pupil, and in such cases a slight cause will suffice to rekindle the inflammation. During the recurrence of the inflammation, fresh lymph will be effused, and the posterior synechiæ will increase still further in number and firmness, until finally, after perhaps frequent relapses, the whole circumference of the pupil is firmly tied down to the capsule, and the communication between the anterior and posterior chamber is completely interrupted. It will be seen hereafter that such an exclusion of the pupil (circular synechia) is one of the most frequent causes of irido-choroiditis.

[The pathological changes in the iris as the result of chronic inflammation are: extensive hyaline thickening of the endothelium; detachment of the epithelium; proliferation of the nuclei of the endothelium in those parts which are described as reticulated glandular tissue; frequent disease of the lymphoid apparatus of the iris, with disease of the general lymphatic apparatus of the body. The vessels also are almost always affected by the pathological changes in their vicinity. (See "Klinische Monatsblätter für Augenheilkunde," Beiträge, 1881.)—B.]

The prognosis of iritis will depend very much upon the severity and the cause of the inflammation. If the disease be seen at a very early stage, before any adhesions have been formed between the edge of the pupil and the capsule of the lens, or whilst these are yet so slight and brittle as to be readily torn through by the energetic use of atropine, the prognosis is in every way very much more favorable, than if numerous firm posterior synechiæ have already been established, and resist the action of atropine. Parenchymatous and syphilitic iritis afford a less favorable prognosis than the simple or the serous form, as they are generally accompanied by very considerable exudations of lymph at the edge of the pupil, on the surface and into the structure of the iris, and into the anterior chamber. The tendency to implication of the cornea, or the deeper tunics of the eyeball must also be borne in mind. In traumatic iritis, the nature and extent of the injury, the presence of traumatic cataract, or the existence of inflammation of the ciliary body or choroid must all be taken into consideration in framing the prognosis.

Treatment.—The patient should be carefully guarded against the injurious influences of bright light, and sudden changes of temperature, as well as cold and wet. Perfect rest of both eyes must also be enjoined, and if the patient has to leave the house, a bandage should be placed over the affected eye, and a shade over the other, or goggles should be worn. But if the disease is very severe, strict orders must be given that the patient is to keep in a darkened room. We are, however, very frequently obliged to treat even severe cases of iritis as out-patients, and may, even in such instances, frequently succeed in effecting an excellent cure. This mode of treatment should, however, only be adopted from necessity, and not from choice, and strict injunctions should be given to the patients to guard their eyes as much as possible against all noxious influences during the intervals of their visits.

The point of the very greatest importance in the treatment of iritis is to obtain a wide dilatation of the pupil as soon as possible, and hence a strong solution of atropine should be at once energetically applied to the eye. The beneficial effect of atropine is three-fold: 1. Wide dilatation of the pupil is produced, and the iris is, therefore, removed from contact with the anterior capsule of the lens, so that no adhesions can be formed between them at the edge of the pupil, or on the posterior surface of the iris. Thus one of the chief dangers of iritis, the formation of extensive posterior synechiæ, is prevented, and the numerous evil consequences or dangerous complications to which they may give rise are obviated. 2. Rest will be afforded to the inflamed muscular tissue of the iris by a wide dilatation of the pupil; for if the constrictor pupillæ is not paralyzed, its constant action in endeavoring to regulate the size of the pupil according to the stimulus of light, must of necessity tend to increase the inflammation, just as would be the case in any other inflamed muscular tissue, if this could not be kept perfectly at rest. 3. The vascular tension of the eye will be diminished, and the intra-ocular circulation relieved, which will diminish the state of congestion of the iris and ciliary body. Moreover, the irritation of the eye and the ciliary neuralgia will generally be alleviated in a very marked manner. It is, however, absolutely necessary that the solution of atropine should be of a sufficient strength, and should be energetically employed. In the normal condition of the eye, an extremely weak solution (gr. j ad f ℥ viij of water) will suffice to produce a wide dilatation of the pupil, but in iritis it is very different. On account of the inflamed and swollen condition of the tissue of the iris, of the lymph effused into its meshes, and of the hyperæmia, great resistance is offered to the action of the atropine; hence a very strong solution must be used, and the application repeated very frequently, before we can thoroughly overcome this resistance. I am in the habit of employing a solution of from four to six grains of atropine to the fluidounce of water, and of applying it at the interval of five minutes for half an hour at a time, this being repeated, if necessary, three or four times a day; so that altogether the atropine may have to be applied from eighteen to twenty-four times a day, in order to produce and maintain a sufficient dilatation of the pupil. If the case is seen early, before any adhesions, or only very slight and brittle ones, are formed, we may generally succeed in producing a wide dilatation at the end of a few hours, and then it is not difficult to maintain it. I find that patients apply the atropine with much greater regularity and exactitude if they are told to use it for half an hour at a time, at intervals of five minutes, and to repeat this at stated periods three times a day, than if they are only directed in general terms to apply it fifteen or eighteen times a day. As we have frequently at the hospital to treat even severe cases of iritis as out-patients, I invariably apply the atropine myself at the interval of a few minutes, until either a decided effect has been produced upon the pupil, or the result is negative. In the former case, the patient will himself experience the great relief to the pain and irritability of the eye which has been produced by the instillations, and will readily and gladly carry out the treatment at home. Moreover, the dilatation thus effected can generally be maintained until the next visit, even if the remedy is not applied in the interval quite as frequently as directed. I have often been able to treat even severe cases of iritis with great success by this simple means, without the employment of almost any other remedy, except perhaps the use of warm poppy fomentations; the result being a perfectly circular pupil, without any, or only the slightest, adhesions. I would again, therefore, urge in the very strongest terms the energetic use of atropine in iritis, a line of treatment at present, unfortunately, but too much neglected in English ophthalmic practice, the evil results of which neglect are constantly evidenced by the numerous cases of recurrent iritis, chronic irido-choroiditis, etc., which we but too frequently meet with, and which might have been to a very great extent prevented by the early and efficient use of atropine. It is quite useless to prescribe a weak solution of atropine (gr. ss–j ad f ℥j) to be used a few times in the course of the day; this cannot produce a dilatation of the pupil when the tissue of the iris is inflamed, its effect will be *nil*, as can be easily seen by watching the state of the pupil in cases where such weak solutions are employed.

But we sometimes find that the action of even a strong solution of atropine, frequently applied, is resisted, and that it produces little or no effect, and increases rather than diminishes the irritability of the eye. In such cases, its use must be desisted from until the irritation is relieved by the application of a few leeches to the temple, or perhaps by paracentesis of the anterior chamber. This relief of the inflammatory irritation and intra-ocular tension, permits of a freer absorption through the cornea, and hence the effect of the atropine will now be often very marked and rapid. This effect, as Von Graefe has pointed out, is sometimes noticed without the reapplication of the remedy. Thus atropine may have been applied in cases of iritis or keratitis without producing any dilatation of the pupil, but many hours afterwards this has ensued after the application of leeches. We sometimes notice, also, that although dilatation of the pupil may have been produced, yet that it cannot be thoroughly maintained, the atropine appearing to lose its effect. In such cases, it will be found that this is likewise due to the great irritation of the eye and the increase in the intra-ocular tension, which prevent the absorption of the remedy through the cornea. Whereas after the application of leeches or the performance of paracentesis, the atropine will again regain its power over the iris. I need hardly mention, that if the pupil is firmly tied down by numerous and thick adhesions, the atropine should be applied only in moderation, in order to soothe the irritability and diminish the tension of the eye. But if the posterior synechiæ are of recent date, and not very broad and firm, but narrow and tongue-like, the long-continued use of atropine succeeds in tearing them through. It is often found, however, that when this remedy is employed for a considerable length of time, it increases, instead of allaying the irritability of the eye, and may even induce conjunctivitis or acute granulations. The latter are, however, less frequently met with than a vascular condition of the lids, accompanied by swelling of the conjunctiva and great irritation of the eye. In such cases, the atropine must be stopped at once, and a mild astringent collyrium substituted for it. The strength and nature of the latter must vary with the degree of conjunctivitis. A solution of one grain of alum, zinc, or nitrate of silver to the fluidounce of water will be found the best. In vesicular granulations, a collyrium of from six to ten grains of borax to one fluidounce of water proves of much service. The irritability of the eye may also be allayed and the dilatation of the pupil tolerably maintained by the use of a collyrium of belladonna (Ext. bellad. Ʒss, Aq. dest. f Ʒj), which is to be applied frequently in the course of the day. It is sometimes found that posterior synechiæ, which resist the action of atropine, soon tear through upon the application of Calabar bean. Hence this remedy may be tried alternately with the atropine.

The use of atropine is to be continued even for some weeks after the subsidence of the iritis, so that the wide dilatation of the pupil may be maintained and the iris be kept in a state of rest. It has been urged by some, that the long-continued use of a strong solution of atropine is apt to produce a permanent dilatation of the pupil from paralysis of the sphincter pupillæ. But this is a most rare and exceptional occurrence, and if any tendency to dilatation should remain, it may be easily overcome by the occasional use of the Calabar bean, which excites the action of this muscle. Although I am in the habit of using atropine most extensively in the treatment of iritis and other affections of the eye, I have never met with a case in which this condition of permanent dilatation was produced, nor have I ever observed a case of poisoning from the excessive use of atropine. Such cases do, however, sometimes occur, and are evidently produced by the passage of the atropine through the lachrymal puncta to the throat. The principal symptoms of poisoning by atropine are: great increase in the frequency of the pulse, dryness of the throat, dysphagia, great irritability of the bladder and genital organs, impairment of memory, hallucinations, and exciting dreams. The pupils of the eyes are very widely dilated. Generally, these symptoms are only moderate in character when the poisoning has occurred in the mode above described, but their severity is very great if the atropine has been swallowed by mistake, and a considerable dose has thus been taken. The best and most rapid antidote is the subcutaneous injection of morphia[1] (one-fifth or one-fourth of a grain), to be repeated, if necessary—even several times—at intervals of a few hours. The effect of the remedy is very marked and rapid; within a few minutes the violence of the symptoms has greatly subsided and the patient is calm and quiet. To avoid the danger of poisoning, when strong collyria of atropine are used with great frequency, Von Graefe recommends the patient to close the eye directly after the application, and subsequently on reopening the eye to wash it well. He also sometimes employs a subcutaneous injection of morphia at night, in order to prevent all risk. Liebreich[2] has devised a small instrument, like a serre-fine, which is attached to the lower punctum, and this produces a slight ectropium of this part of the lid, thus preventing the entrance of the atropine into the punctum.

[1] Vide Dr. Bell, "Trans. Edin. Med.-Chir. Society," 1867, and Von Graefe's article, "A. f. O.," ix. 2, 70; also a very interesting case of severe "Poisoning by Atropine," reported by Dr. Schmid, "Kl. Monatsbl.," 1864, p. 158.
[2] "Kl. Monatsbl.," 1864, 411.

I have already stated that we occasionally meet with persons whose eyes show an extraordinary antipathy to the use of atropine, and in whom even a drop of a very weak solution suffices to produce great irritation of the eye, and perhaps severe erysipelas of the lids and face. In such cases it should be stopped at once. My friend Dr. Seeley, of Cincinnati, has informed me that he has found in such idiosyncrasies much benefit from combining the atropine with a weak solution of sulphate of zinc. [When atropine acts as an irritant in the ordinary solution, it is sometimes advisable to use a preparation of atropine dissolved in refined castor oil, in which the oil acts as a lubricant to the irritated conjunctiva; or solutions of daturine or duboisine may be employed for a change. In cases of extraordinary antipathy to atropine, both the latter drugs, however, would probably give rise to the same unpleasant symptoms.—B.]

The severe ciliary neuralgia which so often accompanies iritis is most relieved by the application of leeches to the temple, and the use of hot poppy or laudanum fomentations. The leeches should be applied towards evening, so that the nocturnal exacerbations may be relieved. Free after-bleeding is to be encouraged by the use of hot fomentations or poultices. [The use of Heurteloup's artificial leech has some advantages over the live leech, and a recent modification of the apparatus by Dr. F. B. Loring, of Washington, is an improvement upon the old instrument. Local depletion in iritis is a very valuable remedy, and should be frequently repeated when the indications require it.—B.] The nocturnal pain and restlessness of the patient are also much alleviated by the use of opium, and this remedy should never be omitted in such cases, as it is of much consequence that the patient should enjoy a good night's rest. I myself often employ the subcutaneous injection of morphia for this purpose.

A blister may be applied behind the ear, and kept open for a few days, and the compound belladonna ointment should be rubbed into the forehead. [It is sometimes necessary to frequently repeat the blisters, and they may be applied over the eyebrow and on the temple, placing a small one, one inch square, and repeating it by one of the same size on sound skin next it.—B.]

If there is a considerable tendency to exudation of lymph or pus at the edge of the pupil, so that atropine does not act on the latter, into the anterior chamber, on the surface of the iris, or into its structure, the patient should be put rapidly under the influence of mercury. One grain of calomel in combination with one-fourth or one-fifth of a grain of opium should be given every two or three hours, until salivation is produced, which will generally occur in from thirty to forty hours; even when this is produced, a slight degree of tenderness of the gums should be maintained. I, however, greatly prefer the treatment by inunction, as the digestive powers are thus not impaired, and the constitutional effects of the drug are, moreover, more rapidly and surely obtained. Indeed I have met with instances in which mercury had been given by the mouth for some time without producing any constitutional effect, and where this rapidly supervened upon inunction. Half a drachm or a drachm of the strong mercurial ointment should be rubbed into the inside of the arms and thighs two or three times daily, until the mouth becomes slightly affected, the gums showing an indication of the bluish line; when it is to be applied once daily in much smaller quantity. In order to prevent the staining of the skin, the ointment may also be rubbed into the bottom of the feet, but here it is absorbed with less rapidity on account of the greater thickness of the skin. Mr. Pridgin Teale[1] recommends that the

---

[1] Vide Mr. Teale's interesting paper "On the Relative Value of Atropine and of Mercury in the Treatment of Acute Iritis." "R. L. O. H. Reports," v. 166.

mercurial ointment should be smeared on a broad piece of flannel which is to be wrapped round each arm of the patient, who should remain in bed ; a small quantity of fresh ointment should be added every night. In syphilitic iritis, with well-marked nodules, the use of mercury should never be omitted. and I have also found much benefit in such cases from the constant use of hot-water compresses, continued without intermission night and day for several days. I first saw this mode of treatment employed two years ago, by De Wecker, and soon afterwards had the opportunity of trying it in a case of syphilitic iritis with numerous gummata of considerable size, which had to a great extent resisted the action of mercury. I ordered hot-water com-presses to be applied to the eye of as high a temperature as the patient could bear, and these were changed every few minutes, and continued for a great part of the day and night. Within the course of two days the gummata had diminished considerably in size, and within four or five days they had almost entirely disappeared. In another instance, the effect of the com-presses was equally favorable. Of course, it is only in exceptional cases that this mode of treatment can be employed, for it requires the constant and undivided attention of a nurse; moreover, few patients will submit to the trouble and inconvenience. This remedy also greatly hastens the absorption of hypopyon. Hot bread-and-water or linseed-meal poultices also prove very beneficial in allaying the pain, hastening the absorption of exudation, and facilitating the action of atropine. They should be changed every fifteen to twenty minutes; at first they may be continued all day, and in severe cases at night; as the case progresses more or less considerable intervals may intervene between their application.[1] In the rheumatico-gouty form, prepa-rations of guaiacum are often very serviceable.

Formerly it was very much the custom to place all cases of iritis under the influence of mercury, quite irrespective of the fact whether the necessity for its use really existed or not. Now, however, a more rational mode of treatment obtains, and mercury is only used in those cases in which there is much effusion of lymph. In specific cases, the iodide and bromide of potas-sium, together with the decoction of bark, should be administered after the use of mercury. Whilst the latter remedy is being employed, it is also wise to maintain the patient's strength by the use of tonics, more especially prep-arations of steel and quinine.

In the rheumatic form of iritis, benefit is often experienced from the use of oil of turpentine internally, as was first recommended by Dr. Carmichael. Although I have often employed it with advantage, I have frequently been obliged to give up its use on account of the derangement of the stomach which it produces. It should be given in doses of from half a drachm to one drachm two or three times daily, made into an emulsion, to which a little carbonate of soda is added to prevent the derangement of the digestive organs. Mr. Pridgin Teale uses this remedy very extensively in kerato-iritis, as well as in low forms of iritis or keratitis, and speaks most strongly in its favor. [The arthritic varieties of iritis are always very obstinate in resisting treatment. It is necessary in these cases to pay special attention to the free action of the skin, bowels, and kidneys. Frequent small doses of Rochelle salts, the regular use of the Turkish bath every day, or alternating with a general " massage " of the entire body, and the prolonged administra-tion of either salicylic acid or the salicylate of soda, are all necessary and valuable remedial rgents.—B.]

If the aqueous humor is very cloudy, or a considerable hypopyon is

---

[1] *Vide* Mooren, "Ophthalmiatrische Beobachtungen," p. 134, and Schiess-Gemueus, "Kl. Monatsbl.," 1870, p. 198.

formed, paracentesis should be performed, and, if necessary, repeated several times. The same should be done if the pain is very severe and does not yield to the usual remedies. The broad needle should be very slowly removed from the anterior chamber, so that the escape of the aqueous humor may not be very sudden, otherwise there may occur great *hyperæmia ex vacuo* of the inner tunics of the eye. In order to facilitate the escape of the stringy portion of lymph, the needle should be slightly tilted sideways, so as to cause the section to gape, or the same may be done with a small curette or probe.

If the iritis is very intense and obstinate, resisting all our remedies, and more especially if the sight is much impaired; if the synechiæ are numerous and firm, or there is complete exclusion of the pupil; and if the intra-ocular tension is markedly increased, a large iridectomy should be made at once. I have often seen this produce the most striking benefit, although it must be remembered that if the adhesions between the pupil and capsule are at all considerable and broad, or if there is occlusion of the pupil from deposit of lymph within its area, an iridectomy will subsequently be necessary, and the condition of the eye will in all probability be much worse when the inflammation has run its course; and hence the result of an iridectomy be far less favorable than if it had been made at an earlier period, before the changes of structure had attained any considerable degree. Moreover, the iridectomy generally acts as the best antiphlogistic; the inflammation, which had before resisted all our remedial measures, rapidly subsiding after the operation.

In *iritis serosa*, much benefit is often experienced from exciting the free action of the skin and kidneys by diaphoretic and diuretic remedies. Atropine should also be applied, as well as a suppurating blister behind the ear; but it must be confessed that local remedies often prove of little avail. The state of the intra-ocular tension, of the sight, and of the field of vision must be narrowly watched, and if symptoms of glaucoma supervene, no time should be lost in making a large iridectomy.

The treatment of *traumatic* iritis must vary according to the nature of the injury. If a foreign body has become implanted in the iris, it must be carefully extracted, with or without the excision of the corresponding segment of the iris. If the lens has also been injured and a traumatic cataract has been formed, linear extraction, perhaps combined with iridectomy, should be at once performed; as the lens may become much swollen, setting up great irritation, and thus increasing intra-ocular tension. If a portion of the iris prolapses through a small wound in the cornea, it should be pricked, so that the aqueous humor may flow off, and the collapsed protruding portion of iris should then be excised, and a firm compress applied. After an injury to the iris, the inflammation should be combated, according to circumstances, by cold or hot compresses, leeches, and atropine; and, if necessary, rapid salivation should be induced.

In order to prevent, if possible, the recurrence of the inflammation, more especially in cases of chronic iritis, the patients should be warned against undue exposure to cold winds, draughts, bright light, etc., and should be ordered to wear the blue eye-protectors. Nor should they be permitted to strain their eyes with fine needle-work or very small print, particularly by artificial light. Their diet must also be carefully regulated, and every over-indulgence in wine or alcohol strictly forbidden. Inattention to these different points frequently causes the recurrence of the inflammation.

19

3.—FUNCTIONAL DISTURBANCES OF THE IRIS.

(1) Mydriasis.

Although the dilatation of the pupil is generally considerable, it is not so extreme as that produced by a strong solution of atropine, where the iris is contracted to a very narrow, hardly perceptible rim. The dilatation of the pupil may be uniform and regular, so that the pupil retains its circular form, or it may be partial and irregular, the pupil thus acquiring a somewhat ovoid shape. The pupil, besides being dilated, is more or less immovable, acting but slightly, or not at all, under the influence of light, the effort of accommodation, or the convergence of the visual lines. The sight is also somewhat affected, which is due in part to the bright glare which is experienced on account of the wideness of the pupil, and also in part to the circles of diffusion formed upon the retina. If the impairment of sight be simply due to the mydriasis, it will be remedied if the patient looks through a small circular opening in a card, or through the stenopæic apparatus, for then the glare will be diminished, and the formation of circles of diffusion prevented. But very frequently paralysis of the ciliary muscle coexists with the dilatation of the pupil, and the impairment of vision is chiefly due to the loss of accommodation. The features which distinguish the symptoms due to loss of accommodation from those which are simply caused by mydriasis, are frequently overlooked by medical men, and thus much confusion is often produced in the narration of cases. Nor is it of unfrequent occurrence that the symptoms of amblyopia, produced by paralysis of accommodation, are referred to some serious intra-ocular or cerebral lesion. There is not, however, a necessary relation between the degree of dilatation of the pupil and the paralysis of the ciliary muscle, for the pupil may be widely dilated and the ciliary muscle but slightly, if at all, affected; the converse is, however, of less frequent occurrence.

When the pupil is widely dilated, it no longer presents its usual brilliantly black appearance, but assumes a somewhat grayish tint, which is due to the greater amount of light reflected from the lens and the fundus of the eye.

Mydriasis is generally monocular, unless it is due to some cerebral cause, or to a deep-seated intra-ocular lesion affecting both eyes. Monocular mydriasis often produces considerable disturbance of sight, on account of the difference in the brightness of the two retinal images, and the presence of circles of diffusion. For the purpose of accurately measuring the size of the pupil, Mr. Zachariah Laurence's "pupillometer" [Fig. 108] will be found very useful.

["The pupillometer consists essentially of two parts: 1, a pair of indices or 'sights;' and 2, a graduated scale. The sights are formed by two vertical, knife-edged, brass bars (indices); the one (m) fixed; the second (f) movable by means of a screw (s), the head of which (h) is furnished with several small projecting spokes, by which the screw may be turned with great delicacy by the tip of the finger. The horizontal plate (p), the scale to which these indices are attached, is of white metal, and is graduated into whole, half, and quarter lines. The scale is graduated on both sides, so that, by simply reversing the instrument, the pupil of each eye may be successively measured. The application of the pupillometer is obvious, from the annexed figure. The edge of the fixed index (m) is held in a line with the inner edge of the pupil, and then the movable one (f) is gradually screwed up till its edge

corresponds exactly with the outer edge of the pupil. The i|
the two indices represents the diameter of the pupil.'"—H.]

Causes.—Before entering upon the different causes whic|
mydriasis, it will be well briefly to consider the action of ce|
upon the condition of the pupil, either in increasing or in|
size. Certain substances, more especially belladonna, hyoscy|
monium, have the power of producing a marked dilatation of the pupil, and
are hence termed *mydriatics.* We shall here, however, confine our attention
to the action of atropine upon the pupil and the accommodation. In
numerous experiments made by Donders,[2] it was found that if a solution of
four grains of sulphate of atropine to a fluidounce of water was applied to the

[Fig. 108.]

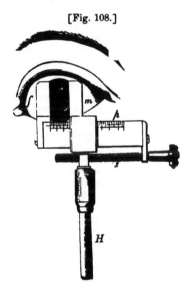

eye, the pupil began to dilate within fifteen minutes, arriving at the maximum degree of dilatation in from twenty to thirty-five minutes, and finally
complete immobility ensued. The younger the individual and the thinner
the cornea, the more rapid was the action. The diminution in the power of
accommodation commences somewhat later than the dilatation of the pupil,
but gradually returns, together with the mobility of the pupil, after some
days. After the lapse of forty-two hours there is generally a slight diminution in the size of the pupil, accompanied by some accommodation, which
increases with tolerable rapidity up to the fourth day, but does not become
perfect till about the eleventh day. The weaker the solution of atropine,
the longer will it take to act, and the less and more transitory will be its
effect. By employing an extremely weak solution (one grain to eight or ten
fluidounces of water), we may dilate the pupil without affecting the accommodation. That the action of the atropine is due to its absorption through the
cornea, is proved by the experiments of Von Graefe,[3] who withdrew some of

[1 Laurence and Moon's "Handy-Book of Ophthalmic Surgery," p. 20.]
[2 Donders, "Anomalies of Refraction and Accommodation," p. 585.]
[3 "A. f. O.," i. 1, 462, note.]

[During the last two years numerous experiments have been made as to the physiological and therapeutical value of the various mydriatics, such as duboisia, hyoscyamia, and the hydrobromate of homatropia. Ladenburg's experiments upon the mydriatic alkaloids show conclusively that hyoscyamia, daturia, and duboisia are identical with each other, and not merely closely related; and that atropia and hyoscyamia, though not actually identical, are isomeric in composition. He concludes, therefore, that there are only two mydriatic alkaloids, atropia and hyoscyamia. He also has succeeded in converting hyoscyamia into atropia. (See "Bericht über d. dtsch. Chem. Gesellsch.," xiii., 1880.) Pautynski employed a one-half per cent. solution of hydrobromate homatropine, and found that dilatation of the pupil began in nineteen and one one-hundreth minutes, reached its maximum in from thirty minutes to two hours, and disappeared in twenty-three and seventy-five one-hundreths hours. He asserts that there is less antagonism between pilocar-pine and homatropine than between pilocarpine and atropine. ("Klinische Monatsblätter für Augenheilkunde," Sept. 1880.) Risley's experiments upon hydrobromate homatropine resulted in the following conclusions: In solutions of two, four, and six grains to the fluidounce, it paralyzes the ac-commodation, and this paralysis disappears entirely in from sixteen to thirty hours. Dilatation of the pupil accompanies the paralysis and is more persistent. The drug is no more liable to produce conjunctival irritation than atropia or duboisia, and it produces far less constitutional disturbance than either of them. ("Am. Journ. Med. Sci.," Jan. 1881.) Schaefer finds that atropia dilates the pupil more slowly than duboisia, but its effect lasts longer. Homatropia dilates the pupil more quickly than either of the two other drugs, but the dilatation is less, and its duration is shorter. The strength of the solution of homatropia exerts no apparent influence upon the duration of its effect. The accommodation is most quickly paralyzed by duboisia and next by homatropia; but the effect of the latter lasts only about twenty-four hours, while that of duboisia lasts three or four days. Homatropia is to be preferred for simple dilatation of the pupil or for par-alyzing the accommodation preparatory to determining the refraction; but as a therapeutic agent it is inferior to both duboisia and atropia. ("Archiv für Augenheilkunde," x. 2.) As regards the comparative therapeutical value of these drugs, Risley concludes: 1st. That the sulphates of atropia, duboisia, and hyoscyamia, and the hydrobromate of homatropia, are efficient

[1] "Klin. Beitrage z. Pathol. und Physiol. der Augen und Ohren." Braunschweig, 1843.

its for paralyzing the accommodative function, and in the treatment of
enopic eyes. 2d. In the employment of the last three named, the dura-
of the treatment is very much shortened. 3d. For the correction of
unlies of refraction in otherwise normal eyes, the homatropia is to be
'erred. 4th. If retino-choroidal disturbance is also present, hyoscyamia
uboisia is preferable to atropia because of the shorter duration of the
tment, and to homatropia because of their most persistent control over
ciliary muscle. 5th. Hyoscyamia is preferable to duboisia, since the
lency to systemic poisoning is not so great. ("Trans. Amer. Ophth. Soc.,"
l.) See also papers by Oliver, in "Amer. Journ. Med. Sci.," July, 1881,
July, 1882; and by Galezowski, in the "Recueil d'ophthalmologie,"
, 1881. Also, a paper upon the "Physiological Action of mydriatics
Myotics," by Fitz Gérald and Laborde, in the "Tribune médicale" for
21, Dec. 5 and 19, 1880; and Jan. 6 and March 20, 1881.—B.]
alabar bean produces excessive contraction of the pupil, together with a
ruction of the ciliary muscle, and an artificial myopia. Its action will
more fully explained in the article upon the "Affections of the Accom-
ation." I think there can be no doubt that it chiefly produces its effect
n the pupil by exciting the nerves to the sphincter pupillæ, although the
mis may also be in part due to the paralysis of the radiating fibres of
iris supplied by the sympathetic. But the spasmodic contraction of the
iry muscle speaks strongly in favor of the excitation of the third nerve.
iiopathic mydriasis is not unfrequently due to rheumatic origin, the
ent having been exposed to cold or wet, and it is in such cases probably
ied by rheumatic inflammation of the nerve sheaths. It is generally
mpanied by more or less complete paralysis of some or all the muscles
plied by the third nerve. It may be also due to syphilis. I have met
a few instances in which a varying degree of mydriasis appeared in one
and in which all the ocular muscles were unaffected; the ciliary muscle
being either not at all, or only very slightly affected. In these cases,
affection could be traced to no other cause than syphilis, and the
friasis had occurred some time after the secondary symptoms. The dila-
on of the pupil yielded gradually, but slowly, to the administration of
de of potassium, and the occasional application of a blister behind the
esponding ear. Mr. De Méric, in an interesting paper read before
British Medical Association at Leeds (1869), reports several cases of
ilitic mydriasis. In one case, all the ocular muscles were paralyzed,
the mydriasis was considerable; there had, however, been caries of the
t. In two other cases, the mydriasis was accompanied by ptosis, in
ther the latter was absent, but the dilatation of the pupil very obstinate.
two cases the secondary symptoms had quite vanished, in another the
iaries were on the wane.
Iydriasis may likewise be caused by direct injury to, or compression of
nerves supplying the constrictor pupillæ, as, for instance, in consequence
evere blows upon the eye, or of an increase in the intra-ocular tension.
hose cases in which it is caused by a blow, the mydriasis is not unfre-
ntly partial, only a certain portion of the sphincter pupillæ being affected.
Further remarks upon the causation of mydriasis will be found under
head of "Anomalies of Accommodation."—B.]
Iydriasis may also be due to irritation of the sympathetic, as may be
in certain spinal diseases. The ephemeral dilatation of the pupil,
ph occasionally occurs for a short time at different periods of the day, is
ably due to this cause. Von Graefe has called attention to the inter-
ig and important fact that this ephemeral mydriasis is sometimes a

premonitory symptom of insanity, more especially of ambitious monomania. The dilatation met with in helminthiasis may also be ascribed to irritation of the sympathetic.

[Complete mydriasis, with unimpaired accommodation, may appear after violent periorbital pain, and in these cases a careful ophthalmoscopic examination should be made, for a glaucomatous condition may lie at the bottom. Sometimes mydriasis, with other signs of paralysis of the third nerve, precedes locomotor ataxia. Monocular mydriasis, with sluggish action of the iris, is to be regarded as a suspicious brain symptom in suspected disease of the nerve-centres, as pointing to beginning paralysis; though Arndt regards it as a sign of spinal irritation. Mydriasis is a frequent symptom in hysteria, and during epileptic attacks. Partial mydriasis is generally due to compression or injury of the ciliary nerves, as may be observed in division of the optic nerve, or in the more modern operation of optico-ciliary neurotomy without enucleation.—B.]

Dilatation of the pupil is also a common symptom in certain diseases of the brain, e. g., meningitis, hydrocephalus, and diseases of the cerebellum, also in many intra-ocular diseases, in which the sensitiveness of the retina is much diminished. In exceptional instances, the pupil may still act perfectly, even although the eye is absolutely blind. In such cases, the conductibility of the optic nerve, and the reflex action which it produces on the ciliary nerves are unimpaired, but the image is not perceived by the brain.

Treatment.—In the rheumatic form of mydriasis a blister should be applied behind the ear, and iodide of potassium, or a preparation of guaiacum, should be administered internally. I have, however, often found a more marked and rapid effect to result upon the paralysis of the accommodation from the application of the blister, than upon the mydriasis. If the dilatation of the pupil does not yield to these remedies, but shows a tendency to become chronic, tincture of opium should be dropped into the eye, electricity should be applied, and instillations of solutions of Calabar bean may be tried. The latter remedy should not, however, be applied of too great a strength, or too frequently, otherwise it will produce much fatigue of the sphincter pupillæ, instead of simply moderately stimulating it. Frequent and firm closure of the eyelids, convergence of the visual lines, and repeated exercise in reading, etc., are also of advantage in stimulating the contraction of the pupil. [Sulphate of eserine is a more active and less irritating myotic than the mother-drug Calabar bean. A solution (one centigramme to five millilitres) should be dropped into the eye as often as necessary, unless it occasions too much conjunctival and ciliary irritation. If the mydriasis is accompanied by paralysis of accommodation, the constant current of electricity should be resorted to, or subcutaneous injections of strychnia may be given.—B.]

In very rare instances, the faculty exists of voluntarily dilating the pupil. Seitz[1] mentions a case of a young student, who was able voluntarily to produce a dilatation of about three millimetres by taking a deep inspiration, and then holding his breath, at the same time making a strong effort, during which the muscles of the neck and back became very tense. The experiment succeeded best when he regarded an object lying but a short distance from the eye.

(2) MYOSIS.

Idiopathic myosis is of rare occurrence. The pupil is in such cases often extremely contracted, perhaps to the size of a pin's head, or even less, and

---

[1] "Augenheilkunde," p. 315.

ery slightly on the stimulus of light. Even strong solutions of
produce but a very moderate degree of dilatation. On account of
ne minuteness of the pupil, but little light is admitted into the
stinal images are consequently but slightly illuminated, and the
his account more or less impaired. The small size of the pupil also
nsiderable contraction of the peripheral part of the field of vision.
may be caused by a spastic affection of the sphincter pupillæ, or
ysis of the radiating fibres of the iris. The irritation of the branch
d nerve, which supplies the sphincter pupillæ, may be due to some
use, or to reflex action from the fifth nerve. It may also be pro-
too great and long-continued use of the eyes at very minute objects,
tch-making, engraving, etc.; in consequence of which, the sphincter
time acquires a preponderating power over the dilator. The
to paralysis of the dilator muscle is met with in those spinal lesions
the sympathetic nerve is affected, so that its influence upon the
es of the iris is impaired. Dr. Argyll Robertson reports[1] a very
case of spinal affection, in which there was marked myosis in
the pupils being about the size of a pin's point. Even a strong
atropine had but an imperfect and transient effect, but Calabar
acted the pupil still more, to about one-fourth of a line. A tumor[2]
mal swelling[3] pressing upon the cervical portion of the sympathetic
produce myosis.
peculiar condition termed *hippus*, there is a chronic spasm of the
cing rapid contractions and dilatations of the pupil, which follow
in quick succession, and are independent of the influence of light.
ally allied with nystagmus.
atment of myosis must of course vary with the cause, which is
ied at a distance from the eye. Periodic instillations of atropine
tried, although they generally have but a slight and only tem-
ct upon the myosis.
dle or spastic myosis is of cerebral origin, and is met with in
ng meningitis, in cases of poisoning by alcohol, opium, nicotine, etc.,
mes at the beginning of an hysterical convulsion. The paralytic
yosis is much commoner, and is often due to direct compression of
nd sympathetic, or to injury of the spinal cord in the cervical
or inflammatory diseases of the spinal cord. Monocular and
myosis is observed as a very early symptom of ataxy, and some-
pears when other symptoms begin. Even in cases of marked
rophy in ataxy, there may be no myosis. In the myosis due
atropine produces only partial and transient dilatation, while
the myosis. When the myosis is of the spastic variety,
ally more or less spasm of the accommodation; but when the
paralytic, the accommodation is almost always intact.—B.]

4.—TREMULOUS IRIS (IRIDODONESIS).

st frequent cause of this condition is absence of the lens, or its
complete dislocation. In such cases, the iris will be observed dis-
oscillate and tremble when the eye is moved in different directions.
f partial dislocation of the lens, the tremulousness will be confined
rtion of the iris which has lost the support of the lens.

* Edinburgh Med. Journal," Feb. 1869.
Willebrand "A. f. O.," i. 1, 319.
Lairdner, "Monthly Journal of Medicine," 1855 (vol. xx. p. 75).

In such cases the lens has generally been found partially dislocated, or much diminished in size.

The treatment of injuries to the iris must be directed to diminishing any inflammatory symptoms which may supervene. Atropine should be frequently dropped into the eye; leeches should, if necessary, be applied to the temple, and, for the first few hours after the accident, cold compresses will afford great relief, and assist in checking a tendency to inflammation. If there is any prolapse of the iris through the corneal wound, or if the lens has been injured, the treatment laid down in the articles upon "Wounds of the Cornea," and "Traumatic Cataract," must be pursued.

Small foreign bodies, such as splinters of steel or glass, portions of guncap, etc., may become lodged in the iris, or may injure it in their passage to the back of the eye. The presence of even a minute foreign body in the tissue of the iris is a source of constant irritation, and consequently soon sets up more or less severe inflammatory complications, giving rise to corneo-iritis, or perhaps suppurative irido-choroiditis. It is, therefore, most advisable to extract a foreign body in the iris as soon as possible. The best mode of doing this is by an iridectomy, the segment of iris in which the foreign body is lodged being excised.

[For further consideration of this subject, see section 9 of this chapter.—B.]

6.—TUMORS OF THE IRIS, ETC.

[Tumors of the iris may be divided into two classes: benign and malignant. Among the first class are to be placed the epidermoid growths and the cysts, the pigmented nævi, and the granulation tumors. In the second group belong the sarcomatous and carcinomatous growths, and tubercles of the iris.—B.]

Cysts of the iris are comparatively a rare affection, and are almost always the result of some injury to the iris. Thus they have been met with after the lodgement of foreign bodies in the iris, penetrating or incised wounds of the latter, blows upon the eye, or even after operations for cataract, such as the operation of division, or the common flap extraction. Sometimes it is difficult to discover the exact cause, or to ascertain with certainty that any accident has ever occurred to the eye. In such cases, a very careful examination may, however, sometimes lead us to detect a slight opacity of the cornea, the remains of a former perforation.

[Fig. 112.

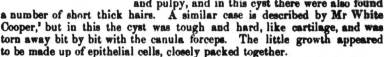

After Mackenzie.]

The cysts generally appear in the form of small transparent vesicles, situated on the surface of the iris, from which they may spring from a broadish base [Fig. 112] or a little pedicle. Their contents, instead of being limpid and transparent, may be opaque, causing the cyst to assume the appearance of a little pearl. Von Graefe[1] records a case in which the contents were sebaceous, soft, and pulpy, and in this cyst there were also found a number of short thick hairs. A similar case is described by Mr White Cooper,[2] but in this the cyst was tough and hard, like cartilage, and was torn away bit by bit with the canula forceps. The little growth appeared to be made up of epithelial cells, closely packed together.

The presence of the cyst may not be productive of any particular inconvenience or impairment of the sight, except inasmuch as the latter may be interfered with by the cyst protruding more or less into the area of the pupil. But in other cases, it sets up a considerable degree of irritation, accompanied by ciliary injection, photophobia, lachrymation, etc., or it may give rise to iritis. In a case narrated by Mr. Hulke,[1] sympathetic inflammation of the other eye was set up, which yielded rapidly after the excision of the cyst.

[The development of a cyst in the iris must be regarded as generally destructive to the functions of the eye, though cases are on record where the disease has come to a stand-still with partial preservation of vision.—B.]

In an interesting paper upon cysts of the iris, Mr. Hulke says: "An examination of all the cases which I have been able to collect shows: I. that cysts, in relation with the iris projecting into the anterior chamber, originate in two situations—1, in the iris; and 2, in connection with the ciliary processes. The first lie between the uveal and the muscular stratum of the iris, and are distinguished by the presence of muscular fibres upon their anterior wall; the second lie behind the iris, and bear the uveal as well as the muscular strata on their front. II. It also shows that these cysts are of more than one kind; that there are—1, delicate membranous cysts, with an epithelial lining, and clear limpid contents; 2, thick-walled cysts, with opaque thicker contents (whether these are generally distinct from 1 we are not yet in a position to determine, but it seems probable that they are so); 3, solid cystic collections of epithelium, wens or dermoid cysts; 4, cysts formed by deliquescence in myxomata."

De Wecker[2] believes that serous cysts are never developed in the iris, but that they are the result of sacculation of the latter; and that the formation of the cyst does not take place by the distention of a pre-existing space in the tissue of the iris, but that this space (a fold or sacculation of the iris) is caused either by injury or inflammation, the serous contents being the aqueous humor. [De Wecker's view of the cystoid degeneration of a portion of the iris, has been confirmed in part by Knapp, Alt, and others. There seems to be no doubt that sacculation of the iris through injury may lead to total cystoid degeneration of the iris. Yet De Wecker thinks it possible that, including these cases, and all epidermoid growths, real retention cysts may be developed in the tissue of the iris. Rothmund's idea, that serous cysts are caused by a hyperplasia of the epithelium on Descemet's membrane, has no positive basis to rest upon.—B.]

The tissue of the iris covering the anterior cyst-wall generally becomes so stretched and attenuated, that the limpid contents of the latter are perfectly distinguishable, and we can often see quite through it to the posterior wall. [The inner surface of the cyst is usually covered by delicate epithelium, and destitute of pigment.

The latest classification of cysts of the iris is by Girard-Teulon, who divides them into, 1, cysts with an internal epithelial wall and serous contents; 2, dermoid cysts, sometimes containing fine hairs; 3, white or pearly cysts, which however, properly speaking, are not cysts, but tumors of the structure of the pearly epithelioma. The very rare instances of cysts occurring in very young children are probably due to a congenital alteration. The anterior surface of the pupillary membrane and the posterior surface of the cornea, which at first are in contact, probably become in these cases adherent, so as to circumscribe a sort of cavity, limited behind by the pupillary mem-

[1] "R. L. O. H. Rep.," 6, 12.
[2] Knapp and Moos' "Archives of Ophthalmology and Otology," i. 1, p. 89.

contracted. There was slight excavation of the optic nerve. The patient again refused an iridectomy. Some months later, the glaucomatous changes having led to a complete loss of sight, the patient submitted to an iridectomy, on account of the very severe ciliary neuralgia which had supervened. The little shrunken tumor was sent to Dr. Schweigger for examination, who, as Mooren says, doubtlessly did not receive it, as its receipt was never acknowledged by him. The other eye was subsequently affected with sympathetic irido-choroiditis, which yielded to an iridectomy.

[The simple *granuloma* has only of late years been recognized as a distinct growth. It is a rare tumor, and hence was confounded clinically with fungoid malignant neoplasms, and histologically with gummata. Microscopically, there is very little difference between the granuloma and certain sarcomata, for it consists of a vascular fibroid tissue with small, round, and fusiform cells. De Wecker describes three varieties: 1. Simple idiopathic granuloma, occurring almost exclusively in children. 2. Teleangiectatic, often leading to spontaneous hemorrhage into the anterior chamber, and hence differing hardly at all from vascular nævi. 3. Traumatic granuloma, the most frequent, and not uncommonly occurring after abscission of a corneal staphyloma. During the past three or four years there have been published a number of articles upon *tubercles* of the iris, in which these tubercles have been considered as histologically the same as granuloma, and one author, Dr. Haab, of Zurich, does not hesitate to describe tubercle of the iris as granuloma iridis. They may occur in the iris alone, or in the conjunctiva and choroid as well, and, *Haab* thinks, may be regarded as the local manifestation of general miliary tuberculosis. This question as to the real nature of the tuberculous nodules in the iris is still unsettled. They certainly are very rare, and, moreover, do not occur in the choroid with anything like the frequency stated. *Haab* prefers to use the term "iritis tuberculosa" for this disease. (See "Annales d'oculistique," vol. lxiv.; "Archiv für Ophthalmologie," Bd. xix. 1—xxv. 4; "Archiv für Augen- und Ohrenheilkunde," Bd. i.; "Annali di ottalmologia," iv.; De Wecker, in Graefe und Saemisch's "Hdb. der Augenheilk.," Bd. iv.) A case of tuberculosis of the iris in a child is reported by Ritter. The child was two years old, and the mother had noticed a gray spot in the pupil for three weeks. An attempt was made by an iridectomy to remove the mass, which filled the external half of the anterior chamber. This proved unsuccessful; and as a granulating mass began to grow from the scleral wound, the eye was enucleated. Two months later the child had a violent attack of convulsions, with left hemiplegia. A microscopical examination of the eye showed tuberculosis of the iris, which had begun in the form of nodules, and had gradually led to tubercular infiltration of the entire iris and sclero-corneal wound. There were also the signs of cyclitis and partial opacity of the lens. ("Archiv für Augenheil.")—B.]

Cancer [Sarcoma.—B.] of the iris is almost always due to an extension of the disease from the deeper tunics of the eye; it is extremely rare as a primary affection of the iris, and is then generally melanotic in character. It appears in the form of a small, dark, yellowish-brown elevation or tubercle at some point of the iris, perhaps somewhat resembling a little syphilitic button or condyloma. The tumor may remain stationary for a length of time, or rapidly increase more and more in size, and protrude into the anterior chamber in the form of a dark-brown or blackish mass, which either perforates the cornea or the anterior portion of the sclerotic, which becomes staphylomatous at this point, and, gradually yielding, the tumor sprouts forth. As soon as the true nature of the disease is recognized, no time should be lost in excising the eyeball. This is much wiser than removing only the anterior half of the eye, as a similar disease may exist in the deeper tunica. Hirschberg[1] records a case of primary melano-sarcoma of the iris, in which the iris was alone implicated, the tumor having been developed from its anterior portion, the elements of the ciliary body being perfectly unchanged. He moreover points out with regard to the diagnosis between the simple and sarcomatous (malignant) tumors of the iris, that they first occur in children between the ages of one and twelve, and are of a light yellowish-white color, and often very vascular, their surface being uneven and somewhat ragged; whereas the sarcomata have a darker color and a smooth surface.

[Primary sarcoma of the iris, though a comparatively rare disease, is not so uncommon as was formerly supposed. Within the last five or six years quite a number of cases have been reported, the most recent of which are by Kipp, three by Knapp, one by Lebrun, one by Roosa, and one by Carter, of London. (See "Archives of Ophthalmology," vol. v.; "Annales d'oculistique," vol. lx., 1869; "Archives of Ophthalmology," vol. viii.; "Trans. of Amer. Ophthal. Soc.," 1869; Carter's Treatise on "Diseases of the Eye," Amer. ed., p. 273.)

Sarcoma of the iris may be removed by means of a lance-knife or a narrow cataract-knife. The incision should be in the sclero-corneal margin, and should be curved, so that the wound may gape and allow the tumor and iris to prolapse on pressure of one lip of the wound. In making the incision, the tumor should not be wounded, as profuse hemorrhage may result and render the further steps of the operation very difficult. Iritis or irido-cyclitis may result from the operation, but, even with this possibility, the removal of the tumor should always be preferred to enucleation of the eye, provided that the neoplasm involves the iris only.

Lepra of the iris, in which a degeneration of the iris with the formation of nodules occurs, has received the faulty name of tubercle of the iris. It has been observed in Brazil by Pedraglia, who thinks the uveal tract is only involved secondarily to the other parts of the eye. Bull and Hansen have observed it in Norway, and consider that the nodules begin in the corneal margin and then spread to the iris. In the latter, the nodules always develop from the periphery, and generally in the lower half of the iris. They may grow so large as to fill the anterior chamber. They consider that iritis with the formation of nodules, produced by the leprous dyscrasia, occurs very often in those who suffer from the tuberous form of the disease. (See "Klin. Monatsbl.," Bd. x.; Bull and Hansen, "The Leprous Diseases of the Eye," 1873.)—B.]

7.—CONGENITAL ANOMALIES OF THE IRIS.

Congenital Irideremia [Aniridia.[1]—B.], or absence of the iris, is occasionally hereditary. I have seen one instance in which the iris was completely wanting in both eyes of the father, this condition being accompanied by a partial luxation and opacity of the crystalline lenses; and in the son (an infant a few months old) there was total irideremia in both eyes, but the latter appeared otherwise quite normal. Sometimes the iris is not completely wanting; a small rudimentary portion, of varying size, being apparent at

---

[1] "A. f. O.," **14, 3, 235.**
[2] See Manz in Graefe und Saemisch's "Hdb. der Augenheilkunde," Bd. i.; Zehender's "Monatsbl.," **1871.**—B.]

the periphery. Absence of the iris is often accompanied by opacity or displacement of the lens, nystagmus, and imperfect development of the cornea, which perhaps does not acquire its normal size. The power of accommodation may also be impaired, but this is not due, as was formerly supposed, to the absence of the iris, but may be caused by an arrest in the development of the ciliary body. In those cases in which irideremia is not accompanied by any other affection, the sight may be very good, more especially if the glare of the light and the circles of diffusion upon the retina are diminished by the use of stenopæic spectacles.

[Manz regards aniridia as the result of a check in development, and thinks the cause should be sought for in the lens, which plays an analogous *rôle* here to that played by the embryonic vitreous in coloboma of the choroid.—B.]

Coloboma, or partial deficiency of the iris (cleft iris), is almost always accompanied by a cleft in the ciliary body and choroid. It is due to an arrest in the development of the iris, and may vary very much in size and shape. The coloboma is generally situated at the lower, or lower and inner, portion of the iris, and is irregularly triangular or pyriform in shape, the base of the triangle being turned towards the pupil, the apex towards the periphery. [Fig. 113.] Coloboma of the iris generally affects both eyes; sometimes it is confined to one, generally the left, and is often accompanied by other congenital anomalies of the eye, such as cleft of the eyelids, congenital cataract, microphthalmos, nystagmus, cleft palate, etc. The fissure in the iris does not necessarily extend quite up to the periphery, but at the latter point a margin of iris may exist, uniting the two edges of the cleft. Moreover, the area of the coloboma may be closed by a rudimentary, darkly pigmented membrane, which might cause the deficiency of the iris at this point to be altogether overlooked by a superficial observer (Seitz). If the fibrous layer of the iris is deficient to a greater extent than the uveal layer, the edge of the cleft is fringed with a distinct black margin. In simple coloboma iridis, the acuity of vision is generally not at all affected; it may be very different, however, if the affection is associated with a considerable cleft in the ciliary body and choroid.

[Fig. 113.

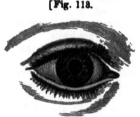

After T. W. Jones.]

[A defect of the iris known as pseudo-coloboma has been investigated by Von Mittelstädt, whose opinions as to its morphology and genesis are as follows: The difference between a pseudo-coloboma and a complete coloboma is one of degree, both defects being brought about by the same process, viz., a total or partial failure in the closing of the embryonic ocular fissure. He considers pseudo-coloboma, not as the first processes in the formation of coloboma, but as the last remains of the embryonic ocular fissure which is tending towards closure. (See "Archives of Ophthalmology," ix. 4.)

The so-called bridge-coloboma consists in the pillars of the coloboma being united by a narrow transverse band of fibres, which may be pigmented, though it is generally not.—B.]

Amongst the other congenital anomalies of the iris, we must call attention to the eccentric position of the pupil (*corectopia*), and to the cases in which there exists more than one pupil (*polycoria*). The eccentric displacement of the pupil may sometimes be so slight that it is hardly observable, but in other cases it is well marked, there being only perhaps a small rim of iris at the side towards which the pupil is displaced. Sometimes both eyes are affected, and then the displacement of the pupil may be symmetrical. I had, some time ago, under my care at the Royal London Ophthalmic Hospital, two very interesting cases of corectopia, occurring in two sisters. In each eye the pupil was displaced, and the lens dislocated, both these conditions being congenital. The eyes of the parents were quite normal.

In cases of *polycoria*, a second pupil may exist at some little distance from the original one, being separated from it by a more or less considerable band of iris, the second pupil being, in fact, a partial coloboma (annular) of the iris. In other cases, several small pupils exist near the normal one, being separated from it and each other by narrow trabeculæ of iris, and this condition is evidently closely allied to that of persistent pupillary membrane. The existence of two or more pupils does not generally produce any impairment of sight, or give rise to monocular diplopia or polyopia.

[*Dyscoria* is the name given to that condition of the iris in which the pupil has not the normal circular form.—B.]

Persistence of the pupillary membrane is a rare affection, and is characterized by the presence of one or more delicate fibrillar bands, springing from the larger circle of the iris, and passing over the smaller circle into the pupil, which they may either cross to be inserted at the other side into the larger circle of the iris, or they may pass over into a thin, pigmented, circumscribed membrane, situated in the area of the pupil, and perhaps attached to the capsule of the lens. These large trabeculæ are often connected to each other by numerous crossbars of delicate fibrillæ.[1] Weber[2] has described a very interesting case, in which the fibres formed a series of arcades. The fibrillæ were very thin and delicate, and were about eighteen or twenty in number, and united by numerous thin fibrillar crossbars. They sprung from the larger circle of the iris, and passed straight over the lesser circle to the centre of the pupil, which was occupied by a circumscribed, pigmented, membranous patch, firmly attached to the capsule of the lens. Into this membrane the fibrillæ were inserted. The remaining portions of the capsule, as well as the edge of the pupil, were quite free from any deposits or adhesions, and the pupil acted perfectly under the influence of light. It appears probable that these remains of the pupillary membrane are more frequent in young children, giving way and disappearing as the person gets older. Their true nature is, moreover, sometimes overlooked, they being mistaken for simple adhesions between the pupil and the capsule of the lens.

8.—OPERATIONS FOR ARTIFICIAL PUPIL.

It is unnecessary to enter into a description of the various modes of making an artificial pupil which have been in vogue at different times, as they have now been all abandoned in favor of the following operations, of which that of iridectomy enjoys by far the widest and most varied application, and hence demands at our hands the most full and exact description.

(1) IRIDECTOMY.

The following instruments are required for the operation:

1. A silver wire speculum for keeping open the eyelids. Weiss' stop-speculum (Fig. 114) will be found the best, as, by means of an easily ad-

---

[1] For several interesting cases of this affection, as well as for a brief *résumé* of the cases hitherto described in ophthalmic literature, *vide* two articles of Cohn's in "Kl. Monatsbl.," 1867, pp. 62 and 119.

[2] "A. f. O.," viii. 1, 337.

justable screw, it permits the eyelids to be kept fixedly apart at any desired distance, so that they cannot press the branches together, and thus narrow. the aperture. This form of speculum is seen in Fig. 114. If the patient should strain very much, and the speculum presses upon the eyeball, an assistant should lift it forward a little, so as to remove it from the globe.

2. A pair of fixation-forceps for steadying the eyeball. They must catch accurately, and the tooth should not be too sharp and pointed, otherwise it

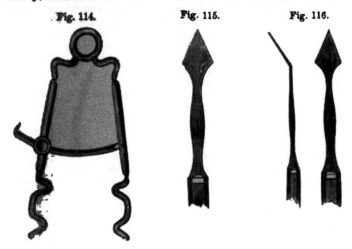

Fig. 114.   Fig. 115.   Fig. 116.

will easily tear through the conjunctiva. If the latter is thin and rotten (as is often the case in elderly persons), Waldau's fixation-forceps are to be preferred, which, instead of being toothed, are finely serrated, so that they obtain a firm hold of the conjunctiva without tearing through it.

3. A broad lance-shaped knife. It should be about the same width as that represented in Fig. 115. If it is much broader, the internal wound will be considerably smaller than the external, and in order to enlarge it to the same size as the latter, the edge of the knife must be much tilted in withdrawing the instrument from the anterior chamber; but this proceeding is often somewhat difficult, and may prove dangerous in the hands of an inexperienced operator. The shape of the knife must vary with the direction in which the iridectomy is to be made. If it is made outwards (to the temporal side) the straight knife is to be used; but if the iridectomy is made inwards or upwards, the blade must be bent at a more or less acute angle (Fig. 116), according to the prominence of the nose or of the upper edge of the orbit. If the anterior chamber is extremely shallow, so that the iris is nearly in contact with the cornea, and especially if the pupil is at the same time dilated, it will be better to make the incision with Von Graefe's narrow cataract-knife, than with the lance-shaped one; for with the former we can skirt the edge of the anterior chamber, and make a large incision without any risk of wounding the lens.

4. The iris forceps should catch most accurately, and, when closed, should be perfectly smooth at the extremity; for if they are rough and irregular, they will scratch and tear the iris and the lips of the incision, and thus perhaps set up some irritation. They may be straight (Fig. 117) when the iridectomy is made outwards, although I, even here, prefer to have them

20

slightly bent. For the upward or inward operation they must be at a still more acute angle (Fig. 118).

5. The iris scissors (Fig. 119) should be bent at an angle, and, though sharp, should not be too finely pointed. Care should be taken that the blades close tightly, and do not override each other, which may easily occur in such slight scissors, if the joint is not sufficiently strong and firm. Instead of these, a pair of scissors curved on the flat [Fig. 120] may also be used.

The operation is to be performed in the following manner: The patient is to be placed in the recumbent position, either in bed or on a couch, the head

Fig. 117.   Fig. 118.   Fig. 119.   Fig. 120.

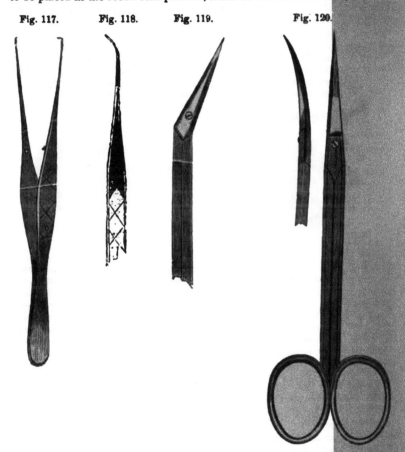

being slightly elevated. Unless there be very exceptional reasons to the contrary, an anæsthetic should always be administered. I prefer anæsthesia in all cases of iridectomy, especially if the eye is acutely inflamed, for the operation is then often very painful; and, however courageous and determined the patient may be, he may find it impossible to control some sudden, involuntary movement of the eye or head, which may endanger the result of the operation, or even imperil the safety of the eye. If an anæsthetic is employed, it should be given so as to anæsthetize the patient completely, and render him quite passive, otherwise he may prove far more unruly than if none had been administered, as the operation is of so delicate a nature that absolute quietude of the eye is necessary. If sickness should supervene, the further steps of the operation must be delayed until this has passed away.

Let us now suppose that an outward iridectomy is to be performed upon the right eye for the cure of glaucoma. If the operator is ambidextrous, he may seat himself upon the couch or bed in front of the patient, and make the incision with his left hand. If not, he should place himself behind the patient. The eyelids having been opened to the desired extent by the stop-speculum, the operator should seize the conjunctiva near the inner side of the cornea with a pair of fixation-forceps, exactly opposite to the place where the incision is to be made. The straight iridectomy knife is then to be thrust into the sclerotic, about half a line from the sclero-corneal conjunctiva (Fig. 121), and, the handle of the instrument being laid well back towards

Fig. 121.   Fig. 122.

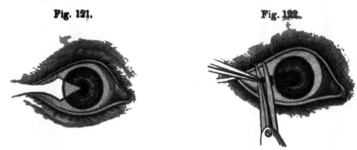

the temple, the point is to be passed into the anterior chamber at its very rim, and carried on slowly and steadily towards the opposite side until the incision is of the desired extent. The knife is then to be slowly and gently withdrawn, the aqueous humor being allowed to flow off as slowly as possible, so that the relief of the intra-ocular pressure may not be sudden; otherwise this will cause a rapid overfilling of the intra-ocular bloodvessels, and perhaps a rupture of the capillaries of the retina and choroid, producing sometimes very extensive hemorrhage. When the knife has been nearly withdrawn from the anterior chamber, the handle is to be somewhat depressed, so that the upper edge of the blade is slightly elevated, and the upper angle of the internal incision should then be enlarged to a size corresponding to the external incision. The same proceeding may be repeated downwards, or the incision may be enlarged to the required extent with a pair of blunt-pointed scissors curved on the flat, the one point being introduced just within the anterior chamber, and the incision then enlarged upwards and downwards.

On the completion of the section, the forceps are to be handed over to an assistant, who should, if necessary, fix the eye, being careful at the same time not to press or drag upon the eyeball, but simply to rotate it gently in its bed. If the iris does not protrude through the lips of the wound, the operator should pass the iris forceps (closed) into the anterior chamber, and then, opening them somewhat widely, he should seize a fold of the iris, and draw it gently through the incision to the requisite extent, and cut it off with the scissors quite close to the lips of the wound (Fig. 122). The excision of the iris may be done either by the operator himself, or by an assistant. In the former case, the iris forceps should be held in the left hand, and the scissors in the right, as it requires some practice to use the latter well with

the left hand.   If a portion of the iris protrudes into the incision, there will
be no occasion to introduce the forceps into the anterior chamber, but the
prolapsed portion is to be seized, and, if necessary, drawn forth somewhat
further and divided.

The portion of iris may be excised with one cut, or else this may be done
according to either of the following modifications introduced by Mr. Bowman.

The protruding portion of iris may be drawn to the right-hand angle of
the incision, and partly divided close up to the angle, the other portion being
then gently torn from its ciliary insertion (slight snips of the scissors aiding
in the division), and drawn to the opposite angle, to be there completely cut
off.   This mode of operating is illustrated in Fig. 123, a, the prolapse drawn

Fig. 123.

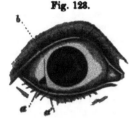

Fig. 124.

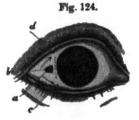

down to the lower (right-hand) angle, a', of the incision, where the inferior
portion is to be divided, and the other drawn up in the direction of b, to the
upper angle of the incision.

Or again, the prolapse (Fig. 124, a) may be divided into two portions at b.
The lower portion is to be drawn in the direction of c, to the lower angle of
the incision, and snipped off.   The upper portion is then to be drawn in the
direction of d, and also divided.   There is, however, this disadvantage in
this mode of operating, that, if there is much hemorrhage, the upper portion
of iris is somewhat hidden, or it may slip back into the anterior chamber,
and have to be searched for.

But either method, if well accomplished, will yield an excellent artificial pupil.   The iris will be torn away quite up to its ciliary attachment,
and the pupil will consequently reach quite up to the periphery (Fig. 125).

Fig. 125.

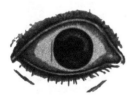

If there is any hemorrhage into the anterior
chamber, the blood should be permitted to escape
before coagulation.   A small curette is to be inserted between the lips of the wound, slight pressure being at the same time made upon the eyeball with the fixation-forceps, so as to facilitate the
escape of the blood.   But if the latter does not
escape readily, it should not be forced out, but be
permitted to remain, as it will soon be absorbed,
especially if a compress bandage is applied.

[Rubbing the closed lids over the eyeball from
side to side or in a rotatory manner often facilitates the escape of the blood
from the anterior chamber, and also assists in smoothing the pillars of the
coloboma.—B.]

I have described the mode of performing iridectomy in the outward direction, as this is the easiest, and it may therefore be wise for an unskilled
operator to make it at first in this direction, until he has gained a certain
degree of practice and dexterity, and then to pass over to the upward or
inward incision.   The operation in either of the latter directions is cer-

tainly more difficult than the temporal, on account of the prominence of the nose or upper edge of the orbit, and the consequent necessity of employing a knife bent at a more or less acute angle, which an unskilled operator may find somewhat difficult to keep quite flat.

The size of the iridectomy and the direction in which it is to be made, should vary with the purpose for which the operation is performed. Thus, if it be done solely for the purpose of arresting inflammation, or of diminishing intra-ocular tension, it should, if possible, always be made directly upwards, for then the upper lid will cover the greater portion of the artificial pupil, and thus not only hide the slight deformity, but also cut off much of the irregularly refracted light. In these cases, more especially in glaucoma, the incision should be made somewhat in the sclerotic, so that the iris may be removed quite up to the ciliary insertion, and should be of a sufficient size to permit of the excision of about one-fifth of the iris. We find that if both these requirements are not fulfilled, the beneficial effect of the iridectomy in checking the inflammation and the increase in the tension is either greatly diminished or not permanent.

But when iridectomy is performed simply for the purpose of making an artificial pupil through which to admit the light, as in opacity of the cornea, lamellar cataract, etc., it should be made of a much smaller size, and, if possible, inwards, as the visual line cuts the cornea slightly towards the inner side of the centre. But with regard to the position, we must be guided by the condition of the cornea, endeavoring to make the artificial pupil opposite to that portion of the cornea which is most transparent, and most true in its curvature. The incision should in these cases be slightly in the cornea, and a narrow belt of iris may be left standing, so that the irregular refraction produced by the periphery of the cornea and of the lens, with its consequent confusion of sight, may be diminished. For [Fig. 126.] the same reason, the iridectomy should not be large, otherwise its base will expose a considerable portion of the edge of the lens. Hence the incision should be made with a narrow iridectomy knife, or even with a broad needle. [Fig. 126.] If a very small incision is made, the iris may be drawn out with a blunt silver or platinum iris hook, instead of the forceps, just as in the operation of iridodesis. This mode of operating is also indicated in those cases in which there are extensive adhesions between the edge of the pupil and the anterior capsule. In such cases, the incision should, if possible, be made at a spot corresponding to a point at which the edge of the pupil is not adherent, so that the hook may seize this portion of the iris. If the whole edge of the pupil is adherent, and the iris is thin and rotten, it is often impossible to obtain a good-sized pupil, for the iris breaks down, and tears between the forceps, and only small portions can be removed piece-meal. Or again, the adhesions of the pupil to the capsule may be so firm, that they resist the traction of the forceps, and this portion of the iris remains standing. In fact we have performed the operation, which Desmarres has recommended in such cases, and has termed "iridorhexis." A portion of the iris is excised, leaving the adherent pupillary edge standing. In order to overcome this difficulty in seizing the iris, Liebreich[1] has devised a pair of iridectomy forceps, in which the teeth are so situated that the surface in which they grasp is turned at a right angle; in this way they can firmly seize the iris, just as a pair of fixation forceps.

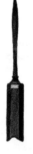

[1] "Knapp and Moos' Archives," i. 1, 22.

[It is sometimes necessary to make an artificial pupil in cases of adhesion of the pupillary margin of the iris to the cornea, and here the anterior chamber is usually so shallow that the incision is best made with a narrow cataract-knife, as there is thus less danger of lacerating the iris.—B.]

(2) Iridodesis.

This valuable and ingenious operation was devised by Mr. Critchett,[1] and is very useful in all cases in which we desire to obtain an artificial pupil for optical purposes only, as, for instance, in cases of opacity or conicity of the cornea, or of lamellar cataract, etc.

The operation is to be performed in the following manner: The patient having been placed under the influence of an anæsthetic, and the eyelids kept apart with the stop-speculum, the operator fixes the eyeball with a pair of forceps, and makes an incision with a broad needle in the sclero-corneal junction, slightly encroaching upon the cornea. If the incision is made inwards (which is the best direction) and the nose is prominent, Mr. Critchett employs a broad needle bent at an angle on the flat. With regard to the size of the incision, it is of importance to remember, that whilst, on the one hand, it should be sufficiently large to admit of the easy introduction of the hook or forceps, it must not, on the other, be too wide, otherwise the strangulated portion of the iris, with the ligature, may be drawn into the anterior chamber when the aqueous humor reaccumulates. The incision having been completed, and the broad needle removed, a small loop [A, Fig. 127] of very

[Fig. 127.]

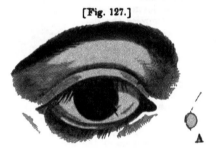

A

fine black silk is to be placed directly over the wound. A blunt platinum or silver hook (bent at the requisite angle) is then to be introduced through the loop into the anterior chamber to the proximate edge of the pupil, which is to be caught up by it, and then the portion of iris thus secured is to be carefully and gently drawn forth into the loop. If it is desired to stretch the opposite portion of the iris, so as to bring it opposite an opacity in the cornea or lens, and thus to displace the pupil considerably to the side of the incision, the operator must be extremely careful that, whilst drawing forth the iris, he does not cause a separation of the opposite border from its ciliary attachment (coredialysis), which may be easily done if the iris be put too much upon the stretch, or drawn forth somewhat roughly. As soon as a sufficient portion of iris lies within the loop, an assistant, with a pair of broad cilia forceps [Fig. 128] in each hand, seizes the two free ends and ties them tightly, so as to include the prolapsed iris firmly within the loop.

[1] "R. L. O. H. Rep.," i. 220.

In tightening the ligature, he should not draw the ends of the loop away from the eye, but should follow the curvature of the sclerotic. The ends of the ligature are then to be cut off, the one being left somewhat longer than the other, in order that it may be readily seized with the forceps, if the loop should show a tendency to be drawn into the anterior chamber. The little strangulated portion of iris quickly shrinks, and the loop may be removed on the second or third day. But instead of the hook, the canula forceps

[Fig. 128.]

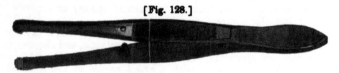

[Fig. 130] may be employed, the iris being seized by them, about midway between the edge of the pupil and its ciliary attachment. The hook is, however, to be preferred.

I have above described the operation which is to be performed when the artificial pupil is to extend to the periphery. But if we desire simply to displace and enlarge the original pupil from its central position towards one side, preserving at the same time the constrictor pupillæ intact, the peripheral portion of the iris must be seized with the canula forceps, and drawn forth through the loop until the pupil occupies the desired position [Fig. 129], when the ligature is to be tightened.

[Fig. 129.]   [Fig. 130.]

It may occasionally occur that, although the sight is considerably improved by the iridodesis, the patient greatly feels the want of more light, and a stronger illumination of the retinal image. In such cases, Mr. Critchett has succeeded admirably by making a second iridodesis in the same eye, in such a manner as to enlarge the pupil and alter its shape, giving it a somewhat crescentic form, with the two corners of the crescent cut off.

The operation of iridodesis is, as a rule, quite free from danger, and productive of but very little irritation. In very rare instances it may, however, give rise to iritis, or even suppurative irido-cyclitis. Such cases have been recorded by Alfred von Graefe,[1] Steffan,[2] etc., but although I have a large experience of the operation, both in the hands of others and in my own, I have never met with a single case in which it caused inflammatory complications. In order to avoid the risk of irritation, and also to simplify the operation, De Wecker has suggested that the prolapse of the iris, instead of being tied, should be allowed to heal in the wound. He makes the incision rather further in the sclerotic, so as to obtain a long track; he then seizes the iris with a very fine pair of iridectomy forceps, and draws it out into the incision. To maintain it in this position, and to accelerate the healing of the wound, a firm compress bandage is applied. The prolapse becomes firmly adherent in the track of the wound, and the little protruding portion soon drops off. This operation is termed "Iridencleisis."

[1] "A. f. O.," ix. 8, 199.   [2] Ibid., x. 1, 128.

[These two operations, iridodesis and iridencleisis, have been almost entirely discarded. Not only have purulent iritis and irido-cyelitis been observed to proceed from the cicatrix, but even sympathetic irido-cyelitis of the other eye has been observed on account of the extreme peripheral nature of the wound in iridencleisis. This danger is less in the operation of iridodesis. (See Arlt in Graefe und Saemisch's "Hdbch. der Augenheilkunde," iii. p. 424.)—B.]

[(8) IRIDOTOMY.

The operation of division of the sphincter through a corneal incision was proposed by De Wecker as a substitute for iridodesis and iridencleisis. He recommends it especially in small central opacities of the cornea or lens. He makes an incision in the cornea, midway between limbus and centre, about four millimetres long. He then introduces a small pair of forceps-scissors through the wound as far as the pupillary margin of the iris, passes one blade of the scissors behind the iris, so as to include the sphincter between the blades, and divides it rapidly. If the iris prolapses into the corneal wound, it must be replaced by a spatula, and atropine at once instilled. This operation has also fallen into disuse in the United States.

The term iridotomy, as now used, includes any incision into the iris, not only in the sphincter, but elsewhere. Mr. Carter cuts out a V-shaped bit of iris by means of De Wecker's iridotomy scissors. This gives an excellent pupil in those cases where the lens has been either extracted or where it disappeared in the course of an atrophic inflammation, and the iris has been changed into a dense membrane, stretching all across the anterior chamber.—B.]

[Fig. 131.   Fig. 132.]

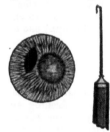

We sometimes find, after a perforating wound or ulcer of the cornea, or the common flap operation for cataract with extensive prolapse, that the iris presents a plane surface tightly stretched from the cicatrix to the periphery of the cornea, and that there is no trace of a pupil. If the lens is absent, a very fair artificial pupil may often be obtained in these cases by simply splitting the fibres of the iris across with a broad needle. The edges of the incision will generally retract, and a very good-sized pupil be left [Fig. 131]; if this is not the case, a Tyrrel's hook [Fig. 132] may be passed through the corneal incision, and one edge of the incised portion of the iris be caught, drawn forth, and excised.

(4) CORELYSIS.

The detachment of adhesions between the edge of the pupil and the anterior capsule of the lens by operative interference, was first extensively practised by Mr. Streatfeild[1] and subsequently also by Weber.[2] The patient having been anæsthetized, and the lids fixed with the stop-speculum, an incision is to be made in the cornea with a broad needle, of sufficient size readily to admit the spatula-hook into the anterior chamber. Prior to the operation, a strong solution of atropine should be applied to the eye, so that any unadherent portions of the pupil may become dilated. The exact posi-

---

[1] "R. L. O. H. Rep.," i. 6, and 2, 309.   [2] "A. f. O.," vii. 1, and viii. 1, 854.

several adhesions and one broad unattached portion of the pupil, the incision should be made opposite the latter. Mr. Streatfeild recommends that the broad needle should be rapidly withdrawn from the anterior chamber, so as to allow as little of the aqueous humor to escape as possible; whereas Weber prefers to withdraw the instrument very slowly, so as to permit the gradual escape of the aqueous humor, in order that the crystalline lens may come in contact with the cornea, and thus be steadied; the spatula will glide over the former, and there is less chance of injuring the capsule.

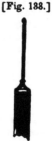

[Fig. 133.]

The incision having been finished, a small spatula-hook [Fig. 133] is introduced into the anterior chamber, and, with a somewhat lateral "wriggling" movement, the instrument is passed slightly beneath the iris, at a point free of adhesions, and is then passed behind the nearest adhesion, and drawn gently and slowly toward the operator; so that it breaks down the band before it, care being taken to keep it quite parallel with the iris, lest the capsule of the lens should be injured. The adhesion may yield at once before the pressure of the spatula, but if it resists, it may be caught in the hook, and thus torn through.

Dr. Passavant[1] does not use the hook in performing corelysis, but after having made the opening in the cornea with the broad needle, seizes the iris with a pair of iridectomy forceps, and, gently drawing it somewhat towards the incision, thus detaches the adhesion. Where several posterior synechiæ exist, he repeats the operation after a day or two. He has thus operated with success on more than fifty cases.

[Neither of these methods has met with much favor at the hands of ophthalmic surgeons. Dr. B. Joy Jeffries, of Boston, has practised Passavant's operation somewhat extensively, and reports favorably upon it. A small iridectomy is on the whole a better operation for these cases. In performing corelysis, Mr. Carter's cutting hook is probably better than the blunt one of Mr. Streatfeild.—B.]

(5) Iridodialysis.

If nearly the whole cornea is opaque, and there is only a narrow transparent rim left, it may be advisable to adopt this mode of forming an artificial pupil, for if the incision is made, as in iridectomy, in the sclero-corneal junction, it is sometimes followed by some opacity of the cornea close to the incision, and this would prove very disadvantageous where the rim of clear cornea is but very narrow. An incision is made in the cornea with a broad needle, at a sufficient distance from the point where the iris is to be removed from its ciliary attachment for the forceps or hook to be easily managed. A fine pair of iridectomy (or canula) forceps is passed into the anterior chamber, a fold of iris seized, gently torn from its insertion, and a portion drawn forth through the incision and snipped off. Thus a marginal pupil can be made opposite the transparent edge of the cornea. Should the vicinity of the incision become a little clouded, this will be at some distance from the new pupil.

I must now briefly enumerate the different diseases in which an iridectomy is indicated. These may be divided into two groups, viz., those affections in which the operation is performed for the purpose of diminishing inflammatory symptoms and an increase in the eye-tension, and those in which the object is simply to make an artificial pupil.

In the first group it is indicated—1. In ulcers of the cornea which threaten extensive perforation, or cases of suppurative keratitis. The iridectomy diminishes the intra-ocular tension, and thus affords a favorable opportunity for the process of reparation, and also improves the nutrition of the parts. 2. If the cornea, after perforation, shows a tendency to become prominent and staphylomatous at this point, and more especially if there is any increase in the intra-ocular tension. 3. In obstinate fistula of the cornea, and in prolapse of the iris. 4. In recurrent or chronic iritis and irido-choroiditis, particularly if the communication between the anterior and posterior chambers is interrupted by circular synechia. Also in cases in which a foreign body has become lodged in the iris, or a tumor or cyst exists in the latter. 5. In traumatic cataract accompanied by much swelling of the lens-substance, great irritation of the eye, and augmented tension. Also in various operations for cataract, the object being partly to prevent bruising of the iris during the extraction of the lens, and partly to diminish the tendency to subsequent inflammatory complications. 6. In the extensive group of glaucomatous diseases, in which there is increase of the intra-ocular tension, leading finally to excavation of the optic nerve and blindness. The importance of an early operation in such cases cannot be over-estimated.

In the *second class* of cases, in which the object of the iridectomy is simply to afford an artificial pupil, it is indicated in the following affections: 1. In opacities of the cornea, also in conical cornea. In the latter case, the object of the operation is, however, strictly speaking, twofold, viz., to diminish the intra-ocular tension, and also to make a pupil opposite a portion of the cornea whose curvature is but slightly, if at all, altered. 2. In occlusion of the pupil after iritis. 3. In lamellar cataract, and in dislocation of the lens.

[In iridectomy for artificial pupil, the coloboma should be small, so as to avoid dazzling the eye, and diminish the resulting circles of dispersion on the retina. Small pupils have the advantage of stenopæic glasses, without their disadvantages. If in corneal opacities, the iris is found to be adherent completely to the posterior surface of the cornea, the formation of an artificial pupil is impossible.

In anterior central capsular cataract, and in the secondary membrani-form cataract after extraction or irido-choroiditis, an iridectomy is often very useful in improving the vision.—B.]

9.—CHANGES IN THE FORM AND CONTENTS OF THE ANTERIOR CHAMBER.

The size of the anterior chamber may undergo considerable alteration. Thus, if the intra-ocular tension be much augmented, or the iris is bulged forward by a collection of fluid, or by exudation-masses between the posterior surface of the iris and the capsule of the lens, the anterior chamber may be extremely shallow, the iris being perhaps almost in contact with the posterior surface of the cornea. Whereas, when the anterior portion of the eyeball is distended and enlarged (hydrophthalmos), or when the crystalline lens is absent or displaced, the anterior chamber increases in depth. The size of the latter also varies according to the age, and the state of refraction. It diminishes with advancing years, and is deeper in myopic and more shallow in hypermetropic persons.

Effusions of lymph and pus may take place into the anterior chamber, and sink down to the bottom in the form of hypopyon, which may attain a considerable size, and even fill the whole of the anterior chamber. The lymph or pus may be effused either from the cornea, the iris, or the ciliary body, as has been described at length in the articles upon the diseases of these parts.

Blood may also be effused into the anterior chamber, this condition being termed "hyperæmia." The hemorrhage may be either spontaneous or traumatic in its origin. In the latter case, it may be due to a wound of the cornea, iris, ciliary body, etc., or it may be produced by a simple blow or fall upon the eye (as from a cricket or racket ball, a "cat," or a blow from the fist), without any rupture of the external coats of the eye. The anterior chamber is filled with blood, and when this has become partially absorbed, we find perhaps that the lens has been dislocated, and that there is also hemorrhage into the vitreous humor. Spontaneous hyperæmia is of rare occurrence. It has been known to occur periodically during the time of menstruation, perhaps vicariously, or after the catamenia have ceased. Cases have been recorded in which the patient could voluntarily produce an effusion of blood into the anterior chamber by stooping or rapidly shaking his head.[1] The best treatment is the application of a firm compress bandage to the eye, for this accelerates the absorption of the blood more than any other remedy. If there is much irritability of the eye or any iritis, atropine drops should be frequently applied.

Foreign bodies, such as portions of metal, gun-cap, splinters of glass, eyelashes, etc., may penetrate the cornea and become lodged in the anterior chamber, lying either free in it, or being perhaps partly adherent to the cornea or the iris, and partly situated in the anterior chamber. Their presence in the latter frequently sets up severe iritis or irido-choroiditis. But in other cases, after the immediate effects of the injury have passed away, the foreign body may remain for many years innocuous in the anterior chamber, without either provoking any serious injury to the affected eye, or symptoms of sympathetic disease in the other. Thus Saemisch[2] records a case in which a fragment of stone remained twelve years in the anterior chamber without exciting any serious injury. The foreign body had originally become lodged in the lens, the latter became absorbed, and then the fragment of stone fell into the anterior chamber, remaining attached to the secondary cataract by a fine filament. As it had set up some irritation a fortnight before the patient consulted Saemisch, the latter extracted it successfully by a large linear incision in the cornea combined with an iridectomy. De Wecker[3] extracted, with success, a fragment of stone which had remained fourteen years in the anterior chamber, without causing any irritation.

In removing these foreign bodies from the anterior chamber, care must be taken that the incision in the cornea is of a sufficient size, and so situated

[1] For cases of this kind, *vide* "A. f. O.," vii. 1, 65; Walther, "System der Chirurgie," 1848; also Mooren, op. cit.
[2] "Klin. Monatsblätter," 1865, 46.   [3] "Klin. Monatsbl.," 1867, 36.

that the foreign body can be easily reached; a large iridectomy should then be made, and the foreign body seized with the iridectomy forceps, or an iris hook, and extracted. If the foreign body (e. g., a splinter of steel) is partly in the cornea and partly in the anterior chamber, the blade of the iridectomy knife or of the broad needle should be passed behind it, so as to steady it and push it forward through the cornea, when its anterior extremity should be seized with a pair of forceps, and then it can be readily extracted.

[Foreign bodies, not prone to decomposition, may remain encapsulated for a long time in the anterior chamber without causing any irritation. The encapsulating wall may consist merely of connective tissue, or it may be lined by epithelium, and should be carefully distinguished from an iris-cyst. Living organisms, as epidermis, hairs, etc., introduced through injury into the anterior chamber, may lead to the formation of epidermoid tumors. Splinters of metal or of wood, which so frequently penetrate into the anterior chamber, very often in so doing wound the iris or the lens, or both, and thus the accident becomes complicated. These should not be allowed to remain. If their presence is suspected, but they cannot be seen owing to extravasated blood or pus, means should be taken to promote absorption of the latter, and when the foreign body becomes visible, the anterior chamber should be opened below, and the particle seized with forceps and withdrawn.

The presence of a foreign body on or in the iris is not a common occurrence. It produces great and constant irritation, leading often to violent inflammation, and this of a purulent character. Its encapsulation here cannot be thought of, and its removal should be attempted at once. The incision may be made with a lance-knife, or, better, with a narrow cataract-knife, upwards or downwards in the sclero-corneal margin, as the case may best indicate. If the particle is not firmly embedded in the iris tissue, it is better to grasp it with a pair of grooved forceps, or attempt to lift it out of its bed by introducing a Daviel's spoon underneath it; if this succeeds, then remove the lacerated portion of iris by an iridectomy. If the particle is firmly embedded, remove a broad piece of iris containing it at once, and thus cut short the operation. Great care should be taken to prevent the foreign body dropping into the posterior chamber, where it would occasion serious trouble, and from which it would be difficult to remove it.

If the foreign body has penetrated the iris and lens, the latter will become more or less completely opaque, and if the particle is small it will be concealed from view. If the iris has been wounded, an iridectomy should be done at once, and the lacerated portion of iris removed. If the foreign particle can then be seen in the lens, or if there is reason to think that it is there, as complete an extraction as possible should be made of the injured lens, and for this reason it is better that the original incision should be made with a narrow knife, so as to insure a sufficiently large wound. It is sometimes possible, after the iridectomy, to remove a foreign body from the lens by means of a curette or spoon, and then extract the lens afterwards. Cases have been known in which small particles have become encapsulated in the lens, and surrounded by a circumscribed opacity, while the rest of the lens has remained transparent. The danger here is that the particle may subsequently sink through the lens, perforate the posterior capsule, and fall either into the vitreous or upon the ciliary processes, where it is sure to excite destructive inflammation.

In rare cases, where the foreign body is of iron or steel, and lying in the anterior chamber or on the iris, it may be extracted by employing a powerful magnet. Cases have been reported in which the poles of the magnet have been introduced into the anterior chamber, and the particle successfully removed. ("Trans. N. Y. State Medical Society," 1880; "Archives of Ophthalmology," vol. ix.)—B.]

Cysticerci are sometimes met with in the anterior chamber, and about twenty cases of this kind have been recorded by different authors. The diagnosis is not difficult, for the little animal is noticed in the form of a small transparent vesicle, generally lying upon the surface of the iris. The vesicle shows at times very decided movements, more especially when the pupil is stimulated to active contraction by the action of strong light, the head and neck of the animal being then perhaps stretched out and moved about. The cysticercus may either lie free in the anterior chamber, or be partly adherent to the iris or cornea. The following case of Mr. Pridgin Teale's,[1] illustrates admirably the symptoms presented by the presence of a cysticercus, and the mode of treatment to be adopted: "Mary Isabel Bateman, æt. 10, living at Anerley, was brought to me on June 2, in consequence of tenderness of the right eye. On examining the eye there was seen (vide Fig. 134) on the surface of the lower part of the iris, an opaque body, constricted in the middle, and rather longer than a hemp-seed, which was evidently causing some distress to the eye. The conjunctiva was slightly injected, the cornea was bright, but dotted on its posterior surface with minute spots, as in kerato-iritis; the iris was active, except at the situation of the white body, near which it was adherent to the capsule of the lens. Tension normal. Reading No. 16 Jäger." The mother stated that for two or three years the eye had been occasionally inflamed. Six weeks

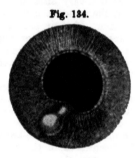

Fig. 134.

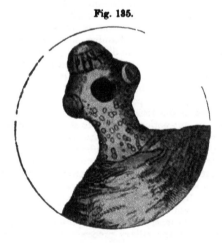

Fig. 135.

ago she first noticed a speck on the iris, about the size of a pin's head, which became doubled in size at the end of five weeks. The child had always been delicate, and had long suffered from threadworms, but never from tape-

[1] "R. L. O. H. Rep.," v. 320.

worm. On June 9, Mr. Teale made an incision at the margin of the cornea with a cataract-knife, and withdrew the piece of iris on which the animal was fixed, and cut it off without destroying the cysticercus. When removed from the eye, the slow movements of the body and changes of shape were easily detected. On examination with the microscope, the head and neck, surmounted by the circle of hooklets and four suckers, were seen to project from the side of the body (vide Fig. 135).

The removal of the cysticercus was soon followed by the disappearance of all symptoms of inflammation and irritability of the eye, and four months afterwards the patient was able to read Jäger No. 1.

[In England and the United States, cysticercus in the eye is exceedingly rare, but on the continent, and especially in Germany, these cases are not very uncommon. The passage of the larva of a tænia into the bloodvessels of the eye through the medium of the blood-current, is easily understood. All parts of the uveal tract may thus prove a resting-place for the cysticercus. If the worm is in the anterior chamber, and not adherent to the iris, it is better to make the incision through the cornea, three or four millimetres from the margin, so as to avoid prolapse of the iris. If it is attached to the iris, an iridectomy must always be done.

A worm known by the name of Filaria medinensis is known to be a not uncommon animal parasite in the eye of the horse, and cases of its occurrence in the anterior chamber of man have been reported by Barkan, Kipp, and others in the United States, and by Argyll Robertson. (See "Trans. Fifth Internat. Ophthal. Congress," New York, 1876.)—B.]

10.—IRIDO-CHOROIDITIS. [IRIDO-CYCLITIS.—B.]

I have already pointed out, when speaking of iritis, that on account of the close relationship between the iris, ciliary body, and the choroid (which in truth form one continuous tissue, the uveal tract), any inflammation commencing in the iris is very prone to extend to the ciliary body and choroid, or vice versâ. The most frequent cause of such an extension of the inflammation of the iris to the choroid is to be sought in the presence of considerable posterior synechiæ, or still more in complete exclusion [seclusion—B.] of the pupil.[1] In such cases, the recurrence of the inflammation and its extension to the ciliary body and choroid are partly due to the constant irritation and teasing kept up by the adhesions at the edge of the pupil, preventing the normal dilatation and contraction of the pupil, which take place in accordance with any alteration in the degree of illumination, the movements of the eye, and the changes in the accommodation. But it is still more caused by the interruption in the communication between the anterior and posterior chamber (in cases of exclusion of the pupil), which prevents that regulation and just balance of the intra-ocular tension in front of and behind the iris, which always exists in the healthy eye. Thus, if there is any increase in the vitreous humor, the anterior chamber becomes narrower, and contains less aqueous humor; if, on the other hand, the quantity of the aqueous humor is increased, the iris is somewhat cupped backwards, and the

---

[1] I must remind the reader that by this term "exclusion of the pupil" is meant, that the adhesion between the edge of the pupil and the capsule of the lens extends completely round the circumference of the pupil, and thus shuts off the communication between the anterior and posterior chamber. The area of the pupil may, in such a case, be perfectly clear and unoccupied by lymph. If this is not the case, but it is filled with a deposit or plug of lymph, it is termed "occlusion" of the pupil, and this involves also exclusion.

laid in the posterior chamber diminished in quantity. In this way, changes in the amount of the fluids in different parts of the eye are prevented from exercising any deleterious influence, if their augmentation does not exceed a certain degree. For on account of the regulation between the anterior, and posterior chamber no harm accrues. But it is quite different when this communication is stopped, and the iris forms, so to say, a firm barrier between the anterior and posterior chamber. For, if there is any increase of tension in the posterior portion of the eye, it cannot then be relieved at the expense of fluid in the anterior chamber, consequently a stasis occurs in the circulation of the inner tunics of the eyeball, which is soon followed by inflammatory complications of a serious nature.

[It is highly probable that the endothelial membrane lying upon and in between the ciliary process, lately described by Kuhnt, plays an important part in the changes in the amount of fluid in different parts of the eye in health and disease, especially in connection with changes in the vicinity of Fontana's space. (See "Bericht der Ophthal. Gesellsch.," 1879, Heidelberg).

As in iritis, so in irido-choroiditis, the inflammation may be either *plastic*, *serous*, or *parenchymatous;* and the latter may be suppurative, or the tissues may be the seat of diffuse gummy infiltration. Etiologically, the disease may be either secondary to an inflammation in the iris, which is by far the more common; or it may be primary or spontaneous; or, finally, it may be sympathetic from injury to the fellow eye; the latter will be considered in a separate section.

Plastic irido-choroiditis, which may be either primary or secondary, in addition to the ordinary signs of plastic iritis, is accompanied by extreme tenderness in the ciliary region, turbidity of the vitreous humor with floating flocculi, and a more or less marked recession of the iris.

The serous form of inflammation is much more insidious and slow, the symptoms of irritation being much less marked. The pupils may be moderately wide and sluggish, but the vitreous from the beginning, especially near the lens, is filled with flocculi and generally turbid. The intra-ocular tension is almost always increased, and the corneal surface is apt to assume an appearance like ground glass. The deposit on the posterior surface of the cornea becomes much thicker, and may be so extensive as to reach continuously from cornea to anterior surface of the iris, and occasionally this deposit is seen upon the capsule. The vitreous opacities may become like long threads, or even membraniform. With all these changes, the circumcorneal injection may be very slight. A mixed form of serous and plastic inflammation is much more frequently met with than a purely serous form. This form of inflammation is generally chronic, and, when well marked, gives all the characteristic signs of chronic inflammatory glaucoma.

Purulent irido-choroiditis, though usually of traumatic origin, may occur primarily as the result of a thrombotic process in the vascular distribution of the eyeball or choroid; or, better, as a metastatic process; or, still more rarely, as a not uncommon complication of cerebro-spinal meningitis. In this form of inflammation, the process usually starts in the choroid and spreads to the ciliary body and iris secondarily. The anterior chamber may be in a short time filled with pus from the inflamed ciliary body, which may entirely disappear in the course of a few hours. The tension of the eye is usually diminished. The process is very apt to end in a panophthalmitis.

Irido-choroiditis gummosa or *syphilitica* is a rather rare disease. Though in all probability beginning in the iris and subsequently extending to the ciliary body and possibly to the choroid, yet there are cases on record in which the gummy nodules occurred in the ciliary body, coalesced, and gave rise to a diffuse infiltration of both iris and choroid. The progress is usually very rapid and the symptoms very violent, and, in spite of treatment, is very apt to end in destruction of the eye; though, if rupture of the sclera can be prevented, the result may be more favorable. (For recent observations, see, 1, "Trans. Amer. Ophthal. Soc.," 1874, and, 2, "Graefe und Saemisch's Hdb. der Augenheilk.," Bd. iv. p. 516. Also "Archives of Ophthalmology," ix. 4.)—B.]

In practice, we can distinguish two principal forms of irido-choroiditis, presenting certain characteristic differences, which it is of consequence to observe, not only with regard to the prognosis, but also with regard to the line of operative treatment which is required in each.

In the *first* form the disease commences with iritis, and if the pupil is not kept widely dilated with atropine, posterior synechiæ soon form and rapidly lead to exclusion of the pupil from circular synechia. The pupil may remain clear excepting just at its edge, where it shows a well-marked border of pigmented exudation. Gradually we notice that small, knob-like bulgings show themselves in the iris, which may remain chiefly confined to one portion, or extend more or less to the whole of it, so that the iris is bulged forward into numerous prominences, like sails before the wind. This bulging is not due to any firm exudation on the posterior surface of the iris, but to a serous effusion behind it; and the partial bulging is due to the fact that some portions of the iris resist the pressure of the fluid more than others. The appearance presented by such cases is very peculiar and characteristic.

On account of the firm adhesion of the whole circumference of the pupil to the capsule, the iris cannot at this point yield to the pressure of the fluid behind it, but bulges out between the pupil and its ciliary adhesion into more or less numerous, knob-like protuberances, which are sometimes so considerable in size as to come in contact here and there with the posterior surface of the cornea. The bulge slopes gradually down towards the circumference of the cornea, but passes steeply down to the pupil, which lies in a crater-like depression.

The iris is mostly very much discolored, and of a gray, ash-like, or greenish tint. On closer examination, more especially with the oblique illumination, it will be seen that its fibrillæ are somewhat opened up and stretched apart, and that it is traversed by a few dilated tortuous veins.

The tension of the eye is generally at first normal, but may then become considerably increased; finally, however, it diminishes more and more as the eye becomes atrophied. If the pupil is clear, the sight may at the outset be good, but when the bulging of the iris occurs, it rapidly deteriorates. If the refractive media and the pupil are sufficiently clear to permit of an ophthalmoscopic examination, the vitreous humor is often seen to be diffusely clouded, with delicate, floating, or fixed opacities suspended in it, proving that the disease is no longer confined to the iris, but has extended to the ciliary body and choroid. If an iridectomy is made in such a case, we notice that when the knife is withdrawn, some aqueous humor escapes from the anterior chamber; but that the latter is not emptied completely, in consequence of the intra-ocular pressure not being able to affect the anterior chamber on account of the exclusion of the pupil. A sufficiently large piece of iris can generally be seized with the forceps and excised, a copious stream of watery yellow fluid simultaneously escaping from behind it. The iris now at once recedes to its normal plane, even although, as Von Graefe points out, the bulging part itself has not been excised, but only a neighboring portion of iris. The artificial pupil thus obtained may be almost entirely clear, excepting just at the edge of the pupil; or, as frequently occurs, a more or less considerable portion of the uvea is found to be left behind in it; the uvea having been separated from the iris proper by the fluid, and become attached to the capsule of the lens.

The second form of irido-choroiditis presents very different appearances. The iris, instead of being arched forward in little knob-like projections, is perfectly straight and even on its surface, although it is pressed forward towards the cornea, producing great shallowness of the anterior chamber, but the pupil is not drawn back. There is complete exclusion of the pupil, and its area is generally occupied by a more or less dense false membrane, or by a thick plug of lymph [seclusion and occlusion.—B.]. The tissue of the iris looks stretched, its fibrillæ are indistinct, its surface discolored, and of a dirty reddish tint, which is partly due to the cloudiness of the aqueous humor, but chiefly to the numerous large tortuous bloodvessels which traverse its surface; there being a considerable stasis in the venous circulation and mechanical hyperæmia, on account of the inflammatory affection of the ciliary body and choroid. The pressing forward of the iris is not due to a collection of fluid behind it, but to the pushing forward of the lens (with the capsule of which the iris is intimately connected by means of extensive, thick masses of exudation), which yields to the intra-ocular pressure. The false membrane behind the iris is generally very considerable, consisting of a thick, organized, felt-like mass of exudation, which adheres closely to the capsule of the lens, and perhaps fills up a great portion of the posterior chamber. The intra-capsular cells generally proliferate, and become clouded, but the lens itself often remains transparent.

In these cases a simple iridectomy is of no avail, for even if we can remove a portion of the iris (which is often very difficult), the opening thus made is again rapidly closed by exudation, for the operation excites a fresh attack of inflammation, and finally such eyes will undergo gradual destruction from atrophy, if they are not operated upon in the manner described below.

I must state that the distinctive characters of these two forms of irido-choroiditis are not always so strongly marked, for we often meet with mixed forms; or, again, the second may supervene upon the first, forming, so to say, a more advanced and hopeless stage.

It has been stated above, that irido-choroiditis may ensue upon an inflammation which primarily affected the iris and then extended to the ciliary body and choroid; or that it may begin in the latter, and only subsequently attack the iris. It is sometimes difficult, at a late stage of the disease, to ascertain with anything like certainty, which course the disease had originally pursued. The following facts, will, however, afford us some guidance. When the disease originated in the iris, we find that there were well-marked symptoms of recurrent inflammation, and that the structure of the iris is considerably changed, being much discolored, thinned, and atrophied. The lens also becomes less frequently opaque, and only at a much later period. The dimness of sight is likewise less considerable, and depends at first chiefly upon the deposit of lymph in the pupil, and only subsequently upon the cloudiness of the lens or vitreous humor. Whereas, if the inflammation commenced in the choroid, the train of symptoms is different. There are marked symptoms of [plastic] choroiditis, with opacity of the vitreous humor, followed very generally by detachment of the retina, from a serous or hemorrhagic effusion. The tension of the eyeball diminishes. Then an opacity of the lens supervenes, very frequently commencing at its posterior pole, and gradually extending thence to the whole lens-substance. At a later stage,

21

the lens undergoes further degenerative changes, becoming chalky, and transformed into a "cataracta secreta." The iris may not be affected until a late period of the disease, and not until some time after the formation of cataract, or it may become inflamed at an earlier stage; but the iritis is generally insidious, and not accompanied by any marked inflammatory symptoms. The pupil becomes adherent, lymph is effused in its area and on the posterior surface of the iris, which may become bulged forward by fluid, or pressed forward by dense masses of exudation. Two very important guides by which to distinguish between this form of irido-choroiditis and that commencing with an inflammation in the iris, are the degree of sight and the state of the field of vision. The perception of light will be far less in the former case, and there will be a marked contraction or absence of that part of the field (the upper) which corresponds to the detached portion of the retina. Thus, if the light from the lamp is distinguished when it is held in the lower half of the field, but becomes invisible when it is removed into the upper half, it indicates a detachment of the lower portion of the retina.

The sight is generally very much impaired in cases of irido-choroiditis, so that the patient can only perhaps distinguish large letters, count fingers, or has only simple perception of light. In irido-choroiditis uncomplicated by detachment of the retina, or glaucomatous or atrophic changes in the retina and optic nerve, the quantitative field of vision should be good.

The *prognosis* is, of course, very variable, according to the stage and form of the disease. If a case of irido-choroiditis (uncomplicated with extensive lesions of the choroid, detachment of the retina, or opacity of the lens) be seen at the outset, whilst the changes in the iris are still but slight, the area of the pupil clear, or only occupied by a film of exudation, and there are no masses of exudation-membranes behind the iris, the prognosis may be favorable if the sight be still tolerably good, and the field of vision normal.

The first form of irido-choroiditis, in which the iris is bulged forwards by fluid, affords a much better prognosis than the second. The most hopeless of all are, of course, the cases of irido-choroiditis with detachment of the retina. In such a case, or if there is no perception of light left, no operation should be attempted excepting for the sake of relieving pain, or diminishing the risk of sympathetic ophthalmia. A certain degree of atrophy of the eye (if it be not too far advanced, and the perception of light and field of vision are good) does not contra-indicate an operation, for we find that the iridectomy often arrests the atrophy, and that the eye regains its plumpness, and a normal degree of tension. [Plastic and parenchymatous irido-choroiditis greatly endanger the eye at all times, and the formation of a wide pupil by no means brings the process to a standstill or prevents relapses. The serous form of inflammation admits of a more favorable prognosis. The most destructive of all is the purulent, for it almost always attacks the choroid throughout, and leads to panophthalmitis. The non-traumatic purulent form of inflammation is perhaps less destructive, though even here not much hope can be entertained of any useful vision.—B.]

The most frequent *cause* of irido-choroiditis is the presence of posterior synechiæ, above all, the circular form. The presence of adhesions between the edge of the pupil and the capsule of the lens leads to frequent recurrences of the iritis, more lymph is effused, more synechiæ formed, until finally the pupil is excluded, and then, if this has not already occurred, future inflammations are sure to extend from the iris to the ciliary body and the choroid. The best safeguard against a recurrence of the iritis and the supervention of irido-choroiditis, is to cure a case of iritis without the formation of any posterior synechiæ. Of course, such eyes do not enjoy a perfect immunity from a recurrence of iritis if a sufficient exciting cause should arise, but they are far less prone to it than if adhesions have remained behind. Irido-choroiditis may also be caused by injuries and wounds of the eye, by the lodgement of foreign bodies (more especially splinters of metal, gun-caps, or glass) within the eye, and by operations, particularly those for cataract. It may likewise arise in consequence of an injury to the other eye, thus constituting "sympathetic ophthalmia.".

If the adhesions between the iris and capsule of the lens are not considerable, and are thin and "tongued," it may be possible to tear them through by the prolonged use of a strong solution of atropine, or to separate them by operative interference (corelysis). But if they are firm and broad, and especially if they extend all around the edge of the pupil, and thus cut off the communication between the anterior and posterior chamber, we must have recourse to iridectomy; for no other means will suffice to guard the eye against the dangers of irido-choroiditis, or to stay the progress of this disease if it is already present.

In the early stage, when the adhesions are not very extensive and firm, and the tissue of the iris has not yet undergone atrophic changes, it is generally not difficult to obtain a tolerably good artificial pupil, by means of an iridectomy. Frequently, however, a small rim of iris, at the edge of the pupil, is so firmly attached to the capsule as not to yield to the traction of the forceps, but is left standing. This does not invalidate the result, if a tolerable sized piece of iris is removed, and a clear artificial pupil and a free communication between the two chambers are established. If the pupil is only adherent at certain points, it will be best to employ a fine blunt hook, instead of the iris forceps, for catching up the iris. The hook is to be passed carefully along to the edge of the pupil (the portion where there are no synechiae), gently turned over the margin, and the iris then drawn out and snipped off. In this way, we may often succeed in excising a considerable segment of the iris, whereas from the rottenness of its structure and the firmness of the adhesions, it would probably have resisted the grasp of the forceps, and only small shreds have been removed. Care must be taken never to employ too much force in the removal of the iris, otherwise a dialysis may be easily produced at the opposite circumference of the iris.

We generally find that after the operation, the inflammatory symptoms quickly subside, that the sight improves, and that the recurrence of inflammation is arrested. In some cases, however, this is not the case. Exposure to cold, bright light, continued use of the eyes, easily reproduce an inflammation. If these recurrences are frequent and obstinate, much benefit is often derived from a second iridectomy, made in an opposite direction, so that the two halves of the iris are completely cut off from each other. This operation has been practised with much success by Von Graefe and Critchett (independently of each other), and I have often found much benefit from its performance in cases of obstinate recurrent iritis. The line of the double iridectomy may be either horizontal or vertical. The advantage of the latter is, that a more or less considerable portion of the upper part of the artificial pupil is covered by the upper lid, which diminishes the circles of diffusion upon the retina.

In that form of irido-choroiditis, in which the iris is bulged forward by knob-like protuberances, and the edge of the pupil is tied down tightly by a firm circular synechia, it is generally not difficult to grasp and remove a considerable piece of iris, and thus to form a good-sized artificial pupil.

On account of the great shallowness of the anterior chamber and the proximity of the bulging iris to the posterior portion of the cornea, it is often very difficult to avoid cutting the iris with the common iridectomy knife.   It is better, therefore, to make the incision with Von Graefe's long, narrow cataract-knife, for with it we can skirt the edge of the chamber, and gain a large incision without fear of injuring the iris.

We unfortunately not unfrequently find that, although the iridectomy is large, the sight is but little if at all improved, for the artificial pupil is occupied by a thick uveal membrane detached by the fluid from the iris.   It is of practical importance to remember the probability of this occurrence on forming our prognosis as to the effect of the operation; hence we should never definitely promise the patient great improvement of sight after the first operation, but prepare him for the probable necessity of a second.   The uveal pigment is so intimately connected with the capsule of the lens, that it is generally unwise to attempt to scrape a portion of it off, as rupture of the capsule and traumatic cataract might ensue.   If we therefore find that so considerable a portion of the artificial pupil (the natural one being also blocked up by lymph) is occupied by the uvea as greatly to impair the sight, it will be best, at a later period, to make another iridectomy in a different direction, in the hope that at this point there may be less deposit upon the capsule.   By this means, or even by a third iridectomy, we may succeed in finally giving the patient a good clear pupil and a considerable degree of sight.   A most interesting and instructive example of this kind occurred amongst the patients at Moorfields, where Mr. Bowman repeated the operation; performing iridectomy twice upon the right eye and three times upon the left.   The result was most successful.   On the patient's admission his sight was as follows: Right eye, letters of 20 (Jäger) with difficulty, counts fingers within eighteen inches.   Left eye, counts fingers with uncertainty within three feet.   Seven weeks afterwards, on his discharge from the hospital, he could read No. 2 with the right eye, and No. 12 with the left.[1]

Even although the first iridectomy may not materially improve the sight, we find that it generally exerts a beneficial influence upon the tissue of the iris and the general condition of the eye; the iris gradually gaining a more normal color and appearance.   Von Graefe was the first to call attention to the fact that a certain degree of atrophy of the eye, consequent upon iridochoroiditis, may be arrested by the performance of iridectomy, and the eye regain its normal tension.   This fact has since been widely acknowledged by all surgeons who have much experience on this subject.   Of course, the atrophy must not have advanced too far, otherwise its arrest will be impossible, the same being the case if detachment of the retina has occurred. The benefit derived from iridectomy (perhaps repeated several times) in these cases, is that the stasis and congestion in the choroidal vessels are relieved, which not only causes an improvement in the choroidal circulation, but also in the nutrition of the vitreous humor.

If we cannot succeed in finding a portion of capsule sufficiently clear of uveal pigment to allow of much improvement of sight, or if the lens is opaque, it will be best to remove the latter.

In certain cases of irido-choroiditis, demanding, in his opinion, an unusually large iridectomy, Mr. Bowman effects this through an incision of moderate extent by seizing the iris at a point beyond the incision and detaching it from its ciliary border beyond the ordinary limits before dividing it.   The same being then done at the opposite side of the incision, the removal of

[1] I have reported this case at length in the "Royal London Ophthal. Hosp. Reports," vol. III.

even half the iris may be accomplished by an incision only extending to one-fourth or one-third of the corneal margin. Slight movements of the curette effectually cause the cut ends of the iris to retract within the chamber, and the blood effused is expelled by gentle pressure or traction made on the eyeball, while the edges of the incision are slightly separated by depressing the posterior lip.

In other instances, Mr. Bowman makes an iridectomy at two opposite points at the same time, by introducing two triangular knives simultaneously, either above and below, or to the right and left; the latter mode being the more easy in manipulation, the former preferable cosmetically and optically. One at least of the two iridectomy knives is a *stop-knife, i. e.*, is provided with a ledge preventing its penetration beyond a certain extent. The knife first introduced a little way will hold the eye, so as to give the surgeon command over the subsequent introduction of the second knife, and the due completion of the incision effected by both. The points of the knives are directed slightly forwards, so as to avoid the lens if transparent, and they are never suffered to be at all retracted until both incisions are complete, so that the aqueous may not prematurely escape. Some manipulative practice is requisite for this proceeding, but it is not difficult to avoid any injury to a transparent lens. The object here is to avoid the necessity of a second iridectomy at a future time, and the method is, according to Mr. Bowman, especially applicable to certain cases of glaucoma, where either a very large iridectomy is desirable, or where there is reason to fear that a single iridectomy practised in the ordinary fashion may be insufficient to completely abate the tension, and where consequently the need of a supplementary repetition of the iridectomy at a future period, and at an opposite point, may be apprehended as likely to arise. Mr. Bowman applies to this double simultaneous iridectomy at opposite parts the term "*diametric*."

Whilst we may afford considerable improvement in the above class of cases from repeated iridectomies, this is by no means the rule in the second kind of irido-choroiditis. Although in the former case the first artificial pupil often becomes narrowed or even closed, yet the texture of the iris improves; at a second operation we mostly succeed in gaining a larger pupil, and at a subsequent one, a tolerably good result as to the sight. But when thick, felt-like masses of exudation exist between the iris and capsule, we fail to remove a considerable portion of the rotten iris, and this attempt, moreover, sets up renewed inflammation, increased proliferation of the exudation-masses, and we thus, instead of improving the condition, hasten the atrophy of the eye. It will therefore be necessary, in order to benefit such cases, to remove not only the iris, but the dense masses behind it; but they are generally so firmly adherent to the capsule that we are almost sure to rupture the latter in our endeavor to remove them. A traumatic cataract is formed, if the lens is not already opaque, and this complicates matters still more. But Von Graefe had an opportunity of seeing that these false membranes could be removed with comparative facility and success when the lens was absent.[1] This led him to remove the lens, prior to attempting the withdrawal of the iris and exudation-masses. In these cases, Von Graefe now operates in the following manner:[2] With his narrow cataract-knife he makes the section just as in his operation for cataract, with the exception that, directly the puncture is made, the blade is passed straight through the iris, and brought

[1] "A. f. O.," vi. 2, 97. *Vide* also the author's abstract of this paper, "R. L. O. H. Rep.," iii. 224.
[2] "A. f. O.," xiv. 3, 141.

out at the counter-puncture, thus freely dividing the iris. This generally causes such a wide laceration of the capsule that the lens-matter exudes even while the section is being made. A pair of firmly catching, cross-grooved forceps is then passed into the incision, and one blade pushed boldly forward between the iris and cornea, and the other behind the retro-iritic masses of exudation; the iris and portions of false membrane which are thus grasped are then to be gently drawn out. If they do not come readily, their removal may be facilitated by making a cut with the scissors at each extremity of the linear incision, which had been made through the iris with the knife. The removal of the iris and false membrane is often followed by the escape of the remaining portion of the lens, in which case the operation may be regarded as completed. If this does not take place, the capsule should be freely lacerated with the pricker (cystitome), and the lens evacuated by a slight pressure of the curette on the cornea, just as in Von Graefe's operation of extraction of cataract. Should some opaque portions of capsule remain behind in the lower portion of the pupil after the removal of the lens, they are to be seized with the grooved forceps and gently removed, if they are not too firmly adherent to the iris or ciliary processes. If the lens is chalky, Von Graefe passes in a curved hook, and pressing this somewhat on the anterior capsule, endeavors to free the lens from any adhesions, and thus make it sufficiently movable to escape through the section by a little pressure of the curette on the cornea. He, however, strongly objects, even in these cases, to the introduction of any instrument (e. g., a scoop) behind the lens.

As the success of the iridectomy and of the extraction of the lens in cases of irido-choroiditis is often invalidated by the contraction and subsequent closure of the artificial pupil, Mr. Bowman has devised the following operation, termed by him "excision of the pupil," which has afforded favorable results: The puncture and counter-puncture may be made as in Von Graefe's operation for extraction of cataract (and with the same knife). The incision is not, however, concluded, but a narrow bridge is left standing at its apex, which aids in preventing the escape of the vitreous. The blades of a pair of fine scissors are then introduced through the first incision (the puncture), and the one blade (blunt-pointed) passed in front of the iris; the other, which is sharp, pierces the iris and anterior capsule of the lens, and entering down in front of the nucleus, and without moving it from its bed, a cut is made diagonally downwards as far as the centre of the lower part of the iris. The scissors are then withdrawn, and next introduced through the counter-puncture, and a similar incision made on this side, so that the two incisions meet at the lower part of the iris, including between them a large triangular piece of iris as well as the constrictor pupillæ. Finally, the base of the triangle is divided by cutting through the upper portion of the iris lying between the puncture and counter-puncture, and the whole triangular piece is then removed, as well as any false membrane attached to it, with a pair of forceps. The bridge of cornea is then divided, and the lens removed in the usual manner. The operation has been varied by Mr. Bowman in two or three ways, according to the cases dealt with. When there is no lens to be removed, the bridge of cornea is not divided, as the operation is already complete. Sometimes the cut across the base of the iris or the third above described, is not necessary, as the triangular portion of iris, including the pupil and capsule, admits of being easily torn off along the ciliary attachment. It is when there is a very dense and tough capsule of false membrane behind the iris, that the third incision with scissors is chiefly required, as avoiding the dangerous dragging of the ciliary structures. In other instances, the entire section of the cornea has been made at one stroke, without leaving the temporary bridge.

Mr. Bowman has also applied the same mode of operating to cases of dense membranous obstruction of the iris region, where the lens has been previously removed, and to these he considers it to be particularly applicable, especially if its performance be delayed until all signs of inflammatory tendency have entirely disappeared.

[In the treatment of plastic irido-choroiditis, atropia should be used frequently and in strong solutions, unless contraindicated. Local bleeding from the temples by means of the natural or artificial leech, and a thorough course of mercurial treatment by inunction or the mercurial vapor bath, should be persisted in. Another valuable remedy is jaborandi or its alkaloid pilocarpine. A hypodermic injection of ten or twenty minims of a four grain solution of the muriate of pilocarpine, every day or twice a day, is very often of great value in cases of a low grade of chronic irido-choroiditis, especially in clearing up the vitreous. Its effects should be carefully watched, for it occasionally causes unpleasant symptoms of collapse in cardiac complications. Very often a smaller dose causes more profuse perspiration and salivation.

In serous irido-choroiditis, frequent paracentesis of the cornea is sometimes of use.

In purulent irido-choroiditis no treatment seems to be of any avail, though large doses of quinine would seem to be indicated.—B.]

Mr. Bowman has made a further modification of the method described on page 326, adapted to remove a larger area of the pupillary structures, and indeed nearly the whole iris, without any traction on the ciliary body. He makes an incision on two opposite sides of the cornea, as for *diametric iridectomy*, and then from the two ends of each incision, with the previously described scissors, incises the iris in such a way as to mark out an irregularly rhomboidal or square portion of the iris and attached structures, the points of the scissors-cut meeting at the margin of the anterior chamber midway between the two corneal incisions. The square portion thus defined is removed by forceps, after the base of it has been cut across as above; or, if the scissors commence their cut at the same point opposite the centre of the corneal wound, the portion removed would be about square, and four movements of the scissors would effect it.

For these operations within the anterior chamber, De Wecker's new and ingenious "forceps-scissors" will be found admirably adapted. They, and the mode of using them, are fully described in the section on "Secondary Cataract."

DISEASES OF THE CILIARY BODY.

INFLAMMATION OF THE CILIARY BODY (CYCLITIS), ETC.

The congestion and hyperæmia of the ciliary body which are met with in cases of iritis accompanied by extensive posterior synechiæ, soon give rise to cyclitis, the inflammation but too frequently extending to the choroid. Again, the reverse may obtain, the inflammation may commence in the choroid, and extend thence to the ciliary body, and perhaps to the iris. But idiopathic cyclitis may also be met with, more especially after injuries to the ciliary region, such as contusions, incised or punctured wounds, or the lodgement in it of a foreign body. The presence of cyclitis is in such cases recognized by the fact that, together with the presence of photophobia, lachrymation, and very marked subconjunctival injection in the form of a bright zone of vessels round the cornea, there is acute, often indeed intense pain, on pressure of the ciliary region, great ciliary neuralgia, and perhaps hypopyon. [Three forms of cyclitis may be recognized, the *plastic*, the *serous*, and the *purulent*. The first form will be somewhat exhaustively treated in the chapter on "Sympathetic Ophthalmia," and, though occurring spontaneously, is not common as a primary inflammation unless from injury of the ciliary body.—B.]

Serous cyclitis often supervenes in the course of serous iritis, more especially if the latter is severe in character, and has been negligently or injudiciously treated with astringent or caustic collyria. The coexistence of serous cyclitis must be suspected if, together with the symptoms of serous iritis, there is acute pain when the ciliary region is pressed with the end of a probe or a curette. This tenderness is very frequently situated at the upper or inner portion of the ciliary region, but where cyclitis is suspected it is always best to test the sensibility of the whole ciliary body. Also, if the tension of the eyeball is increased, accompanied by dilatation of the pupil and shallowness of the anterior chamber; and if the vitreous becomes diffusely clouded, having also large fixed or floating opacities suspended in it. The veins of the iris are likewise often dilated and tortuous. Another very important symptom is the retraction of the ciliary margin of the iris, which is due to its being glued at this point to the ciliary by an effusion of lymph. This retraction causes the anterior chamber to be abnormally deep, and the ligamentum pectinatum to spring forward like a ledge, giving the appearance (as Mooren aptly says) as if the iris were set like a watch-glass in a rim. He has observed this retraction even in quite acute cases of cyclitis.[1] There is at the same time marked and rapid deterioration of the sight, which is in part dependent upon the opacity of the vitreous humor, and in part upon the increase of the eye-tension, which causes compression of the retina. The accommodation and field of vision are also more or less impaired. The supervention of cyclitis in cases of serous iritis is always to be regarded with apprehension, and the state of the sight, of the field of vision, and of the tension of the eye, should be watched with great anxiety, for if the symptoms do not yield to the usual remedies, but rather increase in severity, no time should be lost in performing iridectomy. Still graver is the danger in *purulent cyclitis*, which is characterized by the following symptoms: There is very marked subconjunctival injection, together with great ciliary neuralgia, photophobia, and lachrymation. The color of the iris is somewhat changed, and, if there is considerable iritis, it may be greatly altered. The veins of the iris are dilated. This, indeed, is a very pathognomonic symptom of cyclitis, and it is due to the following cause: On account of the inflammatory changes in the ciliary body and the retraction of the iris, the venous efflux from the iris is more or less impeded, and the blood does not readily flow off from the veinlets of the iris, which, therefore, become dilated and engorged. The region of the ciliary body is very tender to the touch, sometimes the pain thus produced is so exquisitely acute, that the patient shrinks back with apprehension. Pus makes its appearance in the anterior chamber, and sinks down to the bottom in the form of a more or less extensive hypopyon. It should be remembered that hypopyon may be due to a purulent exudation from the ciliary body; for at the rim of the anterior cham-

[1] "Ueber Sympathische Gesichtsstörungen," p. 16.

ber the ciliary body is only separated from the latter by the delicate division of the membrane of Descemet, through which pus may easily exude into the anterior chamber, and then become precipitated in the form of hypopyon. If we can, therefore, exclude the origin of the latter from the cornea and iris, we may be certain, even apart from other symptoms, that it is due to cyclitis. The edge of the pupil is often adherent, its area blocked up with a dense plug of lymph, and a purulent exudation is but too frequently poured out behind the iris, and also perhaps into the vitreous humor. Purulent cyclitis is very apt to occur after injuries to the ciliary body, operations for cataract, and as sympathetic ophthalmia; indeed, it is, as we have seen, the form under which the latter most frequently makes its appearance.

[An important exciting cause of idiopathic cyclitis, especially of the serous form, is found in diseases of the uterus accompanied by disturbance of the menstrual function. De Wecker thinks this is the reason why spontaneous irido-cyclitis occurs with so much greater frequency among women than among men. The restoration of the menstrual flow in these cases exerts a beneficial influence upon the ciliary inflammation. Pregnancy often causes relapses in cases of old chronic cyclitis. In girls from sixteen to twenty years of age, a mixed form of serous and plastic irido-cyclitis or choroiditis is frequently encountered, almost constantly associated with either amenorrhœa or irregular menstruation and chlorosis. This form of inflammation is also not an uncommon complication of the menopause, especially in those women in whom the climacteric period comes on unusually early. (See "Graefe und Saemisch's Hdb. der Augenheilkunde," p. 531.)—B.]

At the commencement, the constant application of hot poppy fomentations frequently affords very marked relief to the severe ciliary neuralgia, and sensitiveness of the ciliary region. Mooren strongly recommends the continuous use of warm poultices, which he applies for four, six, ten, or even twenty-four hours en suite if there is intense pain; but great care must be taken that they are kept at an equal temperature, and at once renewed when the patient complains of their being cold. If the pain continues, and if there is great hyperæmia and congestion of the subconjunctival vessels, as also of those of the iris, leeches should be applied, and when they have drawn very freely, a strong solution of atropine should be employed, in order to produce dilatation of the pupil as soon as possible. If there is much nocturnal pain, or the patient is restless, a subcutaneous injection of morphia is indicated. If the pain shows a marked periodic character, full doses of quinine should be given. When a considerable exudation of lymph occurs into the anterior chamber, or into the vitreous humor, salivation should be induced as rapidly as possible by the inunction of mercurial ointment. It must be confessed, however, that in spite of every care, we are often quite unable to stay the progress of the disease, and prevent the loss of the eye from suppurative irido-cyclitis, terminating in atrophy of the globe. As any accommodative effort of the healthy eye increases the pain in the affected one, it is best to forbid all use of the former, or even to cover it with a bandage, so as to keep it quite at rest.

An extensive iridectomy, if performed at an early stage of the disease, often exerts a very beneficial influence upon the course of the latter. At a later period it is but too frequently followed by a recurrence of severe inflammation, with a fresh exudation of pus, which completely blocks up the artificial pupil. Mooren[1] strongly objects to any operative interference

[1] "Ueber Sympathische Gesichtsstörungen," p. 21.

(especially an iridectomy), for he considers its action not only of doubtful benefit, but even in some cases very dangerous. Only in rare instances does he perform paracentesis. [The general testimony of ophthalmic surgeons is against iridectomy in this disease, and it might almost be said, against all operative interference; though favorable results have been reported from a sclerotomy through the sensitive region; at least so far as the pain is concerned. No operation in this region seems to exert any influence upon the course or duration of the inflammation.—B.]

Injuries implicating the ciliary region are not only dangerous on account of the inflammatory complications to which they may give rise in the injured eye, but also on account of the risk of sympathetic ophthalmia, which they are very prone to excite. Simple incised wounds of the sclerotic at or near the edge of the cornea will often rapidly unite, on the insertion of a fine suture, if they are not extensive in size, and have not penetrated too deeply, and thus caused severe injury to the ciliary body, lens, etc. Such wounds may be produced by fragments of glass or steel, or by a clean cut from a small sharp instrument. In the former case, a careful examination should always be made as to the presence of the foreign body, which may either have fallen out after having wounded the sclerotic, have entered the eyeball, or be lying in the lips of the wound, whence it may be readily extracted. A bead of vitreous is seen protruding between the lips of the little wound, and this constant oozing greatly diminishes the intra-ocular tension, the eye being generally extremely soft. But whilst the tension in the vitreous humor is much diminished, that in the anterior chamber may be augmented, the iris being cupped backwards and the depth of the anterior chamber much increased, and being occupied by yellowish serum. This causes a peculiar and markedly greenish discoloration of the iris, more especially if the latter is normally of a blue or bluish-gray tint. In such cases, by far the best treatment consists in bringing the lips of the little scleral wound together with a fine suture. This is best and most safely done by attaching a curved needle to each end of a very fine silk thread, and passing one needle through the one edge of the wound from *within outwards*, and the other needle through the opposite edge also from within outwards. In this way we shall avoid all danger of injuring the ciliary body or lens from a sudden jerk of the point of the needle deeply into the eye. The suture generally produces little or no irritation, and may be left for eight or ten days, until the wound is firmly united. As soon as the oozing of the vitreous is arrested, the intra-ocular tension increases, and in the course of a day or two it generally reaches the normal standard. If the depth of the anterior chamber is much increased by the accumulation of serum, an iridectomy should be made to re-establish the communication between the anterior and posterior chambers.

[In traumatic irido-cyclo-choroiditis from a perforating wound, it may be generally said that if the eye is not lost by suppuration, it will be by progressive atrophy of the globe. The danger of this result is the greater, the larger the wound has been, the more extensively the ciliary region has been injured, and the greater the probability of a foreign body being in the eye. If the wound gapes, the symptoms of cyclitis generally develop very rapidly; hence the wounds in this region parallel to the corneal margin are much more dangerous than vertical wounds. The presence of a foreign body in the eye posterior to the lens is in almost all cases very difficult to make out. Unfortunately, the cases of such foreign bodies becoming encapsulated are rare; and even when this has occurred, some subsequent shock may dislodge the particle from its resting-place, and a cyclitis or choroiditis is set up which leads to destruction of the eye. The main symptoms which lead the surgeon to suspect the presence of a foreign body are: 1st. The persistence of the pericorneal injection and of a marked tenderness on pressure even when phthisis bulbi has begun; and 2d. The increase of tension with the presence of cyclitis, instead of a diminution of tension as we should naturally expect. A consideration of the removal of such foreign bodies by operation from the eye will be found in the chapter on the " Vitreous Humor."—B.]

A description of the *tumors* met with in the ciliary region will be found in the article upon " Tumors of the Choroid."

CHAPTER VI.

SYMPATHETIC OPHTHALMIA.

THE name "sympathetic ophthalmia" was first applied by Mackenzie to those cases in which an injury of the one eye was followed by a peculiar inflammation in the other, which generally ensues within a short time of the accident, and proves extremely dangerous and intractable. That such sympathy exists between the two eyes had, however, been previously pointed out by Himly and Beer.

The character of sympathetic inflammation is so extremely dangerous and insidious, that if it has once been lit up, we are but seldom able to stay its progress before great, and often irreparable, mischief has been done. In the great majority of cases, the disease shows itself in the form of a very malignant irido-cyclitis, accompanied by great degeneration of the iris, total exclusion [and occlusion] of the pupil, and the formation of dense masses of exudation between the posterior surface of the iris and the capsule of the lens. This is the "sympathetic ophthalmia" *par excellence*, but it occasionally appears in a more tractable and benign form, assuming the character of serous iritis [or irido-choroiditis]. Von Graefe has, moreover, observed a third and still more rare affection, viz., sympathetic choroido-retinitis [in which the inflammatory process occurs exclusively in the posterior part of the eyeball. A fourth form of sympathetic inflammation, rarer than any of the others, is neuro-retinitis or neuritis. (See Abadie and Dansart, "Documents pour servir à l'histoire des affections sympathiques de l'Œil," Paris, 1873; "Trans. Fifth Internat. Ophth. Congress," 1876, paper by Alt.)—B.]

It is of practical importance to distinguish the condition of sympathetic irritation, which sometimes ensues upon an injury or inflammation of the one eye, from sympathetic inflammation. In the former case, the patient finds that any inflammatory exacerbation of the injured eye is accompanied by more or less irritability of the other. He is unable to employ the latter in reading or fine work, without its becoming tired and strained, owing to an impairment of the power of accommodation. The range of accommodation is generally also markedly diminished, the near point being removed further from the eye. Every accommodative effort causes the eye to flush up and become irritable, a bright rosy zone appears around the cornea, and photophobia and lachrymation soon supervene, together with more or less ciliary neuralgia. These symptoms generally subside, more especially at the commencement, as soon as the work is laid aside, but quickly reappear on its being resumed, or when the eye is exposed to cold, bright light, etc. The injured eye, moreover, often also becomes painful and irritable when the other is used for near work. Donders describes a form of severe sympathetic irritation under the name of "sympathetic neurosis." It is particularly distinguished by the intensity of the photophobia and lachrymation, these symptoms being often so severe as to cause a violent spasm of the lids, and directly any attempt is made to open the eye, a stream of scalding tears pours over the cheek. There is, however, no impairment of sight, although from its great irritability the eye is quite unfit for use. Donders considers that this neurosis never passes over into sympathetic inflammation, and yields in a very rapid and marked manner to the removal of the injured eye. Whether or not cases of sympathetic irritation are to be regarded in the light of a premonitory stage of sympathetic inflammation, or whether they are to be looked upon as completely differing from it in character, and as never liable to pass over into it, is at present, I think, an open question. Whilst, on the one hand, it must be admitted that we occasionally meet with instances in which a state of great irritability has existed for a long time without setting up sympathetic inflammation, yet, on the other, it must also be conceded that the attack of inflammation is often shown to have been clearly preceded by symptoms of irritation. Although this question is one of much interest and importance in the study of the true nature of sympathetic inflammation, it is fortunately but of little consequence in the treatment; for I think there can be no doubt that the proper mode of dealing with a case in which marked and persistent symptoms of sympathetic irritability appear, is the immediate removal of the injured eye, more especially if its sight is lost or very much impaired. Indeed, it would be incurring unnecessary risk to neglect doing so, on the supposition that the state of irritation would never pass over into that of inflammation.

Sympathetic irido-cyclitis is characterized by all the symptoms of a severe intra-ocular inflammation. The eyelids are somewhat red and swollen, and there is more or less photophobia, lachrymation, and ciliary neuralgia. Sometimes, however, there is not the slightest pain, so that even in children

[Fig. 186.

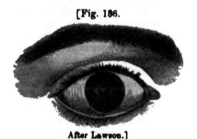

After Lawson.]

we hear no complaint, and this invests the disease with a peculiarly dangerous character, as it is very apt to be long unnoticed by the parents. The ciliary region is generally sensitive to the touch, and often acutely so. Soon there appear some circumcorneal vascularity and chemosis, the iris becomes discolored, and of a yellowish-red tint, the aqueous humor is clouded, and the anterior chamber perhaps diminished in depth. There is a rapid effusion of lymph at the edge of the pupil, soon leading to its complete exclusion [Fig. 136]; indeed, the action of atropine exerts but little influence upon the pupil. The exudation is not, however, confined to the pupillary edge, but extends to the posterior surface of the iris and the ciliary processes. The iris becomes firmly glued down to the capsule of the lens, and, as the disease advances, these exudations assume a very dense, firm, and organized character. Lymph is also effused upon the surface and into the stroma of the iris, often to such an extent that the latter appears soaked in it. The pupil is either covered by a film of exudation, or may be completely occluded by a dense yellow nodule. On account of the inflammatory swelling of the ciliary body, this region is very sensitive to the touch, and the circulation of the iris is greatly impeded, and the venous efflux obstructed; hence we soon notice the appearance of large tortuous veins upon the iris. Its structure soon becomes degenerated and changed into a firm, tense, fibrillar tissue, which cannot be caught up in a fold by the iridectomy forceps, but is so friable and rotten that it tears and breaks down under their grasp. Hence if an iridectomy is attempted, we shall only succeed in tearing away a small portion of the iris, and probably set up fresh inflammation, which will lead to a rapid increase in the density and extent of the exudation-masses. If the pupil and refracting media are sufficiently clear to permit of the use of the ophthalmoscope, we may notice opacities in the vitreous humor, and inflammatory changes in the choroid and retina. Or there may be dense masses of exudation in the anterior portion of the vitreous humor, giving rise to a peculiar yellow, lustrous reflex. At a later stage of the disease, when the morbid products have become more consolidated, the periphery of the iris is often drawn back, which is due to a direct retraction caused by the adhesion of its posterior surface to the ciliary processes (Von Graefe[1]). Whereas, on account of the increase in the exudation behind the iris, the latter, and with it the lens, is moved forward, so that the more central portion of the iris and the pupil are approached nearer the cornea, and the anterior chamber narrowed, whilst the periphery of the iris may be drawn back towards the ciliary body. In other cases, fluid is effused behind the iris, and the latter becomes bulged out into little protuberances. The attack is often so insidious and painless, that the patient pays but little heed to the first stage of the inflammation, thinking perhaps that he has only caught a slight "cold" in the eye; and it is not till the sight becomes materially affected, that he is frightened and seeks medical aid. In children especially (from their taking but little heed of the impairment of sight and from the absence of pain) the disease is sometimes allowed to proceed very far indeed before much attention is paid to it by the parents. But although the spontaneous pain is often absent, we find that the region of the ciliary body is generally very sensitive to the touch, and sometimes, as has been pointed out by Bowman and Von Graefe, at a spot corresponding symmetrically to the point at which the other eye has been injured, or where it still remains tender to the touch.

The tension of the eye varies considerably; at first, it is generally more or less increased, but then it gradually diminishes until the eye becomes quite soft, being still, however, liable to considerable fluctuation in consistence. It is, moreover, a fact of great practical importance, that, if such eyes are left alone, and the acme of the inflammatory process is allowed to subside, and the eye to become quiet, gradually and slowly its condition often begins to improve. The tension becomes better, and gradually augments until it may even reach the normal standard; the tissue of the iris improves greatly in appearance, loses its dirty-yellow hue, and assumes a fresher and more normal tint. [It is probable that pure sympathetic plastic irido-cyclitis is rare, and that the choroid is involved in the inflammatory process, if not throughout its whole extent, at least in its anterior portions; though the most destructive changes are found in the ciliary body. From statistics of one hundred and ten cases compiled by Alt, pure irido-cyclitis was found in only four cases, or only three and three-quarters per cent. (See "Archives of Ophthalmology," v. parts 3 and 4.)—B.]

[1] "A. f. O.," xii. 2, 151.

In the sympathetic serous iritis we find that the symptoms are very different, and closely resemble those of serous iritis, or serous irido-cyclitis. Together with a certain degree of ciliary injection, we notice that the iris is somewhat discolored, the pupil perhaps dilated, the aqueous humor faintly clouded, and the posterior surface of the cornea dotted by innumerable, small, puncti-form opacities, which are perhaps arranged in the form of a pyramid, having its base downwards. The depth of the anterior chamber may be increased. If the inflammation has extended to the ciliary body, this is sensitive to the touch, and the vitreous humor is likewise clouded, more especially if there is also choroiditis. The intra-ocular tension is often augmented. This form is much less common, and much less dangerous than sympathetic irido-cyclitis, but it may pass over into the latter.

According to Mooren,[1] the cases in which the sympathetic inflammation commences in the iris afford a more favorable prognosis than if it starts from the choroid, the worst form being where it begins in the ciliary body.

Von Graefe[2] describes another and very rare form of sympathetic inflam-mation, under the name of "*sympathetic choroido-retinitis*," and narrates two cases, illustrative of the symptoms presented by it. In one of these, the patient had a dislocated chalky lens lying in the anterior chamber of a perfectly blind, and somewhat atrophied left eye. The lens was removed with facility by Von Graefe, but the operation was accompanied by a considerable loss of fluid, yellow vitreous humor. The eye remained irri-table, and, and very sensitive to the touch for several weeks, and there were, moreover, symptoms of plastic cyclitis. Six weeks after the operation, when these symptoms had somewhat subsided, sensibility to the touch still remained; but the sight of the right eye, which had hitherto been perfectly good, began suddenly to be impaired, this being unaccompanied by any pain. The acuity of vision had already on the second day after the attack sunk to one-fifth, and there was considerable torpor of the retina, with indistinctness of eccentric vision in the whole of the temporal half of the visual field. With the ophthalmoscope, the retinal veins were seen to be very tortuous and dilated, more especially on the inner side. The retina also showed a delicate and diffuse cloudiness, which not only veiled the choroidal ring of the optic nerve, but extended to certain portions of the retina, especially along the course of some of the larger retinal vessels. Slight symptoms of iritis soon supervened, and very delicate punctiform opacities were observed on the membrane of Descemet. The power of accommodation was almost completely paralyzed. These symptoms gradually subsided, and the sight became finally quite restored. Whether this favorable result was chiefly due to the remedial measures employed (local depletion, bichloride of mercury, and afterwards iodide of potassium), or to the extinction of the sensibility of the left eye to the touch, was uncertain. Von Graefe himself lays the greater stress upon the last fact. The morbid appearances of the retina disappeared less rapidly than the functional disturbances, and then there were noticed patches of choroiditis. [Probably a still rarer form of sympathetic inflammation is pure and simple *neuro-retinitis*. Inflammation of the nerve and retina no doubt very often exists in cases of sympathetic in-flammation, but it is concealed by the products of irido-cyclitis or choroiditis. In a report of seven cases of sympathetic neuro-retinitis by Alt, irido-cho-roiditis existed in six. In five of the cases complete recovery occurred, and in two the second eye was lost. In the tabulated statistics of one hundred

---

[1] *Vide* Mooren's very interesting and valuable work, "Ueber Sympathische Gesichts-störungen," p. 82. Berlin, Hirschwold, 1869.
[2] "Archiv f. O.," xii. 2, 171.

and ten cases by Alt, before referred to (l. c. p. 473), simple neuro-retinitis occurred in five eyes, or four and one-half per cent., and in these five cases, in the eyes enucleated, the uveal tract was affected in all, and the optic nerve and retina in three cases. The percentage of affections of the optic nerve and retina coincident with sympathetic irido-choroiditis is very large, Alt having found it to reach seventy-nine per cent. This is certainly worthy of consideration, as is also the fact that in the five cases of pure neuro-retinitis the retina was detached in three.

Of late years, mention has been occasionally made of *sympathetic inflammation* affecting the *cornea*, or sympathetic keratitis. There are, however, as yet no sufficient facts, not enough actual observations to substantiate this statement. A case is reported by Maats, from the Utrecht clinic, in which the so-called sympathetic corneal trouble was the appearance of phlyctenula on one cornea ten months after an injury to the other eye. Another case is reported by Pagenstecher, in which there was an obstinate superficial keratitis in one eye, after removal of a corneal staphyloma in the other eye. Both cases are referred to by Alt (l. c. p. 458).—B.]

The *causes of sympathetic inflammation* are to be sought in those lesions which may set up a plastic inflammation of the ciliary body. 1. Amongst the most frequent causes are injuries to the eye, such as punctured and incised wounds, more especially in the region of the ciliary body. If such wounds are extensive, the lens has generally escaped, accompanied perhaps by considerable loss of vitreous and extensive intra-ocular hemorrhage. Small incised wounds of the ciliary region, or situated partly in the latter and partly in the cornea, are not necessarily of so dangerous a character, more especially if they have only penetrated the coats of the eye, without injury of the lens or vitreous humor. In such cases, no time should be lost in bringing the lips of the little wound together with a suture. [It usually suffices to bring the lips of the conjunctival wound together, without passing the suture into or through the sclera.—B.] Union by the first intention will take place, and many an eye will thus be saved, which might otherwise have not only been itself lost from choroiditis, but might have also proved a source of danger to the other eye. In wounds which implicate the cornea alone, there is generally not so much danger of sympathetic inflammation; although, if they are accompanied by a considerable prolapse of the iris, and this is situated near the periphery, it may, by dragging upon and irritating the ciliary processes, set up sympathetic inflammation. But when there has been a penetrating wound of the cornea (such as may be produced by a pair of scissors), and the iris and lens have been also injured, there is always some risk. The disease may, moreover, be likewise produced by severe contusions of the eye.

2. Foreign bodies lodged within the eye, are a most frequent cause. Amongst these we must especially enumerate portions of gun-cap or of metal, and splinters of glass or stone. They prove a source of constant irritation to the eye, more especially if they are considerable in size, and differ in their chemical constituents from the structures in which they are embedded. Inflammation of the iris and choroid supervenes, and the eye may become gradually atrophied, shrinking down to a small shrivelled stump. But even then, all danger to the other eye, if this has hitherto escaped, is by no means passed, for such stumps are a source of constant risk, as long as they remain *painful to the touch*, and show signs of irritability. Years may elapse after the injury, and the patient have long since forgotten his surgeon's admonition as to the danger to the other eye, when suddenly the latter becomes sympathetically inflamed, and, in spite of all our efforts, perhaps destroyed.

[The explanation of an outbreak of sympathetic trouble in an eye, occurring many years after an injury to the other eye, is no doubt to be found in a change of position of chalky or ossified exudations which have irritated parts of the uveal tract hitherto undisturbed and possibly normal. This may be occasioned by a fall or a blow on the head, even without direct injury of the diseased eye. Or even without this injury by contre-coup, a slight hemorrhage from some atrophic vessel may light up a fresh cyclitis and lead to sympathetic irritation.—B.] The longest time which I have known to elapse between the injury of one eye and sympathetic inflammation in the other is twenty-six years, which occurred in the following case:[1] J. K., æt. 42, an ironfounder, came under my care at the Royal London Ophthalmic Hospital, on March 2, 1869. He had lost the left eye twenty-six years ago through an injury from a piece of metal; the globe had shrunk to one-quarter of its normal size, and was very painful on pressure. The right eye remained perfectly well after the accident until 1860, when it was attacked with iritis, for which an iridectomy was performed at that time; it being, however, deemed unadvisable to do anything to the left eye. Since the iridectomy in 1860, he had been able to follow his occupation up to Christmas, 1868, when this eye again became inflamed, and its sight failed more and more. On March 2, 1869, it presented the following symptoms: The eye-tension is normal, the field of vision complete, but the sight so much impaired that he cannot decipher letters of Jäger twenty, but only see their black outline. The cornea is somewhat hazy, the iris inflamed, the pupil clouded, and with the ophthalmoscope hardly any reflex can be obtained from the fundus. No relief being experienced from the application of atropine and warm fomentations, I urgently advised the removal of the left eyeball, to which the patient submitted on March 19. A piece of metal was found in it, firmly embedded in a mass of exudation matter (on the inner side of the sclerotic), in the centre of a firm fibrous cord, which appeared to be the shrunken and disorganized retina. March 23: The right eye has improved so much since the extirpation of the other, four days ago, that the patient is now able to read words of Jäger sixteen. The inflammatory symptoms have greatly subsided; the cornea and pupil are clearer; there is still, however, but little reflex from the fundus. March 30: He now reads words of Jäger ten. The refracting media are much clearer and the outline of the optic disk can be indistinctly seen with the ophthalmoscope. The patient ceased to attend the hospital after this date, and returned to Yorkshire. He writes, however, in the middle of October, that the right eye is strong and well, and its sight so much improved, that he is able to follow his employment (superintendent of an iron forge). Mr. Lawson, in his valuable work,[2] also narrates[3] two interesting cases in which sympathetic mischief did not occur for many years after an injury from a foreign body.

3. Sympathetic inflammation may also be caused by internal inflammations of the eye, more especially if they are accompanied by hemorrhagic effusions, either considerable in quantity, or of frequent recurrence, together with rapid fluctuations in the intra-ocular tension. Also if a bony deposit in the choroid has occurred, and the eye remains irritable to the touch. Indeed the continuance of sensibility in the region of the ciliary body in cases of irido-choroiditis, or in eyes which have undergone atrophy after internal inflammation, is one of the most dangerous symptoms, as such eyes

[1] "Lancet," December 18, 1869.
[2] "Injuries of the Eye, Orbit, and Eyelids," by George Lawson, 1867, 8vo. pp. 405.
[3] Idem, pp. 321–823.

are extremely prone to set up sympathetic inflammation. The latter may also arise in cases of spontaneous detachment of the retina; dislocation, or reclination of the lens; intra-ocular tumors, if secondary irido-cyclitis supervenes; intra-ocular cysticerci; also in prolapse of the iris causing great traction on the ciliary body, and consequently irritation of the ciliary nerves. Hence some surgeons never perform iridodesis, for fear of setting up cyclitis, and thus perhaps inducing sympathetic inflammation. If any of these causes set up plastic cyclitis, they may give rise to sympathetic inflammation.[1] Indeed, Mooren goes so far as to believe "that every inflammation in the course of the uveal tract, quite apart from the primary cause of its origin, is capable of setting up sympathetic disturbances if it manifests itself as a cyclitis from the outset, or as soon as it, in the course of time, assumes this character."[2] [It is necessary here to indicate the importance of recognizing the influence of traction upon the ciliary region in producing irritation. This may come from prolapse and encapsulation of the iris or ciliary processes in a wound; or from a contracting cicatrix in the ciliary region; or from contracting inflammatory exudations behind the iris and on the ciliary processes, which exert a very dangerous traction on the ciliary nerves. This traction may go so far as to cause detachment of the ciliary body from the sclera. Of course, the more ciliary nerves are involved in the process, the greater are the chances of irritation.—B.]

It is a very interesting and important fact that Iwanoff,[3] Hirschberg,[4] etc., found, on examination of some eyes which had been excised for setting up sympathetic inflammation, that the ciliary body had not only undergone inflammation, but had become detached from the sclerotic, thus causing great stretching and irritation of the ciliary nerves, and forming the starting-point of the sympathetic affection of the other eye.

Mooren[5] also mentions a very interesting case in which the sympathetic inflammation was apparently produced by the contusion of the optic nerve in dividing it with the scissors in excision of the eye.

It was formerly generally supposed that sympathetic inflammation was propagated from the injured eye to its fellow through the optic nerves by way of the optic commissure. But this view has been long abandoned as untenable, for cases of sympathetic inflammation have occurred in eyes in which the optic nerves were not only completely atrophied, but had even undergone extensive chalky degeneration. It is now generally held that the sympathy is propagated by the ciliary nerves, and this view certainly receives the strongest support from many clinical facts. Thus we not unfrequently meet with cases, as has been especially pointed out by Bowman and Von Graefe, in which the starting-point of the sympathetic irritation or inflammation in the second eye occurs at a spot of the ciliary region which corresponds symmetrically to that at which the injured eye was hurt, or at which the ciliary region still retains its sensibility to the touch. Moreover, as Von Graefe strongly insists, the danger of the sympathetic inflammation should never be considered as passed, as long as the ciliary region of the injured eye, or its stump, remains sensitive to the touch, more especially if it is accompanied by diminished tension, for it is then a symptom of plastic cyclitis.

[1] Vide also Dr. Laqueur's brochure on "Les Affections sympathiques de l'Œil." Baillière et Fils. Paris, 1869.
[2] Op cit., p. 58.   [3] Mooren's "Sympathische Gesichtsörungen," p. 161.
[4] "Kl. Monatsbl.," Oct. 1869, p. 297.
[5] "Ophthalmiatrische Beobachtungen," p. 160.

[Our knowledge of the nature and etiology of sympathetic inflammation has of late years become more minute and satisfactory through the labors of Meyer, Alt, De Wecker, and others, but especially through the masterly monograph of Mauthner, entitled "Die Sympathischen Augenleiden."[1] The marked characteristic of sympathetic irido-cyclo-choroiditis is the tendency to the rapid development of thick membranous exudations upon the posterior surfaces of the iris and the ciliary processes, which rapidly become organized and form dense and broad adhesions of the iris and ciliary processes to the lens-capsule. Complete posterior synechiæ develop very rapidly after the outbreak of the disease, and the iris bulges at its periphery towards the cornea, while the pupillary margin seems retracted. After a short period the lens, pushed forward again, becomes adherent more or less completely to the iris, and, these being pushed forwards towards the cornea, the anterior chamber is really shallowest at its centre, while the peripheral parts, owing to the retraction of the inflammatory exudation upon the ciliary processes, are deeper. The pupil is usually completely blocked by an exudation. At this stage of the process the tension, which at first was raised, is very much diminished, and the disease may end in two ways. Either progressive phthisis bulbi, secondary cataract with cretaceous deposits in the lens and capsule, and even ossification of the choroid may ensue; or a condition of complete quiescence with even some slight improvement in vision, through gaping of the pupillary membrane, may result. This latter termination is, however, uncommon, and may even be succeeded by total loss of sight. One fact, which should be remembered, is that a serous cyclitis of idiopathic origin accompanying a glaucomatous process with development of a ciliary staphyloma, scarcely ever leads to sympathetic irritation; owing, as De Wecker thinks, to destruction of the ciliary nerves by pressure. ("Graefe und Saemisch's Hdb. der Augenheilk.," iv. pp. 520–530.)

As regards the method of propagation of irritation from the injured eye to the sound eye, until recently there was no manner of doubt that this is done through the medium of the ciliary nerves. Many examinations have been made by numerous observers of eyes enucleated for sympathetic irritation or inflammation in the fellow eye, in which the ciliary nerves have shown signs of inflammation. They have been found torn and compressed; they have been found embedded in the traumatic cicatrix; they have been found inflamed, atrophied, and the seat of fatty degeneration; Schwann's sheath has been found thickened for a long distance from the seat of injury (Alt, l. c. p. 471). These changes are, however, by no means always met with, for in Alt's statistics of one hundred and ten cases, alterations of the ciliary nerves were found in but sixteen and two-thirds per cent. The old view that the optic nerve was the channel of propagation has been again advanced and defended by Alt, as more probable than that by the ciliary nerves; but for this idea to become a working hypothesis, we must have more observations. His modified statement, that the entire nervous apparatus of the eye takes part in the transmission of the irritation, may perhaps be accepted until our knowledge becomes more satisfactory.

This question of the nerve transmission of sympathetic inflammation is one of profound interest. Many curious phenomena have been noticed in cases of injury of the ciliary region, with or without the presence of a foreign body. Obstinate peri-orbital pains, shooting upward along the course and distribution of the supra-orbital nerve, are not uncommonly ob-

[1] "Vorträge aus dem Gesamtgebiete der Augenheilkunde," von Dr. Ludwig Mauthner, 1878–1881, 8vo. s. 600 (Erst. und Zweit. Heft).

served even in pronounced phthisis bulbi. In this latter class of cases the
shrunken eyeball is usually very sensitive, though this is not always so. The
circum-orbital pain on the injured side may be accompanied by the same
pain on the other side, which of course is a prodromal symptom.

Mooren makes a strong plea for the possibility, and in many cases the
probability, that the optic nerve is the seat of the lesion, and that the disease is propagated to the fellow eye along the course of the optic nerve
fibres. (See "Klin. Monatsbl. für Angenheilk.," August, 1881.) Leber has
considered the subject of an infectious origin of sympathetic inflammation.
In four eyes enucleated for sympathetic trouble, he found pronounced hyperplasia of the intervaginal connective tissue of the optic nerve, with proliferation of the endothelium. He refers to the fact that acute panophthalmitis
is not usually productive of sympathetic inflammation, because the inflammatory seeds are partly gotten rid of by purulent perforation of the eyeball,
and partly destroyed or rendered inert by the enormous development of pus.
In his experience, the outbreak of a sympathetic inflammation is not preceded by any marked irritability of the ciliary nerves, and sensitiveness of
the ciliary region he does not regard as sufficient proof of this irritability.
One difficulty in the way of accepting this propagation theory is that the
first manifestation of the inflammatory process in the second eye appears
always in the uveal tract, whereas we should expect an inflammation of the
optic papilla. Leber thinks that the latter may always be present without
being distinctly seen, owing to the sinister character of the inflammatory
process and the turbidity of the vitreous humor. He thinks it both possible
and probable that sympathetic iritis is an inflammation that has extended
from the optic nerve sheath to the eye. (See "Archiv für Ophthalmologie,"
xxvii. 1.)

The discussion on sympathetic ophthalmia, before the International Medical Congress, in London, in 1881, led to the following formal statement of
belief: Sympathetic inflammation, which should be carefully distinguished
from sympathetic neurosis, never occurs before a characteristic process has
developed itself in the eye first injured, the principal symptoms of which
are—1. Dilatation of the posterior lymphatic spaces, with closure of the
anterior lymphatics of the globe. 1. An infective plastic inflammation of the
uveal tissue. The iris becomes infiltrated and covered by solid exudations;
the anterior chamber is lessened; the vitreous humor, and often also the
retina, is drawn forward into a funnel shape; the tension, diminished at first,
is always increased beyond the normal before the transmitted affection appears; the peri-choroidal lymph-space and the peri-neural lymph-sheaths
of the optic nerve are dilated. In sympathetic disease, the choroid shows
an impregnation with lymphoid cells, and there is always more or less
neuritis. Microphytic organisms are also found. The eye secondarily
affected shows corresponding changes of nervous tissue and choroid. The
hypothesis that sympathetic ophthalmitis is explained by the reflex action
through the ciliary nerves is devoid of all convincing proof. Sympathetic
ophthalmitis is to be looked upon as proceeding from a septic choroiditis of
definite type, not improbably resulting from an abnormal continuity between
the external tissue and the uvea. The morbid changes of the vessels, the
increase of the lymphoid cells, and the accumulation of microphytal organisms, are the guiding signs that may indicate the direction in which the
morbid process is propagated. The path of the transmission is most probably
through the lymphatic spaces of the optic nerve.—B.]

The *prognosis* of sympathetic inflammation is most unfavorable, if the
disease has once fairly broken out. In the stage of sympathetic irritation,

the removal of the injured eye arrests the progress; but it is quite different if the inflammation has already set in, more especially if it assumes the character of plastic irido-cyclitis; for then, even the immediate enuclea-tion of the other eye generally fails to have any, or any but a temporary beneficial effect. For a few days or weeks the inflammation appears to be diminished, but then it breaks out again with all its former severity. The serous sympathetic iritis, being more benign in character and more amenable to treatment, affords a more favorable prognosis.

Sympathetic inflammation is more prone to attack youthful individuals than middle-aged or elderly persons. Its course also appears to be more rapid in the young. It generally occurs within a few weeks of the injury, but a long period, even many years, may elapse before it is excited.

Treatment.—With regard to the general treatment of sympathetic inflam-mation, I must strongly insist upon the necessity of complete rest of the eye for a prolonged period and this is to be continued for some length of time after the eye appears to have recovered from the inflammatory attack. Otherwise, there is the greatest risk of a recurrence, which may prove most dangerous and intractable. Whilst the eye remains irritable, the patient should be confined to a darkened room, and if he has to go into the open air, the eye should either be protected by a bandage, or by a pair of dark-blue eye-protectors, or the wire goggles. [In cases of sympathetic inflammation in which the chronicity and slowness of the process is marked, and especially in children, the patients cannot be kept confined to a dark room. The treat-ment succeeds better if the patients are sent out regularly twice a day in the open air. Very often a sweat-bath becomes absolutely necessary in these cases.—B.] In order to allay the irritability of the eye, poppy or belladonna fomentations may be applied, as also a solution of atropine (varying from two to four grains to the fluidounce of water), which should be dropped into the eye several times a day. At the very outset of the disease, we should endeavor to gain, if possible, a wide dilatation of the pupil, and hence apply it more frequently and in a strong solution; but, as has already been stated above, the pupil is generally very imperfectly acted upon by atropine, and at a later stage the adhesions to the capsule are so firm and extensive as completely to resist its action.

The diet should be nutritious and generous, more especially if the patient is feeble and ill-nourished. Tonics, more particularly quinine and prepara-tions of steel, should also be administered.

We have now to consider, in the first place, whether we are enabled by any operative interference to prevent the occurrence of sympathetic inflam-mation; and, secondly, whether we can arrest its progress when it has once broken out.

With regard to the first point, I may state that, as far as I am aware, no instance has been recorded in which sympathetic inflammation ever attacked an eye after the injured eye had been removed, if at the time the other was still quite unaffected. [This statement is proved erroneous in the light of recent observations (see below).—B.] This being so, there cannot be the slightest doubt as to the imperative advisability of the immediate removal of an eye which has been so greatly injured as to have quite lost its sight, or at all events to leave no hope of any restoration of a useful degree of vision. This is still more the case, if the injury has been of a kind which is prone to be followed by sympathetic irritation; for we have no guarantee that we shall have time to check the sympathetic inflammation, if it has once broken out, even by a speedy removal of the injured eye. For although symptoms of sympathetic irritation not unfrequently usher in the inflammation, and the latter may be prevented by the excision of the injured eye at this premonitory stage, yet this is not always the case. The inflammation may occur without any premonitory symptoms, and advance so rapidly, that in the course of a few days the integrity of the eye may be greatly, and perhaps permanently, impaired. Thus, a case is narrated by Mann, in which within four days (and without any premonitory symptoms) an eye became so affected by sympathetic irido-cyclitis, that there was nearly a complete posterior synechia, and the sight had sunk to $\frac{3}{\infty}$. In spite of the immediate removal of the injured eye, and of every endeavor to improve the condition of the other by iridectomy, and subsequently by a second iridectomy with removal of the lens, the eye became atrophied, and only retained perception of light. Such a case should warn us of the danger of procrastination in excision of the blind injured eye, in the hope that there will always be time enough for this when symptoms of sympathetic irritation manifest themselves or during the earliest stage of sympathetic inflammation; for the former may never occur, and the latter may be so rapid in its development and course, that great and irremediable mischief may be done before we can enucleate the other eye. Moreover, there is another point which weighs heavily in the scale amongst persons whose livelihood depends upon their work, and that is, the long time that is lost by them during the treatment of the injured eye; for it may remain painful and irritable for many months, and thus render the patient quite unfit to use the sound eye. It may be laid down as a fundamental rule, that as long as the injured eye remains painful to the touch it is always a source of danger, and may at any moment set up sympathetic inflammation. It should consequently be removed if its sight is lost, or greatly and irremediably impaired, this being particularly indicated if a foreign body remains within the eye. For thus only can we insure the patient against the dangers of sympathetic inflammation. The question as to whether the injured eye should be removed if it still retains some degree of vision is, of course, much more difficult and embarrassing. In deciding upon this point, we must be chiefly guided by the nature and extent of the injury. Thus, if it is a small incised wound of the cornea or sclerotic, and the iris, lens, and vitreous humor have escaped any severe injury, we may by careful and judicious treatment avoid the danger of sympathetic inflammation, and ultimately, perhaps, restore excellent vision. But if the wound is very extensive, and implicates the ciliary region and sclerotic; if the lens has been lost or is injured, a considerable amount of vitreous has escaped, or intra-ocular hemorrhage has occurred; and if, consequently, the injuries are so great that but very little, if any, sight can possibly be saved, it is much better to remove the eye at once, even although some degree of vision may still exist. Still more imperative is such a course, if these extensive injuries are due to a foreign body which has become lodged in the eye, and cannot be removed by operation, for although rare instances occur in which foreign bodies remain encapsulated and quiescent within the eye, such cases form, unfortunately, the great exception. I would especially urge the necessity for the operation if the patient resides at a distance from medical aid, so that a careful watch cannot be kept over the eye, and the first symptoms of sympathetic irritation or inflammation be at once detected. question in all such cases is, whether it is not better to sustain a small than to run the risk of a very great danger. I, however, fully feel and the heavy responsibility which rests upon the surgeon who shall advise removal of an eye which still possesses some sight, and when, as yet, no oms of sympathetic disease have appeared. We can, in such cases, only carefully and conscientiously weigh the different bearings of the case, and place them clearly and forcibly before the patient and his friends, and leave the decision in their hands. I have entered somewhat at length upon this part of the subject, because I feel it to be of great importance to all medical men, and one upon which they should hold strong and decided views. For we never know at what moment we may be called upon to decide a question of this kind, and what reproaches we may not have to make ourselves, if by our procrastination and indecision the second eye is lost from sympathetic inflammation.

We must now pass on to the consideration of the question, as to whether we have any power of checking the progress of sympathetic inflammation if it has once broken out. If the sight of the injured eye is lost, it should be at once removed, for even although this proceeding may not always stop the progress of the sympathetic disease, but only perhaps arrest it for a time, it will probably at least exert a favorable influence upon its course, from the removal of the primary source of irritation. But it will be different if some degree of sight still lingers in the injured eye, more especially if the sympathetic inflammation has already produced extensive injury, for then it must be borne in mind that in some similar cases the injured eye eventually proved of the most use to the patient, he having more sight in it than in the other. It appears certain, from the experience of all authorities upon the subject of sympathetic ophthalmia (amongst whom I would especially enumerate Mackenzie, Bowman, Critchett, Von Graefe, Lawson, Donders, Pagenstecher), that any operative interference upon the second eye during the progress of the sympathetic inflammation is not only not beneficial, but even does positive harm, in increasing the inflammatory proliferation of the exudation-masses behind the iris, and thus hastening instead of arresting the progress of the disease. Von Graefe, however, mentions a case in which the performance of an early iridectomy exerted a beneficial influence upon the course of the inflammation. He employed his narrow cataract-knife, and made the incision very peripheral (just, in fact, as for the operation for cataract), and thus succeeded in seizing and excising a portion of iris. He, however, strongly advises that the iridectomy should be made as early as possible; as soon, in fact, as the ominous character of the disease manifests itself. But, when the disease has become fully established, the pupil and posterior surface of the iris being tied down to the capsule of the lens by firm masses of exudation, and the tissue of the iris shows symptoms of disorganization, no operation should be performed. It is then far wiser to wait until the active inflammatory symptoms have subsided. Von Graefe thinks that we should wait until the tenderness of the ciliary region has diminished, the development of the large venous trunks in the disorganized iris become arrested or retrograding, the exudations in the pupil have changed their yellow color for a more bluish-gray tint, the intra-ocular tension (which is generally distinctly diminished) shows no fluctuations, and, finally, until at least three or four months have elapsed since the outbreak of the disease. In opposition to this, it might be urged that if the disease is thus allowed to run its course unchecked, the eye might become so atrophied, and its functions so much impaired, as to be beyond all hope of improvement. But, in such malignant cases, any operative interference only accelerates this result, and then, again, these are, according to Von Graefe, quite exceptional cases, for generally the atrophy of the eyeball becomes arrested at a certain point, not reaching perhaps a high degree, and the quantitative perception of light remains good. Under such circumstances, much advantage is gained by waiting as long as possible with the operation, because, as he states, "the vascularization and irritability of the exudation masses diminish when the acme of the disease is passed, and besides, the extensive operative interferences which will have to be undertaken will be borne much better; whilst at an earlier period, hemorrhagic effusions from the delicate and newly developed vessels, and the proliferation of the neoplastic formations, again destroy the result of the operation. Moreover, the whole tendency of the diffusion of the traumatic irritation upon the choroidal tract, diminishes with the prolonged existence of the disease; and not unfrequently the tension of the eyeball becomes increased."[1]

The operation which should be performed in such a case is the removal of the lens, together with an extensive iridectomy, and a dilaceration of the masses of exudation. This may be performed according to Von Graefe's method, described at page 325, or to that practised by Bowman.

The mode of performing the operation of excision of the eyeball will be described in the chapter on " Diseases of the Orbit."

The belief that the sympathetic irritation is evidently propagated by the ciliary nerves, led Von Graefe to suggest the division of these nerves at the point where the ciliary region of the injured eye remains sensitive to the touch. Dr. Meyer,[2] of Paris, has performed this operation with marked success in several cases of sympathetic neurosis. After having raised and incised the conjunctival and subconjunctival tissue over the painful portion of the ciliary region, just as in the operation for strabismus, he introduces a squint-hook underneath the tendon of the nearest rectus muscle, so that the eye may be well steadied. He then obliquely punctures the sclerotic at the painful point of the ciliary region with Von Graefe's narrow cataract-knife, in such a manner that the wound lies parallel to the edge of the cornea. The vitreous humor is at once exposed by the incision. The hook being carefully removed, the conjunctival wound is to be closed by a suture, the sclerotic incision healing in the course of a few days. [But little reaction follows the operation, and the only after-treatment required is rest, the hypodermic injection of morphia into the temporal region, and, when there are pain and restlessness, the application of a pressure-bandage.

This operation has been performed by Prof. Secondi, of Genoa, and by Mr. J. Z. Laurence,[3] of London, and with a satisfactory result in each case.—H.]

[As it has been proven that purulent panophthalmitis may give rise to sympathetic inflammation in the other eye, the plan of destroying the injured eye by passing a seton through it, as a prophylactic measure, must of course be abandoned. The experience of modern ophthalmology would seem to limit the performance of enucleation to the following cases: 1. When prodromal symptoms of sympathetic irritation have appeared in the sound eye. 2. When the injured or inflamed eye is the seat of violent pain, which cannot be allayed, and the vision is lost, or nearly so. 3. When there is a foreign body in the eye, and the eye is sensitive and the seat of frequent exacerbations of inflammation, provided the foreign body cannot be removed. (See chapter on " Diseases of the Vitreous.")

There is one class of cases in which the responsibility resting upon the surgeon is very grave. Is an eye to be enucleated which has already caused sympathetic inflammation, but which retains a greater or more useful degree of vision than the sympathetically affected eye? In other words, are we in

---

[1] " A. f. O.," xii. 2, 165.
[2] " Annales d'oculistique," Sept. 1867, p. 129.
[3] " The Lancet," 1868, II. 633; also, " Amer. Journ. of Med. Sci.," Jan. 1869, p. 271.—H.]

such a case to enucleate a still partially useful eye in the hopes of putting a stop to an inflammation which almost invariably resists all treatment? The enucleation of the injured eye in such a case does not exert any good effect upon the other eye, unless, perhaps, in cases of severe pain, while some observers have stated that it increases the sympathetic inflammation. (See Graefe und Saemisch's "Hdb. der Augenheilk.," iv. p. 527.)

To avoid enucleating such an eye, and at the same time allay irritation, it has been recommended by Von Graefe to divide the ciliary nerves near the seat of injury through the sclera; but experience has shown that this operation gives no complete security against the propagation of the irritation. In cases where it results favorably, this is probably due to a diminution of the intra-ocular tension by the sclerotomy. Snellen proposed to cut these nerves externally to the eyeball, by first dividing either the external or internal rectus muscle, and then with a pair of scissors curved on the flat and kept close to the eyeball, and passed backward beneath the conjunctiva until the optic nerve is reached, snip the ciliary nerves as far round as can be reached without injuring the optic nerve. Thus the existing amount of sight is undisturbed.

The operation known as optico-ciliary neurotomy has been proposed recently as a substitute for enucleation, in the class of cases in which the latter operation is indicated, but in which it is desired to avoid the deformity of an empty orbit, or the annoyance of an artificial eye. The operation is performed very much as Snellen's, except that when the entrance of the optic nerve is reached, the blades of the scissors are opened widely and the optic nerve divided, as well as the ciliary nerves, as they enter the sclera near the posterior pole of the eye. All the ciliary nerves are to be divided, and of this the surgeon must assure himself by dislocating the eye forward and inward. The reports of the results of this operation, both as a prophylactic against sympathetic inflammation, and as a means of quelling pain in the injured eye, are very contradictory. It has one great disadvantage: the retro-bulbar hemorrhage is generally profuse, and may produce such a degree of exophthalmos and such severe pain as to necessitate a subsequent enucleation. The operation cannot be regarded as a certain preventive of sympathetic ophthalmia, for the ciliary nerves may be already in a state of irritation posterior to the eye; a condition of affairs very familiar to all ophthalmic surgeons, as existing often in the stump after enucleation. This irritable condition of the stump necessitates an excision of as long a piece as may be reached, and if the eye were still in place, enucleation would first be necessary before the irritable stump could be seized and excised. The operation of optico-ciliary neurotomy has not yet had a sufficiently extensive trial to enable us to judge of it fairly.

The tenotomy of one of the straight muscles is not a necessary step in the operation. The optic and ciliary nerves may be divided through a wound in the conjunctiva between the superior and internal recti muscles and parallel to the corneal margin, by means of a pair of enucleation scissors with long blades.

During the last two years the literature of optico-ciliary neurotomy and neurectomy has become very extensive. Dianoux recommends dividing the conjunctiva and capsule of Tenon between the internal and the inferior recti, and then dividing the tissues next the eye, as in strabotomy. He then introduces his little finger through the wound until he touches the optic nerve, and then divides this nerve and the ciliary nerves on his finger as a guide. He next denudes the posterior part of the eye with scissors, and then closes with a simple dressing. Abadie advises opening the conjunctiva on the outside, divides the tendon of the external rectus, rotates the eye inwards, and divides the optic nerve and ciliary nerves with great care. The eye is then replaced and the muscle stitched in place again. Both Dianoux and Abadie claim that the operation itself is not severe; that the eye preserves its mobility, nutrition, shape, and transparency; and that the pain and irritation being stopped, all sympathetic or reflex action is also arrested or prevented. Girard–Teulon, in reviewing the subject, rejects these claims as valueless. Knapp thinks it possible that the severed ciliary nerves may reunite, and that the sensibility of the cornea should be tested not only immediately after the operation, but also months and even years afterwards, in order to see whether the nervous conduction has remained permanently interrupted.

The worst feature in the operation is the partial or total return of the corneal sensibility. In this regard, Redard's experiments upon animals are interesting. He found that after complete section of all the ciliary nerves, the cornea immediately loses its transparent and glistening appearance, and becomes insensible, and the pupil dilates. The circulation of the optic disk is interfered with and the vision is diminished. The dilatation of the pupil lasts for five or six months. The corneal sensibility returns towards the end of the third month. The cornea frequently becomes perforated, the iris prolapses, and the eyeball rapidly atrophies. Meyer employs the division of the ciliary and optic nerves for cases of neurosis only. He believes in neurectomy rather than in neurotomy. His mode of operating consists in dividing the tendons of the external and internal recti muscles, and also of the two oblique. The fibrous capsule of the globe being then completely detached, he divides and exsects the optic and ciliary nerves, and then reattaches the tendons of the divided muscles. It should be remembered, however, that there are two or three direct ciliary nerves which penetrate the anterior portion of the sclera beneath the recti muscles, and which might remain unsevered by the usual optico-ciliary neurotomy. Krause has examined the ciliary nerves after optico-ciliary neurotomy, and found the nerves in the retro-bulbar tissue normal. The intra-ocular nerves began to be regenerated at the point of division. He does not believe that the central and peripheral ends of the divided nerves unite directly, because the immediate peripheral end undergoes degeneration. The regenerated nerve-fibres were at first small in size and few in number, but eventually they pursue the same course as the original fibres, and in some cases attained the size of the normal ciliary nerves.

On the assumption that the nerves of the cornea are derived in part from the conjunctival nerves, Wadsworth ventures to suppose that in some cases, after division of the ciliary nerves, an increased development of the branches from the conjunctiva occurs. On the other hand, he admits that, if the corneal nerves are derived partly from the conjunctiva, it is difficult to understand how the whole cornea could remain anæsthetic for a long time or even permanently, when only a limited portion of the connection between conjunctiva and cornea has been severed by the operation.

("Bull. et mém. Soc. de chir.," Jan. 5, 1880. "Arch. of Ophth.," ix. 1 and 2. "Roy. Lond. Ophth. Hosp. Rep.," August, 1880. "La France médicale," Aug. 14, 1880. "La Progrés médicale," Sept. 11, 1880; Dec. 25, 1880. "Arch. of Ophth.," ix. 4. "Trans. Amer. Ophth. Soc.," 1880. "Roy. Lond. Ophth. Hosp. Rep.," x. 2. "Arch. für Ophthal.," xxvii. 1. "Klin. Monatsblätter für Augenheilk.," August, 1881; and "Beiträge für 1881." "Trans. Amer. Ophth. Soc.," 1881. Also a long and interesting paper by Knies, in the "Beitr. zur Ophth. als Festgabe Friedrich Horner," Wiesbaden, 1881.)

If sympathetic inflammation has once begun, and the question of the removal of the injured eye has been decided, it remains to determine what are the means at our command for allaying the inflammation in the second eye. These are unfortunately very few. In addition to the frequent, steady, and long-continued use of atropia, hot applications are always agreeable and often beneficial. Leeches or Heurteloup's apparatus, applied to the temple every second or third day, are very often useful. Most observers strongly recommend a thorough course of mercurial treatment, pushed to rapid salivation, with frequent recurrence to the use of the drug. In some cases this no doubt does good, but in many cases it exerts no appreciable beneficial effect upon the disease, and in some instances does positive harm. No operation should, under any circumstances, be done during the height of the inflammation, for it would inevitably increase the trouble. After months, or perhaps years, an operation may be done for artificial pupil provided the quantitative perception of light is good, and the globe not markedly atrophied. The operation should combine the extraction of the lens with the removal of a broad piece of iris, membraniform exudation, and lens-capsule. If this space closes again by exudation, no operative interference should be attempted until the eye is perfectly quiet, and then an iridotomy may be done.

(Mauthner's "Die Sympathischen Augenleiden," 1878 and 1879. "Graefe und Saemisch's Hdb. der Augenheilkunde," iv. pp. 520–530. Carter's "Treatise on Diseases of the Eye," 1876. Nettleship's "Guide to Diseases of the Eye," 1880.)—B.]

CHAPTER VII.

DISEASES OF THE CHOROID.

HYPERÆMIA OF THE CHOROID.

A HYPERÆMIC condition of the choroid is by no means so easy to diagnose with the ophthalmoscope as is often asserted; indeed, it is frequently quite impossible to do so. On the other hand, the epithelial layer of the choroid may be so dense as completely to hide the choroidal vessels; on the other, the diversities, both in the amount and distribution of the pigment in the stroma of the choroid, are so various, as often to render it quite impossible to decide whether or not there is any hyperæmia. It is especially difficult, if both eyes present the same appearances, for we then lose the opportunity of comparing the affected with the healthy eye. Hyperæmia of the choroid may be suspected, if we notice at one portion of the fundus, that the size and redness of the choroidal vessels, more especially of the smaller branches, seem to be increased, so that the intra-vascular spaces appear encroached upon and somewhat crowded together; and more particularly if these symptoms have come on rather rapidly. The disk may also look somewhat flushed and hyperæmic. The external symptoms (*e. g.*, ciliary injection, dilated and tortuous ciliary veins, etc.) which have often been quoted as being indicative of hyperæmia of the choroid, are quite unreliable.

[CHOROIDITIS.

It is by no means easy to separate the pathological processes in the choroid from those in the retina, because of the close relation of the two membranes. Hence it is often necessary to employ the term chorio-retinitis or retino-choroiditis to describe the process going on in the posterior segment of the eyeball. It is, perhaps, well to distinguish the varieties of inflammation in the choroid, as has been done with the iris, viz.: 1st. Serous choroiditis; 2d. Plastic choroiditis; 3d. Parenchymatous or suppurative choroiditis. Various subdivisions of these three main varieties of inflammation are in common use, which will be considered under the proper heads.—B.]

1.—SEROUS CHOROIDITIS.

We may distinguish two principal forms of serous choroiditis, the one constituting acute inflammatory glaucoma, which will be described in the chapter on "Glaucoma;" the other is more simple in its course, and involves the tissues to a far less extent. In the latter form, there are generally hardly any symptoms of irritation, the eyeball being perhaps only very slightly injected, without any photophobia, lachrymation, or spontaneous pain. But the sight is often greatly impaired, on account of the diffuse cloudiness of the vitreous humor, in which may also be noticed, here and there, a few delicate, filiform opacities, or these may assume a firmer and more membranous character. The vitreous opacities, moreover, do not disappear with such rapidity or completeness as in the acute inflammatory glaucoma, but implicate the structure of the vitreous humor (producing synchysis) to a more considerable extent, destroying its septa, and causing relaxation, or even dissolution, of the zonula of Zinn, which is followed by a more or less considerable displacement of the lens (Von Graefe). Symptoms of serous iritis often supervene in the course of the disease; the iris becomes slightly discolored, the pupil somewhat dilated and perhaps slightly adherent, the aqueous humor is secreted in larger quantity and becomes clouded, having small particles of lymph suspended in it, or deposited on the posterior surface of the cornea, and generally assuming a pyramidal arrangement. The state of the intra-ocular tension varies considerably; in some cases it remains normal, or may gradually diminish, the eye becoming softer and softer, and finally atrophic. In other instances we find that, together with an increase in the cloudiness of the vitreous and aqueous humors, the eye-tension augments, or undergoes marked fluctuations. If this increase becomes persistent, glaucomatous complications may soon supervene. Von Graefe[1] thinks that this depends partly upon the age of the patient, and partly on the fact whether the lens is somewhat displaced or not. In simple serous choroiditis or choroido-iritis, we find that when the vitreous and aqueous humors have again become transparent, hardly any (if any) changes in the choroid are to be detected with the ophthalmoscope; and even in the severe forms they are but slight and generally limited to the equatorial region. But there is often noticed a punctated opacity of the posterior pole of the lens.[2]

The treatment of the simpler forms of serous choroiditis must consist chiefly in the application of atropine, of a blister behind the ear, or the artificial leech to the temple; and the eye should be kept perfectly at rest, and guarded against exposure to cold or bright light. Derivatives acting on the skin and kidneys often prove useful, as also the administration of the iodide of potassium, which hastens the absorption of the vitreous opacities. If the eye-tension is increased, paracentesis is to be performed, and repeated, perhaps several times, at intervals of three or four days. Von Graefe recommends that the needle should be extremely fine, and that the puncture should not be made in the sclero-corneal junction, but in the cornea, about one line from its margin, in order to avoid the risk of an adhesion of the iris to the inner wound. Even if secondary glaucoma supervenes, repeated paracentesis may be tried, but if it proves of no avail, iridectomy should be performed. In those very obstinate cases, in which the tension becomes again increased in spite of the iridectomy, and repeated paracentesis does not permanently diminish it, a second iridectomy, in an opposite direction to the first, will be indicated.

---

[1] "A. f. O.," xv. 3, 166.

[2] Von Graefe calls attention to the fact (l. c. p. 168) that eyes affected with posterior polar cataract, but which do not show the slightest traces of any affection of the vitreous, are not unfrequently attacked by secondary glaucoma. He believes that in such cases these lenticular opacities are the residue of a former choroiditis which leaves such eyes, even after the apparent termination of the original disease, very subject to an insidious latent form of inflammation of the choroid; which, if opportunity serves, manifests itself and gives rise to secondary glaucoma. The peculiar vulnerability which exists in eyes affected with posterior polar cataract (and which manifests itself especially in the great and exceptional reaction after any operation), he is also inclined to attribute to a persistent state of irritation of the choroid.

2.—PLASTIC CHOROIDITIS (Plate II., Fig. 4).

[Most modern authorities speak of three varieties of plastic choroiditis, viz.: 1st. Choroiditis disseminata simplex; 2d. Choroiditis areolaris; 3d. Chorio-retinitis circumscripta or centralis; and a fourth—chorio-retinitis disseminata syphilitica—is sometimes added.—B.]

When this disease is at all advanced, it presents most characteristic and striking ophthalmoscopic appearances, which cannot fail to arrest the attention of the most superficial observer. But in the earliest stages it may easily be overlooked, more especially if it commences, as is very frequently the case, in the form of small circumscribed exudations, situated quite at the periphery of the fundus. These little, round, grayish-white spots of exudation vary much in size and shape. In some cases they may not be larger than a millet-seed, in others they attain a considerable magnitude. The larger ones are, however, generally met with in the centre of the fundus. The exudations occur both on the inner surface of the choroid and in its stroma. They are of a dull, whitish-yellow, or creamy tint; the epithelium around them being either normal, or but slightly thinned. At a later stage the exudations become absorbed, and the choroid perhaps undergoes some atrophic changes, becoming thinned and permitting the white sclerotic to shine through, which gives a peculiarly white and glistening appearance to the patch. On the expanse of the latter, we may also sometimes be able to trace the outlines of the faint choroidal vessels which traverse it. Around these atrophic patches the epithelium does not retain its normal appearance, but its cells proliferate, increase in size, and contain a great quantity of pigment, which becomes collected around the margin of the white figure, in the form of a more or less broad, irregular, black girdle. The individual exudations often increase in size and coalesce one with another, thus giving rise to larger patches, which finally attain, perhaps, a considerable magnitude. From the periphery of the fundus, the disease extends more and more towards the posterior pole of the eye, so that at last the whole background of the eye may be thickly studded with innumerable white or yellowish-white patches of varying size and shape surrounded by a deep black fringe, and perhaps divided from each other by strips of healthy choroid. In such cases we often have an excellent opportunity of watching side by side the various changes which the exudations undergo; from their first appearance, as opaque, creamy-white spots, surrounded by unchanged epithelium, to the last stage of glistening-white, atrophic patches, embraced by a deep black circlet of pigment.

In other cases the disease commences in the region of the yellow spot, sometimes in its very centre. One or more small specks are noticed, the centre of which is of a paler red than the surrounding choroid; or the patch may be of a grayish-white or creamy color, with perhaps a faint, pale-red areola round it. The choroid in the region of the yellow spot is generally in such cases of a somewhat deeper tint. The white spots soon increase in number and size, are arranged perhaps in groups, and gradually extend towards their circumference. The periphery of the choroid may remain unaffected, or show only a few scattered groups of exudation.

Although we cannot with certainty diagnose the syphilitic character of the disease simply by the ophthalmoscopic symptoms, as we find that sometimes the most varied forms of this affection are due to syphilis, yet some authors consider that certain appearances are more especially symptomatic of the specific disseminated choroiditis. Thus Liebreich thinks that the latter is distinguished by the fact that the little masses of exudation are small, circumscribed, isolated, and do not show any tendency to coalesce, even when they are grouped closely together. The tissue changes extend deeply into the stroma of the choroid. These appearances are well illustrated in the ophthalmoscopic plate (Plate II., Fig. 4). Von Graefe thinks that syphilitic disseminated choroiditis shows itself most frequently in the form of numerous circumscribed white patches, with a pale-red zone round them, and occurring at the posterior pole of the eye; and which but rarely pass over into any other form of choroiditis. I have also found this form of choroiditis more frequently associated with syphilis than any other. But yet, it must be admitted that the disease may assume most varying appearances. Thus I have seen cases of syphilitic choroiditis in which a large bluish-gray exudation has occupied the region of the yellow spot, and around this were scattered to a considerable distance numerous smaller exudations and atrophic patches, the periphery of the fundus being almost free from any exudations. These appearances (more especially the gray, nebulous effusion) at the yellow spot were almost identical in both eyes.

[In syphilitic choroiditis there is said to be a peculiar dust-like punctate opacity of the vitreous, which at first is movable, but later the particles become aggregated into masses of irregular shape and sometimes having thread-like processes. These opacities are sometimes so dense as to com-

[Fig. 137.

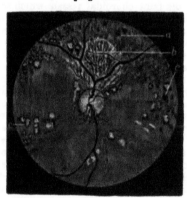

Atrophy after syphilitic choroiditis, showing various degrees of wasting. a. Atrophy of pigment epithelium. b. Atrophy of epithelium and chorio-capillaris; the large vessels exposed. c. Spots of complete atrophy, many with pigment accumulation. (Hutchinson.)—Nettleship.]

pletely conceal the fundus, and generally last for a long period. Where the retina can be seen, it is seen to be cloudy along the course of the vessels. There are no coarse changes in the choroid in this form of inflammation, according to Förster, unless the disease assume the form of simple choroiditis disseminata. It is usually a late manifestation of syphilis, though it may accompany an early iritis, and it often affects only one eye. It is probable that this is merely one stage of the chorio-retinitis disseminata with marked changes in the choroid. (See "Arch. f. Ophth.," xx. 1, p. 33; "Graefe und Saemisch," pp. 606 to 631.)—B.]

The *areolar choroiditis* of Förster[1] is distinguished by certain peculiar features, which show under what different forms the disseminated choroiditis may present itself. I would, therefore, rather consider it as a subdivision of this affection, than as a special disease. [The starting-point in this form of choroiditis seems to be the region of the macula and papilla. The patches first appear as masses of pigment, which grow thinner at the centre; the exudation makes its appearance; and the more this extends, the more the pigment is reduced in extent, till it forms a narrow border around the yellow exudation. In this disease, comparatively good central vision may exist for a long period, until suddenly it diminishes very rapidly and markedly without there being ophthalmoscopically any special cause for it.—B.] The spots are large, oval, or circular, sharply defined, and of a white or yellowish-white color, having traces of faintly marked choroidal vessels in their area. They are separated from each other here and there by strips of normal choroid. They are chiefly grouped around the yellow spot, but are divided from it by a portion of healthy choroid, so that they do not reach up to it. Their size varies considerably, some being nearly as large as the optic disk, others about the size of a pea: they always diminish, however, towards the periphery. The patches are surrounded by a dark zone of pigment, which is the more broad and marked the smaller the central white spot is. Quite at the periphery of the group of white patches are noticed dark-black spots, having no white centre.

[One form of choroiditis disseminata, which, though not so frequent as those hitherto described, is by no means rare, consists in single or conglomerate exudations from the vitreous lamina of the choroid. These nodules grow towards the retina, press it and push it aside, and occasionally become detached from the choroid, and are met with in the innermost layers of the retina. These are not met with near the macula or disk. Though in the beginning isolated, they may coalesce with each other and form "plaques." Clinically, this variety is of no importance.—B.]

The diagnosis of disseminated choroiditis is not difficult, and it could not very easily be mistaken for any other disease. The fact that the little white exudations are situated in the choroid, and not in the retina, may be easily ascertained by attention to the following points, viz., the retinal vessels can be traced distinctly over them, and are not the least interrupted or rendered indistinct in their course; there are no appearances of blood effusions into the retina, which generally occur together with exudations into the latter; the retina is also transparent, and of normal appearance around the exudations, and the retinal veins are not dilated or tortuous. When the exudations are absorbed and the choroid undergoes atrophy, the patches become fringed with pigment and upon their expanse can be noticed remains of the choroidal tissue and of the vessels. Care should be taken to distinguish this form of pigmentation, from the deposits of pigment in the retina which may occur in various forms of choroido-retinitis, as also in the disseminated choroiditis, in which the external layer of the retina becomes more or less glued against the choroid, and destroyed or atrophied, or the pigment of the epithelial layer of the choroid becomes infiltrated into the retina. In such cases, the rods and cones are especially apt to suffer, but the changes may extend deeper, and even involve the ganglion cells.

Again, the retina may suffer by becoming compressed by the exudations and aggregations of the pigment cells, and if this lasts for any length of time, the retina generally becomes thinned and atrophied, being changed

[1] Förster, "Ophthalmologische Beiträge," p. 99. Berlin, 1862.

into a kind of fibrillar tissue, and its normal elements rendered quite indistinguishable. Thus consecutive atrophy of the retina and optic nerve not unfrequently ensue upon disseminated choroiditis. In Plate II., Fig. 4, these appearances are illustrated. The optic disk is seen to be perfectly atrophied, of a bluish-gray tint, and utterly devoid of bloodvessels, excepting the two little twigs which can just be discerned running over its edge. Not a single retinal vessel can be distinguished over the whole fundus. It is but very seldom that we meet with so extreme a case of atrophy, and Liebreich supposes that in all probability a syphilitic retinitis had coexisted with the disseminated choroiditis.

The vitreous humor also frequently becomes affected during the progress of the disease; indeed floating or fixed opacities in it are sometimes the first, or even the only, premonitory symptoms, which call the patient's attention to his eye. I have met with several cases, in which a few small floating opacities in the vitreous humor formed the first symptom, there being at that time no trace of disseminated choroiditis to be detected by the most careful ophthalmoscopic examination. But some time afterwards, small circular patches made their appearance in the choroid. Sometimes, however, the vitreous does not become affected till a late stage of the disease, and it may then be so diffusely clouded as to render the details of the fundus quite indistinct, or be traversed by large, dark, floating or fixed membranous filaments. Subsequently, a posterior polar cataract is often formed.

The iris sometimes becomes inflamed, but hardly ever to a considerable degree, there being only a few delicate adhesions, and very little alteration in the structure of the iris. The inflammation often assumes a serous character, and small opacities are noticed on the posterior wall of the cornea. The external appearance of the eye is generally quite normal; there is hardly any conjunctival or subconjunctival injection, photophobia, or lachrymation, and little or no pain; the pupil being often of a normal size, or but little dilated; and yet the sight may be greatly impaired; and it is only with the ophthalmoscope that we detect the great and striking changes in the fundus.

The sight is often very considerably affected, the patient complaining of a dark cloud, or of black, fixed, and floating objects before his eyes. These scotomata are either due to diffuse and floating opacities in the vitreous humor, or to injuries which the retina has sustained by compression or destruction of some of its elements. The impairment of vision will, of course, be proportionately greater, if the disease is situated at the posterior pole of the eye, than if it be confined to the periphery of the fundus. In the former situation, a very small and circumscribed group of exudations may suffice to destroy central vision; in the latter, even considerable deposits may not materially affect the sight, except in the outline of the field. Not only does the central vision suffer as regards distinctness, when the exudations occur in the region of the yellow spot, but the objects appear distorted and crooked (metamorphopsia), on account of the compression and alteration in the arrangement of the retinal elements. We sometimes notice a marked improvement in the sight, when the exudations are absorbed and the pressure diminished, but, of course, this can only occur if the retinal elements have not suffered too much, or for too long a period.

The field of vision is frequently considerably contracted, and shows more or less extensive interruptions (scotomata) within its area. [With the appearance of the scotomata, may be noticed in many cases hemeralopia; that is, the patient's vision fails when the light fails. Micropsia is another common symptom, which may be explained by the metamorphopsia above alluded to. According to Förster, the range of accommodation is also limited;

23

though it would be difficult to ascertain this fact, owing to the dis
of vision.   Glittering scotomata are also complained of by patie
describe them as bluish-yellow or reddish-yellow spots, which dan
like the particles of the atmosphere over a hot surface.   These a
are a species of photopsia.—B.]

The *prognosis* of the disease must always be extremely guarde
especially if the exudations appear in the region of the yellow s
these, the little spots surrounded by a pale-red rim, which are so cl
istic of syphilis, afford comparatively the best prognosis.

In the most favorable cases the exudations may become absorbed,
behind them only faint traces of a change in the epithelial layer, in
of light-red patches, in which the choroidal vessels can be distinctly
or they may give rise to somewhat deeper cicatrices.   More frequent
ever, they produce extensive atrophy of the stroma of the choroid,
especially apt to be injurious to the sight if the exudations are large,
in the region of the yellow spot, and coalesce together, so as to forn
sive atrophic patches.   Moreover, in forming our prognosis, we mus
bear in mind that the retina is very prone to suffer, both from dir
pression of its elements and from their destruction (more especially
and bulbs) by their becoming glued to the choroid, and pigment bei
trated thence into the retina.   Atrophies of the retina and optic ne
therefore, not unfrequent consequences of disseminated choroiditis.

The causes of this disease are often obscure, but by far the most :
is syphilis.   The insidious choroiditis, which is accompanied by sero
is sometimes observed in delicate, scrofulous, or consumptive individ

The *treatment* must consist chiefly in the administration of me
Indeed, the inflammatory diseases of the choroid appear to be most
cially influenced by small doses (one-twentieth or one-sixteenth of a g
or three times daily) of the bichloride of mercury, continued for a v
period.   If there are distinct evidences of syphilis, and if the disease
in its progress, salivation should be quickly induced, so as, if possible,
the further effusion of lymph and hasten the absorption of that alr
uded.   If this be not done, larger doses of the bichloride, in combinati
the iodide of potassium, should be given.   The artificial leech shoul
plied occasionally; but, if the patient is very feeble, but little blood
be taken, or dry cupping should be substituted.   He must be strictly
to abstain from all use of the eyes in reading, etc., and they sh
guarded against bright light by the employment of dark glasses.
functions of the liver, uterus, or digestive organs are out of orde
should be attended to; and much benefit is often experienced from
of mildly purgative mineral waters, such as Pullna, Marienbad, K
etc.   [The frequent employment of the Turkish bath, or a thorougl
of Zittmann's decoction, or the hypodermatic injection of the hydro
of pilocarpine, are all remedies of great value in this disease.—B.]

3.—SCLERECTASIA POSTERIOR (SCLEROTICO-CHOROIDITIS I RIOR, POSTERIOR STAPHYLOMA). Plate II., Fig. 3.

[The process which leads to the formation of a posterior staphy
different from the process which is at work in an anterior sclerectasia.
an inflammatory process is generally at the bottom of an anterior
loma of the sclera, in the development of a posterior sclerectasia it i
ally conspicuous by its absence.—B.]

This disease is but seldom absent in the more considerable degrees of myopia, and must be regarded as a grave complication.

Eyes affected with sclerectasia posterior generally appear to be abnormally large, prominent, and ovoid in shape. The palpebral aperture is widely open, which is especially conspicuous if only one eye is affected. [These pronounced signs are only present when the posterior staphyloma is very highly developed.—B.] The eyeball also appears lengthened in its antero-posterior diameter, and the infundibulum or hollow, which is seen in the normal eye (when it is much turned in) between the outer canthus and the globe, has disappeared; so that the posterior segment of the eyeball appears lengthened and square, and perhaps of a slightly bluish tint. The lateral movements of the eye may be somewhat curtailed if the disease is extensive. The patients often complain of a feeling of tension and fulness of the eyeball, as if the latter were too large for the socket, and there also may be pain in and around the eye.

The ophthalmoscopic symptoms are generally very marked and unmistakable. The characteristic symptom is a brilliant white or pale yellow crescent at the edge of the optic disk, generally at the outer side (in the reverse image it will, of course, appear towards the nasal side). This crescent may vary much in size, from a small white arc to a large zone, and extends perhaps all round the disk and embraces even the region of the yellow spot, its greatest extent being always in the direction of the latter.[1] Its edges may be either sharply and distinctly defined, or may be irregular, and partially lost in the surrounding healthy structures; irregular patches of pigment are strewn about its margin, and also, perhaps, on its surface, so that little dark islets of varying size and form appear in its expanse. The crescent itself is of a brilliant white, so much so indeed, that the disk, by contrast, appears to be abnormally pink. On account of the white background, the small retinal vessels can be traced more distinctly, and their minute branches be more easily followed, over this patch than in the neighboring fundus. This white crescent is due to a thinning and atrophy of the stroma of the choroid; indeed, the latter has occasionally been found quite wanting in this situation. The pigment cells are not necessarily destroyed, but there is an absence of pigment molecules, for the irregular black patches mentioned above are pathological agglomerations of pigment. On account of the loss of pigment and the atrophy or thinning of the stroma of the choroid, the glistening sclerotic shines through the latter, and lends the brilliant white appearance to the figure. This want of pigment also gives rise to the sense of glare, which the patient experiences in a bright light. The amblyopia which frequently exists in this disease, is also undoubtedly partly due to this fact, for we find that the sight of such patients is often remarkably benefited by blue spectacles. The amblyopia, however, as a rule, depends chiefly upon the disturbance in the intra-ocular circulation, produced by the state of chronic congestion of the venous system of the eye. Hence we find that vision is generally greatly improved by depletion, and more especially by the artificial leech.

The retina generally suffers only in so far from this loss of pigment in the

[1] We must, however, be careful not to call every little white rim at the edge of the disk "sclerectasia posterior," for this may be caused simply by the choroid receding somewhat from the optic nerve, and permitting the light to fall at this spot through the retina upon the denuded sclerotic, thus affording the appearance of a white glistening rim. But this arc is narrow, its edges are sharply defined, and there are no atrophic changes of the choroid around it. This condition may occur in myopic, emmetropic, and hypermetropic eyes.

processes may gradually extend towards each other (leaving less and less healthy structures between them, until they finally pass into each other, and form one large white figure.

The occurrence of inflammatory changes in the choroid and retina in the region of the yellow spot, generally causes great impairment of vision, and the patient also complains of the constant appearance of one or more central, fixed, dark spots (scotomata) in the field of vision. It should be mentioned that they may be apparent to the patient long before we are able to detect with the ophthalmoscope any changes in the region of the macula lutea.

Von Graefe[1] long ago called attention to the important fact that secondary glaucoma may supervene upon sclerectasia posterior, and lead to great impairment of vision, or even blindness, if the true character of the complication is not recognized sufficiently early and a timely iridectomy performed. It always attacks both eyes sooner or later. He states that this secondary glaucoma may either assume the character of glaucoma simplex, or that of the inflammatory form. Glaucoma simplex occurs chiefly in those cases of sclerectasia posterior in which inflammatory symptoms are absent, and all the tissues are normal, excepting, of course, as regards the changes produced by the elongation of the optic axis, and the attenuation of the sclerotic and choroid at the posterior hemisphere of the eyeball. If in such eyes glaucoma simplex supervenes, we find that the tension of the eyeball increases, the optic disk becomes excavated, the visual field impaired, and the sight deteriorated, but generally only after the field has already become greatly contracted; the refracting media, as a rule, remain transparent. According to Von Graefe, the glaucoma simplex would appear, in such cases, to be partly due to the advancing age of the patient, for then the sclerotic becomes firmer and less elastic, thus offering a greater resistance to the process of bulging (ectasia), which causes a tendency to retardation in the venous circulation, and also compresses and irritates the ciliary nerves which pass through it here. This tendency to glaucoma may also be hereditary, showing itself in several members of the same family. In such instances, the myopia has generally reached a considerable degree in childhood, and then, between the ages of twelve and eighteen years, glaucoma simplex supervenes. When, in middle age, the latter attacks eyes which are only moderately myopic, Von Graefe thinks that the combination is accidental.

Frequently, however, secondary glaucoma does not manifest itself in sclerectasia posterior until symptoms of sclerotico-choroiditis posterior have supervened, and then it mostly assumes the character of irido-choroiditis serosa, with periodic cloudiness of the aqueous humor, and effusions into the vitreous.

With regard to the excavation of the optic nerve which is met with in the cases of glaucoma complicating sclerectasia posterior, it must be observed that it does not always present the very marked features of the glaucomatous or pressure cup. This is especially the case if the atrophy of the choroid encircles the disk, for the steepness of the excavation will then be less evident, as also the bending of the vessels. Hence, as Von Graefe points out, we must consider every excavation in sclerectasia posterior as being glaucomatous in character, if the edge of the disk is tolerably distinctly cupped, if the larger veins show a difference in their fulness at its margin, and if, together with these symptoms, the eye-tension is increased, and there are corresponding functional disturbances in the eye (e. g., contraction of

[1] "A. f. O.," iv. 2, 153; ibid., viii. 2, 304. The reader should especially consult his last observations upon this point in the article recently published ("A. f. O.," xv. 3, 178).

the field).   In some of these cases the sight remains wonderfully good, considering the great contraction of the field, and we may find that when the
contraction has gradually extended from the inner side till it has nearly
reached the centre, it passes upwards and downwards, leaving the central
part unimpaired, to meet again on the other side, and thus a small islet of
the field may be left in the centre of the blank.

Sometimes the excavation is, so to speak, double, the margin of the disk
being cupped, and a second (perhaps steeper) excavation existing in the
sclerotic at a distance of from one-quarter to one-half millimetre from the
edge of the disk.   In other cases the excavation is extremely steep, presenting all the features of a very marked glaucomatous or pressure cup; one
peculiarity being that the sight remains relatively remarkably good.

Iridectomy must be performed as early as possible, for paracentesis proves
of no permanent relief.   It must be mentioned, however, that in some
instances, where the contraction of the field already encroaches closely on
the centre, the operation sometimes causes a deterioration of the sight (Von
Graefe).

Complications.—When inflammatory symptoms have supervened and the
disease has assumed the character of sclerotico-choroiditis posterior, the
vitreous humor often becomes clouded, and its posterior portion even perhaps
fluid or detached.   The vitreous opacities may be dark fixed specks, or floating membranous films of varying size and shape, and are often a source of
great anxiety to the patient, for even the physiological motes are rendered
very distinct in short-sighted eyes, on account of the circles of diffusion upon
the retina (*vide* article on "Opacities of the Vitreous Humor").   The most
dangerous form of opacity of the vitreous is that which comes on very suddenly, is confined to the posterior segment of the vitreous humor, uniform in
character, and sharply defined against the transparent vitreous.   It, moreover, shows a slight tendency to oscillate or tremble, and affords a faint gray
reflex, which may easily cause it to be mistaken for detachment of the retina,
until a close examination of its margins shows that the retina is in perfect
apposition with the choroid.   This form of opacity is generally the precursor
of detachment of the retina, and Von Graefe[1] thinks that the following
reasons speak for its being, in all probability, a detachment of the vitreous.
1. Its sudden appearance, whereas the majority of opacities of the vitreous,
with the exception of the hemorrhagic, are more gradual in their development.   2. Its sharply defined limitation, in spite of its considerable extent;
whereas we find that infiltrations of the vitreous of like magnitude generally
pass over gradually into the healthy portion of vitreous.   3. The almost
constant supervention of detachment of the retina.

In speaking of detachment of the vitreous I mention that Iwanoff had
observed it sometimes in sclerectasia posterior, and he thinks that in such
cases it is produced in the following manner:[2] "The vitreous humor does
not grow in proportion to the gradually increasing size of the eye, and the
serous exudation is not at the same time converted into the tissue constituting the vitreous humor, nor does it dissolve it, both remaining indifferent
to each other; the connection between the vitreous and retina becoming,
however, loosened, according to the amount of effusion.   Now in the space
which is thus formed between the vitreous and retina we find that, in proportion to the development of staphyloma, more and more serous effusion
is collected, detaching the vitreous more and more from the retina."

[1] "Kl. Monatsbl.," 1868, p. 301.   [2] "A. f. O.," xv. 2, 57.

Detachment of the retina is unfortunately another not unfrequent complication of the more considerable degrees of sclerotico-choroiditis posterior. Its extent may be at first but slight, and be produced by a serous or hemorrhagic effusion between the choroid and retina; or it may be caused by the contraction of some of the exudations in the vitreous humor exerting traction upon the retina, and thus detaching it[1] (*vide* article on "Detachment of Retina)."

Opacity at the posterior pole of the lens sometimes occurs in the later stages of the disease. The opacity is generally situated very close to the turning-point of the eye, and hence remains immovable when the eye is turned in a different direction. Cataracta accreta, irido-choroiditis, and atrophy of the globe may close the scene.

Causes.—The origin of the affection is still a matter of controversy. [In certain eyes, the insertion of the choroid around the optic nerve entrance is of such a nature that the capability of resistance of the choroid in cases of increasing extension of the growing eye, and in the varying tension of the coats of the eye in the developed organ, is less than it should be. In these eyes also the attachment of the sheath of the optic nerve deviates from the normal, and this influences the power of the resistance of the sclera. In such an eye the posterior staphyloma must be regarded either as the complete development of a congenital malformation, or as the result of a pathological process engrafted on a congenitally weak spot. A second factor which enters into the causation of a posterior staphyloma is an abnormal action of the external muscles of the eyeball. The insufficiency of the internal recti muscles, so often seen in progressive myopia with posterior staphyloma, postulates a previous straining of these muscles.—B.] Without doubt, there generally exists a congenital (and often hereditary) tendency to elongation of the eyeball in the optic axis; and this must necessarily cause a stretching and thinning of the sclerotic and choroid in this direction, which is generally soon followed by consecutive atrophy of the latter. The development of this prolongation of the optic axis is greatly favored by the strong convergence of the visual lines and the state of congestion of the eye which occur during accommodation for near objects, more particularly if these are small and insufficiently illuminated. For during such accommodation, a certain pressure upon the eye always occurs, accompanied by increased intra-ocular tension; in consequence of which, the venous circulation within the eye becomes retarded, and a more or less considerable state of mechanical congestion is produced. Instances of such intra-ocular congestion are furnished by cases of amblyopia due to opacities of the cornea or lens, in which the myopia is caused by the patient's bringing small objects very near to the eye, in order to gain larger retinal images. A similar thing may occur if the patient, whilst using concave spectacles for reading, gradually approaches the book too near to his eyes. We occasionally find that vitreous opacities, and even detachment of the retina, occur in such cases soon after long-continued reading or working with spectacles.

This state of congestion and increased pressure of the intra-ocular fluids leads to softening and extension of the tunics of the eyeball. As the latter receives no support at the posterior pole from the muscles, the prolongation occurs chiefly at this point, the choroid being stretched and generally undergoing consecutive atrophy. At a later stage symptoms of inflammation may arise, and the disease assume the character of sclerotico-choroiditis posterior. The changes in the choroid are then no longer simply due to extension of

---

[1] Heinrich Müller, "A. f. O.," vi, 1, 372.

the eyeball, but to inflammation. Small circumscribed patches of choroiditis appear at the margin of the original white figure, or show themselves in the form of choroido-retinitis in the region of the yellow spot, and the vitreous humor becomes clouded; so that we have in fact more or less pronounced symptoms of choroiditis.

This choroidal atrophy may, however, exist without any posterior staphyloma. Indeed, Schweigger states that a real staphyloma posticum, i. e., a more or less sharply defined local ectasia of the walls of the eyeball, does not take place in the majority of cases of myopia. The presence of a posterior staphyloma may be diagnosed by means of the ophthalmoscope, particularly with the binocular, for we then see that the white, shining portion of the sclerotic exposed through the thinning of the choroid is not of normal curvature, but is peculiarly cupped backwards, giving rise at this part to a slanting position of the optic disk. Schweigger, moreover, thinks that the acuteness of vision is diminished to an unusual degree in those cases of myopia in which posterior staphyloma exists beside the optic nerve. This is the more likely to happen, as he has observed that in cases in which the existence of a posterior staphyloma was proved anatomically, the retina in the expanse of the bulging portion was generally found to be more or less changed in structure, and even atrophied and adherent to the remains of the choroid and sclerotic. [The visible gaping of the intervaginal space of the optic nerve is a constant accompaniment of the development of a posterior staphyloma, and increases with the growth of the latter. This separation of the sheath, together with the necessary displacement of the posterior ciliary vessels, causes disturbances in the circulation in this region of the eyeball, and may explain why, in advanced posterior staphyloma, the optic nerve is so often partially atrophic.—B.]

When the sclerectasia and atrophy of the choroid are considerable, and the myopia high in degree, symptoms of irritation and inflammation almost always supervene. Donders[1] thinks, "that almost without exception, the predisposition to the development of staphyloma posticum exists at birth; that it is developed with symptoms of irritation, which, in moderate degrees of staphyloma, do not attain any great clinical importance; but that in the higher degrees an inflammatory state almost always occurs, at least at a somewhat more advanced time of life, as a result, and as a coöperative cause of the development of the distention and of the atrophy."

Jaeger[2] considers that this crescent or posterior staphyloma, as he terms it, is almost always congenital and often hereditary. It may, indeed, exist for many years, or even throughout life, without increasing in size, or without the occurrence of any choroidal changes in its vicinity, its margin remaining distinctly and sharply defined. But we more frequently find, if the eyes are much used and the myopia increases at all considerably in degree, that the edge of the crescent becomes somewhat irregular and broken, and gradually increases in size; this being evidently due to inflammatory changes in the choroid.

Prognosis.—This should be always very guarded when the disease is at all advanced, when the myopia is progressive, and when the opacities in the vitreous humor are considerable. It becomes still more questionable if the vitreous opacities are diffuse, or large and numerous, if the upper or lower portion of the visual field becomes clouded, which is premonitory or symptomatic of detachment of the retina; and, lastly, if the choroidal changes

[1] "Annals of Refraction and Accommodation," p. 384.
[2] Ueber die Einstellungen des Dioptrischen Apparatus in Menschlichen Auge." 1861, 8vo., S. 252.

their appearance in the region of the macula lutea. They show them-
in the form of small, isolated whitish spots, around the edges of which
are little accumulations of pigment ; these small whitish spots increase
te, and coalesce, and then the atrophy of the choroid becomes very
rent. During this process, the retina is more or less irritated, and this
ices dimness of vision, which, however, disappears again when the retinal
tion subsides. These atrophic changes in the region of the yellow spot
rise to fixed black spots in the visual field, which, if considerable, may
ir working at small objects impossible. The alterations in the macula
generally commence first in one eye, and may for a time be confined
but sooner or later they mostly extend also to the other eye.

eatment.—Patients suffering from sclerotico-choroiditis posterior should
articularly warned against working for any length of time at near
ts, or with their head bent forward, for intra-ocular venous congestion
is easily produced. It is also very injurious to read in a recumbent
ion. The best posture for reading is, to sit with the head thrown back,
o have the light falling on the book from behind, so that the page may
all illuminated, but the eye not exposed to the direct glare of the light.
riting, it is advantageous to use a sloping desk, so that the person need
oop. If such persons are permitted the use of spectacles for reading
vriting, we must particularly point out the danger of bringing the object
ear when the eye becomes somewhat fatigued, as this will cause a strain
accommodation. The work or book should then be laid aside, until
es have been thoroughly rested. In extreme cases, we should strictly
l all work at near objects, either with or without spectacles.

e irritation of the retina which gives rise to the appearance of flashes
lored light, or showers of bright stars, etc., is best relieved by the
ation of flying blisters to the temple or behind the ear. They may be
advantage repeated at intervals of six or eight days.

e feeling of glare and dazzling, of which many of these patients com-
when they are in a bright light, and which often produces severe
y neuralgia and headache, is effectually alleviated by the use of blue
icles.

he inflammatory changes in the choroid are at all considerable or
ssive, we should always prescribe a prolonged course of small doses
bichloride of mercury (one-sixteenth or one-twentieth of a grain).
atives acting on the skin and kidneys, and hot stimulating foot-baths
ht, also prove beneficial.

he eye is very irritable, the external tunics of the eyeball injected, the
disk reddened and hyperæmic, and if the patient experiences pain in
round the eye, together with a feeling of weight and heaviness in the
ll, as if he can hardly keep his eyelids open, we must insist upon a
lete rest of the eyes, and an absolute cessation, for some length of time,
all working at near objects. We must be extremely stringent in the
rcement of such directions, as the patients are apt to resume work as
as their eyes feel a little better, and then at once to call up again all
mptoms of irritation and congestion, which may cause a rapid increase
e myopia and of any existing sclerotico-choroiditis posterior. Such
are also much benefited by the use of stimulating lotions to the closed
nd its vicinity, by the eye-douche, and by the application of the arti-
leech. If there is any spasm of the ciliary muscle, atropine must be
dically employed. The artificial leech generally relieves the irritation
eye and the peculiar and very distressing feeling of heaviness and
g in the eyeball, when all other forms of treatment have proved of no

avail. But when the disease is very considerable, and when there is any fear of a detachment of the retina, its use is often dangerous, for the sudden relief of the intra-ocular circulation is followed by severe reaction, and temporary hyperæmia of the vessels of the choroid and retina; and hence an effusion of blood may take place and produce detachment of the retina.

4.—[PARENCHYMATOUS OR METASTATIC CHOROIDITIS.—B.] SUPPURATIVE CHOROIDITIS. (PANOPHTHALMITIS.)

The course of this disease is generally very rapid and severe. It commences in the form of an acute and violent inflammation of the eye. The eyelids become very swollen, red, and œdematous, the upper lid hanging down in a large massive fold. The conjunctiva and subconjunctival tissue become injected, and there is a considerable, firm gelatinous chemosis, which surrounds the cornea like a dusky-red girdle, and perhaps protrudes between the aperture of the eyelids when they are slightly opened. A thin muco-purulent discharge oozes out between the lids, but sometimes it is absent, and the edges of the lids and the chemotic swelling look dry and crusted. On opening the eye, we may find that the cornea is quite clear, but the anterior chamber is diminished in size; and occupied, perhaps, by a more or less considerable hypopyon; the aqueous humor is clouded, the iris pushed forward, discolored, and of a yellowish hue; the pupil is sometimes dilated, in other cases it is of a normal size or slightly contracted and tied down by lymph, or its area occluded. The tension is often increased, and the eye is acutely sensitive to the touch; it is also prominent and its movements are greatly impeded, on account of the infiltration into the subconjunctival tissue. If the refractive media and the pupil are sufficiently clear, we observe a peculiar yellowish, golden reflex from behind the lens, in the anterior portion of the vitreous humor, which is due to a purulent infiltration of the latter. The retina may become infiltrated with serum, or undergo suppurative changes, and the latter also extensively affect the choroid and ciliary body. The changes cannot be seen with the ophthalmoscope, on account of the exudation into the pupil, or the opaque condition of the vitreous humor. There is often a serous effusion from the choroid, which causes either a circumscribed or complete detachment of the retina, or this may be produced by hemorrhagic effusion from the choroid. Moreover, it must be remembered that, together with this pressure of serum or blood behind the retina, the contraction and shrinking of the exudations in the vitreous humor, and the consequent traction upon the retina from in front, tend to produce a very extensive detachment, generally of a funnel shape. Indeed, although the detachment may for a time remain partial and circumscribed, it almost always becomes complete as the disease advances.

The cornea may remain transparent throughout; but as a rule, it becomes clouded, infiltrated with pus, and then gives way, shrivelling up into a little yellowish membrane, like wash-leather; or it may remain entire, and a spontaneous perforation of the eyeball occur through the sclerotic, generally at or between the insertion of the recti muscles. The disease is mostly accompanied by very intense pain in and around the eye, which often extends over the corresponding side of the head and face. It is frequently most agonizing, until the eyeball perforates, or paracentesis is performed, on which it rapidly subsides. There are often also marked febrile symptoms, accompanied, perhaps, by severe vomiting. In other cases, the inflammatory symptoms and the pain are far less pronounced, and the whole course of the disease is more insidious and of a milder type, although its results may be just as disastrous. The sight becomes rapidly and very greatly impaired, so that the patient may only be just able to distinguish between light and dark, or not even this. He is, moreover, much troubled by subjective flashes of light, showers of bright stars, etc.

Among the most frequent causes of suppurative choroiditis are injuries[1] and wounds of the eye, and the lodgement of foreign bodies, more especially portions of gun-cap or metal, within the eyeball, particularly in the ciliary region and vitreous humor; such cases being often accompanied by very severe inflammatory symptoms and intense pain. Although foreign bodies may remain for a length of time suspended in the vitreous humor without doing much harm, or may become surrounded by lymph, and be thus encysted or encapsulated, yet this is only of very exceptional and rare occurrence, more particularly if they are considerable in size, and of a nature to set up irritation by undergoing chemical changes. Inflammation of the vitreous humor supervenes, extending to the retina and choroid, and the eye becomes destroyed by plastic irido-choroiditis, or suppurative panophthalmitis.

The disease may also ensue upon operations, such as those for the removal of cataract, either by extraction, or still more frequently after couching (vide the article upon "Cataract"). It occurs most frequently in old and decrepit individuals, or in instances in which the patients are exposed after the operation to bad ventilation, overcrowded rooms, or other influences which impair the purity of the air (pyæmia in a hospital, typhoid fever, etc.). It is an interesting and important fact, that eyes operated upon for chronic irido-choroiditis show very little tendency indeed to take on suppurative inflammation, even although the lens may have been removed, together with a portion of the iris and dense masses of exudation. Indeed, such eyes bear a great deal of operative interference with impunity.

Suppurative inflammation of the cornea and iris (as, for instance, in purulent and diphtheritic conjunctivitis) may also be followed by panophthalmitis.

It may likewise be produced by a direct extension of the inflammation from the meninges to the eye, as in cases of typhus, cerebro-spinal meningitis, etc.; but it may also in such instances be due to metastasis, examples of which are not unfrequently seen in puerperal fever. A very short time after the occurrence of the embolism suffices to set up secondary metastatic foci of disease in even distant organs. According to O. Weber,[2] two days will suffice for this. This metastatic form of the disease may either assume a very severe and acutely inflammatory type, rapidly leading to suppurative disorganization of the globe; or it may run a more insidious but equally destructive course. It is chiefly met with in cerebro-spinal meningitis, puerperal fever and pyæmia; and then almost invariably attacks both eyes.[3] In a case of double metastatic choroiditis in a puerperal woman, reported by Hosch, the microscope showed the vitreous of each eye filled with leptothrix fibres, showing the abundant development of a fungoid growth. There were also great numbers of micrococci in the retinal vessels, which corresponded exactly with the fungous thrombi found in other septic processes. The rapid development of pus through the entire retina, uveal tract, vitreous,

[1] Vide Arlt's "Bericht der Wiener Augenklinik," 1867.
[2] Billroth, "Handbuch der Chirurgie."
[3] Vide Dr. Knapp's article on "Metastatic Choroiditis," "Archiv f. O.," xiii. 1, 127; also Dr. Wilson's paper on "Diseases of the Eye in Cerebro-spinal Meningitis," "Dub. Quart. Journ.," May, 1867 [also "Amer. Journ. Med. Sci.," January, 1878].

cornea, and lens, he regards as due to the diapedesis of the white-blood corpuscles under the influence of infectious substances in the blood, which act
upon the vascular walls. It has also been met with in inflammation of the
umbilical cord in the new-born child, in scarlet fever, smallpox, malignant
pustule, phlegmonous erysipelas, and cholera. Schmidt-Rimpler has seen it
in rheumatism without cardiac complication, and in general tuberculosis.[1]—
B.] According to some writers, an important symptom, as showing the implication of the eye in cases of meningitis, cerebro-spinal meningitis, or
thrombus of a cerebral sinus, etc., is œdema of the conjunctiva, eyelids, and
orbital cellular tissue, accompanied by more or less considerable exophthalmos. This fact, which shows the direct connection between the ocular
and cerebral affection, has assumed special interest and importance since
Schwalbe has found that fluid injected into the arachnoid space passes (by
the lymph paths) through the optic foramen into the capsule of Tenon, orbit,
and also between the sheaths of the optic nerve. These experiments of
Schwalbe, as well as those of Schmidt and Manze, will be referred to in the
chapter upon the optic nerve. From these researches it appears that the connection between the cerebral and ocular affection is, as Berthold[2] has lately
pointed out, as follows: He believes—" 1. That the affection of the eye in the
different forms of meningitis is due to an extension of the inflammation of the
meninges to the eyeball. 2. That this extension of the inflammation occurs
through the optic canal by means of the lymph paths. 3. According to the
intensity of the inflammation and the exudations poured out by it into the
lymph spaces of the eye, there is either a filling of the capsule of Tenon
accompanied by conjunctival chemosis, or a filling of the subvaginal space
(between the two sheaths of the optic nerve), causing engorged papilla or
optic neuritis; or again, in the severest cases there is suppurative inflammation of the retina and vitreous. 4. The iritis and irido-choroiditis occurring
in meningitis are always consecutive." It is a question whether it may not,
in cerebro-spinal meningitis, be sometimes due to the exposure of the cornea
to injuries, on account of the great lagophthalmos.

Dr. Estlander[3] describes the choroiditis which is met with in relapsing
fever, and generally occurs from the second to the fourth week. The first
symptom is a more or less diffuse cloudiness of the vitreous humor, which
veils the details of the fundus oculi, and then floating or fixed opacities
appear. Generally iritis supervenes, posterior synechiæ are formed, and at
a later stage hypopyon and chemosis. He considers the disease to be an inflammation of the ciliary body due to a disturbance in the nutrition of the
eye, which is produced by the changes in the blood in this kind of fever;
and points out that it is quite different from the suppurative, metastatic
choroiditis, which is observed in severe cases of typhus and is due to embolism.

The *prognosis* of suppurative choroiditis is most unfavorable, for this is
one of the most destructive and intractable diseases of the eye. It is but
seldom that we can arrest its progress in time to save any useful degree of
sight. In most cases it soon ends in atrophy of the eyeball, either with or
without a previous perforation of the cornea or sclerotic and escape of some
of the contents of the eye. The dangerous nature of the disease is especially
terrible in cases of metastatic choroiditis, for instance in puerperal fever, or
cerebro-spinal meningitis, as both eyes are generally affected, and then, if

[1 "Graefe und Saemisch," iv. p. 633.]
[2 "A. f. O.," xvi, 1, 169; *vide* also articles by Schmidt, "A. f. O.," xviii. 1, 18, and
by Michel, ib., p. 127.
[3 "A. f. O.," xv. 2, 108.

the patient should survive, it will be only to pass his days in utter blindness. But in some cases, the danger is not confined to the loss of sight, for even life may become imperilled, as Von Graefe has shown, by the extension of the suppurative inflammation to the brain, there setting up suppurative meningitis, which may prove fatal.

After perforation of the cornea or sclerotic has taken place, the intense pain and inflammatory symptoms generally at once subside to a very considerable degree. The eye diminishes in size, and gradually becomes shrivelled up and changed into a small contracted stump, which, as a rule, does not remain painful, and is not prone to give rise to sympathetic inflammation, except indeed it contains a foreign body, which keeps up a considerable degree of irritation, and is always a source of danger to the other eye. Sometimes, however, the eye retains a certain size and consistence, not becoming more completely atrophied, and on the aqueous and vitreous humor becoming more transparent, we may be able to examine them with the ophthalmoscope, and find that fresh masses of exudation are effused; the latter subsequently becoming opaque.

The treatment must in the first place be directed to saving, if possible, some amount of sight, and then, if this be out of the question, to mitigating the great sufferings of the patient. Thus, if it be produced by a foreign body which it is possible to seize and extract, this should be done without loss of time, even although it may be necessary to pass the instrument into the vitreous humor (vide article upon "The Presence of Foreign Bodies in the Vitreous Humor"). If the lens is injured and swollen, it should be at once removed, together with a considerable portion of the iris, if symptoms of severe inflammation supervene.

If there is a perforating ulcer of the cornea with hypopyon, either paracentesis (perhaps frequently repeated) or iridectomy should be performed.

If a foreign body has entered the vitreous humor and lies beyond our reach, and if it be small and has not injured the lens or committed any considerable mischief in its course, we must endeavor by the strictest antiphlogistic treatment to subdue the inflammatory complications, and if possible, to prevent suppurative choroiditis. Indeed, in some of these cases, the foreign body becomes encapsulated and remains innocuous, an excellent degree of vision being perhaps restored. But when a foreign body remains in the eye, we must always keep in mind the great danger of sympathetic inflammation. If the eye is hopelessly destroyed by the accident, it will be far the wisest and safest course to remove it at once, so as not only to avoid all danger of sympathetic irritation, but also the occurrence of suppurative choroiditis. For when symptoms of panophthalmitis have supervened, it will be no longer safe to do so, because there is imminent risk of the suppuration extending to the brain and producing fatal suppurative meningitis. Cases, in which this has occurred after excision of the eyeball during acute panophthalmitis, have been recorded by Von Graefe, Knapp, Manhardt, etc.[1]

If the inflammatory symptoms are very severe, and of a sthenic character, iced compresses should be constantly applied as long as they prove agreeable to the patient. Leeches should be placed on the temple, and if the patient is strong, and the suppuration has not already become too extensive, so as to afford little or no chance of arresting it, rapid salivation should be induced, in the hopes of checking the inflammation and preserving some degree of sight. Generally, however, this proves futile. The severe pain in and around the eye is often most relieved by hot poppy fomentations or

[1] "Kl. Monatsbl.," 1863, p. 456.

poultices, and by the subcutaneous injection of morphia at the temple. If there is hypopyon, or the tension of the eye is much increased, paracentesis of the anterior chamber should be performed, and repeated at intervals of a day or two, or even less. If the eye is very distended, and causes great suffering to the patient, the paracentesis may be made into the vitreous humor instead, which often affords great relief.

The patient's strength must be sustained by a very nourishing diet, the free use of stimulants, and by the administration of tonics.

If the pain and inflammation are very severe and protracted, and so greatly enfeeble the patient as even to endanger life, it will be best to remove the eye at all hazards, even at the risk of an extension of the disease to the brain, in order at once to remove all source of pain, and thus enable the patient to regain his strength.

[This procedure is still regarded by many as questionable surgery. There are too many cases on record of a fatal termination by the extension backwards of the inflammation to the meninges. In most of the severer cases there is more or less inflammation of the orbital cellular tissue, and relief may sometimes be obtained by incising the orbital tissue as well as the eyeball, for the purpose of lessening the tension.—B.]

Knapp[1] has described two very interesting cases of embolism of the choroidal vessels. In each patient there existed well-marked cardiac disease (in the one endo-carditis, in the other insufficiency and stenosis of the aortic valves with hypertrophy of the left ventricle). The affection of the sight was quite sudden, the patients noticing a dark cloud before the eye, which at first pervaded the whole visual field, but then became concentrated in the central portion. The impairment of vision does not occur with such great suddenness as in embolism of the central artery of the retina, nor to such an extent, for in the one case V = one-tenth, in the other the patient could read the finest print, and only noticed a large scotoma lying near the axis of vision. There were marked chromopsy and photopsy. The ophthalmoscope revealed a circumscribed cloud or veil in the central portion of the fundus (and corresponding to the scotoma), which was due to a serous effusion into the retina which extended to the disk. The vessels were also hyperæmic in this clouded portion of the retina. These conditions were evidently those of collateral effusion and hyperæmia, and due to embolism of some of the choroidal vessels at this point. These phenomena are easily explained when we remember the anastomosis between the central artery of the retina, and those ciliary arteries which perforate the sclerotic in the vicinity of the disk. The patients subsequently quite regained their sight, and the fundus resumed its normal appearance.

5.—[WARTY OUTGROWTHS OF THE CHOROID.—B.] COLLOID DISEASE OF THE CHOROID.

This affection was first described by Wedl,[2] and consists in the formation of peculiar, transparent, bead-like globules on the inner surface of the choroid. Donders[3] supposed them to be due to senile changes, dependent upon a colloid metamorphosis of the nuclei of the hexagonal pigment cells, whereas H. Müller[4] thought that these little bodies lie horizontally behind the pigment cells, and are due to an adventitious thickening of the elastic

[1] "A. f. O.," xiv. 1.   [2] "Grundzüge der Histologie," 1854.
[3] "A. f. O.," i. 2, 107.   [4] Ibid., ii. 2, 1.

lamina. From the researches of Mr. Hulke, the latter view appears to be the true one;[1] he moreover found that the capillary vessels of the choroid do not appear to be primarily affected, as the blood corpuscles could be distinctly seen gliding along the capillary vessels in unbroken column *beneath* the globules, *i. e.*, to the outer side of them.

The colloid globules are highly refracting, and are arranged singly, or in little groups or clusters. They assume various shapes, being globular, oval, or club-shaped. They are but slightly, if at all, affected by reagents. Their size varies from one twelve hundred and fiftieth to one four hundred and thirtieth of an inch (Hulke). They are very apt to undergo chalky and fatty degeneration, and then present a finely granular appearance. [They often present a concentric lamellar structure. The retinal epithelium is not directly involved in their growth.—B.]

On account of the colloid masses pushing aside, or even destroying, the hexagonal pigment cells, the latter are crowded together, so as to form a narrow, dark rim or fringe around the single or aggregated globules. Hence, the choroidal epithelium presents here and there a somewhat variegated, patchy appearance. Indeed this is about the only sign by which the presence of colloid disease of the choroid can be recognized with the ophthalmoscope. We notice[2] small, faintly pigmented pale patches, surrounded by a dark fringe of pigment cells, the choroidal vessels being hidden by the chalky deposits. These patches may be strewn about at small intervals over a considerable portion of the choroid, more especially towards the equator of the fundus.

It was supposed that these colloid formations were due to some senile changes, as they are most frequently met with in old persons. But Hulke[3] has seen them also occur in quite young individuals, and considers that inflammation is the cause of these adventitous thickenings of the elastic lamina, as he has frequently found colloid disease associated with inflammatory changes. He states that it is almost always present in shrunken globes which have been repeatedly inflamed, and he has also seen it several times in acute traumatic inflammation.

On account of the atrophy of the choroidal epithelium, and consequent injury to the rods and bulbs of the retina, the sight is often much impaired at an advanced stage of the disease, and if the latter has invaded the posterior pole of the eye. Fortunately, however, it frequently remains confined to the periphery of the fundus (the vicinity of the ora serrata), and then of course only the outline of the visual field will be affected.

6.—TUBERCLES OF THE CHOROID [CHOROIDITIS TUBERCULOSA.—B.].

It was formerly supposed by some surgeons that a peculiar form of plastic choroiditis was sometimes met with in the later stages of chronic tuberculosis, and was consequently termed "tubercular choroiditis." The extensive and very careful researches of Cohnheim have shown, however, that this is not the case, for he has failed to detect the presence of tubercular deposits in the choroid in any case of localized tuberculosis of the lungs or intestines.[4] Manz,[5] however, discovered anatomically, in three instances, the important and interesting fact of the presence of tubercles in the choroid in acute

---

[1] "R. L. O. H. Rep.," i. pp. 70 and 180. [2] Liebreich, "A. f. O.," iv. 2, 290.
[3] "R. L. O. H. Rep.," i. 181. [4] "A. f. O.," xiv. 1, 188, note.
[5] Ib., iv. 2, 120, and ix. 3, 133.

choroidal vessels; Busch thought that they were formed from the colorless cells of the stroma of the choroid; whereas Cohnheim considers that they are developed from peculiar migratory cells (Wanderzellen) resembling lymph-corpuscles, which lie strewn about in the choroid.

Soon after the publication of Cohnheim's paper, I was fortunate enough to diagnose, with the ophthalmoscope, the presence of tubercles in the choroid, and submitted the preparation to the Pathological Society.

As this is the first case in which tubercles of the choroid have been met with in England, and as it illustrates well their ophthalmoscopic characteristics, I give it in extenso.

M. J. P., a little girl, æt. eight, was admitted on November 5, 1867, into King's College Hospital, under the care of Dr. Garrod, with symptoms of acute tuberculosis. She had become rapidly emaciated during the last month, and had during that time suffered from dyspnœa and dry cough. On admission there was great febrile disturbance, pulse 132, respirations 66, temperature 101°. Slight dulness of left side of chest, and crepitation about the second intercostal space. November 6th: Temperature 106°, pulse 148, respiration 96. Urine acid, no albumen. Puerile respiration on right side, slightly tubular on left. I examined the eyes with the ophthalmoscope, and diagnosed the presence of tubercles in the choroid. November 11th: The patient grew rapidly worse and died on this day.

Post-mortem examination by Dr. Kelly:

The brain substance was apparently normal, but on the superior aspect of the left hemisphere were seen two or three small opacities in the pia mater. Both lungs were filled with miliary tubercle. Liver and heart healthy, kidneys contained tubercles in their cortical substances and were congested throughout. Capsule of spleen had some tubercular (?) deposits, the organ itself being healthy. The mesenteric glands were somewhat increased in size and number, and some solitary glands of the small intestines were enlarged. The surface of the peritoneum was healthy.

Examination of the eyes during life:

I found that the eyes appeared externally quite normal. The sight was perfect (No. 1 Jaeger). The field of vision normal. The refracting media perfectly transparent. With the ophthalmoscope, it was found that the optic nerve and retina were healthy, the retinal veins slightly dilated; the outline of the disk perfect. In the choroid—which was otherwise perfectly normal—were noticed numerous small, circular, prominent, grayish-white nodules, which were chiefly situated in the vicinity of the optic disk, more especially in the region of the yellow spot. Towards the periphery of the fundus they were more sparsely scattered. The epithelium of the choroid around the nodules was only very slightly altered in appearance, the cells being evidently opened up or pushed aside by the nodules, and there was no agglomeration of pigment around the latter, but the thinned portion of the epithelium passed insensibly over into the normal condition. At some points, a nodule could be seen lying beneath a retinal vessel which passed distinctly over it. The nodules were prominent, but whether or not the retinal vessel was arched forward by the tubercle could not be accurately determined, as it was quite impossible, on account of the restless movements of the patient's eye, to distinguish with certainty as to the presence of a parallax. The condition was very similar in both eyes.

The diagnosis of tubercular deposits in the choroid was verified by a careful dissection made by Mr. Bowater Vernon, the curator of the Moorfields Hospital, an account of which will be found in the "R. L. O. H. Reports," vi. 2, 168.

Other interesting facts in connection with this subject are, that Cohnheim found that the thyroid gland, which was supposed to enjoy a special immunity from tubercular deposits, was in most cases implicated. In Guinea-pigs he has, moreover, succeeded in producing tubercles in the choroid by inoculation. The matter was taken from a tuberculous lymphatic gland, and the animal died five weeks after the inoculation, when, besides those in the choroid, miliary tubercles were met with in all the organs, viz., in the lungs, liver, kidneys, spleen, serous membrane, etc."[1]

7.—TUMORS OF THE CHOROID.

[The choroid is very often the seat of tumors, most of which belong to the class of melano-sarcoma. Much more rare are the unpigmented fibro-sarcomata, and the rarest of all are the myomata or fibromata.—B.] But in many instances the tumor presents a mixed character, being partly sarcomatous and partly carcinomatous. According to Von Graefe,[2] the great majority of choroidal tumors are of a sarcomatous nature; a much smaller proportion are of a mixed character; and only in exceptional instances are they carcinomatous. These differences in the nature of the tumor are, however, only recognizable with the microscope, as the eye does not present any special symptoms which would enable us to decide whether or not a given case of intra-ocular tumor is of a sarcomatous or carcinomatous nature.

[The melanotic sarcoma is the most common of all choroidal tumors, and is generally situated in the equatorial or ciliary regions, though it is occasionally met with in the posterior part of the eye in the neighborhood of the optic nerve.

The unpigmented or leuco-sarcoma is much less common than the pigmented, and is generally composed of round cells, though occasionally there are found large numbers of very large fusiform cells. According to Knapp, the sarcomata which are composed to a large extent of these elongated cells probably proceed from the external layers of the choroid, while the small round-cell tumor arises from the chorio-capillaris. The former variety, resembling fibro-sarcoma, have a much slower course, and are not so much inclined to produce metastatic deposits as the small-cell variety.

The term *cavernous sarcoma* is used to describe a form of growth in which there is an enormous development of vessels.

In rare cases a sarcoma may undergo partial ossification, and these tumors are known histologically as osteo-sarcoma.

Among the more rare mixed forms of tumor may be mentioned the sarcoma-carcinomatosum, the glio-sarcoma, and the myxo-sarcoma.—B.]

(1) SARCOMA OF THE CHOROID.

The disease presents itself at the outset, as a small nodule in the [anterior] or lateral portion of the choroid, being developed from the pigmented connective tissue of the latter. During the earliest stage, the choroidal epithelium and the retina may remain unaffected, passing intact over the little nodule; but, as the latter increases in size, the retina generally becomes

[1] "A. f. O.," xiv. 1, 205.
[2] "A. f. O.," xiv. 2, 115. The reader will find in this article a very interesting and valuable account of the chief differences between the symptoms, development, and course of sarcoma of the choroid and glioma retinæ.

more or less detached by the effusion of a serous or hemorrhagic reddish-brown fluid, which causes the detached portion of the retina to fluctuate and tremble on every movement of the eye. According to Iwanoff,[1] detachment of the vitreous precedes that of the retina in tumors of the choroid. Subsequently the retina mostly becomes completely detached (the vitreous humor undergoing corresponding diminution in volume), giving rise to the well-known funnel-shaped detachment, the apex of which is situated at the optic nerve, the base at the ora serrata; the space external to the detached retina being occupied by the tumor, and more or less fluid. The lens now soon becomes cataractous, if this has not already occurred, more especially at its posterior pole. The vitreous humor may lose its transparency at an earlier stage of the disease, whilst the detachment is still but partial, so that the details of the fundus are, perhaps, obscured by a diffuse haziness of the vitreous, intermixed with more or less filiform or membranous opacities. If the retina retains its transparency and lies in close contact with the tumor, it may be possible, in some cases, to recognize the latter with the ophthalmoscope, as it presents the appearance of a distinct, smooth, or slightly nodulated swelling, the color of which may vary from a pale-brown to a dark coffee-colored tint, according to the amount of pigment which it contains. If the detached retina should undergo inflammatory or fatty changes and become thickened, a yellow reflex may take the place of the brown color of the tumor. But this reflex differs from that met with in glioma, by not being of such a brilliantly white or whitish-yellow tint, or so brightly opalescent (Von Graefe).[2] As a rule, the early stage of the disease is accompanied by a serous detachment of the retina, which will completely hide the presence of the tumor; and it is only when the latter increases in size and reaches up close to the detached retina, that small, dark, knob-like protuberances may appear beneath the latter, side by side, perhaps, with portions of detached retina, which show a distinct tremulousness when the eye is moved. I may as well now call attention to the fact that the degree of the intra-ocular tension is of great diagnostic importance in cases of detachment of the retina; for whilst it is, as a rule, diminished in cases of simple detachment, it either remains normal or is more or less increased when the latter is due to the presence of an intra-ocular tumor. Indeed, in the more advanced stages of sarcoma, the disease often assumes marked glaucomatous symptoms. The tension of the eye is greatly increased, the cornea perhaps steamy, roughened, and anæsthetic, the anterior chamber very shallow, the iris pushed forward and its tissue atrophied, the pupil dilated (often irregularly), the lens perhaps opaque, the sight lost. The patient complains of great ciliary neuralgia, extending, may be, to the corresponding side of the head and face. The sufferings are especially acute and sudden if intra-ocular hemorrhage has occurred. At a later date staphylomatous bulgings may appear in the ciliary region, and might be mistaken for masses of tumor; their transparency, when a strong light is thrown upon them, will, however, guard us against such an error (Von Graefe). After the increased tension has existed for some length of time, a severe attack of acute glaucomatous inflammation may supervene. Von Graefe calls attention to the fact that he has several times noticed this occurrence after atropine had been applied for the purpose of facilitating the ophthalmoscopic examination. Now, if we do not know the history of the case (the prior detachment of the retina, etc.) and the media are too clouded to permit of an ophthalmoscopic examination, it may be very difficult to recognize the true nature of the disease, and it

[1] "A. f. O.," xv. 2, 69.   [2] "A. f. O.," xiv. 2, 109.

will be perhaps considered a simple case of glaucoma. An iridectomy is made, and the pain temporarily relieved by the diminution of the tension. But it soon recurs with all its former violence, the eye again becomes hard, our suspicions are aroused as to the presence of an intra-ocular tumor, the eyeball is enucleated, and our conjectures are verified. This fact has led some surgeons to the belief that melanotic sarcoma is very prone to become developed in glaucomatous eyes. But this does not appear to be the case, the glaucomatous condition being simply one phase of the disease. Such cases of supposed glaucoma in which intra-ocular tumors were subsequently found, have been observed by Bowman,[1] Von Graefe,[2] Hutchinson,[3] Dor,[4] etc.

Sometimes, however, the presence of the tumor sets up great irritation, and finally gives rise to a plastic form of irido-choroiditis, which leads to a more or less considerable temporary atrophy of the eyeball. The shrunken globe becomes the seat of intense, persistent pain, for the relief of which enuclea-tion is performed, and then the tumor, the real source of the mischief, is dis-covered. It must be mentioned, however, that whilst temporary atrophy of the globe is not unfrequently observed in the course of glioma retinæ, this is only exceptionally the case in sarcoma of the choroid; as the choroidal in-flammation generally assumes a secretory or serous-hemorrhagic character, indeed the glaucomatous condition may even continue after the extra-ocular development of the disease. The atrophy generally depends upon sloughing of the cornea from paralysis of the corneal nerves, which is followed by more or less severe suppurative panophthalmitis (Von Graefe).[5] Attention has been called by Von Graefe[6] to several points which may enable us to distin-guish between simple atrophy of the eyeball, and that which is dependent upon intra-ocular sarcoma. In the latter case, very severe spontaneous par-oxysms of pain occur, whilst the ciliary region is hardly, if at all, sensitive to the touch; whereas, in the atrophy ensuing upon irido-cyclitis, the reverse obtains, there being but little, if any, spontaneous pain, but the eye remaining for a long time sensitive to the touch. Moreover, if a sarcoma is present in the atrophied globe, the diminution in size, or flattening of the eyeball, occurs in the antero-posterior axis, the equatorial region not contracting to the same extent. The depressions caused by the four recti muscles are, therefore, unusually apparent upon the anterior surface of the globe. Again, on account of the subsequent contraction of the connective-tissue elements, which have been formed within the eye in the course of the panophthalmitis, a barrier is, to a certain extent, placed against the development of the tumor in front. Hence, although the latter increases in size, the collapsed eyeball does not fill out and become plumper, but remains flattened, and a retro-ocular exten-sion of the morbid growth occurs, pushing the eyeball forward, and thus causing a certain degree of exophthalmos. In estimating the degree of the latter, we must not forget that the eyeball is diminished in size, otherwise we may easily undervalue the extent of the protrusion.

The progress of sarcoma of the choroid is generally slow as long as it is confined by the firm sclerotic within the cavity of the eye, and it may remain stationary for a considerable length of time; but if it has once per-forated the coats of the eyeball, its progress is very rapid. Its exposed sur-face becomes ulcerated, and covered by a dark-red crust of blood, and ichorous discharge, upon the laceration of which it bleeds freely, often very profusely. Perforation may take place through the cornea, (generally at or

[1] " R. L. O. H. Rep.," iv. 81.
[2] " R. L. O. H. Rep.," v. 88.
[3] " A. f. O.," xiv. 2, 120.
[4] " A. f. O.," x. 1, 179.
[5] " A. f. O.," vi. 2, 244.
[6] Ibid.

near the sclero-corneal junction), at the front part of the sclerotic, or at its posterior portion, close to the optic nerve. The disease may also extend into the optic nerve; small, dark, stringy patches being found to pass backwards from the lamina cribrosa between the nerve tubules, and thus causing an extension of the disease into the orbit, or towards the brain. With regard to the implication of the optic nerve, Von Graefe is of opinion that the disease at the outset extends from the lamina cribrosa along the inner surface of the nerve-sheath, or along the septa of the perineaurium. Whereas in glioma, the whole thickness of the nerve is simultaneously affected. Or again, small, circumscribed, black patches make their appearance on the sclerotic, being apparently independent of the disease, and their presence is generally prognostic of a rapid extension of the tumor. According to Virchow, the microscope, as a rule, reveals a progressive implication of the sclerotic.

The appearance which the tumor presents on section, varies with the amount of pigment which it contains. It is generally marbled or speckled, some portions being pale, others of a more or less deep brown tint. These melanotic-sarcomatous tumors may, however, be of a uniform, black, inky color. But according to Virchow,[1] sarcoma of the choroid may, in very exceptional cases, be quite colorless. It has hence been termed "leuco-sarcoma;" and this is probably due to some local cause, it being perhaps primarily developed from the less pigmented inner portion of the choroid. [These teleangiectatic forms of sarcoma are not very uncommon, and generally occur in unpigmented tumors.—B.]

Sarcoma is characterized, microscopically, the presence of cells of varying size and shape. They may be stellate, spindle-shaped, oval, or round, having, perhaps, well-marked prolongations. They contain nuclei and nucleoli. Sometimes the cells are of an extremely large size (giant cells of Virchow), and contain a great number of nuclei. Between the cells is observed a variable quantity of scanty, fibrillated, intercellular tissue. But there is a complete absence of an areolar mode of arrangement, and in the pure form of sarcoma the cells are not collected into groups or nests within large meshes of connective tissue. Where the latter arrangement prevails in a portion of the tumor, it proves that it is not a simple sarcoma, but of a mixed nature, viz., carcinomatous sarcoma. The cells often contain a considerable amount of pigment, and the disease is then termed melanotic sarcoma. This is v ry frequently the structure of intra-ocular tumors. [The mode of origin of the various forms of sarcoma is not entirely known. It is still undecided whether they arise from proliferating cells which have exuded from the vessels, or whether they originate in the stroma of the adventitia of the vessels.—B.]

With regard to the prognosis of simple sarcomatous tumors, there is no doubt that they are decidedly malignant, and manifest a great tendency to metastasis. According to Virchow, the degree of malignancy varies with their structure. Thus he states[2] that those sarcomata which contain small cells (quite irrespective of the shape of the cell) are far more dangerous than those in which the cells are large. On account of the small size and vast quantity of the cells, such tumors are generally soft, and should be viewed with every great suspicion, whereas the giant cell (myeloid) sarcomata afford a relatively favorable prognosis.

There can be no doubt of the fact that the intra-ocular growth is the

---

[1] "Die Krankheiten Geschwülste," ii. 284; vide also Hulke, "R. L. O. H. Rep.," ii. 283, and iv. 85, and Knapp, "Intraoculare Geschwülste," p. 126.
[2] "Die Krankheiten Geschwülste," ii. 269.

primary affection, and that the metastatic tumors are secondary. They occur chiefly in the liver, lungs, brain, and kidney. A peculiarity of the sarcomatous tumors, which distinguishes them from the carcinomatous, is, that they show little or no tendency to affect the lymphatic glands, and hence it is more than probable that the infection of distant organs is caused through the blood, and not through the lymphatic system.

The causes of intra-ocular sarcoma are yet uncertain, but there is no doubt that it not unfrequently becomes developed after injuries of the eye. It may also be formed in eyes which have undergone atrophy after irido-choroiditis, etc. Here, however, we must be upon our guard not to mistake cause and effect. But if the eye has been for many years lost from irido-choroiditis, before symptoms of an intra-ocular growth reveal themselves, it may, I think, be fairly assumed that the latter is a secondary affection. Thus, Mr. Bowman removed an eye affected with melanotic sarcoma, which had been lost from acute inflammation twenty years previously.[1]

Sarcoma of the choroid occurs most frequently after the age of thirty, being but very rarely seen under the age of fifteen;[2] Hirschberg, however, records a case in which a colorless sarcoma of the choroid, with secondary nodules in the retina, occurred in a girl aged twelve.[3] Von Graefe has never observed a single instance in which choroidal sarcoma affected both eyes, although he has met with cases in which the second eye became amaurotic; the ophthalmoscopic examination yielding at first a perfectly negative result, but at a later period, atrophy of the optic nerve set in. In two of these cases, melanotic nodules were found at the base of the brain, reacting on the chiasma and the optic nerve of the other side.

[*Cystoid formations* are mentioned by Alt. They are situated in the equatorial region and have an endothelial lining. Alt saw them in only one case.

Granuloma of the choroid is sometimes met with after injuries. This tumor never attains any great size, and seems eventually to be changed into cicatricial tissue. There is a case reported by Leber of a granuloma of the choroid from a patient who had suffered from trachoma.

Enchondroma of the choroid has been reported by Knapp. It was probably in the beginning a sarcoma which had subsequently undergone cartilaginous degeneration. Alt thinks that the hyaline cartilage is developed from the remains of the vitreous inclosed in the tumor. (See "Comp. der Histologie des Auges.")

The treatment consists in enucleation of the ball as soon as possible, and before the glaucomatous symptoms have set in, or the intra-ocular growth has become also extra-ocular.—B.]

Sarcoma of the ciliary body[4] is also sometimes met with, and when it has acquired some size, it can be distinctly observed protruding into the anterior chamber. The iris is, at this point, pushed aside from its ciliary insertion by a dark-brown tumor, which more or less fills up the anterior chamber, its apex perhaps lying in contact with the cornea; the pupil is at the same time irregularly distorted. On examining the position of the morbid growth behind the iris, with the oblique illumination, we may perhaps observe it encroaching upon the area of the pupil, and extending backwards into the vitreous humor, the lens being generally displaced to a corresponding degree backwards or upwards. The surface presents a dark-brown appearance, being either quite smooth or somewhat lobulated.

---

[1] "R. L. O. H. Rep.," iii. 279. [2] "A. f. O.," xiv. 2, 106. [3] Ibid., xvi. 302.
[4] *Vide* Von Graefe's cases, "A. f. O.," xii. 2, 233; also one reported by the author in "Lancet," January 22, 1870.

[The case of De Wecker's reported as myoma of the choroid, probably began in the ciliary body. Primary sarcoma of the ciliary body is certainly very rare, the growths involving this region usually spreading from the choroid.—B.]

(2) CARCINOMA OF THE CHOROID.

We may distinguish two forms of cancer of the choroid, viz., the medullary and the melanotic. I have, however, already stated that we cannot with any degree of certainty diagnose the true nature of these tumors, except by an examination of their minute structure. We may, however, find some assistance in framing our diagnosis, by remembering that cancerous tumors show a more rapid progress than simple sarcoma, leading at an earlier period to metastatic affections, and manifesting a great tendency to implicate the lymphatic glands.

On a microscopic examination of *medullary carcinoma*, we notice large areolar spaces, formed by fibrillæ of connective tissue; and within these spaces are contained nests of variously shaped cancer-cells. The latter may be stellate, fusiform, ovoid, or round, and closely resemble epithelial and ganglion cells. They contain a large nucleus, and within this there are numerous nucleoli.

The *melanotic carcinoma* is only distinguished from the medullary by the more or less considerable amount of pigment contained in the cells and the trabeculæ forming the areolæ. It may be so great as to give a dark inky color to the tumor. In the melanotic cancer there are also large areolæ enclosing nests of pigmented cancer-cells.

The melanotic cancer is extremely dangerous, and is very prone to recur at an early date. Von Graefe states that he does not remember any case in which the apparent cure exceeded four years. In the majority of cases the disease recurred locally or in other organs within three, six, or twelve months.

Sometimes the tumor presents a mixed character, being in part sarcomatous, in part carcinomatous, and the relative predominance of the one over the other may influence the rapidity of the progress and of the recurrence. More probably, however, the sarcoma may have existed for some time, when the cancer elements become developed and greatly hasten the growth. Virchow does not believe that the sarcomatous elements pass over into those of cancer, so that the latter is developed from the sarcoma, but that the two conditions exist side by side, arising out of the same primary structure, and growing together like two branches from one stem.[1]

The treatment to be adopted for these tumors (both the sarcomatous and carcinomatous) is the same, viz., the extirpation of the eye as soon as the diagnosis can be established with anything like certainty. The early removal of the eye is indicated, not only because we may thus perhaps be in time to prevent the infection of other organs, but also to prevent the extension of the disease to the optic nerve. In removing the eyeball, the optic nerve should be cut very far back, so that we may, if possible, get beyond the seat of the disease.

If, on removal of the eye, the cut end of the optic nerve looks swollen and dark, it should be pulled out as far as possible with a pair of forceps, and divided close to the orbit. This is often very difficult if we endeavor to look for the nerve, and hence it is best, as Mr. Hutchinson[2] suggests, to

---

[1] "Die Krankheiten Geschwülste," N. 182.   [2] "R. L. O. H. Rep.," v. 1, 92.

feel for its trunk with our forefinger, and, when it is thus found, to seize its extremity with a pair of strongly toothed forceps, and drawing it forth, divide it.

When the optic nerve is found to be diseased, or the tumor has extended into the orbit, the chloride of zinc paste should always be employed (*vide* "Tumors of Orbit").

De Wecker[1] describes a unique case of *myoma* of the choroid which occurred in his practice. The patient's left eye was hard, the anterior ciliary vessels dilated and tortuous, and he suffered from severe paroxysms of pain. Nearly the whole of the internal half of the iris was pressed forward towards the cornea by a reddish-brown tumor, which also occupied the greater portion of the pupil. The vitreous humor was clear, the optic disk somewhat hyperæmic. The eye was enucleated, and the microscopic examination of the tumor was made by Iwanoff, who found that it was a myo-sarcoma, there being in it distinct unstriped muscular fibres.

Leber,[2] again, describes a very interesting and peculiar case in which the sarcoma of the choroid assumed a distinctly cavernous character.

8.—FORMATION OF BONE IN THE CHOROID.

A formation of true bone is not unfrequently met with[3] on the inner surface of the choroid, in eyes which have undergone atrophy and become shrunken. True osseous tissue occurs, according to Knapp,[4] in the eye only in consequence of plastic inflammation of the capillary layer of the choroid; whereas cretefaction may occur in all the tissues of the eye. The nature of the process of ossification is identical with the formation of bone in periosteum. These osseous deposits may appear in the form of small circumscribed spots or plates, or they may be so extensive as to form a complete hollow cup, reaching from the ciliary processes to the optic nerve, and being perforated by the latter. In close apposition to this formation of bone may often be noticed cartilaginous tissue.

The shrunken eyeball in which a deposit of bone has taken place, is not unfrequently very painful, both to the touch and spontaneously, and may give rise to sympathetic inflammation.

9.—COLOBOMA OF THE CHOROID.

The ophthalmoscopic symptoms presented by this condition are very striking and characteristic, and show a remarkable similarity in all cases, although, of course, the extent of the coloboma and of the bulging backwards of the sclerotic greatly influence these appearances. Liebreich gives an admirable illustration of this condition in his "Atlas."[5]

With the ophthalmoscope there is observed a most peculiar, large, white figure at the lower part of the fundus, extending perhaps nearly up to the disk, or even embracing this in its expanse. Anteriorly it may reach more or less closely up to the ciliary processes, or even quite up to the corresponding coloboma of the iris. In some rare instances, however, the colo-

---

[1] "Traité Theorique et Pratique des Maladies des Yeux" (2d edition), 1, 545.
[2] "A. f. O.," xiv. 2, 221.
[3] *Vide* Wedl's "Atlas der Pathologische-Histologie des Auges.".
[4] Knapp's "Archives," ii. 1.
[5] Plate xii. Fig. 5. [See also Schiess-Gemuseus, "A. f. O.," xix. 1, p. 219.—B.]

homa of the choroid exists without there being any cleft in the iris. I had lately under my care at Moorfields, a patient in whose right eye there was a coloboma of the iris and choroid, whereas in the left eye there was only a coloboma of the choroid. It is also very rare to meet with a coloboma of the choroid confined to the region of the yellow spot.[1] Together with the coloboma of the choroid, there always exists a staphylomatous bulging backwards of the sclerotic. This may be nearly of the same depth throughout, or suddenly and abruptly increase in depth, which can be distinctly observed with the ophthalmoscope, as it produces a peculiar appearance in the course of the retinal vessels, which will be seen suddenly to dip round this edge and be slightly interrupted in their course, thus giving rise to a marked parallax. These appearances can be well studied in Liebreich's illustration.

On the white expanse are noticed the retinal vessels, which do not, however, pursue their regular course, but undergo peculiar windings, some twisting and curling round over the edge of the coloboma. The presence of the retina, or at least of some attenuated, vicarious membrane, is proved by the appearance of the retinal vessels on the surface of the coloboma. The retina may either lie in apposition with the sclerotic, or be stretched across the bulge in the latter, and in this case it is often slightly folded, so that branches of its vessels may appear to spring directly from the sclerotic, on account of their continuity with the other retinal vessels being hidden by the folds. Traces of choroidal vessels may also be noticed upon the white figure. The margin of the latter is very sharply defined, of a dark reddish-brown or coffee-colored tint, and strongly pigmented. If the cleft stops short of the disk, it will be divided from the latter by a sharp line of demarcation, and a more or less normal portion of fundus; whereas, if the disk is included in the coloboma, its appearance is remarkably changed, for it can hardly be distinguished from the rest of the white figure except by its more deep gray tint; its form being elliptic, with its long diameter placed horizontally.

If the anterior extremity of the coloboma does not reach up to the cleft in the iris, there are noticed small rudimentary ciliary processes, and it is divided from the coloboma of the iris by a more or less extensive portion of perhaps darkly pigmented fundus, traversed by a kind of raphe, or white stripe (sometimes there are two or three). Where the coloboma of the choroid touches that of the iris, the ciliary processes may be completely wanting. Saemisch[2] narrates a very interesting case of coloboma of the iris and choroid, in which the former was divided from the pupil by a narrow band, which was probably a remnant of the pupillary membrane. Baumler[3] has also noticed such little bands traversing the area of the pupil in cases of coloboma.

If the region of the yellow spot is not involved, the sight may be tolerably good, but there is always an interruption in the field of vision (scotoma), corresponding in size and situation to the coloboma of the choroid. Liebreich has also observed and figured ("Atlas," Pl. xii. Fig. 4) the very singular and curious condition of a coloboma of the sheath of the optic nerve.

[1] Vide De Wecker, "Traité des Maladies du Fond de l'Œil," p. 207; also "Kl. Monatsbl." 1872, p. 56.

[2] Vide Arlt, "Krankheiten des Auges," ii. 128; also Saemisch, "Kl. Monatsbl.," 1867, p. 69.

[3] L. c., p. 87.   [4] "Wurzburger Med. Zeitschrift," iii. 84.

cases. The field of vision is sometimes contracted at the periphery, and there may also be interruptions (*scotomata*) in it, corresponding in situation to the rupture in the choroid.

Although, in favorable cases, the cicatrization of the rupture in the choroid is not followed by any subsequent affection of the retina or optic nerve, yet the former may afterwards become detached.[1] Dr. Frank[2] also narrates a case in which rupture of the choroid was followed by atrophy of the optic nerve.

The treatment must principally consist in hastening the absorption of the hemorrhagic effusions into the choroid and vitreous humor, and for this purpose the compress bandage and the repeated application of the artificial leech will be found most serviceable.

Incised wounds of the sclerotic and choroid are not generally accompanied by a protrusion (hernia) of the choroid, but the edge of the wounded choroid may be forced out between the lips of the sclerotic incision by the exuding vitreous humor. In wounds of the choroid there is often a considerable effusion of blood into the choroid and vitreous humor.

II.—HEMORRHAGE FROM THE CHOROID.

Extravasation of blood from the choroid may be produced by an accident, such as a blow upon the eye, or a wound implicating the sclerotic and choroid. But it also occurs in diseases of the eye which influence the intra-ocular circulation—as for instance glaucoma, sclerotico-choroiditis posterior, etc.—and produce a congestion of the choroidal vessels, more especially if the latter should be diseased. [Occasionally well-marked signs of perivasculitis choroidea have been observed in these cases.—B.] In such cases, any sudden strain, such as violent vomiting or retching, or the sudden relief of the intra-ocular tension by paracentesis or iridectomy, may cause a rupture of some of the smaller choroidal vessels, and perhaps considerable hemorrhage. It may also occur spontaneously, or after severe and protracted exertion of the eye, as in engraving, sewing, prolonged use of the microscope, etc.

The blood may be effused between the choroid and sclerotic, into the tissue of the choroid, or between the latter and the retina. If the hemorrhage is but slight, it will simply produce small circumscribed ecchymoses in the choroid, but if it is considerable in quantity, it may cause detachment of the retina, or perforate the latter, and escape into the vitreous humor. This, as will be stated in the article upon hemorrhage into the vitreous humor, chiefly depends upon the situation of the hemorrhage, for if the latter takes place near the *ora serrata*, it is more likely to perforate the retina (on account of the thinness of the latter at this point), and to escape into the vitreous humor. Whereas, if the extravasation occurs near the posterior pole of the eye, it is more apt to produce detachment of the retina. Esmarch[3] has narrated a very interesting case of extravasation of blood from the choroid, with perforation of the retina in the region of the yellow spot and escape of the blood into the vitreous humor, where it gradually underwent absorption, until nothing remained but a small dark speck about the size of a pin's head, the perforation in the retina having healed without leaving any trace behind it. Sometimes, however, the position of the little cicatrix may remain recognizable as a small black pigment spot.

[1] "Kl. Monatsbl.," 1866, p. 111.   [2] "R. L. O. H. Reports," iii. 84.
[3] "A. f. O.," iv. 1, 350.

Effusion of blood between the sclerotic and choroid may produce detachment of the latter.

With the ophthalmoscope, effusions of blood into the choroid may be recognized by their presenting the appearance of uniform, dark, cherry-colored patches, of varying size and shape, being irregular, circular, oval, etc. Their edges may be sharply defined, or somewhat indistinct and irregular. The color of the apoplexy is uniformly red, and not striated, nor are its edges serrated or "feathery," as is the case when blood is effused into the inner layers of the retina, and follows the course of the optic nerve fibres. Again, the retinal vessels can be distinctly seen to pass straight over the effusion, without being interrupted or hidden by it. If no retinal vessels should be situated over, or in very close proximity to the hemorrhage, the situation of the latter, upon a plane deeper than that of the retina, is best recognized by means of the binocular ophthalmoscope. If the disease has lasted some little time, some of the neighboring extravasations have probably undergone partial absorption, and given rise to peculiar appearances in the choroid, which will aid us in our diagnosis of the exact situation of any special ecchymoses. During the process of absorption, the effusion gradually assumes a paler and more yellowish-white tint, and becomes fringed by a circlet of pigment. The smaller ecchymoses may leave no trace behind them, or only a small pigment spot.

If the hemorrhage is but slight, and is situated at the periphery of the fundus, it may produce no impairment of vision, or only a small scotoma; but it is very different when it is situated at or near the yellow spot, for then it may very greatly affect the sight, and render the patient unable to read even large type; a more or less dense cloud or spot covering the letters and rendering them indistinct.

The treatment must be the same as that which is adopted for hyperæmia of the choroid and retina, and hemorrhagic effusions into the latter.

[Embolus of one of the ciliary arteries or of one or more of the choroidal vessels has been found in the eyes, but there is no special ophthalmoscopic sign of its presence.—B.]

12.—DETACHMENT OF THE CHOROID FROM THE SCLEROTIC.

A few cases of this very rare affection have been described, more especially by Von Graefe and Liebreich,[1] and a very beautiful illustration of this condition will be found in the latter's "Atlas."[2] Iwanoff[3] has also given a very careful description of the dissection of an eye affected with detachment of the choroid.

The ophthalmoscopic symptoms of this disease are very marked and characteristic. A more or less considerable globular protrusion is observed in the vitreous humor. Its outline is sharply defined, its surface tense and smooth, and devoid of all wrinkles or foldings, and upon it the retinal vessels can be distinctly traced as they pass over it from the normal fundus. But the most characteristic symptom of all, is the appearance of the choroidal vessels and intra-vascular spaces lying close beneath the retina. At the angle where the protrusion springs from the normal fundus, the retina is not unfrequently somewhat detached, becoming still more so at a later date. The color of the protrusion varies from a pale yellowish-gray tint to a darker red, according as the fluid causing the detachment is of a serous or hemor-

[1] "A. f. O.," iv. 2, 226; Liebreich, ibid., v. 2, 259.
[2] Pl. vii. Fig. 4.   [3] "A. f. O.," xi. 1, 191.

rhagic nature. Its surface is not unfrequently studded with small ecchymoses. On account of the protrusion being situated so far in front of the focal length of the eye, it can be distinctly seen in the erect image at some distance from the eye, affording a faint yellow reflex in place of the bright red glow of the normal fundus. The retinal vessels can also be distinctly observed to traverse its surface. It may be especially distinguished from simple detachment of the retina, by the fact that it does not oscillate, tremble, or fall into small wavy folds when the eye is moved in different directions, but retains its tense, smooth, bladder-like appearance.

It may be difficult, or indeed quite impossible, to determine whether the detachment of the choroid is due to a serous or hemorrhagic effusion, or to some morbid growth pressing it forward. And only as the disease progresses shall we be able to decide this question with certainty, for simple detachment of the choroid by fluid always ends in irido-choroiditis, and softening and atrophy of the eyeball; whereas, in intra-ocular tumors, symptoms of increased tension and glaucomatous inflammation generally supervene as the disease progresses.

[Detachment of the choroid has been known to follow cataract extraction. ("Archiv f. Augen- und Ohrenheilkunde," Bd. i. S. 186.)

That part of the choroid next the ciliary body is most apt to be detached, and here it is most likely to be mistaken for a sarcoma. But in the latter the tension is increased, while in detachment of the choroid the tension is diminished.

The subject of treatment has not received any attention, probably on account of the extreme rarity of the disease. Whether the scleral puncture or the method by drainage, as pursued in detachment of the retina, would prove of any use, can only be determined by trial.—B.]

1. *Increased Tension of the Eyeball.*[1]—This is generally not very considerable, and never reaches the highest degree. [It is remarkable that with a very considerable degree of increased tension, the vision remains normal.—B.] In families in which glaucoma is hereditary, a marked increase of tension is often met with, even in early life, although the disease may not break out till a much later period, or even not at all. In such cases, there can be no objection to look upon this abnormal tension as a predisposing element of glaucoma, more particularly if it be accompanied by hypermetropia, and a disproportionate diminution of the range of accommodation. It has been supposed by some, that the increased degree of tension always precedes, for a longer or shorter period, the other symptoms of glaucoma; Von Graefe has, however, met with several marked exceptions to this rule. In some cases in which he operated for glaucoma in the one eye, the other was found to be of a perfectly normal tension at the time of operation, but was soon after attacked by glaucoma, in one case even by glaucoma fulminans. But an increase in the tension of the eyeball should always excite our suspicions, and should at once lead us to examine as to the presence of other symptoms of glaucoma; if we find none, we should still watch the eye with care, and warn the patient carefully to observe whether any other symptoms begin to show themselves, e. g., rainbows around a candle, rapidly increasing presbyopia, periodic dimness of vision, etc. We must be upon our guard against the but too frequent error, that a sense of fulness or tension within the eye experienced by the patient, is any proof of the increased hardness in the eyeball; for this feeling of fulness may exist without the slightest increase of tension. Another frequent error is, to suppose that all acute inflammations of the eye are accompanied by an increase in the intra-ocular pressure. A careful examination of ordinary cases of acute inflammation of the conjunctiva, cornea, iris, etc., will at once prove the fallacy of this opinion, for the tension will be found normal. If the degree of tension is increased, we must regard it as a dangerous complication, which is to be carefully watched, lest it be the precursor of other glaucomatous symptoms.

2. *Rapid Increase of any pre-existing Presbyopia.*—[A better expression is "recession of the near-point" and diminution of the range of accommodation; or the refraction may be diminished; the latter is not a common anomaly, and Laqueur even denies it. Helmholtz explains it by the eyeball having become more nearly a sphere under the influence of the increased intra-ocular tension; and this has been proven by measurements of the corneal radius.—B.] As the persons attacked by glaucoma are mostly beyond forty-five or fifty years of age, some degree of presbyopia is generally already present, but it is found that this often increases in a very rapid and marked manner during the premonitory stage of glaucoma; so that the patient may be obliged, in the course of a few months, frequently to change his reading-glasses for stronger and stronger ones. This rapid increase in the presbyopia appears to be not so much due to a flattening of the cornea through an increase in the intra-ocular tension, as to the action of this pressure upon the nerves supplying the ciliary muscle, thus causing paralysis of the latter. Haffmans has called particular attention to the fact that hypermetropia very frequently occurs together with glaucoma. It appears probable that hypermetropic eyes are more prone to glaucoma than others; but hypermetropia may also be developed in the course of the disease. The cause of this is, however, still quite uncertain; it is probably to be sought

---

[1] The method of ascertaining and noting the degree of intra-ocular tension is fully explained in the Introduction, p. 35.

for in some changes in the crystalline lens (rapidly progressive senile involution), by which the refractive power of the latter is considerably diminished.

3. *Venous Hyperæmia.*—The congestion of the anterior ciliary veins is generally slight during the premonitory stage, and they never present that peculiar tortuous, dilated appearance, so characteristic of chronic glaucoma. Generally, only a few scattered, dilated veins are seen running over the sclerotic. On examination with the ophthalmoscope, the retinal veins are also found to be dilated and tortuous, there may be likewise spontaneous venous pulsation, or this may be produced by slight pressure upon the eyeball. [It should not be forgotten that spontaneous venous pulsation also occurs in perfectly normal eyes. The narrowing of the veins begins at the porus opticus, and the dilatation follows from the periphery towards the centre, immediately succeeding the radial pulse.

4. *Arterial Pulsation.*—This is first seen on the disk, and is always pathological. It can be produced in the normal eye by firm pressure with the finger, and can be increased in the glaucomatous eye in the same way. The arterial branches on the disk, one or all, contract and dilate, but the pulsation is not noticed beyond the margin of the disk. This spontaneous pulsation is of great diagnostic importance. Von Graefe saw it twice in orbital tumors, and once in descending neuritis, in neither of which cases was there any glaucoma.—B.]

5. *Cloudiness of the Aqueous and Vitreous Humors.*—The aqueous humor is often found slightly but uniformly hazy, rendering the structure of the iris somewhat indistinct, and causing a slight change in its color. The vitreous humor also becomes a little clouded, but uniformly so, for on ophthalmoscopic examination, we do not find dark masses floating about in the vitreous humor, but only a diffused cloudiness, which renders the details of the fundus more or less indistinct. This haziness of the humors is very variable in its degree and duration; sometimes it is so slight as to be hardly perceptible, at others it is so considerable as to prevent any ophthalmoscopic examination. In the majority of cases, however, it is but moderate in the premonitory stage. It may come on several times a day, lasting but for a few minutes at a time, or it may be less frequent, or of longer duration. [The cause of the cloudiness is an exudation, which is either inflammatory in its character or the consequence of venous stasis. In some cases, the cornea is also diffusely cloudy in its parenchyma. Oblique illumination will also in some cases render visible a punctate, gray precipitate upon the membrane of Descemet.—B.]

6. *Dilatation and Sluggishness of the Pupil.*—On comparing the pupil of the eye affected with premonitory symptoms of glaucoma, with that of the other (supposing this to be healthy), the former will be found somewhat dilated and sluggish, reacting but slightly on the stimulus of light. The dilatation is never so considerable as in the advanced stages of glaucoma, when we often find the pupil widely dilated and quite immovable; its sluggishness is, however, generally well marked. [This condition of the pupil is probably not due to diminution of function in the retina, but to an iridoplegia caused by paralysis of the ciliary nerves going to the iris, the direct result of the increased tension.—B.]

7. *Periodic Dimness of Sight.*—The patient is troubled by occasional intermittent dimness of sight. At such times, surrounding objects appear veiled and indistinct, as if they were shrouded in a gray fog or smoke. The degree of dimness varies considerably, as does also the duration of these attacks; sometimes they may last for several hours, at others, only for a few minutes. At such a time there may only exist a slight contraction of the field of

vision; generally, however, there is only indistinctness of eccentric impressions in certain directions. Although these obscurations may be due to transitory cloudiness of the aqueous and vitreous humors, they are generally caused by disturbances in the circulation of the eye. The character of these obscurations may be imitated by pressure upon the healthy eye, and Donders has found that the dimness of vision shows itself as soon as retinal arterial pulsation is produced by this pressure upon the eyeball. I have experimented a good deal upon this point, and have arrived at the same results. I have also found, by experiments upon myself, that by regulating the amount of pressure, I have been able to produce any kind of obscuration, from the slightest, in which only the objects lying quite at the periphery of the field of vision appeared somewhat clouded, to that excessive dimness in which the light of a bright lamp was rendered quite unapparent. The increased intra-ocular pressure, acting directly upon the retina, does not, therefore, appear to be so much the cause of these obscurations; but we must seek for it rather in the impairment of the circulation, the stagnation and fulness of the veins, and, perhaps, the emptying of the arteries (ischæmia retinæ). The increased pressure produces the changes in the circulation, and the latter causes the obscurations. The truth of this assertion is also proved by the fact that these attacks of dimness are generally brought on by anything that causes congestion of the bloodvessels of the eye—for instance, a full meal, great excitement, long-continued stooping, violent exercise, etc.

8. *The appearance of a halo or rainbow around a candle.*—This is also a very constant symptom of the premonitory stage. On looking at a candle, the patient sees a colored halo, or rainbow, around the light. The outer side of the ring is red, the inner bluish-green. This has been supposed by some to be a mere physical phenomenon, due to a diffraction (interference) of the rays of light, owing to some change in the refractive media, especially the peripheral portion of the lens.

It is seen when the pupil is dilated, but disappears when the patient is directed to look through a small opening. It may, however, be also due to congestion of the vessels, for I have seen it sometimes brought on by stooping.

9. *Ciliary Neuralgia*, i. e., pains, more or less acute, in the forehead and temples and passing down the side of the nose, occur occasionally at an early period, but sometimes only at a later part of the premonitory stage, at the same time with the intermittent obscurations. In some instances they are, however, quite absent. [The sudden increase of tension will in some cases explain this neuralgia by pressure upon the ciliary nerves in the sclera. When the neuralgia involves several branches of nerves, we must assume some irritation of the trigeminus.—B.]

10. *The field of vision* is occasionally somewhat contracted; generally, however, there is only some indistinctness of eccentric impressions in certain directions, more particulorly if the illumination is but moderate. In glaucoma, the contraction of the field, as a rule, commences at the inner (nasal) side, and extends thence towards the centre, as well as above and below, until, at a later stage of the disease perhaps, only a small slit-shaped field is left at the outer side.

The intensity of these symptoms varies with the severity of the attack. They may be so slight as to escape all observation, or they may be very marked if the attack is severe, and then there are often added to the symptoms above enumerated, diminution in the size of the anterior chamber, arterial pulsation, and indistinctness of eccentric vision. The latter symptom

may be absent if the illumination is very bright, but becomes evident if it
be moderated.

At the commencement, these premonitory symptoms only show themselves
at long intervals, of perhaps several months, but gradually they become
more frequent. At first, months may elapse between each attack, then
weeks, then days, and when they occur at intervals of a few days, the second
stage, the glaucoma evolutum, may be expected, although this may even
occur when a long interval exists. This stage may also be suspected as
close at hand, if the premonitory symptoms do not disappear after sleep,
even of short duration (Von Graefe). If the periodic attacks no longer leave
behind them a normal pupil, and a normal acuteness of vision, still more, if
the optic nerve is already cupped, we must no longer designate it as the
premonitory stage, but as a case of glaucoma evolutum, with periodic increase of the symptoms.

The premonitory stage may last for an indefinite period; years may even
elapse before it leads to confirmed glaucoma; but in the majority of cases it
does not extend beyond a few months, or it may pass over into glaucoma
even after the second or third attack, there being only remissions, and not
clear and well-defined intervals between the attacks. Sometimes, as has
been mentioned above, the premonitory symptoms are so slight as quite to
escape the notice of the patient, particularly if the other eye is still perfectly
healthy. It is different, however, when one eye has already been lost by
glaucoma, for then the patient's attention and anxiety are at once aroused
by any of the premonitory symptoms, and he early consults his medical
attendant, fearful lest he should also lose the sight of the second eye.

[Laqueur's observations upon the prodromal stage of glaucoma are interesting. He thinks that the influence of advanced years in the etiology of
glaucoma has been over-estimated, and that the climacteric period in women
has no influence at all in its production. A very common cause of the
appearance of the prodromal symptoms is intense hunger. In other patients
the symptoms appear after sudden attacks of fright or anger, after sleeples-
ness, violent and exhausting exercise, etc. The well-known symptoms of
colored rings or circles, which are most distinct at the centre of the field,
are also visible to the patient as far as the extreme periphery of the field,
though less distinctly; and an observant patient will also see a faint, colorless, diffuse ring outside of the colored ones. The prodromal stage may
either disappear of itself, or during sleep, or as a consequence of the instillation of eserine. Under the action of the latter remedy the vision becomes
perfectly clear, the tension diminishes, the cloudy and colored rings disappear. Laqueur attributes the production of the latter symptoms to the
diffuse corneal opacity. He considers that eserine simply postpones an
attack of glaucoma, and that it never exercises any influence on the ultimate
course of the disease.—B.]

In the great majority of cases, as already stated, acute inflammatory
glaucoma is preceded by a more or less marked premonitory stage of varying
duration. The intervals between the premonitory attacks become less and
less frequent, until the latter recur perhaps every two or three days, or even
every day. The patient is then suddenly seized, frequently at night-time
and after having passed perhaps several sleepless nights, by a severe, often
excruciating, pain in and around the eye, which extends to the forehead,
temple, and down the corresponding side of the nose, as far as the extremity
of the bone. Sometimes this pain reaches also to the corresponding half of

the head, and even to the occiput, which causes it often to be mistaken for an attack of rheumatism. At the same time there may be considerable constitutional disturbance, febrile excitement, and severe nausea and vomiting, and these symptoms may be of such prominence that the patient is supposed to be suffering from a severe bilious attack, and the affection of the eye is either overlooked, or is thought to be dependent upon this, But the eye shows marked symptoms of acute internal inflammation. The eyelids may be much swollen, red, and puffy. The conjunctival and subconjunctival vessels are injected, the veins in particular being dilated and gorged. There may also be very considerable serous chemosis, which completely hides the deeper subconjunctival vascularity and the rosy zone around the cornea. There are also much photophobia and lachrymation, but they are accompanied by very little mucous discharge, and this chiefly of a thin frothy character. The cornea is clouded on its posterior surface, being perhaps studded with minute opacities, deposited from the aqueous humor. [There may be loss of the epithelium of its anterior surface and circumscribed opacities. Fuchs describes this cloudiness of the cornea as an œdema. The cornea is equally œdematous in all its layers in but a few cases, the anterior layers being usually the most œdematous. The œdema also collects between the anterior layers and Bowman's membrane. Very marked changes in the anterior epithelium are occasionally met with, such as very small drops lying upon Bowman's membrane between the feet of the basic cells, their contents being either homogeneous or granular. These drops are usually situated at the anterior end of the nerve-channels. All these changes are nothing but an œdematous condition, which is the immediate cause of the corneal opacity. (See "Archiv für Ophthalmologie," xxvii. 3.)—B.] The sensibility of the cornea may be also somewhat diminished, but this anæsthesia never attains the same degree as in chronic glaucoma, where it is often so great, that the cornea may be touched or even rubbed with a roll of paper or the brush of a quill pen, without its being felt. Occasionally, the anæsthesia is only partial, being confined to a certain portion of the cornea. This loss or diminution in the sensibility is due to the compression of the nerves supplying the cornea by the increased intra-ocular tension, as is proved in cases of acute glaucoma, where the sensibility at once returns after diminution of the tension by iridectomy or paracentesis. The sensibility of the cornea is best tested by touching it delicately with a finely rolled spill of silk paper, care being taken to keep the eyelids well apart, so that the conjunctiva is not touched. In healthy eyes, the cornea is so exquisitely sensitive that the slightest touch of a foreign body will be felt and resented.

The anterior chamber is found to be somewhat more shallow, the [lens and] iris being pressed forward, and even, perhaps, in contact with the cornea, the aqueous humor is clouded, the iris somewhat discolored and of a dirty hue—in some cases there may even be acute iritis, with deposits of lymph at the edge of the pupil—the pupil is dilated and sluggish, and in elderly people a peculiar green reflex is often seen, coming apparently from the back of the eye.

It has already been stated that this green reflex was formerly considered as the principal and pathognomonic symptom of glaucoma. It is due to the following cause: The lens undergoes certain physiological changes after the age of forty, amongst others assuming a yellowish tint. Now, if the eye of an elderly person (and they are the most prone to the disease) is attacked by glaucoma, the aqueous humor becomes turbid and of a dirty, bluish-gray color, and this bluish-gray tint, mixing with the yellow of the lens, gives rise to this peculiar green reflex. The latter is the more marked on account of the dilatation of the pupil which exists in glaucoma, as more light is thus reflected from the lens, more particularly its periphery, than when the pupil is of the normal size. The grayish haziness of the vitreous humor, moreover, also tends to increase the intensity of the reflected light. Two facts prove that this is the true explanation of this green reflex. 1st. If the anterior chamber is tapped, and the aqueous humor flows off, the green reflex at once disappears. 2d. If a youthful eye is attacked by glaucoma, this reflex is not visible, for at this period of life the lens has not yet acquired a yellow tint, and in such a case the pupil looks, therefore, only of a dirty, bluish-gray color.

The eyeball will be found abnormally hard. The refractive media are generally so clouded as to render an ophthalmoscopic examination impossible. If they are, however, sufficiently clear to permit of the details of the fundus being seen, we find the retinal veins dilated, tortuous, and perhaps pulsating; the optic disk may be slightly reddened or of a dirty-yellow appearance, and there is either spontaneous arterial pulsation, or this may be readily produced by slight pressure on the eyeball. In the first attack of acute glaucoma, no cupping of the optic nerve is found, for this only occurs when the increased tension has lasted for some time.

After iridectomy, we generally find more or less extensive hemorrhagic effusions into the retina and choroid. It was formerly supposed that they often exist prior to the operation, but, according to Von Graefe, this is not the case, except the glaucoma is secondary to some hemorrhagic affection of the retina (e. g., retinitis apoplectica).

Vision may be either greatly impaired, so that the patient is only able to distinguish letters of the largest type or to count fingers, or it may be lost completely and suddenly, as at one stroke, being diminished to a mere quantitative perception of light, i. e., to a mere distinction between light and dark, not an appreciation of colors and objects. In some very severe cases even this is lost. The field of vision is generally somewhat contracted, often concentrically. The patient is in most cases also troubled with subjective appearances of light, balls of fire, showers of bright stars, etc.

The impairment of sight is evidently not so much due to direct compression of the nerve-fibres of the retina by the increased tension, as to the impediment of the arterial blood supply (ischæmia retinæ) which is produced by the latter. Moreover, Von Graefe[1] thinks it probable that when the impairment of vision is very great, as in cases of acute inflammatory glaucoma, in which of course there is no excavation of the optic nerve, the tissue of the retina is also specially affected. This supposition is, moreover, supported by the fact that retinal hemorrhages are of constant occurrence after the iridectomy, if there has been, together with considerable increase of tension, marked cloudiness of the refracting media. Von Graefe formerly explained the occurrence of these ecchymoses as being due to the sudden diminution of the morbidly increased tension; but this explanation, as he now points out, appears to be insufficient, more especially when we remember that in cases of glaucoma simplex these retinal hemorrhages do not occur after iridectomy, even although the tension had been greatly increased. Hence he thinks it probable that the interrupted, and therefore defective, supply of arterial blood (which is evidenced by the spontaneous arterial pulsation which is but seldom absent during the glaucomatous attack), the impediment of the venous circulation, and, finally, the inundation of the retinal tissue by the fluids effused from the uveal tract, lead to a state of frangibility (softening) of the retinal tissue, which favors the occurrence of these hemorrhages.

---

[1] "A. f. O.," xv. 8, 109; vide also Rydel, ib., xviii. 1, 1.

The inflammatory symptoms may gradually subside, but the blindness continue; this is, however, very exceptional. In most cases, the inflammatory attack passes off after a few days or weeks, having, perhaps, undergone during this time several remissions, and vision may be entirely restored.[1] Such a temporary recovery may occur spontaneously, or after the use of antiphlogistics, mercury, opium, leeches, etc. But the eye does not return to its normal condition; the anterior chamber mostly remains somewhat shallow, the iris discolored, the pupil dilated and sluggish, the field of vision somewhat contracted, and the tension of the eyeball more or less augmented. But the disease is not arrested. The acute inflammatory attacks may recur again and again, leaving the vision each time in a worse condition, and the visual field more contracted, until the sight is finally completely destroyed. In other cases, no further acute inflammatory attacks occur, but chronic inflammatory exacerbations take place. Or the disease may progress insidiously, without any apparent recurrence of the inflammatory symptoms. The eyeball becomes more and more tense, the field of vision more contracted, often to a slit-shape, the sight gradually lost, the fixation perhaps eccentric,[2] the cornea roughened and anæsthetic, the anterior chamber very small, the pupil greatly dilated and fixed, the iris discolored, atrophied, and shrivelled up to a narrow rim, the subconjunctival veins turgid and tortuous, forming large round the cornea. If the refractive media are sufficiently clear to permit of an ophthalmoscopic examination, we then find that there is a progressive excavation of the optic nerve, that the retinal veins are dilated and tortuous, and that there is either a spontaneous or easily producible arterial pulsation. We not unfrequently find, even after the disease has thus insidiously run its course without any inflammatory exacerbation since the first acute attack, that at a later stage these inflammatory attacks, even of a very acute kind, may again occur. When the disease has run its course, and all, even quantitative, perception of light is lost, Von Graefe calls it "glaucoma consummatum," or "absolutum."

Sometimes we meet with a *subacute* form of glaucoma, in which all the inflammatory symptoms are much diminished in intensity; the pain is also less, nor is the sight so much impaired as in the acute cases.

The very dangerous disease which has often been termed "hemorrhagic glaucoma," is really a secondary glaucoma supervening on some of the hemorrhagic affections of the retina, especially retinitis apoplectica, and will therefore be described in the section on "Secondary Glaucoma."

Von Graefe[3] has called attention to a class of cases in which the course of acute glaucoma is most rapid, so that the sight, even all quantitative perception of light, of a previously perfectly healthy eye, may be entirely lost within a few hours, or even within half an hour, of the outbreak of the dis-

---

[1] Mr. Pridgin Teale has informed me of the interesting fact that increased glaucomatous tension may be relieved by morphia. He was called to a patient suffering from acute glaucoma of a few hours' duration, and being unable to iridectomize for some hours later, he injected one-eighth of a grain of morphia under the skin in order to relieve the pain. In half an hour the pain had gone, the dimness of sight almost amounting to blindness had disappeared, and on his seeing the patient four hours afterwards, the tension (+2) had become normal. He at once deferred the operation until glaucoma supervened a fortnight later.

[2] By the term "central fixation" is meant, that a line drawn from the object through the centre of the cornea of the observer would strike his yellow spot; his visual line being in fact fixed upon the object. Eccentric fixation, therefore, means that some other portion than the yellow spot is directed to the object, having retained more sensibility than the macula lutea.

[3] "A. f. O," 7, viii. 2.

ease. He has termed this *glaucoma fulminans*. It is, however, a very rare form indeed, in comparison with the common acute glaucoma.

He has found that cases of glaucoma fulminans are also occasionally distinguished by a very rapid development of the other symptoms of increased intra-ocular pressure, viz., intense ciliary neuralgia, rapid dilatation of the pupil, soon reaching its maximum extent, rapid diminution in the size of the anterior chamber, anæsthesia of the cornea, and stony hardness of the eyeball. Sometimes, however, these symptoms are not more pronounced than in the common form of acute glaucoma, and yet the sight may be completely destroyed within an hour or two. The phenomena of vascular excitement may appear simultaneously with the loss of sight, but they occasionally lag behind in a peculiar manner. On microscopic examination, the aqueous and vitreous will be found to be diffusely clouded, but if they are sufficiently clear to permit the details of the fundus to be seen, a considerable overfulness of the retinal veins will be observed. Diminution in the size of the arteries and excavation of the optic nerve appear, comparatively, very rapidly. Von Graefe has in one case noticed the latter in a very deep form, even within a few weeks after the outbreak of the disease. He thinks we must assume that, in this form, the increase in the tension is either more considerable or more sudden than in the ordinary cases. On account of the great stagnation in the venous circulation of the eye in these cases, iridectomy is often followed by extensive hemorrhage into the retina and choroid.

2.—CHRONIC INFLAMMATORY GLAUCOMA.

This disease may be insidiously developed from the premonitory stage. The premonitory symptoms become more frequent, and continue for a longer period; the intermissions are of less duration, until there are no longer any distinct intermissions, but only remissions, and the disease gradually and almost imperceptibly passes over into chronic glaucoma; the eye assuming the same condition as it did in the acute form, after the conclusion of the inflammatory process. It becomes more and more tense, until it may at last assume a stony hardness ($+$ T. 3), so that it cannot be dimpled by even a firm pressure of our finger. The subconjunctival veins become dilated and tortuous, the sclerotic assuming in the late stages of the disease a peculiar waxy hue, which is due to atrophy of the subconjunctival tissue, and to a diminution in the calibre of the subconjunctival arteries. The cornea gradually loses its sensibility more and more, frequently, however, only in certain portions. It also becomes flatter. The anterior chamber becomes shallow, the aqueous humor clouded, and this turbidity may change with great rapidity, occurring, perhaps, several times a day. It may be produced by any excitement or fatigue, often coming on after a full meal, excessive exercise, etc. The iris is pushed forward, so as to be perhaps almost in contact with the cornea. It is dull and discolored, its fibrillæ being more or less obliterated, and not showing a clear and distinct outline. The pupil is widely dilated, and either immovable or extremely sluggish to the stimulus of light. The field of vision becomes greatly contracted, assuming, perhaps, a slit shape. As has been before pointed out, the contraction of the field in glaucoma begins, as a rule, at the inner side, extending from thence upwards and downwards, so that the outer portion is the last to become affected. Vision progressively deteriorates, the fixation often becomes eccentric, and finally the sight may be completely destroyed, so that not even a remnant of quantitative perception of light is left, even although the light be intensified by means of a powerful biconvex lens.   On ophthalmoscopic examination, we find that the fundus always appears more or less clouded, often to such an extent as to prevent our distinguishing the details of the background of the eye. This haziness is due to opacity of the aqueous and vitreous humors, and in some cases also of the cornea and lens. But if the media remain sufficiently clear to permit of an examination, we find the retinal veins widely dilate and tortuous, the arteries diminished in calibre, and presenting either ad spontaneous or easily producible pulsation; the optic nerve more or less deeply cupped, and the vessels displaced at its periphery. The chief and characteristic difference between the acute and the chronic inflammatory glaucoma is, that the latter may lead to even complete destruction of sight, without any symptoms of severe inflammation or great pain.   There may only be insidious attacks of chronic, frequently recurring inflammation, leading gradually to loss of sight. At first these inflammatory attacks may be intermittent, occurring at considerable intervals, whereas later they may only show remissions. In other cases again, after the eye has been suffering for some time from these insidious chronic inflammations, it may be suddenly attacked by a severe acute exacerbation, causing very great pain and suffering.   These acute exacerbations may recur again and again, and the pain may be so severe that recourse must be had to an iridectomy for its relief, even although there is no chance of restoring any sight. In such instances, the patient and his friends must be warned beforehand that the operation is not performed for the sake of giving any sight, but only in order, if possible, to relieve the pain.   In many cases, particularly if the iridectomy be made sufficiently large, the relief may be permanent; in others it is only temporary.   When speaking of acute glaucoma, it was mentioned that after the first acute attack, the disease might gradually pass over into chronic inflammatory glaucoma, no fresh acute attack occurring, but only chronic, latent, inflammatory exacerbations.

When the disease has run its course, and all sight is lost, Von Graefe terms it "glaucoma absolutum." Then any chance of benefiting the sight by an operation is past. [Bluish-red vessels run over the dense white sclera, the limbus assumes a bluish tint, the cornea becomes cloudy in spots, and if the lens is transparent the optic disk is seen to be dense white.—B.] The lens frequently becomes opaque, assuming the peculiar greenish hue so characteristic of glaucomatous cataract. The glaucoma absolutum may exist for a length of time without the eye undergoing any changes, except that atrophies of the iris, choroid, and optic nerve become more and more apparent. In other cases, frequent—often very acute and violent—inflammatory symptoms show themselves, accompanied by intense ciliary neuralgia and headache. In the last stages of the disease other changes occur; the eye becomes reduced to a narrow streak, the cornea opaque and softened, more particularly in its central portion, and hemorrhagic effusions take place in the anterior chamber, the vitreous humor, and the inner tissues of the eyeball.   Sclerotic staphylomata are formed, and suppurative inflammation may even occur, leading to atrophy of the globe. Von Graefe calls this the stage of glaucomatous degeneration. In it, iridectomy no longer proves a sure remedy for the inflammatory complications.   Generally, the sight is entirely lost. Sometimes the one eye may be lost from chronic inflammatory glaucoma, or from the apparently non-inflammatory form (glaucoma simplex), and the other be attacked by acute glaucoma.

3.—GLAUCOMA SIMPLEX (DONDERS).[1]

This disease was for a long time considered as distinctive from glaucoma, with which it was supposed to have nothing in common but the excavation of the optic nerve, and was originally described by Von Graefe under the title of "Amaurosis with excavation of the optic nerve."

The course of the disease is often exceedingly insidious, so that it may be considerably advanced before the patients pay any particular attention to it, supposing, but too frequently, that the increasing weakness of sight is simply owing to old age. Though this impairment of vision may be noticed also for distance, it makes itself particularly felt in reading, writing, sewing, etc., and convex glasses are found but of slight assistance. There is generally no premonitory stage, for the intermittent obscurations, rainbows around a candle, etc., are mostly due to some slight inflammatory attack, accompanied by cloudiness of the refractive media.

The external appearance of the eye may be perfectly healthy. The refractive media may be quite clear, the cornea sensitive, the anterior chamber of the normal size, the iris healthy and not discolored, or but very slightly so, this being only apparent on comparison with the iris of the other, healthy eye; the pupil perhaps slightly dilated and a little sluggish. But the eyeball is generally found to be abnormally tense, and with the ophthalmoscope we observe that the optic nerve shows a glaucomatous excavation. Sometimes this increase in tension varies greatly, being very marked at one time, and hardly, if at all, apparent at another; it is of great consequence, therefore, to examine such eyes frequently, and at different periods of the day. There is still a good deal of discrepancy of opinion as to the invariable presence of increased tension of the eyeball in this form of glaucoma. Some assert that tension is always increased in all cases of glaucoma simplex; others, again, think that although this undoubtedly does occur in the majority of cases, yet that in others it is absent. Von Graefe, in particular, maintains that the intra-ocular tension is not in all cases increased in a marked manner. He thinks that the occurrence of glaucomatous excavation of the optic nerve, without any marked increase in the tension of the eyeball, may be explained thus: That perhaps the resisting power of the optic papilla varies in different individuals, perhaps also at different ages. Just as iritis and irido-cyclitis serosa may occasionally be observed, particularly in young individuals, to exist for some length of time with an unmistakable increase of tension, without any excavation; may not, on the other hand, the power of resistance of the optic papilla be absolutely (?) or relatively so diminished that an exceedingly slight increase of tension, not exceeding the normal range of variation of tension, may already cause an excavation? But every, even the most considerable increase of tension, requires to act some time before it leads to cupping. The truth of this is shown in cases of acute glaucoma, where there is no cup directly after the first acute attack, although this may have lasted for some weeks, during which the intra-ocular tension was greatly increased. In glaucoma fulminans it is somewhat different, for there it appears to supervene early. It a long-continued, though slight, increase of tension will lead gradually an excavation of the optic nerve, which increases more and more in depth; vessels then become interrupted at its edge, and there is spontaneous or ly producible arterial pulsation. The veins appear dilated, and perhaps

[1] Haffmans, "Archiv," viii. 2.

somewhat tortuous. If the tension continues, the optic nerve gradually atrophies, the arteries become diminished in calibre, and complete blindness may supervene. It is found that if the increase in tension is very slow and gradual, the excavation of the optic nerve may become very considerable in depth, without the sight or field of vision being markedly impaired. Increased intra-ocular tension is, therefore, generally the first symptom of glaucoma simplex, being accompanied perhaps by a relatively rapid increase of presbyopia, and some hypermetropia; gradually, however, the optic nerve becomes cupped, and these symptoms may last for a considerable time without others supervening. In some cases, however, the augmented tension may exist for a long period without the presence of other glaucomatous symptoms.

Occasionally glaucoma simplex may run its course, even to complete blindness, without the appearance of any inflammatory symptoms. The disease slowly but surely progresses, the eyeball becomes more and more hard, the cornea anæsthetic, the anterior chamber narrower, the vessels more turgid and congested, the pupil dilated and sluggish, the retinal veins engorged, the arteries diminished in calibre, and perhaps pulsating, the optic nerve deeply cupped and whitish in color, the visual field more and more contracted, and the sight finally destroyed. [Beginning glaucomatous cupping may be diagnosticated when a vessel makes a distinct bend at the margin of the disk, and when its papillary end lies deeper than its retinal end. As the excavation increases in depth, and the wall becomes steeper, the apparent displacement of the vessels becomes more marked, until finally they appear interrupted, the portion between the margin of the cup and its bottom being lost to sight.—B.]

In such instances, the course of the disease may be so insidious that the sight of the eye (if the other is perfect) may be completely lost, without the patient being aware that there is anything the matter with it. Perchance he closes the good eye, and then he discovers the blindness of the other, and thus often supposes that the vision has been suddenly lost. On being questioned, he may perhaps remember that he occasionally experienced slight pain in and around the eye, which was supposed to be rheumatic; that it sometimes became a little flushed and watery, which was attributed to a cold; but otherwise he noticed nothing peculiar. This may not only occur amongst the humbler classes, following pursuits which require but little employment of the sight in reading, sewing, etc., as amongst laborers; but it may even occur amongst men of literary habits and avocations, employed for many hours daily in reading and writing.

But, in the majority of cases, inflammatory symptoms show themselves during the progress of the disease, and these may assume an acute, a chronic, or an intermittent type. They present the same character as in acute or chronic inflammatory glaucoma; rapid diminution of vision, obscurations, rainbows around a candle, augmentation of tension, dulness of the aqueous and vitreous humors, etc. Sometimes, however, these inflammatory symptoms may not appear until the disease has long run its course, and the sight has been completely lost. In other cases, they may be so transitory as to escape our observation, and their previous existence may not be ascertained, except by a very close examination into the history of the case. Where manifest symptoms of inflammation are apparently wanting in a case of glaucoma simplex, the condition of the other eye, if healthy, should be ascertained; and then, on a comparison of the two, we may often detect slight changes in the color and structure of the iris, and slight haziness of the aqueous humor of the affected eye, which, but for this comparison, would have escaped our attention. Von Graefe also points out the necessity of examining such patients at a period of the day most favorable for the observance of any inflammatory symptoms, and points out the fact that whilst the inflammatory symptoms in iritis, etc., particularly the deeper injection, become commonly more apparent soon after sleep, the reverse obtains in glaucoma, for here they become the more prominent the longer the patient keeps awake, more particularly if he remains up beyond his customary time for retiring to bed. He mentions an interesting case, illustrative of the peculiar transitory character which the inflammatory symptoms may occasionally assume. The right eye of the patient in question ordinarily presents a perfectly healthy appearance, but for several years past it assumes a well-marked glaucomatous condition when he has been playing cards for some length of time, and only then. On such occasions, the anterior chamber becomes shallower, the aqueous humor diffusely clouded, the pupil somewhat dilated and sluggish, the retinal veins dilated, particularly towards the edge of the optic disk, and arterial pulsation may be produced by the faintest pressure upon the eyeball; together with these symptoms, there is indistinctness of vision, surrounding objects appearing to be covered by a veil or cloud. Not till the following morning have all these symptoms disappeared, then the sight is again normal (No. 1 of Jäger's types at twelve inches), and the increase in the tension of the eyeball, which was very manifest during the attack, is no longer appreciable.

Glaucoma simplex, as a rule, attacks both eyes, almost symmetrically, but at a more or less considerable interval.

[With the failure in central vision is connected also some indistinctness in eccentric vision, and even a pronounced defect in the field. In fact, the latter may precede the former, begins at the periphery, and extends on the nasal side towards the centre, the temporal side being the longest preserved.—B.]

Haffmans considers that glaucoma simplex is identical with the premonitory stage of glaucoma of Von Graefe, and maintains that all the symptoms enumerated as existing in the premonitory stage are present in glaucoma simplex; but I think it of the greatest practical importance to maintain the existence of a premonitory stage, for we find, after all, that its course is generally very different from that of glaucoma simplex. The premonitory stage may exist even for many years without producing any glaucomatous changes in the eye, the symptoms may only show themselves at long intervals, and in their intermissions the eye may be perfectly healthy; or they may recur at more frequent intervals, and pass over into acute or chronic glaucoma. In other cases, they may pass over into developed glaucoma after only a few premonitory attacks. Besides this, we find that the most brilliant results of iridectomy are to be expected in the premonitory stage; but this is by no means the case in glaucoma simplex, for here the results of iridectomy differ in a very peculiar and important manner.

4.—SECONDARY OR CONSECUTIVE GLAUCOMA.

latter is not affected. Thus diffuse keratitis becomes more frequently complicated with secondary glaucoma than the circumscribed infiltration of the cornea; and the equatorial choroiditis accompanied with vitreous opacities, than the disseminated choroiditis.[1] Amongst the diseases in which secondary glaucoma most frequently supervenes are: 1. Diffuse keratitis and anterior staphyloma of the cornea. 2. Iritis serosa, and iritis complicated with considerable posterior synechiæ. 3. Traumatic cataract. 4. Dislocation of the lens. 5. Serous choroiditis. 6. Sclerectasia posterior. 7. Intra-ocular tumors. 8. Hemorrhagic affections of the retina.

A fuller account of this subject will, however, be found in the sections in which these different diseases are treated. [Cicatricial ectasia of the cornea is probably the most frequent cause of secondary glaucoma, especially if there are extensive adhesions of the iris to the cornea. Whether the secondary increase of tension in these cases is in consequence of an increase of secretion within the eye due to a stretching of the ciliary nerves, or to the collection of fluid behind the iris causing venous stasis in the ciliary body, is still a moot point.—B.] With regard to the secondary glaucoma supervening upon retinitis apoplectica, I must, however, briefly call the attention of the reader to some of the most important points. This complication is particularly met with in persons beyond middle age, of a very full habit, and affected with more or less extensive sclerosis of the coats of the arteries. The disease commences as retinitis apoplectica, and after this has existed for from one to six months (Von Graefe), secondary glaucoma supervenes, which may assume a very pronounced and acutely inflammatory character, in which case it is often accompanied by the most intense ciliary neuralgia. The field of vision is but slightly, or not at all, contracted, and there is no glaucomatous excavation, nor, as a rule, arterial pulsation. Dr. Hermann Pagenstecher[2] has found on microscopical examination that in these cases the walls of the retinal vessels are greatly thickened (sclerosis), and show considerable varicosities. This sclerosis of the walls of the vessels and their consequent loss of elasticity must, as he points out, have an important effect in disturbing the circulation of this part of the eye. He mentions one curious case of hemorrhagic glaucoma which was evidently of sympathetic origin, as it improved very greatly and rapidly after excision of the other eye. Or it may appear in the form of glaucoma simplex, the increase in the tension being very gradual, acute inflammatory exacerbations occurring only at a later stage. The disease is often accompanied by hemorrhagic effusions into the vitreous and aqueous humors; and during an acute paroxysm the sight may be suddenly lost, this being probably due to a hemorrhagic detachment of the retina. Von Graefe points out the fact, that in such cases the application of atropine may accelerate the outbreak of the glaucoma.[3] He also states that in two-thirds of the cases of glaucoma supervening on hemor-

---

[1] "A. f. O.," xv. 3, 121.   [2] "A. f. O.," xvii. 2, 98.

[3] That atropine will sometimes cause an outbreak of glaucoma in cases of intra-ocular tumor, and acute exacerbations in chronic glaucoma, was pointed out by Von Graefe, in "A. f. O.," xiv. 2, 117. Dr. Derby, of Boston, has also related two cases in which the instillation of atropine was directly followed by an outbreak of acute glaucoma ("Transactions of American Ophthalmological Society," 1869). I have likewise met with a few such instances. In one case, the patient had lost the left eye from chronic glaucoma, and, complaining of slight premonitory symptoms in the right, atropine was applied to the latter. I briefly examined the eye with the ophthalmoscope, and within twenty-four hours a severe attack of acute glaucoma occurred. These facts should warn us not to employ atropine unnecessarily, to be careful as to its extreme purity, and to make any ophthalmoscopic examination as brief and as little trying to the eye as possible.

rhagic retinitis, the outbreak occurred between the fourth and the tenth week after the first functional disturbance of the eye. Hence, the longer the tenth week has passed, the less chance is there of secondary glaucoma.

But glaucoma may also complicate diseases which stand in no causal relation to it. Thus it may supervene upon senile cataract or upon cerebral amaurosis. In the former case, the cataract should never be removed at the same time that the iridectomy is made for the relief of the glaucoma, for in case any vitreous humor should be lost during the extraction of the lens, it might very easily give rise to severe intra-ocular hemorrhage. Some months should elapse between the two operations, in order that the improvement in the circulation, tension, and nutrition of the eye may become thoroughly established.[1]
[In a few rare cases secondary glaucoma has been known to complicate detachment of the retina, in which there is usually diminution of intra-ocular tension; and in one case reported by Desmarres it appeared in a typical case of retinitis pigmentosa. Finally, several observers, among them Quaglino, have observed glaucoma supervene in eyes with congenital coloboma iridis and total irideremia.—B.]

5.—OPHTHALMOSCOPIC SYMPTOMS OF GLAUCOMA.

The characteristic ophthalmoscopic symptoms of glaucoma are—pulsation of the central vessels of the retina (vide p. 386), and excavation of the optic nerve.
The stasis in the venous circulation of the retina is often very considerable, the veins are dilated and tortuous, the smaller veinlets assuming a corkscrew appearance; if the stasis be very great, the larger venous branches may even show peculiar bead-like swellings. This is, however, very rare. I have seen one case in which there was a distinct tendency to these swellings, but Liebreich figures a case, in his "Atlas d'Ophthalmoscopie," in which it existed in the most marked manner. After diminution of the pathological increase in the intra-ocular tension, the stagnation in the venous circulation ceases, the calibre of the veins diminishes in size, and they lose their tortuosity. For instance, after the performance of iridectomy and the consequent diminution in the tension of the eyeball, we frequently have an opportunity of observing the change in the venous circulation. Thus, extensive retinal ecchymoses are perhaps met with, and the veins, which, before the operation, were very dilated and swollen, are now much diminished in size and paler. The retinal arteries in glaucoma appear very thin and small, and much paler than in the normal eye.
Whilst spontaneous venous pulsation may occur in normal eyes, spontaneous arterial pulsation is only observed if the intra-ocular tension is markedly increased, or in cases of insufficiency of the aortic valves. The

---

[1] It is an interesting fact that glaucoma may also, in rare instances, become developed in an eye in which the lens is absent, and this, as has been pointed out by Rydel ("Bericht über die Wiener Augenklinik," p. 155), is an important point with regard to the theory that the beneficial effect of the iridectomy in glaucoma is due to its relief of the irritation and teasing of the iris, which occur when the latter, together with the lens, is pressed forwards owing to the increased intra-ocular tension. Now, in two cases of glaucoma in eyes without a lens, the anterior chamber was deep and the iris lying in its normal plane, so that there could be no question of its being teased or irritated by anything. Heymann also reports some cases of glaucoma becoming developed in eyes in which the lens was absent ("Kl. Monats.," 1867).

arterial pulsation is synchronous with the radial pulse, but slightly later than the carotid pulsation. It is confined to the disk, and presents a rapid to-and-fro movement, and a rhythmical filling and emptying of the arteries. The arterial diastole takes less time than the systole, and is characterized by a rapid, jerky entrance of a column of blood into a previously empty vessel.

6.—ON THE NATURE AND CAUSES OF THE GLAUCOMATOUS PROCESS.

The true nature and cause of the glaucomatous process are still involved in some obscurity and doubt. In the great majority of cases of glaucoma there are marked inflammatory symptoms, but it must be freely admitted that we do sometimes, although far more rarely, meet with cases of glaucoma simplex, in which no inflammatory symptoms can be detected. Indeed it is the latter fact which causes all the difficulty, for we can easily explain the increased tension, and all the symptoms which follow in its train, as due to an inflammatory origin; but we cannot as satisfactorily explain what constitutes the primary cause of the increased tension in glaucoma simplex, which leads to the gradual loss of sight from excavation and degeneration of the optic nerve without any appearance of inflammation. In the inflammatory forms of glaucoma, the seat of the inflammation is chiefly in the uveal tract, the choroid, ciliary body, and the iris. But other structures, such as the cornea, sclerotic, and retina may subsequently become involved. This irido-choroiditis causes an increase of serosity, more especially in the vitreous humor, and an augmentation of the intra-ocular tension; the latter giving rise to all the glaucomatous symptoms described above. Together with this increase in the volume of the vitreous humor, there exists in glaucoma a diminution in the power of absorption, and this may explain why these serous effusions are not removed, as in other forms of choroiditis, by an increased activity of the absorbents. Attention has been called by some writers to the fact, that the sclerotic appears peculiarly rigid and unyielding in glaucoma, and it has been supposed that this is not unfrequently congenital or hereditary, and may form a predisposing element to glaucoma. Now, if such an abnormal rigidity of the sclerotic exists, we can easily understand how any rapid, though slight augmentation in volume of the contents of the eyeball, must not only give rise to a disproportionate increase in the intra-ocular tension, but must also augment the tendency to stagnation in the bloodvessels. Coccius has found in a case of glaucoma, that the sclerotic had undergone fatty metamorphosis, and he thinks that the affection of the sclerotic may perhaps have been the cause of the increased intra-ocular tension. There can be no doubt that the rigidity of the sclerotic plays a very important part in glaucoma; for we find that in youthful individuals, in whom the sclerotic is more elastic and yielding, an increase of the intra-ocular tension, dependent upon some inflammation of the uveal tract, may exist for some time without exerting any deleterious effect upon the optic nerve or retina. The sclerotic perhaps yields a little, as a whole, before this increased tension and adapts itself to it, or it may become slightly bulged at a certain point; whereas in older persons, in whom the sclerotic is more firm, rigid, and unyielding, the existence of an increase in the intra-ocular tension is much more dangerous, for it soon causes the least resistant tissue (in this case the optic nerve) to yield before it, and become excavated. Von Graefe attaches very great importance to the part played by the sclerotic in the pathogenesis of glaucoma, especially glaucoma simplex.

When considering the different forms of glaucoma, we had frequent occasion to point out the great variations in the intensity of the inflammatory symptoms. We saw that in acute glaucoma, the inflammation might be very severe during the first attack, but that after its subsidence, the inflammatory exacerbations might assume an insidious, chronic character, and the disease gradually pass over into glaucoma absolutum, without the recurrence of any acute attack. Again, that in the chronic form the inflammatory symptoms might, at the outset, be but little marked, but that in the course of the disease acute exacerbations, even of a very severe character, might show themselves. In the third form (glaucoma simplex), it was stated that the disease might occasionally run its course without the apparent occurrence of any inflammatory symptoms—the eyeball becoming stony-hard, the optic nerve deeply excavated, the sight destroyed—but the refractive media remaining perfectly clear. But in the vast majority of cases of glaucoma simplex, inflammatory symptoms, of varying severity, do show themselves during the progress of the disease. Now, on account of the fact that glaucoma simplex may occasionally run its course without the apparent presence of any inflammatory symptoms, and on account of the increased tension being sometimes the first manifest symptom of the disease, it has been supposed by Donders that the inflammation is not the integral part of the glaucomatous process, but only a complication, which, though occurring in the majority of cases, need not necessarily be always present. He considers the increase in the intra-ocular tension as the essence of the disease, and therefore, the glaucoma simplex, which runs its course without any inflammatory symptoms, as the primordial type of the disease; and he thinks that the acute or chronic inflammation which shows itself in the majority of cases of glaucoma is but a complication, which is of secondary importance, and not necessary to the glaucomatous process. He, therefore, speaks of glaucoma simplex, and glaucoma cum ophthalmiä. The anomaly in the secretion of the fluids of the eye, he thinks due to an abnormal irritation of the nerves regulating the intra-ocular secretion. Now from some very interesting and ingenious experiments made by Dr. Wegner ("A. f. O.," xii. 2, 1), it appears certain that the vaso-motor nerves of the iris, and in all probability those of the choroid also, are furnished by the sympathetic. He found in experiments upon rabbits that a division of the sympathetic in the neck leads to a dilatation of the vessels of the iris and choroid, and a diminution of the intra-ocular pressure. It may consequently be assumed that irritation of the vaso-motor nerves would produce an increase in the intra-ocular pressure. But, as Wegner states, the latter experiment is extremely difficult and uncertain, on account of the impossibility of regulating the degree of irritation with sufficient delicacy. The intimate relation between the branches of the fifth nerve supplying the eyeball and the sympathetic, easily explains how an irritation of the former may be reflected to the sympathetic, and thus cause hyper-secretion of fluid within the eye, and an increase in the intra-ocular pressure. In this way the cases of glaucoma complex are readily explained. Such cases have been observed by Hutchinson[1] and Horner.[2] In one case of Horner's, the attacks of neuralgia were simultaneously accompanied by glaucomatous symptoms. The numerous and very interesting experiments performed by Drs. v. Hippel and Grünhagen[3] on animals, chiefly rabbits and cats, have shown that the fifth nerve exercises the greatest influence on the intra-ocular tension, and it would appear that its

---

[1] "R. L. O. H. Rep.," iv. and v.   [2] "A. f. O.," xii. 2.
[3] "Kl. Monatsbl.," 1868, 884; vide also "A. f. O.," xiv. 3, 219, and xv. 1, 265 [and

action is twofold: 1. It directly dilates the vessels going to the eye; 2. It gives rise to an increased effusion of fluid in the posterior portion of the eye-ball, a fact which is proved by the persistent increase in the eye-tension. They found that the third nerve only in so far influences the intra-ocular tension, as it causes contraction of the external muscles of the eye; and that the sympathetic exerts no influence whatever.

Dr. Adamük,[1] on the other hand, maintains very strongly the opinion that the intra-ocular tension depends upon the lateral pressure in the vascular system, and is solely influenced by the sympathetic.

It has also been urged that inflammatory glaucoma cannot occur primarily in a hitherto healthy eye, that an increase in the tension of the eyeball pre-existed; that, in fact, glaucoma simplex had existed, perhaps quite unknown to the patient, and that the inflammation supervened upon this. But we sometimes meet with cases of acute glaucoma in which there was no trace of increased tension, or any other glaucomatous symptom, prior to the outbreak of the disease. Thus Von Graefe mentions cases in which he has operated for glaucoma upon the one eye, the other being at the time of operation of quite a normal degree of tension; and yet the latter was soon after attacked by glaucoma, in one case even by glaucoma fulminans. He thinks, more-over, that the mere increase of tension should not be allowed to constitute a premonitory stage, for even a considerable increase of tension may exist for an indefinite period without the appearance of other glaucomatous symp-toms. In families in which glaucoma is hereditary, an increased resistance, often of a marked degree, exists even in infancy, and the disease may not show itself till middle age, or even not at all.

The question whether the inflammation be but of secondary importance or not, is one of much consequence. The great difficulty lies in those cases (although they are but rare) in which we find the glaucomatous disease running its course without any, even the slightest, symptom of inflamma-tion; for if this be possible, then, indeed, we cannot look upon the inflam-matory symptoms as the sine qua non of the disease.

With regard to this subject of the origin of glaucoma simplex, Von Graefe[2] has recently expressed his opinion in the following terms: " If the principal doubts as to the theory of glaucoma formerly found their chief support in the supposition that the same cause which kindles the inflammatory changes of the typical glaucoma, also gives rise to the simple increase of tension, these doubts have now fallen into the background, partly on account of our more extended knowledge of the evolution of secondary glaucoma, and partly in consequence of the modifications which have very lately been made in the theory of inflammation. For if we observe in a certain form of secondary glaucoma, for instance after dislocation of the lens, to-day a simple increase of the tension, to-morrow inflammatory cloudiness of the refracting media, and thus both appearing alternately, according to the more energetic action of the cause (e. g., the more considerable movements of the lens), we must surely be convinced of the identity in the nature of both forms, and of the existence of differences varying simply in degree, according to the intensity and duration of the cause; for if it is admitted that the form of glaucoma which commences with opacity of the media is inflammatory, I think we cannot deny this nature to the other, which goes hand in hand with it, although for the sake of distinction this may very well be termed 'the non-inflammatory' or 'simple secretory.' But still more is the supposition of a difference purely of degree strengthened by the theory of inflammation

[1] " Kl. Monatsbl.," 1868, 392.   [2] "A. f. O.," xv. 3, 198.

advanced by Cohnheim, which once more brings the essence of inflammation within the territory of abnormal secretion. If, through the influence of some cause which suddenly and powerfully affects the vascular system, a considerable effusion of cell elements takes place into the fluids of the eye, a visible opacity is thereby produced; whereas if the admixture is less considerable, and takes place under a more tardy and less intense action of the cause, the transparency of the media need not be visibly affected. In such instances it often only requires a very slight additional impulse, e. g., the congestion arising during the process of digestion, to increase the opacity to such a degree as to render it apparent." He is, therefore, of opinion that we must presume that in glaucoma simplex there exists in the eye a *permanent stimulus*, and must consider it to be—from the exact similarity of its course and of the results of treatment—a *secondary glaucoma* dependent upon a varying, or at least not uniformly localized intra-ocular cause. This intra-ocular cause is, however, still shrouded in obscurity, but it seems that special attention ought to be paid to the condition of the sclerotic, both in clinical and anatomical investigations.[1]

He thinks that in the cases of glaucoma simplex, a lengthened observation will generally show us that transitory inflammatory exacerbations (perhaps of a very ephemeral nature) do mostly occur. Such exacerbations may be but very slightly marked, and easily escape the attention of the patient or his medical attendant; or they may but occur at certain periods, or be produced only by certain causes, as, for example, in the case mentioned above, in which they only came on whenever the patient played at cards. The absence of any externally visible symptoms of vascularity is no proof of the non-existence of internal inflammation, for the ophthalmoscope constantly reveals to us the presence of even considerable inflammation of the choroid and retina, without the existence of any increased vascularity of the external tunics of the eyeball. The haziness of the aqueous and vitreous humors, which may arise during such an ephemeral exacerbation, may likewise be so slight and delicate as to escape detection with the ophthalmoscope, for we know that fine diffuse opacities of the aqueous humor are often quite invisible by transmitted light.[2]

[During the past three or four years, the nature and causation of glaucoma have occupied very largely the attention of ophthalmic surgeons, especially in Germany, and a number of observers have published extensive papers as the results of their experiments and observations upon the subject. Though some light has been thrown upon the nature of the disease by these studies, the pathology, and to a certain extent the causation also, of glaucoma is still obscure. The two great theories now, as heretofore, are the inflammatory and the neurotic or irritative. In 1876 Knies published an article upon glaucoma, followed by a second one in 1877, based upon a careful examination of twenty-two glaucomatous eyes, which had been enucleated for various reasons. (See "Arch. f. Ophth.," xxii. 3, and xxiii. 2.) The most frequent, and, as he thinks, the most important pathological change found in these eyes was the obliteration of Fontana's space, for he reasons that the obliteration of this space must cause an increase of the intra-ocular tension. Furthermore, he does not think that the flattening of the anterior chamber from advance of the iris and lens, must necessarily be regarded as a sign of increased tension. In every eye examined, indubitable signs of inflammation or its consequences were found in the neighborhood of Schlemm's canal; and

---

[1] "A. f. O.," xv. 211.

[2] For further information upon this interesting and important subject, I must refer the reader to Von Graefe's and Dr. Haffmans' paper on "Glaucoma," "A. f. O.," viii. 2.

this held good as well for cases of secondary glaucoma as for the primary form. His investigations led him to the following conclusions:

1. The most important change in real glaucoma, is the annular adhesion of the periphery of the iris with the cornea or the obliteration of Fontana's space; the excavation of the optic nerve is a secondary matter.

2. The same relation exists also in secondary glaucoma.

3. Iridectomy cannot be replaced by the use of eserine, nor by the other methods of operating proposed.

4. Sclerotomy is an exception to the preceding, as the excision of a piece of iris is unimportant; it may therefore be substituted for an iridectomy.

5. The relationship between many staphylomatous processes and glaucoma, is proven by pathological examinations.

About the same period Ad. Weber published the results of his own investigations upon glaucoma. (See the "Arch. f. Ophth.," xxiii. 1.) He came to the conclusion that a pure theoretical analysis of the physical features of glaucoma leads to the conviction that the cause can only be a purely mechanical one, that of a gradual narrowing of the filtration channels of the fluids contained within the eye. In all forms of glaucoma, the inflammatory as well as the non-inflammatory, the primary as well as the secondary, these channels are narrowed and finally obliterated. Weber hesitates to accept the view that the swelling of the ciliary processes is the cause of glaucoma. It is true that the group of symptoms known as glaucoma appear when this mechanical obliteration has taken place, and that the exciting cause of the so-called primary glaucoma is the swelling of the ciliary processes. But this pathological condition is not confined to glaucoma, but is met with in other diseases; neither is it, even in connection with a certain rigidity of the sclera, the only cause for the development of the glaucomatous condition. Weber's paper is a very long and interesting discussion of the subject, but does not easily admit of a satisfactory abstract being made.

Next in order of importance appeared a lengthy paper by Schnabel, entitled "Contributions to the Knowledge of Glaucoma." (See "Archives of Ophthalmology," vii. 1, 2, 3, and 4.) In a previous paper published in vol. v. 1, of the same journal, he pronounced the opinion that it had not yet been proven that the clinical picture of inflammatory glaucoma was the consequence of a choroidal inflammation. In this second paper he discusses and combats Knies' interpretations of the pathological changes found in the anterior chamber. The same changes he found himself in glaucomatous eyes, but he does not accept Knies' views. His own conclusions are based upon an examination of thirty-nine eyes examined by himself. He holds that the pathological changes in the periphery of the anterior chamber, do not necessarily present the peculiar clinical picture of the glaucomatous process. What functional disturbances of the eye are caused by the obliteration of the angle of the anterior chamber, he is not sure of, but this obliteration does frequently exist without being clinically observed. He does not consider that the existence of corneal cicatrices with incarcerated iris endangers the eye. The peril of increase of tension and of consecutive excavation of the optic nerve occurs only when the cicatrix begins to bulge. The obliteration of the angle of the anterior chamber alone is harmless; the traction on the origin of the iris and the stretching of the sclero-corneal margin cause the increase of tension. He thinks it erroneous to suppose that iridectomy in glaucoma acts by establishing the communication between the anterior chamber and Fontana's spaces, and denies that the scleral cicatrix possesses any peculiarity of structure by which its imputed function as a filtration tissue could be accounted for. He calls special attention to

Brailey's discovery of the atrophy of the ciliary muscle in glaucomatous eyes. He regards it as the only anomaly demonstrated hitherto by the anatomical examination, which has undoubtedly a relation to the glaucomatous process, and is not merely a consequence of it. It exists before the glaucoma can be clinically demonstrated, as he proves by a case. The highest degree of atrophy is certainly only found in eyes in which the glaucoma had existed for a long time; but the increase of the atrophy does not stand in a direct proportion to the duration and degree of the increased tension.

Later observations of importance are contained in a most admirable paper by Mauthner, entitled "Glaucoma Aphorisms" (see "Archives of Ophthalmology," vii. 2, 3, and 4, and viii. 1). His views are very different from those of Schnabel and others, in that he accepts unequivocally the inflammatory theory of the disease. He first considers the cupping of the optic disk, summing up the evidence derived from the observations of Müller, Mooren, Brailey, and Schnabel, with special reference to the condition of the optic nerve fibres. These have shown that all anatomical examinations of glaucomatous eyes in which the layer of nerve fibres has been preserved, never give, in spite of the yielding of the lamina cribrosa, any other picture than that of a partial funnel-shaped excavation; a picture from which it is possible to explain, according to our present views, the ophthalmoscopic appearance of a "pressure" excavation extending to the margin of the disk. Mauthner holds that the total excavation is not a pressure excavation so long as the function of the nerve is preserved; in this agreeing with Von Jaeger and Klein, and differing from Schnabel. From the sum total of facts presented by himself and other authorities, he believes that glaucoma is a choroiditis, complicated with inflammatory symptoms also in the anterior segment of the eyeball, which as a rule begins with increase of tension but also progresses without this, and is accompanied by the development of an affection of the optic nerve, which is dependent on the process in the choroid, but is not always present. The functional disturbance in glaucoma cannot be explained by a primary affection of the light-conducting apparatus; it depends upon some injury done by the choroiditis to the function of the light-perceiving apparatus. Increase of tension and glaucomatous affection of the optic nerve are neither the cause nor the beginning of blindness. There are real glaucomatous processes which lead to blindness without increase of pressure and without excavation. The nature of the choroidal process which lies at the bottom of glaucoma is still but little understood. Its products are poor in new-formed elements, but it may be, and that not remotely, connected with choroiditis serosa. It begins in the anterior segment of the eyeball as atrophic choroiditis. In the beginning, the pigment epithelium in the erect image shows some delicate alterations, and slight as these are, the process which lies at their foundation is threatening to destroy the layer of rods and cones. Mauthner also differs from Brailey and Schnabel in regarding the atrophy of the ciliary muscle, not as the cause, but as the result of the glaucomatous process. He leaves entirely untouched, however, the subject of the causes of glaucoma, and says nothing of the theory of the impeded outlet at the iris-angle, which has occasioned so much discussion.

Priestley Smith regards the fundamental and essential cause of primary glaucoma to be an insufficiency of space between the ciliary processes and the lens. All conditions which tend to promote venous turgescence, arterial hyperaemia, or increased secretion within the eye, might become exciting causes of glaucoma, provided this abnormality were present. He suggests that the starting-point of glaucoma is some condition which raises the vitreous pressure slightly above the aqueous pressure. Narrowing of the circumlental space would tend to raise the vitreous pressure, and circumstantial evidence favors the idea that narrowing of this space is actually the starting-point of primary glaucoma. Examination of a large number of eyes has convinced him that the diameter of the lens increases with age; that its whole bulk is increased with the advance of life. He has found in glaucomatous eyes, after enucleation, that the circumlental space was sometimes widely open; but there was usually evidence to show that it had previously been abnormally narrow. As the diameter of the lens increased, the distance which separated it from the ciliary process decreased, and that the circumlental space diminished with age.

Brailey's theory of glaucoma starts out with the axiom that the amount of transudation varies with the blood pressure, which pressure is increased locally whenever any artery is dilated up to its origin from a arger trunk. This enlargement of the vessels is seen within the eye, and affects almost solely the bloodvessels of the ciliary region and iris. This enlargement is probably the consequence of an affection of the vaso-motor nerves. The existence of arterial dilatation may be due in some cases of glaucoma to irritation of the nerves of the ciliary body consequent on the extreme stretching of the fibres of the suspensory apparatus of the lens. Brailey infers that arterial enlargement, if not found on enucleation, has never existed; though he admits that, if the disease has not lasted long enough for atrophy of the arterial walls to have supervened, it may have existed and then afterward subsided. This might explain the phenomena of intermittent glaucoma, and the occasional cure of glaucoma by paracentesis alone. He believes that atrophy with sclerosis of the ciliary body and iris is always preceded by some inflammation, and when these are once established, there will be an actual diminution of the fluids normally recruiting the vitreous and aqueous, unless an enlarged arterial supply exists. He recognizes the existence of an intra-ocular current, passing from the vitreous through the canal of Petit into the posterior chamber of the aqueous humor, then through the pupil into the anterior chamber and thence out. A slightly increased pressure from vitreous to aqueous might carry the periphery of the iris forward and aid in blocking further exit through the ligamentum pectinatum. In cases of advanced and applied iris, he attributes the position of the iris to an increased flow of fluid towards Schlemm's canal from the ciliary body, due either to its inflammation or to the increased vascular supply. Whenever the canal of Schlemm is blocked by the iris, this condition is accompanied, as be found in a large number of cases, either by perforated corneal ulcer, or by an acute inflammation of the ciliary body and usually with extreme atrophy of the latter. It is thus clear that obstruction at the canal of Schlemm is sufficient to maintain a glaucomatous condition, and even to originate one, provided the iris has been brought into the required position. In a still more recent paper, Brailey holds that in glaucoma inflammation of the iris, ciliary body, and optic nerve is always present, and that it is one of the earliest symptoms of primary glaucoma, being developed previous to the tension. It is usually most pronounced in the ciliary body. The advanced position of the iris is caused in the first instance by an enlargement of the ciliary folds, due to their vascular turgescence, but afterwards its application is rendered more close and extensive by the pressure of fluid behind it. Later there occurs very rapid atrophy of the ciliary muscular fibres with dense connective-tissue formation between them and in the optic nerve. The choroid is compressed and atrophic, but rarely presents any trace of inflammation. The cause of the increased intra-ocular fluid is in the first instance an inflammatory hyper-secretion of fluid from the ciliary body and iris.

But when the atrophic changes have occurred in the ciliary body and iris, the occlusion of the entrance to Schlemm's canal is the sole agent in keeping up the tension.—B.]

Glaucoma is a disease of old age, being most frequently met with between the ages of fifty and sixty, but it may occur even at a much later period; it is but seldom observed in early life or before the age of thirty. [It has been known, however, to occur in young persons, Stellwag having seen a case in a girl of twelve, Schirmer in a boy of twelve, and Laqueur in a boy of twelve. Glaucoma occurs in about one per cent. of all eye diseases, and with about the same frequency in the two sexes, though the acute inflammatory form is met with oftener in women, and the simple non-inflammatory in men. In a certain proportion of cases the disease is hereditary.—B.] Von Graefe believes that the predisposition of old age to glaucoma is chiefly due to two causes:[1] 1. The same degree of increased tension more quickly produces an excavation of the optic nerve in old persons; which is probably owing to the diminution of the resistance of the papilla. 2. The increase of tension becomes, *cæteris paribus*, more quickly developed in old age, which is very likely due to the fact that the secretory filaments contained in the ciliary nerves are in a condition more prone to irritation, when they pass through a rigid senile sclerotic, than when they traverse a more youthfully yielding sclerotic. This hypothesis would also tend to explain the fact that glaucoma occurs more frequently in hypermetropic than in myopic eyes, as without doubt the sclerotic is more rigid, especially at the point where the ciliary nerves pass through it, in hypermetropes than myopes.

In females it is most apt to occur soon after the cessation of menstruation. We find that the males who are attacked by glaucoma frequently suffer from gout or disorders of the digestive organs, and are often subject to hæmorrhoids. There is no doubt that glaucoma, especially the inflammatory, may be hereditary, and, as has been already mentioned, the eyes of the individual members of the families in which this disease is hereditary, often show, even in early life, a peculiar increase in the tension, and rigidity of the sclerotic; and these symptoms may exist for many years without any glaucomatous outbreak. Von Graefe[2] has remarked the interesting fact that when already several generations have been affected with glaucoma, the outbreak occurs earlier, in the middle or even the first period of life. In some of these cases of hereditary glaucoma, the premonitory stage may last for eight, ten, or even sixteen years.

We have stated that glaucoma may appear as a primary or secondary disease. In the former case, it may occur after severe external injuries, or without any apparent external or internal cause. It always attacks one eye first, and may remain confined to this; but when once the one eye has become affected by glaucoma, there is a great tendency in the disease to invade the other also. We must, therefore, always prepare such a patient for the eventuality—the great likelihood even—of the other eye becoming also affected. By careful and judicious treatment, and by abstinence from excessive fatigue and exertion of the eye, much may be done to retard the attack, and break its force. The nature of the glaucomatous process in the first eye is generally no criterion as to the form which may occur in the other. We find, for instance, that the first eye may be suffering from glaucoma simplex, or chronic inflammatory glaucoma, and the other be attacked by the acute form, or even by glaucoma fulminans. The time which may intervene before the second eye becomes affected varies greatly; sometimes a few

[1] "A. f. O.," xv. 8, 230.   [2] "A. f. O.," xv. 8, 228.

days only elapse, in other cases many months, or even years. In the secondary glaucoma, which may supervene upon another affection (traumatic cataract, irido-choroiditis, etc.), this disposition to extension of the disease to the other eye is far less than in the primary form; but still such a tendency does exist, and may be called into activity by any injury to, or operation upon, the sound eye.

7.—PROGNOSIS AND TREATMENT OF GLAUCOMA, ETC.

If the disease be left to itself, or be treated by inefficient remedies, the prognosis is most unfavorable, as it leads sooner or later to destruction of sight. The old treatment, which consisted in leeching, cupping, mercury, opium, etc., fails, and is sure to fail, in staying the progress of the disease. The acute inflammatory attack may subside under the use of these remedies, or even without any treatment whatever; the inflammatory symptoms may diminish, the refractive media again become transparent, the sight restored, and the patient and his medical attendant may deceive themselves with the fond hope that the dangerous disease has passed away and is cured. But this is not so. Sooner or later the eye again becomes attacked, perhaps by acute exacerbations, perhaps by insidious chronic inflammations, which gradually lead to total and irremediable blindness.

[It should be especially remembered that all mydriatics, particularly atropia, are to be avoided; for an acute attack of glaucoma has been repeatedly known to occur after instillation of atropia.—B.]

The chief and most important indication in the treatment is the diminution of the abnormally increased intra-ocular tension, for as long as this exists we cannot hope to arrest the progress of the disease. Paracentesis of the cornea has long ago been tried in the treatment of glaucoma, and has lately been again strongly recommended as a cure for this disease; but we know that its effect is but transient, that it relieves the intra-ocular tension for a short time, but that this relief is not permanent, for the latter (as well as other glaucomatous symptoms) soon manifest themselves again. [Sperino has most strongly advocated paracentesis of the cornea, but has come to the conclusion that in the advanced stages of glaucoma it cannot rival iridectomy. —B.] Division of the ciliary muscle (as it has been termed) has also been much vaunted as a cure for glaucoma. That it may temporarily relieve tension by causing the escape of the aqueous and perhaps of some of the vitreous humor, cannot be denied; but tapping the anterior chamber will do the same thing. If a considerable amount of vitreous humor flows off, the tension may even be permanently diminished. But the escape of vitreous in glaucoma is a thing to be avoided, if possible, and not to be desired or courted; for we find that the loss of vitreous (for instance, in the operation of extraction of cataract) generally renders the eye more prone to chronic inflammatory affections of the choroid, accompanied by opacities of the vitreous humor, etc. At present no evidence has been brought forward by the supporters of this operation that would permit of our placing it side by side with iridectomy in the treatment of glaucoma. [Hancock first proposed intra-ocular myotomy, thinking that glaucoma was caused by a spasm of the ciliary muscle. He introduced a Beer's cataract-knife in the sclero-corneal margin between rectus externus and inferior, and cut through sclera and ciliary muscle for about one-eighth of an inch in a direction from above and forwards, outwards and backwards. Various modifications of this operation have been proposed by Solomon, Heiberg, and Prichard. It is said to be without danger, and to give the best results in acute glaucoma.—B.]

More recently the incision of the sclerotic (sclerotomy) has been brought forward as a substitute for iridectomy in some cases of glaucoma, and has been chiefly recommended by De Wecker[1] and Quaglino.[2] The former now performs the operation as follows: With a narrow Von Graefe's knife he makes the puncture and counter-puncture exactly as in his operation for extraction of cataract; but in withdrawing the knife, he leaves the central part of the flap standing, which diminishes the tendency to prolapse of the iris. He has tried it seven times in cases of absolute glaucoma accompanied by intense pain; the latter was stopped and the eye-tension diminished. Quaglino makes the incision in the sclerotic (about two millimetres from the cornea) with a very wide iridectomy knife, and in withdrawing it very slowly, he presses the back of the blade somewhat against the iris, so as to prevent prolapse of the latter. If a portion of iris should protrude, it must be gently replaced; but if it should protrude again, I think it would be better to excise it than to irritate the iris by repeated attempts to replace it. I think that the operation must be tried much more extensively before we can arrive at any just conclusion as to its relative value. [For a full and complete history of the operation of sclerotomy, the reader is referred to Mauthner's pa er on "Glaucoma Aphorisms," already quoted. (See "Archives of Ophth.," vii. 2, 3, and 4.) Both De Wecker and Quaglino think it offers better results in acute glaucoma than in any other form of the disease, but Schmidt thinks it is to be preferred to iridectomy only in those cases where the iris is so atrophied that its excision is rendered very difficult. Mauthner believes that even simple and chronic glaucoma, as well as the acute inflammatory form, can be cured by sclerotomy; but the scleral wound must be made in the proper way, and must not be too small. He lays down the following rules for the technique of the operation: 1st. A one per cent. solution of sulphate of eserine must be dropped into the eye before the operation. 2d. The operation should, if possible, be performed without narcosis. 3d. The section, if possible, should be made upwards. 4th. Enter with Von Graefe's narrow knife at one millimetre from the edge of the cornea, as if about to make a scleral flap. 5th. When the knife has made the counter-puncture, it is to be pushed slowly forward, and the operation is to be ended in the slowest possible manner, and with a sawing motion of the knife. 6th. The flap is not to be completed, but the apex is to be left as De Wecker advised. 7th. The sum of the length of the two incisions should exceed the length of the incision in simple iridectomy. 8th. The knife is not to be removed from the eye until the aqueous has entirely escaped. 9th. Eserine is again to be instilled, and a tight bandage applied. Mauthner thinks that sclerotomy should unconditionally replace iridectomy in the following cases: 1st. In the so-called prodromal stages of glaucoma. 2d. In glaucoma simplex, where central and peripheral vision are still almost normal. 3d. In chronic glaucoma, when the defect in the field has drawn extremely near to the point of fixation. 4th. In congenital hydrophthalmos. The operation, however, has not yet been done with sufficient frequency to allow of its ultimate value to be fixed. Glaucoma, in the United States, is a rare disease, and though sclerotomy has been done a number of times, the statistics are too small to be of any value. Galezowski recommends crucial sclerotomy in glaucoma. He divides the sclera and cornea with a narrow knife, for a distance of half a centimetre in each, in the horizontal meridian, on both sides of the cornea, and also in the vertical meridian, on both sides. Eserine

---

[1] "Kl. Monatsbl.," 1871, p. 805; and "Annales d'oculistique," Mars–Avril, 1872.
[2] "Annali di ottalmologia," 1871, p. 200; vide also a paper read at the Ophthalmological Congress held in London, 1872.

is then instilled, and a press re-bandage appplied.   The anterior chamber is reëstablished in five or six days.

The general opinion expressed at the Ophthalmological Section of the London International Medical Congress was, that iridectomy still remains the best operation for most cases, notably for cases of acute glaucoma. When myotics produce no effect on the pupil, sclerotomy is inadmissible, on account of entanglement of the iris, which is sure to ensue.   Sclerotomy may be resorted to in buphthalmos, in simple chronic glaucoma, in hemorrhagic glaucoma, and in cases where the field of vision is contracted nearly to the point of fixation.—B.]

Iridectomy, on the other hand, has been proved to diminish (and in the vast majority of cases permanently) the abnormally increased intra-ocular tension.   The admirable results of this operation in the treatment of glaucoma have long admitted of no doubt, tested and endorsed as they have been by most of the distinguished oculists of Europe.

Some opposers of the operation have, apparently, thought that its supporters claimed for it the power of restoring sight in all cases of glaucoma, whatever their stage or nature might be.   But none of its advocates have ever done this; they have only upheld its curative powers in those cases in which irreparable changes in the structure of the eye had not yet taken place.   The extent of the benefit which may be expected from iridectomy will, therefore, depend upon the stage and form of the disease in which it is had recourse to.   It may be laid down as an axiom, that the sooner the operation is performed when the premonitory symptoms have become marked and frequent, or after the outbreak of the disease, the better; so that the affection has not yet had time to produce material changes in the structures of the organ.   Let us now shortly consider what prognosis may generally be given of the beneficial effects of iridectomy in the various stages and forms of glaucoma.

The Premonitory Stage.—As long as the premonitory symptoms only occur at distant intervals, and the intermissions are complete, the eye returning to its normal condition during the intervals, we may postpone the operation with safety.   We should, however, warn the patient against any excessive fatigue or exertion of the eyes, and their exposure to very bright light or rapid changes of temperature; against everything, in fact, that may produce hyperæmia and irritation of the organ, and which may thus hasten the outbreak of the disease.   He must also abstain from excesses of every kind. But the system of lowering and starving patients suffering from glaucoma is not advisable, indeed often most injurious, more particularly if they are elderly, and have been very free livers.   Such patients should be placed upon an easily digestible, nourishing, and even perhaps generous diet, and should be permitted a moderate allowance of stimulants, the quantity being regulated by their former habits and the condition of their general health.

[Adamük reports a case occurring in the practice of Iwanoff, of a lady who for nearly three years kept the premonitory symptoms of glaucoma in abeyance by small doses of quinine, never amounting to more than twelve grains in the day.—B.]

If the intermissions are no longer complete, but there are only remissions of the symptoms; if the periodic obscurations, the ciliary neuralgia, the iridisations occur at short intervals of a day or two; if the eccentric vision becomes impaired and the field contracted, the vessels congested, and the eyeball tense, it would be dangerous to delay the operation any longer.   The acute attack is then probably imminent, and we cannot foretell what its severity may be, and whether it may not burst forth in a very acute form, even that of glaucoma fulminans, and rapidly lead to such serious lesions of the structures as greatly to im ril, or even to spoil, the integrity of the organ, before operative aid can be obtained. But there is another reason why we should not wait for the acute outbreak of the disease, for we cannot be certain that it will occur, as the affection may gradually, and perhaps almost imperceptibly, pass over into the chronic glaucoma, with excavation of the optic nerve, accompanied by such a deterioration of the retina and other tissues that the operation may then prove of but little avail. If iridectomy is performed during the premonitory stage, when the symptoms become marked and the attacks frequent, but before any structural changes have taken place, the prognosis is most favorable, for the progress of the disease is arrested, and the sight of the eye saved.

In *acute inflammatory glaucoma* the prognosis is also favorable, if the operation is only performed sufficiently early. If the impairment of vision increases very rapidly, if the sight is already diminished to a mere quantitative perception of light, or if the visual field is much contracted, the delay of the operation would be most dangerous, and it should be performed at once. We may generally expect a nearly perfect result if iridectomy be had recourse to within a fortnight after the outbreak of acute glaucoma; always remembering, however, that at least good quantitative perception of light must still be present. But we should never voluntarily wait so long, as there is always a risk that during the delay the tissues may undergo serious changes. Von Graefe lays particular stress upon the fact, that the immediate necessity for the operation depends less upon the intensity of the inflammatory symptoms, the acuteness of pain, or the amount of increased tension, than upon the state of vision. If this be not greatly impaired, if the patient is still able to read large type, the operation may be postponed, if it be necessary, for a day or two. But in the interim, the patient must be closely and anxiously watched, and if rapid diminution of vision occurs, no further delay must be permitted. Sometimes the question may arise, whether a patient suffering from an attack of acute glaucoma may be permitted, if necessary, to undertake a journey in order to have the operation performed, or whether he may be safely allowed to wait until the inflammation has subsided, and the eye has again become "quiet." Here I must strongly urge the necessity of not delaying, for if the journey be postponed until the inflammation is allayed, the eye may be found to be irretrievably lost. The journey would have proved far less dangerous than the delay. But even if the most favorable event should occur, if the inflammation should subside, and the eye apparently regain its former condition, we know but too well that the disease is not cured, that it will sooner or later recur, either in the acute form or as chronic glaucoma. In the latter case, the progress may be so insidious that serious and irreparable changes in the optic nerve, the retina, and the coats of the vessels may have occurred, before the patient's attention is attracted to the state of his   e.

In *glaucoma fulminans the operation must be performed as soon as possible.* The structures undergo such great and rapid changes that the effect of the operation may not be perfect even when it is performed within three days after the outbreak of the disease, as was shown in a case of Von Graefe's.

In those cases of acute glaucoma in which the pain is very intense, and there is much inclination to vomit, but the impairment of vision is only moderate, Von Graefe thinks it may be better to wait a day or two before performing iridectomy. Here he employs the subcutaneous injection of morphia (one-eighth to one-third of a grain), in the region of the temple, in order to procure a good night's rest, and to quiet the nervous system before operating. But if we give chloroform, the operation need not, I think, be postponed on this account. In fact, iridectomy proves the best antiphlo-gistic, and its beneficial effects in acute glaucoma are most marked and bril-liant if it be performed sufficiently early. The tension is generally greatly diminished directly after the operation. In the next few days it may increase again a little, but then it subsides spontaneously to the normal standard. The anterior chamber is either re-formed very shortly after the iridectomy, or in the first few days. The relief of the often agonizing pain is generally immediate; patients soon fall into a tranquil and refreshing sleep, after having perhaps passed several sleepless, miserable nights; the inflammatory symptoms rapidly subside; the sight is greatly improved, partly from the diminution in the intra-ocular tension, and partly from the escape of the turbid aqueous humor. This improvement rapidly increases during the first fortnight, and is generally due to the absorption of the retinal ecchymoses which occurred during the operation. The improvement of sight reaches its maximum extent about two months after the operation. If the latter has been performed sufficiently early, vision is generally perfectly restored, the patient being able to read the very finest print (with, of course, the proper glasses, if he is presbyopic), and this improvement is, in the vast majority of cases, permanent. Such a result may even be expected up to within a fort-night after the outbreak, if, at the time of the operation, there was still good perception of light and no considerable contraction of the field.

In the late stages of acute glaucoma the results of the operation vary. In such cases, the prognosis will depend upon the extent to which the degenera-tive alterations in the tissue have already advanced. The prognosis may be favorable if the visual field is only moderately contracted, more particularly if the contraction is not slit-shaped but concentric, the fixation central, and vision not vary greatly impaired, especially if the impairment depends upon cloudiness of the refractive media and increased intra-ocular tension. The operation will generally not only restore an excellent and useful amount of vision, but this improvement will mostly be permanent. It is different, however, if the field is greatly contracted, especially if it be slit-shaped, if the fixation is eccentric, vision much impaired, and the latter due, not to opacity of the refractive media, but to an already considerable excavation of the optic nerve and deterioration of the retina. Here the prognosis must be guarded, for although the operation may do much even in such cases, the good results may sometimes not be permanent, but the sight be gradually lost again, either through recurrence of inflammatory attacks, or through progressive excavation and atrophy of the optic nerve.

The prognosis of the effect of iridectomy is extremely bad in the secondary glaucoma supervening upon hemorrhagic affections of the retina (the so-called hemorrhagic glaucoma). Only in very rare instances is there any permanent improvement; generally the operation gives rise to a great increase in hem-orrhagic effusions, which may burst through into the vitreous, rapidly destroy the last glimmer of sight, and produce such excruciating pain, that the eyeball has to be excised as the only mode of relieving the patient from his agony. Von Graefe has quite abandoned the operation in this form of glaucoma. It may be a question, however, whether, in those cases in which the patient has already lost the other eye, we may not afford him the last chance and operate, warning him well, however, of the but too probable un-fortunate result.

In *chronic inflammatory glaucoma*, the prognosis must also be guarded. The progress of the disease is but too often so insidious, that the patients do not apply for medical aid until very considerable changes have taken place in the tissues, more particularly the optic nerve and retina. Iridectomy

will, however, generally arrest the disease, and preserve the existing amount
of vision, or even improve it. This is particularly the case if the fixation is
still central, the sight not too much impaired, the optic nerve not deeply
excavated, and the field of vision not slit-shaped, but contracted laterally
or concentrically. In such cases, the progress of the disease and of the
structural changes is generally stayed, and the existing amount of vision
permanently preserved. The beneficial effects of the operation are, however,
far more slowly developed than in acute glaucoma. Months elapse before
the improvement has reached its maximum degree, or before we can be
certain that the effect will be permanent. But even when the field is greatly
contracted and the fixation very eccentric, we may yet occasionally be able
permanently to preserve a certain amount of sight, enough perhaps to enable
the patient to find his way about. And even this little must be looked upon
as a great boon in comparison with total blindness. But in such cases, the
effect of the operation is sometimes only temporary, the tension of the eye
again increases, the vision slowly but steadily deteriorates, leading at last to
complete loss of sight. This is far more frequently due to progressive atrophy
of the optic nerve, than to a recurrence of the glaucomatous symptoms.

Should a recurrence of the glaucomatous inflammatory symptoms with
increased tension, take place after an iridectomy, the operation may be
repeated with benefit; before doing so, the effect of repeated paracentesis
should however be tried. This is particularly the case when the original
iridectomy has not been sufficiently large, or the iris has not been removed
quite up to its ciliary insertion. The second iridectomy should be made
diametrically opposite the first, so as to cut off the two halves of the iris
from each other; I have often performed this second operation with much
advantage in obstinate cases of glaucoma, and it appears to have more effect
than if the second iridectomy is made beside the first. In those cases of
glaucoma where it seems likely that the first iridectomy will not suffice to
diminish the tension permanently, and that a second one will probably be
required, the two opposite iridectomies may be made simultaneously with
Mr. Bowman's stop-knives, as described in the chapter on "Cataract." If the
tension still increases again in spite of the second iridectomy, paracentesis
should be again repeatedly tried. Should the other eye be hopelessly blind,
either from glaucoma or some other cause, and especially if it is subject to
inflammatory attacks and is painful to the touch, it would be advisable to
remove it, as the obstinate return of tension may be due to sympathetic irritation caused by the lost eye.

Von Graefe has called attention to the fact, that a whitish discoloration
of the optic nerve (which is generally a symptom of progressive atrophy)
sometimes occurs in glaucoma, and even increases in intensity for some
months after the operation (particularly in cases of some standing) without
endangering the sight. The discoloration progresses up to a certain point,
and then remains stationary. It is only dangerous when this increasing
whiteness is accompanied by a simultaneous deterioration of vision.

Even in those cases of glaucoma which are not accompanied by manifest
inflammatory symptoms (glaucoma simplex), we find that mostly iridectomy
proves of service. Here, as in chronic glaucoma, the misfortune often is,
that the patient does not apply until the disease has far progressed. If only
one eye is affected, this may be nearly lost before the patient even discovers
that anything is the matter with it, and then on examination we find that
the disease has nearly, if not completely, run its course, and that there are
such serious changes in the structures that the operation can prove but of
little if any avail. It is otherwise if the second eye becomes affected with

the same form of disease; for then the patients speedily seek medical aid, and will consent to a timely operation, even although their sight may still be good. In order to arrest the disease permanently, the operation must be performed early, before irreparable changes in the tissues have been produced. Von Graefe particularly urges that the operation should be performed in time, and should not be delayed until considerable impairment of vision or inflammatory symptoms manifest themselves. Here also the beneficial effects of the iridectomy show themselves slowly and gradually. If the atrophy of the optic nerve has not proceeded too far, a steady, though slow, improvement will take place. He has seen cases in which, during a period varying from half a year to three years, the field of vision and the sight had gradually but persistently deteriorated, and where after iridectomy (during a period of observation extending from one to three years), either a complete arrest, or even a considerable improvement occurred. Such improvement also occurred in two cases in which, together with a perfectly typical excavation, all appreciable increase of tension was absent. He considers that the improvement is the more likely if the impairment of sight depends not only upon the condition of the optic nerve, but is also due to a still evident impediment in the conducting power of the retina.

Fig. 188.

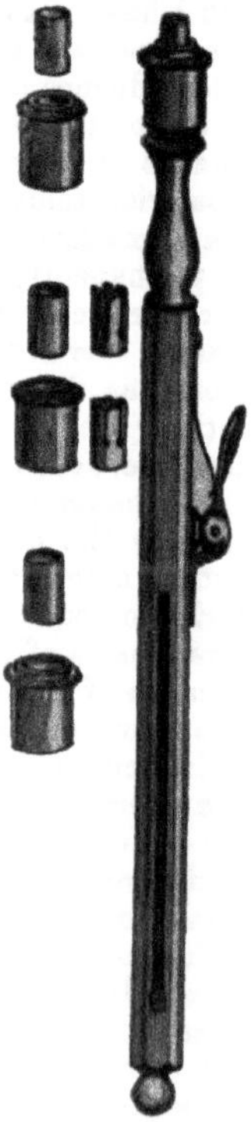

I have already mentioned that the results of iridectomy vary greatly and peculiarly in glaucoma simplex. In the great majority of cases the tension is diminished to a normal standard, and the effect of the operation permanent. In others, the tension still remains somewhat too considerable after the operation, and may gradually increase more and more. In such cases repeated paracentesis, at intervals of two or three days, may be tried, and if this fails, a second iridectomy should be made diametrically opposite to the first, which generally has the desired effect. Finally, in a very small number of cases, Von Graefe' has found that the iridectomy, instead of diminishing the tension, is followed by an increase of tension, and by a rapidly progressive or sudden loss of sight, just as if an acute attack of glaucoma had supervened.

In *glaucoma absolutum* in which all sight, even the quantitative perception of light, is lost, iridectomy is never indicated except to diminish the inflammatory symptoms or severe pain. For these purposes it is to be performed, care being taken to impress upon the patient and his friends that the object of the operation is to ameliorate his sufferings, and not to restore the sight. The iridectomy should always be of a large size. In cases of glaucomatous degeneration it may also be necessary to employ it for the same purpose. Should it prove unable to arrest the inflammatory exacerbations, should it be followed by extensive hemorrhages, or should these occur spontaneously, and all sight is lost, the question may arise whether it would not be better to remove the eye altogether; for there may be fear of the other eye sympathizing.

De Wecker[2] recommends his trephine in those cases of absolute glaucoma

[1] "A. f. O.," xv. 3, 202.
[2] 'Annales d'oculistique," 1872, Septembre–Octobre, p. 137.

in which a satisfactory iridectomy cannot be made on account of the advanced atrophy of the iris, and a simple sclerotomy would not suffice. In such cases the object is to relieve the patient of the often intense pain without submitting him to the operation of excision of the eyeball. De Wecker therefore removes with the trephine a circular portion of from one to one and one-half millimetre in diameter at the edge of the cornea, in such a way as to avoid all risk of injuring the lens, or of approaching too closely to the ciliary body. In this way a large filtrating cicatrix is established. The instrument is constructed on the same principle as Heurteloup's artificial leech. The cutting cylindrical blade is enclosed in a solid tube, from which it does not protrude, except upon the pressure of a spring. The instrument is fitted with four hollow cutting cylinders of one, two, two and one-half, and three millimetres in diameter, so that the size of the incision can be varied according to circumstances. Moreover, by means of a screw the depth of the incision can also be determined and regulated to a nicety.

I have endeavored to point out as plainly and simply as possible the facts which should guide us in forming a prognosis of the beneficial effects to be expected from iridectomy. Nor have I made any statement the accuracy of which I have not myself frequently tested. This part of the subject demands the most earnest attention, as too slight a regard for the different facts which should influence our prognosis of the effect of iridectomy in glaucoma, has been one of the chief reasons why this operation has proved unsuccessful in the hands of some practitioners.

How iridectomy diminishes the abnormally increased intra-ocular pressure in glaucoma has not yet been decided. That it does in the vast majority of cases permanently relieve the tension is, however, an undoubted and incontrovertible fact. Various theories have been advanced in order to explain the *modus operandi.* Amongst other hypotheses, some have thought that the tension was diminished by the excision of a considerable portion of the secreting (iris) surface; others, that the removal of the iris quite up to its ciliary insertion, and the consequent exposure of the zonula Zinnii, facilitates the interchange of fluid between the vitreous and aqueous humors, and thus diminishes the difference in the degrees of tension between these humors. We must admit, however, that this problem has not at present been satisfactorily solved. [A recent statement of Exner's, based on anatomical investigations, is of some importance here. Assuming that, with the increase or decrease of the intra-vascular tension is connected a corresponding change in the intra-ocular tension, he found that iridectomy lessened the intra-vascular tension as follows. The excised iris contains the smaller branches of the arteries and veins with the connecting capillaries; there remain behind in the eye only the larger arterial and venous trunks. Between these are formed direct anastomoses, as injected preparations show, by which the arterial blood passes directly into the veins. Thus a lessening of tension is brought about in the arteries of the iris, and indirectly in the choroidal arteries.—B.] Now some opponents of the operation apparently reject it, because the solution of the *modus operandi* has not yet been found. They would rather deprive their hapless patients of the benefits of iridectomy, which would, in all probability, either restore or preserve vision; they would rather permit them to lose their sight, than perform an operation, the effect of which in diminishing tension, though fully proved, they cannot at present satisfactorily explain.

Some writers have stated that the operation of iridectomy, as it is to be performed in glaucoma, is just the same as the old operation for artificial pupil. Nothing could be more erroneous. The principle of the two opera-

tions is entirely different.   In the old operation, an opening was made in the cornea, and a small portion of iris, in proportion to the desired size of the pupil, excised.   In the modern operation of iridectomy for glaucoma, the chief point is to make the incision in the sclerotic, or at the sclero-corneal
junctio
of the
intense tl
tension, t
partial
tomy i
forman
or it was

tomy is made, more especially in an opposite direction, and the iris removed quite up to its ciliary attachment, the beneficial effects at once become apparent, the tension diminishes, the inflammation subsides, and the vision improves.   The iridectomy should be made upwards, for the upper lid generally covers the greater portion of the artificial pupil, and thus not only hides the slight deformity, but also cuts off much of the irregularly refracted light. But this operation is somewhat more difficult than that in the horizontal direction, and consequently the beginner will do well, at first, to perform the operation outwards or inwards.   For a full description of the mode of performing iridectomy, I must refer the reader to p. 307.

In these cases of fully developed glaucoma, in which iridectomy has only been able to preserve a certain amount of sight, considerable benefit is often experienced from the application of the artificial leech to the temple some months afterwards.

I must, in conclusion, call attention to certain disadvantages which may ensue upon iridectomy, but these are slight indeed when compared with the inestimable boon which the operation affords in this disease.

[When an iridectomy has been done on an eye during an acute attack of glaucoma, if the eye is examined some days later when the media have become clearer, retinal hemorrhages may, as a rule, be seen, generally in the vicinity of the disk and macula, though they may reach to the equator. Hemorrhages into the vitreous have also been met with.   The vascular walls are here probably very fragile, and when the tension is relieved by the operation, they are not strong enough to resist the vascular pressure.—B.]

There cannot be any doubt that the performance of iridectomy during the period of irritation of primary inflammatory glaucoma of the one eye predisposes to, or accelerates, the outbreak of the disease in the other.   This, according to Von Graefe,[1] is probably due to the traumatic irritation produced by the operation in the one eye, being reflected to the other and there awakening a pre-existing disposition to glaucoma.   This predisposition of the second eye to glaucoma chiefly manifests itself during the first four days. Von Graefe, however, never observed this tendency in glaucoma simplex or secondary glaucoma.   It is especially frequent if the second eye has already shown premonitory symptoms, for he has in such cases found that a marked glaucomatous attack occurred within a fortnight after the operation in

[1] "A. f. O.," xv. 8, 117.

lens, with equally good results. The drug worked well in cases of recurring glaucoma after iridectomy, and in some cases of glaucoma simplex. He does not, however, advise eserine as a substitute for glaucoma, but thinks it brings the eye into a more favorable condition for the successful performance of the operation. The eserine probably acts as an irritant to the muscular tissue of the vessels as well as upon the iris and ciliary muscle; contracting the calibre of the vessels and thus reducing the intra-ocular pressure.

Knapp states that he has used eserine methodically in the majority of cases of glaucoma, and gives some striking results. In one case of acute glaucoma eserine was instilled from the second day of the disease, and the patient was permanently cured. In another case of acute glaucoma, which set in seventeen days after an iridectomy for chronic glaucoma on the other eye, eserine produced a temporary improvement only, and an iridectomy had to be done. In chronic glaucoma the results were either negative or unfavorable, and in no case did he see any benefit from eserine. He endorses De Wecker's proposition of the prophylactic use of eserine in the healthy eye after an iridectomy for glaucoma in the other. He, however, recognizes that the indiscriminate use of eserine is to be avoided, owing to its tendency to produce congestion and inflammation of the iris; for it may cause an acute attack in a case of chronic glaucoma. Knapp thinks that if the pupil fully contracts and the attack is completely cured, an operation may perhaps never be necessary; but if the remedy produces incomplete myosis and incomplete reduction of tension, or if relapses occur, iridectomy should not be delayed.[1]

According to Priestley Smith, the very pronounced changes which atropine and eserine cause in the tension of glaucoma, must be connected with some abnormality in the glaucomatous eye, and this lies in the mechanical relations of the iris. Whenever a myotic or mydriatic lowers or raises the tension of an eye in a marked degree, it does so by altering the position of the iris in such a manner as to hinder or promote the escape of the intra-ocular fluid. Atropine is potent for mischief chiefly in the primary form of glaucoma and in its earlier stages. In the earlier stages the periphery of the iris is pressed upon behind by the ciliary processes, and is very nearly in contact in front with the cornea; hence any thickening of this portion of it is apt to cause a sudden blocking of the angle of the chamber, and consequently a sudden aggravation of the glaucomatous state. In the later stages, atropine can hardly increase the obstruction at the outlet of the eye, for the periphery of the iris is already adherent to the cornea, and the ciliary processes are atrophied and retracted. When an eye of normal tension is rendered glaucomatous by atropine, it is reasonable to suppose that the angle of the chamber was already dangerously narrow, and therefore prone to obstruction whenever any unusual dilatation of the pupil should occur. Occasionally the use of eserine in primary glaucoma will completely reduce the tension and permanently cure the glaucoma. When the eyeball becomes, as it were, locked and is unable to recover of its own accord, eserine unlocks the outlet for the pent-up fluid, the turgid ciliary processes subside, and everything returns to its previous condition. It is in the sudden but comparatively mild attacks, which come and go at intervals during the premonitory stage of the disease, when the outlet of the chamber appears to be

---

[1] [For a consideration of the effects of eserine on the eye and its mode of action, see a paper by Mohr in the "A. f. O.," xxiii. 2; by De Wecker in the "Bericht über die Verhandl. der Ophtho.-gesellsch.," Heidelb., 1875. Weber, "A. f. O.," xxiii. 1.]

constantly on the brink of danger, but never occluded for any length of time, that eserine acts with the greatest promptness and certainty. In simple chronic glaucoma, eserine will sometimes cause a temporary reduction of tension and corresponding improvement of vision, but the improvement is never permanent. In the advanced stages of glaucoma, when the periphery of the iris is adherent to the cornea, eserine cannot in any way relieve the obstructed outlet. When eserine fails to do good, it is very likely to do harm. When the mechanical effect upon the iris is unattainable, then the vascular effect induced by eserine is distinctly injurious. ("Ophthalmic Review," February and March, 1882.)—B.]

CHAPTER IX.

DISEASES OF THE CRYSTALLINE LENS.

1.—CATARACT.

BY the general term "cataract" is understood an opacity situated in the crystallin lens: to such only should it be applied. When the opacity is in the capsule, it is termed "capsular cataract;" whereas, when both the capsule and lens are involved, it is designated "capsulo-lenticular cataract." The term "spurious cataract" of old authors, which was the name given to deposits of lymph in the pupil, should be altogether abolished.

Etiology.—It must be frankly admitted that the etiology of cataract is still shrouded in much obscurity and doubt. It appears most probable that the principal causes of the loss of transparency of the lens are to be sought in an impairment of its nutrition, due to some morbid alteration in the vitreous humor, and in inflammatory changes within the lens itself. The defect in the nutrition may be due to certain alterations in the condition of the blood, to senile involution, or to inflammatory lesions of the neighboring tunics (*e. g.*, irido-choroiditis, sclerotico-choroiditis posterior, retinitis pigmentosa, etc.). [The uncomplicated senile cataract is the prototype of the primary cataract, that is, of that form of lens opacity not the consequence of some demonstrable disease of the eye. The lens depends for its nutrition upon the aqueous humor and vitreous humor. It is also possible that the fluid found between the folds of the suspensory ligament is of importance also for its nutrition. A simple osmotic process not only takes place through the zonule, but also through the spaces between the epithelial cells of Descemet's membrane. Any disturbance in the osmotic action of these parts affects the nutrition of the lens, and any disturbance in the nutrition of the lens is shown by a cloudiness. Hence from a cloudy lens may be inferred with some probability a pathological change in the vitreous or aqueous humors. Becker thinks that we may indirectly infer some disease of the general organism from the occurrence of binocular non-senile cataract, and refers especially to the double soft cataract of young people, and to the posterior cortical cataract of both eyes. The occurrence of retinitis pigmentosa with this form of cataract points unmistakably to disease of the vascular system, and the same may be said of the binocular cataract occurring with some obscure forms of choroiditis.—B.] According to Mooren[1] the formation of cataract is always a secondary, never a primary phenomenon; its origin being always due to certain inflammatory or atrophic changes in some portion of the uveal tract. Simple affections of the optic nerve or retina, which are unaccompanied by any changes in the vitreous, do not exert any influence on the development of cataract.

[1] " Ophthalmiatrische Beobachtungen," p. 208.

The presence of secale cornutum in the system may produce cataract. Thus, Dr. Ignaz Meyer[1] has shown that the consumption of bread containing ergot of rye may give rise to it. The ergotism has lasted in some of these cases for two or three months, the principal symptoms being the fits. The development of the cataract was very slow, and always occurred in both eyes. The mode in which the ergotism gives rise to cataract is still very uncertain, but is probably due to some impairment of the nutrition of the lens. De Wecker thinks that this mal-nutrition may, perhaps, be owing to a diminution in the blood supply to the anterior portion of the uveal tract, on account of the prolonged spasmodic contraction of the ciliary muscle. Rothmund[2] has observed a rapid development of cataract in children who were affected with a very peculiar disease of the skin, which somewhat resembled ichthyosis.

[This is considered doubtful by Becker, as the facts advanced are not convincing. He also doubts the connection between rapidly developed cataract and ichthyosis. He thinks there is more reason for recognizing rickets as a cause of cataracta zonularis. (See "Graefe u. Saemisch's Handb. der Augenheilkunde," Bd. v. S. 226.)—B.]

Cataract is, as a rule, a disease of old age, and the loss of transparency of the lens is probably chiefly due to its deficient nutrition, dependent upon an inefficient blood supply, and consequent diminution of the watery constituents of the crystalline. We must not, however, mistake for this condition the small punctate opacities which are due to senile fatty degeneration of the fibrillæ of the lens, and which sometimes appear in old persons in the form of a fringe of small, yellowish-gray dots, situated quite at the periphery of the lens, where they remain stationary for a very long period. It is an interesting fa t that Iwanoff[3] has often found œdema of the retina in the eyes of old persons affected with cataract, and it is a question, as he points out, in how far this morbid process in the retina may have been the cause of the cataract, by producing some changes in the vitreous humor.

Inflammations of the inner tunics of the eye, more especially of the iris, choroid, and vitreous humor, may give rise to cataract, not only by an impairment of the nutrition of the lens, but also by the inflammatory changes implicating the intra-capsular cells, and even the lens itself. Again, the cataract may be due to the presence of extensive deposits of lymph upon the capsule, which prevent the osmotic interchange of material between the lens and aqueous humor. If these exudations cover the greater portion of the anterior capsule, the opacity of the lens generally soon becomes complete; whereas, if the exudation is confined to the area of the pupil, the cataract is often only partial. In the former case, the watery constituents of the lens soon become absorbed, the lens becomes diminished in size and shrivelled up, and may in time be almost entirely absorbed, there being only an opaque, white, chalky disk left behind.

[There is a form of opacity occurring in the anterior cortex or in the anterior capsule in the immediate equator of the lens, which is not progressive, and which is met with very frequently in young persons in chronic ill-health or who are suffering from some slowly wasting disease. These opacities never encroach upon the centre of the lens, and cannot be seen except when the pupil is widely dilated. They appear in the form of dots or striæ, and generally are spread regularly all around the equator of the lens. They never increase, though watched for years, and do not interfere with vision.

---

[1] " A. f. O.," viii. 2, 120.   [2] Ibid., xiv. 1, 159.   [3] Ibid., xv. 2, 90.

Another form of immovable or very slowly progressive opacity is met with in patients who are highly myopic. This is a cortical opacity, generally of the striated variety: though sometimes many of these opaque striæ coalesce and then the opacity becomes much denser, and vision is markedly affected. Though this form of cataract is generally progressive, its progress is very slow, and though vision may be much interfered with, the clear portions of the lens may be often made useful by occasional instillations of atropia, thus keeping the pupil dilated.—B.]

[Streatfeild thinks it important to draw a line of separation between cataract and other opacities of the lens. He would not include as cataracts any of those cases in which, by the ophthalmoscope, no opacity or striæ can be seen in the pupillary space of the lens If the lens opacity is perfectly penetrable by the light from the mirror, he would call the case one of lens opacity, and not cataract. Such opacities do not necessarily imply incipient cataract and should not be confounded with it. (See " British Med. Journ.," June 25, 1881.)—B.]

Cataract is very frequently due to some injury to the lens, but this form will be considered more at length under the head of " Traumatic Cataract."

[Before describing the various forms of cataract, mention should be made of some rare anomalies which have been described among the congenital defects of the lens.

1st. *Congenital aphakia* or complete absence of the lens. Such an anomaly, existing alone in the eye, has never yet been described: but there are cases on record where from some intra-uterine process, an anterior staphyloma has been developed with total loss of the lens. (See " Graefe u. Saemisch's Handb.," p. 229.)

2d. *Coloboma Lentis.*—This defect in the lens may extend more or less into the substance of the lens from the periphery; may occur with or without defect in other parts of the eye, as in the uveal tract; and may be either monocular or binocular. Cases are reported by Hirschberg, Bresgen, Becker, Heyl, and others. (See "Graefe u. Saemisch," l. c.; " Archives of Ophthal.," iv. 1; " Trans. of Fifth Internat. Ophthal. Congress," 1876.)—B.]

Considerable difficulty is experienced in attempting to classify the principal forms of cataract in such a manner that their distinctive features shall be easily recognized and remembered. Not only are the minor varieties numerous, but some of them do not present any marked characteristics, so that their description often proves somewhat confusing and unintelligible to the novice.

I think it most practical to divide lenticular cataracts into two principal classes: 1. The cortical, or soft cataract; 2. The nuclear, or hard cataract. The former is the most frequent kind of congenital cataract, and is met with in various forms up to the age of thirty or thirty-five, and is chiefly characterized by the fact that, although the whole lens may be involved in the process, there is no hard nucleus. The nuclear cataract occurs generally after the age of thirty-five or forty, and is distinguished by the presence of a more or less large, yellow, hard nucleus. I am well aware that so general a division is open to the objection that exceptional cases are not unfrequently met with, so that all varieties cannot be embraced in it. Yet in a practical point of view I believe it to be the best, as it enables us to lay down broad rules as to the modes of operation to be selected. For instance, the cortical cataract may be operated upon by division with the needle, by suction, or by linear extraction; whereas, the nuclear cataract, on account of the presence of a hard nucleus, demands extraction either through a corneal or scleral flap, or by the assistance of some form of traction instrument.

But there is one form of soft cataract which requires a special description, as, on account of its peculiar structure, it may often be best treated by an operation which does not interfere with the lens itself. I mean the lamellar or zonular cataract. Cataracts produced by injuries to the lens, and opacities in the capsule, will be considered under the heads of " Traumatic Cataract " and "Capsular Cataract."

Formerly, much attention was paid to the symptoms which distinguished cataract from glaucoma and amaurosis. But since the discovery of the ophthalmoscope, these diseases could not be mistaken for cataract, except through the grossest ignorance or carelessness.

A fully formed, mature cataract may be at once recognized even with the naked eye. The pupil is no longer dark and clear, but is occupied by a whitish opalescent body, which lies close behind it. [Fig. 139.] It is diffi-

[Fig. 139.]

cult, however, when the affection is incipient and but slightly advanced, more especially when the opacity commences at the edge of the lens, for it may then be easily overlooked except the eye is carefully examined with the ophthalmoscope and the oblique illumination. If elderly persons complain somewhat of dimness of sight, the condition of the lens should always be examined, even although they may apparently be only suffering from presbyopia and are able to read the smallest print with suitable convex glasses; for amongst the aged, cataract is most common, and often commences at the very edge of the lens in the form of small spicular opacities, which might easily escape detection. Wherever incipient cataract is suspected, the pupil should be dilated by a weak solution of atropine, and the lens examined with the ophthalmoscope and the oblique illumination. If there is any objection to dilating the pupil, a very fair view may, however, be obtained even of the margin of the lens, by directing the patient to turn his eye to one side, and then looking very slantingly behind the iris.

Care must, however, be taken not to mistake the physiological changes which occur in the lens in old age, for commencing cataract. These changes consist in a thickening and consolidation of the lens-substance, especially of the nucleus, which assumes a yellow tint. If this physiological cloudiness is very marked, it might easily be mistaken for incipient cataract. The chief distinctive features are, that in the former case the sight is perfect (any existing presbyopia being corrected by suitable glasses), the opacity remains absolutely or almost entirely stationary for a very long period, and the cloudiness is not observable with the ophthalmoscope, although perhaps very evident with the oblique illumination.

The catoptric test, which was formerly much employed in the diagnosis of cataract, has fallen into complete disuse since the discovery of the ophthalmoscope, and the introduction of the oblique illumination. The catoptrical examination depended upon the three images which may be observed in a healthy eye when a lighted taper is moved before it. Two of these images are erect, the third is inverted. The first is an erect image of the candle, and is produced by reflection from the surface of the cornea; the second is also erect, and is produced by reflection from the anterior surface of the lens; the third is inverted, and is due to reflection from the concave posterior surface of the lens. The first two images move in the same direction as the candle, the third in the opposite direction. If the lens becomes opaque, of course the image from the posterior surface is lost, and that from the anterior surface also soon becomes indistinct.

With the oblique illumination, opacities in the lens will appear of a light-gray, or whitish color. The slighter forms are best seen by only a moderate amount of light.

In employing the ophthalmoscope for the diagnosis of cataract, the mirror alone is to be used (without any lens in front). To gain a larger image, a convex lens may be placed behind the mirror. The illumination is to be weak. Incipient cortical cataract, composed of centripetal stripes, will appear in the form of well-defined dark streaks upon a red background. Punctiform opacities also appear as dark spots, but are often not so observable as with the oblique illumination.

I will now briefly describe the characteristic appearances presented by the different forms of cataract.

I. *Lamellar or zonular cataract* (*Schichtstaar*) is generally congenital or developed in early infancy [and is one form of partial cataract.—B.]. Von Arlt originally called attention to the fact that it often occurs in children who have suffered from convulsions, but the connection between the two has not yet received a satisfactory explanation; for it is difficult to understand why only certain peri-nuclear layers of the lens-fibres should be affected by the mal-nutrition or succussion consequent upon the violent muscular spasms during the convulsions.

As lamellar cataract does not materially impair the sight, it often escapes detection until much later in life. Its appearance is very characteristic, and its diagnosis easy. On dilating the pupil with atropine, we observe an opacity of the lens measuring from two to three and a half lines in diameter. It is quite uniform from the periphery to the centre, and is sharply defined against the transparent margin of the lens. The cataract consists, in short, of a layer of opaque lens-substance lying between the nucleus and a transparent portion of the cortical substance. Hence it has been designated "Schichtstaar," or lamellar cataract. The nucleus of the lens is transparent, which is proved by the uniform character of the opacity, which is not more dense in the centre than at the periphery, and by the relatively fair sight which such patients enjoy even when the pupil is dilated. Moreover, with the ophthalmoscope, a reddish-brown reflex shines through the central portion of the lens.

With the oblique illumination, the opacity appears of a uniform light-gray color, sharply defined, and surrounded by a more or less broad margin of transparent cortical substance. It will now also be seen that there is a clear portion of cortical substance between the opacity and the anterior capsule. In the centre of the opacity may often be remarked one or more small white spots. With the ophthalmoscope, the opacity has the appearance of a well-defined dark disk, the centre of which affords a reddish-brown reflex. If the margin of the cortical substance be clear, the details of the fundus will be visible through it. If there are opacities in it, they will appear as fine dark stripes or specks upon a red background. Some of the varieties of lamellar cataract are very pretty. For instance, I have seen cases in which little stripes ran from the opacity into the cortex, their extremities being studded with small pearl-like opacities. Lamellar cataract is either stationary or very slowly progressive. It is, therefore, of consequence, before deciding upon an operation, to determine whether the cataract be progressive or not. In deciding this, we must be chiefly guided by the condition of the marginal cortical substance. If the latter is perfectly clear and transparent, the cataract is stationary; if it is diffusely clouded or presents punctiform or striped opacities, it is progressive. Von Graefe thinks that its progress is most rapid when the stripes are broad, and the interjacent lenticular substance is somewhat opaque and studded with coarse specks. If the opacities consist only of very fine dots, or a few delicate narrow stripes, the progress is very slow.

According to Von Graefe, lamellar cataract may also be formed later in life in dislocated lenses, and after iritis.

Vision may be relatively good if the opacity is not dense; for instance, large print may be read. But the sight is always improved by dilatation of the pupil with atropine, for this permits the rays from the object to pass through the clear marginal portion of the lens. I have seen cases in which the difference in the sight before and after dilatation of the pupil, has been most marked; so that persons who, prior to it, could with difficulty decipher large letters, were afterwards able to read the smallest print. The accompanying diagrams (Figs. 140 and 141) will explain this. Fig. 140 (a), the

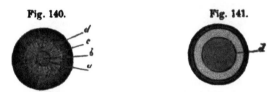

Fig. 140.   Fig. 141.

undilated pupil occupied by the opacity (b), which extends beneath the iris as far as the dotted line (c), where the transparent margin (d) commences. As the latter is completely covered by the iris, the rays can only pass through the central opaque portion; hence the indistinctness of sight. But on dilatation of the pupil (Fig. 141) the transparent margin (d) is exposed, and the rays can now pass through it to the retina. The solution of atropine to be used for dilating the pupil should be extremely weak (one grain to eight or twelve fluidounces of water), so that we may obtain complete dilatation of the pupil without any paralysis of the accommodation. If this point is not attended to, we may easily be misled by the fact of the patient's complaining that after the dilatation the sight is dim and misty, which may be due simply to the fact that the accommodation is paralyzed by the atropine, which was too strong.

Persons suffering from lamellar cataract are often supposed to be shortsighted, as they hold small objects (a book, for instance) very close to the eye, in order to gain larger retinal images. In time, however, this constant accommodation for very near objects may really give rise to myopia of even a considerable degree.

In practice, it is important to remember two facts with regard to lamellar cataract: 1. That the opacity is surrounded by a more or less clear margin of cortical substance, which, if it be sufficiently wide and transparent, may admit of excellent sight when the pupil is dilated. 2. That the greater portion of the lens is transparent and in a normal condition, and will, therefore, swell up far more than a cataractous lens, after laceration of the capsule and the admission of the aqueous humor, as, for instance, in a needle operation.

[II. Another very rare form is the *spindle-shaped* or *fusiform* cataract, which is the most typical form of the axial cataract, running through the entire diameter of the lens. It may be congenital or acquired, and has been met with in connection with lamellar cataract.—B.]

III. *Cortical Cataract.*—The opacity generally commences at the margin. All grayish-white stripes are observed running towards the centre of the lens. At the very commencement, the interjacent lens substance is either perfectly transparent, or but sparsely studded with little opaque dots. Soon, however, the cloudiness becomes more general and diffuse, until the whole lens is involved. Sometimes the stripes may be observed both on the anterior and posterior cortical substance, the lens between them being transparent. The difference in their position may be easily recognized with the oblique illumination. The anterior stripes are close behind the pupil, whereas the others are far back in the eye, and appear concave, the concavity being turned towards the observer.

[Fig. 142.

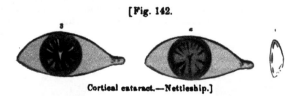

Cortical cataract.—Nettleship.]

On examining an incipient cortical cataract with the ophthalmoscope, we notice dark, well-defined stripes intersecting the red background, and radiating from the margin of the lens to the centre. Between them, at the very edge of the lens, there is often a fringe of short, stunted stripes. Punctiform opacities, which with the oblique illumination appeared of a gray color, now look like little dark dots strewn about on and between the stripes.

In rare instances the opacity, instead of being striped, consists of innumerable little dots with clear portions of lens-substance between them. With the naked eye, it looks like a diffuse uniform opacity.

The following symptoms are characteristic of a fully formed, mature cortical cataract: The opacity is of a gray or bluish-white color, which increases somewhat in density towards the centre. On account of this white tint, the movements of the pupil appear peculiarly marked and distinct. If the volume of the lens be increased through the imbibition of fluid, the iris may be slightly arched forward, and the pupil somewhat dilated and sluggish. The stripes are broad, white, and often very opalescent, like mother-of-pearl. There is no admixture of yellow in the color of the opacity, which proves at once that the nucleus is not hard. With the oblique illumination, we notice that the outer layers of the cortical substance, although opaque, are somewhat translucent, so that we can see through them into the deeper layers. This is of importance with regard to the consistence, for in the very soft or the fluid cataract the dense white opacity reaches quite up to the capsule, and is not at all diaphanous.

Von Graefe[1] calls attention to a peculiar cataract which is sometimes met with in early infancy. Its diagnosis is of special importance, as it is very frequently complicated with lesions of the deeper structures of the eyeball. It commences as a milky-white cloud in the outer portions of the cortical substance, and soon reaches quite up to the capsule. The opacity is either completely homogeneous, or studded with small white dots which extend close up to the capsule. The lens, which is at first somewhat increased in volume, soon diminishes again in size on account of the absorption of its fluid constituents. In cases, therefore, in which the volume of the lens is much diminished, and considerable opacities are lodged in the central portions of the anterior capsule, the degree of sight and the state of the field of vision, should always be carefully tested prior to an operation, in order that

[1] "A. f. O.," i. 2, p. 256.

may be d

generally

nature in the
increase but slowly,
stripes an
cataract is not of
always asc
cause, such
both eyes are
as diabetes is

In children
increases with advancin
age of thirty or
linear extraction.
has existed
Its fluid a
substance beco
the cataract sh
breaks from the p

like a little wrin
very young subje
that finally t
a hard, chalky
of old writers.
absorption of t
frequently met
r instance, i
nts, instead
breaking dow
which is e
the age of t
which can t

[143]

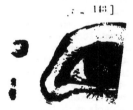

such cases
sink d
duced.
fluid cata
it is
the im
coalescer

IV. Cataract is not unfrequently met with in those conditions of the blood in which its watery constituents are very deficient, so that it assumes great density (as, for instance, in diabetes). This gives rise to an exosmosis of the watery constituents of the lens, a loss of transparency in its fibres, and a deposit of calcareous and other salts. In diabetes, the cataract does not generally appear until a late stage of the disease, when the patient is greatly emaciated and enfeebled, and his health much broken. I have, however, met with some cases in which the opacity of the lens appeared whilst the general health was still good. The diabetic cataract is mostly met with about or before middle age, and does not present any peculiar or characteristic symptoms. It generally affects both eyes, and is mostly of a soft consistence, and rapid in its formation. In elderly persons, however, it will be more firm, and contain a more or less hard nucleus. The perception of light, and the condition of the field of vision should always be very carefully examined in such cases, as affections of the retina and optic nerve not unfrequently occur in the course of diabetes, and may, therefore, coexist with the cataract, and thus render the prognosis of the operation unfavorable. Another fact which should be remembered in operating for diabetic cataract is, that the iris is often very susceptible of irritation, so that iritis is exceptionally easily set up. The amblyopia which is sometimes met with in persons affected with diabetes may, however, be simply due to paralysis of the accommodation.

[From recent chemical investigations there is no doubt that the diabetic cataract sometimes contains sugar, and probably always does, though the quantity may be so small as not to be detected. From statistics the percentage of cataract in diabetic patients is small, varying from four and twenty-eight one-hundredths per cent. to nine and five-tenths per cent. Becker regards the prognosis of operations for the removal of a diabetic cataract as favorable. He has never observed suppuration of the cornea following an extraction, and plastic iritis only occurred once. Galezowski thinks that in diabetic cataract the liquids of the eye are saturated with glucose, which causes more or less interference with the nutrition of the lens. The origin of the cataract is traceable directly to the faulty composition of the aqueous humor. Glycosuric cataract occurs more frequently among fat diabetic individuals than among thin ones. It begins almost always in the posterior laminæ of the lens, and generally advances very rapidly; hence there is no time for the cataract to become hard and voluminous. Diabetic cataracts may be simple and entirely uncomplicated by any other alteration in the eyes, or there may also be present amblyopia, with or without hemiopia, retinal hemorrhages, etc. (See "Recueil d'ophthalmologie," August, 1880.)—B.]

V. *The nuclear or hard senile cataract.*—It has been already stated that after the age of from thirty to thirty-five the lens undergoes certain physiological changes. The nuclear portion becomes firmer and more consolidated, and assumes a yellow tint. This condition may exist for many years without any marked increase, without deterioration of sight, or without any opacity being observable with the ophthalmoscope; but the division between the physiological and pathological consolidation and cloudiness is only one of degree. When these senile changes increase to such an extent that the sight is perceptibly impaired, and when the opacity of the lens is progressive and becomes marked even by transmitted light, I think that we must then no longer consider it as a physiological condition, but as commencing nuclear cataract. In the latter case, the nucleus presents a marked yellow or yellowish-brown tinge, and is easily distinguishable from the cortical substance, which may remain clear, except perhaps in the immediate vicinity of the nucleus. With the oblique illumination, the cataract will appear as a round yellow opacity, situated at some distance behind the pupil. The anterior layers of the cortical substance are translucent and transparent, so that we can see through them into the centre of the lens, and the pupil throws a deep shadow upon the surface of the opacity. The nuclear cataract may be very dark, even black in color, which is due to the imbibition of hæmatine. The "black cataract" may easily be overlooked if the eye is not examined with the ophthalmoscope or the oblique illumination. In black cataract the prognosis of the success must be somewhat guarded, as it is not unfrequently complicated with inflammatory lesions of the deeper tunics of the eye, and a fluid condition of the vitreous humor.

Pure nuclear cataract is but rarely met with. In the great majority of cases of senile cataract the cortex is also affected, so that we have in truth a mixed form, viz., a hard yellow nucleus with a more or less firm cortical substance. I think it well, however, to retain the name of "nuclear" cataract for the senile form, as indicating the presence of a hard nucleus.

Senile cataract generally commences at the periphery of the lens in the form of small centripetal stripes, between which we may often notice smaller and shorter spikes, situated at the very margin of the lens. The stripes may run along the anterior or posterior surface of the lens, the interjacent substance being clear. The opacity gradually becomes more general, and involves more and more the centre of the lens; the intervals between the stripes becoming clouded and perhaps studded with small opaque dots or patches. As the cataract progresses, the distinction between the nucleus and the cortex becomes more marked, the former showing a distinct yellow tint.

Sometimes the stripes commence in the posterior cortex, extending from the margin to the posterior pole of the lens, where they coalesce; the opacity thus assuming a stellate appearance. The intervals between the stripes may remain transparent for some time, as also the nuclear portion of the lens, so that we can see quite to the back of the latter. The view of the background of the eye is of course obscured in the centre by the confluence of the stripes, but if the segments between them are clear, we may yet at the periphery distinguish the details of the fundus; such forms are often extremely slow in their progress. When opacities commence at the posterior pole of the lens, either in the form of centripetal stripes or of circumscribed spots or patches, the general condition of the eye should be carefully examined, as this form of cataract (posterior polar cataract) not unfrequently shows itself in the later stages of sclerotico-choroiditis posterior, retinitis pigmentosa, detachment of the retina, and other deep-seated lesions. The coexistence of any such complication would, of course, materially affect our prognosis of the result of an operation.

We occasionally meet with incipient cataracts in which there is a marked difference between the amount of the opacity, according to whether the oblique illumination or the ophthalmoscope be used for examination. On account of the great opalescence of the stripes, the opacity is very apparent to the naked eye and with the oblique illumination; yet, on testing the vision, we find it surprisingly good, and with the ophthalmoscope we can, with a little management, clearly distinguish the details of the fundus. I have noticed this peculiarity several times in myopic patients; the progress has generally been very slow.

In the majority of cases, one of the first symptoms noticed by a person affected with incipient cataract is, that distant objects appear somewhat indistinct and hazy, or as if surrounded by a halo. After a time, near objects also become indistinct, and in reading, the print has to be approximated closer to the eye or observed through a strong convex lens, in order that a larger retinal image may be gained. If the opacity is chiefly or entirely confined to the centre of the lens, the margin being clear, the patient will see best when his back is turned to the light, or when he shades the eye with his hand, so that the pupil becomes somewhat enlarged. Dilatation of the pupil by a very weak solution of atropine will have the same effect. If the cloudiness be confined to the margin of the lens, the reverse will obtain; the sight will be best when the pupil is small.

Sometimes, persons suffering from incipient senile cataract complain that they are getting myopic, requiring the aid of a concave glass in order to distinguish distant objects. The reason of this fact is somewhat doubtful, and can only be explained upon the supposition that there is some increase in the volume of the lens, which gives it a higher refractive power.

[Cases occasionally come within the experience of ophthalmic surgeons in which the presence of cataract has been diagnosticated and its progress predicted, and in which after a varying time, extending sometimes to years, the opacities have receded and grown less, and finally entirely disappear. The reports of the cure of lenticular cataract by internal medication and by electricity, which have become of late quite frequent, no doubt may be referred to this natural disappearance of the opacities. An actual progressive cataract, especially one well advanced to maturity, can of course be removed in one way only, that is, by operation. In some of these reported cures, a subsequent examination by a competent ophthalmoscopist would no doubt reveal the presence of the same opacities that were recognized before.

In the equatorial region of the lens we sometimes see in persons, who have reached the middle period of life or have passed beyond it, certain bifurcated linear opacities, which may extend entirely around the lens, though usually they are more marked above or below. These may exist for years unchanged, but are certainly the beginning of a cataract. They have been called gerontoxon lentis or arcus senilis lentis, but a better name is incipient cataract.—B.]

It was formerly thought that senile cataract almost always commenced at the centre of the lens, and extended thence towards the margin. This opinion led to great mistakes, and caused incipient cataract to be often entirely overlooked.

On examining a mature senile cataract with the oblique illumination, we at once notice the presence of a yellow nucleus. Its size may be estimated from the extent of the yellow reflex, its hardness from the depth of the color. The darker the yellow tint, the harder and more compact will the nucleus be. The cortical substance is of a gray or bluish-white color, traversed by numerous centripetal opalescent stripes, and studded perhaps with small white dots or patches.

The rate of progress of senile cataract is very difficult to determine with accuracy. It is far more rapid in the cortex than in the nucleus. Sometimes years may elapse before it arrives at maturity. It may remain at an incipient stage for a very long time without apparently making any progress, and then suddenly advance very rapidly, arriving at maturity within a few months or even weeks. We must, therefore, always be upon our guard against giving a decided opinion as to when any given case of incipient cataract will be fully formed, and fit for operation. Patients are sure to ask this question, and we may fall into great mistakes by giving a decided answer. This can only be predicted with anything like certainty, when the progress of the case has been constantly watched. As a general rule, I may state that if the cortical substance presents broad, white opalescent stripes and large flakes or spots, the progress is more rapid than if the stripes or spots are small and narrow, and the intermediate lens-substance clear.

Senile cataract occurs most frequently after the age of fifty or fifty-five, and sooner or later generally affects both eyes.

When a mature senile cataract has existed for some length of time, it may also undergo some retrogressive changes; but these are far less than in the cortical cataract, for they only affect the cortical substance and not the nucleus, which becomes harder and firmer. The fluid constituents may be partially absorbed, and some of the elements may undergo a fatty or chalky degeneration, so that the cataract diminishes in thickness and becomes flatter, but is very coherent. The molecules are aggregated together into small masses, which become adherent to the inner surface of the capsule, or are often collected at the margin of the lens. They may prove in so far dangerous, that they are very apt to remain behind in the capsule when the cataract is extracted, and give rise to secondary cataract. In very rare instances, a great portion of the cataract may be absorbed, and the sight of the patient materially improved. In the majority of such cases, the yellow nucleus may still be seen shining through the cortical substance, but now, however, no longer in the centre, but sunk down to the bottom of the capsule (Morgagnian cataract). If the cortical substance is gray, very opaque, and pretty uniformly studded with fine dots or patches, it may be considered as soft; not, however, pulpy or diffluent, but friable, so that small coherent portions are apt to remain behind, and adhere to the pupil or the corneal section after the chief portion of the cataract is removed.

2.—TRAUMATIC CATARACT.

When the capsule is perforated or torn by a sharp instrument, the aqueous humor is admitted to the lens-substance, which may become rapidly opaque. If the perforation is extremely small and superficial, such as might be produced by a very fine needle, the danger may be but slight. The lips of the wound in the capsule may unite, and no permanent, or only a very limited, opacity may remain; but if the wound is larger, much aqueous humor is admitted, and the lens will swell up very rapidly, and press upon the iris and ciliary body. The iris is often considerably lacerated, or protrudes through the corneal wound, and this greatly increases the irritation and danger of severe inflammation. Flakes of softened lens-matter, or broken portions of lens, fall into the anterior chamber, and, coming in contact with the anterior surface of the iris, produce great irritation; or portions of lens-matter may exude through or become entangled in the wound. The inflammation, which may involve the iris, ciliary body, and choroid, may assume either a purulent or serous character. In the latter case, there may be more or less increase in the intra-ocular tension, with the attendant train of glaucomatous symptoms. In children the danger of secondary inflammation is less than in adults, as the lens is softer, the iris less impatient of pressure, and absorption more rapid; in fact, the lens may be almost entirely absorbed, so that finally there only remains a small, hard, white disk. The lens becomes more rapidly opaque in the young than in elderly persons. I have occasionally met with cases in youthful individuals, in which, a few days after the injury to the lens, the latter had become almost completely cataractous. The swelling of the lens is often very considerable, so that its volume is much increased; the iris is consequently pushed forward and the anterior chamber diminished in size. This pressure of the swollen lens upon the iris and ciliary body produces great irritation, and may give rise to severe irido-cyclitis. The danger is very great when a foreign body—*e. g.*, a piece of gun-cap or a chip of steel—is lodged in the lens, or having passed through it, is fixed in the deeper tissues of the eye, as it is frequently followed by a most destructive inflammation. After any injury to the lens, the history of the accident should be inquired into, and if it was caused by a chip of steal, a shot, etc., the condition of the eye must be carefully examined, in order that we may, if possible, ascertain whether the foreign body be still in the eye, and whereabouts it is situated. [It is well known that small foreign bodies may perforate the capsule, enter the lens, and become embedded there for a varying time, sometimes without causing any special irritation. Generally their presence leads to clouding of the entire lens, but this is not always so, as the opacity may be limited to the immediate vicinity of the foreign particle. The capsule may close completely by first intention, and the cicatrix becomes scarcely perceptible. If, however, some of the lens-matter has exuded and been absorbed by the aqueous, the wound in the capsule unites irregularly, so as to throw the capsule into small folds. The appearance of a traumatic cataract is that of the soft, cortical cataract. For a consideration of the subject, see paragraph upon the removal of foreign bodies from the lens—also " Archives of Ophthalmology," vii. Nos. 2, 3, 4; ix. No. 1.—B.] After an injury to the lens, the condition of the eye must be anxiously watched. The tension of the eyeball, the state of the sight and of the field of vision must be frequently examined, so that the earliest symptoms of any glaucomatous complication may be detected, and, if possible, cut short. The danger of sympathetic inflammation must likewise be kept in mind. A traumatic cataract may also be produced through a simple contusion of the eye, without any laceration or rupture of the external coats of the eye. Thus a blow upon the eye or over the head from the fist, or some blunt body (a piece of wood, whip, etc.), may give rise to traumatic cataract. Special attention was called by Mr. Lawson to this fact some years ago, who recorded several instances of this kind.[1] In such cases, however, the capsule is generally ruptured, in most instances, as was pointed out by Von Graefe,[2] at the periphery of the lens, just where the thick anterior passes into the thin posterior capsule. Sometimes, however, no tear in the capsule can be detected. [Cases of rupture of the posterior capsule alone have been reported by Knapp and Aub (" Archives of Ophthalmology," i. 1), and an isolated rupture of the anterior capsule from contusion has been reported by Becker. (" Graefe u. Saemisch's Hdb.," p. 276.)—B.]

3.—CAPSULAR CATARACT, ETC.

Capsular cataract presents a white, somewhat chalky appearance, and is situated in the area of the pupil. Strictly speaking, this term is inaccurate, for it would appear that the capsule itself does not become opaque, for although it may become wrinkled and changed in thickness, it retains its transparency, as has been shown by H. Müller[3] and Schweigger.[4] According to Müller, these opacities are not owing to any changes in the structure

---

[1] *Vide* " R. L. O. H. Rep.," iv. 179; also Mr. Lawson's book, " On Wounds and Injuries of the Eye," p. 130.

[2] " Berliner klinische Wochenschrift," 1864, 19. A translation of this Lecture upon "Traumatic Cataract " will be found in the " Ophth. Review," ii. 137.

[3] " A. f. O.," ii. 2, 58, and iii. 1, 55.   [4] Ibid. viii. 1, 227.

of the capsule itself, but are due to the deposition on its inner surface of new layers of a substance which is often much akin in its structure to that of the capsule, but is in other cases of a fibrous character. Certain hyaline changes also occur in the capsules of old persons, which are chiefly situated at the inner surface of the anterior capsule. If these transparent hyaline deposits should undergo here and there chalky degeneration, they become manifest to the observer, appearing as small whitish deposits on the anterior surface of the lens.

Schweigger insists strongly on the fact that capsular cataract only occurs as a complication of a previous cataractous opacity of the lens. Thus, when the fluid constituents become absorbed in a retrograding cataract, the harder portions may become adherent to the inner portion of the capsule, and thus produce an opacity at the inner side of the latter, the capsule being here also somewhat wrinkled and perhaps thinned. This opacity is chiefly situated in the area of the pupil, and is of a whitish or whitish-brown tint, and incrusted with chalky deposits or fragments of cholesterine crystals, and its situation close behind the anterior capsule becomes very evident with the oblique illumination. The intra-capsular cells are generally unchanged, excepting they have become destroyed during the process of adhesion between the inner surface of the capsule and the lens-substance. The diagnosis of this form of capsular cataract in retrogressive lenticular cataract is of much practical importance in performing the operation of extraction, for, on account of the toughness and adhesion of the capsule to the subjacent lens-substance, sufficient laceration with the cystitome will be very difficult, and a displacement of the lens may easily occcur. In such cases, it is better, therefore, instead of endeavoring to divide the capsule with the pricker, to seize its anterior layer with a pair of fine iridectomy forceps, and gently withdraw it, which will not only afford a sufficient opening for the ready exit of the lens, but also remove the opaque thickened capsule, which would have subsequently materially interfered with the sight. Or again, in such a case the extraction of the lens in its capsule may be indicated, for in these retrogressive cataracts the adhesion between the capsule and the zonula of Zinn is generally so much loosened that the lens escapes very readily in its capsule, there being the less fear of a rupture of the latter as it is generally abnormally tough and adherent to the lens.

[Becker holds that capsular cataract may be primary and remain so for years before a lenticular cataract makes its appearance. This is pure phakitis, and consists mainly in a proliferation of cells upon the inner cells of the anterior capsule. It is not limited here, however, but spreads to the equator, and even to the posterior capsule. Not only is there proliferation of the intra-capsular cells, but these cells become opaque. Such a pure phakitis proves that the eye is elsewhere diseased, and explains why these eyes are more prone to severe reaction after operations. That capsular cataract may be primary, that is, independent of lenticular cataract, is certainly true, and capable of clinical demonstration.—B.]

Capsular cataract is found most frequently in those opacities of the lens which are complicated with irido-choroiditis, and here great proliferation of the intra-capsular cells occurs; they may subsequently undergo fatty degeneration, and finally disappear and be replaced by calcareous deposits; the chalky degeneration of the lens not unfrequently taking its start from the capsule (Schweigger).[1] As capsular cataract occurs most frequently in the later stages of irido-choroiditis, the history of the case and the general con-

<hr>

[1] Loc. cit., p. 236.

dition of the eye, as well as the degree of sight and the extent of the visual field, must be carefully examined before any operation is undertaken, in order that the presence of any deep-seated lesions (e. g., detachment of the retina) may not be overlooked.

Anterior central capsular cataract may be congenital, but is more frequently formed in early childhood, in consequence of a perforating ulcer of the cornea. If it is congenital, and there are no traces of iritis or of an ulcer of the cornea, it is probably due to some intra-uterine arrest of development. But it is generally caused by an ulcer in the cornea, and occurs in this way: if an ulcer, which is situated at or near the centre of the cornea, perforates the latter, the aqueous humor escapes, the iris and lens fall forward, and come in contact with the cornea. Plastic lymph is effused in the ulcer, and a little nodule of this is deposited upon the centre of the capsule. As the pupil contracts on the escape of the aqueous humor, only the central portion of the capsule remains uncovered by the iris, and this is, therefore, the place where the cataract is formed. As the nutrition of the lens is impaired near the deposit of lymph from the disturbance in the osmosis, the superficial layers of the cortical substance in its vicinity become somewhat opaque, the intra-capsular cells perhaps also undergoing proliferation, etc. The ulceration of the cornea heals, and on the aqueous humor becoming again retained, it tears through the adhesion between the cornea and the capsule, the iris and lens recede to their former position, but the capsular opacity remains. Frequently the deposit of lymph on the capsule becomes absorbed, and only the opacity on the inner surface of the capsule and the contiguous portion of the lens remains behind, the capsule, though changed in its thickness, being transparent. Now, if the cornea subsequently clears, the true origin of the capsular cataract may remain unsuspected. But even in an apparently transparent cornea I have often, with the oblique illumination, been able to discover a trace of a central opacity, showing the seat of a former ulcer. Even, however, if the cornea should in after-years be quite clear, this would not be a proof that there had not been a small central perforating ulcer, for we constantly find extensive and deeply situated corneal opacities clearing away perfectly in the course of time. Another objection which is sometimes urged against this view of the origin of central anterior capsular cataract is, that there could have been no perforation if no anterior synechia remains. But the very fact of the formation of the capsular cataract in this way, precludes the existence of an anterior synechia (at least in the centre), for the adhesion between the anterior surface of the capsule and the cornea must be so slight that the reaccumulation of the aqueous humor is sufficient to tear it through; which could not occur if so much lymph was effused as to produce an anterior synechia.

Moreover, in very rare instances, of which I saw one several years ago at Prof. Von Arlt's clinic in Vienna, we may trace a very delicate thread of lymph from the anterior capsule to the posterior portion of the cornea. When the central capsular cataract is very prominent, and elevated above the surface of the capsule, it is termed "*pyramidal cataract*" [Figs. 144 and 145]; but even in such cases Müller has found it covered by transparent capsule.

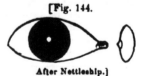

[Fig. 144.

After Nettleship.]

Very superficial wounds of the lens may also produce anterior capsular cataract, if, together with the cataractous changes in the lens-substance, the intra-capsular cells undergo proliferation. Mr. Hulke[1] thinks that it is pro-

---

[1] "R. L. O. H.," i. 188

duced in ophthalmia neonatorum in the following manner, it being remembered that the space between the cornea and the lens is only very slight: "In ophthalmia neonatorum, when the cornea becomes inflamed and swollen, its posterior surface may actually come in contact with the front of the lens, and then a dot of lymph poured out upon the latter by the inflamed cornea, or even the mere pressure contact, may give rise to opacity by preventing the proper nutritional osmosis through the capsule." Mr. Hutchinson,[1] on the other hand, supposes that "the mere proximity of the inflammatory action on the surface of the conjunctiva and cornea suffices to disturb the nutrition of the lens-capsule, and to produce deposits." It is difficult to

[Fig. 145.

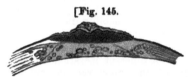

Magnified section of a pyramidal cataract. The parallel shading represents the thickness of the opacity, the double (black and white) outline is the capsule; on each side are the cortical lens fibres, many being broken up into globules beneath the opacity. Lying upon the puckered capsule over the opacity is a little fibrous tissue, the result of iritis.—Nettleship.]

understand, however, why, if this were so, the disturbance of the nutrition, and the deposit should always be confined to a small portion of the capsule in the centre of the pupil, and should not also affect the more peripheral parts.

Anterior capsular cataract may also appear after iritis, if an effusion of lymph has taken place into the area of the pupil, and the posterior synechiæ subsequently yield to the action of atropine, etc., the adhesions and deposits of lymph at the edge of the pupil may gradually disappear, while the central nodule of exudation in its area remains, and, on account of the disturbance of the nutrition of the lens at this point, may give rise to cataractous changes in the subjacent lens-matter.

Changes in the posterior portion of the capsule are of far less frequent occurrence than in the anterior. The opacities which are met with at the posterior pole of the lens (hence termed posterior polar cataract) are gener-

[Fig. 146.

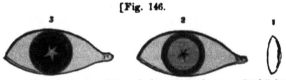

Posterior polar cataract. 1. Section of lens; 2. Opacity seen by transmitted light; 3. Opacity seen by reflected light.—Nettleship.]

ally due to changes in the cataractous portions of the neighboring cortical substance, which may become intimately adherent to the capsule, or hyaline deposits may be formed upon the latter. In rarer instances, a new formation of cells is observed on the inner surface of the posterior capsule, being due to a proliferation of the intra-capsular cells which have extended themselves to the posterior capsule (Schweigger).[2] But the posterior polar opacities may be situated in the most anterior portion of the vitreous humor close to the posterior capsule, being due to inflammatory or nutritive changes in the vitreous. In such cases, as Stellwag[1] points out, the opacity presents a smooth and somewhat glistening aspect, whereas that dependent on deposits on the inner surface of the capsule is generally rough and granular, projecting perhaps somewhat into the lens-substance. I have already called attention to the fact that these opacities, situated at or near the central portion of the posterior capsule, are most frequently due to some disturbance in the nutrition of the lens or vitreous humor, dependent upon chronic inflammations of the deeper tunics of the eyeball, and are often met with in the later stages of sclerotico-choroiditis posterior, retinitis pigmentosa, detachment of the retina, or remain after serous choroiditis.

In very rare instances the opacity at the posterior pole of the lens may be congenital, and is then in all probability due to the imperfect retrogression of the hyaloid artery (Ammon).[2]

I will now pass on to the different operations suitable to various forms of cataract, commencing with the flap extraction; but before so doing, I must touch upon certain important preliminary considerations.

It is generally deemed important that a cataract, especially the senile form, should be mature before it is submitted to an operation. In mature cataract the opacity involves the whole lens, and the iris throws little or no shadow upon it. The sight is so much impaired that the patient is unable to distinguish the largest print, or to count fingers. If the cataract is immature, it will not come out *en masse*, but the transparent portions of lens-substance are stripped off, and remain adherent to the capsule or the ledge of the pupil. They swell up very considerably, and may produce great inflammation or a dense secondary cataract. These observations do not of course apply to zonular cataract, which may never become mature. The question now arises, what should be done if the cataract remains immature for a long time, yet is so advanced as greatly to impair vision? Can we hasten its progress? Undoubtedly, but we run some risk' in so doing—a risk which should not, I think, be incurred except under peculiar circumstances. If, for instance, a person who is entirely dependent upon his sight for his means of subsistence is affected with double cataract, whose progress is extremely slow, and which, though very immature, is sufficiently dense to prevent his following his customary occupation, it may be advisable to hasten the progress of the cataract. This is to be done by gently pricking the lens with a fine needle, so as to slightly divide the capsule and the lens-substance, and admit a little aqueous humor. This may be repeated several times, care being taken not to divide the lens too freely at one sitting, lest a severe iritis or irido-choroiditis be set up. The pupil is to be kept widely dilated with atropine, and the state of the eye narrowly watched, for fear of any severe inflammatory symptoms ensuing. It is safer still, as was recommended by Von Graefe, to make a preliminary iridectomy, so as to afford more room for the swelling of the lens; moreover, the existence of an iridectomy would prove of advantage when the final operation of removal of the lens is performed. This proceeding is, however, accompanied by the disadvantage that it necessitates two operations, with an interval of some weeks between them; which often proves of much inconvenience and anxiety to patients who come from a distance, or to those who are of a very timid and nervous character. Indeed, not many patients will submit to such repeated operations. Since the introduction of Von Graefe's new operation, I must

[1] "Augenheilkunde," 3d edition, p. 153.　　[2] "A. f. O.," iv. 1, 59.

confess that I have paid less heed to the necessity of waiting with the operation until the cataract is quite mature, for I have obtained excellent results where this has not been the case; indeed, I have removed with perfect success lamellar cataracts in persons above the age of twenty-five. As a rule, I should, however, *prefer* to operate on a cataract which is quite mature, as it affords a better chance of complete removal. Again, instead of hastening the progress of the cataract, the lens may be removed in its capsule, which obviates the danger of unripe portions being left behind. Whilst on the one hand, it is dangerous to operate too early, it may also be wrong to wait too long after the cataract is fully formed. In children especially, we should operate early, for otherwise the sight and the sensibility of the retina may permanently suffer, and oscillation of the eyeball (nystagmus) may also be produced. Later in life, a mature cataract may exist for many years without the sensibility of the retina being affected by this passive exclusion from the act of vision. But in children it is different; in them the passive suppression of the retinal image produced by the cataract, appears to exert a similar influence upon the sensibility of the retina, as the active suppression which occurs in cases of squint, and which often rapidly leads to great amblyopia. Again, we have seen that when a mature cataract has existed for some time, it may undergo certain retrogressive changes, its fluid constituents may become absorbed, fatty or calcareous masses may be collected at its margin or adhere to the capsule, and remain behind when the lens is removed, giving rise to inflammatory complications and secondary cataract. It is wiser, therefore, to operate before such secondary changes have set in.

Should we operate upon the one eye if the other is quite free from cataract? I think it is advisable, where the operation is almost certain of succeeding, as, for instance, in the division or linear extraction of cataract of young individuals; for the operated eye, although differing greatly in its state of refraction from the other, will assist somewhat in the act of vision. The visual field will be extended, and the fear of amblyopia will be removed, as the eye may be separately practised with suitable convex glasses. Moreover, the personal appearance will be improved.

Should both eyes be operated upon at the same time in cases of double cataract? It is doubtless safer to operate only on one eye at a time. Unsuspected peculiarities in the constitution or the temperament may show themselves in the course of the treatment, a prior knowledge of which may prove of great value in the treatment of the other eye, and lead us, perhaps, to select a different mode of operation. On the other hand, it has been urged that it is very rare to see a bad result (*e. g.*, suppuration of the cornea) in both eyes, if they have been operated upon at one sitting. In this point we must be much guided by personal circumstances. It may be very inconvenient for the patient to have the operations divided, and the treatment thus extended over a long period; or, if he be in a weak and nervous condition, it may be unwise to submit him to the anxiety of two operations. If one cataract is mature and the other only partially formed, but yet sufficiently opaque to prevent the patient from following his customary employment, it may be necessary to operate upon the former, so as to enable him speedily to resume his avocations whilst the other is advancing to maturity. If no such necessity exist, we generally wait till both cataracts are mature.

It is of little consequence at what time of the year extraction is performed. Formerly, it was thought advisable to operate chiefly in the spring and early summer, but we now operate all the year round, except during intensely hot or cold weather, for extremes of temperature are not favorable for the progress of the case. If the weather is hot and oppressive, the patients become very restless, irritable, and exhausted. The time of day is also of little or no moment, although I myself prefer the morning, for we can then judge by the evening whether or not any primary inflammatory reaction is likely to set in, and if so, we can without loss of time endeavor to check it.

Before an operation is decided upon, the general health must be examined, and if this be at all impaired we must endeavor to improve it as much as possible prior to operating. It is of the greatest advantage for the result of the operation to have the patient in perfect health. The chief fear is, that in a weak and decrepit person the vitality of the cornea may be so low that its healing power is greatly impaired, or that it may even slough after the operation. A symptom of some importance, as being indicative of this low vitality, is the loss of elasticity of the skin, so that if we pinch up a fold of skin on the back of the hand, it does not fall back at once, but remains wrinkled. Severe cough or chronic bronchitis contra-indicate flap extraction. If double cataract occurs in youth or early middle age (before the age of forty-five), and if its formation is rapid, we must examine whether the patient is suffering from diabetes, for this is a not unfrequent cause of cataract. The lens becomes affected chiefly in the later stages of the disease, when the health is much broken. The cataract is generally soft, and its formation rapid. In old persons a more or less large and hard nucleus will be present, but diabetic cataract does not show any special characteristics. If diabetes is found to exist, special care must be taken to examine the sight and the field of vision, as affections of the retina and optic nerve not unfrequently occur in the course of the disease, and may therefore coexist with the cataract and render the prognosis of the result of an operation unfavorable.

The general condition of the eye should always be carefully examined before an operation for cataract is determined upon. The tension of the eyeball, the degree of sight, and the state of the field of vision must be ascertained, so that the presence of any deep-seated lesion may not escape detection. Otherwise, we might fall into the reprehensible and unjustifiable error of operating upon an amaurotic eye.

Should the patient be suffering from epiphora, dependent upon some affection of the lachrymal apparatus, or from inflammation of the eyelids or the conjunctiva, this should, if possible, be cured prior to the operation, as any such complication not only enhances the difficulties of the after-treatment, but may even endanger the result of the operation.

The method to be pursued in examining the perception of light and the condition of the field of vision, in a person affected with mature cataract, has been already explained in the Introduction (p. 41). Such a person should be able to distinguish a low-burning lamp at a distance of ten or fourteen feet, if his perception of light is good, and there is no lesion of the deeper tunics of the eye. If there is any marked deterioration of the perception of light, or of the field of vision, the history of the case must be carefully inquired into, in order that we may detect the presence of any complication. If the upper or lower half of the field is lost, we must suspect detachment of the retina; if the lateral halves are wanting, an affection of the optic nerves. Cerebral amaurosis generally causes a concentric contraction of the field, or the latter may commence at the temporal side. In glaucoma, the contraction of the field begins almost invariably at the nasal side. If such a contraction of the field exists, the tension of the eyeball must be ascertained, and the other symptoms of glaucoma searched for. If glaucoma attacks an eye affected with mature senile cataract, the glaucoma must first be cured by an iridectomy, and then subsequently, at the interval of several months, the cataract should be removed. But this must not be done until all symptoms of irritation and increased tension have subsided, and the improvement in the nutrition and circulation of the eye has been firmly reëstablished. (*Vide* the article on "Glaucoma.")

The pupil should be dilated by atropine before the operation. In a very presbyopic eye, with an exceedingly shallow anterior chamber, there is always some danger, even to an expert operator, of wounding the iris either before the counter-puncture is made, or whilst the flap is being formed. Wide dilatation of the pupil is the best safeguard against such a danger, for the iris will be removed out of the way of the puncture, the counter-puncture, and the line of incision. When the aqueous humor flows off, the pupil again contracts somewhat; but this will not be of much consequence, as the section should by this time be nearly completed. The degree of rapidity with which the pupil dilates under the influence of atropine also affords us a hint as to the probability of iritis. Von Graefe has called attention to the fact that, if the iris is easily and quickly affected by atropine, there is less tendency to subsequent iritis than if its action is tardy and imperfect.

The patient should be operated upon in the recumbent position, being placed either on a couch or in his bed. In the hospital I prefer operating in the ward, as there is considerable risk of the dressing being disturbed in the removal of the patient from the operating theatre. The light should, if possible, come from the side, for this dazzles the patient less, and causes much less reflection upon the cornea than when it comes from the foot of the bed or from a skylight. The latter, indeed, is the worst light of all for eye operations, more especially those of a very delicate nature.

The position which the operator is to assume with regard to the patient will depend upon which eye is to be operated on, and upon the fact whether the surgeon is ambidextrous or not. Some think it a *sine quâ non* that an oculist should be able to use both hands equally well; but this is not the case. By changing his position, he may always operate with the right hand upon either eye, either by the upper or lower section. Yet I strongly advise every surgeon to practise operating with the left hand, for he will constantly find it a great advantage to be able to use it well. For instance, in performing iridectomy, it is very desirable that he should be able to grasp the iris with the forceps held in the left hand, and snip it off with the scissors in the right, or *vice versâ*. Still, if he finds, after much practice on the dead subject, that he cannot operate for extraction nearly so well with the left hand as with the right, he should not endanger the result of the operation by using the left hand. If the left eye is to be operated on (either by the upper or lower section), the surgeon, if he is not ambidextrous, is to seat himself on the couch in front of the patient, and on his left side. If he operates with his left hand, he will stand behind the patient. The latter position is also to be assumed when the right eye is to be operated on.

[Since the general introduction of Lister's antiseptic method of operation and treatment into general surgery, attempts have been made to introduce this method or some modification of it into the field of ophthalmic surgery. Various operators have practised antiseptic operating for cataract, and some have convinced themselves that the results thus obtained were more favorable than by the old method. Still the method has not met with general adoption, owing to some points of difficulty. The incautious sponging with solutions of carbolic acid cannot be allowed on such a delicate organ as the eye. A complete closure of the wound against all contact with atmospheric air is not possible, owing to the connection between the conjunctival sac and the nasal duct. The application of a constant spray of carbolic acid during the operation is very irritating to the eye, and also tends to dull the edge of the knife. The use of boracic acid solutions, in place of either carbolic or salicylic acids, is less open to these objections; and the dipping of the instruments into absolute alcohol previous to operating is, perhaps, to be recommended. Von Graefe, of Halle, has practised the antiseptic method extensively, and gives the following directions in operating for cataract: The day before the operation he uses a one per cent. solution of atropine in the eye, and shortly before the operation he washes the conjunctival sac carefully with a two per cent. solution of carbolic acid, as well as the external surface of the lids and surrounding orbital region. The eye is then closed, and kept covered till the commencement of the operation with a sponge soaked in the same solution. The instruments are then dipped in absolute alcohol, and carefully wiped with a clean soft cloth. The sponges used during the operation are all moistened with the same solution. The spray in ordinary use is not employed at all. After the operation is completed, and all coagula are removed, the eye is again carefully washed with the carbolized sponge, and atropine is instilled. As soon as the sponge is removed from the closed lids, the whole region is covered with a piece of boracic lint, freshly soaked in a four per cent. solution of boracic acid. This is covered by a piece of waxed cloth soaked in the same solution. The hollow is then filled up with picked lint, over which, as well as the other eye, a flannel bandage is carefully rolled. This bandage is changed every day for three days, and replaced in the same careful manner by a similar dressing. Von Graefe thinks that by this method his percentage of loss has been less, and the general results have been better. In the United States, the antiseptic method in ophthalmic surgery has not found as yet many adherents, probably because the additional trouble and care have not been answered by the expected improvement in results.—B.]

4.—FLAP EXTRACTION.

[In this operation the entire section is within the limits of the cornea.—B.] The section may be made either upwards or downwards, as the advantages are pretty evenly balanced. The downward section is, however, the easier of the two. There is often, moreover, an uncontrollable tendency for the eye to roll upwards beneath the lid, which materially enhances the difficulties of the operation, and may greatly embarrass the operator, especially during the laceration of the capsule and the exit of the lens. The chief advantages

[Fig. 147.]

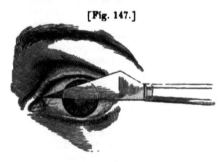

of each mode of operating may be briefly stated to be as follows: In favor of the upper section [Fig. 147], it may be urged that the broad smooth surface of the inside of the upper lid will lie in contact with the section and support it, and thus facilitate the union; whereas the edge of the lower lid may rub against the lips of the incision, or even get between them, set up considerable irritation, and prevent union by first intention. Again, if in the upper section the wound does not unite by first intention, either from the occurrence of prolapse of the iris, or suppuration of the edge of incision, the cicatrix thus produced will be hidden by the upper lid. But to this it may be objected, that if the prolapse has produced much distortion of the pupil, the latter may be so much covered by the upper lid as greatly to impair the vision; so that it will be necessary to make an artificial pupil in another direction. The advantages offered by the lower section [Fig. 148]

[Fig. 148.]

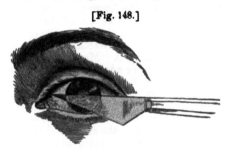

are, that it is more easy of performance; as are also the division of the capsule, the exit of the cataract, and the removal of the remains of cortical substance. The cornea is, moreover, less liable to be bruised, and should suppuration of the cornea occur, it is more likely to limit itself than in the upper section. Bearing these points in mind, I should advise the beginner at first to perform the lower section, until he has acquired sufficient dexterity and experience in operating to give each method a fair trial.

The instruments required for flap extraction are: 1. An extraction knife. 2. A pair of forceps for fixing the eyeball. 3. A pricker, or Von Graefe's cystitome, for dividing the capsule. 4. A curette, which, for convenience sake, is fixed to the other end of the pricker. 5. A blunt-pointed secondary knife. 6. A blunt-pointed pair of scissors.

Various forms of extraction knives are recommended by different operators. I myself prefer Sichel's knife (Fig. 149). It is rather long and narrow,

Fig. 149.

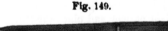

and increases regularly, but not too abruptly, from point to heel, so that the flap is formed by simply pushing the blade on through the anterior chamber until the section is completed. Its wedge shape fills up the gap, and prevents the premature escape of the aqueous humor. The handle is to be lightly held between the thumb, fore and middle fingers, the thumb being slightly bent outwards at the joint. The elbow must be kept close to the side and the wrist steady, so that all movements are made from the fingers and hand.

I will now proceed to a description of the operation, and I shall throughout suppose that the right eye is to be operated upon by the upper section.

I shall enter somewhat at length into the description of the mode of operating, the accidents which may occur, and the principles which should guide us in the after-treatment, because most of these questions are of importance in every mode of operating for the extraction of cataract; hence it is absolutely necessary that the surgeon should be acquainted with them, even although he may entirely abandon the common flap extraction for Von Graefe's new operation.

The operator should stand or sit behind the patient, who is to be placed in the recumbent position. If he is about to operate without fixation, he will hold the upper eyelid with the forefinger of his left hand, drawing it upwards and away from the eye. The tip of the second finger is to be placed gently against the sclerotic on the nasal side of the cornea, so as to prevent the eye from rolling too far inwards. An assistant is to draw the lower eyelid down without everting it. Many of our best operators do not employ fixation, and generally make admirable sections; but yet cases will occur in which even the most skilled operator does not make the counter-puncture just at the desired point. The chief difficulty in operating without fixation is, that the eye may roll swiftly inwards directly the puncture is made, or even before, so that the cornea becomes almost hidden in the inner canthus, and the knife has to traverse the anterior chamber and to make the counter-puncture, without the operator being able to see its course. This will prove extremely embarrassing to the beginner, and may even unnerve him for the remainder of the operation. I should, therefore, strongly recommend him to fix the eyeball, as this greatly facilitates the first part of the operation, and as there is not the slightest objection to his doing so. It has been objected that the fixation often produces pain and much irritation, but this will hardly occur, if it be gently and carefully done. Moreover, so sensitive an eye would prove most difficult to operate upon without fixation. Afterwards, when the operator has gained more confidence and dexterity, he may do without it, if he chooses. Various instruments have been devised for this purpose, but the common fixation-forceps are the best. Their use in this operation has long been advocated by Von Graefe, and more lately by Mr. France. As soon as the counter-puncture is made, they are to be removed, for the eye is then completely under our control. The operator should rather fix the eye himself than entrust this to an assistant, for it is impossible that their hands can work together with such unanimity as if both hands are guided by the same volition. If fixation be employed, an assistant must hold the lids. If the right eye is to be operated on, he should stand on the left side of the patient, and place the tips of the fore and second fingers of his right hand upon the edge of the upper lid (without touching the lashes), and draw it gently upwards and a little inwards, away from the eyeball. If the lids are at all moist, a piece of linen may be folded round the fingers, so as to prevent their slipping. The lower lid is to be held with the forefinger of his left hand. But if the assistant is not dexterous and trustworthy, and the surgeon cannot operate well without fixation, the spring speculum may be employed to keep the lids apart, but I am rather afraid of it, as it is apt to irritate the eye, and to press upon the eyeball.

The operation is divided into three periods—1st. The formation of the flap; 2. The laceration of the capsule; 3. The removal of the lens.

First Period.—Let us again assume that the right eye is to be operated upon by the upper section, and that the operator will fix the eye. Holding the forceps in his left hand, he seizes a fold of conjunctiva and subconjunctival tissue near the lower edge of the cornea (as in Fig. 150, after France), or, as I prefer it, rather more to the nasal side, and draws the eyeball gently down, so as to bring the cornea well into view. Then, holding the knife lightly in his right hand, and steadying the latter by placing his ring or little finger against the temple, he enters the point at the outer side of the cornea about a quarter of a line from its edge, and just at its transverse diameter, and then carries the blade steadily and rather slowly across the anterior chamber to the point of counter-puncture, keeping it quite parallel to the iris. Special care must be taken not to rotate it or to press upon its

Fig. 150.

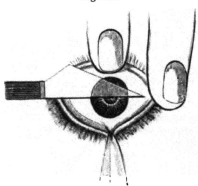

edge, but rather to press upon the back of the blade, as if, in fact, he were wishing to cut with this. If this be done, the blade will be pushed steadily on and fill up the gap, thus preventing the premature escape of the aqueous humor. I find this pressing upon the back of the blade one of the most difficult things for the young operator to acquire. The eye of the operator is not to be kept fixed upon the point of the knife, but upon the point where he wishes to make the counter-puncture, for this will insure the knife being brought out at the desired spot, which should lie slightly in the upper half of the cornea, about a quarter of a line from its edge. As soon as the counter-puncture is made, the forceps are to be removed and the handle of the knife turned back towards the temple, the blade being pushed steadily on until the section is all but finished. When only a small bridge of cornea remains undivided, the section is to be slowly completed by turning the edge of the knife a little forwards, and, instead of carrying it straight on, drawing it back from heel to point until the section is finished. Von Graefe insists especially upon the advantage of doing this, for as the narrowest part of the blade thus issues last from the incision, the flap will be less elevated than by the broad part; moreover, the altered position and direction of the knife cause a relaxation in the tension of the muscles of the eye, and thus diminish straining. When the incision is completed, the upper lid is to be gently and carefully dropped, so that it may not catch in between the lips of the wound and evert the flap. The patient having been calmed by a few words of encouragement, we pass on to the

Second Period, the Opening of the Capsule.—This may be done either with a pricker (Fig. 151, which represents this instrument, together with the curette, which is placed at the other end of the handle), or with Von Graefe's cystitome. The patient is directed to look well down to his feet, and the upper lid being slightly lifted, the pricker is introduced with its blunt angle downwards. When arrived at the inner side of the pupil, it is slightly rotated, so as to turn its point against the capsule, which is to be divided across as far as the outer edge of the pupil by one or more incisions. The

Fig. 151.   Fig. 152.

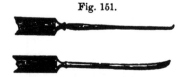

point is then turned downwards, and the instrument carefully removed, so as not to entangle it in the iris or cornea. For flap extraction, I prefer Von Graefe's cystitome (Fig. 152—beside it is an enlarged view), as it makes a freer opening, and as we need not change its horizontal position in lacerating the capsule; whereas the handle of the pricker requires to be a little elevated, which causes more or less gaping of the section. Care must be taken not to press the point of the pricker or cystitome against the lens in dividing the capsule, otherwise we may cause a displacement of the lens into the vitreous humor.

Third Period, Removal of the Lens.—The patient being again directed to look downwards, the point of the forefinger, or the end of the curette, is to be placed against the lower lid, and gentle, but steady, pressure made upon the globe [Fig. 153]. The point of the other forefinger may be placed on the upper portion of the eyeball, so as to regulate and alternate the pressure to a nicety. The pressure on the lower lid should be at first backward, in order that the upper edge of the lens may be tilted slightly forward against the upper portion of the pupil, which gradually dilates and permits the presentation of the lens. The pressure is then directed a little more upwards and backwards, so that the lens advances through the pupil into the anterior chamber, and makes its exit through the incision. If it halts a little in its course through the section, it may be extracted with the curette. The pressure throughout should be steady, but very gentle, in order that the lens may not be violently jerked out, which is generally accompanied by rupture of the hyaloid membrane and an escape of vitreous humor. When the lens has been removed, we should examine its outline to see whether this is perfect, or whether it is irregular or notched, as the latter shows at once that portions of the cortical substance have remained behind. If the cataract is not quite mature, fragments of cortex are apt to remain in the capsule, or are stripped off during the passage of the lens through the pupil or the corneal incision, to either of which they may cling. These portions should, if possible, be removed, as they are apt to set up iritis or to give rise to secondary cataract. The lids are, therefore, to be closed and lightly rubbed in a circular direction, so that any little flakes remaining behind the iris may be brought into the area of the pupil, whence they are to be gently removed with the curette, as likewise any portions adhering to the lips of the wound. The vision of the patient may also be tested by trying if he can count fingers, and if it is not as good as might be expected, we may examine again as to whether remnants of lens-substance still linger behind.

We must now briefly consider what course is to be pursued if any untowa circumstances arise during the different steps of the operation.

Under the following circumstances, it is advisable to withdraw the knife at once, and to postpone the operation until the wound is united: 1. If the puncture is too near the edge of the cornea, or in the sclerotic. 2. If it is too far in the cornea, so that the flap would be too small. 3. If the aqueous humor spirts out when the point of the knife has only just entered the an-

[Fig. 153.]

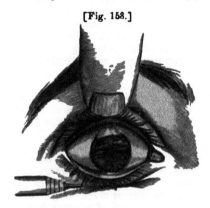

terior chamber, for the iris will then fall forward upon the knife, which would become entangled in it, so that it would he impossible to finish the section without lacerating the iris considerably. 4. If the point of the knife is so blunt that it will not readily make the counter-puncture.

Fig. 154.   Fig. 155.

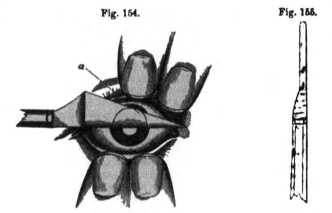

Should the aqueous humor escape directly the counter-puncture has been made, the section may yet be finished without wounding the iris, by placing the point of the fore or middle finger of the other hand upon the edge of the blade, and pushing the iris off from it as the section is being slowly completed. If, however, it is impossible to avoid wounding the iris, it is better to cut boldly through it, as this is far less apt to excite iritis than if the knife becomes entangled in it. If the counter-puncture is too close to the sclerotic, the knife must be slightly drawn back, and another counter-puncture made, or the size of the section be diminished by turning the edge of the blade slightly forwards in finishing the flap. This should also be done when the counter-puncture is too low. If it be too high, the flap will be too small, and this may be remedied (1) by making another counter-puncture a little lower down, (2) by turning the edge of the blade back in cutting out, or (3) by enlarging the section downwards with a secondary knife or a pair of blunt-pointed scissors. The last proceeding is to be preferred if the counter-puncture is much too high. If we purpose doing this, the section is to be continued until only a little bridge of cornea is left standing (Fig. 154, a). The knife is then to be withdrawn, and the section enlarged by dividing the cornea to the required extent at the counter-puncture with the probe-pointed secondary knife (Fig. 155), or with blunt-pointed scissors. The advantage of leaving the little bridge standing is, that it will keep the cornea tense, and prevent its yielding before the knife or scissors. The bridge is then to be divided, or, before so doing, the capsule may be opened. The size of the flap should always be noted before the section is completed, so that we may enlarge it in the above manner if necessary. If the section is too small to permit the ready exit of the lens, there is much danger of rupture of the hyaloid membrane and escape of vitreous humor, and of bruising the iris and cornea. It is also advisable to leave the bridge standing if the patient is very unruly, and strains greatly as we are making the section. A few moments' rest will generally suffice to restore his quietude, and then the bridge may be divided.

[Fig. 156.]

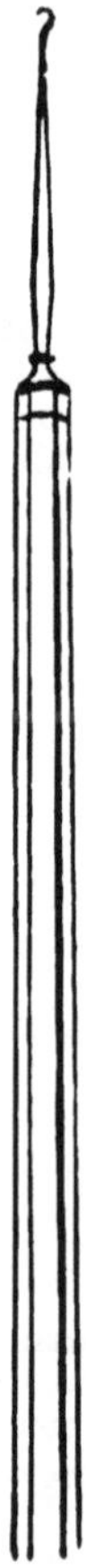

If the lens does not, at the third period, readily present itself in the pupil, we must on no account attempt to force this by pressing strongly on the eye; but we must lacerate the capsule again, and more freely than before. If the capsule be so tough as not to be readily torn with the cystitome, it sometimes comes away with the lens, or it may be divided with the point of the knife, or be afterwards removed with a hook or a pair of iris forceps.

If a little vitreous humor escapes with the lens, it is but of slight consequence as far as the immediate result of the operation is concerned. Some operators snip off the protruding portion of vitreous close to the incision, but I think it best not to do so, as it is simply followed by a fresh oozing out of vitreous; I therefore close the eye at once, and apply a firm compress bandage over it. But it is very different if it escapes before the lens, for then it will push the latter aside, so that it may even fall to the bottom of the vitreous humor. If this accident should occur, a hook [Fig. 156] or scoop should be passed behind the lens, and the latter gently "fished out." It should be extracted at all hazards, for if it remains behind it is but too likely to set up a most destructive and painful pan-ophthalmitis. Many operators do not consider it of much consequence, if even a considerable amount of vitreous is lost in an operation of extraction of cataract. But there is no doubt that it is always a source of great danger to the future safety of the eye, for it not only frequently induces an insidious form of irido-choroiditis, or inflammatory or suppurative changes in the vitreous, but it is also, according to Iwanoff,[1] generally followed by detachment of vitreous, which may lead to detachment of the retina. This is likewise proved by the interesting and important experiments of Gouvea[2] on the eyes of animals.

After the exit of the lens, the corneal flap sometimes becomes wrinkled and collapsed, so that it falls away from the line of incision. This wrinkling is due either to increase of the intra-ocular tension, or to a diminution in the elasticity of the cornea. Von Graefe lays great stress upon the importance of this symptom, considering it unfavorable if the collapse be at all considerable, for he has found that suppuration of the cornea often occurs in such cases. If we therefore find, in a case of double cataract which is to be operated on at one sitting, that the cornea of the first eye becomes much wrinkled after extraction, it will be wise to submit the other eye to a different mode of operation. In such cases, also, great care must be taken that the flap is not turned back when the upper lid is let down. If the iris protrudes between the lips of the wound after removal of the lens, or if the pupil is distorted, the lids should be closed and lightly rubbed in a circular direction, so as to replace the iris, and restore the regularity of the pupil. If the prolapse still persists, it may be gently replaced with the curette. But if all our efforts prove unavailing, it is by far the best course to draw it out a little further and snip it off. The iridectomy will not be of the slightest disadvantage, more especially in the upper section; in fact, it may prove of positive advantage, not only in favoring the cure, but also in exposing remnants of lens-substance which may be situated behind the iris, and have, perhaps, caused the prolapse; whereas the occurrence of prolapse after extraction is one of the chief dangers and annoyances of this operation. The protruding portion of iris sets up considerable irritation, and prevents, perhaps, the union of the section, the aqueous humor flowing off through the fistulous opening; and this constant irritation may set up iritis or irido-cyclitis. Even if the iris unites with the section, a broad unsightly cicatrix will be left, the pupil being, perhaps, greatly distorted or almost obliterated. To prevent all these untoward complications, I strongly advise the removal of a portion of the iris if the prolapse cannot be easily returned, or if the iris has been much contused by the exit of the lens, or by our endeavors to restore the prolapsed portion. Dr. Williams, of Boston, U. S. A., unites the edges of the corneal wound by a very delicate suture, which keeps the lips of the incision in contact, facilitates the union, and diminishes the risk of prolapse. [In the United States the flap operation has been very generally discarded for either the peripherical linear operation of Von Graefe or some modification of it.—B.]

Hemorrhage into the vitreous humor is a disastrous occurrence. It may take place either at the time of the operation, or some hours afterwards. The patient complains of a sudden sharp pain, a gush of vitreous takes place, followed by blood, and the eye is lost. In such cases there generally exists a diseased condition of the choroidal and retinal vessels, detachment of the retina, etc.

The after-treatment of flap extraction is a subject of great importance, as much may be done by timely care and attention. As the rules with regard to the after-treatment of cases of flap extraction also apply more or less to those in which some other mode of extraction is performed, I shall enter somewhat at length upon this subject; and as the after-treatment of the different operations for cataract involves the same principles, I shall lay

[1] "A. f. O.," xv. 2.   [2] Ibid., xv. 1.

down certain broad general rules of treatment, which will, however, require modification according to the exigencies of particular cases. It being of consequence to detect and combat any unfavorable symptoms at the earliest stage, the surgeon should visit the patient very frequently during the first few days after the operation, and, if possible, change the dressings himself, so that he may watch the condition of the lids, the quantity and character of the discharge, etc. At one time the antiphlogistic treatment was in great repute. Local and general depletion were had recourse to, and perhaps repeated several times, upon the slightest appearance of pain or inflammatory symptoms. But now this mode of treatment has justly fallen into disuse. Our primary object is to obtain adhesion of the corneal flap by the first intention, and this will take place far more readily in a strong, healthy person, than in one who is weak and decrepit; nearly one-half of the cornea has been divided, and for a time the other half has to carry on the nutrition of the whole, and to assist in the process of union. It must also be remembered that this operation is generally performed in persons above the age of fifty or fifty-five, and even indeed in the very aged, whose vital powers will not bear depression. The general health and the reparative powers of the system must therefore be sustained. The better and stronger the patient's constitution is, the more favorable may be the prognosis of the result of the operation. Even the florid, turgid, apoplectic-looking individual warrants a better prognosis than the very aged, decrepit person, whose general health is poor and feeble, whose cheeks are pale and shrunken, whose arteries are rigid and skin unelastic. Von Graefe also considers the prognosis less favorable if the eyeball is deep-set and sunken, and the diameter of the cornea short; for in such cases flaccidity and wrinkling of the corneal flap, and suppuration of the cornea, are of not unfrequent occurrence on account of its feeble nutrition.

The after-treatment must be varied according to the general health, constitution, and habits of the patient. The diet should from the commencement be light, nutritious, and easily digestible. Meat may be allowed once daily; it should, however, be finely minced, so that there is no need for mastication, which would disturb the quietude of the eye. Good beef tea or mutton broth may be given occasionally during the day, but slops are, as a rule, to be avoided. But whilst we endeavor to sustain the patient's strength, we must not fall into the opposite error of over-feeding him. In a very plethoric and full-blooded individual, especially if marked inflammatory and febrile symptoms manifest themselves, a strictly antiphlogistic regimen must be observed. With regard to stimulants and beer, we must be entirely guided by the patient's constitution and habits. It is very unwise to cut off all stimulants from an individual who has always, and perhaps largely, indulged in their use; we should allow him a moderate amount of his customary beverage, watching the while its effect, and diminishing or increasing the quantity as the case may demand. In feeble, decrepit persons, stimulants and malt liquor, together with a good nutritious diet, often prove of great service; quinine and ammonia being also given.

It is well to administer a gentle purgative the day before the operation, so that the bowels may not require to be opened for a day or two after the latter. A mild dose of castor oil should then be given, in order to prevent any straining; and this may be repeated if necessary.

When the operation has been concluded, the patient is to be placed in bed in a darkened room. At night, his hands should be tied to the side of the bed, to prevent his touching his eyes during sleep. The lids of both eyes may be fastened with a strip or two of sticking plaster, although this is apt to irritate from its shrinking and hardening. I myself prefer a light bandage, especially Liebreich's, which is the most convenient for this purpose. If this is found to be too hot, I employ a very thin gauze bandage. A piece of soft linen is to be applied over the eyelid to soak up any discharge, and prevent its clogging and hardening the charpie, a little pad of which is to be next applied, the whole being kept in place by the bandage. But if we desire to exert more pressure upon the eye, we must employ Von Graefe's compress bandage, the application of which, however, demands far more care and practice.

So much nicety and attention are required in the application of these bandages, and in the regulation of the amount of pressure, that we are but seldom able to entrust this to a nurse. If we cannot change the compress ourselves, or leave this duty to a practised and trustworthy assistant, it is far better to abstain altogether from its use. It should be changed night and morning, and, if the eye feels uncomfortable, even more frequently. The quantity and character of the discharge upon the linen and charpie should be examined, as it affords a clue to the condition of the eye. The edges of the lids should be gently sponged with lukewarm water, so as to remove any hardened discharge from the eyelashes, which may also be smeared with a little cold cream or simple cerate. This will prevent their sticking together, and thus interfering with the ready escape of tears or discharge. Great care must, however, be taken not to rub or press upon the upper eyelid, otherwise the coaptation of the flap may be disturbed and union prevented. Much comfort and relief are afforded by the sponging and cleansing of the eyelids and the change of the compress. The eye should not, however, be opened or examined unless we specially desire to ascertain its condition. Union of the flap generally takes place within the first forty-eight hours, or even sooner. Then it is advisable to apply a drop of atropine once or twice daily to the inside of the lower lid, without widely opening the eye. This soothes the eye and dilates the pupil, so that there is less chance of a secondary cataract, and the torn edges of the capsule, having no chance to adhere to each other or to the iris, will readily retract and shrivel, and thus leave a good free opening. Moreover, should iritis occur, it will be of great advantage to have the pupil already widely dilated. It is an interesting fact that if atropine was applied before the operation, its effect upon the pupil partially returns when the section is united, and the aqueous humor reaccumulated. Should the atropine cause any irritation, a solution of belladonna should be substituted. A few hours after the operation, the patient generally experiences a slight sensation of pressure and smarting in the eye, which lasts for a few minutes, but reappears at intervals of an hour or two. It is due to an accumulation of tears and aqueous humor. If the pain increases toward night and becomes continuous, and the eye is hot, and the patient restless and uncomfortable, morphia should be administered either internally or endermically. I generally employ the subcutaneous injection, varying in strength from one-sixth to one-fourth of a grain. It may be repeated if necessary. If the eye is very hot and painful, much relief is often experienced from cold-water compresses. But their use requires much care and discretion, for if they are applied for too long a time, they may depress the circulation of the part too much, and thus increase the danger of suppuration of the cornea. I have also sometimes found great relief from the application of two or three leeches to the temple, especially in plethoric individuals. I must, however, state that Von Graefe, after having for many years employed leeches, has now entirely abandoned their use during the first three days after the operation. He thinks that they prove injurious, inasmuch as they produce in the first instance an increased congestion of the infiltrated structures, and thus favor suppuration of the edges of the wound.[1] In such cases he much prefers, if the patient be plethoric and robust, a small venesection of from four to eight fluidounces; also if there is much pain accompanied by considerable lachrymation and swelling of the lids during the first thirty-six hours after the operation, for during this period suppurative inflammation generally commences. But it is not to be employed if suppuration has already set in.

If the case goes on well, without the appearance of any unfavorable symptoms, such as severe pain in and around the eye, swelling of the lids, muco-purulent discharge, or copious lachrymation, the eye should not be opened during the first five or six days. Nothing is so bad as being too curious as to the result, and opening the eye too early to assure ourselves that everything is going on well, for this may easily set up iritis. It is very different if unfavorable symptoms arise, for then it is best to open the lids and carefully examine the condition of the eye, so that we may know what is really the matter, and what treatment should be adopted. The upper lid should be gently lifted, and the state of the cornea and iris examined. This is best done by the light of a candle, which should be shaded by the hand of the nurse or assistant until the moment that the surgeon is ready to examine the eye. In this way, the latter is exposed only for a few seconds to the light, and the glare and intensity of the illumination are far less than if daylight is admitted into the room.

But the case may not run so favorable a course. The thinly cicatrized wound may yield, and a portion of the iris protrude through it. This frequently happens a few days after the operation. The patient experiences a feeling of grit or sand in the eye, as if a foreign body were lodged under the eyelid. The lids become swollen, the eye painful, and there is a copious, clear, watery discharge, which, after a time, assumes more of a muco-purulent character. These symptoms may arise suddenly, perhaps after a fit of coughing or sneezing, which has caused the section to yield. If the prolapse is large, and produces a wide gaping of the wound, the pain and irritation are often very great. The eye should be opened and the real condition ascertained. If protrusion of the iris has occurred, the lids must be gently closed again, and a firm compress applied, which will not only favor the consolidation of the wound by the formation of a layer of lymph over the prolapse, but will prevent its increasing in size; and by the continuance of gentle pressure will even cause it to shrink. Afterwards, when the wound is quite consolidated, and a firm layer of exudation covers the prolapse, the latter may be pricked with a fine needle, as has been recommended by Mr. Bowman, so as to let the aqueous humor, which is distending it, flow off. The prolapse then shrinks and dwindles down. This pricking may be repeated several times. If the prolapse is large and widely distends the section, it may be necessary to remove it, either with scissors or with the extraction knife, a compress being afterwards applied. Some surgeons touch the prolapse with a stick of nitrate of silver, but this often produces great irritation. The prolapse may have so drawn up the pupil that it is quite covered by the upper lid, or even involved in the section, which will afterwards necessitate the formation of an artificial pupil, and this will often cause the prolapse to shrink. Prolapse of the iris, occurring after extraction, is not only a source of long-continued trouble to the patient, but may even prove very dangerous, by setting up protracted inflammatory complications —e. g., irido-choroiditis—which may eventually destroy the eye.

[1] Von Graefe's Clinical Lecture, "Kl. Monatsbl.," 1863, translated in "Ophthalmic Review," No. 8.

may be due to the bruising or contusion of the iris by the instruments, or by the passage of the lens through the pupil, or it may be set up by the irritation produced by portions of lens-substance which have remained behind. The patient experiences pain in and around the eye; the lids become swollen, and there is more or less photophobia and lachrymation. On opening the eye, we may find a considerable amount of chemosis surrounding the cornea, which is clear, but the aqueous humor is somewhat clouded, the iris discolored, and the pupil contracted. If the patient is sufficiently strong, much benefit is derived from the application of leeches to the temples. A strong solution of atropine (four grains to the fluidounce of water) should be frequently applied, so that the pupil may be widely dilated. Belladonna ointment should be rubbed over the forehead three or four times daily.

If, after flap extraction, the case has throughout progressed favorably, the patient may be permitted to leave his bed for an hour or two at the end of the fifth or sixth day. He should, however, wear a light bandage, and the room be somewhat darkened, but it should at the same time be kept cool and well ventilated. If remaining in bed proves very irksome, which is apt to be the case in country people accustomed to an active life, it may be well to permit the patient to get up even on the third or fourth day. But then he must be very carefully watched. In a hospital in which there are no special eye wards, the bed should have dark-blue curtains round its head, so as to afford a protection against cold and draught, and the bright light of the ward. In such a case, I think it also very advisable to keep the patient in bed some days longer than would be necessary in a private room or a special ward. At the end of the first week, the bandage may generally be exchanged for a shade, and the patient be gradually accustomed to the light. Should, however, any inflammatory symptoms appear, such as photophobia, lachrymation, swelling of the lids, etc., the bandage should be reapplied, and increased care be taken of the eye. If the weather is favorable, the patient may go out into the air at the end of a fortnight. This often proves of great benefit, especially if there is any conjunctivitis, which is apt to become chronic if the confinement to the house has been long. In such a case a weak astringent collyrium should be prescribed. [Von Arlt prefers the flap operation for cataracta aecreta, with annular or total posterior synechiæ, whether there are extensive post-iritic membranes or not, and has never observed suppuration of the cornea in these cases after such an operation.—B.]

I have already mentioned that, in certain cases of immature senile cataract, in which the progress is extremely slow, and the opacity so advanced or situated (e. g., at the posterior pole of the lens) as to impair vision considerably, it may be advisable to hasten the progress of the cataract by pricking the capsule and admitting the aqueous humor to the lens-substance. Great care must, however, be taken not to divide the capsule too freely, as this may cause considerable swelling of the lens-substance, and give rise to severe iritis or irido-cyclitis. It is much better to make only a small opening in the capsule, and to repeat the operation if necessary, several times, more especially if a considerable portion of the lens is still transparent. If severe inflammation supervenes, and if it does not yield rapidly to antiphlogistics, it is advisable, more especially if the tension of the eye is increased, to remove the lens at once, either by the flap extraction or Von Graefe's operation; in the former case it would be well to make at the same time a large iridectomy.

Von Graefe[1] has recommended that a downward iridectomy should precede the laceration of the capsule. About five or six weeks afterwards a superficial crucial incision is made in the capsule with a fine needle (the pupil having been previously widely dilated by atropine). This wide dilatation is to be maintained in order to afford plenty of room for the swelling of the lens, and prevent its pressing upon the iris and ciliary body. Generally, but very slight irritation follows the laceration of the capsule, and flap extraction may be performed from about six to twelve days afterwards, when the cataract will readily escape. For reasons already stated, I should prefer to make the iridectomy upwards.

I have before mentioned that the chief dangers to be feared after flap extraction are suppuration of the cornea, prolapse of the iris, and iritis. The principal causes which may produce the latter are: 1. Bruising of the iris by the instruments and by the passage of the cataract through the pupil, more especially if the latter is somewhat small and rigid, so that it dilates with difficulty. 2. The contusion and irritation which the iris may suffer in the attempts to replace a prolapse. 3. The irritation set up by portions of lens-matter remaining behind the iris or adhering to the pupil, which is especially apt to occur if the pupil is small and rigid and the cataract immature, or if it possesses a small nucleus, with a considerable portion of soft cortical substance. Now, in accordance with the fact that the segment of the iris corresponding to the corneal section is the portion most exposed to these different influences, we find that this almost always forms the starting-point of the inflammation (iritis). In order to diminish these dangers, it has been proposed to remove this portion of the iris prior to the extraction of the cataract—to perform, in fact, a preliminary iridectomy. Von Graefe originally pointed out that such a proceeding might be advantageous in some cases, and Dr. Mooren[2] subsequently submitted this plan to an extensive trial, with marked success. Mooren makes the iridectomy about two to six weeks before the extraction. But it must be admitted that few persons are willing to undergo two separate operations for the extraction of cataract, except this be absolutely necessary. To avoid this inconvenience, the iridectomy may be combined with the operation of flap extraction, as was advised by Jacobson, who introduced the following modification of the flap extraction.[3] The patient having been placed under chloroform, the lower flap extraction is to be performed, the puncture and counter-puncture, however, lying about half a line below the horizontal meridian of the cornea, and not in the substance of the latter, but in the sclero-corneal junction, as he believes that union takes place more readily here than in the cornea. The lens having been removed in the usual manner, he excises the corresponding segment of iris, in order to diminish the risk of iritis, prolapse of the iris, and suppuration of the cornea.

I have mentioned that Professor Jacobson places the patient thoroughly under the influence of chloroform. Most operators (amongst whom I must include myself) have hitherto been afraid of giving chloroform in flap extraction, on account of the danger of vomiting or retching during or after the operation. The wound is so large (embracing nearly half the cornea) that a fit of vomiting or severe retching may cause a great loss of vitreous

---

[1] "Archiv f. Ophthalmologie," x. 2, 209; vide also a paper upon this subject by Dr. Mannhardt in the "Sitzungsberichte der Ophthalmologischen Gesellschaft," 1864.
[2] "Die vermindesten Gefahren einer Hornhautveseiterung bei der Staarextraction," by Dr. Mooren. Hirschwald, Berlin, 1862.
[3] "Ein neues und gefahrloses Operations-Verfahren zur Heilung des Grauen Staares," von Dr. Jacobson, Petersb., Berlin, 1868.

humor, and may even force out the retina and choroid. Professor Jacobson states, however, that there is no danger of vomiting if the patient be thoroughly narcotised, and Mr. Windsor, of Manchester, has published[1] a series of twenty cases of flap extraction successfully performed under chloroform. If chloroform is given in eye operations, the patient should be placed thoroughly under its influence; otherwise it is better to abstain altogether from its use. These operations, more especially those upon the iris and for cataract, are of so delicate a nature, that a sudden start of the patient's head, or a fit of vomiting or retching, may not only endanger the result of the operation, but even the safety of the eye. When the patient is so deeply narcotized, the sudden inhalation of a strong dose of chloroform may prove very dangerous; and it is therefore of great importance to know exactly what percentage of chloroform the patient is breathing. For this reason I greatly prefer Clover's apparatus for administering chloroform. It is not only the safest method, but by no other have I uniformly seen such perfect tranquility and unconsciousness produced, without there being any cause for fear. There is little or no struggling or straining; the patient breathes calmly and quietly; and when he is thoroughly under its influence, the most difficult and delicate ophthalmic operations may be performed without fear or risk. In order that there may be no vomiting or retching, strict orders should be given that the patient does not take any food or drink for three or four hours prior to the operation.

[Edward von Jaeger has recently invented a knife which, from its shape, effects what Lebrun has sought to obtain by the gradual rotation of the blade. The knife looks like a Beer's cataract-knife, has one surface of the blade concave with a radius of six or seven millimetres, the other convex with a radius of five millimetres. The back is straight, thin, and blunt. The knife is introduced with its convex side towards the globe, and is pushed forward horizontally like Beer's knife. Von Jaeger makes the section upwards, and hence, owing to the curvature of the blade, there must be a different knife for each eye. The operation is completed without an iridectomy. (See Von Jaeger, "Der Hoheschnitt, eine neue Staar-Extractions-Methode," 1873.)—B.]

5.—EXTRACTION OF THE LENS IN ITS CAPSULE.

This operation was first practised by Richter and Beer, but fell into disuse until it was some years ago reintroduced, amongst others by Sperino, Pagenstecher, and De Wecker. Dr. Pagenstecher[2] originally removed the lens in its capsule with much success by the lower flap operation (the section lying, however, in the sclerotic), combined with a large iridectomy, the patient being anaesthetized. He has favored me with the following description of his present mode of operating, for during the last eighteen months he has adopted Von Graefe's upward linear incision, and he has found that the delivery of the lens in its capsule is (cœteris paribus) as easy as with the flap operation. Indeed, he has observed, that loss of vitreous is less frequent, and if it does happen, less copious than with the flap incision. In those cases in which the connection between the capsule and the suspensory ligament is not sufficiently relaxed to permit of the easy extraction of the lens in its capsule by slight pressure of the curette on the lower part of the cornea, he employs a large, but very shallow, round curette (made by Messrs. Weiss).

[1] "Ophthalmic Review," vol. ii. 365.
[2] "Klinische Beobachtungen," Wiesbaden, 1866.

This is to be very carefully passed behind the equator of the lens[1] and slid downwards along the posterior capsule, until its free margin embraces the lower circumference of the equator of the lens. After a slight rotation, produced by turning the handle from the centre towards one angle of the incision, the lens is gently drawn upwards, the handle of the curette being at the same time somewhat depressed towards the edge of the orbit, thus pressing the lens slightly against the cornea and preventing its slipping out of the cavity of the curette. Since employing the linear incision, he has abandoned the use of anæsthesia, as there is generally a great tendency for the eye to roll upwards during the narcosis, which, of course, renders the manipulation of the curette very difficult. The eyeball, even if the curette is used, is to be steadily fixed with the forceps, which are to be applied at that point of the sclerotic which lies exactly in the same meridian as the centre of the linear incision. After having practised the extraction of the lens in its capsule for a period of five years, Dr. Pagenstecher has arrived at the following conclusions as to the cases in which it is indicated: 1. He prefers the extraction of the lens in its capsule to that with laceration of the latter, in all those cases in which it may be presumed that the capsule is firmer than its attachment with the zonula of Zinn. This generally occurs in cases of over-ripe cataract, both in those which are hard and somewhat shrunken, and those which are softish or partly fluid (Morgagnian cataract). 2. It is also very suitable in those cases in which the progress of the opacity is extremely slow, and certain portions of the lens always remain transparent, so that the cataract never becomes perfectly mature. Such cataracts are generally small in size, and the capsule is but very slightly attached to the zonula. 3. It will, as a rule, be found suitable in those cases of cataract which have become developed after irido-choroiditis, and iritis with posterior circular synechia. The adhesions between the capsule and the iris must, of course, be detached prior to the extraction of the cataract, for which purpose a small, blunt-pointed silver hook is to be employed. 4. It may be recommended where, together with the cataract, there is a tremulous iris; for it will often be found that the latter is caused by a shrinking in the size of the lens, or a diminution of the vitreous humor, which should generally lead us to suspect atrophy of the zonula. The last two categories are, moreover, also suitable for this mode of operation, because of the tendency to inflammatory complications of the iris which exists in them; in consequence of which, it is a matter of much importance to guard the iris against the irritation produced by remnants of cortical substance or portions of capsule.

[The advantages claimed by Pagenstecher for this method are: 1. The gain of a perfectly clear pupil. 2. The absence of plastic and recurrent iritis. 3. No danger of any diminution of the resulting vision through clouding of the capsule, and consequently no necessity for any secondary operation. 4. The very best degree of visual acuity. 5. Recurrent hemorrhages are much rarer than when the capsule is left behind. 6. The dazzling sensations due to diffusion of light through the capsule are done away with. 7. There is no prolapse and cicatrization of the capsule in the wound. The disadvantages admitted are: 1. The healing of the wound is in some cases somewhat slower than by other methods. 2. Vitreous opacities are more frequent. 3. The average resulting astigmatism is somewhat greater than after extraction without the capsule. (See "Archiv für Augenheilkunde," x. 2.)

---

[1] This manœuvre is facilitated, as Dr. Pagenstecher points out, if a little pressure is exerted on the lower portion of the lens, which causes the summit of its equator to be tilted forwards, and frequently detaches the zonula from the periphery of the lens.

Jacobson's operation closely resembles Pagenstecher's. Macnamara has lately advocated for this operation the use of a broad keratome in making the incision, and extracts the lens and capsule without an iridectomy. This is the model operation in theory.—B.]

Mr. Bowman has also occasionally extracted the lens in its capsule by Von Graefe's operation in cases of over-ripe cataract, in which the connection between the capsule and the suspensory ligament was relaxed.

De Weoker[1] performs the lower flap operation; the incision does not, however, lie far in the sclerotic, nor does he leave a conjunctival bridge standing. A portion of iris having been excised, he passes a curette behind the lens and draws it out in its capsule. When the lens has reached the incision, an assistant, grasping its edge with a Daviel's curette, extracts it. His results have also been very favorable, and he has often succeeded in extracting the lens without any loss of vitreous humor.

[The desire to have a clear, movable pupil has led many surgeons to attempt the removal of the lens and capsule in various ways. Küchler undertook to extract lens and capsule by splitting the cornea in its horizontal meridian, as in his operation for the cure of corneal staphyloma, and then removing the lens without an iridectomy. ("Graefe u. Saemisch's Hdb. der Augenheilk.," iii. p. 314.) Gioppi makes the peripherical linear incision as Von Graefe did, but the resemblance ceases here. He neither performs an iridectomy nor opens the capsule, but removes lens and capsule with an instrument resembling Waldau's spoon.

In all these cases, the operator should satisfy himself that the connection between capsule and zonula is a loose one before attempting the dislocation of the lens and capsule en masse.—B.]

6.—LINEAR EXTRACTION.

Before describing this mode of operating, I will glance for a moment at its history.[2] In 1811, Gibson introduced it as supplementary to the needle operation, in those cases of soft cataract in which the lens (after having been divided) was not absorbed with the desired rapidity or success. He also employed it in capsular and membranaceous cataract. His mode of operating consisted in removing the lens through a small corneal section, which was about three lines in extent, and was situated about one line from the sclerotic. In 1814, Travers, after dividing the capsule, displaced the lens in the anterior chamber, and then removed it through a small corneal section. He, however, subsequently gave up this method, and, making a quarter section of the cornea, divided the capsule with the point of the knife, and if the lens was sufficiently soft, let it escape through the section, but if it was too firm for this, he introduced a curette into the anterior chamber, and by its aid removed the lens piecemeal. Both the operations of Gibson and Travers fell into disuse, until about 1851, when Bowman and Von Graefe, quite independently of each other, reintroduced linear extraction. Von Graefe, having worked out the subject extensively and with great care, states, in his first essay upon it,[3] that the linear extraction is especially indicated in the cortical cataract of youthful individuals, and also in those cases in which there is so much swelling up of the lens-substance (either in con-

---

[1] "Maladies des Yeux," 2d edit., p. 225.
[2] For an interesting historical sketch of this operation, I must refer the reader to Von Graefe's paper on "Modified Linear Extraction," "Arch. f. Ophthalm.," xi. 8.
[3] "Arch. f. Ophthal.," i. 2.

sequence of a needle operation, or of some injury to the lens) as to threaten the safety of the eye. But he thinks it unsuitable if the lens retains its normal consistence, and still more so, if there is a hard nucleus. As a general rule, linear extraction is, therefore, indicated in cases of cortical cataract occurring between the age of ten and thirty, or even thirty-five. It is also often employed with advantage as supplementary to the needle operation. Linear extraction is to be performed in the following manner: The pupil having been previously well dilated with atropine, and the patient placed under the influence of an anæsthetic, the eyelids are to be kept apart by Weiss's spring speculum, and the eye steadied with a pair of forceps. An incision is then to be made in the cornea, at its temporal side, and about one line from the sclerotic, with a broad straight iridectomy knife. The incision should be from two to two and a half lines in extent. The capsule is then to be divided with the cystitome, and the lens removed. In order to facilitate the exit of the cataract, the convexity of the curette is to be placed against the edge of the cornea, which causes the section to gape; a slight counter-pressure being at the same time exerted by the forefinger of the left hand against the inner side of the eyeball. By alternately pressing with the curette and the finger, the soft lens-substance will readily exude through the incision. If portions of cortical substance remain behind the iris, the lids are to be closed, and the globe lightly rubbed in a circular direction to bring these flakes into the pupil or anterior chamber, whence they may be readily removed. Or Mr. Bowman's suction syringe may be employed for this purpose. Should the iris protrude through the incision it must be gently replaced, but if it has been much bruised by the exit of the lens or the movements of the curette, it will be wiser to excise a portion of it. A light compress bandage is to be applied after the operation, and the pupil should be kept well dilated with atropine.

Von Graefe found that, although occasionally a cataract possessing a firm nucleus may be removed through a linear incision without danger, this operation is, as a rule, inapplicable when the nucleus is hard, for the iris must then be more or less bruised by the passage of the lens through the narrow section. The scoop may also have to be introduced into the anterior chamber behind the lens, so as to facilitate its removal, and this, of course, adds to the contusion of the iris. Great irritation of the latter is likewise often produced by portions of hard lens-substance remaining behind the iris or in the pupil. Now, as the segment of the iris which corresponds to the incision is the most exposed to bruising, and interferes the most with the ready use of the scoop, we find that this is almost always the starting-point of any subsequent iritis. In those cases in which there was a somewhat firm nucleus, Von Graefe was therefore led to modify the linear extraction, and to excise a portion of iris prior to the laceration of the capsule, and then to remove the lens with a broad flat scoop.[1] The stages of this operation were as follows: 1. The incision was made at the edge of the cornea (temporal side), and embraced about a quarter of its circumference. 2. A portion of iris was removed, the size of which did not, however, quite equal the extent of the incision. 3. The capsule was freely divided quite up to the margin of the lens. 4. A scoop was then introduced at the free edge of the lens and gently inserted between the posterior cortical substance and the nucleus, and the cataract lifted into the anterior chamber and extracted. The scoop which he employed for this purpose was shallower, broader, and sharper at the extremity than Daviel's curette. Thus originated the "modified linear"

[1] "Archiv f. Ophthalm.," v. 1.

or "scoop" extraction—an operation which afterwards assumed so important a position in ophthalmic surgery. By this modification Von Graefe greatly extended the applicability of the linear extraction, for he was now able to remove through a linear incision cataracts whose cortex was of a pulpy consistence, and the nucleus moderately large and hard; a form of cataract which would otherwise have necessitated the flap extraction. I would here remark that to Von Graefe belongs the credit of having first suggested, in some cases, the combination of an iridectomy with flap extraction, and also of having introduced the modified linear or scoop extraction. The principle of the latter operation is essentially his, whatever changes may be made in the shape of the scoop, and it is worthy of remark that the latest operations assimilate it more to that originally used by him. Mr. Critchett has already pointed out these facts in his admirable paper upon scoop extraction,[1] in which he says: "Thus there suddenly appeared three new methods of operating for cataract, bearing the name of their several champions—the method of Mooren, of Jacobson, and that of Schuft (Waldau); but justice compels me to state that these gentlemen lighted their tapers at the torch of their great master, Professor Von Graefe. Each of these methods had been previously suggested and practised by him, but only in exceptional cases, instead of as a general rule."

Waldau shortly afterwards contrived a different form of scoop, of varying size, which was deeper, broader, and flatter at the bottom than Von Graefe's. Its edges were, moreover, high and thin, so as to bite into the lens, the anterior lip being the highest, and thus facilitating the removal of the cataract by pressing after it. By its aid he proposed to remove even the hard senile cataract. It was soon found, however, that this form of scoop was too large and cumbersome, and its edges too high and sharp, and that it was therefore difficult to introduce it readily behind the lens, more especially in hard senile cataract, in which it may very easily cause displacement of the lens or rupture of the hyaloid membrane. Mr. Bowman and Mr. Critchett have since devised some forms of scoop which are far better and in all cases preferable to Waldau's. The scoop operation, as performed at Moorfields, has proved remarkably successful in the hands of some of our English ophthalmic surgeons, more especially in those of Messrs. Bowman and Critchett, who have worked out the subject most thoroughly, and have done the most to bring this operation to perfection. As my description of it must be necessarily brief, I would refer the reader to their admirable articles u on this s j ct in the "Royal London Ophthalmic Hospital Reports," vpl. iv. p. 4.ub e

Dr. Adolph Weber has lately introduced a mode of extracting hard cataracts through a linear incision made with a lance-shaped knife, without any excision of the iris or the employment of a traction instrument. He speaks in the highest terms of its success in one hundred and three cases in which he has performed it, and some other operators are also very warm in its praise. Dr. Weber has favored me with the following outline of his present mode of operating; for a fuller description of his operation, I must refer the reader to his valuable and very interesting article in "Von Graefe's Archiv." He employs a large lance-shaped knife[2] (Fig. 157), which is ten and twenty-five one-hundredth millimetres in length, and ten millimetres broad at a distance of six and five-tenths millimetres from its point; and

[1] "Royal London Ophthalmic Hospital Reports," iv. 319.
[2] "A. f. O., xiii. 187.
[3] When the cataract is not very large and hard, Weber uses a somewhat smaller knife, which is however constructed on the same principle.

Fig. 157.

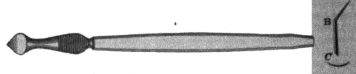

the centre of the upper margin of the cornea, just in the sclero-corneal junction; if the diameter of the cornea is less than twelve millimetres, the incision is to lie a little further away from the edge of the cornea. The blade is to be carried slowly and steadily forwards across the anterior chamber as far as the base of the instrument; its point will then have nearly reached the opposite (lower) margin of the cornea. The knife is then to be *very slowly* withdrawn. This will prevent the sudden escape of the aqueous humor, which, from its stimulating the constrictor pupillæ, would cause the pupil to contract. Moreover, during the slow and gradual withdrawal of the knife we can press the back of the blade somewhat against the edge of the section, and thus prevent prolapse of the iris. The capsule is then to be very freely lacerated, for which purpose **Weber** uses a very minute double hook, the stem being bent at an angle, so as to permit of its being readily turned. The capsule is to be divided in the following way, the lines of incision lying somewhat beneath the iris, as shown in Fig. 158, where the dotted line indicates the pupil. The hook having been passed down

Fig. 158.

to *a*, Fig. 158, the capsule is to be divided from *a* to *b*, and thence to *c*; then the instrument is to be again passed to *a*, and the capsule divided from *a* to *d*, and thence to *c*, the last incision lying, of course, along the inner margin of the section. If, on the withdrawal of the hook, the capsule does not present in the section, the instrument is to be reintroduced, passed down to *c*, and the square, torn portion of capsule drawn out in the direction of *f*; or it may be extracted with a small pair of iridectomy forceps. The anterior thin lip of a peculiarly constructed curette is then to be placed on the external lip of the wound, so as to press this back a little, and thus facilitate the presentation of the equator of the lens in the incision, the exit of the cataract being assisted by a slight simultaneous pressure of the fixation-forceps below the cornea. During the exit of the lens, the iris generally protrudes a little into the wound, and if it does not retract at once when the cataract has escaped, it should be replaced by applying Von Graefe's vulcanite curette, and gently moving this from the angles towards the centre of the section. This will soon cause the iris to retract, and the pupil resume its normal position, a point which should be always carefully attended to before the operation is considered as finished. ["Graefe u. Saemisch Handb. der Augenheilk.," iii. pp. 309-314.—B.]

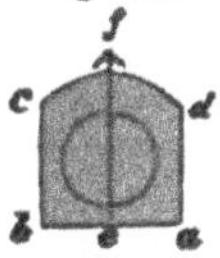

7.—SCOOP EXTRACTION.[1]

Prior to this operation the pupil should be widely dilated with atropine, and the cataract examined with the oblique illumination, so that the size and hardness of the nucleus, and the consistence of the cortical substance, may be ascertained; for the size of the incision should be apportioned to that of the nucleus, and to the extent and consistence of the cortical substance.   The patient should be placed thoroughly under the influence of an anæsthetic, for any sudden start may endanger the safety of the eye, more especially during the period of the introduction of the scoop.   The incision is to be made in the upward direction with a broad lance-shaped knife in the sclero-corneal junction, and should average from four to four and one-half lines in extent. A corresponding portion of the iris having been removed, the capsule is to be freely divided with the pricker.   The next and most difficult step of the operation is the removal of the lens with the scoop, for which purpose either Mr. Critchett's (Fig. 159) or one of Mr. Bowman's (Figs. 160 and 161) scoops may be employed.   The eye having been fixed with the forceps, the scoop is

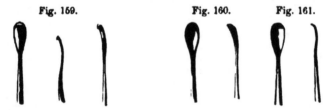

Fig. 159.   Fig. 160.   Fig. 161.

to be introduced into the section, being turned directly towards the back of the eye, so that its anterior lip may glide past the free upper margin of the lens exposed by the iridectomy.   When the edge of the scoop has passed the margin of the lens, it is to be turned quite flat, and slowly and gently insinuated with a delicate, somewhat wriggling movement into the posterior cortical substance between the capsule and the nucleus, until its further end has passed the margin of the latter.   When the lens is well grasped by the scoop, it should be slowly removed, care being taken that its anterior surface is not pressed too much forward, otherwise it will bruise the iris and cornea.

8.—VON GRAEFE'S MODIFIED LINEAR EXTRACTION.

Von Graefe has lately devised a very important modification of the linear extraction, which combines the advantages of the flap with the scoop extraction.   For whilst the section lies almost entirely in the sclero-corneal junction, it yet, on account of its shape and mode of formation, gapes sufficiently to permit the ready exit of even a hard senile cataract without the aid of any traction instrument.   The success of this operation has been so great that most ophthalmologists, amongst whom I may mention Mr. Bowman, have entirely abandoned the scoop extraction, and even to a great extent the flap operation.   My own experience of it has also been extremely

[1] For a full description of this operation, *vide* the valuable articles by Mr. Critchett and Mr. Bowman, "R. L. O. H. Rep.," iv. 4, pp. 316 and 332.   [Also "Annales d'oculistique," lii. p. 115; and "Klin. Monatsbl. f. Augenheilk.," 1864, p. 349.—B.]

favorable, and I prefer it greatly to every other mode of extraction for senile cataract.

The operation is divided into four periods: 1. *The incision;* 2. *The iridectomy;* 3. *The laceration of the capsule;* 4. *The removal of the lens.*

1. The patient having been placed under the influence of an anæsthetic, the eyelids are to be kept apart with the stop-speculum and the eye fixed and gently drawn down with a pair of forceps, which are to be applied close beneath the centre of the cornea. For this operation I prefer Dr. Noyes' (of New York) speculum, the rack and screw of which are on the nasal side, thus leaving the temporal side of the eye quite free for the manipulation of the knife in forming the section. Another advantage of this form of speculum is, that it does not press upon the eyeball, but lifts the lids away from it. One and the same speculum does not, however, suit both eyes, but it must be made right and left. The same is the case with Weiss' stop-speculum, for the knob of the screw should always be on the lower branch (if the upper section is made), for if it is on the upper branch its projection will considerably incommode the operator during the making of the incision. If it is found during any part of the operation that the patient is straining a good deal and that the speculum is pressing on the globe, an assistant should be directed to lift it forward a little away from the eyeball, and keep it thus until the operation is completed.

The point of a long narrow knife[1] (Fig. 162), with its cutting edge upwards, is then to be entered in the sclerotic near the upper and outer portion of the cornea (at the point *A*, Fig. 163, which represents the left cornea), about

Fig. 162.   Fig. 163.

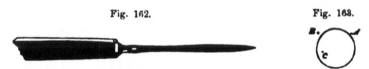

one-third of a line from its edge, so that it may enter the anterior chamber quite at the periphery. The point of the knife should be at first directed downwards and inwards towards *c*, so as to enlarge the inner incision, and then, when the blade has advanced about three and one-half lines into the anterior chamber, the handle is to be depressed and the point carried up and along to *B*, where the counter-puncture is to be made, at a point lying opposite to that of the puncture (*A*). Great care must be taken that the counter-puncture does not lie too far in the sclerotic, which may easily occur if the presentation of the point of the knife is not carefully watched, or the blade is passed too far downwards and inwards before it is turned upwards to make the counter-puncture.

Such an error will give rise to a wide gaping wound, and in all probability, if the patient strains at all or the speculum presses on the globe, to great loss of vitreous, even perhaps before the iris has been excised, and almost with certainty during the pressure which has to be made on the eyeball to facilitate the escape of the lens. In order to avoid any irregularity in the height of the corneal flap (Lappenhöhe), Von Graefe recommends that when the point of the knife is carried downwards and inwards (towards *c*, Fig. 163),

---

[1] The knife should be very narrow. Gradually some instrument-makers have departed more and more from the original model, and have made it much too broad. Von Graefe lays great stress upon the advantages of having the instrument very narrow, as its manipulation at the extreme periphery of the anterior chamber is much more easy, and the facility of turning it much greater than when the blade is broad.

through the anterior chamber, its edge should not be kept quite parallel to the iris, but turned a little forward. By so doing, we give to the temporal portion of the wound a more horizontal direction, so that it lies in almost the exact continuation of the remainder of the section.

As soon as the counter-puncture has been made, the edge of the blade is to be turned somewhat obliquely upwards and forwards, and the knife pushed straight on until its length is nearly exhausted, when the section is to be finished by drawing it slowly and gently backwards from heel to point. [In Fig. 164, the section is represented by the uppermost undotted line.—H.] The knife will now be beneath the con-junctiva, which is next to be divided in such a manner as to leave a conjunctival flap of from one to one and one-half lines in height. In order that it may not exceed this extent, the edge of the blade must be turned horizontally forwards or even downwards. If the cataract is hard and the nucleus very large, it is advisable to make the points of puncture and counter-puncture about one-third of a line lower, so as to obtain a somewhat larger section. Directly the counter-puncture is made, the aqueous humor escapes beneath the conjunctiva and bulges this out, giving rise to a considerable thrombus, which somewhat hides the exact point of counter-puncture and the line of section. This is often very embarrassing to the young operator, and apt to mislead him as to the true course of the section he is making.

[Fig. 164.]

By this incision, the track of the wound lies almost perpendicular to the surface of the cornea, and is more steep (less slanting) than that made by the lance-shaped iridectomy knife. Thus the exit of the lens is much facilitated, for its equator passes more readily into the track of the wound, and the cortical substance also exudes more easily. T e is, however, the disadvantage that if the section is made too steep the suspensory ligament loses its support, and hence there is a greater tendency to loss of vitreous humor than if the incision is made with the lance-shaped knife. Von Graefe[1] does not now give the knife so steep a direction in making the section as originally, but turns its edge somewhat more obliquely upwards and forwards; in this way the external wound lies throughout in the sclero-corneal junction, the conjunctival flap is more easily formed, and the section gapes less than if it be made more steeply.

If the cataract has a big, firm nucleus, care must be taken that the incision is sufficiently large to permit of the ready exit of the lens without the necessity of employing much pressure upon the eye, or the use of a scoop. In such cases I always make the puncture and counter-puncture somewhat lower down, and a little nearer the horizontal diameter of the cornea, which is, I think, to be preferred to a more peripheral position of the section. For a large, hard cataract, the incision should measure about five lines ; but if the cataract, though perfectly hard, is somewhat flattened, one of about four and three-quarter lines will suffice. This will permit of the easy exit of the cataract, a very gentle pressure with a curette upon the lower portion of the cornea sufficing to "coax" it out. If it is found, however, during the fourth stage that the section is a little too small, it is better to enlarge it somewhat at each angle with a pair of blunt-pointed scissors, than to endeavor to *force out* the lens by an extra degree of pressure on the cornea, as this will be almost sure to cause rupture of the hyaloid, and an escape of the vitreous humor perhaps even before the exit of the lens, in which case we shall be obliged to pass in a scoop behind the cataract and thus remove it.

[1] "A. f. O.," xiii. 2, p. 559, and "A. f. O.," xiv. 3, 109.

Mr. Critchett prefers to make the section throughout in the cornea close to its edge, as he thinks that this diminishes the chance of vitreous and of prolapse of the iris. He also makes but a small incision.

2. *The iridectomy.*—If the section does not come well into view, somewhat hidden by the upper lid, an assistant is to draw the eye down with a pair of forceps, taking great care not to press upon or down the eyeball. The operator should then turn down the little conjunctival flap over the cornea with a pair of very small iris forceps, so that prolapsed portion of the iris will be laid quite bare; the iris should then, if necessary, be drawn forth a little more, and excised to the required extent quite close to its ciliary insertion. This is not, however, to be done by one cut, but by three or four successive snips, the scissors being slightly turned so as to follow the curvature of the eyeball, which allows of the blades being applied quite close to the section, or even perhaps a little between its lips. As it is particularly at the angles of the wound that little portions of iris are apt to remain involved in the section, special attention should always be directed to these situations, and any little protrusion be snipped carefully off. For if little portions of iris remain in the incision, they may retard the firm union of the section, be productive of much irritation, and give rise to a cystoid cicatrix, or to a more or less considerable prolapse of the iris, which may not only prove very troublesome by keeping up a long-continued state of irritation, but even dangerous to the eye, by giving rise to inflammatory complications, such as iritis serosa. Another point to which Von Graefe calls particular attention[1] is the position of the cut angles of the sphincter pupillæ after the excision of the iris, and he always looks, before he passes on to the laceration of the capsule, whether or not the sphincter has retracted to its proper position. If one or both angles of the sphincter are displaced upwards or involved in the section, the convex surface of the vulcanite curette should be placed on the cornea close to the angle of the wound towards which the pupil is displaced, and then gently passed from the periphery towards the centre of the cornea: this will not only tend to push the iris down, but will also stimulate the action of the constrictor pupillæ, and thus assist in causing the retraction of the angle of the sphincter. If only the nasal angle of the latter is involved, we may push this gently down, and smooth the iris with the back of the cystitome before we proceed to lacerate the capsule.

The extent of the iridectomy must vary somewhat according to the size and hardness of the nucleus, and also according to the position of the upper lid. If the nucleus is large and hard, I think it better to remove a considerable portion of iris, even perhaps almost corresponding to the size of the incision; for this will permit of the ready exit of even a large hard cataract, without any bruising of the iris. Moreover, if the upper lid hangs down sufficiently to cover the upper third of the cornea, no unsightliness or inconvenience will be produced by so wide an iridectomy, But it will be different if the palpebral aperture is wide, so that the whole cornea is exposed, for then the large artificial pupil may give rise to a considerable and annoying sensation of glare, and also diminish the acuity of vision by producing circles of diffusion upon the retina, on account of the irregular refraction at this portion of the periphery of the cornea.

3. *Laceration of the capsule.*—The operator, steadily fixing the eyeball with the forceps, next freely divides the capsule with the pricker or Von Graefe's cystitome by three successive incisions. The one is to com-

[1] "A. f. O.," xiv. 8, 186.

mence at the lower edge of the pupil, or even a little below it beneath the iris, and extend upwards along its inner side, the other passing to the same extent along the outer margin of the pupil. Both incisions should reach quite up to the periphery of the lens exposed by the iridectomy. An expert operator may even carry the incision beneath the iris nearer the periphery of the capsule, so as to obtain a very free laceration of the latter. But this requires considerable dexterity and delicacy of manipulation, otherwise the pricker may easily bruise the iris, or press so much upon the lens as to displace it. If there are slight adhesions between the iris and the capsule, they should be divided by passing the instrument a little beneath the edge of the pupil. Finally, the capsule should be lacerated at its periphery in a line corresponding to that of the incision. In using the pricker, its edge should always be turned in a slanting direction and not be pressed firmly backwards, otherwise the cataract may be dislocated into the vitreous humor, or its upper margin displaced behind the upper edge of the incision.

De Wecker has lately devised an instrument for lacerating the capsule, which he terms a "pince-cystitome." It closely resembles a pair of curved iridectomy forceps, each branch of which is furnished with a small triangular cutting blade (like Von Graefe's cystitome), situated on the extremity, and extending for a little distance along the convex or outer side. It is to be used in the following manner: The branches having been introduced closed and that as far as the lower border of the pupil, it is to be turned so as to bring the triangular extremity of the cystitome in contact with the anterior capsule ; the branches are then to be opened (whilst they incise the capsule along the lower edge of the pupil) to the width of about four millimetres; being kept thus opened, the capsule is to be incised by them from below upwards, parallel to the margin of the artificial pupil as far as the upper edge of the lens, when they are to be closed, so as to seize the flap of the capsule thus formed, and then the closed forceps are to be removed in the same way as an ordinary cystitome. We can thus excise a square flap of the capsule.

[Peripheral cystotomy for cataracts in general has now been practised somewhat extensively for about two years, both in France and the United States. Dr. Gruening first applied the peripheral division of the capsule to the extraction of a Morgagnian cataract in 1877, and since then Knapp and others have employed it for all hard cataracts. (See a paper by Martin in the "Annales d'oculistique," Janvier-Fevrier, 1878 ; and, also, articles by Gruening and Knapp in the "Archives of Ophthalmology," vii.)

Watson advises opening the capsule before making the corneal section in the operation for cataract. (See "Med. Times and Gazette, May 7, 1881.)—B.]

4. *Removal of the lens.*—During the earlier period of performing his new operation, Von Graefe was in the habit of assisting the exit of the lens by pressing upon the upper portion of the sclerotic with a broad curette, and aiding this by counter-pressure with the forceps below the cornea. When the edge of the lens had once presented itself in the section, its delivery was still more assisted by gliding the curette in a lateral direction along the sclerotic to the angles of the incision (this was termed the *Schlitten-manœuvre*). It was found, however, that the removal of the lens was often difficult, without exerting a dangerous degree of pressure, and that, occasionally, it was necessary, in order to extract the lens, to pass in a scoop, or a peculiarly shaped hook devised by Von Graefe.

He has now, however, substituted for this manœuvre the use of a vulcanite curette, which he presses against the lower portion of the cornea, and thus aids the removal of the cataract. It is to be used in the following manner: The eye is to be fixed with the forceps, which are not to be placed directly below the cornea, as they would then interfere somewhat with the manipulation of the curette, but slightly to the inner or outer side of the centre. The curette is then to be placed upon the lower margin of the cornea, and pressed slightly backwards and upwards, so as to cause the upper edge of the lens to present itself in the section; and then the pressure is to be made directly backwards, in order that the lens may be rotated round its transverse axis and tilted well forward into the wound. When this has occurred, its exit is to be gently aided by pushing the curette slowly upwards over the surface of the cornea, so that it follows step by step the delivery of the lens. If the upper margin of the lens does not present in the section, but shows a tendency to get behind its upper edge, the latter should be gently pressed back with the edge of a curette by an assistant, which will generally cause the lens to enter the incision; or the operator may do this himself, and exert the counter-pressure just beneath the cornea with the forceps. Or, again, the lens may be gently pushed back a little with the pricker, until its upper margin again lies opposite the incision. If it is found that portions of the lower cortical substance are stripped off and are inclined to lag behind, the curette should be drawn a little back again, and the fragments of cortex pushed along after the body of the lens, and in this way the whole cataract may generally be removed. If the appearance of the cataract indicates the presence of a good deal of soft matter, it is well to work this gently towards the centre, by pressing the curette lightly from the lower and lateral margin of the cornea towards its centre, before attempting to remove the lens, for thus we may often succeed in getting the soft matter to exude, together with the firmer nuclear portions. If small fragments of lens-matter still linger behind after the body of the cataract has been removed, they should be coaxed out by again passing the curette over the cornea, and pushing them in front of the instrument. Or, as Von Graefe advises, the lid-holder having been removed, the operator should gently rub the lids, more especially the lower one, in a circular direction, and thus loosen the marginal portions of cortex from behind the iris, and bring them into the area of the pupil, and thence out through the wound. Von Graefe attaches great importance to the removal of remnants of cortical substance, and often devotes some length of time to this purpose.

The object of making the curette of vulcanite instead of silver is that it is more resilient, and the degree of pressure can, therefore, be regulated with the greatest nicety, and its touch is moreover more agreeable to the cornea. The vulcanite has, however, the disadvantage of being very brittle, so that it breaks very readily. For this reason I have lately preferred Weiss' tortoise-shell curette, which offers all the advantages of the vulcanite, without its brittleness.

The loss of vitreous humor has diminished very considerably since Von Graefe substituted the latter mode of removing the lens (by pressing from below) for the "Schlitten-manœuvre;" indeed, in the last two hundred and thirty operations, he only lost vitreous humor in nine cases, which gives less than four per cent.[1] In three of these the vitreous humor was, moreover, fluid. If this occurs, the vitreous may escape directly the section is finished, and even before it is attempted to excise a portion of iris. In such a case it is best to excise a portion of iris, if this can be done without very great loss of vitreous, and then to remove the lens in its capsule by passing Critchett's scoop behind it into the vitreous humor, and lifting it out. A considerable quantity of vitreous will, of course, escape, but any subsequent

---

[1] "A. f. O.," xiii. 2, 556.

inflammation is likely to be far less severe, if the entire lens is removed in its capsule, than if more or less considerable fragments of lens-substance and capsule remain behind.

Several of the best operators still differ in opinion as to the advantage of making the section in the sclerotic or in the cornea, for whilst Von Graefe prefers the former, Critchett and Von Arlt are in favor of the latter proceeding. I think that the exact line and extent of the incision should vary with the size and hardness of the nucleus, and the dimensions of the cornea. If the nucleus is large and firm, and the diameter of the cornea small, the section should be made slightly more in the sclerotic, the puncture and counter-puncture being also somewhat lower, for we shall thus gain a larger section, and the delivery of the lens will be easy, and free from all squeezing and bruising of the parts. If the section is made in the cornea, and more espe-cially if a portion of cornea is left standing at the top, the exit of the lens is often difficult and labored, and accompanied by a good deal of bruising of the parts and stripping off of the surface matter of the lens, which, if it remains behind, may set up very considerable irritation. Moreover, the upper edge of the lens may be caught behind the portion of the cornea which has been left standing, and be firmly wedged in between it, or the lens may even be displaced upwards behind the sclerotic. This is the more apt to occur if the first pressure, which is made with the curette upon the lower portion of the cornea, is not made backwards and upwards, but only upwards, for then the lens will be pushed directly upwards, and may become lodged behind the upper portion of the cornea. The object of the backward pressure upon the lower portion of the lens is to tilt its upper edge into the section, for when it has once gained this position the escape of the lens is easy enough, provided the section be of a sufficient size. My own experience, I must admit, is greatly in favor of the sclerotic section lying in the sclero-corneal junction, or very slightly beyond it. But where a considerable section is required, I prefer to obtain this rather by making the puncture and counter-puncture lower, than by making the incision more in the sclerotic, for in the latter case there is always a greater risk of loss of vitreous.

For a long time I made the section strictly according to Von Graefe's directions, but I found occasionally that, in spite of every care, vitreous was lost if the patient suddenly strained very much, or nipped his eyelids firmly together, or if he retched or vomited from the chloroform. For from the very peripheral position of the incision rupture of the hyaloid and escape of the vitreous are but too prone to occur under the above circumstances; more-over, there is also a greater risk of prolapse of the iris at the angles of the incision. Hence I have gradually come to adopt a less peripheral section, and now generally make the puncture and counter-puncture just external to (about one-half a line from) the sclero-corneal junction, and about one and one-quarter or one and one-half lines below the summit of the cornea, but the centre of the section lies at the upper edge of the cornea. I, however, vary the situation of the puncture and counter-puncture, according to the size of the cornea and the size and hardness of the nucleus. If the cornea is large and the nucleus but moderate in size, I make both the punctures nearer the cornea, and a little higher than when the cornea is small and the nucleus big and firm. I think it better somewhat to vary the shape, position, and size of the section, according to the peculiarities of the case, than to lay down a hard and fast rule as to these points. Since I have made the section less peripheral, I have certainly lost vitreous much less frequently than formerly. De Wecker

Fig. 165.

likewise advocates a very similar section, although he makes the puncture and counter-puncture slightly more in the sclerotic than I am in the habit of doing. In his operation "The puncture and counter-puncture lie in the sclerotic one millimetre outside the edge of the cornea, in a horizontal line, passing two millimetres from the upper margin of the cornea; the exit of the instrument corresponding with the upper margin of the cornea."[1] Whilst Von Graefe's incision (if the cornea has a diameter of twelve millimetres) is ten millimetres in extent, De Wecker's is about eleven and one-half millimetres, the size of the cornea being the same (*vide* Fig. 165). OB equals six millimetres, OC equals seven millimetres, OE equals four millimetres, (EB equals two millimetres), RC equals nine and twenty-five one-hundreths millimetres, CD equals eleven and forty-eight hundred and ninety-one ten-thousandths of a millimetre, or nearly eleven and a half millimetres.

The after-treatment of this operation is generally extremely simple. Liebreich's bandage should be applied directly after the operation, and if any severe pain should arise in the course of the day, cold-water dressing (frequently changed) should be applied, care being taken that it is not persisted in too long. If the pain does not yield to this treatment, a leech or two should be applied to the temple. On the second day atropine drops should be prescribed. The patient may generally leave his bed on the second or third day, but this will depend upon individual circumstances, and upon the fact as to whether he can have proper supervision. With some patients it is advisable to permit their leaving the bed even the day after the operation, but it is always wiser to err on the side of safety. The general rules laid down for the after-treatment of flap extraction also apply to Von Graefe's operation. [Bribosia proposes two modifications of the peripherical linear operation. He advises, as the first step, the laceration of the capsule by a stop-needle through the cornea. He then introduces the narrow knife, and in passing it across the anterior chamber, rotates it slightly, so as to cause a prolapse of the iris upon the knife, which he thus excises. This is not to be recommended.'—B.]

Dr. Taylor, of Nottingham, has operated by a method somewhat similar to that of Von Graefe (but quite independently of him) since the summer of 1865, indeed both appear to have begun about the same time.[3] He more lately, however, substituted the following operation:[4] The eye having been fixed with a pair of sharp forceps at the upper and middle third of the margin of the cornea, he enters a pointed knife (a line in width and bent at an angle) in the sclero-corneal junction, one or two lines from the forceps at the summit of the cornea, and this, being passed well into the anterior chamber, is pushed, with a sawing movement, along the summit, for a distance of three lines. If no iridectomy is to be made, the capsule is now to be opened with the pricker; otherwise a portion of the iris, having been drawn out of the wound, is to be excised, and the capsule then lacerated. Finally the section is to be sufficiently enlarged with a narrow, blunt-pointed knife, to permit of the ready exit of the lens by simple pressure on the lower part of the cornea.

[Dr. Taylor[5] has lately modified the above method, by excising a small portion of the periphery of the iris instead of its whole breadth, the pupillary margin and portion of iris attached to it being left untouched and free the anterior chamber; the lens is then extruded through the gap in the

Annales d'oculistique," Mars–Avril, 1872.
Report of Fourth Internat. Ophthal. Congress," London, 1872.—B.]
Ophthalmic Review," No. 9.   [4] "R. L. O. H. Rep.," vi. 3, 197.
The Lancet," Nov. 4, 1871.

ordinary way, gliding behind the pupil so that there is no stretching of the sphincter. In this way Dr. Taylor believes he has secured all the advantages in the way of safety and certainty of an associated iridectomy, and at the same time attained the grand desideratum, a central and movable pupil.

To avoid the disadvantages in Von Graefe's operation arising out of the peripheral position of the wound, and the disadvantages in flap extraction arising out of the height of the flap, Dr. Liebreich was led to devise a new method of extraction.[1] He found that without actual formation of a flap, that mechanism can be brought about, by means of which the advancing equator of the lens overcomes the obstacles of the iris and of the sphincter pupillæ in order to enter the wound. Avoiding iridectomy, he found he could do without elevators and forceps, "and thus change the whole operation into a less violent and almost painless one."

The incision is situated entirely within the cornea, with the exception of the points of puncture and counter-puncture, which are placed about one millimetre beyond it in the sclerotic[2]—the whole remaining incision passing with a very slight curve through the cornea, so that the centre of it is about one and one-half or two millimetres within the margin of the cornea (Fig. 166). All the instruments required are two, namely, a very small Von Graefe's

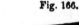

Fig. 166.

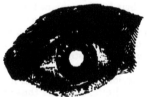

knife, and a cystitome which has a common Daviel's spoon at the other end. Supposing the right eye is to be operated upon; the operator, standing behind the patient, takes hold of the upper eyelid with the index finger of his left hand, whilst he slightly presses the middle finger against the inner canthus of the eye. The knife, held in the right hand with its back horizontal and backwards, the plane of the blade making with the horizontal meridian of the eye an angle of about 45°, enters the sclerotic at the point indicated. "Without altering the direction, the knife passes through the anterior chamber in order to make the counter-puncture on the opposite side, so that the point of the knife becomes visible in the sclerotic about one millimetre (or less) distant from the cornea. The knife is now pushed forwards, and its retraction finishes the incision. As soon as the incision is made, the eyelid is to be dropped.

The second part of the operation consists in the careful opening of the

In the third part, Daviel's spoon is slightly pressed against the inferior margin of the cornea, and the index finger of the left hand, which holds the eyelid, through it exerts a very slight pressure on the highest point of the cornea. Thus the lens is made to rotate a little, its lower margin presses,

[1] "Thomas' Hospital Reports," New Series, vol. ii. p. 259.

[2] This is true only as regards the outside of the wound; in reference to the inside, all the wound, even the puncture, is situated in the cornea, the peripheral part of which cannot be reached by a knife introduced in the indicated position without previously passing through a small portion of the sclerotic.

in the manner already described, against the posterior surface of the iris, pushes the iris forward, passes along it to the margin of the pupil, overcomes the obstacle and places itself freely in the wound, which is made to gape by Daviel's spoon pressing against it. A slight pressing movement of the index finger of the left hand, by means of which the upper eyelid is shifted from above downwards over the cornea, serves to expel the lens. Similar movements of the lids are employed for the purpose of forcing out any *débris* of the cortical substance, after pushing them from behind the iris towards the pupil, by gently rubbing the shut eyelids. Should the pupil then not appear round, but its margin drawn towards the wound, it regains its normal position by an outward shifting of the lower lid ; or, if that be not sufficient, by the introduction of Daviel's spoon. Immediately afterwards I put some atropia into the eye, and close it by my compressive bandage."

This operation is well adapted, Dr. Liebreich says, for the different cataracts, with the exception of—"1. Those laminar cataracts, which need only be treated by iridectomy. 2. Cataracts which in earliest childhood have to be operated upon by repeated division. 3. Perfectly liquid cataracts (division with a broad needle). 4. Partial cataracts, without a nucleus, already absorbed to a great extent, and therefore chiefly traumatic cataracts, for which also division suffices."—H.]

More recently several new methods of operating for the extraction of cataract have been introduced, of which I will briefly describe the following:

Dr. Lebrun's operation[1] closely resembles Liebreich's, except that the puncture and counter-puncture lie at the edge of the cornea ; that the section forms somewhat more of a flap, and lies in the upper half of the cornea. The operation is to be performed as follows: The lids being kept apart by the speculum and the eyeball fixed, Von Graefe's knife is introduced one or two millimetres below the external extremity of the transverse diameter of the cornea, Fig. 167, the cutting edge being turned upwards and slightly forwards, so that the plane of the blade forms an angle of about 30° with that of the iris. The anterior chamber is to be traversed rapidly and the counter-puncture made at a corresponding point of the opposite side of the cornea. The incision is then to be continued upwards in such a manner that it describes a circular curve, the summit of which lies slightly below the upper edge of the pupil when in a medium state of dilatation, *vide* Fig. 167.

Fig. 167.

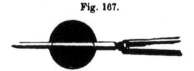

Dr. Lebrun terms this "extraction by a small medium flap." [See "Report of Fourth Internat. Ophthal. Congress," p. 205, London, 1872.—B.]

The following are some of the advantages claimed for the operations of Liebreich and Lebrun: That they are easy to execute; that no iridectomy is made, and that the pupil, therefore, remains central and movable; that there is no risk of loss of vitreous, at least prior to the exit of the lens, or of suppuration of the flap; and that the wound heals very readily. Of the two, Liebreich's is the easier, as the section is made downwards, and, consequently, both the speculum and the fixation of the eyeball by an instrument

[1] " De la Cataracte," par le Dr. Warlomont. Paris, 1872.

may be more readily dispensed with. Amongst the disadvantages which may be urged against both proceedings, the chief are: The tendency to a more or less considerable adhesion of the iris to the edges of the incision, producing, perhaps, an extensive anterior synechia with all its attending evils—evils not confined to the present, but which may prove a source of danger to the eye hereafter, just the same as in cases of leucoma adhærens; or a prolapse may occur. Again, if the section does not heal kindly, but its lips become clouded and somewhat infiltrated, an ugly cicatrix is left, giving rise, perhaps, to an irregular curvature of the cornea with more or less astigmatism and impairment of vision. Moreover, if the nucleus is small and there is much soft matter, it may be difficult to get the latter away on account of the iris falling into the section, and we must then either leave more or less of the soft matter, or repeatedly irritate and bruise the iris by pushing it back with the curette, or we must excise a portion of the iris. Some of the above disadvantages are of less moment in Lebrun's operation than in Liebreich's, as an anterior synechia, a whitish cicatrix, or an irregular curvature of the cornea, would fall in the upper segment of the cornea. It is evident, however, that no true estimate of the real value of these operations can be arrived at, until we are furnished with full and accurate statistics of the results achieved by them.

I will now briefly mention the principal arguments which may be advanced in favor of, or against, the different operations for senile cataract. In doing this, I shall confine myself to the flap extraction, the scoop operation, and Von Graefe's new modified linear extraction.

There cannot be any doubt that the common flap extraction is the most perfect operation of all, when it turns out perfectly successful. It is nearly free from pain; it does not in the least interfere with the appearance of the eye; the pupil remains central and movable; the sight is perfect, and is not at all deteriorated and confused by circles of diffusion upon the retina, which are always more or less present when an iridectomy has been performed. It must, however, be confessed that these great advantages are often more than counter-balanced by the considerable dangers which beset the operation. On account of the great size of the flap, there is much risk of the vitality of the cornea becoming impaired, and of its undergoing partial or even diffuse suppuration, which may be accompanied by suppurative iritis or irido-choroiditis. Again, prolapse of the iris is a not unfrequent complication, proving a source not only of great annoyance and irritation, but even of danger to the eye. The after-treatment also demands much care and attention—more, indeed, than can generally be bestowed in an hospital, especially in a general one, with no special nurses or ophthalmic wards. Now, in the scoop extraction, these two principal dangers—suppuration of the cornea and prolapse of the iris—are nearly completely eliminated. On account of the position and shape of the incision, suppuration of the cornea, even of limited extent, is rare, and a prolapse of the iris can only be slight, and is confined to the angles of the section. Moreover, an anæsthetic may be administered without any fear. But it must be admitted that iritis, chronic and insidious irido-choroiditis, inflammation of the intra-capsular cells, and secondary cataract are more common than in flap extraction. Von Graefe's operation, however, offers all the advantages of the scoop extraction, viz., administration of an anæsthetic, linear shape of the incision, involving but a small portion of the cornea, and iridectomy, and yet one more most important one, power of removing the lens without any traction instrument. It is in my opinion to be preferred, as a rule, to any other mode of extraction, more especially in hospital practice, as the patient requires far less watching and attendance, and the after-treatment is extremely simple. The confinement to the bed and house is also much shorter than in flap extraction. I think it is especially indicated in very feeble, decrepit, nervous, and unmanageable patients, or those suffering from severe cough, or bronchitis; also if the pupil is adherent, or small and rigid, so that it dilates but imperfectly under the influence of atropine, or if the cataract is complicated with some choroidal or retinal lesion. It is also the safer operation for diabetic cataract, for in the flap extraction (even with a preliminary iridectomy), there is always some risk of suppuration of the cornea in these patients, as they are generally in a very feeble state of health. As the iris is exceptionally impatient of irritation, and bruising in cases of diabetes, it may be advisable, in order to secure the greatest immunity from this danger, to make a double iridectomy, viz., upwards and downwards, so as to get a broad vertical pupil, the two opposite portions of the iris being thus completely cut off from each other. I am sometimes asked by medical practitioners and students which operation I consider the easier and safer for an inexperienced operator. I think that, all things considered, the downward flap operation is the easier, for when the section has been successfully completed, the chief danger and difficulty are past; whereas in the modified linear extraction the iridectomy is superadded. I should, therefore, recommend that when the surgeon has operated several times by the lower flap extraction, and has acquired some experience and dexterity, he should pass on to the upper flap extraction, and Von Graefe's operation. The only two points in the latter which demand practice, care, and dexterity, are the incision and the removal of the lens. If the section is too small, the delivery of the lens will be difficult and forced, and will necessitate enlargement of the incision, considerable pressure upon the eyeball, or the introduction of some form of traction instrument. If, on the other hand, it is too large and lies too far in the sclerotic, there is imminent risk of losing much vitreous humor, perhaps even before the removal of the lens is attempted. Considerable nicety and care are also required in coaxing out the lens by pressing upon the cornea with the curette; for if this is roughly and clumsily done, the hyaloid may be ruptured, the vitreous escape, and the lens will probably be pushed somewhat aside, and a scoop will have to be employed for its removal.

[The model operation, towards which the efforts of every ophthalmic surgeon are directed, is the removal of the lens and capsule through a corneal or sclero-corneal incision, and without an iridectomy, so that the patient may possess a circular and movable pupil. The peripherical linear incision, slightly modified to suit the special case, gives, all things considered, the best results, though it necessitates an iridectomy, which, of course, is a disadvantage. It has been suggested that the iris should be detached from its peripheral attachment for a space corresponding to the sclero-corneal incision, instead of excising a piece of it; and that through this dialysis the capsule may be opened, and the lens extruded. This has been done by several surgeons, but owing to bruising of the iris tissue, the success has not been such as to warrant its continuance.—B.]

9.—RECLINATION OR COUCHING.

I only mention this operation to state that, in my opinion, it should be completely abandoned. Although it may appear to be temporarily successful, it has been found that ultimately about fifty per cent. of the eyes have been lost from chronic irido-choroiditis, etc.

10.—DIVISION OR SOLUTION OF CATARACT. [DISCISSION.—B.]

This operation is more especially indicated in the cortical cataract of children and of young persons up to the age of twenty, or even twenty-five; also in those forms of lamellar cataract in which the opacity is too extensive to allow of much benefit being derived from an artificial pupil. After the age of thirty-five or forty, the lens is generally too hard to undergo anything but very slow absorption, even after frequent repetitions of the operation; the iris is also more impatient of irritation and pressure, so that the danger of setting up iritis is much increased; and there are other operations which are much to be preferred for cataracts occurring at this time of life. In infants and young children, an operation for cataract should not be unnecessarily postponed, as the presence of the cataract is very apt in infancy to give rise to nystagmus, and to that form of amblyopia which is dependent upon non-use of the eyes, and which is similar in character to that so often met with in strabismus.

The object of the operation of division is to lacerate the anterior capsule with a fine needle, so as slightly to break up the surface of the lens and to permit the aqueous humor to come into contact with the lens-substance, which, imbibing the fluid, softens, and becomes gradually absorbed. The time required for the absorption varies with the age of the patient and the consistence of the cataract. In infants and young children, the lens is often absorbed in from six to ten weeks, and one operation may suffice for this purpose; but in adults it may have to be repeated several times, and in them great care should be taken not to divide the capsule and the lens too freely at one sitting, for this will cause great swelling of the lens-substance, or the exit of considerable flakes into the anterior chamber, and either of these causes may set up severe iritis or irido-cyclitis. The same caution is necessary in cases of lamellar cataract, because in these a large portion of the lens is transparent and of normal consistence, and will therefore imbibe much aqueous humor and swell up very considerably.

[There are two operations for division of cataract, viz.: Division through the cornea, or the anterior operation for absorption; and division through the sclerotic, or the posterior operation for absorption.

[*Keratonyxis.*—B.] *Division through the Cornea.*—H.]—Prior to the operation, the pupil should be widely dilated with atropine. The patient, more especially if a child, should be placed under the influence of an anæsthetic. Infants should be firmly rolled in a blanket or sheet so that their movements may be controlled. The eyelids are to be kept apart with the spring speculum, and the eye fixed with a pair of forceps. A very fine needle is then to be passed somewhat obliquely through the outer and lower quadrant of the cornea, at a point lying well within the dilated pupil, so that the iris may not be touched by the stem of the needle during the breaking up of the lens. The track of the corneal wound must not be too slanting, otherwise its channel will be too long, and the tissue of the cornea will be stretched and bruised during the working of the needle, and this may produce an opacity in the cornea; nor must it be too straight, otherwise the aqueous humor might easily escape. The size and number of the incisions in the capsule must vary with the amount of effect that we desire. If the latter is to be but very slight, a single small horizontal or vertical tear may suffice, or a crucial incision of limited extent may be made. But if we desire a more considerable effect, more especially in the cortical cataract of children, the incisions must be more extensive, or the superficial portion of the lens is to be gently broken up or comminuted by a series of short superficial incisions, which converge towards the centre of the cataract. In infants and young children the needle may be far more freely used than in adults, or in cases of lamellar or partial cataract. In such, it is always safer to repeat the operation, even several times, than to do too much at one sitting. It may be repeated at intervals of three or four weeks, if it is found that the absorption has become arrested or progresses but very slowly; but all irritability and redness of the eye should have disappeared before the needle is again introduced. If the opening in the capsule is too large, or the cataract broken up too freely, the lens will imbibe much aqueous humor, and, swelling up very considerably, will press upon the iris and ciliary body, and may thus set up severe iritis or irido-cyclitis; or if the incisions in the capsule are too extensive, fragments of lens-substance may fall into the anterior chamber, and there set up great irritation.

Fig. 168.

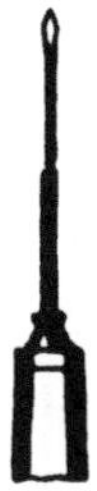

The needle used for this operation should be very small; its cutting, spear-shaped point should only extend to about one-fifteenth or one-twentieth of an inch from the end, and the stem should be cylindrical, so that the aqueous humor may be retained throughout the operation. I always use Bowman's fine stop-needle (Fig. 168), which fulfils all these indications.

[*Scleronyxis.*—B.] [*Division through the Sclerotic.*—The pupil should be widely dilated with atropia, and the patient prepared for the operation precisely as for the anterior puncture. The knife-needle (Fig. 169), with its cutting edge looking upwards, is then passed through the sclerotic at a point on its transverse diameter a line and a half or two lines from the temporal margin of the cornea, and perpendicularly to the surface of the eyeball. "The puncturation should be made quickly, and the needle introduced only a short distance. This accomplished, the surgeon should steady the eye with the needle, and wait an instant until the patient has recovered from the shock. The direction of the needle should then be changed, so that its point may be advanced between the iris and the lens; then the instrument should be steadily pushed on until its point reaches the opposite pupillary margin of the iris. In executing this step, care must be taken neither to wound the ciliary body or iris, nor to spit the lens on the needle. If the former accident happens, injurious inflammation may result; if the latter, especially if the lens be hard, it will probably be dislocated, and in this case it should be at once extracted. When the needle is pushed into the lens without dislocating it, the instrument should be carefully withdrawn until its point is free, and then pushed on again in the proper direction.

"This step being accomplished, the needle should be rotated one-quarter round its axis, so as to present its cutting edge towards and exactly over the diameter of the lens. This last movement is highly important, as the lens will thus offer the firmest resistance, and will not tilt over and be dislocated in being cut; a free incision should then be made by withdrawing the needle a short distance, pressing firmly its edge against the cataract. If the lens be hard, several incisions should be made in the anterior capsule, and then this membrane freely lacerated crosswise with the point of the instrument; this accomplished, the instrument should be withdrawn. The lens exposed to the aqueous humor will become softened, partly absorbed, and at a subsequent period the operation may be repeated, and the lens completely broken up."[1]

[1] "Laurence on the Eye," edited by Hays, Phila., 1854, p. 727.

The instrument recommended for this operation is the knife-needle, devised by Dr. Isaac Hays,[1] of Philadelphia. The common straight needle does not cut well beyond a short distance from the point, unless it be made so thin as to endanger its breaking; and with a curved needle it is impossible to divide up the lens. By means, however, of the knife-needle the division of a lens of even considerable hardness can be satisfactorily accomplished.

Figs. 169, 170.

The actual size of the knife-needle is represented in the accompanying cut (Fig. 169). "This instrument, from the point to the bead near the handle (a to b, Fig. 170), is six-tenths of an inch, its cutting edge (a to c) is nearly four-tenths of an inch. The back is straight to near the point, where it is truncated, so as to make the point stronger, but at the same time leaving it very acute; and the edge of this truncated portion of the back is made to cut. The remainder of the back is simply rounded off. The cutting edge is straight, and is made to cut up to the part where the instrument becomes round, c. This portion requires to be carefully constructed, so that as the instrument enters the eye it shall fill up the incision, and thus prevent the escape of the humors. In the magnified view of the instrument (Fig. 170) the proportions of the blade are not very accurately represented, the rounded part being rather too slender, and the handle should be octagonal, with equal sides, and of the same thickness its whole length."—H.] [Scleronyxis is a more serious operation than keratonyxis, and is really only applicable to partially absorbed cataracts, which lie more deeply behind the iris.—B.]

The after-treatment is generally very simple. The pupil should be kept widely dilated with atropine, so that the iris cannot be pressed upon by the swollen lens or any flakes that may have fallen into the anterior chamber. A bandage should be worn for the first twenty-four hours, and the patient should be kept in a somewhat darkened room for the first day or two, especially if there is much reaction. Generally, however, this is but slight, the eye only looking flushed, and watering somewhat on exposure to bright light. My friend, Mr. Lawson, has even successfully operated by this method upon some cases of monocular cortical cataract in adults (between the ages of twenty and thirty), and treated them throughout as out-patients. These were, however, exceptional cases, in which it was absolutely necessary that the patients should follow their employment. In order to expedite the cure, which is often of consequence in patients from the country, it is a very good plan, after the lens-matter has become softened by the admission of the aqueous, to remove the whole cataract by a broad linear incision. In children this may generally be done within a week after the division, and thus the sight may be restored in a few days; whereas, otherwise, many weeks or even months would have elapsed before the cataract would have been entirely absorbed. The same proceeding may be employed in cases of partial cataract, the transparent portion of the lens being made opaque, and softened by the introduction of the needle. This mode of operation has been very successfully practised and much advocated by Mr. Bowman, who also often

[1] "American Journ. of the Med. Sciences," July, 1855, p. 81.

advantageously employs the suction syringe for the removal of the lens after it has been previously broken up by the needle.

[In performing discission from behind, Jones uses a curved, spea: cataract-needle, and pierces the sclera on the temporal side, about c of an inch back of the corneal margin, and half-way between the in of the external and the inferior recti muscles. He pushes the needle vitreous toward the centre of the globe, and then turns its point agi posterior capsule, and freely lacerates it. The needle is then wit He performs the operation in all sorts of cases, even in those of sen ract in very old people, and without any bad results. ("The Lance 12, 1880.)—B.]

If symptoms of irritation and inflammation should set in after th tion of division, and they do not readily yield to antiphlogistics, but in severity, and more especially if the tension of the eyeball is aug the cataract should be at once removed through a good-sized linear made near the periphery of the cornea with an iridectomy knife. also to be done if the capsule has been too freely divided, and the or considerable portions of lens-substance have fallen into the chamber, and are setting up much irritation. If the lens is so firm cannot all be readily removed through the linear section, it will be combine an iridectomy with it, than to endeavor to remove the poi lens by repeated introductions of the curette into the anterior chamb iridectomy is also indicated if an increase of tension has existed i little time, and if the perception of light and the extent of the field (are markedly deteriorated.

Two special forms of inflammation may follow the operation, and e the safety of the eye. In the one, the inflammation is chiefly plastic lent in character. The iritis or irido-cyclitis is accompanied by pla: dations behind the iris, and into the vitreous humor, leading event all probability to chronic irido-choroiditis and atrophy of the globe. other form, the inflammation is of a serous nature, giving rise to an in secretion of the vitreous humor, and an augmentation of the intr tension—in a word, to a glaucomatous condition of the eyeball, whi cause irretrievable destruction of the sight if timely relief be not af

As these imflammatory complications are most apt to occur in adul the age of fifteen or twenty, more especially if the cataract is only p of a lamellar nature, Von Graefe advises that in such cases, or if ; terior synechiæ exist, an upward iridectomy should be made a fev before the operation of division. By so doing, plenty of room afforded for the swelling up of the lens, and if fragments have fal the anterior chamber, they will produce far less irritation.

11.—OPERATIONS FOR LAMELLAR OR ZONULAR CATAR.

When describing the nature of lamellar cataract, I mentioned those cases in which a sufficiently broad margin of transparent lens-su exists, great improvement of vision may often be attained by dila pupil by atropine. A glance at the accompanying figures will explain In Fig. 171, a represents the undilated pupil occupied by the op which extends beneath the iris as far as the dotted line c, where tl parent margin d commences. As the latter is completely covered iris, the rays of light can only pass through the central opaque hence the indistinctness of vision. But when the pupil is dilated (F the transparent margin of the lens *d* is uncovered, and the rays can now pass through it to the retina. This fact is of great practical importance, for it furnishes us with a very valuable indication as to the treatment of such cases of lamellar cataract, for we may often succeed in restoring excellent vision by simply making an artificial pupil, without operating upon the lens itself.

Fig. 171.   Fig. 172.

Such a proceeding possesses very marked advantages over any operation for the removal of the lens, for the patient retains the power of accommodation, and is freed from the necessity of wearing cataract glasses, which are not only inconvenient, but also unsightly, more especially in youthful individuals. The artificial pupil may be made either by means of an iridectomy or an iridodesis. The former operation has the disadvantage that the base of the artificial pupil (Fig. 174) is opposite the periphery of the lens *d*, and may therefore give rise to a certain indistinctness of vision, on account of the rays being irregularly refracted by the edge of the cornea and lens, circles of diffusion on the retina being thus produced. In order to diminish this defect, the iridectomy should be but small. In most cases, I think, Mr. Critchett's operation of iridodesis is to be preferred. A considerable portion of iris should be drawn out, in order that the entire pupil may be drawn near the margin of the cornea, for the iris will thus cover a large extent of the opaque portion of the lens. There will thus result a pupil like that in Fig. 173, having its apex, and not its base, opposite the clear portion of the lens. Mr. Critchett has also in some cases obtained great improvement of sight by making a second iridodesis close to the other, thus gaining a somewhat broader pupil, and admitting more light.

Fig. 173.

Fig. 174.

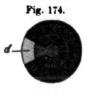

If the transparent margin in lamellar cataract is not sufficiently broad or clear to admit of much improvement of vision by an artificial pupil, the lens itself must be operated upon, either by division with or without iridectomy, or by Von Graefe's operation.

In persons under twenty-five, I think it best slightly to divide the lens with a needle, and to repeat this several times, and then, when the whole lens has become opaque and softened, to remove it through a large linear incision, or with the suction curette. It is never wise to operate on both eyes at the same time, for in some cases eyes affected with lamellar cataract are extremely irritable, and considerable irido-choroiditis, with or without sloughing of the cornea may supervene and destroy the eye. If this has occurred in the one eye, we should be greatly upon our guard in operating upon the second at a subsequent period, or devise some other mode of operating. In persons above the age of twenty-five, I have succeeded very well in removing the lens by Von Graefe's operation.

12.—OPERATIONS FOR TRAUMATIC CATARACT.

If the wound in the lens is of but slight extent, and the patient young, the cataract may be left to absorption if no symptoms of inflammation set in. The pupil should be kept widely dilated with atropine, and the condition of the eye carefully watched. If inflammatory symptoms supervene, it may be necessary to remove the lens by linear extraction, more especially if it swells up considerably, or large portions have fallen into the anterior chamber and are setting up irritation. This operation should also be at once performed if the wound in the lens has been considerable, so that the latter, imbibing much aqueous humor, becomes rapidly swollen and presses upon the iris and ciliary body. The simple linear extraction will generally suffice if the lens is so softened that it will readily escape through the incision. But if the nucleus or the greater portion of the lens is still firm, it may be more advisable to make a large iridectomy, in order to afford more room for the swelling of the lens, and then to leave the latter to undergo absorption, which will now be attended by far less risk. In those cases in which great swelling of the lens is accompanied by severe inflammation, it will be best to make a large iridectomy, and remove the cataract, either with or without the aid of the scoop. If there is much soft matter, this may be removed with the suction syringe, although I am rather afraid of its use in such cases, especially if there is any iritis or irido-choroiditis, as it may easily produce hyperæmia *ex vacuo* of the inner tunics of the eyeball. If a foreign body—*e. g.*, a chip of steel, glass, or gun-cap—is lodged in the lens, it is wiser to endeavor to remove it, together with the lens. This should be done by introducing a scoop well behind the foreign body and lifting it out; for if we permit the lens to undergo absorption, the foreign body will at last become disengaged and fall down into the anterior or posterior chamber, and probably set up severe and even perhaps destructive inflammation. The situation of a bit of metal in the lens may often be recognized by the aid of the oblique illumination, when we may observe a little brown spot in the lens, or a little dark line showing the track of the foreign body.

If the foreign body has passed through the lens and is lodged in the vitreous humor, retina, or choroid, great attention must be paid to the condition of the eye, as severe and destructive inflammation is but too likely to ensue. The degree of sight, the state of the field of vision, and the tension of the eyeball, should be especially watched. If in such a case the lens swells up very considerably, it may be wise to perform linear or scoop extraction combined with a large iridectomy, in the hope that the absence of the lens may diminish the inflammation, although it must be remembered that the chief exciting cause—the foreign body—still remains behind, and may at any time, even after the lapse of years, again set up inflammation. In all such cases of injury, the condition of the other eye must also be anxiously watched. At the earliest symptoms of sympathetic irritation, the wounded eye should be at once removed, for only thus can we insure the safety of the other. If the injury is so severe that the sight is greatly, and probably permanently, impaired, the immediate removal of the eye may be indicated, even although the eye does not sympathize. This is especially the case amongst the laboring classes, who cannot be under our immediate supervision, or cannot afford the time to undergo a lengthened course of treatment without the hope of regaining any useful degree of vision. The same course may be advisable amongst the higher classes, if from circumstances—such as officers being ordered abroad, necessity for a long voyage, etc.—they cannot be under constant supervision, so that the earliest symptoms of sympathetic inflammation may be detected.

18.—REMOVAL OF SOFT CATARACT BY A SUCTION INSTRUMENT.

In the extraction of soft cataract through a simple linear incision, some difficulty is occasionally experienced in removing the firmer portions without exerting a certain amount of pressure upon the globe, or introducing the curette into the anterior chamber. This difficulty has led Mr. Pridgin Teale[1] to the ingenious employment of a suction curette for the more easy and complete extraction of soft cataract.

The instrument now used by Mr. Teale is almost identical with the one described in his original paper. It is represented in Fig. 175, and consists

Fig. 175.

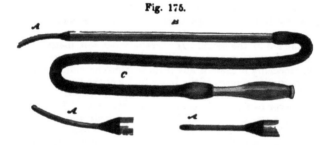

of three parts: (*B*) a stem, formed of a glass tube, with (*A*) a tubular curette at one end, and (*C*) an India-rubber tube with a mouth-piece at the other end. (1) The *hollow* glass stem (*B*) is five inches in length, and allows the operator to watch the progress of the suction as the material is drawn into the transparent tube. (2) The India-rubber tube (*C*) is about twelve inches in length, and furnished with a mouth-piece which enables the operator to apply the suction either with considerable force or the most exquisite gentleness, using his tongue as a piston, under the most perfect control. (3) The curette (*A*) is about five-eighths of an inch in length and of the same size as an ordinary curette; it is slightly convex on its upper surface and not flat, and its whole calibre does not require a larger opening in the cornea than the common curette. The point should be as round and blunt as possible, and the opening on the upper surface should be equal in size to the section of the tube, and as near to the extremity as the required bluntness will permit. Mr. Teale performs the operation in the following manner: The pupil having been well dilated by atropine, a puncture is to be made in the cornea with a broad needle at a point opposite the margin of the fully dilated pupil, and, passing obliquely through the substance of the cornea, the instrument should enter the anterior chamber at a point opposite the margin of the pupil when of medium size. Such a valvular opening will prevent any scar in front of the pupil, and diminish the risk of prolapse or an anterior synechia. The capsule having been freely divided, the curette should be carefully introduced through the corneal wound, and its end (the opening looking towards the cornea) held steadily in the area of the pupil and gently buried in the opaque matter, the convex surface being pressed

<hr>

[1] "R. L. O. H. Rep.," iv. 2, 197.

somewhat back towards the posterior capsule. The suction power should then be carefully applied and continued in gentle inspirations as long as any opaque matter comes forward into the pupil, and, when the latter is quite clear, the instrument is to be withdrawn. On no account is the curette to sweep either in front of or behind the iris in search of opaque matter.

Fig. 176.

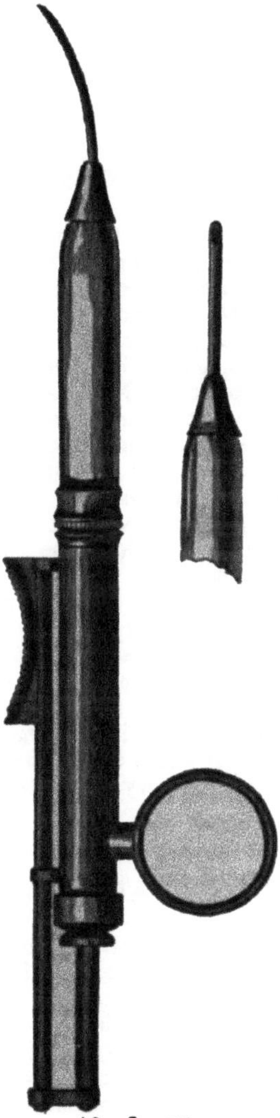

After Lawson.

Mr. Teale has found this mode of operating extremely successful, the recovery being very speedy, and the operation followed by little or no irritation. He considers it *applicable* in all full-bodied complete cataracts in persons under the age of forty; including in this category spontaneous, diabetic, and those traumatic cataracts in which, from the rent in the capsule being of moderate extent, the eye remains quiescent until the cataract is completely formed; and finally, incomplete cataracts which have been rendered complete by division of the capsule. He thinks it *unsuitable* in those forms of complete or immature cataracts in which portions are transparent and glutinous, and require great force to draw them into the curette; also in traumatic cataract, if there is much irritability or iritis, if there has been rupture of the posterior capsule, or if so much of the lens has been absorbed that the anterior and posterior capsule are nearly in contact; or in degenerate cataract.

Mr. Bowman has devised an excellent suction syringe (Fig. 176), the use of which is very easy, and which can be regulated with great nicety.[1] The operator, having made an incision in the cornea with the broad needle, and freely divided the lens, can introduce the nozzle of the instrument (which is to be held in the right hand) in the corneal aperture, and gently "suck out" the soft lens-substance.

Although it appears that the idea of employing suction for the removal of cataract dates back as far as the fourth century, and that it has since been advocated by several authors, more especially in later years, by Blanchet and Langier, it never attained a recognized position until it was introduced by Mr. Teale. This operation has now met with much and deserved favor, more especially at the Royal London Ophthalmic Hospital, Moorfields, where it has been employed with marked success. It is especially indicated in soft cortical cataract, which may generally be very readily and completely removed by the suction instrument. If the cataract be somewhat more firm in consistence, it will be well to break it up with the needle a few days previously. I have also used it with much advantage in removing portions of

---

[1] Both Mr. Teale's and Mr. Bowman's instruments are made by Messrs. Weiss.

soft cortical substance which have remained behind in the pupil in the operations for senile cataract, either in the common flap or Von Graefe's operations, for such portions may often be more readily and thoroughly removed in this way than by rubbing the eyeball or the reintroduction of the scoop. Some care and delicacy are, however, required in the use of this instrument, for, if too great a suction power is employed, hyperæmia (*ex vacuo*) of the iris and the deeper tunics of the eyeball may easily be produced.

14—SPERINO'S TREATMENT OF CATARACT BY PARACENTESIS.[1]

This mode of treatment is chiefly based upon the theory that the impairment of vision in cataract is partly dependent upon a temporary disturbance in the intra-ocular circulation, especially an occasional state of congestion of the choroid, and partly upon the opacity of the lens. Dr. Sperino holds that the opaque lens-fibres may regain their transparency as long as their intimate structure is not disorganized, which always follows, more or less rapidly, upon the opacity, but less so in old than in young persons. Now, as the operation of tapping the anterior chamber relieves the intra-ocular circulation, it often produces a marked and immediate improvement in the sight, and in some cases often-repeated tappings have at last effected a complete cure. In others their effect has been but moderate, or even negative. The operation consists in making a small puncture with a broad needle at the edge of the cornea or slightly in the sclerotic; a blunt probe is then inserted between the lips of the wound, and the aqueous humor slowly evacuated. The evacuations by the same opening may be made repeatedly during a single sitting, followed by an interval of several days, or singly at an interval of a day or two. The operations in cataract were repeated a great number of times. In one case one hundred and sixty-seven tappings were made, and finally linear extraction was performed. I am not aware that this treatment has been adopted by any other surgeon on a sufficiently large scale to warrant any exact conclusion as to its efficacy. It would be, I think, very difficult to find patients who would submit to such a very protracted course of treatment and such numerous operations.

15.—OPERATIONS FOR CAPSULAR AND SECONDARY CATARACT.

I have already stated that capsular cataract often occurs in retrogressive lenticular cataract, and that in such cases it may be advisable to remove the lens in its capsule. If, in an operation for senile cataract, the capsule is found so tough and thickened that it resists the pricker, it should be torn across with a sharp hook, and then, after the extraction of the lens, the capsule should be removed by the hook or a pair of forceps. In such cases, the connection between the posterior capsule and the hyaloid is not unfrequently loosened, and the lens may often be readily extracted in its capsule by the hook. Some operators, in making the section, divide the tough capsule across with the point of the knife.

Secondary cataracts vary much in thickness and opacity. They may be produced by portions of lens-substance remaining behind and becoming en-

---

[1] *Vide* a most interesting work by Dr. Sperino, entitled "Etudes Cliniques sur l'Evacuation répétée de l'Humeur aqueuse dans les Maladies de l'Œil," Turin, 1862. Also a review of this work in the "Ophthalmic Review," ii. p. 294.

tangled in the capsule, by the deposition of lymph upon the latter, or by the proliferation of the intra-capsular cells.

Again, if the more fluid constituents of a cataract become absorbed and the cortical substance undergoes chalky or fatty degeneration, the lens gradually dwindles down, and assumes the appearance of a flattened, shrivelled disk.

Mr. Bowman[1] has also called special attention to another form of secondary cataract, in which the capsule, though quite transparent, is crumpled or wrinkled, and thus produces much confusion of vision by irregularly refracting the rays of light.   This condition of the capsule may easily escape detection, even although the eye be examined with the oblique illumination, and is not perhaps noticed until the ophthalmoscope is employed, when the observer finds that he cannot obtain a clear and distinct view of the optic disk, but that it looks somewhat distorted.   On then getting the capsule itself into focus, the wrinkles may be readily observed.

No operation for secondary cataract should be performed until the eye has quite recovered from the cataract operation, and is entirely free from all irritation.   Generally three or four months should be allowed to elapse between the two operations.   Nor should it be done if the area of the pupil is not of a good size.   If it has become contracted, or is partially occupied by lymph, or if there are extensive posterior synechiæ, a preliminary iridectomy should be made, and then, when the eye has become quiescent, the operation upon the capsule may be performed.

Formerly, the favorite mode of operating was by the removal of the obstructing membrane.   But this is falling more and more into disuse, as it often proves a very dangerous operation, and is far less safe than opening up the membrane by the needle, which is attended by much less risk of setting up inflammation.   Moreover, it is a well-established fact that a small, clear aperture in the opaque membrane will afford most excellent sight.

For the needle operation, anæsthesia is hardly necessary, unless the patient proves very unmanageable.   The eyelids should be kept apart with the stop-speculum, and the eye may be steadied with the forceps.   Bowman's fine stop-needle should then be passed through the cornea at a short distance from the margin, and the operator should endeavor to tear a hole in the centre of the opaque membrane.   The portion which is thinnest, least opaque, and consists chiefly of wrinkled capsule, should be selected for this purpose. It is to be torn across in different directions, the point of the needle comminuting the membrane, without, however, being allowed to go deeply into the vitreous humor.   If the operator finds, after one or two ineffectual attempts to transfix it and tear it through, that the false membrane yields before the needle and eludes it, or if it is too tough and firm to be torn through, he should at once have recourse to a second needle.   This is to be passed into the anterior chamber from an opposite point of the cornea. Transfixing and steadying the false membrane with the needle held in his left hand, the operator employs the other needle to tear the membrane and open it up.   Or the points of the needles may be made to cross each other, and then, after being revolved a few times round each other, be separated, which will cause the membrane to be torn across.   Great care must be taken to use the needles with extreme delicacy, and not to drag roughly upon the adhesions between the capsule and the iris, otherwise severe inflammation may be set up.   If any portion of the iris should have been considerably dragged upon during the use of the needles, it may be advisable to excise

[1] "R. L. O. H. Rep.," iv.

this segment, in order to allay any tendency to inflammatory reaction. This ingenious double-needle operation was first devised by Mr. Bowman,[1] and has proved a most valuable addition to ophthalmic surgery. Should the false membrane be found but slightly adherent to the iris, so that it floats almost freely in the pupil, the adhesions may be torn through by the needle, and the whole membrane extracted through a linear incision by the canula or small iris forceps. If the adhesions are found to be so firm that a good deal of force would have to be employed to break them down or to divide them, these should on no account be attempted: but the free portion should be caught by a sharp hook, gently drawn through the linear incision, and snipped off, which will leave a good-sized opening in the capsule.

In cases of chalky or siliculose cataract, in which the capsule looks like a little wrinkled bag containing small chalky chips of lens, it may be possible to remove the whole capsule with a sharp hook through a good-sized linear incision, as in Fig. 177. But it is often a very dangerous operation, setting

Fig. 177.

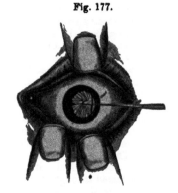

After Stellwag.

up perhaps severe irido-choroiditis, which may even lead to atrophy of the eyeball.

After an operation for secondary cataract, atropine should be applied, the patient be kept in a somewhat darkened room for a few days, and carefully watched, in order that the first symptoms of inflammatory reaction, accompanied perhaps, by increased intra-ocular tension, may be detected. Within from twelve to twenty-four hours after the operation, the patient may experience a good deal of pain in and around the eye, and down the corresponding side of the nose (ciliary neuralgia); there is perhaps some subconjunctival injection and lachrymation, and the sight appears somewhat cloudy. Great benefit is often experienced from the use of very cold (iced) compresses after this operation, as they diminish the irritation, and often cut short an attack of severe inflammation. On trying the tension of the eyeball it is found increased, and the iris pushed forward (sometimes partially), so that the anterior chamber is narrowed. If the intra-ocular tension is considerably increased ($+$ T 2), and this persists for twelve hours from the commencement, Mr. Bowman[2] strongly advises that the bulging part of the iris should be punctured with a broad needle, thus establishing a communication between

---

[1] "Med.-Chir. Trans.," 1858, p. 315. [2] "R. L. O. H. Rep.," iv. 366.

the anterior and posterior chambers, which will generally diminish the intra-ocular pressure and cut short the inflammation.

Dr. Agnew,[1] of New York, has devised the following operation: He passes a stop-needle through the centre of the membrane, thus fixing both the eye and the latter; he then makes a linear incision on the temporal side of the cornea, through which he passes a small sharp-pointed hook, the point of which is passed into the same opening in the membrane as the needle. He now tears the membrane, and by a rotatory movement of the hook rolls it up round the latter, and then either draws it out altogether, or, if this cannot be done, he tears it widely open.

For those cases in which severe and protracted inflammation has followed the removal of cataract, giving rise to a dense secondary cataract, Dr. Noyes,

Fig. 178.

Fig. 179.

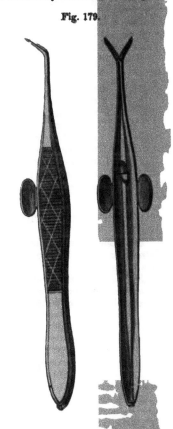

of New York, has devised the following operation,[2] which he has performed with much success: He makes a puncture at the centre of the outer margin of the cornea, with Von Graefe's cataract-knife, carries it across the anterior chamber, and makes the counter-puncture at a corresponding point on the opposite side; he then partially withdraws the knife until its point arrives opposite the middle of the iris, when he plunges it backwards through the false membrane into the vitreous, making the wound as large as possible. After withdrawal of the knife, a small blunt hook is to be passed in through each corneal wound, and caught in the wound made in the iris (false membrane?), and traction made in opposite directions, so as to drag out a portion of tissue at each corneal wound, where it is to be snipped off. Thus a large central pupil will be made.

When the natural or artificial pupil becomes closed by dense false membrane through the occurrence of irido-choroiditis after extraction of cataract, we must endeavor to make a new artificial pupil, and to remove portions of the false membrane by one of the operations described at pp. 325, 326. De Wecker operates in such cases in the following manner, employing his new forceps scissors: Let us suppose that Von Graefe's operation has been performed, and the pupil closed by false membranes. An incision of eight millimetres is to be made with a Von Graefe's knife through the cornea and iris, about two millimetres from the lower margin

[1] "Kl. Monatsbl.," 1865, p. 389.   [2] "R. L. O. H. Rep.," vi. 2, 200.

of the cornea, *vide* Fig. 178. The forceps scissors, Fig. 179, are then to be so introduced that one blade passes behind the iris and exudation masses, the other along the posterior surface of the cornea. With two incisions which meet at the apex, a triangular portion of the iris is to be excised. The forceps scissors are bent at an angle, and can be passed through a small corneal opening, and yet be widely opened in the anterior chamber, and are therefore of the greatest use for any operation with the latter. The *iridotomy*, or incision of the iris to produce an artificial pupil for optical purposes, may also be made with De Wecker's new forceps scissors, which would, I think, be very useful for this purpose.

[Streatfeild employs for this purpose two "needle-hooks," made of two cataract-needles bent at their ends into two small hooks. The hook part is three-twentieths of a centimetre in extent, and should make but a small section of a large circle. He places the sharp parts of the hooks one on each side of the cornea near its margin, presses them into the cornea, and on towards the centre of the anterior chamber. The hooked extremities are then turned down into the membranous septum, and then drawn slowly in opposite ways. By this method the lateral and backwards dragging are both obviated, and the aqueous humor is retained, while the iris is unaffected. (See " Report of Fourth Internat. Ophthal. Congress," London, 1872.)

Weber, in these cases of secondary membraniform obstruction, uses a two-edged lance-shaped knife, four millimetres wide. This he plunges through the cornea and membrane on the temporal side; passes it behind the obstruction and then out again on the nasal side. Then with a pair of De Wecker's forceps scissors he cuts through the membrane above and below, and thus excises a quadrilateral piece.—B.]

14.—DISLOCATION OF THE LENS (ECTOPIA LENTIS).

The dislocation of the lens may either be partial or complete. In the latter case it may be displaced into the vitreous or aqueous humors, or beneath the conjunctiva.

Partial Dislocation.—In the slightest degree of partial displacement, the lens is simply turned somewhat upon its axis, one portion of its periphery being tilted obliquely forwards against the iris, the other backwards and

[Fig. 180.

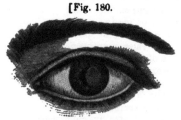

After Lawson.]

away from the latter. Or again, the dislocation may be eccentric, the lens being somewhat shifted towards a certain direction, so that its centre no longer corresponds to the optic axis, but lies more or less considerably to one side of it; the periphery of the lens may even lie across the normal pupil. [Fig. 180.] This form of displacement generally occurs in a downward direction: but it may also take place upwards and inwards, or upwards and outwards. Such partial displacement of the lens may be occasioned by various causes, amongst others by anterior synechia, for if in such a case an adhesion exists between the iris and the capsule of the lens, the latter is drawn forwards with the iris at this point, and therefore somewhat displaced or tilted. It may also occur, as Stellwag has pointed out, in cases of anterior scleral staphyloma.

On examining an eye affected with partial displacement of the lens, we find that when it is moved rapidly about in different directions, the iris is slightly tremulous at the point where it has lost the support of the lens, where the latter has receded from it. Moreover, it is here also somewhat cupped or curved back, being on the other hand pushed forward and prominent at the point where the edge of the lens is tilted forward against it. In the former situation, the anterior chamber will consequently be slightly deepened, in the latter narrowed. If the pupil is widely dilated with atropine, we can easily recognize the altered position of the lens by the aid of the oblique illumination, or, still better, by the direct examination with the ophthalmoscope. With the latter, the free edge of the lens will be noticed as a sharply defined, dark curved line, traversing the red fundus, and forming the outline of a transparent or opaque lenticular disk. If the displacement is so great that a considerable portion of the background of the eye can be examined through that part of the pupil in which the lens is absent, a distinct erect image of the details of the fundus will be obtained. In the reverse image, the prismatic action of the edge of the lens can be easily observed, for then the double image of the fundus will appear, and the two images cannot be simultaneously distinctly seen; for whilst the one is clearly defined, the other will appear hazy, and in order to render the latter distinct, either the position of the observer's eye or of the ocular lens must be changed. Such a partial displacement of the lens will also have a peculiar effect upon the patient's sight, for he will generally be affected with monocular diplopia, or polyopia, which is due to the difference in the refraction of the two portions of the pupil, and to the prismatic action of the peripheral portion of lens which lies across it. The state of refraction will also differ in the two portions of the pupil, for in that in which the lens is absent, a very considerable degree of hypermetropia will exist. Von Graefe[1] mentions a case of displacement of the lens, in which, when the patient was endeavoring to distinguish a small object, the eye deviated in a certain direction, in order that the rays might impinge upon the central portion of the lens. If the pupil is small, the patient may observe the edge of the displaced lens entoptically, or the same phenomenon may be produced with a dilated pupil, if he looks through a minute aperture in a card or a stenopæic apparatus.

If the dislocation of the lens is due to an accident, etc., e. g., a severe blow upon the eye, the sight is often greatly impaired directly afterwards by hemorrhage into the aqueous and vitreous humors. As the blood becomes absorbed the sight may gradually improve, if there is no other deep-seated lesion.

17.—COMPLETE DISLOCATION OF THE LENS.

Into the Vitreous Humor.—The iris will be observed to be markedly tremulous when the eye is moved in different directions, and the anterior chamber will be somewhat deepened. If the catoptric test be employed, it

[1] "A. f. O.," i. 2, 291.

will be found that the lenticular reflections are wanting. On examining the eye with the oblique illumination, the absence of the reflection from the anterior capsule will also be noticed, and the position of the displaced lens will in most cases be easily recognized, more especially if the pupil is dilated, as a portion of the lens generally occupies some part of the pupil, or floats across it when the eye is moved. If the lens is opaque, the sight will of course be temporarily lost when the lens lies across the pupil. The position of the lens will vary with that of the head. If the latter is held erect, it will sink down into the vitreous humor; if the head is bent forward, the lens will fall against the pupil, or may even pass through it into the anterior chamber. With the ophthalmoscope, the situation of the lens in the vitreous humor can be very easily ascertained, for it will appear as a black lenticular body, generally lying in the lower portion of the vitreous humor. The latter is of course more or less fluid, generally entirely so. In spontaneous luxations, the lens is frequently opaque, and in such cases the sight will be greatly improved. Even if it is transparent at the time of the displacement, it generally becomes opaque in the course of a few months. In such cases the cataract may assume the lamellar form, only some layers around the nucleus becoming clouded. But a dislocated lens may retain its transparency for very many years, if its capsule is uninjured. Mooren has

[Fig. 181.

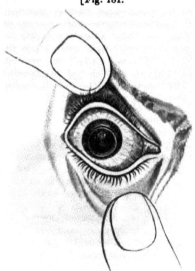

After T. W. Jones.]

seen a case in which the lens remained clear for thirty-six years.[1] When the lens has sunk into the vitreous humor out of the area of the pupil, the eye will be extremely hypermetropic; in fact, in a similar condition to one operated on for cataract.

Dislocation of the Lens into the Anterior Chamber.—Although this condition may occur in a transparent lens, it is more frequent when the latter is

---

[1] Ophthalmiatrische Beobachtungen, 257.

chalky, and perhaps diminished in size.   The displacement is moreover erally spontaneous and gradual, and not due to an accident.   There is no difficulty in recognizing the affection, for in the anterior chamber will observed a lenticular disk, either transparent and diaphanous, or white opaque. [Fig. 181.]

If the lens is in its capsule, a sharply defined yellow border will be not encircling the disk (Von Graefe).   The lens may be either entirely in anterior chamber, or a part may lie in and behind the pupil.   The l condition is especially dangerous, as the presence of the lens in the pup apt to set up irritation and inflammation of the iris, from maintaining a stant "teasing" and contusion of the edges of the pupil.   In some case lens does not retain its position in the anterior chamber, but falls back in into the vitreous humor, and it may thus frequently alternate in its posi being sometimes found in the anterior chamber, at others in the vitr Its presence in the anterior chamber will cause a considerable deepeni the latter, and a cupping back of the iris.   Adhesions are sometimes fo between the capsule and the cornea; the latter may even ulcerate an lens escape through the perforation (Von Graefe).[1]

Severe inflammatory symptoms may also supervene, implicating the co iris, and the deeper structures of the eyeball, and accompanied perhaps l increase in the intra-ocular tension.   There is often also very severe per ciliary neuralgia.   But the inflammation may even extend sympatheti to the other eye.   On the other hand, the lens may remain for a very period in the anterior chamber without producing any irritation or pail

Dislocation of the Lens under the Conjunctiva.—This is always due t accident, generally to a heavy blow from some blunt substance, hitting eye below, and knocking it forcibly against the roof or upper edge of orbit, hence the most frequent seat of this displacement is upwards inwards, or upwards and outwards.   The rupture in the choroid gene occurs quite anteriorly, between or in front of the insertion of the

[Fig. 182.

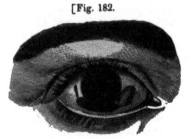

After Lawson.]

muscles.   The form of dislocation is most frequently met with in pe after the age of thirty or forty, when the sclerotic has lost its elasticity is characterized by the following appearances: Beneath the conjuncti noticed a small, well-marked, prominent tumor [Fig. 182], which may cause a little circumscribed prominence of the lid.   The color of the t varies, it may be dark from the presence of effused blood in and beneath conjunctiva, or of a portion of prolapsed iris; or the conjunctiva ma transparent, and only slightly injected, and then the grayish-white len

[1] "A. f. O.," i. 1, 348.

be easily recognised. But in some cases only a part of the lens has escaped beneath the conjunctiva, the rest remaining within the eye. Whilst the sclerotic has been ruptured, the conjunctiva, on account of its laxity and elasticity, has generally yielded before the lens, and has not given way or been torn, but covers the displaced lens. The pupil is mostly irregular and drawn up, and there is a more or less considerable prolapse of the iris. If the capsule has been ruptured and the lens escaped from it, the remains of the torn shreds of capsule will be seen with the ophthalmoscope, just as after an operation for cataract.

Dislocation of the lens may be spontaneous, and is then generally due to a gradual relaxation or elongation of the suspensory ligament, or its partial rupture. In such cases the lens is often opaque, and the vitreous humor perhaps fluid. Moreover, in such a condition a very slight shock to the eye, which has perhaps been unnoticed by the patient, will produce dislocation of the lens. The affection may also be congenital, and even hereditary, occurring in several members of the same family. Thus, Mr. Dixon[1] mentions a case in which a partial displacement of the lens existed in a mother and three sons. Mr. Bowman narrates a case in which a patient, suffering from dislocation of the lens, had two uncles affected with the same disease. If the affection is congenital, it is generally accompanied by more or less amblyopia, and perhaps nystagmus, and such eyes are as a rule also very myopic. In such cases the dislocation mostly exists in both eyes. But the most frequent cause is an injury to the eye from blows or falls upon this organ, which cause a rupture of the suspensory ligament, and a more or less complete dislocation of the lens. Mr. Bowman[2] has called attention to the fact that glaucomatous symptoms occasionally arise in cases of dislocation of the lens.

According to Von Graefe,[3] partial displacements of the lens, depending upon relaxation or rupture of the zonula, appear to be more prone to excite an increase of the eye-tension, than if the dislocation is complete, and the lens is freed from its attachment and floats about; for in the latter instances, glaucomatous symptoms generally only supervene if the lens periodically pushes the iris forward or becomes jammed in the pupil, or between the iris and the cornea. As long as the capsule remains entire, we must assume that the secondary glaucoma which sometimes supervenes on displacement of the lens is partly due to a stretching of the zonula and ciliary processes, and partly to the pressure of the lens upon the iris and ciliary region, which sets up irritation. The glaucoma sometimes assumes the simple form, in other cases the inflammatory, accompanied by serous iritis.

The treatment of dislocation of the lens must vary according to the exigencies of the case. Where it is but slight, the sight may not be materially affected, and no operative interference may be indicated. If, however, the displacement is so considerable that the free edge of the lens lies in the pupil, and thus gives rise to great impairment of the sight, and very annoying diplopia, an endeavor should be made to remedy this defect. The best mode of treatment is that originally adopted by De Wecker,[4] viz., an iridodesis made in the opposite direction to that in which the lens is displaced, so that the artificial pupil will be brought opposite that portion of the eye in which the lens is deficient, and the iris will be drawn over the displaced lens, and cover the latter to a more or less considerable extent. The patient will then be in the condition of a person whose lens has been extracted, and he will be

[1] "R. L. O. H. Reports," i. 54.   [2] "R. L. O. H. R.," v. 1.
[3] "A. f. O.," xv. 3, 136.   [4] "Maladies des Yeux," 2d edition, p. 94.

able to see well both at a distance and near at hand through suitable convex glasses. For obvious reasons, iridodesis is in such cases to be preferred to an iridectomy. If the lens is completely dislocated into the vitreous humor, and is setting up no disturbance, it is wiser not to interfere. But if inflammatory complications arise, or the sight is much impaired by the lens floating about across the pupil when the eye is moved, it will be best to remove it. An iridectomy should be made opposite the point towards which the lens is displaced, and the latter is then to be removed by Critchett's scoop. The operation is, however, often very dangerous, for a considerable amount of fluid vitreous will be lost, and severe irido-choroiditis, with subsequent atrophy of the globe, may supervene.

When the lens is luxated into the anterior chamber, we may endeavor to obtain its reposition into the vitreous humor, by making the patient assume the horizontal posture, and applying a compress bandage. If it falls back into the vitreous humor, its maintenance in this situation may be assisted by an iridodesis, or temporarily by the application of a solution of Calabar bean. If the presence of the lens in the anterior chamber sets up inflammatory reaction, or impairs the sight, it should be extracted with the scoop, and it will be better to combine an iridectomy with this operation. The incision should be made in the lower part of the cornea with a Von Graefe's cataract-knife. To prevent the escape of the lens into the vitreous humor, De Wecker advises that it should be transfixed with a needle, and kept in its position in the anterior chamber, until the scoop can be introduced beneath it. If the lens simply disturbs the sight without setting up any inflammation, we may endeavor to gain its absorption by the operation of division, care being taken not to lacerate the capsule too freely, but rather to repeat the operation several times.

In the subconjunctival dislocation, an incision should be made, and the lens removed; and the prolapsed portion excised, so that the wound may be quite smooth. If a tolerably firm union of the lips of the wound has already taken place, it will suffice to apply a compress bandage; but if the rupture in the sclerotic is gaping, it will be better to unite its edges with one or two fine sutures, in the same manner as has been advised for incised wounds in this region.

With regard to the treatment which is to be pursued if symptoms of glaucoma arise in cases of displacement of the lens, Von Graefe[1] advises that where the displacement is moderate, and the iris partially pushed forward, an iridectomy should be made, and the portion of iris which is pushed forward removed. It is of importance that the incision should be very peripheral, for otherwise the entrance of the vitreous humor into the anterior chamber pushes back the iris, and renders its excision very difficult. He points out, moreover, that the removal of the lens is apt, in such cases, to prove especially dangerous, for as there is a free communication between the anterior chamber and vitreous space, and the intra-ocular tension is increased, it is impossible to prevent a great escape of vitreous humor, which may be accompanied by serious intra-ocular hemorrhage. But if the iridectomy proves insufficient to stay the glaucomatous symptoms, or if the lens is completely luxated, it will be necessary to remove the latter.

[It has been asserted by several observers that in death by hanging rupture of the capsule or fracture of the lens is occasioned by the shock. Dyer has published the results of observations upon ten eyes of five criminals executed by hanging. In one eye, where the lens was opaque, it was

[1] "A. f. O.," xv. 3, p. 157.

dislocated downwards and outwards.   In six eyes either the anterior capsule was ruptured or the lens was fractured.   In two cases this occurred in both eyes.   In experiments u on dogs by hanging, the first dog presented the same lesion in both eyes; the second dog in neither eye; and the third dog in one eye only.   (See "Trans. Amer. Ophthal. Soc.," 1866 and 1869.) D'Œnch has made some investigations into the subject of congenital dislocation of the lens.   He finds that it always affects both eyes, generally in a symmetrical manner.   The direction of the displacement is almost always either upward, upward and inward, or upward and outward.   The lenses are generally transparent; sometimes their size is below the mean.   The suspensory ligament is sometimes found, and sometimes not.   In about one-fourth of all the cases there is myopia.   The position of the lenses may remain unchanged throughout life.   Heredity has been proved in some of the cases.   (See "Archives of Ophthalmology," x. 1.)—B.]

CHAPTER X.

DISEASES OF THE VITREOUS HUMOR.

1.—INFLAMMATION OF THE VITREOUS HUMOR.—HYALITIS.

IT was formerly supposed that the vitreous humor was incapable of undergoing inflammation, on account of the absence of nerves and bloodvessels in its structure. Thanks, however, to the researches of Virchow and Weber, it has been proved beyond doubt that the vitreous humor has become inflamed. Although these inflammatory changes generally either accompany or supervene upon inflammation of the deeper tunics of the eyeball, viz., the retina and choroid, yet many believe that idiopathic hyalitis may occur, and that it may be quite impossible to trace any participation of the other tunics of the eye. Dr. Hermann Pagenstecher has, however, made a series of very interesting experiments upon rabbits, by introducing various foreign bodies into the vitreous, watching with the ophthalmoscope the changes thus produced, and finally examining the eyes microscopically. These experiments have led him to the opinion that the vitreous cannot undergo primary inflammation, but that it is always secondary and dependent on changes in the neighboring tissues.[1]

The inflammatory changes consist chiefly in a proliferation or hyperplasia of the cells of the vitreous humor, which become opaque and granular, and undergo, perhaps, fatty degeneration. Sometimes, there is a considerable development of connective-tissue elements, or there may be a great tendency to suppuration, and large quantities of pus cells be formed. [De Wecker thinks that the difference between the inflammation of any dense tissue and that of the vitreous humor is, that while purulent infiltration of the former causes destruction of the inflamed tissue, in the vitreous there is a displacement of the structure, with rapid absorption of the watery constituents.—B.]

The progress of hyalitis is best studied by watching what changes occur when a foreign body (e. g., a piece of gun-cap, steel, etc., or a displaced lens) is lodged in the vitreous humor. If the refracting media are sufficiently clear to permit of an ophthalmoscopic examination, we find that soon after the accident, the vitreous humor in the vicinity of the foreign body loses its transparency, and becomes somewhat hazy, which is due to the proliferation of the vitreous cells, and an increase of their nuclei and molecular contents. The foreign body appears to be enveloped in a thin mist or cloud of bluish-gray tint, which assumes a more dense and firm appearance if much connective tissue is developed, and a creamy-yellow color if suppuration sets in. The track of the foreign body is often visible, in the form of a thin whitish-

---

[1] A brief summary of his views will be found in the "Centralblatt für die medicinischen Wissenschaften," 1869, No. 48; but a full account of the experiments, etc. is published in Knapp's "Archives of Ophthalmology and Otology," 1869, vol. i. 2.

gray opacity, like a thread running towards it. We sometimes find that these inflammatory changes in the vitreous humor, consequent upon the lodgement of a foreign body within it, are idiopathic, no trace of inflammation of the other structures of the eye being visible, either externally or with the ophthalmoscope. Generally, however, this is not the case, for symptoms of irido-cyclitis or choroiditis soon supervene, and the eye is but too frequently lost through suppuration.

The simple (non-suppurative) form of hyalitis may be either acute or chronic, and the opacity of the vitreous be either diffused or circumscribed. On ophthalmoscopic examination, we may find the whole vitreous humor diffusely clouded, which renders the details of the fundus either completely invisible or very indistinct, so that they appear to be covered by a thin gray film or veil. In this diffuse opacity may be noticed dark, thread-like films, of varying size and shape, which may be either fixed, or float about when the eye is quickly moved. Neoplastic formations of connective tissue are often met with at the anterior portion of the vitreous humor, close to the posterior pole of the lens. They give rise to a more or less extensive opacity, which is sometimes termed posterior polar cataract. But connective tissue is also formed in other portions of the vitreous humor, often in very considerable quantities, giving rise to membranous and filamentous opacities, which, traversing the vitreous in different directions, may perhaps even divide it into fibrillar compartments. The true cellular gelatinous substance of the vitreous humor disappears in proportion to the development of the connective tissue, and generally becomes fluid (synchysis). In such cases the retina is often found to be extensively detached, and the vitreous humor shrivelled up to a very small space; and chiefly consisting of connective tissue, of an almost tendinous structure, interspersed with flocculi containing cells which have undergone various changes, and not unfrequently pigment molecules.

Although simple hyalitis sometimes occurs idiopathically, yet generally it is dependent upon an inflammation of the retina, choroid, or ciliary body. [Serous hyalitis, with liquefaction of the vitreous humor, and more or less opacity, is met with most frequently in serous inflammations of the eye, like glaucoma, or with progressive staphyloma posticum.—B.]

Still more so is this the case in the suppurative form of hyalitis, which is but seldom idiopathic, being mostly associated with purulent irido-cyclitis or irido-choroiditis, which supervenes perhaps upon operations for cataract, injuries, etc. As the cornea is but too frequently opaque, or the pupil blocked up with lymph, it is often impossible to trace the course of the disease with the ophthalmoscope. If we are, however, able to do so, we sometimes find that the anterior portion of the vitreous humor, close to the lens, yields a yellow, creamy reflex, which may be very well seen with the oblique illumination. It is called posterior hypopyon, and is due to pus in the anterior portion of the vitreous, which may have made its way from the ciliary body or anterior segment of choroid, having burst through the retina. In such a case, the other portions of the vitreous may be found comparatively, or even completely, healthy. In other instances, the suppuration occurs at the posterior or lateral portions of the vitreous, to which it may remain chiefly confined, but it may also become general, and involve the whole of the vitreous humor. Panophthalmitis generally ensues, and the globe gradually becomes atrophied, with or without previous perforation of the cornea or sclerotic.

[See a paper "On the Phenomena of Suppurative Hyalitis," by Heff and Brailey, in the "Royal London Ophthalmic Hospital Reports," x. 2.

When purulent hyalitis is circumscribed, in other words, forms an abscess, the contents of this abscess may eventually be absorbed, the walls of the abscess collapse, and by their traction occasion partial or total detachment of the vitreous. The same may occur from the contraction of membranous bands in the vitreous which have become organised.—B.]

The prognosis of inflammation of the vitreous humor will depend chiefly upon the cause, and the extent to which the deeper tissues of the eye are implicated. I must therefore refer the reader for a consideration of these points, as well as the question of treatment, to the diseases of the choroid and retina. With regard to the treatment, I may, however, state, that in acute cases of diffuse hyalitis, much benefit is often experienced from salivation and the periodic application of the artificial leech to the temple.

2.—OPACITIES OF THE VITREOUS HUMOR.

[Syn. Myodesopsia.—B.]

The presence of opacities in the vitreous humor is easily detected with the ophthalmoscope in the direct mode of examination. The patient should be ordered to move his eye quickly and repeatedly in various directions, and then hold it still. These movements will cause the opacities to be shaken up, and they will float about in the field of vision, and we shall thus be enabled to judge of their size and density and to distinguish between the fixed and movable ones. When the eye is held still, the latter soon sink again to the lower portion of the vitreous. The excursions which these opacities make are often very considerable, and allow us to estimate approximately the degree of fluidity of the vitreous. The binocular ophthalmoscope is particularly useful in the examination of vitreous opacities, and in determining the different depths at which they are situated.

[Vitreous opacities are of two kinds: 1st, those which have migrated into the vitreous with subsequent transformation of the cellular elements; 2d, those which are the results of disintegration of the normal elements of the vitreous. The first is represented by purulent infiltration and by hemorrhage; the latter of which is shown by the presence of crystals, doubtless hematine crystals, the residuum of old hemorrhages. The opacities may be very fine, almost molecular; or they may have the form of fine lines and threads; or they may be membraniform. ("Graefe und Saemisch's Handb. der Augenheilk.," iv. S. 678–699.—B.]

We have seen that in simple hyalitis the opacity of the vitreous assumes a diffuse gray appearance, shrouding the whole fundus in a fine veil, the sight being at the same time greatly affected. Sometimes the opacity is chiefly confined to one portion, perhaps the central, in which case the yellow spot and the retina in its vicinity will appear hazy, whilst the details at the periphery of the fundus can be clearly seen. This partial uniform opacity may shift somewhat when the eye is moved. A peculiarly dangerous form of diffuse opacity of the vitreous is that which occurs suddenly, and, after clearing somewhat, recurs perhaps several times, for it is but too often followed by detachment of the retina. We must not, however, confound with this the temporary cloudiness of the vitreous which occurs in glaucoma, and which is due to a serous hypersecretion, evidently dependent upon irritation of the ciliary nerves.

Together with a more or less diffuse opacity, we often meet with various circular, membranous, or filiform opacities which are due to the remains of blood-effusions, or alterations in the cells of the vitreous humor, which may have undergone fatty, purulent, or pigmentary changes; or connective-tissue elements may have been formed. These opacities assume very various shapes and forms. At first, perhaps, the patient only notices a dark speck before his eyes, which he cannot wipe away; then thin, flaky membranes may appear, which float about and assume different forms and positions with every movement of the eye. Between these opacities, the field of vision may either appear clear or be more or less diffusely clouded. The nearer the opacities are to the retina, the more will they throw a shadow upon it. If they are some distance from it, they may not throw individual shadows, but only give rise to a general dimness of vision. The patients, as Von Graefe has pointed out, often throw their eyes periodically upwards in reading, etc., in order to cause the opacities to move and shift their position, so that the field of vision may be momentarily cleared, which, of course, enables them to see more distinctly. This periodic upward movement of the eye is accompanied by an elevation of the upper lid, and gives a peculiar and characteristic appearance to the patient.

With the ophthalmoscope, we can readily distinguish these opacities as dark, fixed, or floating bodies, assuming various shapes, like dark spots, threads, or reticulated fibrillæ; sometimes, however, they are so delicate and fine that we cannot individualize them, and the whole fundus only appears to be hazy and veiled.

The disease in which opacities of the vitreous are by far most frequently met with is sclerotico-choroiditis posterior. The posterior portion of the vitreous frequently becomes fluid, and the opacities may be seen floating very freely about in it. Sometimes, however, the synchysis extends to the greater portion or even the whole of the vitreous humor.

Extravasation of blood into the vitreous humor is a very frequent cause of these opacities. The hemorrhage is generally due to a rupture of some of the vessels of the choroid, more especially at its anterior portion, where it is most vascular, and at which situation the retina is thinnest, and therefore most readily gives way; whereas, when the effusion takes place in the posterior portion of the choroid, it is more prone to cause detachment of the retina than to perforate the latter and make its way into the vitreous. This is due to the fact that the connection between the choroid and retina is at this point very lax, and the retina thicker than in the region of the ora serrata. Hence a more or less considerable detachment of the retina is generally produced at the posterior portion of the fundus before perforation takes place. When the blood has become absorbed, and the vitreous is again transparent, we can always discover changes in the choroid, such as exudations, etc., showing whence the hemorrhage has proceeded, and we are also sometimes able to detect a cicatrix in the retina, where the latter has been ruptured by the extravasation of blood. Schweigger[1] has pointed out that hemorrhage into the vitreous humor occurs far more frequently from the choroidal vessels than from those of the retina, for the latter are not only smaller in size, but on account of the peculiar arrangement of the connective-tissue fibrills (Stützfasern) of the retina, and the resistance offered by the membrana limitans interna, hemorrhage from the retina extends generally towards the choroid, and not into the vitreous.

We are generally able, with the ophthalmoscope, to easily distinguish extravasations of blood into the vitreous, as they yield a peculiar bright-red color. But if the hemorrhage is very extensive and diffuse, it may not be possible to light up the eye at all, the fundus looking quite dark, and not

---

[1] "A. f. O.," vi. 2, 269.

affording the least reflex. The sight is generally very greatly suddenly impaired, the patient having the sensation as if there was a dense red mist or veil before his eye. When the blood is beginning to be absorbed, fixed and floating opacities of a filiform, reticulated, or membranous character make their appearance, and become rolled up into dark, fantastically-shaped masses when the eye is moved. Sometimes when the absorption has gone on for some time, and the vitreous has regained much of its transparency, a fresh extravasation takes place, and this may recur several times. Although the patient may regain a considerable amount of sight during these intervals, the recurrence of hemorrhage is always to be regarded with great anxiety, as it but too frequently leads to detachment of the retina, glaucomatous complications, or atrophy of the eyeball.

When the hemorrhage has been at all considerable, permanent opacities are generally left behind, and may produce great impairment of vision and even detachment of the retina by traction. H. Müller[1] was the first to show that the latter is a not unfrequent consequence of opacities in the vitreous.

Extravasations of blood into the vitreous humor are very often of traumatic origin, being produced, for instance, by severe blows upon the eye, causing a rupture of the bloodvessels of the choroid or retina. They may, however, arise independently of this, if there is much congestion of the internal tunics of the eyeball, or if the coats of the vessels are diseased.

In the treatment of opacities of the vitreous humor, we must be especially guided by the cause, and whether they are due to, and a part symptom of, inflammatory affections of the deeper tunics of the eyeball, or, perhaps, to intra-ocular hemorrhages caused by rupture of some of the choroidal vessels. In the former case, our attention must be chiefly directed to the treatment of the primary disease. The absorption of the vitreous opacities may, however, be greatly aided by preventing all congestion of the choroidal or retinal vessels by the application of the artificial leech. I have often gained great benefit from its use, as it facilitates and hastens the absorption, and relieves the intra-ocular bloodvessels. If the patient is weak and anæmic, I generally prefer dry cupping at the temple, making use only of the glass cylinder of Heurteloup. This may be repeated once or twice a week, according to circumstances. But if the patient is strong and plethoric, I invariably take blood away by means of the artificial leech, one cylinder full being the usual quantity. In those cases in which the affection of the vitreous is dependent upon derangement of the functions of the uterus or liver, the general health must be strictly attended to. Much benefit is experienced from the use of saline mineral waters, as the Pullna, Kissingen, Kreuznach, etc., and the tendency to congestion and hyperæmia of the vessels of the eye should be relieved by hot pediluvia or hip-baths. The absorption of blood into the vitreous may also be hastened by the application of a firm compress bandage. In case of dense membranous opacities of the vitreous which had resisted all efforts of absorption, Von Graefe has derived much benefit from tearing them through with a fine needle.[2] This produces not only an improvement in the sight, but renders the opacities more amenable to treatment, and prevents their exercising any deleterious influence upon the retina by traction.

[If the opacity is recent, the patient should be kept in bed, with a compress bandage and the use of atropine and leeches to the temple. In the more chronic forms, good results have occasionally been obtained from hypodermic injections of the hydrochlorate of pilocarpine, beginning with a small

---

[1] "A. f. O.," iv. 1, 372.   [2] Ibid., ix. 2, 101.

dose and increasing it to toleration, but being careful to produce no cardiac collapse. The infusion of jaborandi may be given by the mouth in its place. (See "Trans. N. Y. State Med. Soc.," 1879, and "N. Y. Med. Journ.," April, 1879.) Le Fort and Onimus have advised the use of the constant current, as an aid in clearing up vitreous opacities, and have spoken highly of the results obtained. ("Gaz. méd. de Paris," July 11, 1874; "La France méd.," 1874, No. 33.) De Wecker has never seen any rapid results from this treatment, and thinks there is danger of increasing the opacities by a too careless use of the current.—B.]

It is of much practical importance to distinguish between the pathological opacities of the vitreous humor and the subjective physiological musæ volitantes (*Myodesopsia*) which are met with in perfectly healthy eyes. These assume the most various shapes and appearances. Sometimes they look like small transparent disks or circles, which may be isolated or arranged in groups; or they may resemble strings of bright beads, or filamentous bands, which float about in all directions through the field of vision. They are generally due to minute beaded filaments or groups of granules in the vitreous humor, and are quite physiological, occurring more or less in all eyes. They are so minute that they are perfectly invisible with the ophthalmoscope, and this instrument is, therefore, of the greatest use in enabling us to distinguish between the physiological and pathological *muscæ volitantes* for directly it reveals to us the presence of opacities in the vitreous, however, slight they may be, we must regard them as pathological products. I must, however, mention in passing, that certain changes in the choroid and retina may give rise to fixed dark spots in the visual field (so-called "scotomata"). No careful observer could, however, confound these with the opacities in question.

Muscæ become very evident when the person regards some light and highly illuminated object, as, for instance, the bright clear sky, a very white wall, or the brightly illuminated field of the microscope; whereas in a subdued light, the floating bodies may be hardly, if at all, observable. They are also increased by fatigue of the eye from overwork, or when the retina is very sensitive and irritable; the same often occurs if there is any derangement of the nervous system or of the digestive organs. The situation of the muscæ may be approximately ascertained, as was shown by Listing, by making the patient look through one of the minute apertures of the stenopæic apparatus, or a pin-hole in a card. Now, if the card is moved in a certain direction (e. g., upwards), and the objects also move upwards, they are situated behind the pupil; whereas, if they move in the opposite direction, they lie in front of the pupil. The greater the degree of movement, the further does the object lie from the pupil.[1] The position of the objects can be estimated with still greater accuracy by Donders' mode of examination à double vue. He employs a diaphragm pierced by two small apertures situated about one line from each other, so that two shadows are thrown upon the retina, and cover one another by nearly one-half.[2] We must distinguish the muscæ which have their seat in the vitreous humor from the appearances produced by eyelashes, muco-lachrymal drops on the conjunctiva and cornea, and the radii and spots situated in the lens. For full information upon this interesting subject of "Entoptics," I would refer the reader to Dr. Jago's excellent and exhaustive treatise[3]

---

[1] Helmholtz, "Handbuch der Physiologischen Optik," 150.
[2] Donders, "On the Anomalies of Accommodation and Refraction of the Eye," 201.
[3] "Entoptics, with its Uses in Physiology and Medicine," by James Jago, M.D., 1864 (Churchill).

Short-sighted persons are especially troubled by muscæ, for even the physiological motes are rendered peculiarly marked and distinct by the size of the circles of diffusion upon the retina. In consequence of this, they often prove a source of the greatest anxiety and trouble to the patient. Already, perhaps, in constant dread that his myopia should rapidly increase, and lead eventually to great impairment of vision, or even total blindness, the appearance of these muscæ often frightens him greatly, and causes him to yield undivided attention to his eyesight, and to watch every symptom with anxiety. This is more particularly the case with those persons who are dependent upon their sight for their livelihood, or are naturally of a nervous and anxious temperament. Even although we may earnestly and repeatedly assure them that these physiological motes are not of the slightest importance, and are a source of no danger, we but too frequently fail to alleviate their mental distress. They seek advice from others who, in their opinion, are more competent and willing to understand the nature of their complaint. Amongst such patients the charlatan finds his most fervid and profitable followers. I have met with several most distressing cases in which advertising quacks have greatly frightened patients who complained of these motes, assuring them that they depended upon some secret disorder, and if not speedily and properly treated, that they would lead to amaurosis, of which, indeed they were the sure precursory symptoms. Such patients must be cheered up, and prevented as much as possible from thinking of their ailments. Their general health must be strengthened, and any irregularities of the circulation or digestive organs removed. Much benefit is often also produced by the use of dark-blue or neutral tint eye-protectors, as they diminish the intensity of the light, and thus render the muscæ less visible.

It has been already mentioned, in speaking of the opacities in the vitreous humor, that the latter may lose its normal gelatinous consistence, and become partially or wholly fluid. This condition, which is termed synchysis, cannot be diagnosed with certainty if there are no floating opacities. An erroneous opinion sometimes prevails, that the eye is always soft in all cases of fluid vitreous. But this is not the case, for the tension of the eyeball varies according to the amount of the vitreous humor, and not according to the nature of its consistence. Thus in glaucoma, the tension of the eyeball may be very greatly increased, owing to the hyper-secretion of the vitreous humor, which may be perfecty fluid. Again, diminution of the intra-ocular tension only proves that the contents of the vitreous are diminished in quantity, although it must be allowed that in such cases the vitreous is often fluid. Tremulousness of the iris is also an uncertain symptom. It can exist only when the iris has lost its natural support from the crystalline lens, either through absence of the latter, or through its having become displaced. Together with fluidity of the vitreous, the diameter of the eyeball may have become increased, and the position of the lens with regard to the iris somewhat altered, and therefore, on account of this loss of support, the iris may be tremulous. But the most reliable symptom is the presence of floating opacities. In staphylomatous enlargements of the eyeball, the vitreous is always found more or less fluid. The same occurs if a foreign body or a displaced lens has become lodged in the vitreous. Moreover, when vitreous humor is lost, as for instance during an operation for cataract, or owing to a wound of the eye, this loss is always made up by fluid. It is of importance to be aware, if possible, of the consistence of the vitreous humor before undertaking an operation for cataract, in order that we may take every precaution to limit, as much as possible, the loss of vitreous which must inevitably occur.

[This senile synchysis is often met with in eyes in which the vitreous lamella of the choroid is thickened, or, in other words, glandular degeneration of the choroid.—B.]

According to Iwanoff,[1] fatty degeneration of the stroma and cells of the vitreous humor, with subsequent fluidity of the latter, is not of unfrequent occurrence, more especially in the aged, in whom it is due to senile decay, and is here a quasi-physiological condition.

A most beautiful and striking appearance is presented by the presence of crystals of cholesterine in the vitreous. As this condition generally, if not indeed always, occurs in a fluid state of the vitreous, it has been termed sparkling synchysis (synchysis étincelant). The exact mode of origin of these crystals is not at present known, but it seems that they often occur after hemorrhage into the vitreous, and are therefore very probably deposited from the blood; or they may be due to fatty changes in the vitreous humor. The appearance presented by cholesterine in the vitreous is most characteristic and striking, if the ophthalmoscope is used. On every movement of the eye, a shower of bright, sparkling crystals is seen floating through the field of vision, which gradually sink down to its lower part when the eye is again held still. Sometimes the crystals float about in an otherwise clear vitreous, or they may be intermixed with darker filamentous opacities, to which they may even adhere, fringing them with a sparkling, lustrous border. They have also been met with in the retina and optic nerve, and even between the retina and choroid. When they are situated at the anterior portion of the vitreous, close behind the lens, they may be noticed even with the oblique illumination. Von Graefe mentions a case in which they gradually disappeared.

Detachment of the vitreous humor is altogether pathological in its nature, and is of serious danger to the safety of the eye, as it frequently leads to detachment of the retina. It is mostly due to some injury of the eye, but is also occasionally observed in cases of staphyloma of the cornea, and of posterior staphyloma, as well as in consequence of extraction of cataract with or without loss of vitreous. Iwanoff, however, states that detachment of the vitreous humor is of rare occurrence after extraction of cataract, if no vitreous has been lost; whereas it occurs, as a rule, in all cases in which there has been a considerable loss of vitreous humor.[2] He divides the detachments of the vitreous, which occur after injuries of any kind, into two categories. In one class,[3] the detachment occurs immediately after the injury, in consequence of the diminution in the contents of the eyeball and the vacuum which is thereby produced, and which is immediately filled with a serous fluid. In the other, the detachment is formed gradually, and depends upon slowly progressive changes in the vitreous humor, which may probably be set up by various morbid processes in the other membranes of the eye. The detachment which occurs after extraction of cataract may belong to either category. At present, no exact data can be given for the ophthalmoscopic diagnosis of this detachment of the vitreous. Von Graefe[4] thinks it probable that the suddenly formed, tolerably uniform opacity in the posterior segment of the vitreous, which is sometimes observed in sclerectasia posterior, is a detachment of the vitreous. This opacity is especially characterized by the suddenness of its appearance, by its defined line of demarcation against the healthy vitreous, although it may be of considerable extent, and by the almost constant supervention of detachment of the retina.

---

[1] "A. f. O.," xv. 2, 4
[2] *Vide* also Dr. de Gouvea's article, "A. f. O.," xv. 1, p. 244.
[3] Loc. cit., p. 64.
[4] "Kl. Monatsbl.," 1868, p. 301.

8.—FOREIGN BODIES, ETC., IN THE VITREOUS HUMOR.

If a foreign body becomes lodged in the vitreous humor, it but too frequently excites the most severe and destructive inflammation of the tissues through which it has passed, or with which it lies in contact. Thus if it has entered through the cornea, this and the iris often become violently inflamed; the lens, through which the foreign body has also passed, becomes cataractous and swells up, thus tending to increase still more the severity of the inflammation. If the injury has been severe and the foreign body lies in the vitreous humor close to the retina, it often excites inflammation, perhaps of a suppurative character, in this and the choroid, which may lead perhaps to atrophy of the globe. If the media remain sufficiently clear to permit of an ophthalmoscopic examination of the fundus, we generally find that for the first few days the foreign body may be seen of its natural color, mostly sunk down in the vitreous humor. Then, the latter becomes somewhat clouded in the vicinity of the foreign body, surrounding it with a thin, grayish-blue halo, which, as the plastic nature of the exudation increases, assumes a denser and more opaque yellowish-white appearance, hiding the foreign body from view. It has, in fact, become encysted. At the same time the vitreous humor is often more or less diffusely clouded, and dark, filamentous opacities float about in it. When it regains sufficient transparency to permit of an ophthalmoscopic examination of the fundus, we not unfrequently find that a detachment of the retina has occurred (perhaps to a considerable extent), and that a more or less extensive inflammation of the choroid has taken place. In some rare instances, however, the course may be more favorable; so that, although the injury may be followed by severe inflammation, the foreign body becomes encysted in the vitreous humor, which gradually regains its transparency as the inflammatory symptoms subside, and finally the sight may be restored to its normal condition, the foreign body lying innocuous in the vitreous humor. Such instances are, however, very rare, and can only occur when the foreign body is small. The following is a brief outline of such a case, which came under my care at the Middlesex Hospital, in 1862.[1]

"Samuel P——, aged 20, was wounded in the left eye by a chip of iron flying off a hammer. This was followed by severe inflammatory symptoms, great swelling of the lids, lachrymation, photophobia, iritis. At the outer and upper side of the iris, quite close to the periphery, there was a small triangular opening, showing the passage of the foreign body, and, corresponding to it, there was a small cicatrix in the cornea. On his admission into the hospital (about a week after the accident) he could only count fingers up to a distance of seven or eight feet. The tension of the eye was then, and remained throughout, normal. When the inflammatory symptoms had greatly subsided, a short ophthalmoscopic examination was made, and it was found that the vitreous humor was clouded, with a few filamentous opacities floating about in it. The condition of the eye was soon so much improved that the patient could read No. 1 of Jäger, and No. 19 at eighteen feet; the lens was clear, the vitreous slightly hazy, yet permitting the optic disk to be distinctly seen. At the outer and lower portion of the vitreous was seen a white, opalescent, oval mass, the encysted foreign body, whilst its passage through the vitreous could be traced by a faint bluish line running towards it. A local, circumscribed inflammation in the choroid had occurred in its vicinity, and small portions of choroidal pigment were agglomerated

[1] *Vide* "Lancet," Aug. 23, 1862.

around the foreign body. I saw the patient occasionally for some years after the accident; the last time was about three years ago, and the eye was then in precisely the same condition, and he could use it perfectly."

I must mention, however, that even after a foreign body has lain encysted and dormant for many years in the vitreous humor, it may give rise to severe inflammatory symptoms, which may lead to atrophy of the globe, or awaken sympathetic ophthalmia.

Dr. Berlin, of Stuttgart, has lately called attention to a fact, with regard to the course often taken by foreign bodies in the vitreous, which had hitherto been overlooked.[1] He has found, from his dissection of eyes wounded by foreign bodies, that, when the latter lay in the lower portion of the vitreous humor, they had, in most cases, first struck the retina and choroid, and, having rebounded from the posterior wall of the eye, had then sunk down in the vitreous. This was proved by finding a spot on the retina and choroid where these had been wounded, lying in a straight line with the entrance of the foreign body. Dr. Berlin, moreover, points out the great importance of accurately testing not only the acuteness of vision, but also the condition of the visual field; for a deficiency in a certain portion of the field occurring immediately after the injury, may guide us in discovering the presence of a foreign body in the vitreous, as well as its position. Thus in one case in which the field was wanting outwards and upwards, he diagnosed the foreign body as lying at the inner and lower quadrant of the eyeball. An incision was made at this point, and the edge of the knife struck against a hard body, which, however, eluded the grasp of the forceps. The eye was excised, and then it was found that the incision had actually grazed the bit of steel. If hemorrhage has taken place, the greatest quantity is found about the foreign body. Dr. Berlin[2] now employs, like Von Graefe, the narrow extraction knife, making the section downwards, but otherwise the same as in Von Graefe's operation for extraction of cataract.

The treatment must be chiefly directed to subduing the inflammation. Cold compresses should be applied to the eye, and perhaps leeches to the temple. The pupil must be kept widely dilated by atropine. If suppurative iritis or irido-cyclitis is set up, it may be necessary to put the patient rapidly under the influence of mercury; or, if there is a considerable hypopyon, repeated paracentesis, or a large iridectomy may be indicated. The latter should never be neglected if the tension of the eye is increased.

With regard to removal of the cataractous lens, or of the eyeball, from its setting up sympathetic irritation or inflammation, I must refer the reader to the chapters upon "Traumatic Cataract" and "Sympathetic Ophthalmia." The question may arise as to the advisability of removing a foreign body in the vitreous humor, and we must be principally guided in deciding this by its position and nature. Interesting cases of this kind have been reported, amongst others, by Dixon ("R. L. O. H. Rep.," No. 6) and Critchett ("Lancet," 1854).

[The removal of foreign bodies from the vitreous is a question of great importance in ophthalmic surgery, for two reasons: first, because of the possibility of preserving a certain amount of vision in the wounded eye, in spite of severe inflammation; and secondly, because of the possibility of preventing sympathetic inflammation. The presence of a foreign body in any eye is not only almost certain to cause destructive inflammation of that eye,

---

[1] *Vide* his valuable papers on "Foreign Bodies in the Vitreous," "A. f. O.," xiii. 3, 275, and ib., xiv. 2, 275.
[2] Knapp's "Archives of Ophthalmology and Otology," i. 1, 30.

but is an exceedingly frequent cause of sympathetic inflammation of the fellow-eye. Where the foreign body can be seen with the ophthalmoscope, an attempt should always be made to remove it. Where its presence is suspected, an operation is almost always justifiable. Gently probing a wound through the coats of an eye, from which vitreous is protruding, is under certain circumstances admissible and even wise. Even when a foreign body has become encapsulated in the vitreous, the eye is never safe from dangerous inflammation.

During the last two or three years the application of the magnet to determine the presence of particles of iron or steel within the eye and their extraction, has yielded valuable practical results. Various forms of magnets have been employed, among the best of which may be mentioned the one contrived by Dr. Gruening. This consists of a number of magnetized steel rods arranged in the form of a cylinder, not in contact with each other, but in close proximity, and enclosed at their ends in iron caps, from one of which projects a delicate point of malleable iron, thirty-two millimetres long, one millimetre wide, and three-tenths of a millimetre thick. This point lifts a weight of two hundred and twenty-five grains, and has the power, when introduced between the lips of a wound in the sclera, of attracting particles of iron or steel weighing as high as fifty centigrammes, a distance of several millimetres through the vitreous. Electro-magnets have also been devised by Bradford, Hirschberg, and others. Bradford's consists of a single cell, the fluid being a solution of bichromate of potassa and sulphuric acid, and the induction coil is supplied with several tips, varying in suspensive power from eleven to twenty ounces. This is a much more powerful instrument than any permanent magnet, and may aid in the extraction of large particles of iron or steel by drawing them towards the surface, and thus facilitate their extraction. McHardy calls attention to the pain experienced by some patients when the injured eye is brought well within the range of the pole of the magnet. This pain he regards as a proof of the completion or interruption of the galvanic current which induced the magnetic action, and therefore as furnishing conclusive evidence not only of the lodgement of a particle of iron or steel, but also that the magnet is exercising a sensible traction thereon. It may be generally stated that the smaller a particle is which has lodged in the vitreous, the less likelihood there is of its extraction, especially if it be of such a nature as cannot be acted upon by a magnet. Occasionally a grooved hook, such as has been successfully employed by Knapp, proves of service. But in too many instances all attempts at removal fail, and there is no resource then left but enucleation of the injured eye. In the words of Dr. H. D. Noyes, "an eye enclosing a foreign body is usually doomed." Destructive inflammation may be postponed, but sooner or later it is almost sure to occur, bringing with it in its train, all the dangers of sympathetic inflammation of the fellow eye. The literature of perforating wounds of the eyeball and lodgement of foreign bodies in the eye has grown to extensive proportions within the last two or three years, and the editor would refer to the following sources for more complete information upon the subject: "Medical Record," May 1, 1880. "Archives of Ophthalmology," ix. parts 1, 2, 3, and 4. "Archives of Ophthalmology," vii. 2, 3, and 4; viii. 4; x. 2 and 4. "Centralblatt für prakt. Augenheilk.," June, 1881. "British Med. Journ.," March 26 and May 28, 1881. "Transactions of N. Y. State Med. Soc.," 1881. "Arch. f. klin. Chirurgie," xxvi. 3. "Boston Med. and Surg. Journ.," March 31, 1881. "Crónica oftalmológica," Agosto 12, 1881. "Graefe und Saemisch,

Handb. der Augenheilk.," iii. pp. 392 *et seq.*   H. D. Noyes' "Treatise on Diseases of the Eye," 1881.—B.]

Although cysticerci have been met with in various parts of the eye, as the cornea, anterior chamber, iris, and lens, as well as in the orbit, their most frequent seat appears to be in the background of the eye.   Thus Von Graefe[1] states that among eighty thousand patients, he has found a cysticercus in the deeper tissues of the eye in rather more than eighty cases; in the anterior chamber three times, beneath the conjunctiva five times, in the lens once, and in the orbit once.   The youngest individual was nine years old; about ninety per cent. of the cases occurred between the ages of fifteen and fifty-five, and nearly two-thirds of the cases were met with in men.   In England the disease would seem to be very rare.   I have only met with one case of cysticercus in the vitreous diagnosed with the ophthalmoscope, which occurred in a soldier who was sent to me for examination by Professor Longmore.   If the membrane which envelops the cysticercus in the vitreous humor is not too dense, the entozoon presents a very peculiar and characteristic appearance.   Its original seat appears generally to be beneath the retina, and it is only at a later stage of its existence that it perforates the latter (with its head first), and makes its way into the vitreous humor.   Sometimes it carries the retina with it, and thus produces an extensive detachment, by which it is covered. In other cases, it tears through the retina and lies free in the vitreous humor. Here it frequently becomes encysted, being surrounded by a more or less dense membrane, which may prevent the recognition of the real nature of the affection.   If this is not the case, but the entozoon is without an investing membrane, it presents the appearance of a pale grayish-blue or greenish-blue vesicle, somewhat circular or flask-shaped, with a short neck and round head, on which the suckers may be seen.   If the animal is alive, we may, by closely watching it, observe distinct undulating, tremulous movements of its outline, the head being perhaps alternately stretched out from, or drawn into, the receptaculum.   The position of the latter, in which the head and neck lie when they are retracted, is indicated by a small white spot at one point of the vesicle.   The slightest movement of the head causes a gentle quivering motion of the vesicle, and, on bright illumination of its surface, we notice, especially near the margin, a peculiar bright iridescence, the play of colors constantly changing, but having a decidedly red tint.   All these minutiæ are more easily distinguished when the cysticercus lies free in the vitreous humor, than when it is covered by the retina.   If, in the latter case, its movements are very marked and considerable, the superjacent retina may also undergo a distinctly tremulous motion.   Von Graefe has been able in four cases to watch the development of the entozoon from the very commencement.   At the outset, there appeared a delicate grayish-blue opacity at some portion of the fundus, situated evidently in the retina or between the latter and the choroid.   In the course of three or four weeks, the little cysticercus vesicle escaped, in two cases from the most prominent portion of the opacity into the vitreous humor.   In the other two cases, the outline of the vesicle became gradually more and more apparent from beneath the opacity, and was distinctly situated beneath the retina, the latter lying either in tense and close apposition to the entozoon, or being separated by an effusion of sub-retinal fluid, in which case there exists a greater mobility of the vesicle. The latter gradually glides along further and further beneath the retina, until at last, after perhaps several months have elapsed, it breaks through into the vitreous humor.   The original position of the cysticercus beneath

[1] "A. f. O.," xii. 2, 174.

the retina is indicated by the faintly recognizable
white spot, from which can be traced a distinct g
has made its way for some distance beneath the
Although opacities of the vitreous may appear at
not the rule, but at a later period the vitreous {
and the eye is finally lost from slow and insidic
this occurs within two years of the outset of the d

The presence of a cysticercus being so extre
Von Graefe[1] was led to attempt its extraction,
possible to retain a certain degree of vision, to pr
or at the worst, to diminish the pain and protra
of the eyeball. After a time, however, he alm
former modes of operating, and more recently a
in his operation for cataract.[2] The section was
narrow extraction knife, the iris excised, the cap
removed. He then tore through the hyaloid fc
book which he formerly employed for the remov:
on in the direction of the cysticercus, alternate
towards the section. He watched with great at:
vitreous which are thus brought towards the wou
hook, for as soon as yellowish threads and porti(
them, it is a proof that the close vicinity of the
When the cyst itself appears near the wound,
and the vulcanite curette pressed a little upon tl
lips of the incision slightly to gape, and facilitat
He recommends the same form of incision for th
lying in the vitreous, when such an operation ap

In Plate V., Fig. 9, will be found an excellent
ances presented by a cysticercus in the vitreo
planation of this plate, "The parasite, whicl
beneath the retina, and then, after perforating it
humor, could be seen with such perfect distir
movements and coärctations of the vesicle coul(
outline, but also at the posterior wall, which co-
the anterior wall. This was especially the case
as the red tint in the illustration shows, more l
at the margin, on which the light falls more
suffers greater reflection. The neck, especia.
vesicle, is more opaque, and studded with min-
cles). This more opaque portion, where the
the most firm, and we must endeavor to seiz(
tract the animal. In a case upon which I ope:
in seizing it at this point with the canula for
sclerotic. By means of an ophthalmoscope, wh
I illuminated the animal and the instrument,
curately. In the illustration, we recognize a t
other two being placed posteriorly), and the
directed upwards. The shape of the head did n (
ance depicted in the illustration, but varied in

[The *filaria spiralis* has been observed in t.
De Wecker thinks none of the reports are re

---

[1] "A. f. O.," iii. 2, 230, and ib., iv. 2, 171.
[2] "A. f. O.," xiv. 3, 143. [See also "Gaz. hebdon
und Saemisch," loc. cit., iv. p. 711.—B.]

ophthalmoscopically be easily confounded with a persistent hyaloid artery. See "Graefe u. Saemisch," l. c. p. 714.—B.]

In rare instances, the formation of new bloodvessels in the vitreous may be observed with the ophthalmoscope. Thus Becker[1] saw new vessels formed upon the anterior surface of an abscess in the vitreous humor, and again in purulent infiltration of the vitreous; in the latter case, the vessels were situated close behind the lens, and were distinguishable with the naked eye. Becker,[2] moreover, narrates an extraordinary case of an independent neoplastic formation, in which the connection between the newly formed vessels of the growth and those of the retina could be distinctly traced.

[Though these cases of vascular new formation are rare, yet enough have been reported to admit of a positive opinion as to their occurrence. They almost always occur near the optic disk, are connected with the papilla or the retina, and are developed at the expense of the vitreous. If the latter is hazy, they might be mistaken for a detachment of the retina. There are three interesting cases of this rare lesion reported in the "Royal London Ophthalmic Hospital Reports," x. 2, the most marked feature in all being curiously convoluted bunches of vessels. In one case, the abnormal vessels completely vanished under the administration of mercury.—B.]

4.—PERSISTENT HYALOID ARTERY.

The hyaloid artery generally shrivels up and disappears during the later period of fœtal life. In some rare instances, however, remains of it in the vitreous humor have been subsequently traced with the ophthalmoscope, either in the form of a short, dark stripe, or of a dark thread running through the vitreous humor from the optic disk towards the posterior portion of the lens. If the vessel is still patent and carries blood, as was noticed by Zehender,[3] it appears, by incident light, like a red cord, which, in this case, underwent considerable undulations when the eye was moved, the vitreous humor being evidently fluid.[4] Liebreich records a case in which there existed a physiological cup of the optic nerve, together with the persistent hyaloid artery, and the latter could be distinctly traced up to its point of origin from the central artery of the retina. A remarkable case is reported by De Wecker,[5] in which a transparent hyaloid canal existed in both eyes of a patient. A unique case of persistent hyaloid artery was under my care at Moorfields about two years ago. It occurred in a lad about sixteen years of age. Arising from one of the arteries in the disk, was seen a small arterial twig running with a slight bend for a short distance into the vitreous humor, ending in a loop and passing over at once into a vein, which, twisting itself, like a corkscrew, three times round the artery, terminated in one of the large central veins. An excellent drawing of this case, made by Dr. Liebreich, will be found in the "Transactions of the Pathological Society," 1871, p. 232. Saemisch[6] has recently recorded a very interesting case in which the ophthalmoscope revealed in one eye the presence of a grayish-blue membrane in the vitreous humor, which was connected posteriorly with the retina in the immediate vicinity of the optic disk, veiling the upper third of the latter. More anteriorly, the membrane passed over into a narrow cylindrical canal, which, spreading out again a little, terminated near the posterior pole

---

[1] "Bericht über die Wiener Augenklinik," 114.
[2] "Kl. Monatsbl.," 1868, 259.
[3] Ibid., 1869, p. 210.
[4] Ibid., 106.
[5] Ibid., 1868, 349.
[6] Ibid., 1869, p. 304.

of the lens. Whilst the anterior portion was quite devoid of bloodvessels, the same was not the case with the posterior part, for on the pale-blue membrane near the retina vessels could be observed, which could be distinctly traced as passing directly over into those of the retina. This membrane was probably due to some arrest of development in connection with the hyaloid artery, and resembled closely a case reported by Becker.[1] [A case is also reported by Kipp, of a persistent fœtal artery in each eye. See "Archives of Ophthalmology," iii. 3, p. 190. Tumors occurring in the vitreous primarily, independent of morbid growths elsewhere in the eyeball, have not been reported, if we except a case of teleangiectatic granuloma reported by Vaalais in the "Archives de physiologie," Mai–Juin, 1880.—B.]

[1] "Kl. Monatsbl.," 1868, p. 354.

CHAPTER XI.

DISEASES OF THE RETINA.

1.—HYPERÆMIA OF THE RETINA.

WE may distinguish two forms of hyperæmia of the retina, viz., the arterial or active, and the venous or passive. The former is generally acute, and is characterized by the patient experiencing some symptoms of irritability in the eye, such as photophobia, lachrymation, subconjunctival redness, and an inability to continue for any length of time any work which necessitates a strong effort of the accommodation. There are often also subjective symptoms of an irritable state of the retina, such as flashes of light, etc. On examining the eye with the ophthalmoscope, we find that the optic disk is abnormally red and flushed, on account of the increased injection of the capillary twigs upon its surface. If this increased vascularity is very pronounced at the margin of the disk, its outline becomes somewhat ill-defined from its similarity in tint to the surrounding fundus. The size of the arteries may be slightly increased, and the smaller branches are more numerous and apparent, which is especially observable in the region of the yellow spot. The retinal veins are also somewhat dilated. According to Stellwag, more or less considerable portions of the fundus are rendered almost uniformly red by a very delicate and close-meshed network of vessels. It must always be remembered, that the degree of vascularity of the retina and optic disk varies much in different individuals, and in persons of different complexions. Thus, it is less marked in pale and anæmic individuals than in the florid and plethoric. If only one eye is affected, the appearances presented by it should always be compared with those of the other eye, as this will enable us more accurately to estimate the degree of vascularity of the retina, and guard us against an error in diagnosis.

Arterial hyperæmia of the retina is generally dependent upon causes which excite an increased vascularity of the eye; thus it may be artificially produced by the application of a drop of some astringent collyrium to the conjunctiva. It is often due to prolonged exposure to very bright light, more especially if the eyes are at the same time employed in some small and delicate work, as for instance in microscopizing, engraving, watchmaking, etc., by artificial light. It is also frequently met with in hypermetropic persons who work or read much without the assistance of glasses.

In the venous or passive form of hyperæmia, we notice that the retinal veins are abnormally large, dark, and perhaps tortuous, which is especially marked in the veinlets, which may present a somewhat spiral appearance. There is also either a spontaneous, or a very easily producible, venous pulsation. If the venous congestion has lasted some length of time, we frequently notice a slight œdematous condition of the retina round the optic disk, or along the course of some of the larger vessels, which appear to be fringed by a delicate grayish-blue opacity or halo. Care must be taken not greenish striæ. These were, however, only observable by a weak illumination, and in the direct mode of examination. The opacity shades off towards the periphery, gradually and imperceptibly, into the transparent normal retina, which not unfrequently remains quite unaffected. The serous infiltration is especially marked in the vicinity of the optic disk, but gradually diminishes in intensity towards the region of the yellow spot, on account of the decrease in the thickness of the retina at this point. Hence the choroid also shines through more distinctly here, and thus lends a redder tint to the macula lutea. Indeed this redness is sometimes so very striking, more especially on account of its contrast with the neighboring grayish opacity of the retina, that it might be readily mistaken for an effusion of blood. The periphery of the retina is often quite free from serous infiltration, and the details of the choroid can then be plainly distinguished at this point. The optic disk is always somewhat swollen and œdematous, and its outline indistinct and ill-defined, the choroidal and sclerotic margins being rendered unapparent by the serous infiltration.[1] The retinal arteries generally show but little alteration in their appearance, being, perhaps, only slightly veiled, and a little attenuated. The veins, on the other hand, are strikingly hyperæmic; they are large, dark, and tortuous, this tortuosity being especially marked in the smaller branches. On close examination, we may often notice that the vessels do not, throughout their whole course, lie always on the same level, but here and there dip a little into the effusion, or are pushed a little outwards (towards the vitreous) by it. In the former case, they will seem slightly indistinct and veiled; in the latter, the portion which is nearest to the observer will appear peculiarly dark and visible. These peculiarities are best distinguished with the binocular ophthalmoscope, or in the erect image. Sometimes, also, there are small extravasations of blood on or beside the vessels. The sight is always much affected, sometimes so considerably that the patient cannot distinguish the largest letters, or count fingers. The field of vision is also contracted, but if the peripheral portion of the retina is unaffected, the corresponding portion of the field will not be impaired. The first complaint of the patient is, generally, that he notices a gray film or veil before his eyes, which gradually increases in thickness and surrounds the various objects, hiding them more and more from the sight, until he becomes almost totally blind. With all this, the external appearance of the eye remains normal and healthy, excepting that the pupil generally becomes sluggish and somewhat dilated, but even this is not always very marked, and might be easily overlooked. There is no marked photophobia, lachrymation, ciliary injection, or intense pain; none of the symptoms, in short, which are still so often erroneously described as characteristic of inflammation of the retina, but which are not due to retinitis, but to hyperæsthesia of the

---

[1] Œdema of the retina is chiefly recognized with the ophthalmoscope by the great curves which the retinal veins describe, for, although the retina may be very considerably thickened by serous infiltration, it yet remains transparent, or only shows the faintest veil-like diffuse opacity. Hence œdema of the retina may easily be taken for a very slight detachment of the latter; indeed, it would be almost impossible to distinguish between these conditions; moreover, œdema of the retina may lead to detachment. Iwanoff describes (in a very interesting paper on "Œdema Retinæ," "A. f. O.," xv. 2, 88) the changes which the retina undergoes from these serous infiltrations, and shows how very large lacunæ are formed in it, leading to its becoming very considerably thickened. He found these lacunæ chiefly at the periphery of the retina, at the equator, and quite close to the optic nerve. Vide also a paper by Mr. Nettleship, "R. L. O. H. Rep.," viii. 3. [The dividing line between well-marked œdema of the retina and serous retinitis is very difficult, nay, well-nigh impossible to draw. The infiltration may be circumscribed or diffuse; may be marked in some places and nearly absent in others, and may not involve the optic disk at all.—B.]

retina—two perfectly different affections. We shall see hereafter to what grave errors in treatment a diagnosis of retinitis from these symptoms but too frequently leads. It must be particularly remembered, that in serous retinitis the ophthalmoscopic symptoms are never so marked and striking as might be expected from the great impairment of sight, the latter being probably chiefly due to the compression of the nerve elements by the serous effusion.

The *prognosis* should always be very guarded, because if the affection lasts for some time, the nerve elements of the retina may become atrophied, and the sight be permanently destroyed. Or again, this form may pass over into a more chronic inflammation, affecting chiefly the parenchyma of the retina, and giving rise, perhaps, to diseases of the choroid or of the vitreous humor. The danger of detachment of the retina must also be borne in mind.

The *treatment* should be chiefly directed towards relieving the congestion of the retinal vessels, and for this purpose local depletion by means of the artificial leech will be found most efficacious. The free action of the kidneys and skin should be maintained by saline diuretics and diaphoretics. A pair of dark-blue glasses should be worn, so as to protect the eyes against all glare and bright light. All employment of the eyes must be forbidden until they have quite recovered.

In the *parenchymatous* retinitis, the changes are not confined to a serous infiltration of the connective tissue, but this and the nerve elements of the retina undergo other inflammatory changes, such as proliferation of the cells, hypertrophy, sclerosis, and fatty or colloid degeneration. The sclerosis of the connective tissue may, according to Iwanoff,[1] be chiefly confined to the membrana limitans interna, or affect the basic connective tissue which pervades the retina in a vertical direction, and supports the other elements like a framework. On account of these various changes, the ophthalmoscopic appearances are far more marked and striking than in serous retinitis. [It is more correct to speak of this form of inflammation as neuro-retinitis, as the retina, from its anatomical relations to the optic nerve, is almost never involved alone. This interstitial neuro-retinitis is to be distinguished from the so-called neuro-retinitis descendens, or choked disk; it usually extends but a short distance into the optic nerve, and hence is a purely localized inflammation.—B.] The optic disk is opaque, swollen, somewhat hyperæmic, and of a reddish-gray color; its outline is irregular and indistinct, passing insensibly over into the retina, without any clear line of demarcation. The swelling is due to serous infiltration or inflammatory exudation, which may have extended from the retina to the optic nerve, or *vice versâ*. If the effusion is serous in character, the opacity will be of a pale, grayish-pink, or fawn color; but where there is much exudation of lymph, it will be more opaque, white, and perhaps somewhat glistening. If the exudation occupies the more external layers of the retina, the vessels may be observed to pass distinctly over it without any dipping; whereas, if it is situated in the inner layers of the retina, or quite on the surface of the disk, the vessels will be more or less interrupted and hidden by it. The retinal arteries are sometimes but slightly changed in appearance, in other cases they are more or less diminished in size, and rendered indistinct by the exudations. The veins are increased in size, darker in color, and their tortuosity is generally very marked.

---

[1] *Vide* Iwanoff's very interesting paper on "Retinitis," in the "Kl. Monatsblätter," 1864, 415, and also in the "Archiv f. Ophthalmologie," xi. 1, 136.

often arranged in bundles, and, if they increase very greatly in quantity, they may gradually compress and destroy the nerve fibres. The optic nerve fibres and ganglion cells may also undergo proliferation and sclerosis of their elements, and subsequently, perhaps, fatty degeneration. Another very interesting fact is, that in this form of retinitis the membrana limitans interna becomes thickened, and occasionally shows, at certain points, small excrescences which bulge into the vitreous humor. The latter is often affected, becoming hazy and pervaded by opacities, which are chiefly observable at its posterior portion. Detachment of the retina may also occur. This form of retinitis is very frequently associated with irido-cyclitis or irido-choroiditis, and then it generally commences at the peripheral portion of the retina, near the ora serrata, and extends towards the centre. When these inflammatory exudations are situated in the inner layers of the retina, we find that they are rather striated in appearance, and that the retinal vessels, instead of passing straight and uninterruptedly over them, are seen to dip into them here and there, becoming indistinct or even invisible at these points.

After the disease has lasted for some time, the exudations and hemorrhagic effusions may undergo absorption, the stasis in the circulation be relieved, the bloodvessels assume a more normal appearance, and the swelling and oedema in and around the optic disk subside, so that it regains a more sharply defined outline. The sight at the same time improves considerably, and this amelioration may become permanent. But the disease does not always run so favorable a course, for the nerve elements of the retina may have suffered so considerably as to render any improvement of the sight impossible. This may be due either to the inflammatory changes (sometimes even assuming a purulent character) which they have themselves undergone, or to the great hypertrophy and sclerosis of the connective tissue, which encroaches more and more upon the nerve elements, compresses them, and gradually leads to atrophy of the retina. If the optic nerve has been much implicated in the inflammatory process, the atrophic changes may also commence in it.

The coats of the bloodvessels often undergo sclerosis and fatty degeneration, becoming thickened, and the channel of the vessel perhaps narrowed. The bloodvessels then assume the appearance of whitish bands, with a small central red streak of blood flowing through them. As this change in the coats of the vessels may take place to a greater or less extent in all forms of retinitis, I do not think that it is desirable to make a special form of it, even in those instances in which it assumes a very considerable extent, affecting perhaps nearly all the retinal vessels, as in some rare and very exceptional cases, recorded by De Wecker,[1] Nagel,[2] and Iwanoff. The latter has proposed to call it "Perivascular retinitis." In the case mentioned by Nagel, all the retinal arteries and their branches in both eyes were changed into white bands, which, on closer examination, were observed to be pervaded by a central red line or blood current. Only very few of the small arterial twigs were of a red color. The veins, on the other hand, were normal in appearance, although somewhat narrow and irregular in calibre. At the periphery there were a few fine veinlets changed into white bands. On account of this white appearance of the bloodvessels, it might easily be supposed that they were bloodless, and the case be mistaken for one of embolism of the central artery of the retina. The difference between these two conditions may, however, be best distinguished, as has been shown by Liebreich,

[1] De Wecker, "Études Ophthalmologiques," 2d edit., ii. 318.
[2] "Klinische Monatsblätter," 1864, 394.

Blood extravasations of varying size and extent are strewn about on and around the bloodvessels in different portions of the retina, as well as on the optic disk and its vicinity. If these extravasations are situated in the inner portion of the retina, they will present a peculiarly striped or striated appearance, their edges being irregular; which is due to the radiating course of the optic nerve fibres, between which the blood is effused. If the hemorrhages occupy the more external layers of the retina, the effusions will be round, and have a smooth uniform appearance quite free from stria. [Interstitial neuro-retinitis may proceed from onset to termination without any hemorrhage. In this form of retinitis occurring in syphilitic patients, with or without a coexisting iritis, the occurrence of hemorrhages is a very rare exception. Where hemorrhages occur, they are usually the result of thrombosis of the veins.—B.] The exudations into the retina also vary much in size and appearance. Sometimes they look like small white or grayish-white dots, strewn about singly or in small clusters. In other cases they are larger, and form well-marked white patches or flakes of considerable size, the edges of which are perhaps fringed by the smaller dots. The color of these exudations varies from a grayish-white to a creamy tint, and they often have a peculiar glistening appearance, which is due to their containing fatty elements. They are met with in different parts of the retina, but especially in and around the optic disk, and in the region of the yellow spot.

Although I have used the term exudation for these patches in the retina, I must state that this is not always quite correct in the strict acceptation of the term, for they are often due to inflammatory changes in the connective tissue or nerve elements of the retina, giving rise to a proliferation of the cells and their contents, or they are caused by a degenerative metamorphosis of a fatty or colloid nature. But as it is difficult, and often quite impossible, to distinguish ophthalmoscopically between these different products, and as the term exudation has been generally accepted, I have thought it best to retain it.

When the exudations are situated in the external portion of the retina (in which case, they are generally due to proliferation of the cells, and fatty or colloid degeneration of the external granular layer with sclerosis of the membrana limitans externa; the bacillar layer becoming subsequently affected), we find that they afford the appearance of smooth, grayish-white or cream-colored, perhaps glistening patches, which do not show a striated arrangement, and are evidently situated beneath the retinal vessels, for the latter pass over them without dipping into them, or being interrupted or veiled in their course. We may at the same time often notice that the choroid in the vicinity of the exudations is undergoing certain inflammatory changes, which consist chiefly in a thinning of the epithelium and an absorption of its pigment, so that the choroidal vessels become more apparent. The stroma of the choroid also becomes affected, and it is now no longer a case of simple retinitis, but of choroido-retinitis. When the retinal exudations subsequently become absorbed, we find that extensive changes in the choroid have taken place beneath them. In such cases the inflammation, although apparently chiefly affecting the retina, often commences in the choroid, and extends thence to the retina.

The inflammatory changes may, however, be chiefly confined to the inner portion of the retina, giving rise at first to hypertrophy of the stroma, formation of nuclei in the layer of the optic nerve fibres, and neoplastic formations of connective tissue (Iwanoff).[1] These fibres of connective tissue are

---

[1] "A. f. O.," xi. 1, 189.

objects is mostly indistinct and hazy, the objects appearing to be shrouded in a mist or cloud. In other cases, the impairment of sight is very considerable.

The field of vision may, as far as extent is concerned, be normal, but the perception at the periphery is generally somewhat diminished, often, indeed, considerably so; there may also be gaps in the field, the situations of which correspond to those of the more extensive exudations in the retina.

A peculiar phenomenon is sometimes observed, as consequent upon inflammatory changes in the region of the yellow spot, either dependent upon retinitis or chorio-retinitis; I mean *micropsia*, so that objects appear smaller to the patient than they really are. If he be directed to copy or trace a given figure (such as a circle or quadrant), he will always draw it considerably smaller than it is in reality. The difference in the sizes of the image of the object in the two eyes (if only one is affected with micropsia) may also be estimated, as has been suggested, by holding a prism, with its base downwards, before the affected eye; this will cause its retinal image to lie a little below that of the other eye, and the patient can thus easily estimate their relative sizes. This micropsia is evidently due to the fact, that the position of some of the rods and cones is deranged by the inflammatory changes in the retina. Besides the diminution in the size of the objects, the patients often notice that horizontal lines, instead of appearing straight, seem bent and crooked; this is termed "metamorphopsia,"[1] and is due to an alteration in the position of the rods and cones, which may be caused by the presence and pressure of inflammatory products, or by shrinking and contraction of the retina.

3.—RETINITIS ALBUMINURICA (NEPHRITIC RETINITIS.
Plate III. Fig. 6).

As a certain form of inflammation of the retina is often m t with in Bright's disease of the kidney, and as it presents some special and characteristic symptoms, it has been designated "retinitis albuminurica." The peculiar grouping and localization of the pathological changes in the retina are mostly so marked and constant in this form of retinitis, that, as has been more especially pointed out by Liebreich, the presence of Bright's disease may be diagnosed with certainty by means of the ophthalmoscope alone. [In the light of our present knowledge on this subject, we cannot now speak with equal positiveness in this matter of diagnosis. The same variety of retinal exudation has been observed in certain chronic diseases of the general organism and of the brain and membranes, in which there was no renal disease of any kind, or at least none that could be detected by frequent and careful examinations. Another point to be remembered is that chronic nephritis almost always affects both eyes, though it may not be to the same degree, or exactly at the same time. But cases of this form of retinitis have been repeatedly observed confined exclusively to one eye. Hence it cannot now be said that "the presence of Bright's disease of the kidney may be diagnosed with certainty by means of the ophthalmoscope alone."—B.] At the outset of the disease this is not, however, the case, for then the appearances do not yet afford any special characteristics. The affection commences with a fulness in the retinal veins, which are dilated, darker in color, and more or less tortuous; whereas the arteries are either normal in appearance or but slightly narrower in calibre. The optic disk is hyperæmic, and this

---

[1] *Vide* Förster's very interesting paper upon this subject in his "Ophthalmologische Beiträge." Berlin, 1862.

is soon followed by a faint, bluish-gray, serous infiltration of the optic nerve and the retina in its vicinity. The outline of the disk then becomes somewhat veiled and indistinct, so that the choroidal and sclerotic rings are hidden from view, and the optic nerve appears to pass gradually over into the retina, without any sharply defined line of demarcation. The retinal vessels are also somewhat veiled, and covered by a pale bluish-gray film, which extends to some distance from the disk (perhaps three or four times its diameter), and hides the details of the subjacent choroid. The retinal hyperæmia may extend a considerable distance beyond this serous infiltration, and a few extravasations of blood are often noticed scattered about on different portions of the retina. As the disease advances, the symptoms of venous hyperæmia become much more marked, the veins look turgid, dark, and more tortuous, the veinlets assuming a corkscrew appearance. The arteries, on the other hand, are narrowed and more or less hidden by the infiltration. The optic disk becomes more swollen and infiltrated, and its outline gradually merged into the retina. The infiltration of the disk and of the retina is of a serous character, and gives to these parts a faint grayish-red or fawn-colored appearance, interspersed with delicate grayish-white striæ, which are due to sclerosis of the connective tissue and of the optic nerve fibres. The retinal vessels are frequently interrupted at various points of their course, by being covered and more or less hidden by the exudation. As a rule, the swelling and infiltration of the optic nerve are not very great in retinitis albuminurica; but we occasionally meet with cases in which the reverse obtains, and the disk assumes the peculiar appearance met with in optic neuritis. It is very prominent, swollen, and "woolly," and of a grayish-red and marked striated appearance, which is chiefly due to hypertrophy of the connective-tissue elements of the optic nerve. The outline of the disk is indistinct and irregular, and its bloodvessels more or less completely hidden by the infiltration. According to Liebreich, this form of optic neuritis may occur only in the later stages of nephritic retinitis, after extensive degenerative changes in the retina have existed for some length of time, or it may precede these, or even exist by itself.

Numerous extravasations of blood are noticed in different parts of the retina, and even on the optic disk. They vary much in size and shape, and lie chiefly in the internal layers of the retina, as is shown by their striated appearance, and the fact that they are situated on the same level as the retinal vessels, some of which may even be partly covered and hidden by them. The hemorrhages may, however, also occur in the external layers of the retina, or between the latter and the choroid. These blood extravasations into the retina are often very numerous, and of considerable size, a fact at which we cannot be surprised when we remember that the coats of the retinal vessels are frequently extensively diseased; that there is always a certain degree of stasis in the retinal circulation produced by the swelling of the optic nerve; and, finally, that there is mostly a more or less considerable disturbance in the general circulation, owing to the hypertrophy of the left ventricle, which is so frequently met with in Bright's disease. If the effusions of blood are very extensive, they may alter the appearance of the exudation very considerably, giving to it a dirty, yellowish-red tint.

As the disease of the retina progresses, we notice the appearance of small white spots or larger patches in different portions of the retina, at some little distance from the optic disk. These gradually increase in size, and, coalescing with each other, finally form a broad white mound or wall round the optic disk. The opacity extends especially towards the inner side of the retina, and somewhat further along the sides of the retinal vessels. This white mound does not reach close up to the optic disk, but is always separated from it by a broad zone of the faint gray or fawn-colored infiltration, in the centre of which can be indistinctly traced the outline of the disk. The peripheral portion of the mound is irregular, and broken up here and there into small circumscribed dots of exudation, which form a kind of fringe round the larger figure. In the region of the yellow spot we notice a very peculiar appearance, which, as was first pointed out by Liebreich, is especially characteristic of nephritic retinitis, viz., a collection of small, stellate, white, glistening figures, which look just as if they had been lightly splashed in with a small brush. Subsequently, if the exudation increases in size, these stellate spots may become merged into it, and this peculiar appearance be completely lost. The two ophthalmoscopic symptoms which are most characteristic of retinitis albuminurica are these bright stellate dots in the region of the yellow spot, and the broad glistening white mound which encircles the optic disk. [The term "stellate dots" conveys an erroneous idea. The masses of exudation are yellowish-white, vary very much in extent and prominence, are generally elongated, and are not stellate in shape. They are, however, arranged in a radiating or stellate manner around the macula lutea as a centre, the rays being generally longer towards the temporal side of the retina. They are usually accompanied by hemorrhages, and may even be covered by a large hemorrhage or several smaller ones, though there may be no hemorrhages throughout the entire course of the disease. Neither the general infiltration of the disk and retina, nor this peculiar exudation in the region of the yellow spot, is pathognomonic of chronic renal disease, but, when the two occur together, chronic desquamative nephritis is in the majority of cases the cause.—B.] But it must be stated that similar appearances, especially the stellate dots, may be met with in other forms of retinitis, more particularly in neuro-retinitis; with this difference, however, that the peculiar grouping of the ophthalmoscopic appearances is not the same. In a case of neuro-retinitis recorded by Von Graefe,[1] these peculiar white spots in the macula lutea were very evident, but, as he points out, such cases may be distinguished from nephritic retinitis by the following characteristics: (a) that the white spots due to degenerative changes in the retina (neuro-retinitis) are situated much closer to the optic disk; (b) that the swelling of the retina in the vicinity of the disk is more considerable; (c) that the swelling of the optic nerve is also more pronounced; and (d) that the veins are much more dilated and tortuous, which lends a far more red and vascular appearance to the optic entrance.

Retinitis albuminurica does not always manifest itself so characteristically; for the different symptoms above enumerated may assume considerably less prominence, or some of them may be altogether absent. Thus the optic disk, and the retina in its immediate vicinity, may appear almost normal, and there may be only a slight alteration in the retinal vessels, a few hemorrhagic effusions, and here and there white patches of exudation, lying either isolated or along the coats of the vessels. In the region of the yellow spot, these patches assume a streaky appearance (Mauthner).

Nephritic retinitis may become complicated with inflammatory changes in the choroid and vitreous humor, or with detachment of the retina. At a later stage, atrophy of the optic nerve and of the retina may close the scene.

In favorable cases, the serous infiltration, the effusion of blood, and certain of the white patches may subsequently become absorbed, so that the retinal is soon followed by a faint, bluish-gray, serous infiltration of the optic nerve and the retina in its vicinity. The outline of the disk then becomes somewhat veiled and indistinct, so that the choroidal and sclerotic rings are hidden from view, and the optic nerve appears to pass gradually over into the retina, without any sharply defined line of demarcation. The retinal vessels are also somewhat veiled, and covered by a pale bluish-gray film, which extends to some distance from the disk (perhaps three or four times its diameter), and hides the details of the subjacent choroid. The retinal hyperæmia may extend a considerable distance beyond this serous infiltration, and a few extravasations of blood are often noticed scattered about on different portions of the retina. As the disease advances, the symptoms of venous hyperæmia become much more marked, the veins look turgid, dark, and more tortuous, the veinlets assuming a corkscrew appearance. The arteries, on the other hand, are narrowed and more or less hidden by the infiltration. The optic disk becomes more swollen and infiltrated, and its outline gradually merged into the retina. The infiltration of the disk and of the retina is of a serous character, and gives to these parts a faint grayish-red or fawn-colored appearance, interspersed with delicate grayish-white striæ, which are due to sclerosis of the connective tissue and of the optic nerve fibres. The retinal vessels are frequently interrupted at various points of their course by being covered and more or less hidden by the exudation. As a rule, the swelling and infiltration of the optic nerve are not very great in retinitis albuminurica; but we occasionally meet with cases in which the reverse obtains, and the disk assumes the peculiar appearance met with in optic neuritis. It is very prominent, swollen, and "woolly," and of a grayish-red and marked striated appearance, which is chiefly due to hypertrophy of the connective-tissue elements of the optic nerve. The outline of the disk is indistinct and irregular, and its bloodvessels more or less completely hidden by the infiltration. According to Liebreich, this form of optic neuritis may occur only in the later stages of nephritic retinitis, after extensive degenerative changes in the retina have existed for some length of time, or it may precede these, or even exist by itself.

Numerous extravasations of blood are noticed in different parts of the retina, and even on the optic disk. They vary much in size and shape, and lie chiefly in the internal layers of the retina, as is shown by their striated appearance, and the fact that they are situated on the same level as the retinal vessels, some of which may even be partly covered and hidden by them. The hemorrhages may, however, also occur in the external layers of the retina, or between the latter and the choroid. These blood extravasations into the retina are often very numerous, and of considerable size, a fact at which we cannot be surprised when we remember that the coats of the retinal vessels are frequently extensively diseased; that there is always a certain degree of stasis in the retinal circulation produced by the swelling of the optic nerve; and, finally, that there is mostly a more or less considerable disturbance in the general circulation, owing to the hypertrophy of the left ventricle, which is so frequently met with in Bright's disease. If the effusions of blood are very extensive, they may alter the appearance of the exudation very considerably, giving to it a dirty, yellowish-red tint.

As the disease of the retina progresses, we notice the appearance of small white spots or larger patches in different portions of the retina, at some little distance from the optic disk. These gradually increase in size, and, coalescing with each other, finally form a broad white mound or wall round the optic disk. The opacity extends especially towards the inner side of the retina, and somewhat further along the sides of the retinal vessels. This white mound does not reach close up to the optic disk, but is always separated from it by a broad zone of the faint gray or fawn-colored infiltration, in the centre of which can be indistinctly traced the outline of the disk. The peripheral portion of the mound is irregular, and broken up here and there into small circumscribed dots of exudation, which form a kind of fringe round the larger figure. In the region of the yellow spot we notice a very peculiar appearance, which, as was first pointed out by Liebreich, is especially characteristic of nephritic retinitis, viz., a collection of small, stellate, white, glistening figures, which look just as if they had been lightly splashed in with a small brush. Subsequently, if the exudation increases in size, these stellate spots may become merged into it, and this peculiar appearance be completely lost. The two ophthalmoscopic symptoms which are most characteristic of retinitis albuminurica are these bright stellate dots in the region of the yellow spot, and the broad glistening white mound which encircles the optic disk. [The term "stellate dots" conveys an erroneous idea. The masses of exudation are yellowish-white, vary very much in extent and prominence, are generally elongated, and are not stellate in shape. They are, however, arranged in a radiating or stellate manner around the macula lutea as a centre, the rays being generally longer towards the temporal side of the retina. They are usually accompanied by hemorrhages, and may even be covered by a large hemorrhage or several smaller ones, though there may be no hemorrhages throughout the entire course of the disease. Neither the general infiltration of the disk and retina, nor this peculiar exudation in the region of the yellow spot, is pathognomonic of chronic renal disease, but, when the two occur together, chronic desquamative nephritis is in the majority of cases the cause.—B.] But it must be stated that similar appearances, especially the stellate dots, may be met with in other forms of retinitis, more particularly in neuro-retinitis; with this difference, however, that the peculiar grouping of the ophthalmoscopic appearances is not the same. In a case of neuro-retinitis recorded by Von Graefe,[1] these peculiar white spots in the macula lutea were very evident, but, as he points out, such cases may be distinguished from nephritic retinitis by the following characteristics: (a) that the white spots due to degenerative changes in the retina (neuro-retinitis) are situated much closer to the optic disk; (b) that the swelling of the retina in the vicinity of the disk is more considerable; (c) that the swelling of the optic nerve is also more pronounced; and (d) that the veins are much more dilated and tortuous, which lends a far more red and vascular appearance to the optic entrance.

Retinitis albuminurica does not always manifest itself so characteristically; for the different symptoms above enumerated may assume considerably less prominence, or some of them may be altogether absent. Thus the optic disk, and the retina in its immediate vicinity, may appear almost normal, and there may be only a slight alteration in the retinal vessels, a few hemorrhagic effusions, and here and there white patches of exudation, lying either isolated or along the coats of the vessels. In the region of the yellow spot, these patches assume a streaky appearance (Mauthner).

Nephritic retinitis may become complicated with inflammatory changes in the choroid and vitreous humor, or with detachment of the retina. At a later stage, atrophy of the optic nerve and of the retina may close the scene.

In favorable cases, the serous infiltration, the effusion of blood, and certain of the white patches may subsequently become absorbed, so that the retinal

[1] "A. f. O.," vi. 2.

of the retina, but upon uræmia. In the latter case, the at
startling suddenness, so that the patient may become perfa
a few minutes or hours, the recovery being as rapid. Mc
always present marked general symptoms of uræmic pa
intense headache, vertigo, loss of consciousness, sickness, e
sions, etc. The ophthalmoscopic symptoms in these cases of u
are, moreover, quite negative. But we may not unfrequent
and succession of symptoms of amblyopia dependent upon
upon uræmia. Thus nephritic retinitis has perhaps existed
advanced degree, for some time, giving rise to a certain amo
and suddenly the latter is greatly increased by an attack of t
has noticed the very rapid development of a high degree
in cases of uræmic amblyopia.

It was at one time supposed by some observers (especiall
the amblyopia is sometimes premonitory of, and precedes, t
kidney. But this is not so, the affection of the retina occt
nephritis (either acute or chronic) is already fully develope
later stages, more especially together with the small contra
is, however, also observed in the large flabby kidney.

Sometimes, indeed, the amblyopia is the only marked sy
tion of the kidney being unknown and unsuspected by th
medical adviser. In some of these cases there are, howe
derangement of the digestive functions, nausea, sickness, et
sulted as to the condition of the sight, the ophthalmos
symptoms of retinitis albuminurica, the urine is tested
then it is discovered that the patient is suffering from Brigl
affection of the retina attacks both eyes, either simultaneo
interval.

Hypertrophy and dilatation of the left ventricle are almc
with; indeed, in thirty-two cases Von Graefe found the
The frequent occurrence of extensive retinal hemorrhages
ably due to the disturbance in the circulation caused by
although it must also be remembered that the coats of the
often diseased. That nephritic retinitis may, however, occt
trophy, and dilatation of the left ventricle is proved by a
Mandelstamm and by Horner. The former[2] found that out
of retinitis albuminurica, hypertrophy of the left ventricle
in two. [The retinitis is sometimes complicated by suboon
rhages, and more rarely by extravasations into the capsule
exophthalmos. In these cases there is always a cardiac
possibly also a tendency to the hemorrhagic diathesis.
central retinal artery has been observed by Völckers in two

Great uncertainty still exists as to the connecting link l
tion of the kidney and that of the retina. The cause is ye
together with Bright's disease, we should so frequently m
form of retinitis, the ophthalmoscopic symptoms of whic
and peculiar, both in the grouping and localization, that fr
ance alone we are able to diagnose with certainty the p
minuria.

It has been supposed by some, that the inflammation an
the retina are due to an impairment of the nutrition of the

[1] Mooren, " Ophthalmiatrische Beobachtungen," 1867,
[2] Pagenstecher, " Klinische Beobachtungen," 1866, p.

upon the great amount of urea in the blood. By other observers (especially Traube[1]) it has been thought that the secondary increase in the tension of the aortic system forms the starting-point of the disease. In favor of the latter opinion, we must admit the extreme frequency of hypertrophy and dilatation of the left ventricle as an accompaniment of nephritic retinitis, as also the constant occurrence of more or less extensive extravasations of blood in the retina at the outset of the disease.

The prognosis as to the degree of sight that may be regained by the patient, must depend upon the extent to which the pathological changes in the retina have advanced, and still more upon the degree to which the nervous elements of the retina have suffered. [The fact that vision is very much improved, and even restored in some of these cases, proves that the nerve elements of the retina were but slightly injured, and that the violence of the inflammation was mainly in the connective-tissue elements of the retina. Vision may return to a very marked degree, while ophthalmoscopically the individual spots of exudation show little change, except that they have become more flattened.—B.] It has been already stated that many of the inflammatory products may become absorbed; thus the white patches due to fatty degeneration of the connective-tissue elements of the retina may disappear entirely, and the sight be completely restored. On the other hand, if there is sclerosis of the retinal nerve elements, we find that, even although the large white patches, the serous infiltration, and the blood extravasations become to a great extent absorbed, serious impairment of sight remains behind. Sometimes atrophy of the optic nerve may even ensue, especially if it has been much implicated in the inflammation. As a rule, however, nephritic retinitis leads only very exceptionally to complete blindness. In very rare instances, even very extensive detachments of the retina may entirely disappear if there is no elongation of the optic axis.[1]

There is no direct connection between the improvement in the sight and the absorption of the exudations, etc., and the amount of albumen in the urine, or the condition of the kidney disease; for the former may occur without any amelioration in the constitutional affection. The best prognosis is afforded by those cases in which the albuminuria occurs in advanced pregnancy, after scarlatina, typhoid fever, etc., for here we sometimes find that the pathological changes in the retina may disappear altogether, and the sight be entirely restored.

The treatment must be directed chiefly towards the primary disease. I have found most benefit from the use of tonics, more especially the tincture of the muriate of iron, citrate of quinine and steel. Free action of the skin should be encouraged and maintained. If symptoms of uræmic poisoning supervene, diaphoretics and purgatives should be freely administered. The only local application from which I have found any benefit is the artificial leech. In those cases in which it is unadvisable to abstract blood on account of the anæmic condition of the patient, I apply the dry cup to the temple, and have often seen this followed by marked improvement in the vision. It is to be repeated at intervals of five or six days.

4.—RETINITIS LEUCÆMICA.

Although Liebreich, as far back as 1861, described, and gave an illustration,[2] of a peculiar form of retinitis which sometimes occurs in leucocythemia,

[1] "Deutsche Klinik," 1859, p. 314.   [2] Vide "A. f. O.," xviii. 2, 108.
[3] Liebreich's "Atlas d'Ophthalmoscopie," plate x. Fig. 3.

Blood extravasations of varying size and extent are strewn about on and around the bloodvessels in different portions of the retina, as well as on the optic disk and its vicinity. If these extravasations are situated in the inner portion of the retina, they will present a peculiarly striped or striated appearance, their edges being irregular; which is due to the radiating course of the optic nerve fibres, between which the blood is effused. If the hemorrhages occupy the more external layers of the retina, the effusions will be round, and have a smooth uniform appearance quite free from striæ. [Interstitial neuro-retinitis may proceed from onset to termination without any hemorrhage. In this form of retinitis occurring in syphilitic patients, with or without a coexisting iritis, the occurrence of hemorrhages is a very rare exception. Where hemorrhages occur, they are usually the result of thrombosis of the veins.—B.] The exudations into the retina also vary much in size and appearance. Sometimes they look like small white or grayish-white dots, strewn about singly or in small clusters. In other cases they are larger, and form well-marked white patches or flakes of considerable size, the edges of which are perhaps fringed by the smaller dots. The color of these exudations varies from a grayish-white to a creamy tint, and they often have a peculiar glistening appearance, which is due to their containing fatty elements. They are met with in different parts of the retina, but especially in and around the optic disk, and in the region of the yellow spot.

Although I have used the term exudation for these patches in the retina, I must state that this is not always quite correct in the strict acceptation of the term, for they are often due to inflammatory changes in the connective tissue or nerve elements of the retina, giving rise to a proliferation of the cells and their contents, or they are caused by a degenerative metamorphosis of a fatty or colloid nature. But as it is difficult, and often quite impossible, to distinguish ophthalmoscopically between these different products, and as the term exudation has been generally accepted, I have thought it best to retain it.

When the exudations are situated in the external portion of the retina (in which case, they are generally due to proliferation of the cells, and fatty or colloid degeneration of the external granular layer with sclerosis of the membrana limitans externa; the bacillar layer becoming subsequently affected), we find that they afford the appearance of smooth, grayish-white or cream-colored, perhaps glistening patches, which do not show a striated arrangement, and are evidently situated beneath the retinal vessels, for the latter pass over them without dipping into them, or being interrupted or veiled in their course. We may at the same time often notice that the choroid in the vicinity of the exudations is undergoing certain inflammatory changes, which consist chiefly in a thinning of the epithelium and an absorption of its pigment, so that the choroidal vessels become more apparent. The stroma of the choroid also becomes affected, and it is now no longer a case of simple retinitis, but of choroido-retinitis. When the retinal exudations subsequently become absorbed, we find that extensive changes in the choroid have taken place beneath them. In such cases the inflammation, although apparently chiefly affecting the retina, often commences in the choroid, and extends thence to the retina.

The inflammatory changes may, however, be chiefly confined to the inner portion of the retina, giving rise at first to hypertrophy of the stroma, formation of nuclei in the layer of the optic nerve fibres, and neoplastic formations of connective tissue (Iwanoff).[1] These fibres of connective tissue are

[1] "A. f. O.," xi. 1, 139.

retinal vessels are apparently of about double the size of those of a normal eye, which Heyl thinks is due to the presence of molecular fat in the plasma of the blood, thus causing the full width of the vessel to appear. In leukæmia the veins appear unusually large, and the arteries very narrow. Heyl's explanation of the apparent size of the retinal vessels will not be accepted by all. (See "Trans. Amer. Ophthal. Soc.," 1880.)

In progressive pernicious anæmia, the retina is apt to be the seat of hemorrhages, with more or less pronounced inflammation. In this disease there is a diminution or destruction of the red-blood corpuscles, which is no doubt intimately connected with the hemorrhages. The retinal veins are greatly engorged; there are sometimes small white masses of infiltration. The hemorrhages are always extensive, and the fundus resembles that found in leukæmia and diabetes. The extravasations are in the inner layers of the retina, but there are sometimes hemorrhages between the retina and choroid. The disturbance of vision is very marked in most cases, but does not always occur. ("Graefe und Saemisch's Handb.," v. 8. 604.)

Uhthoff describes three sets of changes which he found in the retina in progressive pernicious anæmia. 1st. In all six cases there were hemorrhages into the different layers of the retina, and in a few spots the entire retina was filled by an extravasation, with more or less destruction of tissue. 2d. He found varicose hypertrophy of the non-medullary nerve fibres in the nerve-fibre layer of the retina. Some nerve fibres showed small varicosities of a finely granular appearance, and without any nucleus. Most of the hemorrhages occurred in the posterior pole of the eye. 3. There was a deposit of glistening colloid, and finely granular masses, of very varying form and size, in the middle granule layer of the retina. (See "Klinische Monatsblätter für Augenheilkunde," December, 1880.)—B.]

6.—RETINITIS SYPHILITICA.

A peculiar form of retinitis is sometimes met with in persons suffering from constitutional syphilis, and it is occasionally possible to diagnose the nature of the malady from the ophthalmoscopic appearances alone. It must be admitted, however, that the latter may in some cases be so slightly marked, that our diagnosis as to the syphilitic nature of the disease must chiefly depend upon the general history of the case, and upon the presence of other symptoms of constitutional syphilis. [Leber[1] thinks that every case of pronounced diffuse retinitis points very strongly to a syphilitic origin.

At the outset, there is simply hyperæmia of the optic disk and retina. The retinal veins are somewhat dilated, dark, and tortuous, but not markedly so, and the venous congestion diminishes as the disease progresses. Sometimes the venous hyperæmia is only partial. The retinal arteries are attenuated and diminished in size. The optic disk is slightly swollen, and its outline hazy and ill-defined. The disk, as well as the surrounding retina, is veiled by a faint bluish-gray film, which is due to a serous transudation of the optic nerve and retina. This film is often extremely delicate and faint, assuming perhaps only the appearance of an exaggeration of the physiological gray reflex which the retina of normal, darkly pigmented eyes presents. This uniform bluish-gray opacity does not extend regularly in all directions from the optic nerve, but is often principally developed in certain parts of the retina, and more especially along the course of the vessels,

[1] ["Kl. Monatsbl.," 1869, p. 610.—B.]

whence it shades off gradually and imperceptibly into the healthy retina. In the vicinity of the disk, the opacity is markedly striated. Although minute punctiform opacities generally occur in the region of the yellow spot, they are not so brightly glistening, or arranged in the peculiar stellate manner as those met with in nephritic retinitis, but are strewn about irregularly. They are, moreover, distinguished from these, by the fact that they undergo very rapid changes, perhaps disappearing and reappearing in the course of a few days, the sight at the same time undergoing corresponding fluctuations. The spots in Bright's disease are, on the other hand, very persistent, and their remains may often be distinctly traced even many months after the acute retinitis has passed away, and its residua alone remain, or atrophy of the disk has set in. We also in syphilitic retinitis sometimes meet with a peculiar tawny, reddish-brown tint in the region of the yellow spot.

The inflammatory changes in syphilitic retinitis consist chiefly in a serous infiltration of the retina, and sclerosis of the connective-tissue elements, more especially of the vertical trabecular fibres (stütz fasern), hence also the striated character of the opacity. The other portions of the retina are generally exempt from inflammatory and degenerative changes; but this is not always the case, and thus may arise a mixed form of syphilitic retinitis, in which the special and pathognomonic symptoms are accompanied, and perhaps somewhat masked, by other changes in the parenchyma, and great swelling of the optic nerve. Thus white spots or patches may be noticed in the retina. These may occur in small isolated patches, or in the form of large striped opacities situated in the innermost layers of the retina; their pressure perhaps causing complete emptiness of some of the vessels, which are changed into white bloodless bands (Liebreich). These, however, are never so brilliantly white as the spots met with in nephritic retinitis.

As a rule, retinal hemorrhages are not usually observed in syphilitic retinitis, or only to a very moderate extent. Sometimes, however, cases occur in which numerous and extensive extravasations of blood are noticed, which may be situated in different layers of the retina, and also between it and the choroid. Syphilitic retinitis is not unfrequently associated with inflammation of the choroid, and occasionally with irido-choroiditis, or iritis. If the symptoms of the inflammation of these tunics are very pronounced, the affection of the retina may be overlooked, more especially if the vitreous humor, as is often the case, is diffusely clouded and traversed by dark flakes, and the details of the fundus are thus rendered indistinct. Care must be taken not to mistake such an indistinctness of the optic disk and retina for that dependent upon retinitis, or to diagnose the presence of the latter simply from the great impairment of vision. A practised and careful ophthalmoscopist would not, however, fall into such errors of diagnosis.

Together with the symptoms of syphilitic retinitis, we often notice certain more or less extensive changes in the choroid. These may occur either in the vicinity of the retinal opacity, or at some distance from it, or be chiefly confined to the periphery of the fundus. These changes consist principally in a thinning and discoloration of the epithelial layer, the pigment cells of which are collected together into small masses, giving rise to more or less considerable groups of small gray dots intermixed with little black spots, which are aggregations of pigment cells. The latter may, perhaps, subsequently invade the retina (Liebreich). In other cases, the inflammatory changes affect the deeper portions of the choroid, and we then notice large gray patches in which the pigment cells of the epithelial layer and stroma of the choroid are absent, so that the choroidal vessels can be distinctly seen ; such patches being generally fringed by a dark zone of pigment.

Syphilitic retinitis generally occurs together with, or shortly after, the appearance of secondary symptoms, and is sometimes, as has already been stated, accompanied by inflammation of other tunics of the eye, such as choroiditis or irido-choroiditis. It may also be due to hereditary syphilis (Hutchinson). [It occurs in the proportion of about three or four in a thousand cases.—B.]

The course of the disease is generally slow, lasting many weeks or even months, and relapses are very apt to occur.

The sight often diminishes rapidly, so that in the course of a few days the patient may be only able to decipher No. 16 or 20 of Jäger, and may become greatly impaired, more especially if the region of the yellow spot is much affected. We find, also, that the condition of the sight fluctuates considerably with the presence or absence of the little punctiform opacities in the macula lutea. [Central scotomata sometimes occur in both eyes, and may be of considerable size, and there is usually qualitative light-perception through them. This scotoma may be annular in shape. The color-sense is at first normal, except in the scotoma ; but if retinal or nerve atrophy begin, color-blindness also appears. Subjective photopsic manifestations are sometimes complained of.—B.] Another interesting phenomenon is the frequency of micropsia in syphilitic retinitis. [This is explained by the fact that the rods and cones are separated more widely from each other, so that the image of an object meets a smaller number of sensitive elements than in the normal condition. Metamorphopsia for parallel lines is explained in the same way. —B. [The field of vision is often either not at all, or only slightly, impaired, but it frequently shows peculiar circumscribed zonular defects in the vicinity of the yellow spot, to which, as well as the frequent presence of photopsies, particular attention has been called by Mooren.

The prognosis of the disease is favorable, more especially if the patient is seen at a very early period of the attack. Although the sight may be considerably impaired, the inflammatory changes in the retina do not, as a rule, affect the nervous elements, but chiefly consist of a serous infiltration of the retina, and hypertrophy and sclerosis of the connective tissue. But if the latter is greatly hypertrophied, it will press upon the nerve elements, and may thus even lead to their atrophy. There is much tendency to relapses, either after the attack has entirely, or nearly completely, subsided, or as the disease is progressing towards recovery. By the recurrence of such relapses, the ultimate functional condition of the retina may, of course, be greatly endangered.

In treating syphilitic retinitis we must place our chief reliance upon mercury, for the greatest benefit is generally experienced from bringing the patient rapidly under its influence. This may be done either by its administration internally, or by inunction. I myself prefer the latter method, and generally prescribe from ʒss to ʒj of the ointment to be rubbed into the inside of the arms and thighs three times daily, and this mostly causes salivation in the course of a few days. If the patient has been recently salivated, a combination of iodide of potassium and bichloride of mercury should be given.

[In all cases of retinitis it is better to use atropia to prevent the ciliary muscle pulling on the choroid and thus indirectly on the retina. The patient should wear dark glasses.—B.]

As hyperæmia and congestion of the retina are generally not marked, the application of the artificial leech is not always indicated.

considerably; in some cases there is only a moderate degree of hyperæmia and serous infiltration, rendering the disk somewhat indistinct, and its outlines irregular; in others, the disk is of a deep red tint, and its margin so ill-defined, that it can only be distinguished from the surrounding retina by the emergence of the retinal vessels. The veins are dark, much dilated, and very tortuous, and along their course, more especially at their points of division, are seen numerous extravasations of blood. The arteries may retain their normal appearance, but generally become attenuated, and sometimes changed into white, bloodless bands. The extravasations of blood vary much in number, extent, and situation. They occur very frequently in the inner layer of the retina, and are then characterized by their peculiarly irregular and striated appearance, and also by the fact that they cover the bloodvessels more or less completely, or that the continuity of the latter is interrupted, the gap being occupied by the hemorrhage. The blood frequently makes its way from the optic nerve layer through the retina, the elements of which it pushes aside, to the outer layers, or even to the choroid, so that the hemorrhages may be situated in the more external portions of the retina, or between this and the choroid. In such cases, the effusions will be more sharply defined, uniform, and circular, and be distinctly situated beneath the retinal vessels. Effusions of blood into the retina always show more tendency to extend outwards towards the choroid, than inwards towards the vitreous humor, where the internal membrana limitans offers a stronger barrier to them. They may, however, break into the vitreous, and produce dense opacities. Sometimes, however, they extend along the inner surface of the retina, and then give rise to large, uniform, smooth-looking red patches, which completely cover and hide the vessels. The hemorrhagic effusions occur in different portions of the retina, and may be chiefly confined to the vicinity of the optic disk or yellow spot, or to the periphery of the fundus. Extravasations may also occur on the disk.

[Retinitis hemorrhagica must not be regarded as a distinct form of inflammation. All varieties of retinitis may be accompanied by hemorrhages, and, with the exception of the syphilitic, they generally are.—B.]

The effusions of blood retain their color for a very long time, more especially in old people, and then, breaking up, they either slowly undergo absorption, or become changed into a dark, crumbling mass (Liebreich). In the former case, they gradually assume a lighter, grayish tint, which, commencing at the edge of the extravasation, slowly extends to the whole, the blood being gradually absorbed. Sometimes these extravasations undergo fatty or pigmentary degeneration, in the latter case giving rise to more or less considerable black patches. The latter occurs sooner in blood effused into the vitreous, than when it is situated in the retina (Liebreich). The disease shows a great tendency to relapses, and in this is to be found one of its chief dangers, for if they occur frequently, or to a considerable extent, the function of the retina may be greatly impaired, and even atrophy of the optic nerve and retina ensue. The prognosis should therefore always be guarded, especially if the extravasations are numerous, and situated in the yellow spot. The sight is in some cases not very markedly affected, or not in a degree corresponding to the striking ophthalmoscopic appearances presented by the numerous and extensive hemorrhages. This depends entirely upon which part of the retina is the seat of the effusions. If the latter have occurred at the periphery, the sight may be quite unaffected; if in the yellow spot, it will be greatly impaired. Sometimes the attack is extremely sudden, a patient finding that in the course of a few moments, or on awakening in the morning, he has become absolutely blind. The patients at the same

time often experience a feeling of dizziness and fa
is not unfrequently somewhat contracted, and al
interruptions or gaps, or there may appear in it
which are in all probability due, as was pointed
shadows thrown by the blood extravasations up
the retina.

Occasionally we find that in the course of ret
of glaucoma supervene, the disease then consti
affection which has been termed "hemorrhagic
which has been given in the chapter on "Glauco

Retinitis apoplectica often occurs together with
circulation, which may be due to affections of th
thus it is not unfrequently seen together with
hypertrophy and dilatation of the left ventricle,
[extensive arterial sclerosis, and aneurisms of t
the large majority of cases hemorrhagic retinit
when cardiac or vascular lesions exist. Cardia
the same trouble in both eyes. Atheroma of the
a supposable lesion. Hence we must look to ar
emboli of the smaller branches of the central ret
appearances; but autopsies of such cases have no
if there exists any impediment to the venous effl
tumors, etc., pressing upon the optic nerve within
the cranium. In such cases, however, the blood
soon followed by œdema and inflammation of th
quent cause is fatty or atheromatous degeneratio
vessels, and it is consequently often met with i
cases it may be of prognostic importance, as it
vessels of the brain may also be degenerated, and
consequently be apprehended. The treatment
tempting to remove the cause, and preventing,
the disease. Diuretics and saline aperients, mor
are often of much benefit. Locally, the artificia

[Attention has of late been called to the s
retinal hemorrhages in young men. In these c
only in proportion to the opacity of the vitreo
blood. The hemorrhages are usually confined t
the retina, are almost always large, and of rou
ultimate result of these repeated extravasation
whitish patches of degeneration at the periphe
degeneration of the chorio-capillaris, and occa
of detachment of the retina. Eales attributes
stances to a neurosis affecting both the circul
leading on the one hand to partial inhibition of
the bowels, and to a vaso-motor contraction of t
canal; and, on the other hand, to a compensato
capillaries, especially those of the head, causing
system and capillaries of the retina with liability
of any intensifying cause, like coughing, laugh
"Ophthalmic Review," January, 1882.)—B.]

7.—RETINITIS PIGMENTOSA (Plate III., Fig. 5).

[Retinitis pigmentosa, or pigmentary degeneration of the retina, consists in a chronic interstitial connective-tissue proliferation of all the layers of the retina, with atrophy of the nerve elements and the development of pigment from a proliferation of the pigment epithelium.—B.]

This disease is principally characterized, as its name suggests, by the presence of pigment in the retina, which gives rise to a most peculiar and unmistakable appearance, more especially when the pigment is deposited in considerable quantity. In the latter case, we notice that the greater portion of the retina is covered by large black masses, which are arranged chiefly along the course of, and in close proximity to, the retinal vessels.

On close examination, we find that these black masses of pigment consist of circular or irregularly shaped spots, often with long narrow prolongations, which are likened to bone corpuscles; and of narrow black lines running along the side of a vessel or completely covering it. On account of the deposits of pigment along the coats of the vessels, the latter often appear, for a certain portion of their course, changed into fine black lines. At the division of the vessels, the pigment deposits assume a peculiarly characteristic stellate appearance. The pigment is sometimes deposited along the course of vessels which are still pervious and carry blood. For an illustration of the ophthalmoscopic appearances of retinitis pigmentosa, *vide* Plate III., Fig. 5.

These deposits of pigment always exist in the greatest number at the periphery of the fundus, where they first make their appearance, and whence they gradually extend towards the posterior pole of the eye, so that they form a more or less broad girdle, which encircles the central portion of the retina; but at a later period, the region of the yellow spot also becomes invaded by the disease. The pigment appears to be, as a rule, first developed at the inner (nasal) side of the retina; indeed, it always remains more extensive on this than on the temporal side. The retinal vessels undergo in this disease certain constant and marked changes, which evidently greatly influence the condition of hemeralopia and the contraction of the field of vision. These changes consist in a hyaline thickening of the coats of the retinal vessels, and a consequent diminution in their calibre; they, however, retain their transparency, and simply appear diminished in size, and this condition is consequently frequently described as being due to atrophy of the optic nerve. The smaller branches are often completely obliterated. Schweigger[1] has more especially pointed out this fact, and considers that the peculiar torpor of the retina, which is noticed when the illumination is moderate, is due to the fact, that on account of the diminution in the calibre of the arteries an insufficient amount of blood is supplied to the retina. At a later stage of the disease, atrophy of the optic nerve and of the retina almost always occurs. Changes in the choroid are also not unfrequently met with. These may be chiefly confined to a thinning and atrophy of the epithelium at certain points, so that the choroidal vessels become apparent, and are seen traversing these lighter patches, which are often fringed by a dark zone of pigment; or the stroma of the choroid may become affected, and, if it be much thinned, the white sclerotic may be seen glistening through it. In such cases, the fundus affords a very marked and striking appearance, being marbled with more or less extensive, reddish-gray, or grayish-white glistening

---

[1] "Vorlesungen über den Gebrauch des Augenspiegels," p. 117.

patches, in the expanse and at the edge of which are agglomerations of pigment. It is now no longer a case of simple retinitis pigmentosa, but of choroido-retinitis.

At a later stage of retinitis pigmentosa, we often find that an opacity makes its appearance at the posterior pole of the lens, which remains either stationary or is but very slowly progressive. The retinitis almost always affects both eyes. In rare instances, the vitreous humor also becomes affected, and small gray, circumscribed flakes are seen floating about in it. Externally the eyes present nothing abnormal, excepting that the pupil is generally small, and the anterior chamber somewhat shallow. [In a few instances defects of development, especially microphthalmos and coloboma of the iris or choroid, have complicated the disease in the retina, though the latter may have been acquired. In congenital retinitis pigmentosa, the eyes are apt to be small, and nystagmus is almost always present.—B.]

Great diversity of opinion still prevails as to the formation of the pigment, and whether it is primarily developed in the retina, or whether it makes its way into the latter from the choroid. Until several eyes, in which the typical form of retinitis pigmentosa has been diagnosed during life with the ophthalmoscope, have been submitted to careful microscopical examination, this cannot be decisively settled. At present, it appears certain that the disease may arise in both ways. Thus Donders found that the pigment may be developed in the retina itself, probably in consequence of a chronic inflammation of this membrane. That such may actually be the case, without any participation of the choroid, is also proved by a case of Schweigger's,[1] in which he found, on microscopical examination, that the deposit of pigment on the retinal vessels may occur quite independently of any changes in the choroid, for in this case the choroidal epithelium was perfectly normal, even in spots where the retina was pigmented. The pigmentation was confined to the retinal vessels, the coats of which were thickened and the smaller branches obliterated, these changes extending beyond the pigmentation. In those cases in which irregular roundish masses of pigment are strewn about the retina, Schweigger thinks that the disease is always due to choroiditis, and that the deposits of pigment partly become developed in the firm exudations which have forced their way into the retina from the choroid, or are due to the fact that the proliferating pigmentary epithelial cells of the choroid are floated into, or grow into the retina. Junge thinks that a deposit of pigment along the retinal vessels can only take place in the retina when the external layers are more or less destroyed, so that the pigment can make its way from the choroid into the retina. Dr. Landolt[2] believes that the disease is due to a very chronic perivasculitis of the retinal vessels.

There is, moreover, another way in which an infiltration of pigment from the choroid into the retina may occur, for an accurate knowledge of which we are chiefly indebted to the valuable researches of H. Müller and Pope.[3] It appears that a proliferation of the granular cells of the retina, similar to that in nephritic retinitis, may take place independently, accompanied by hypertrophy of the radiating connective-tissue fibres in the external granular layers, which become bent in an arcade-like manner. The bacillar layer of the retina becomes destroyed, and the hypertrophied granular layer protrudes above the external layer of the retina; between those protrusions there exist corresponding depressions, into which the pigment cells of the epithelial

[1] "Vorlesungen," p. 113.   [2] "A. f. O.," xviii. 1, 326.
[3] "Wurzb. Med. Zeitschrift," iii.; also "Roy. Lond. Oph. Hosp. Reports," iv. p. 76.

layer of the choroid become pushed and heaped up into little black masses, which lend a peculiarly marbled appearance to the retina. It is doubtful, however, as Schweigger points out, whether this morbid process yields the peculiar ophthalmoscopic appearances characteristic of retinitis pigmentosa.

Leber has quite recently had the opportunity of microscopically examining the eyes of a person affected with retinitis pigmentosa, which he had diagnosed during life with the ophthalmoscope.[1] He found the following changes: 1. Atrophy of the nervous elements of the retina, which was more complete in the external layers than in the nerve-fibre layer, and increased gradually from the centre to the periphery. 2. Hyperplasia of the connective-tissue framework of the retina, together with a neoplastic lamina of connective tissue on the inner surface of the nerve-fibre layer. 3. Thickening and sclerosis of the coats of the bloodvessels. 4. Reticulated pigmentation in all the layers, which follows especially the course of the bloodvessels. 5. Extensive changes in the pigment of the choroidal epithelium. 6. Very numerous excrescences on the elastic lamina. 7. Small, circumscribed exudations (which had undergone fatty degeneration) between the retina and choroid. He points out[2] the probability that the very great development of the excrescences (drüsen) of the elastic lamina (which has been observed in all cases of retinitis pigmentosa accompanied by changes in the pigment epithelium) plays a more important part in this disease than has been hitherto supposed. It may be assumed that their growth causes changes in the epithelial layer of the choroid, proliferation of its cells, and the disappearance or new formation of pigment. Moreover, the destruction of the bacillar layer of the retina, and perhaps even of a part of the external granular layer, might be produced by the same cause.

The earliest and most striking symptom of which the patients complain, is that of hemeralopia, or night-blindness [which may last for years before the limitation of the visual field becomes marked.—B.]. During the day, or in a bright illumination, they may be able to see perfectly well, but as soon as it becomes dark, or they are taken into a dimly lighted room, their sight becomes greatly impaired. I need hardly point out that this peculiar impairment of vision is quite independent of the fact whether it be night or day, and is simply due to the retina being in a condition of torpor, which demands a very bright illumination in order to enable it to distinguish objects which a healthy eye could see with ease even by a moderate amount of illumination. This torpor of the retina is in all probability not due to the pigmentation of the retina, but, as Schweigger insists, to the obliteration of the retinal vessels or to the diminution of their calibre through a hyaline thickening of their coats, so that the retina receives only a diminished and insufficient supply of blood. The truth of this opinion is proved by the fact that Schweigger has noticed the presence of hemeralopia and contraction of the field of vision in children before the appearance of any pigment in the retina; but in all these cases there was a marked contraction of the retinal arteries, whilst the older brothers and sisters had retinitis pigmentosa. He also observed this, in some rare instances, in older persons (between the ages of forty and fifty), who suffered from all the symptoms of retinitis pigmentosa, e. g., hemeralopia from torpor of the retina, great contraction of the visual field, without any trace of pigmentation of the retina or any other symptom except contraction of the arteries and paleness of the disk. In

[1] "A. f. O.," xv. 3, 1 [Graefe u. Saemisch, "Hand. der Augenheilk.," v. p. 638 et seq.—B.].
[2] "A. f. O.," xv. 3, p. 21.

similar cases, Von Graefe has subsequently found a deposit of pigment in the retina.

Although central vision may be excellent, enabling the patient to read the finest type, the field of vision is often so very greatly contracted that but a few inches' area is left, thus rendering the patient almost blind for eccentric objects, and giving him an awkward and restless appearance in his efforts to keep from stumbling and falling. Such patients therefore experience great difficulty in crossing a street or in passing along a crowded thoroughfare, as, although they may see well straight before them, they cannot distinguish that which lies in the lateral parts of the field. [In rare cases, in place of the concentric limitation, there is an annular defect in the visual field. In very rare cases we meet with a central scotoma without any other limitation of the field. The limitation of the field in all cases is due to destruction of the layer of rods and cones, as proved by Leber and Landolt. The condition of the color-sense varies very much.—B.] Even in very high degrees of typical retinitis pigmentosa, Leber has found the appreciation of color normal in the central portion of the retina. But in the mixed forms, in which central vision is greatly impaired at an early stage of the disease, the color-blindness was often very marked.

As long as the region of the yellow spot is not attacked the sight may remain good; but between the ages of thirty-five and fifty the disease almost invariably leads to complete blindness, the retina and optic nerve becoming atrophied. The disease, as already stated, generally attacks both eyes. Pedraglia mentions a case in which it affected only one eye, and I have also met with one among my patients at Moorfields. The affection is frequently congenital and also hereditary. [The congenital form is peculiar in that the pigment is not present at birth, but appears during the first year. This disease may cause congenital blindness from atrophy of the retina or of the optic nerve. In rare cases hemeralopia may be a congenital symptom, without limitation of the field. Acquired retinitis pigmentosa is often also hereditary. —B.] Although it may be present at birth, it always slowly and gradually increases in extent with advancing years. Schweigger has noticed that pigmentation of the retina is not only preceded by contraction of the arteries, but also by small light-colored dots or faint stripes in the choroid, which are closely strewn about the periphery of the fundus; they may be isolated, or coalesce and form larger spots.

The description which I have given here is that of typical retinitis pigmentosa. But we occasionally meet with cases which show marked anomalies in their course: e. g., the impairment of the sight may be typical, but the ophthalmoscopic appearance anomalous, and vice versâ; or again, both the impairment of vision and the ophthalmoscopic appearances may be anomalous, this being especially observed in certain cases of congenital amblyopia and amaurosis. (For further information, see a paper by Leber on "Anomalous Forms of Retinitis Pigmentosa," "Arch. f. Ophth.," xvii. 1, p. 314.) In regard to the spots occasionally observed in the choroid, similar appearances, according to Leber, are observed directly after birth and during the earliest years of infancy in cases of congenital amaurosis or amblyopia, in which symptoms of retinitis pigmentosa afterwards supervene. He thinks that these pale, punctiform spots are probably due to the excrescences of the elastic lamina. (See "Arch. f. Ophth.," xv. 3, p. 23.)

[Etiology.—In the great majority of cases the cause is unknown, but in a small proportion of cases, syphilis seems to be the cause.—B.] The disease may first show itself about the age of eight or ten, or even later in life, at thirty or forty. It frequently occurs in several members of the same family, and is then often hereditary. Such cases are mentioned amongst others by Laurence, Mooren, and Hutchinson. Laurence[1] met with it in four members of the same family (of eight); in this case it was not hereditary. Mooren has also seen it in four persons of the same family. Liebreich has pointed out the important fact that it occurs very frequently in marriages of consanguinity, and often together with deaf-mutism. Other malformations, such as supernumerary fingers and toes, are also sometimes seen, together with retinitis pigmentosa. [According to Leber it also occurs with congenital or acquired defects in the nervous system, as idiocy and melancholia. Direct heredity is not a common cause, as Leber found it only once in sixty-six cases of the disease. About three-fourths of all the cases occur in men. Some authors, as Perrin and Mauthner, are inclined to consider long residence in hot climates a cause. Liebreich asserts that the disease occurs very frequently among the Jews, and attributes it to the great frequency of consanguineous marriage among them.—B.]

The *prognosis* is of course very unfavorable, as these cases always end sooner or later in total blindness. With regard to *treatment*, I can only recommend care of the eyes, more especially against bright glare and over-work, and attention to the general health. Occasionally some temporary improvement of the central vision has taken place after the application of the artificial leech, and the administration of the bichloride of mercury, iodide of potassium [iron and strychnia], etc.; but it has been noticed that this improvement has been followed by a marked and rapid deterioration of the field of vision (Mooren). [Graefe und Saemisch, "Handb. der Augen-heil.," v. S. 658, 659.]

[8.—RETINAL DISEASE IN DIABETES.

The form of lesion in the retina is not always the same. In many cases hemorrhages only are present; in others, in addition to the hemorrhages, there appear white masses of exudation; in others, diffuse hemorrhagic retinitis with exudations strongly resembling the picture of nephritic retinitis. The white spots of exudation are never very large, and do not coalesce. The retinitis is sometimes followed by atrophy of the optic nerve. Opacities of the vitreous are very common, and are probably of hemorrhagic origin. Iritis and hemorrhagic glaucoma are rare complications.

Lesions of the retina are by no means invariable symptoms in diabetes. The prognosis is doubtful or unfavorable. The treatment is solely that of the constitutional disease.

In oxaluria, certain changes have been reported as occurring in the retina, which are probably the remains of hemorrhages ("Graefe u. Saemisch, Handb. der Augenheilk.," v. pp. 593-598). In diseases of the liver accompanied by jaundice, hemorrhages are said to occur in the retina, with degeneration of the granule layers into opalescent bodies, but without any marked disturbance of vision during life.—B.]

[1] "Ophthalmic Review," ii. p. 82.

9.—DETACHMENT OF THE RETINA (Plate V., Fig. 10).

If the detachment of the retina from the choroid is very extensive and reaches far into the vitreous humor, the symptoms presented by it are so marked and characteristic that it may sometimes be recognised with the naked eye, but certainly with the greatest ease by the aid of the ophthalmoscope. On examining in the direct method an eye affected with an extensive detachment of the lower half of the retina, we at once notice that, when the eye is moved in different directions, we see the usual bright-red reflex from the upper part of the fundus, but that in the lower half this is not the case. Here, on the other hand, the reflex has a bluish-gray or greenish tint, and on closer inspection we observe a bluish-gray, floating, wave-like opacity, which is thrown into marked undulating folds with every movement of the eye, and which is traversed by dark, crooked, and distorted vessels. On account of the bulging forward of the detached retina into the vitreous, these details can be readily seen with the direct examination at some little distance from the eye. The detached retina also reflects the light very strongly, which is chiefly due to the difference between the color and refracting power of the fluid situated between the retina and choroid and those of the vitreous humor. The minute details may be examined either in the upright or reverse image, and the extent of the detachment, as well as the course and displacement of the vessels, should be carefully studied. It will be noticed that the vessels are darker than on the normal retina, and that they are very crooked and tortuous, riding, so to speak, on the folds of the retina, between which they may even be completely hidden for a part of their course. They, as well as the undulating gray folds of retina, quiver and tremble with every movement of the eye. On tracing out the limits of the detached portion, we generally find that, even beyond its marked commencement, there is a faint grayish opacity or thickened appearance of the retina, and that the vessels are somewhat darker, and show a slight tendency to be curved. This opacity of the retina is due to serous infiltration. If the detached fold of retina is large and prominent, it throws a distinct dark line of shadow upon the neighboring fundus.

Whilst little or no difficulty can be experienced in recognizing a considerable detachment of the retina, the same cannot always be said of the slighter degrees, the diagnosis of which often demands considerable dexterity and experience on the part of the observer. This is more especially the case if the subretinal fluid is transparent, and the vitreous humor is somewhat clouded. [The condition of the vitreous is of great importance in these cases. Anything which lessens the intra-ocular tension would render a detachment more easy. This would naturally occur after a diminution of the volume of the vitreous in consequence of connective-tissue degeneration and shrinking.—B.] Sometimes, it is only by tracing out most carefully and with the greatest exactitude, the course of each individual retinal vessel from the optic disk towards the periphery of the fundus, that we are enabled to detect a very slight degree of detachment. In such a case, we notice that as the vessels reach the detached portion (which is generally somewhat opaque and thickened, or thrown into a slight fold), they assume a darker tint, and instead of preserving a straight course, they become tortuous and bent, forming a more or less marked deflection.

On close examination, we also notice that the vessels lie on a different level to those which retain their normal position, being closer to the observer, who has consequently slightly to alter his accommodation in order to obtain as distinct an image of them. Indeed, the appreciation of this difference in the plane of the vessels is one of the most delicate aids in the diagnosis of commencing detachment of the retina. We can, moreover, detect a well-marked parallax; for if we make a lateral movement with the object lens, the portion of the vessel which is elevated by the detached retina, will be seen to make a greater movement than that part which lies in the normal retina. The detached portion of retina also reflects the light more strongly, which is especially appreciable in the direct examination.

On tracing the course of the vessels further, we often find that as we approach the periphery of the fundus, the detachment becomes more conspicuous and extensive, the retina being, perhaps, thrown into distinct whitish-gray folds near the equator of the eye. In the portion of retina which is still *in situ* and in close proximity to the detachment, we may sometimes notice small, reddish-white exudations, and also, as was especially pointed out by Von Graefe,[1] small red, isolated patches, which are made up of minutely coiled bloodvessels. Small partial detachments of the retina are often difficult to recognize, as they may simply appear in the form of little, faint, gray streaks. The details are best appreciated with the binocular ophthalmoscope. The color of the detachment depends chiefly upon that of the fluid which lies beneath it; at first, the detached portion of the retina is generally transparent, but at a later period it becomes more or less opaque and clouded. This may, however, be the case from the commencement, if the detachment supervenes upon inflammation of the retina. The subretinal fluid also varies considerably in composition. When recent, it is transparent, or of a faint straw color, and of a serous nature, containing a good deal of albumen (Bowman),[2] which coagulates on exposure to heat, or may even do so in the eye, and then it becomes adherent to the walls of the detached retina in the form of opaque flakes (Liebreich). It may also contain blood, fibrin, nuclei, pigment and fat molecules, or cholesterine.

The detachment most frequently occupies the lower portion of the fundus, and its extent varies considerably. It may for some time remain confined to the periphery of the fundus, and then gradually extend further and further, until it reaches the optic nerve, and thus involves the whole of the lower half of the retina. It often, also, mounts up somewhat on one or both sides of the disk. When the detachment occurs in the upper portion of the retina, it soon extends downwards, which is due to the gravitation of the fluid, and in such a case the greater portion of the retina may become detached all round the optic disk, forming a funnel-shaped detachment, the apex of which is at the optic nerve. But we may sometimes also observe that, as the fluid gravitates downwards, the upper portions of the retina fall again into apposition with the choroid, regaining perhaps a considerable or even normal degree of transparency; this being, moreover, accompanied by a great improvement of vision. This, I may state, in passing, is a most important point with regard to the indications of treatment. [The detached retina shows signs of diffuse inflammation with interstitial connective-tissue hypertrophy, or there may be cystic degeneration of the various layers.

When the retina is entirely detached, as is not unfrequently the case after long-continued intra-ocular inflammation, especially of the ciliary body, there is no reflex from the fundus, and hence no ophthalmoscopic image. Usually in these cases the retina has one point of attachment behind at the optic disk, and anteriorly is adherent all round to the ciliary processes,

---

[1] "A. f. O.," I. 1, 367.
[2] Bowman, "Royal London Ophthalmic Hospital Reports," vol. iv. p. 136. 1864.

though this is not always the case. It is greatly thickened, thrown into folds, very hyperæmic, and sometimes contains hemorrhages.—B.]

Sometimes, if the retina has been tensely stretched by the fluid beneath it, a rent may occur in it, and we can then observe with the ophthalmoscope that there exists a gap, within which the vessels and intra-vascular spaces of the choroid are distinctly apparent;[1] the edges of the torn retina being curled or rolled up into little folds.

The first symptom which the patient generally notices is that of a faint gray cloud floating before him, or of a dark spot, surrounded by a lighter halo. This cloud has a wavy, indistinct outline, and its position in the field of vision corresponds accurately with the situation of the detached portion of retina. Thus, if the detachment be situated at the lower part of the retina, the patient notices a little cloud or curtain hanging down into the upper part of the visual field, like the edge of a veil, or peak of a cap. He also notices that linear objects, instead of preserving a straight outline, appear to be wavy and broken. This metamorphopsia is probably due to a change in the normal position of the nerve elements of the retina in the close vicinity of the detachment, this displacement being, perhaps, caused by a slight dragging upon that portion of the retina which is no longer in situ. Knapp[2] points out that the metamorphopsia due to detachment of the retina, is distinguished by the fact that the objects are fringed with a colored ring, and undergo slight undulating movements. Sometimes, this metamorphopsia is the principal symptom which leads us to detect a small circumscribed detachment of the retina. The patients also often complain of bright flashes of light, bright circles, or stars, etc., these photopsies being due to the irritation and stretching of the retina produced by the change in its position. The black spots and flakes which float about in the field of vision, assuming various peculiar forms, are caused by opacities in the vitreous humor, which are very frequently met with in detachment of the retina, and may even be the cause of it. [Chromatopsia in the region of the detached retina is also complained of by patients: some speaking of a blood-red appearance, others of a dark violet or intense blue.

The detachment generally occurs suddenly, though it may be preceded by floating vitreous opacities, especially in myopic eyes. In some cases, oftener than has hitherto been supposed, the retina becomes reapplied to the choroid without spontaneous perforation, and remains permanently attached. The detachment sometimes complicates a retinitis albuminurica or an orbital abscess, and the prognosis is here more favorable for its reattachment. Sometimes after a detachment has existed for some time, signs of irido-cyclitis appear which usher in a phthisis bulbi. Another complication of chronic detachment is cataract, of somewhat rapid development and soft consistence.—B.]

On examining the field of vision, we find a more or less marked impairment and contraction of certain portions of it, which correspond to the situation of the detachment. Thus, if the latter has occurred below, the upper portion of the field will be impaired, and vice versâ. If the detachment is very irregular in its outline, the field presents corresponding irregularities, the outline of the defective portion rising and falling according to the rise and fall of the detachment. We find that the field of vision is contracted not only quantitatively, but also qualitatively; although there is no doubt that the retina, even when actually raised from the choroid by fluid,

---

[1] Vide Liebreich's "Atlas," Plate VII., Fig. 1.
[2] "Klinische Monatsblätter," 1864, p. 807.

may retain a certain degree of perceptive power, the patient being able to tell the movements of the hand or even to count fingers.

The indistinctness or contraction of a certain portion of the visual field is also seen occasionally to precede the detachment of the retina, and is, therefore, of great prognostic importance. Thus, in cases of extensive sclerectasia posterior, we may sometimes detect a marked contraction of the field in a certain direction (say upwards, or upwards and inwards), but the most careful and accurate ophthalmoscopic examination will fail to discover any detachment. But some time afterwards this may occur, and at a point of the retina corresponding to that portion of the field which was defective.

Etiology.—The causes of detachment are numerous, and sometimes obscure. It may be produced by blows upon the eye, or by penetrating wounds of the posterior portion of the eyeball, in which case there is often a cicatricial contraction of the retina; also by effusions of blood or serum beneath the retina and choroid. In such cases, the hemorrhage generally occurs from the choroid, on account of the greater vascularity of this membrane. When speaking of hemorrhage into the vitreous humor (p. 494), it was mentioned that when the bleeding occurs in the central portion of the fundus, it is prone to lead to detachment of the retina; whereas, in the equatorial region it is more apt to break through into the vitreous humor. But hemorrhage from the retina itself, by making its way outwards between the choroid and retina, may lead to a detachment of the latter.

The serous effusion between the retina and choroid which produces the detachment, may be the product of inflammatory lesions of these tunics, or may be due to a sudden compression of the vessels of the eye and an impediment to the venous reflux, as, for instance, in cases of exophthalmos due to intra-orbital tumors, etc.

[According to Iwanoff[1] œdema of the retina may easily produce detachment of the latter; the serosity of the lacunæ perhaps first separating the retina into two laminæ; and then detaching it.—B.]

The most frequent cause is undoubtedly an elongation of the optic axis, as in cases of sclerectasia posterior, for the elongation of the sclerotic is accompanied by a corresponding stretching of the choroid and retina. The former, on account of its firm union with the sclerotic, and its greater elasticity, follows this gradual distention, but the retina is less elastic, and will, therefore, have a greater difficulty in following the traction of the sclerotic and choroid; its connection with the latter will be rendered lax, and any slight effusion or exudation from the choroid will suffice to produce an extensive detachment. Such effusions are the more likely to occur in these advanced cases of sclerectasia posterior, as there is generally some choroiditis present, or a disturbance of the intra-ocular circulation.

[Another cause for retinal detachment is found in chronic inflammation of the choroid or retina, and in cystic degeneration of the latter.—B.]

A cysticercus, making its way through into the vitreous humor, may give rise to a considerable detachment of the retina, which will be tense, and not undulating or falling into folds. It may also be produced by a tumor springing from the choroid, and here the early diagnosis of the cause of the detachment is of much consequence. This may be difficult when the tumor is small, as the detachment may then be loose and undulating; whereas, when it increases in size, and protrudes more into the vitreous humor, the retina may be stretched tensely over it, and not fall into wrinkles or folds; or distinct nodules, perhaps of a dark, pigmented appearance, are seen stretching

[1 " A. f. O.," xv. 11, 103.]

out the detached retina here and there. The diagnosis of a tumor is still more strengthened, if, with the increase in the size of these nodules, the eye-tension progressively augments (Von Graefe).[1] Indeed, the tension of the eyeball is of great importance in the differential diagnosis between a simple detachment of the retina, and one produced by a subretinal tumor. In the former case, the eye-tension is almost always decidedly diminished; whereas, the reverse obtains in cases of intra-ocular tumor, the tension being either normal, or markedly augmented as the growth advances. Bowman[2] has, however, in a few rare instances met with a tendency to increased tension in cases of simple detachment of the retina.

The retina may be, by traction, also detached in front, through the contraction and shrivelling up of opacities in the vitreous humor, which are by one extremity attached to the retina. In contracting, they draw the latter from the choroid, its connection with which is often already but very slight, as, for instance, in cases of sclerectasia posterior.

The *prognosis* of detachment of the retina is unfavorable. In some very rare instances the disease may remain stationary at an early stage, and whilst the detachment is still but inconsiderable. Or the detachment may even disappear, the subretinal fluid having become absorbed, or penetrated into the vitreous humor after a spontaneous rupture of the retina. In such cases, the retina is reapplied to the choroid, and may regain its functions, even after the detachment has lasted for some time, for the rods and bulbs retain their anatomical characters for a long time. Such cases are, however, very rare. One is described by Von Graefe, in which the detachment occurred in consequence of an orbital abscess, and where, after the escape of the discharge, the retina became reattached to the choroid, and the sight restored.[3] A similar case is recorded by Dr. Berlin.[4]

Mr. Bowman has also mentioned a case to me, in which he has observed the total spontaneous disappearance of a considerable detachment. Other cases have been narrated by Liebreich, Galezowski, Steffan, etc. [Cases have also been reported in this country of spontaneous recovery, both before any treatment had been undertaken and after all treatment had failed. The editor has seen several, notably, one of total detachment in one eye and partial in the other, in a young man of twenty, in whom the retina became almost entirely reattached in the worse eye, and partially in the other, after all treatment, except puncture, had proved futile. The patient was discharged from observation.—B.]

But in the great majority of cases the natural course of the disease is slowly but surely progressive, leading finally to total blindness, sometimes in consequence of irido-choroiditis and atrophy of the globe. Although the detachment generally remains confined to one eye, it may extend to the other, and this is to be especially feared, if the same cause exists in the latter, e. g., extensive sclerectasia.

Until the last few years, the treatment has been entirely directed towards endeavoring to procure the absorption of the subretinal fluid, or to prevent and retard the progress of the detachment. The chief remedies that were employed for this purpose were derivatives, mercury, the application of the artificial leech, etc.; the patients being at the same time strictly ordered to abstain from all employment necessitating any prolonged effort of the accommodation, or that might produce congestion of the eye or head. The results, however, of this mode of treatment were not favorable, and only in

[1] "Arch. f. Ophth.," xii. 2, 289.
[2] "Klin. Monatsblätter.," 1868, p. 49.
[3] "R. L. O. H. Reports," iv. 184.
[4] Ibid., 1866, p. 77.

very rare instances did the detachment disappear. I must confess that I have never succeeded in achieving this result by medicinal means, although I have been sometimes able to retard the progress of the disease by suitable treatment, together with complete rest of the eyes, and the occasional and guarded application of the artificial leech. The latter should, however, be employed with extreme care, as its application is always followed by a certain degree of intra-ocular hyperæmia, which might easily tend to increase the detachment. For this reason, I often prefer dry cupping at the temple or the back of the neck, more especially in those cases in which hyperæmia might prove particularly dangerous, e. g., sclerectasia posterior accompanied by marked symptoms of congestion and vascular excitement. [Diasoux thinks very highly of the methodical hypodermic injection of nitrate of pilocarpine as a curative agent, and says that even its tardy use may be advantageous. All the cases in which he has employed it were favorably affected before the tenth injection. He regards the drug as a special derivative for the eye. (See "Archives d'ophthalmologie," Nov.-Dec., 1880.)—B.]

The fact that the absorption or gravitation of the subretinal fluid, or its escape into the vitreous after spontaneous rupture of the retina, is followed by a marked return of sensibility in the reattached retina, has led some of the most distinguished ophthalmologists, especially Bowman and Von Graefe, to endeavor to gain a similar favorable result by operative treatment, by dividing the retina and permitting the fluid to escape into the vitreous humor.

Von Graefe,[1] in order to gain this end, divided the retina with a peculiar cutting needle having two sharp edges. The eye being steadied with a pair of forceps, the needle is entered in the sclerotic about four or five lines from the edge of the cornea, and in the meridian corresponding to the most prominent part of the detachment, and if the situation of the latter permits it, the puncture should be made in the outer hemisphere. The needle should be passed perpendicularly behind the lens into the vitreous chamber for about six lines, and then, the apex being turned, by a simple lever movement towards the fundus, the one edge is to be pressed against the retina. This movement is to be continued whilst the needle is simultaneously withdrawn. By the latter retracting incision, the continuity of the prominent retina is to be divided. Care must be taken not to bring the point of the needle in contact with the choroid.

[This operation of puncture or laceration of the retina has proved by no means so successful in the hands of other surgeons. Though there is rarely any grave reaction, the improvement in most cases has been but moderate, and a permanent cure has been very rarely reported.—B.]

Mr. Bowman states that his object in operating in detachment of the retina "has never been to give external vent to fluid, though this has almost always been one immediate effect of my punctures, but rather to open a permanent communication inwards from the subretinal space, under the idea of allowing the effused fluid to escape into the vitreous chamber, rather than to spread further between the retina and choroid, thereby further severing their organic connection. So slight is this connection that fluid effused at one part easily gravitates to another more dependent part."[2] At first Mr. Bowman only

---

[1] "Arch. f. Ophthal.," ix. 2, 85 ; vide also Mr. Roger's able translation of this article in "Royal London Ophthal. Hosp. Rep.," vol. iv. p. 218.

[2] Vide Mr. Bowman's very interesting article on "Needle Operations in Cases of Detached Retina," "Royal London Ophth. Hosp. Reports," iv. 184.

used one needle, simply puncturing the retina through the sclerotic, but he now employs two, lacerating the retina in a manner similar to that in his double-needle operation for opaque capsule. This operation is performed in the following manner: The lids are to be kept apart with the spring speculum, and the eye, if necessary, fixed with a pair of forceps. The needles, which should have a fine lancet-point, are then to be introduced separately through the sclerotic at a short distance from each other, and at a point corresponding to the most prominent part of the detachment; the points are then directed towards each other so that they may pierce the retina at the

Fig. 188.

same spot; by then separating their points the retina is torn between them (as in Fig. 188). Generally a little oozing of the subretinal fluid takes place under the conjunctiva, indeed it may even give rise to a small elevation. The vitreous often becomes somewhat turbid after the operation, but soon clears again, and then the small tear in the retina may sometimes be detected. The points of puncture of the sclerotic must vary of course with the position and extent of the detachment, but they will generally lie from one-quarter to one-half an inch from the margin of the cornea, and between the tendons of the recti muscles. As the operation gives but little pain, anæsthesia need not, as a rule, be administered. The operation is generally followed by some, often by very considerable improvement of the sight and the state of the field of vision. It is true that this improvement is mostly but temporary, and that the operation may have to be repeated several times, each repetition being again followed by a diminution of the detachment and amelioration of the sight; such repetitions should not, however, follow too closely upon each other, otherwise serious irritation of the eye may be set up. I have seen instances in which the improvement after one operation has lasted for many months, and Bowman and Von Graefe have observed cases in which it has been maintained for about two years. Von Arlt[1] mentions one in which the cure still continued fourteen months after the operation.

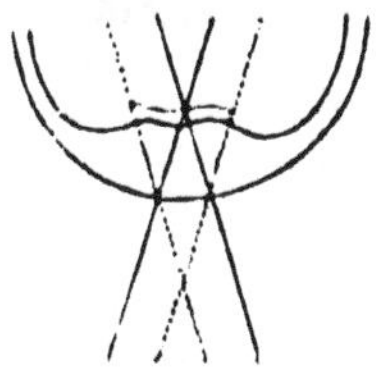

The operation is free from danger, and is generally followed by but slight symptoms of irritation.

If we consider the striking results often obtained by it, and compare these with the want of success accompanying the former plan of treatment, it must be conceded, I think, that its adoption is to be recommended. From my own favorable experience of its results, I have no hesitation in speaking in its favor. We should, however, be careful to distinctly warn our patients that the effect may only be slight and temporary. The operation should, if possible, be done at an early stage, so as to limit the extent of the detachment, and prevent the risk of the retina undergoing organic changes, leading to the permanent impairment of its perceptive functions. For a more complete exposition of these points, I must refer to the articles of Bowman and Von Graefe already quoted.

I should mention that De Wecker employs a small trocar for puncturing the retina, which he enters from the opposite side of the eye, and, after withdrawing the subretinal fluid, tears the retina in removing the instrument.

[The method introduced in 1876 by De Wecker, and called the "system by drainage," consists in the introduction of a loop of very fine gold wire through the sclera and choroid, and leaving it in situ, thus providing for a constant draining of the subretinal fluid. It has not proven particularly

---

[1] "Bericht der Wiener Augenklinik," 1867, s. 86.

successful, and a number of serious losses have been reported from violent choroidal inflammation. Hirschberg speaks highly of a return to the old *scleral puncture*, first practised by Sichel in 1859, and elaborated by Von Graefe, De Wecker, and Von Arlt, and more recently by Wolfe. Hirschberg thinks it may be resorted to in every case of detachment, that a preliminary cure will be obtained as a rule, but that relapses will recur from the nature of the affection. The time at which to perform the operation seems to be a subject of difference among surgeons. Von Arlt favored it in recent cases, while Von Graefe advised waiting until the fluid has descended by its own gravity, and in this Hirschberg agrees with him. In any event, it is not advisable to operate during an attack of retinal or choroidal inflammation (see "Arch. of Ophthal.," viii. 1; "Graefe und Saemisch, Handh. der Augenheil.," v. p. 704). Samelsohn has advised the employment of a pressure bandage with confinement to the bed for a long period (see "Centr. für die med. Wiss.," No. 49, 1875). Abadie recommends galvano-puncture as a method of treatment, in hopes of provoking artificially foci of chorio-retinitis which will attach the retina firmly to the choroid. He plunges the needle through the sclera just at the site of the detachment, of course avoiding the course of the muscles. On examining the eye with the ophthalmoscope, several days afterward, there may be seen a whitish blotch surrounded by a blackish areola, which is the patch of chorio-retinitis desired. In all his cases there was a certain amount of improvement, but the detachment subsequently recurred. (See "Gazette hebdomadaire," Dec. 9, 1881.)—B.]

10.—[OPHTHALMIC MIGRAINE.—B.] EPILEPSY OF THE RETINA.

Dr. Hughlings Jackson has described a very peculiar condition of the retina met with during the epileptic fit, and has given to it the name of "epilepsy of the retina." With regard to it he says:[1] "In one case, however, a case of 'epileptiform convulsions,' I had the opportunity of examining the fundus of the eye, if not during a genuine fit, at least during a condition in which consciousness was lost, and in which the pupils, ordinarily small, were dilated as if under the influence of atropine. The optic disks were extremely pale. Once the vessels disappeared for an appreciable time. After a while, however, they reappeared and were found to vary with the respiration. When the patient in-spired the vessels disappeared, returning again on expiration, like lines of red ink on white paper." It appears to be a temporary complete anæmic condition of the retina, dependent in all probability upon a contraction of the retinal vessels, just as the unconsciousness occurring during the epileptic fit is, according to Brown-Séquard, due to a contraction of the vessels of the brain, and consequent anæmia of the latter.

[This condition has been called *ophthalmic migraine*, or *megrim*. The main symptom is transient loss of sight, which may be attended by other symptoms, such as headache, nausea, and occasionally peripheral anæsthesia. The attack sometimes occasions total blindness in both eyes, and sometimes takes the form of hemianopsia. It involves no permanent danger to the sight, and vision may be very rapidly restored by the inhalation of a few whiffs of nitrite of amyl.

Férd's views upon ophthalmic migraine differ somewhat from those hitherto held. According to him, the ocular trouble may consist of subjective

[1] "Roy. Lond. Ophth. Hosp. Reports," iv. p. 14.

The first case of embolism of the central artery of the retina leading to sudden and complete blindness was diagnosed by Von Graefe.[1]

The patient generally complains that the loss of sight upon the affected side has taken place very suddenly, and is so great that he can hardly distinguish between light and dark. On ophthalmoscopic examination, we notice very marked and characteristic appearances. The optic disk is exceedingly blanched but transparent, the vessels upon it being greatly attenuated. The retinal arteries are thin, resembling small, narrow threads, and are, perhaps, to a greater or less extent, bloodless, and changed here and there, for the whole or a certain part of their course, into white bands. Sometimes small red plugs or coagula may be noticed in the vessels. The retinal veins are also thinner, irregularly filled, and showing in some of the branches a complete emptiness for a part of their course, alternating with a column of blood or plugs of coagula. In Von Graefe's case, a very peculiar condition was observed in a vein, viz., a very irregular movement of the column of blood, which moved with a sudden start towards the optic nerve, and then again became stationary; the alternatingly full and empty portions of the vessels remaining as before, excepting that their situation was changed. The next change is observed in the region of the yellow spot, which some days after the outset of the affection becomes opaque and covered by a faint bluish-gray or bluish-green film, hiding the subjacent choroid, and gradually shading off at the periphery into the normal retina. This opacity is due to a serous infiltration of the retina at this point, and varies considerably in extent, reaching or even exceeding somewhat the size of the optic disk. It is generally ovoid in shape, with its longest diameter horizontal. It often shows a somewhat mottled appearance, being studded with small, gray granules. In the centre of the film, at the foramen centrale, is noticed a marked, bright cherry-red spot, which is not an extravasation of blood, as is often erroneously supposed, but is due, as Liebreich has pointed out, to the fact that at this point the retina is transparent, permitting the choroid to shine through, which assumes a redder tinge on account of the contrast

[1] "Archiv f. Ophthal.," v. 1, 186.

with the surrounding grayish-blue opacity. The vessels running towards the yellow spot are often hyperæmic, so that their finer branchlets can be distinctly traced, and they also often show well-marked blood coagula.

The following case, which came under my care at King's College Hospital, well illustrates the appearances presented by embolism of the central artery of the retina:

W. P., æt. forty-two, married, has always been in good health. About the beginning of April, 1867, he had a severe cold, which kept him in bed. On the second morning he noticed that the right eye was somewhat inflamed, and smarted, and on trying his sight he found that it was much affected. No more reliable history could be obtained. On May 16th he first came under my care. The right eye looked healthy, the pupil somewhat dilated and sluggish, refracting media clear. He was, however, totally blind, being hardly able to distinguish between light and dark. The ophthalmoscope showed that it was a case of embolism of the central artery of the retina. The optic disk was very pale, but transparent, the vessels, on its expanse, much attenuated and anæmic, so that it was somewhat difficult to trace their exact relations to each other. The outline of the disk and the retina in its vicinity were somewhat hazy. This film-like opacity increased in density and extent towards the region of the yellow spot, where it assumed a grayish-blue tint. The vessels running from the disk towards the yellow spot were numerous and somewhat hyperæmic, so that their terminal branches were clearly observable. In some, the blood current was distinctly interrupted, small red portions of the vessel alternating with bloodless ones. I could not, however, on the closest examination, detect any jerky movement of the blood in these vessels; and as the red portions of the vessel did not appreciably alter their position during several weeks, I attributed them to blood coagula in the vessel. In the centre of the yellow spot was noticed a red, cherry-colored irregular patch, which evidently depended upon the contrast in color above referred to. Another smaller red patch was observed somewhat above and to its outer side, resembling it in appearance, but being due to an effusion of blood. The whole aspect of this region otherwise resembled very closely the appearance presented in the figure illustrating embolism of the central artery of the retina (Plate IV., Fig. 8). The appearance of the retinal vessels was also very characteristic of this affection. Thus, from the lower side of the disk a small artery emerged, which was perfectly white in the disk and for some portion of its course over the retina (about twice the diameter of the disk), where it became again filled with blood. It looked, indeed, like a small white band. The accompanying vein was filled for a short distance from the disk, but at its first division there was a well-marked plug, and on the peripheral side of this, it was bloodless for a considerable portion of its course. Some of the other vessels in the vicinity of the disk showed marked irregularities in their fulness, being, at certain points, hardly apparent or resembling small white threads, and at others well filled. These irregularities extended even to some of the peripheral branches. The left eye was quite normal. The heart was examined by Dr. Duffin, and found healthy. Although the patient's health was good, he appeared suffering from some cerebral affection, as he was very forgetful, inconsequent, and somewhat wandering.

The case was kept under constant observation, and examined with the phthalmoscope at intervals of a few days. Although the state of some of the bloodvessels changed somewhat, no marked alteration in the condition things took place until the beginning of June, when the disk became re vascular, but its outline more indistinct, the retina at its margin, more especially upwards, looking œdematous. The vitreous humor became clouded, showing diffuse and floating opacities. At the lower portion of the fundus, small circumscribed specks of disseminated choroiditis were observed. In about a fortnight two large extravasations of blood appeared, one at the periphery of the fundus, the other running from the disk to the upper part of the yellow spot. They were evidently situated in the retina, just beneath the internal elastic lamina, as they covered the retinal vessels, and were uniform and smooth, without any striated appearance. At the commencement of July, he was sent to Walton Convalescent Hospital. In the beginning of October his eye presented the following appearance, which it has retained more or less up to the present time: The vitreous is quite clear, the retina is undergoing transparent atrophy, the vessels are extremely small, and the retina is so thin that the epithelium of the choroid can be abnormally well seen. The inner half of the disk is covered by a thick network of blood-vessels (collateral circulation), which are so closely arranged that they present the appearance of an extravasation of blood, but by pressing upon the eye, they can be emptied, and be observed to refill when the pressure is relaxed. The extravasation running from the disk to the yellow spot has disappeared, but that at the upper part of the fundus, though smaller, is yet very apparent.

[In very rare instances, the embolus is not situated within the central artery of the retina before its entrance into the eyeball, but in one of its branches within the eye. Then, the swelling and œdema of the retina, the alteration of the vessels, and the loss of sight are confined to the affected pigment of the retina. Such cases have been recorded by Saemisch,[1] Hirschman,[2] and Knapp.[3] The latter insists strongly upon the importance of testing whether any pulsation can be induced in the retinal arteries by pressure on the eyeball, for this symptom is of great diagnostic value, indicating the absence or presence of circulation in the retinal vessels; for, if no pulsation can be produced, it shows that the circulation in the artery is arrested. Knapp says, "In such eyes only whose retinal artery was obstructed by embolism or injury, I never could produce a visible beating of the retinal arteries during the first week. As a rule, it is not before the end of the second week that pulsation could again be seen by applying pressure to the globe; and at this time, too, the calibre of the retinal vessels had regained half or two-thirds of its normal size." Where the embolism is confined to one branch of the central artery, we find that the corresponding portion of the retina is more or less œdematous and opaque, this extending, perhaps, to some considerable distance. The calibre of the affected vessel is greatly diminished, and it may, as well as its branches, be partly or entirely bloodless, in the last case looking like a thin white band. In the corresponding portion of the field of vision, the sight is *entirely and suddenly lost*, there being not the faintest glimmering of light-perception; but the central vision may be normal, as also that in the other portions of the visual field. In Knapp's case, there were very extensive venous hemorrhages in the corresponding segment of the retina. It appears that, even although the morbid changes in the retina may disappear, the serous and hemorrhagic effusions becoming absorbed, the retinal veins losing their dilatation and tortuosity, and a collateral circulation being established, this segment of the retina never regains its function, and the corresponding portion of the visual field is entirely wanting.

[1 "Kl. Monatsbl.," 1866, p. 35.   2 Ibid., p. 37.]
[3 "Archives of Ophthal.," i. 1, 64; *vide* also his articles on "Embolism," "A. f. O.," xvi. 1, 207.]

The opacity of the retina may appear within a few hours. Hemorrhages in the retina frequently occur, but are few in number and small in size. Sometimes signs of a returning circulation appear, especially in the veins. When the cloudy infiltration of the region round the macula grows less marked, the red spot in its centre also becomes less noticeable. Eventually the optic papilla becomes white and opaque, and the vessels are in part changed into cords. At this stage, the ophthalmoscopic picture is that of optic nerve atrophy.

Complete embolism of the trunk of the central artery causes total and incurable blindness. The number of eyes that have been examined microscopically is small, and although the presence of the embolus in several of them has been demonstrated, the results of the examination have not been entirely satisfactory.[1]

Etiology.—The most frequent cause is some cardiac disease, especially valvular disease with hypertrophy, or recent endocarditis. Another cause is extensive atheroma of the large vessels, another aneurism of the aorta. Embolus of the central artery of the retina is also met with in the course of febrile diseases, and during pregnancy, and has repeatedly been seen in Bright's disease, and here Leber thinks it might be due to a detached venous thrombus. Embolus of the arteries of the brain with attacks of apoplexy is a not uncommon complication. Secondary glaucoma has repeatedly been observed, in which an iridectomy proved useless, and the eye had to be enucleated to relieve the pain.[2] As regards treatment, little can be done. Paracentesis of the anterior chamber and iridectomy have been recommended, but any benefit resulting from them has been transient, and they have frequently done positive harm. Hence dietetic advice and controlling the action of a diseased heart is about all that can be done.—B.]

[*Thrombosis* of the *central retinal vein* is a subject that has recently excited some attention. Very often there is no assignable cause, though sometimes we may have extensive calcification and sclerosis of the arteries. Angelucci reports four cases, in none of which was there any œdema of the papilla at any time, and no subsequent canalization of the thrombus. Hemorrhages into the retina were few in number, and small in size. In one case there was marked retinal œdema at the macula, atrophy of the papilla, and diminution in calibre of the retinal vessels. The amblyopia in these cases is instantaneous. Subcutaneous injections of strychnia have been recommended by both Angelucci and Michel. (See "Annali di ottalmologia," ix. 2.)—B.]

18.—HYPERÆSTHESIA OF THE RETINA.

Before the discovery of the ophthalmoscope, this affection was generally mistaken for inflammation of the retina, and we still meet with this error in some books treating of diseases of the eye. Such a mistake is a grave one, as it has led to a most injudicious and improper treatment of cases of hyperæsthesia retinæ, viz., by antiphlogistics, depletion, salivation, etc., thus increasing the severity and the duration of the symptoms.

Hyperæsthesia of the retina generally occurs in young persons, especially in females of a very excitable, nervous, and hysterical temperament, and in delicate, feeble health. It is sometimes due to an accident, shock, or a blow on the eye, etc., to exposure to very bright light, such as a flash of lightning,

[1 " R. L. O. H. Rep.," viii. 1 and 2; " Brit. Med. Journ.," April 4, 1874; " Arch. f. Ophth.," xx. 2, 287; "Graefe and Saemish, Handb. des Augenheil.," v. 8, 541.]
[2 " Amer. Journ. Med. Sci.," April, 1874; " R. L. O. H. Rep.," viii. 1 and 2.]

or to prolonged use of the eyes by strong artificial light. It may also occur without any apparent cause, except some derangement in the general health, more especially of the uterine functions.

On examining the eye, we find that there is intense photophobia, together with lachrymation, accompanied, perhaps, by a spasmodic twitching of the eyelids, or even a severe spasm of the orbicularis muscle. There is often great ciliary neuralgia, the pain extending to the face and the corresponding side of the head. The retina is extremely irritable, and the patient is greatly troubled by photopsies, such as bright, dazzling stars, colored rings, etc., before the eyes, these photopsies being either spontaneous, or very easily producible by the slightest pressure upon the eyeball. Moreover, the retina retains impressions for an abnormally long period, so that if any object is regarded, its image is retained for a very appreciable space of time. The eye itself will be found quite normal, the refracting media clear, the fundus perfectly healthy. The sight is but very slightly, if at all impaired, and is always greatly improved when the intensity of the light is diminished by the use of blue glasses, with which the patient will be able to read the smallest print. But whilst the central vision is perfect, the peripheral portion of the retina is anæsthetic, so that the field of vision, as is pointed out by Von Graefe, is markedly concentrically contracted. This fact might easily mislead a superficial observer to mistake it for a case of commencing amaurosis. The phosphenes[1] are, however, very marked in the portion of the retina which is anæsthetic, and are very readily produced by slight pressure upon the eyeball.

The photophobia is often most severe, the patient being quite unable to face the light, or it comes on directly he attempts to use his eyes in reading, etc. It is always greatly relieved by the use of dark-blue glasses. Mooren[2] mentions an extraordinary case of hyperæsthesia, in which the sensibility of the retina was so greatly increased, that the patient could read large print in the dark, in which a normal eye could not distinguish a letter. It was, indeed, a true case of nyctalopia. All these symptoms had become developed in a very short time. The treatment must consist chiefly in improving the general health, encouraging the patient, and diminishing the excitability of the retina. If the photophobia is severe, it may be necessary to confine the patient in complete darkness for six or eight days, and then gradually to accustom him to an increasing amount of light (Von Graefe). In the open air he should wear blue glasses. Internally, tonics should be administered, more especially preparations of zinc or steel, according to the special indications of individual cases. Zinc (either the valerianate or lactate) should be given in increasing doses, commencing with one-half or one grain twice a day, and gradually increasing this to four or even five grains. Subsequently, steel and quinia will be found very useful. Great care must be taken not to weaken the patient, especially by depletion. Although the artificial leech may be occasionally employed with benefit, it must be used with extreme care, otherwise it is apt to increase the severity of the symptoms, and retard the cure. I prefer dry cupping, either at the temple or the back of the neck. If the patient's spirits are much depressed, everything must be done to cheer him up and encourage him in believing in a speedy cure.

---

[1] The luminous rings which appear when the eyeball is firmly pressed.
[2] "Ophthalmiatrische Beobachtungen," p. 271.

14.—TUMORS OF THE RETINA.

[1. *Glioma or Gliosarcoma* (Syn. Fungus Hæmatodes Oculi—Small-cell Sarcoma of Retina).—B.]

According to Virchow, only two kinds of tumor occur in the retina, viz., Glioma and Gliosarcoma. The intra-ocular tumor, generally known as medullary cancer, encephaloid tumor or fungus hæmatodes, is in reality, as Virchow has shown, developed from the retina. As it originates in the interstitial connective tissue (*neuroglia*) of the retina, and in this, as well as in its minute structure, closely resembles cerebral glioma, he has termed it *Glioma retinæ*, a name which has been already extensively adopted by British and foreign pathologists.

[Histologically it is identical with the small round-cell sarcoma, and clinically it is characterized by very rapid growth, great tendency to spread and to the development of metastatic tumors in distant organs. Recent investigations on fresh and hardened specimens have led Delafield to call these tumors sarcomata, and in this opinion Alt and Leber are both inclined to coincide. Microscopically, there is no difference between the two. (For full information on this subject, see Virchow's "Die Krankheiten Geschwülste," Knapp's "Intra-oculare Geschwülste," Alt's "Lectures on the Human Eye," New York, 1880, Hirschberg's "Der Markschwann der Netzhaut," "Graefe und Saemisch's Handb.," v. p. 717 *et seq.*, and the important papers by Von Graefe, Iwanoff, Hirschberg, and others, in the later volumes of the "Archiv f. Ophthal.")—B.]

The symptoms presented by the disease are generally very marked and characteristic. In the earlier stages, the external appearance of the eye is quite healthy and normal, there being, as a rule, no pain or symptoms of inflammation. But the sight is lost. The pupil is more or less widely dilated, and shining, from the bottom of the eye, is noticed a bright, glistening, yellowish-white reflection, which is often already noticeable at some little distance. [Fig. 184.] On account of this yellow luminous reflex, this condition was formerly called "amaurotic cat's-eye." With the ophthalmoscope, the details of the growth can be beautifully seen. At the outset, the disease is limited to one portion of the retina, which becomes opaque, thickened, and somewhat mottled in appearance. The morbid growth gradually increases in extent and prominence, until it protrudes in the form of a yellowish-white nodulated mass into the vitreous humor. According to Virchow, the increase in the size of the tumor is partly due to the growth of the original mass, and partly to the formation of new foci of disease in its vicinity; and hence, on becoming larger, the growth assumes a lobulated appearance, certain portions of the retina being thicker than others. On the expanse of the tumor, we can generally observe with the ophthalmoscope numerous bloodvessels, which anastomose very freely with each other, and between these vessels are often noticed small effusions of blood. Indeed, these tumors are very vascular; and this fact, as Hirschberg[1] points out, is not only valuable in a diagnostic

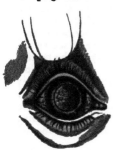

[Fig. 184.

After Von Ammon.]

---

[1] "A. f. O.," xvi. 2, 50.

point of view, but tends to explain the rapidly developed glaucomatous symptoms and the temporary atrophy of the eyeball, which are often noticed in eyes affected with glioma.

The above are the symptoms generally presented by the disease when the surgeon first sees it, for as it occurs in the vast majority of cases in children, little heed is paid to the condition of the sight, and the affection is unnoticed until the attention of the parents is arrested by the bright-yellow reflex coming from the bottom of the eye, and only then is medical aid sought. Hence we but seldom enjoy the opportunity of seeing the earliest development of the disease, and of following its gradual progress. In the very earliest stage, there are noticed, according to Von Graefe,[1] numerous small white patches, of varying size, which lie partly behind the retinal vessels, and partly pervade the retina as far as its inner surface, and then give rise, already at a very early stage, to a marked elevation. They may be distinguished from inflammatory infiltrations of the retina by their circular, sharply defined outline, the periphery of such figures not being broken up into punctated or striated opacities, as occurs in the latter case. Moreover, they are of a decidedly white tint, and not of the creamy yellow hue met with in inflammatory infiltrations. These small patches soon coalesce, and increase in size and thickness, but spread at first only along the surface. But as the disease advances, the posterior surface of the retina bulges forward (Hirschberg),[2] the little individual nodules which are thus formed, coalesce and give rise at a circumscribed spot to a lobulated cauliflower growth of the external surface of the retina (glioma retinæ circumscriptum tuberosum). At this period, there is already noticed a considerable dissemination of secondary foci. The retina is generally already partially detached at a very early stage, and the tension of the eye mostly somewhat increased. The detachment is often peculiarly defined, perhaps forming an acute angle, at the apex of which a white patch may be noticed (Graefe).[3] The peculiar reflex and the details of the tumor are rendered still more marked and conspicuous on the retina becoming detached. When the disease is more advanced, and the whole retina is implicated in it and thickened, the detachment is generally complete and funnel-shaped, the apex being situated at the optic nerve, and the base at the ora serrata. Knapp[4] describes a very curious case in which the glioma sprung from the inner layer of the retina, protruded into the vitreous humor, and was covered not only by the portion of retina which it implicated, but by a second envelope of detached retina, including its ciliary portion. As a rule, the morbid growth can be very readily detached from the choroid, but in some cases the retina is firmly glued to the latter (Virchow),[5] the tumor gradually filling the eyeball and causing the vitreous humor to shrink and become absorbed to a corresponding degree. The retina in such cases becomes folded inwards, so that the different folds are superimposed upon each other.

When the growth enlarges still more, the lens and iris become pushed forward towards the cornea, the lens often becoming opaque and partially or even completely absorbed. The intra-ocular tension, which has generally been for some length of time augmented, becomes now very markedly increased, and this may be accompanied by more or less acute inflammatory symptoms and severe pain. The state of the eye-tension is of consequence with regard to the differential diagnosis between an intra-ocular tumor and a simple detachment of the retina, for in the latter case it is as a rule always

---

[1] " A. f. O.," xvi. p. 129. [2] Ibid., p. 88. [3] Ibid., xvi. p. 129.
[4] Knapp's " Archives," ii. 1, 168. [5] Loc. cit., p. 162.

diminished. As glioma occurs in the vast majority of cases in young children, in whom glaucoma is hardly ever met with as a primary affection, an increase in the intra-ocular tension (other causes for this being absent) should at once arouse our suspicions (Von Graefe).[1]

When the tumor has filled the cavity of the eyeball, the latter generally soon gives way at some point. The perforation takes place at the cornea or near its margin, or at the anterior portion of the sclerotic, and but seldom at its posterior part. Perforation at the latter situation, and the extension of the growth into the orbit must be suspected if the movements of the eyeball are markedly curtailed, and the eye protruded. When the tumor has once burst through the coats of the eyeball, its growth is very rapid. It sprouts forth between the eyelids, which are greatly swollen and often much everted, and acquires, from its exposure to the atmosphere and external irritants, a dusky-red, fleshy, and very vascular appearance, and hence the name "fungus hæmatodes." [Fig. 185.] From it there exudes a sanious fluid, which be-

[Fig. 185.

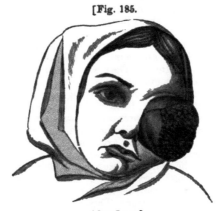

After Gross.]

comes crusted on its surface, and if any excoriation of the latter occurs, the tumor bleeds very freely.

Sometimes, however, the disease does not run so regular a course, for after the tumor has attained a certain size within the eye, symptoms of irido-choroiditis supervene, the pupil becomes blocked up with lymph, the eye-tension falls below the normal standard, and the disease for a time assumes the character of an iride-choroiditis, passing on to temporary atrophy of the eyeball. The latter is generally due to suppurative choroiditis, but may, in rare instances, be also caused by suppuration of the cornea (Von Graefe). Together with this atrophied condition of the eyeball, there are often very intense, spontaneous paroxysms of pain, the eye itself being but slightly, if at all sensitive to the touch; whereas in the atrophy dependent upon irido-cyclitis, the reverse obtains. But the most intense and sudden pain occurs if intra-ocular hemorrhage takes place. At a subsequent period, the symptoms of an intra-ocular tumor again manifest themselves in the partially atrophied eyeball, the tension increases, the tumor augments in size, the cornea or sclerotic gives way, and a rapidly increasing morbid growth sprouts forth.

[1] "A. f. O.," xiv. 2, 130.

Virchow considers that glioma commences in the external layers of the retina, more especially the connective-tissue elements of the granular layers, and Knapp believes that it begins in the external granular layer. Schweigger[1] thought it probable that it originated in the internal granular layer, and Hirschberg[2] has succeeded in proving the truth of this supposition, having found in one case that the disease commenced in a proliferation of the cells in the inner granular layer of the retina. [Leber has found primary tumors at the same time in different layers. The probability is that the tumor, being a connective-tissue growth, may and does spring from the connective-tissue elements of any or all the layers of the retina, as Iwanoff has suggested. The growth may begin in the internal layers, and grow to a considerable size without involving the layer of rods and cones, as in a case reported by Delafield.—B.] At a more advanced stage of the disease, the retinal tissues often disappear almost entirely, so that it is then quite impossible to trace its origin.[3] The membrana limitans interna and the innermost portions of the trabecular connective-tissue fibres (Stützfasern), seem to resist the longest, and may, according to Virchow, be often traced within the tumor, and are seen to divide it into segments. Iwanoff[4] distinguishes two forms of glioma: one, in which the disease commences in the internal granular layer and extends outward; the other, in which it begins in the layer of the optic nerve fibres and extends inwards.

The principal masses of tumor are composed of aggregations of nuclei and cells. [Fig. 186.] The latter are round or oval, small in size, and occasionally have small prolongations. They are sometimes arranged in rows, and contain one or more nuclei. The free nuclei are small and round, and, according to Virchow, correspond exactly to the little light-refracting nuclei of the granular layer. The inter-cellular substance is so scanty that it can be hardly distinguished, but on adding chromic acid it becomes finely granular. In the soft variety of the tumor, the cells are larger than in the hard, and in the latter the cellular tissue is fibrillated.

[Fig. 186.

× 200 diameters.]

[These tumors are sometimes very vascular, the bloodvessels being very large. During their growth, hemorrhages often occur both upon the surface of the retina and within the tumor. These latter are recognized after removal by the patches of blood-pigment, which is sometimes enclosed in cells, and sometimes is found in free crystals.—B.] The tumor may subsequently undergo fatty and chalky degeneration. Sometimes the cells augment in size or assume a spindle shape, and the nuclei increase in number, and then the morbid growth must be considered to be of a sarcomatous nature. Indeed, Virchow has shown that the tumor sometimes assumes a mixed character, one part resembling glioma in structure, another sarcoma, so that it may be termed "glio-sarcoma," and he thinks this to be far more dangerous in character than simple glioma.[5] [This tendency to limit the term "sarcoma" to a large round cell or spindle-cell growth is histologically incorrect, and should not be perpetuated.—B.]

Virchow thinks that a sharp line of demarcation cannot be drawn between glioma and inflammatory neoplasms of the retina, as the former may in its course be accompanied by inflammatory symptoms. He considers "that

[1] "A. f. O.," vi. 2, 326.   [2] Ibid., xiv. 2, 40.
[3] For further information upon the anatomical character of these tumors, I would also refer the reader to Mr. Hulke's valuable papers on "Intra-ocular Cancer," "R. L. O. H. Rep.," iii., iv., and v.
[4] "A. f. O.," xv. 2.   [5] "Die Krankheiten Geschwülste," ii. 167.

the name glioma is apposite, as the neoplastic formation, even if of an inflammatory nature, assumes a more permanent character and tumor-like form, it being, however, of course, always understood that its structure must be composed of homologous elements. A suppurative retinitis can never give rise to glioma."[1]

Von Graefe, however, does not believe that glioma is due to an inflammatory hyperplasia, and thinks that observations which have been advanced in support of such a view, have depended either upon the fact that the sequelæ of intra-ocular inflammations, e. g., plastic inflammations of the vitreous humor, or subretinal deposits, have been mistaken for gliomata ; or that the first period of the tumor has been completely overlooked, and the consecutive inflammatory complications were supposed to form the origin of the disease. Moreover, as he points out, clinical observation shows a marked difference between the first period of glioma and an inflammatory hyperplasia.

The question whether glioma is to be regarded as a malignant disease is still considered doubtful by some observers. Von Graefe,[2] however, speaks in the most decided manner as to its malignancy, and thinks that this increases with the length of its existence and the increase of its development. It has been thought that glioma differs from sarcomatous tumors of the choroid, etc., in this, that it does not appear secondarily to affect distant organs, being only prone to local infection ;[3] but this has been proved to be erroneous. Hulke[4] mentions a case in which the retinal glioma in each eye extended beyond the optic nerves within the skull, and in which he distinctly observed the growth of the glioma in the connective tissue separating the bundles of nerve fibres in the nerve trunk, in front of the optic commissure. The propagation of the disease from the retina occurs in two directions— (1) towards the choroid ; (2) to the optic nerve, and the implication of the latter is, according to Hirschberg, far more frequent than has been generally supposed, occurring almost without an exception and in a tolerably short space of time after the origin of the disease in the retina. Out of the eight cases which he reports,[5] the optic nerve was implicated in six, and in most to a very considerable extent. [Both choroid and optic nerve may be involved very early in the course of the disease, and later, the ciliary body and iris may become infiltrated before the growth perforates the sclera, though this is not common. The optic nerve in rare cases becomes enormously thickened, the infiltration following mainly the medullary sheath of the nerve fibres. Occasionally we meet with small secondary tumors in the sclera, usually on its external surface, which have no connection with the internal growth, or if they have, it is microscopic.—B.] In this tendency to extension of the disease to the optic nerve and thence to the brain, is to be sought the extreme danger of retinal glioma, for a secondary tumor of the brain may be formed, or *encephalitis* ensue. [These intra-cranial tumors may grow to a large size without causing any brain symptoms, though this is not usually the case. The extension to the chiasm and optic nerve of the other eye may lead to complete amaurosis, though there may be no tumor in the second eye itself.—B.] Hence the necessity of excising the eye at the earliest opportunity, and dividing the optic nerve as far back as possible. The first retro-ocular extension of the disease is very difficult to diagnose, but Von Graefe[6] has found that when degeneration of the optic nerve has

[1] Loc. cit., 159.   [2] "A. f. O.," xiv. 2, 110.
[3] Knapp records a case of glioma of the retina in which there were found, after death, secondary gliomata in the liver, lung, and the diploë of the skull. Op. cit., p. 5.
[4] "R. L. O. H. Rep.," v. 172.   [5] "A. f. O.," xiv. 2, 56.   [6] Ibid., xiv. 2, 187.

ensued, the eyeball becomes slightly more prominent, and its lateral movements somewhat curtailed. There is also more resistance felt, if the eye is pressed back into the orbit, and the little furrow between the eyelids and wall of the orbit is obliterated. When the orbital adipose tissue is once implicated, the progress of the disease is very rapid. Knapp[1] has shown that the propagation of the disease to the neighboring tissues occurs in two ways: 1, by dissemination of germs; 2, by direct contact.

[The extension of the growth to the tissues and bones of the face and skull is sometimes very rapid. The parotid and submaxillary glands become infiltrated and form the origin of large secondary tumors. Secondary deposits also occur in the bones of the skull entirely disconnected with the orbital tumor. They originate sometimes in the diploë, sometimes in the periosteum; are very vascular, and are often accompanied by the development of osteophytes. Metastatic growths have been found in the clavicle, the ribs, and the os brachii. The liver is the most frequently involved of all the internal organs, though kidneys, lungs, and ovaries are not uncommonly invaded by the metastatic growth.—B.]

The causes of glioma are quite obscure; but in some cases it appears to be due to a traumatic origin. It occurs in children between the ages of two and eleven, and, according to Hirschberg, no authentic case is recorded in which it was observed after the age of twelve. It may, according to Travers, be sometimes congenital, he having extirpated such an eye in a child of eight months. [When it is congenital its development is very slow, and never goes beyond the first stage during foetal life.—B.] Sometimes both eyes are affected with the disease, and in such cases Von Graefe thinks that we must not consider the affection as having been propagated from one eye to the other by way of the chiasma, for in the cases of Saunders and Hayes, reported by Wardrop, the optic nerve of the secondarily affected eye was found to be quite normal. Nor does the idea of a dyscrasia hold good, on account of the general immunity of other organs from metastatic gliomata. Von Graefe rather seeks the explanation in the peculiar symmetry which exists between the two eyes, the influence of which is so often and very markedly illustrated in inflammatory diseases of the eye. In some instances, glioma appears to be hereditary, and occurs in several members of the same family. Thus Lerche mentions four children being affected with it out of a family of seven; Sichel saw it in four children of the same mother. The children affected with glioma are often of a peculiarly fair and beautiful complexion, although perhaps somewhat delicate in constitution. [The male sex seems somewhat more disposed to be attacked than the female sex. Its frequency, as compared to other eye diseases, varies from four one-hundredths to six one-hundredths per cent.—B.]

The prognosis of the disease is always extremely grave, as the affection is very apt to recur, and we have no guarantee that the optic nerve is not already implicated, even although the intra-ocular tumor may still be very small. For this reason, the immediate removal of the eye should be very strongly urged as soon as the diagnosis of glioma is established, for this is the only chance of saving the patient's life. The opinion that the disease may become spontaneously arrested, or may retrograde, is, according to Von Graefe, quite erroneous. For he[2] has found that the affection progresses steadily and surely, indeed with greater steadiness than sarcoma of the choroid, and that, reckoning from the earliest appearance of the disease,

[1] "A. f. O.," xiv. 2, 187.   [2] "A. f. O.," xiv. 2, 185.

when the tumor still only occupies a small portion of the eye, from one to three years elapse before its extra-ocular development becomes manifest. In those cases in which this occurs at a very early age, e. g., at the termination of the first year of the child's life, he considers it probable that the glioma was congenital.

Treatment.—It has been urged by some surgeons, that the extirpation of the eye is useless, as the disease is sure quickly to recur and end fatally. But cases are on record in which several years have elapsed after the operation, without a return of the disease.[1] The rule is, therefore, to remove the eye at the earliest possible period, so that there may be the chance of the optic nerve being still unaffected.

The chief danger is, that the disease should extend to the brain, or that the tumor, increasing more and more in size, should perforate the eyeball, and from the severe pain, the great enlargement of the tumor, the occurrence of hemorrhage, etc., undermine the patient's health. Cerebral complications should be suspected, if the patient becomes drowsy, languid, and stupid, lying about and sleeping a great deal, if there is great and constant headache, or if symptoms of paralysis manifest themselves. But even when the tumor has burst through the coats of the eyeball, and is fungating extensively, its removal is advisable, more especially if there is much pain and hemorrhage. It must, moreover, be remembered that it is the only chance of prolonging life, and of alleviating the dreadful sufferings of the patient. In excising the eye, the optic nerve should be divided very far back, in order, if possible, to remove all the disease. Von Graefe was in the habit, in such cases, of passing a neurotome (after he has divided the conjunctiva) along the outer wall of the orbit to the bottom of the latter, then pulling the eye as far forwards as possible, and dividing the optic nerve quite close to the optic foramen; he then proceeded with the excision in the usual manner. If the disease has extended to the tissue of the orbit, it will be advisable to apply the chloride of zinc paste after the removal of the eyeball, so as to destroy, if possible, all the morbid tissue. [In removing the contents of the orbit, the periosteum must always be removed as completely as possible. If the eyelids are involved, they are best removed close to the orbital margin, and if the subjacent bone looks diseased, it must be scraped clean. When the disease has not been entirely removed, the growth recurs rapidly, usually within a few weeks.

2. *Sarcoma of the Retina.*—In rare cases sarcoma of the choroid is accompanied by small sarcomatous deposits in the retina, which may be direct prolongations of the choroidal growth, but which occasionally are isolated nodules. Cases have been reported by Klebs, Knapp, and Hirschberg. ("Arch. f. Ophth.," xi. 2, xvi. 1; "Archives of Ophthal.," iv. 1.)

3. *Miliary Tubercles in the Retina.*—Only a single authenticated case of this kind has been reported by Perls, in which the iris and ciliary body were also involved. ("Arch. f. Ophthal.," xix. 1.)

4. *Vascular Growths of the Retina.*—Multiple small vascular tumors, proliferations from the arterial walls, have been met with in the degeneration of the vascular walls occurring in chronic glaucoma. They are said to be transformed later into connective tissue ("Kl. Mon.," Aug. 1871, p. 425).—B.]

[1] *Vide* "R. L. O. H. Rep.," iv. 87; also Von Graefe's article, loc. cit.

16.—CYSTS IN THE RETINA. [CYSTOID DEGENERATION.—B.]

These may occur in varying number, and differ in size from a small pea to a hazel-nut. On a section of the globe, they appear to the naked eye as small transparent vesicles, studded over the outer portion of the retina. They are probably produced by the development of colloid material in the external granular layer, and by a proliferation of the radiating trabecular fibres (Iwanoff).[1] The latter form the outer and lateral walls of the cyst, the inner wall being formed by the internal layers of the retina. Mr. Vernon has met with cysts in the retina in four instances.

[The anterior portion of the retina is in old age the seat of a peculiar cystoid formation, described by Iwanoff as oedema. Between the ora serrata and pars ciliaris retinæ, the retina becomes decidedly thickened, and here spaces develop. The degeneration affects mainly the inner granule layer, and the bacillar layer is generally intact. This cystoid degeneration is also met with in cases of detachment of the retina, both idiopathic and traumatic, and in glaucomatous eyes; and here the degeneration begins generally in the external granule layer, and the cysts sometimes reach a very large size. In some cases there is no trace of any inflammatory origin, though usually this is not so.—B.]

[17.—CONNECTIVE-TISSUE FORMATION IN THE RETINA.

After injuries of the eye with extensive hemorrhages into the vitreous and retina, there sometimes remain dense, pigmented connective-tissue bands in the retina which dip down into the choroid. Occasionally these are met with idiopathically. This condition has been called retinitis proliferans, but Leber thinks the membranes are always the remains of hemorrhages. The retinal vessels sometimes overlie them and sometimes run beneath them, and occasionally the optic disk is entirely concealed by one of these new formations. Usually the vision is markedly affected, but sometimes an amount of vision is retained out of all proportion to the condition revealed by the

---

[1] " Kl. Monatsbl.," 1864, p. 417.

ophthalmoscope. Some of the cases reported in which the membraniform growths appeared to be indirectly caused by extensive retinal hemorrhages, more properly belong to the class of connective-tissue growths within the vitreous. They present a greenish appearance in front of the retina, and extend a varying distance into the vitreous. Parent rejects Manz' theory of the formation of these membranes, and offers as a substitute the theory that the fibrine of the blood in these hemorrhages, being extravasated in too large an amount to be entirely absorbed, becomes organized and is transformed into connective tissue. (See "Recueil d'ophthalmologie," Dec. 1860.)—B.]

[18.—INJURIES OF THE RETINA.

Besides the wounding of the retina which results from rupture of the eyeball, the retina is often wounded by small bits of steel or glass which have penetrated the eyeball. These may remain sticking in the retina, or rebound and fall to the bottom of the vitreous. Foreign bodies may become encapsulated in the retina and remain quiescent for years. Particles of steel have also been removed from the retina. ("Trans. Amer. Ophthal. Soc.," 1878. "Arch. of Ophthal.," vii.) Wounding of the retina is usually accompanied or followed by such destructive inflammation of the other tissues of the eye, that its individual consideration may be omitted.

Rupture of the retina alone and in connection with rupture of the choroid from a blow, has been known to occur, but these cases are extremely rare. Generally the external layers next the choroid are the parts involved. The vision is usually very much disturbed from the effects of such an injury. Blows upon the eye are sometimes followed by loss of vision, where the ophthalmoscope reveals little or no injury. This condition has been called *commotio retinæ* or *concussion* of the *retina*, and there are two varieties of these cases: first, severe cases with entire or almost entire loss of vision, usually of long duration and accompanied with defects of eccentric vision; and second, slighter cases of trivial and brief diminution of central vision alone. When the eye is struck a severe blow, the retinal bloodvessels are instantaneously deprived of their blood, a purely mechanical phenomenon arising from compression of the eyeball, and lasting but a few seconds. The vessels then fill again, apparently to a normal degree. A further direct result of the blow is a distinct diminution in the size of the pupil, and an abnormal resistance to the action of atropia on the part of the sphincter of the iris. Finally, central vision is at once reduced. In about an hour after the injury, changes begin to appear in the retina in the shape of irregular gray dots, which gradually coalesce into a continuous opacity, which slowly changes color, becomes brighter, and sometimes very white. These alterations do not always occur, and Berlin concludes that the disturbance of vision is generally independent of the retinal opacity. Moreover, the disturbance of vision and the retinal lesion do not develop simultaneously; for while vision is at its worst directly after the injury, then improves rapidly for a short time, and finally very slowly, the retinal opacity does not appear until one or two hours after the injury, at a time when vision has already improved. On the other hand, the opacity disappears in a day or two, while it takes a long time for vision to be restored. Finally, observations show that the disturbance affects central vision only, and is entirely independent of the character of the opacity. (See "Archives of Ophthalmology," x. 4.)—B.]

[19.—CYSTICERCUS UNDER THE RETINA.

This was first described by Von Graefe. The worm occurs much oftener between the retina and the choroid than in the vitreous. At first the retina over the bladder is transparent, but it gradually becomes opaque, and the vitreous begins to grow turbid. The visual field is interrupted, and when the animal moves, as it frequently does, it leaves behind it an opaque spot. If the retina becomes totally detached, the cysticercus becomes encapsulated and does not penetrate into the vitreous. When the vitreous remains transparent, the animal may occasionally be seen to move its head and neck. Vision steadily diminishes, and eventually violent inflammatory symptoms supervene, causing acute irido-choroiditis. An attempt should be made to extract the cysticercus by an incision through the sclera in the region of the sac, or by an incision in the sclero-corneal margin, extraction of the lens, and subsequent removal of the entozoon. This latter operation, however, is only suitable when the animal has entered the vitreous. The prognosis in any event is unfavorable.—B.]

CHAPTER XII.

DISEASES OF THE OPTIC NERVE.

1.—HYPERÆMIA OF THE OPTIC NERVE.

HYPERÆMIA of the optic nerve is a part symptom of hyperæmia of the retina and choroid. This condition is characterized by the optic disk being much reddened, its minute vessels fuller and more conspicuous, and its margin indistinct and hazy, so that it is not sharply defined against the surrounding retina; this haziness is least marked at the temporal side. [It should be remembered that the nasal part of the optic disk is naturally redder than the temporal.—B.] In some cases, faint radiating stripes can be seen passing slightly over into the retina. In that form which accompanies hyperæmia of the choroid, the disk is also reddened, but this ceases at the sclerotic ring, and the margin of the disk is everywhere sharply and clearly defined (Mauthner).

2.—INFLAMMATION OF THE OPTIC NERVE (OPTIC NEURITIS, NEURO-RETINITIS), Plate VI., Figs. 13 and 14.

Inflammation of the optic nerve is distinguished by the following ophthalmoscopic symptoms. At the outset, there exists a certain degree of hyperæmia and œdema of the optic nerve entrance and of the retina in its vicinity, so that the disk appears abnormally red and somewhat opaque and swollen, its outlines being hazy and indistinct. In some cases the neuritis is partial, the serous infiltration and swelling being at first chiefly or entirely confined to one portion of the disk. But the inflammatory symptoms soon become more marked. The optic disk becomes enlarged, swollen, and prominent, and its outline irregular and indistinct (from proliferation of the connective-tissue elements), so that it passes over into the retina without any sharp line of demarcation. Moreover, the smooth, transparent, delicate pink appearance of the disk is lost, and it assumes an opaque, reddish-gray tint; the hypertrophy of its connective tissue causing it to appear striated and "woolly." On account of the great swelling and prominence of the disk, it can be seen at some little distance in the erect image: the refraction having in fact become hypermetropic. The inflammation generally extends more or less on to the retina in the vicinity of the disk, rendering the former hazy and indistinct. The appearance of the retinal vessels is also markedly changed. The veins are much dilated, dark, and often very tortuous, dipping here and there into the infiltration, so as to be more or less covered and hidden by it, and interrupted in their course. The arteries may, on the other hand, be so much diminished in calibre as to be hardly distinguishable. On account of the development of numerous small vessels on the disk, the latter is very red and vascular, its edge looking perhaps as if it were covered by a reddish fringe. On and around the disk are scattered numerous striated blood extravasations of varying size and shape. On using a high magnifying power, we are often able to make out that the apparent hemorrhagic effusions in reality consist of minute, closely packed, newly developed bloodvessels. The inflammatory swelling and exudation may, however, be so considerable that the vessels are completely hidden on the disk, and can only be followed up to its margin, and only here and there can the outline of a vessel be faintly traced on its expanse. Although cases of retinitis, more especially the parenchymatous and nephritic, are generally accompanied by a certain degree of inflammation of the optic nerve, I shall here confine myself to the description of optic neuritis as an idiopathic disease, and not as a part symptom of inflammation of the retina.

We may distinguish two principal forms of optic neuritis, viz.: 1. The "*engorged papilla*"[1] (Stauungspapille of Von Graefe), in which the inflammation commences in the papilla (optic disk) and extends upwards along the trunk of the nerve, but generally stopping short at the lamina cribrosa. Hence it might very well be termed "ascending" neuritis. [The term usually employed in the text-books for this form of inflammation has been "choked disk;" but there has recently been introduced into our terminology the word "papillitis," to describe the same ophthalmoscopic symptoms.—B.] 2. The "*descending neuritis*," in which the inflammation commences extra-ocularly, and extends downwards to the optic disk.

The *engorged papilla* is almost always due to an impediment to the circulation within the nerve, which may be caused by an intra-orbital tumor pressing upon the latter, or by an increase in the intra-cranial pressure, and consequent retardation and obstruction to the circulation in the optic nerve. This mechanical obstruction to the circulation in the central vessels of the retina is soon followed by serous infiltration of the optic nerve, and subsequently by inflammatory proliferation of its connective-tissue elements. Hence, there is a considerable swelling of the nerve, and as the firm scleral ring cannot yield, but closely embraces it, the nerve is here more or less strangulated, which impedes the circulation still more. The irritation produced by this compression is soon followed by inflammation. Iwanoff,[2] however, narrates a case of neuritis optica in which the ophthalmoscopic symptoms of engorged papilla and hyperæmia of the optic nerve and retina were very marked, and lasted for more than twelve months; and yet, on microscopical examination, no inflammatory changes were found in the nerve, but only hyperæmia of the vessels, great dilatation of the capillaries, and slight hypertrophy of the connective tissue, but the nerve fibres were quite unaffected.

Von Graefe[3] was the first to recognize the connection between optic neuritis and affections of the brain, as well as certain morbid conditions of the orbit. According to him, the engorged papilla is chiefly distinguished by great, but perhaps partial swelling and prominence of the disk, numerous and considerable hemorrhages on and around the papilla, and great dilatation, darkness, and tortuosity of the veins; the arteries being on the contrary very small, attenuated, and often almost bloodless. The inflammatory infiltration of the retina is confined to the close vicinity of the nerve entrance. [In the choked disk from chronic meningitis, with or without tumors, besides the signs already mentioned, there may also be masses of exudation in the retina between disk and macula, resembling very markedly

---

[1] The "ischæmia of the disk" of Dr. Allbutt, whose work on the ophthalmoscope I would recommend to the attention of the reader.

[2] "Kl. Monatsbl.," 1868, 421.   [3] "A. f. O.," vii. 2, 58.

the appearance hitherto regarded as pathognomonic of Bright's disease. A rare occurrence in papillitis is a spontaneous arterial pulsation from obstructed circulation, due either to neuritis or orbital tumors.—B.]

In the *descending* neuritis the tissue of the nerve is more diffusely clouded, but the swelling and redness of the disk are much less, and its tint is of a faint gray. The opacity of the retina is more diffuse and extensive, and reaches deeper into its structure. The retinal arteries are considerably diminished in calibre, but the veins are less dilated and tortuous than in the engorged papilla. On account of the more extensive implication of the retina, as well as the appearance of white patches on it, the disease sometimes assumes a certain similarity to nephritic retinitis, and might even be mistaken for it by a superficial, careless observer. The chief points in the differential diagnosis of these two diseases have been already mentioned in the article upon "Retinitis Albuminurica" (page 513). On account of its involving so considerable a portion of the retina, this form may be called "neuro-retinitis." As Iwanoff points out,[1] the inflammation of the optic nerve which ensues secondarily upon inflammation of the retina (*e. g.*, nephritic retinitis) or choroid might justly and appropriately be termed "intra-ocular neuritis."

It must be stated, however, that the distinctive characters of these two forms of neuritis are not often so strongly marked, and also that the one may pass over into the other, and thus give rise to a mixed group of ophthalmoscopic appearances. Sometimes in the descending neuritis, the opacity, swelling, and redness are chiefly confined to the periphery of the disk, the central portion being relatively but little involved, and this has hence been called "peri-neuritis."

In some cases of optic neuritis in children, Mr. Hutchinson has met with a peculiar appearance of the retina in the region of the yellow spot, viz., a group of highly refractive globules, resembling at the first glance a cluster of spider's eggs; these groups are almost symmetrical and very definite.[2]

When the inflammatory symptoms subside, the morbid products become gradually absorbed, the swelling and prominence of the papilla diminish, and it gradually becomes flattened; at the same time assuming a paler tint, the neighboring retina remaining perhaps a little clouded. The retinal veins diminish in size and tortuosity, the blood extravasations become absorbed, the opacity of the retina disappears, and the disk may gradually regain a more normal appearance, and vision may be restored. As the swelling and infiltration of the nerve are far more considerable in the engorged papilla than in the descending neuritis, the absorption is also less rapid than in the latter. In severe cases, recovery is, however, the exception, not the rule, for the nerve generally becomes atrophied. Even in those cases in which vision is restored, the disk remains somewhat opaque and of a pale-creamy tint. We are, however, generally able for a long time to distinguish the atrophy ensuing upon optic neuritis from that which is met with in cerebral or cerebro-spinal amaurosis, and which is termed simple or progressive atrophy. In the atrophy consecutive upon optic neuritis, the outline of the disk remains somewhat hazy and indistinct, and does not show the clearly cut, sharply defined contour so characteristic of the other form. The disk may also remain somewhat swollen, and its whiteness lacks transparency and lustre, being dull and of an opaque and somewhat creamy tint. The retinal veins, moreover, retain for a long time a certain degree of dilatation and tortuosity, but, as time passes on, these differences gradually fade away, and finally the disk assumes the appearance of that met with in

[1] "Kl. Monatsbl.," 1868, 423.   [2] "R. L. Ophth. Hosp. Rep.," v. 4., 308.

simple progressive atrophy. When the infiltrations into the optic nerve and retina become absorbed, we often notice a slight thinning and atrophy of the choroid at these points.

The disease generally affects both eyes (especially where it is due to cerebral causes), either simultaneously or at a very short interval, being, according to Bouchut, more marked in the eye corresponding to the hemisphere which is the more severely involved. If the cause is intra-orbital, it is, of course, quite different. I have, however, met with an instance in which the disease (the cause of which could not even be surmised) remained entirely confined to one eye.

The sight is often greatly impaired. Sometimes, the loss of vision is very sudden, the patient becoming perhaps so blind within a few hours or days, as to be quite unable to distinguish between light and dark. But the impairment of vision does not necessarily correspond to the striking morbid alterations presented by the disease; indeed, the sight may even be perfectly normal in cases of marked optic neuritis.

I had lately a case of monocular neuritis under my care, in which the acuity of vision remained perfectly normal throughout, and I have also seen two cases of optic neuritis with Dr. Hughlings Jackson, in each of which the patient could read No. 1 of Jaeger; indeed, Dr. Jackson assures me that such cases are by no means of unfrequent occurrence, but are not often observed by the oculist, simply because the latter is only consulted when the sight is beginning to fail; whereas the physician is called in on account of some other symptom, he suspects cerebral disease, examines the eyes with the ophthalmoscope, discovers optic neuritis, and yet finds that the sight is unimpaired. Mauthner[1] narrates an interesting case, in which a patient affected with optic neuritis retained a normal acuteness of vision up to the time of his death (which was sudden). The post-mortem examination revealed the existence of interstitial optic neuritis, but the retina was healthy quite up to the optic nerve.

The field of vision is generally also more or less affected, and this is a point of much prognostic importance, for, according to Von Graefe,[2] we almost always find that, in those cases of optic neuritis in which the field of vision is contracted, at least a partial atrophy of the optic nerve and retina ensues. The pupil is, as a rule, dilated and sluggish, or even perhaps almost immovable. But, if the sight is good, it may be hardly, if at all, affected. The patient is often much troubled with subjective appearances of light (photopsia and chromotopsia), which, from their fantastic shapes and constant presence, may prove a source of great distress and anxiety. If the neuritis is due to a cerebral cause, it is generally accompanied by more or less marked symptoms of brain disease, such as loss of memory, giddiness, vomiting, impairment of the sense of smell, taste, or hearing, epileptoid fits, paralytic affections, severe headache, etc. The headache is often very great and protracted, the patient being, perhaps, unable to localize it exactly, as it extends over the whole head. Von Graefe calls attention to the fact that in cases of cerebral tumor, the position of the latter may sometimes be ascertained by the acute pain produced by sharply tapping with the finger the corresponding portion of the cranium, which also temporarily increases the severity of the general headache.

Causes.—The engorged papilla may be caused by morbid processes within the orbit, which give rise to great protrusion of the eye, or pressure upon the optic nerve, and consequently impediment of the circulation. Amongst

---

[1] "Lehrbuch der Ophthalmoscopie," p. 293.   [2] "Kl. Monatsbl.," 1863, p. 9.

such causes must be especially instanced tumors, and inflammation of th periosteum or the cellular tissue of the orbit. In such cases we often have an opportunity of watching how the symptoms of optic neuritis disappear and the sight becomes restored, when the tumor has been removed, or the inflammation has subsided and the eye returned to its normal position.

[In "choked disk" due to orbital disease, the lesion is confined to one eye. Though the optic disk may be inflamed here, it is usually compressed by the growth or the exudation; but this may not occur even when the growth large and the exophthalmos pronounced. Inflammation of the capsule of Tenon may produce the same result by causing thrombosis of the vessels of the optic nerve.

Papillitis has also been observed as a result of facial erysipelas, doubtless through the medium of orbital cellulitis. Michel has reported a case of choked disk in a very young child, which was caused, as .the autopsy showed, by hyperostosis of the bones of the skull closing or narrowing the optic foramen ; and several other cases are on record where atrophy resulted from a deformed skull (see "Arch. der Heilk.," xiv.; "Beiträge zur prakt. Augenheilk.," 1876).—B.]

It was for a long time supposed that the engorged papilla is very frequently produced by certain cerebral affections, which either exert a direct pressure upon the cavernous sinus and thus impede the venous circulation in the optic nerve and retina, or effect this by an increase in the intra-cranial tension. It was thought that this impediment of the circulation of the ophthalmic vein gives rise to mechanical congestion of the papilla, which, as has been already mentioned, is soon followed by serous infiltration, and subsequently by inflammatory proliferation of the connective-tissue elements of the optic nerve. The tendency to stasis in the circulation of the nerve is, moreover, increased by the unyielding sclerotic ring, which, as Von Graefe has happily expressed it, acts here the part of a multiplier. But more recent researches appear to entirely disprove this causation of the engorged papilla. Thus Sesemann[1] has found that the superior ophthalmic vein as well as the inferior not only anastomose freely with each other, but also with the facial vein. And, although the central vein of the retina mostly empties itself directly into the cavernous sinus, it anastomoses freely with the superior ophthalmic vein. On account of these numerous anastomoses, an impediment in the cavernous sinus cannot produce stasis (or only a temporary one) in the retinal veins, as they possess other channels for the efflux of the venous blood. The very important researches of Schwalbe, Schmidt, and Manz have, however, thrown a new light upon the subject of optic neuritis in connection with cerebral affections. Schwalbe[2] discovered that a communication exists between the arachnoid space and the optic nerve, for he found that fluid injected into the arachnoid space passed down between the external and internal sheaths of the optic nerve (Schwalbe's subvaginal space) to the ocular extremity of the nerve (optic disk), where the fluid becomes collected, being unable to pass on into the eye. Schmidt[3] verified these facts by further experiments, and found, moreover, that the injection passed into the lamina cribrosa, and hence believes that there exists in the lamina cribrosa a canal-system, which stands in direct communication with the arachnoid space. "Increased intra-cranial tension will therefore press fluid from the arachnoid space into this canal-system. If we suppose that the latter is always filled with fluid, even a slight increase in this from the arachnoid space will pro-

[1] "Archiv für Anatomie, Physiologie," etc., 1869, 2, 154.
[2] "Centralblatt für med. Wissenschaften," 1869, No. 30.
[3] Schmidt, "A. f. O.," xv. 1, 193.

duce a considerable swelling, and extension of the close network in the lamina cribrosa." These facts afford quite a new explanation as to the cause of the incarceration of the intra-ocular extremity of the optic nerve, and its attendant symptoms of engorgement of the disk. If the hydrops of the sheath of the optic nerve becomes considerable, it produces not only a bulging outwards of the sheath, but also, pressing inwards upon the contents of the sheath (optic nerve fibres and bloodvessels), it causes an impediment in the venous efflux, followed by swelling of the disk, dilatation and tortuosity of the retinal veins, diminution in the size of the arteries, etc. If the hydrops of the sheath continues for some time, the œdema may filter through into the retina, and, besides the fluid, formed elements may pass through the walls of the bloodvessels. Manz[1] has found hydrops of the sheath of the optic nerve in so many cases of intra-cranial disease, that he supposes it to be of very frequent occurrence in certain cerebral lesions. From the above facts, it will be evident that hydrops of the sheath of the optic nerve (leading to engorgement of the papilla, etc.) may probably occur, not only in those cerebral diseases which are accompanied by a serous effusion, but it may also accompany intra-cranial affections (e. g., tumors), which increase the intra-cranial tension, displace the normally existing cerebral fluid, and some of this may pass down the sheath of the optic nerve (Manz). Hence this form of optic neuritis (engorged papilla) should make us suspect the presence of a cerebral tumor. But such tumors may also produce simple atrophy of the optic nerve by direct pressure upon it; or they may set up inflammation of the meninges, which, extending to the optic nerve, gives rise to descending neuritis. The latter disease is therefore sometimes met with in cases of meningitis or arachnitis, in which the inflammation extends to the optic nerve, and travels down to the papilla and retina. Optic neuritis has also been met with in cases of cerebro-spinal meningitis.[2] We may, however, have mixed forms of optic neuritis, in which the phenomena presented by the disease are partly due to inflammation of the trunk of the nerve, and partly to obstruction in the circulation.

Microscopical and anatomical researches made upon the human cadaver and experimentally upon animals, have proven to the satisfaction of most ophthalmologists that any disease which causes an increase of the intra-cranial pressure may exert a direct influence upon the optic nerve through the medium of the lymphatic spaces between the sheaths of the optic nerve, which are directly continuous with the subdural and subarachnoidal spaces in the brain. This effect upon the optic nerve, most marked in the intra-ocular part, is a serous exudation into the nerve consequent upon drop-sical distension of the intervaginal space. In addition, there may result a real vaginitis which may lead to obliteration of the intervaginal space, and consequent inflammation of the connective tissue of the optic nerve. The distension of the intervaginal space may be followed by a similar distention of the lymphatic channels within the optic nerve, and if this condition lasts for any considerable time, it always causes atrophy of the nerve fibres. Inflammation of the optic nerve fibres themselves is an exceedingly rare disease.

A few words on the existing views of ophthalmologists as to the connection between intra-cranial tumors and optic neuritis are all-important. Brain tumors are probably the most frequent cause of choked disk. In cases

---

[1] "Deutsches Archiv für Klin. Medicin," ix. 339, 1872; vide also his valuable article, "A. f. O.," xvi. 1, 265.

[2] "A. f. O.," xvii. 1, 178; and "Kl. Monatsbl.," 1865, p. 275 [also, "Amer. Journ. Med. Sciences," Jan. 1873.—B.].

of chronic brain disease, *bilateral choked disk* almost always means either tumor or some other mass of exudation in the cranial cavity. Annuske has concluded, from a very large number of cases, that papillitis is an almost constant symptom of brain tumor. But there are exceptions to this ru and they are not very rare. Cases have been reported where all the symptoms pointed to an intra-cranial growth, and there was no ophthalmoscopic evidence of disease, yet the autopsy revealed a tumor. The reverse is al true, for marked papillitis has existed in both eyes, which the course of disease or an autopsy has proven to be due not to an intra-cranial grow but to an orbital growth, an orbital inflammation, or to a basilar mening with extensive exudation.

Futhermore, let it be distinctly understood that the situation of a tumor cannot be determined with any accuracy by the presence of optic neuri ti Tumors of the cerebellum, of the convexity of the cerebral lobes, and of the base of the skull *may* cause papillitis. Indeed, the latter may by direct compression of the optic nerves or tracts lead to atrophy of the optic nerves without ever causing any papillitis; these cases are, however, rare. Moreover, it should not be forgotten that Bright's disease may cause in the eye an exact picture of choked disk.—B]

In one case of descending neuritis narrated by Von Graefe,[1] the circumscribed basilar meningitis was found to be caused by a peculiar entozoon. situated partly in the right hemisphere and partly at the base of the cranium.

[Seguin and Erb have both reported cases of optic neuritis from transverse myelitis of the cord; Erb's case ended in atrophy and slight concentric limitation of the field of vision. In both of Seguin's cases the neuritis was in the right eye, with irregular defect of the field of vision ("Journ. of Nervous and Mental Diseases," April, 1880).—B.]

Indeed, according to Dr. Hughlings Jackson,[2] who has made so many interesting and valuable researches upon the affections of the eye met with in cerebral diseases, optic neuritis may be produced by "coarse" disease of almost any part of the cerebrum, or cerebellum. This being so, I cannot do better than give the following summary of his experience and views, which appeared in the Hospital Reports of the "British Medical Journal" (March 28, 1868):

"We now report remarks on an acute condition of the optic nerves, which is followed by another kind of atrophy. It is to be kept in mind that the following remarks apply to cases of optic neuritis ('descending neuritis') seen in physicians' practice, and contain an accurate, although a very brief, statement of the chief conclusions at which Dr. Hughlings Jackson has arrived. Optic neuritis from intra-cranial disease is always double, even when the disease giving rise to it is quite limited to a single cerebral hemisphere. Not unfrequently one eye suffers more than the other, but even when one cerebral hemisphere is alone diseased, there does not seem to be any constant relation betwixt the side of the brain affected and the eye more affected. Although, in physicians' practice, the local disease causing optic neuritis is most often of the cerebral hemisphere, it may be in part of either the cerebral or cerebellar hemispheres, or at the base of the skull. Dr. Hughlings Jackson has not yet found optic neuritis, nor indeed optic atrophy of any kind, with disease limited to the optic thalamus, to the pons, or to the medulla oblongata.

---

[1] "Kl. Monatsbl.," 1864, p. 367.
[2] *Vide* Dr. Hughlings Jackson's contributions upon these subjects in the "R. L. O. H. Reports," "The London Hospital Reports," "Med. Times," etc. [See "Graefe und Saemisch's Hdb. der Augenheilk.," v. p. 776–796; "Arch. f. Ophthal.," xix. 8; "Arch. der Heilk.," xiv.; "Roy. Lond. Ophth. Hosp. Rep.," vii. 4.]

The intra-cranial disease is almost always *coarse*. The intra-cranial disease may be of many kinds, probably of any coarse kind. Thus Dr. Hughlings Jackson has found optic neuritis with tumor, with abscess, with blood-clot, with syphilitic 'deposit,' and with hydatid cyst, and all these of the cerebral hemisphere. He has not found, with one exception, any but the most trifling unusual intra-ocular appearances in the chorea of children; a disease which he supposes (*see* 'London Hospital Reports,' vol. i. 1864; 'Lancet,' Nov. 26, 1864; 'Med. Times and Gazette,' Jan. 28, 1865) to depend, at least frequently, on plugging of small branches of the middle cerebral artery. Chorea in children does not at all events depend on *coarse* disease of the brain. From a superficial point of view it is, Dr. Hughlings Jackson thinks, somewhat striking that marked pathological changes in the optic disks are not unfrequently found with unilateral spasm, and with unilateral palsy, and scarcely ever with unilateral irregular movements. Choreiform movements are sometimes observed during recovery from the 'epileptic hemiplegia' which occasionally occurs with optic neuritis. However, the real association is not of optic neuritis with one-sided spasm or palsy, but with intra-cranial coarse disease, which coarse disease, when it is of one cerebral hemisphere, may produce both optic neuritis and the condition (corpus striatum neuritis?) on which the one-sided spasm, or palsy, or both depend. We should not, he thinks—making a mistake analogous to that the old astronomers made—consider amaurosis, from optic neuritis, or the atrophy which follows it, to be the centre-point of a case around which all the other symptoms 'revolve;' but rather try to find the central disease—in physicians' practice often coarse disease of one cerebral hemisphere—to which each of the symptoms (headache, convulsions, amaurosis from optic neuritis) is equally subordinate. He thinks it is not warrantable, even when we find a lump of syphilitic disease in the cerebral hemisphere post-mortem, to say that optic neuritis is 'caused by syphilis,' since just the same ophthalmoscopic appearances may occur with other sorts of 'foreign bodies' in the very same part of the brain. How it happens that a foreign body in the brain sometimes 'excites' changes about itself, and sometimes does not, is the subject of speculations of very different kinds into which we do not now enter. Optic neuritis does not depend on *loss of function* of the part which the coarse disease destroys, as does loss of power of intellectual expression (aphasia). Optic neuritis requires time for its production. Thus, although it occurs with blood-clot, it never, in Dr. Hughlings Jackson's experience at least, occurs with *recent* blood-clot. When coarse disease of one cerebral hemisphere gives rise to headache, vomiting, unilateral spasm, amaurosis from optic neuritis; or, let us say, to the larger uproar called 'cerebral fever,' involving all or most of these, the probability is that there is but one idea throughout, viz., a 'foreign body,' and changes diffused from it in different directions, on which diffused changes the symptoms directly depend. The most important clinical fact about optic neuritis is, that it may exist for a varying time—a few days, a few weeks, or a few months—without any apparent defect of sight. *It must be looked for* in every case of cerebral disease, at all events in every case of cerebral fever. It is necessary to look for it in cases of loss of speech from disease of the hemisphere. As implied in the foregoing, it is only likely to occur in cases where the speech defect depends on *coarse* disease, let us say on a large clot, and then only some time after the seizure. A blood-clot causes loss of speech as a destroyer of an elaborate structure, and subsequently optic neuritis in its character as a foreign body. However, optic neuritis is rarely associated with blood-clot."

[Hughlings Jackson's most recent paper upon optic neuritis in intra-cranial disease is of exceptional interest. He thinks there is but one kind of optic neuritis from intra-cranial disease. Considering it ophthalmoscopically, the most trustworthy localizing symptoms, helping the diagnosis of tumor, are such as convulsions beginning unilaterally, and paralysis of cranial nerves. He doubts whether he has ever seen double optic neuritis from clot. In tubercular meningitis, he believes that swelling of the disk comes on at a time when the diagnosis of meningitis is made from other evidence; it is slight, even, and merges into the fundus like the earliest stage of optic neuritis from intra-cranial tumor. But he admits that intra-cranial tumor sometimes produces an acute illness, not distinguishable by its symptoms from meningitis, tubercular or traumatic. He does not recognize any difference in the kind of disk between cases in which sight is good and those in which it is defective or lost; but only a difference in the stage of changes. He recognizes the difficulty of determining whether a patient has had neuritis from the appearance of the disks at a later period, especially if the patient has never been seen before. He believes that the diagnostic value of optic neuritis is not dependent upon whether the sight be good or lost. He thinks that there is nearly always a stage of neuritis before sight fails, but that sometimes vision is affected before there is any ophthalmoscopic evidence of neuritis. He classes neuritis, headache, and vomiting in one group, depending in very many cases on local gross organic disease within the cranium, but not helping us to determine the locality of the inferred disease. It should be remembered, however, that optic neuritis may occur without any headache or vomiting. Complete recovery with good sight does not negative persisting local gross organic disease within the cranium. Although optic neuritis is so often found with disease of the cerebrum or cerebellum, it does not occur from mere destruction of any particular part of the encephalon. The adventitious mass may be in any part of the encephalon, with the possible exception of the medulla oblongata and may produce double optic neuritis; but on the other hand optic neuritis may not be found with tumors or other masses in different parts of the cranial cavity. It occurs exceedingly rarely in cases of extensive destruction of brain substance by softening or clot. Because, therefore, optic neuritis occurs with tumor of any part, and may not occur with tumors of many parts; because it comes on late in some cases of tumor, and passes off again in some; because it is very rarely found with such widely destructive processes as softening and clot; and because it may not be attended by any defect of sight, it is inferred that it does not depend on destruction of any part of the nervous centres. Hence, Jackson infers that tumor, or any other adventitious product, does not produce optic neuritis in its particular character as this or that kind of pathological product, but in its general character as a foreign body; and then not because it destroys, but by some indirect action. He thinks that optic neuritis results doubly indirectly from intra-cranial tumor by vaso-motor action. At first there are changes of instability about the tumor; next, these promote discharges by the intermediation of vaso-motor nerves, to repeated contractions, with subsequent paralysis of vessels of the optic nerves or centres, and thus at length lead to that trouble of nutrition which is optic neuritis. All the symptoms alluded to are, he considers, signs of an encephalitis provoked by the tumor in its character as a foreign body. He admits that swelling of but one disk is a difficulty in the way of this hypothesis being accepted as satisfactory. (See "Medical Times and Gazette," March 19, 1881.)

Leber's most recent views are as follows: He holds that optic neuritis in cerebral diseases is a true inflammation. It is not caused by stasis in the retinal veins from compression of the cavernous sinus, due to diminished intra-cranial space. It is not the result of irritation of the vaso-motor nerves caused by the cerebral affection. The optic nerve is the path of communication between the affection of the brain and that of the eye. An essential part in this transmission is taken by the effusion of a serous fluid into the sheath of the nerve extruded from the cranium by the increased intra-cranial pressure. This fluid does not act by simple mechanical pressure, and it probably possesses phlogogenic properties.

Hemorrhages at the base of the brain may cause monolateral or bilateral papillitis by the blood passing directly into the intervaginal space.

Cerebral abscess is not infrequently found in cases of double papillitis, but usually there is an injury to the vault of the skull in these cases.

Though "choked disk" occurs in basilar meningitis, whether traumatic or spontaneous, it is especially common in tubercular meningitis, developing sometimes within a few days, but rarely reaching a high degree of swelling of the disk. In some cases, where there was no papillitis, the autopsy revealed dropsy of the sheath of the optic nerve, which accounted for the loss of vision. Cases of choked disk from meningitis of the convexity following injury have also been reported. (See "Amer. Journ. of Med. Sciences," October, 1877.)

In hydrocephalus internus, papillitis has sometimes been met with, and it almost always ends in atrophy of the nerve. Usually, however, the lesion of the optic nerve is a simple atrophy in this disease from the beginning. (See " Graefe und Saemisch," l. c. p. 795.)—B.]

Benedikt[1] considers that, beside the optic neuritis which may be produced by mechanical means (i. e., by an obstruction to the circulation producing the engorged papilla), and that due to a descending inflammation of the optic nerve, we must distinguish a third form, in which the cerebral affection lies altogether out of the course of the optic nerve. In such cases, the symptomatic optic neuritis is due to neurosis of the vaso-motor nerves, causing hyperæmia and swelling of the optic nerve. He points out also that widely extending and periodical symptoms (e. g., intense headache, loss of consciousness, paralysis, amblyopia, amaurosis, etc.), which often appear during the development of a cerebral tumor and correspond to its more rapid growth, are not due to direct irritation produced by the tumor on contiguous parts, but to widespread hyperæmia and swelling dependent on neurosis of the sympathetic fibres, or, so to speak, a local fever. It is just in these cases of symptomatic neuro-retinitis due to neurosis of the sympathetic, that Benedikt has often found great benefit from galvanism of the sympathetic nerve. This theory of Benedikt's receives some support from Leber's[2] observation, that an optic nerve which seems to the naked eye to be perfectly healthy, may show, on microscopic examination, very marked pathological changes, such as interstitial neuritis and perineuritis, fatty degeneration of the bundles of nerve fibres, etc. Now as he has, moreover, met with some of these changes in cases of *quite recent* optic neuritis, in which it was impossible to assume that the inflammatory process had ascended from within the eye to the optic nerve, and the mechanical theory of the causation could not, therefore, hold good, Leber thinks that "in them no other explanation is possible than that which has been already pointed out by Benedikt, viz., that cerebral affections in general may cause direct in-

[1] *Vide* Benedikt's " Electrotherapie," p. 253.
[2] " Kl. Monatsbl.," 1868, p. 302.

flammatory changes in the optic nerve and papilla through irritation of certain nerve-paths (Nerven-bahnen) which are still unknown to us."

Dr. Hermann Pagenstecher believes[1] "that the irritation conveyed through the nerve-tract of the sympathetic to the disk, induces the changes of the nerve fibres, the hyperæmia, and even the development of new vessels, and in this manner, a swelling and cloudiness of the disk and the adjacent parts of the retina are brought about. The latter may then for its part have as a consequence an extreme degree of congestion of the venous system of the retina."

[In many cases, perhaps the majority, of neuro-retinitis with choked disk, and also in cases of descending neuritis, perineuritis is also present. The intervaginal space becomes distended with a cloudy, cellular fluid, and the sheaths themselves infiltrated with lymphoid cells. The interstitial connective framework of the optic nerve is soon involved, and becomes hypertrophied, and the cells and nuclei proliferate. This is the usual result when the cause has been periostitis of the orbit.

Leber also speaks of a medullary neuritis which results in destruction of the medulla by fatty degeneration, and the process ends in gray atrophy. Clinically, this variety of optic nerve inflammation is not to be distinguished from other forms, and it is mainly interesting pathologically. This form of degeneration has been traced back of the chiasm as far as the corpus geniculatum. This inflammation might arise from dropsy of the sheath, or from meningeal inflammation, or be caused by any intra-cranial process, but through the medium, probably, of an interstitial neuritis. This degeneration may affect the chiasm and optic tracts, and leave the optic nerve itself untouched. Some authors mention among the varieties of neuritis without ophthalmoscopic sign, the rheumatic, and this always affects both eyes.

Among children, neuro-retinitis, with all the signs of choked disk in one or both eyes, is sometimes met with, in which it is impossible to determine any cause; the patients being and remaining otherwise perfectly well. In these cases the prognosis is bad.—B.]

But we sometimes meet with cases of optic neuritis, in which it is quite impossible to detect any cause or any impairment of the health, except, perhaps, some derangement of the uterine functions, e. g., insufficiency of the catamenia. I have seen several instances of this kind in young and delicate females, who otherwise enjoyed perfect health. Such cases recover completely, if they are seen at the outset of the disease, and are actively and efficiently treated. [The neuritis in these cases may be caused either by a sudden cessation of the menstrual flow during a period, or by a non-appearance of the flow at the usual period, or, finally, by a condition of metrorrhagia. These cases of neuritis are generally accompanied by headache, with heat and fulness in the head, and sometimes by graver cerebral symptoms. At the climacteric period, also, neuro-retinitis with choked disk is occasionally met with, and Mooren claims to have seen it in cases of uterine displacement, and states that with the cure of the uterine difficulty the neuritis disappears. (See "Ophthal.," Mettheil, 1874.) The prognosis in all these cases depends upon the restoration of the menstrual function promptly, and means should be taken to that end. Where the process is a chronic one, Leber advises a seton in the temple and leeches to the nasal septum; and Mooren advises iced applications to the head.—B.] Mr. Hulke, in an interesting paper on optic neuritis,[2] narrates such cases, and

1 Vide his valuable article, "R. L. O. H. Reports," vol. vii. part 2, 125.
2 " R. L. O. H. Rep.," vi. 2.

also others, in which it occurred in connection with diphtheria, rheumatic fever, etc.

To prove that the distinction between the engorged papilla and the descending neuritis is not a theoretical or arbitrary one, we need only pay attention to the differences in the anatomical changes met with in these two forms. In the engorged papilla, the inflammatory changes are generally chiefly confined to the intra-ocular end of the optic nerve, and do not, as a rule, extend backwards beyond the lamina cribrosa, although the intimate structure of the latter is often greatly changed, and its characteristic features rendered indistinct.[1] Mauthner[2] has seen some preparations of Iwanoff's, in which the proliferation of the connective tissue, instead of stopping short at the lamina cribrosa, had extended somewhat along the trunk of the nerve, and had thus given rise to ascending neuritis.

In descending neuritis, Virchow[3] found that, besides hypertrophy of the vessels and increase in the width of the nerve fibres, the whole trunk of the nerve had undergone inflammatory changes. The neurilemma was thickened, and showed cystoid detachments. Besides this perineuritis, the elements of the interstitial connective tissue had undergone proliferation, producing degeneration and destruction of the nerve tubules.[4]

The *prognosis* must *in all cases* be extremely doubtful and guarded, and in the great majority unfavorable, for, as a rule, optic neuritis ends in more or less complete atrophy of the nerve and loss of sight. Besides the question of vision, it must also be remembered that there arises the still more important one of life, for but two frequently optic neuritis is caused by most dangerous and incurable affections of the brain. The most favorable cases are those in which the disease is due to some temporary and relievable cause, such as irregularities in the catamenia, etc., or a tumor or inflammation in the orbit. But even in these, the morbid changes in the optic nerve may have been so great as to prevent any restitution *ad integrum*, and the end is, more or less atrophy of the nerve. On the whole, the cases in which the progress of the disease and the loss of sight have been very rapid, afford a more favorable prognosis than those in which they have been slow and gradual. In the former instance, a perfect recovery may result, even although all quantitative perception of light has been temporarily lost.[5] According to Von Graefe, the prognosis is also more favorable in children than in adults. The condition of the pupil, with regard to its reacting or not on the admission of light, is of no importance in the prognosis.

With regard to the *treatment*, we can only lay down general rules, as it must be varied according to the nature of the cause and the exigencies and peculiarities of individual cases. If the disease is seen at the outset, the patient should be placed as soon as possible under the influence of mercury (inunction). If the patient is delicate, tonics should be at the same time administered. I have several times observed that this line of treatment has exerted a markedly favorable influence upon the progress of the disease and the morbid effusion, the absorption of which it hastens and facilitates. This is especially the case when the disease occurs without any special intra-orbital or cerebral cause, as in females suffering from derangement of the uterine functions, or persons affected with the suppression of some customary

[1] "Schweigger Vorlesungen," p. 186.
[2] "Lehrbuch der Ophthalmoscopie," p. 289.   [3] "A. f. O.," xii. 2, 117.
[4] *Vide* also Dr. Leber's interesting paper on "Optic Neuritis," "A. f. O.," xiv. 2, 338.
[5] "A. f. O.," xii. 2, 183; *vide* also a case of this kind reported by Hirschberg in the "Berliner Klinische Wochenschrift," September 13, 1869.

discharge, or great inaction of the skin. In some of these cases, I have seen
a complete recovery resulting from the combined influence of mercury and
the local application of the artificial leech. The action of the skin should
be stimulated by diaphoretics, and, if the patient will submit to it, a course
of treatment by Zittman's decoction, which proves especially beneficial in
syphilitic cases. If the disease is not seen till a later stage, when permanent
changes in the nerve have already occurred, I do not think that any benefit
will be derived from salivation, and should prefer the administration of small
doses of the bichloride of mercury, perhaps in combination with the iodide
and bromide of potassium.

The severe and often very violent pain in the head, with which the patients
are frequently affected when the disease depends upon a cerebral lesion, is
generally relieved by a suppurating blister, or, still better, a seton in the
nape of the neck.

To alleviate the congestion of the optic nerve and retina, the artificial
leech should be applied several times, at intervals of a few days, but should
then be desisted from if no benefit results. If the patient is weak and delicate, dry cupping should be substituted.

Galvanization of the sympathetic by means of the continuous current may
also be tried; it is strongly recommended by Benedikt. [This method has
been tried by numerous observers, but there are no records of any favorable
results, and it is now practically given up.—B.]

The fact that hydrops of the sheath of the optic nerve has been so often
found in *post-mortem* examination of cases of optic neuritis, has led De
Wecker to suggest incision of the optic nerve in such cases.[1] For he believes
that according to the theory of Schwalbe and Schmidt, there are two indications to be fulfilled : 1. To give exit to the accumulation of the cerebral
fluid by making an incision into the external coat of the optic nerve. 2. To
relieve strangulation of the nerve by incising the sclerotic ring at the point
where it forms the junction of the sheath with the external enveloping membrane of the eye. He thus hopes to relieve the symptoms of compression,
not only of the nerve itself, but also those of the cerebral centres (headache,
etc.). He tried it first on the dead body, and then in two patients. The
operation was performed thus: An incision was made between the external
and inferior rectus muscle, about one centimetre from the cornea. Then,
cutting through the conjunctiva and subconjunctival tissue, a pair of scissors
(closed) are to penetrate between the eyeball and capsule of Tenon until the
optic nerve is reached. A spatula is then to be introduced and the eyeball
displaced upwards and inwards. After the displacement of the eyeball, it
is easy to feel with the spatula the distended nerve, and to introduce the
sheathed neurotome (an instrument specially made for this purpose by
Mathieu); with this the sheath of the optic nerve and sclerotic ring are to
be incised, the instrument being pressed from behind forwards. In future,
De Wecker purposes introducing the finger up to the nerve, for the purpose
of placing the instrument in its proper position. There was little or no
pain, and although the sight does not seem to have been improved, there
was great relief of the intense headache, especially on the side of the operation.

[Neuritis optica and papillitis are also met with in syphilitic patients,
both in cases of congenital and acquired syphilis. It may be caused by a
gummy tumor in the skull, and is generally a papillitis. This is to be distinguished pathologically from so-called neuritis syphilitica, in which there

---

• International Ophthalmological Congress, London, 1872.

may also be papillitis, but in which the main change is a dense inflammatory thickening of both optic nerves back to the chiasm, and even into the optic tracts. In some cases the starting-point of this change is an intra-cranial gumma which has grown into the optic tracts. Clinically, this form of inflammation cannot be distinguished from other varieties, and hence, correctly speaking, there is no such disease as syphilitic neuritis. The prognosis is moderately favorable if treatment be begun early enough; but if not, the tendency is to atrophy of the nerve.

Leber has reported cases of hereditary neuritis optica, both intra-ocular and retro-bulbar. It manifests itself usually after puberty. Direct heredity as a cause is, however, not common. It attacks the male members of a family almost exclusively. In many of these patients there are other symptoms of nervous disorder. Both eyes are always affected, and the vision is usually markedly interfered with. In most of the cases central vision remains permanently abolished, but eccentric vision is generally restored if treatment is resorted to in time. There is, however, no special treatment indicated in these cases. (See "Graefe und Saemisch," l. c. p. 824. "Archiv f. Ophthal.," xvii. 2, p. 249.)—B.]

Under the head of optic neuritis, Von Graefe[1] has called attention to cases in which there was an extremely sudden loss of sight, the patient becoming, without any clearly defined cause, so absolutely blind in the course of a few hours as to be unable to distinguish between light and darkness. He says: "After constitutional diseases of different kinds (I have observed it occurring after measles, febrile gastric catarrh, and anginæ), but without any marked disturbance of the general health; the field of vision becomes clouded, with or without the presence of chromotopsia and photopsia, and within the course of a few hours or days absolute blindness ensues. Both eyes are generally symmetrically affected, and only in a single case have I seen the disease confined to one eye. This case, however, presented some slightly irregular characters. The pupil generally becomes unusually dilated, and quite inactive to the stimulus of light, retaining but a slight degree of mobility during the movements of the eye or the impulse of accommodation. There is, therefore, reason to assume the existence of a special state of irritation in the fibres of the sympathetic. With the ophthalmoscope may be observed undoubted, though not very conspicuous, changes in the papilla, which are, however, of a markedly transitory character. Its tissue is veiled by a delicate, diffuse opacity, as is also the neighboring retina; the level of the disk is, however, hardly raised, or only in a very slight degree, and only for a few days. The arteries are narrowed, but by pressing upon the eye we can still succeed in producing a slight pulsation (the surest sign of the existence of a continuous circulation),[2] the veins are dilated and tortuous; but their course is tolerably regular on account of the but slight opacity of the tissues." Von Graefe narrates four cases of this kind. In

---

[1] "Archiv f. O.," xii. 2, 135.

[2] If a thrombus in the central artery of the retina has produced ischæmia of the retina, the arteries of the latter will also be extremely small, but even a considerable pressure on the eyeball with the finger will not succeed in producing arterial pulsation or emptying of the arteries. With regard to this subject, Von Graefe says at another place: "If, together with a free venous efflux, thrombosis occurs in the region of the lamina cribrosa or behind it, we must expect to find the retinal arteries empty. But if the venous efflux has been impeded by the swelling of the tissues, either simultaneously or at an earlier date, the arteries may remain partially filled; but on the other hand, pressure upon the eyeball will not produce the usual phenomena, on account of the stoppage in the influx of the blood." ("Arch. f. O.," xii. 2, 134, note.)

two, a complete recovery occurred, although there had been absolute loss of even quantitative perception of light for some little time. In another case, the absolute blindness continued, and the disease passed over into rapid atrophy of the nerve. In the fourth, there was incomplete recovery, with partial atrophy.

Von Graefe considers that in all probability these were cases of retro-ocular neuritis, the swelling and diffuse opacity being due to an interstitial serous infiltration (œdema). The difference between this form and the descending neuritis consists principally in this, that the more marked tissue alterations do not extend to the papilla, that the disease occurs only at certain points, and does not involve continuously the whole trunk of the nerve. In fact, the degree of inflammation is only very moderate, and the disease but seldom depends upon grave intra-cranial lesions. [Retro-bulbar neuritis is now recognized by all ophthalmologists. It is chronic, at first has no ophthalmoscopic symptoms, but generally ends in partial discoloration of the papilla and limitation of central vision, and is almost always bilateral.—B.]

Von Graefe thinks, moreover, that certain cases of ischæmia retinæ, and also perhaps of embolism of the central artery of the retina, may have been in reality instances of retro-ocular neuritis.

The cases of circumscribed central scotoma (interruption of the visual field) combined with amblyopia, which are not unfrequently met with, would appear from recent researches, more especially those of Leber,[1] to be generally due to retro-ocular neuritis, the inflammation being situated in that portion of the nerve which lies between the eyeball and the commissure. From this category must, of course, be excluded the scotomata which are due to changes in the external layers of the retina in the region of the yellow spot. According to Leber, the disease is especially characterized by the following symptoms: At the very outset, there are frequently no abnormal ophthalmoscopic symptoms, excepting perhaps a certain degree of hyperæmia of the optic disk and retina. Soon, however, a faint, somewhat striated cloudiness appears at the margin of the disk, extending more or less on to the neighboring portion of the retina, and resembling somewhat the opacity met with in syphilitic retinitis. Small, white, opaque striæ are noticed on the disk, enveloping and hiding the point of exit of the vessels, and extending perhaps somewhat along their walls on to the retina. These opaque striæ are, according to Von Graefe, especially pathognomonic of the existence of retro-ocular neuritis. [So-called "perivasculitis retinæ."—B.] Here and there small extravasations of blood may be strewn about on the retina in the vicinity of the disk. At a later period, but in some cases even tolerably early, a white or faintly bluish discoloration of the optic disk supervenes, which almost always remains confined to the outer half of the disk, reaching closer up to the edge of the latter than a physiological excavation. Whilst the outer half of the disk becomes blanched, the inner retains its red tint, and this is very characteristic of central scotoma. The disease, which, as a rule, attacks both eyes, either simultaneously or at a short interval, generally becomes gradually developed, progressing slowly but steadily for weeks or months, during which time the partial discoloration of the disk becomes more and more pronounced, and then remains stationary. Sometimes, however, the attack is very sudden, the affection reaching its acme in the course of a few days. This is especially the case in the amblyopia of drunkards. The degree of impairment of vision varies, but, as a rule, a

---

[1] *Vide* Leber's very valuable and interesting paper on "Color-blindness in certain Diseases of the Eye" ("A. f. O.," xv. 8, 26), in which he gives a full and excellent description of this form of amblyopia.

medium amount of sight remains. The disease is almost entirely confined to adults and men, being especially met with in drunkards, heavy smokers, or persons who are much exposed to cold and wet, such as gamekeepers, engine drivers, etc. Out of fifty-six cases which Leber observed, he only met with it three times in women. It is probably, in most instances, due to retro-ocular neuritis; but often also, especially in those cases which occur in drunkards, it is simply produced by hyperæmia, this causing a disturbance in the nutrition of the nerve elements, which may gradually induce atrophic changes.

[The color-scotoma resembles that in the ordinary form of acquired color-blindness. There is no constant relation existing between the amount of central vision and the degree of color-blindness. There may be an extensive central color-scotoma with slight amblyopia, and marked amblyopia with no disturbance of the color-sense at all. The form of the color-scotoma is generally a horizontal oval. These patients see better in a moderate light than in a bright one. The *retinitis nyctalopica* of Von Arlt is probably the same disease as retro-bulbar neuritis. Leber offers the following explanation of this scotoma. Assume that the fibres which supply the macula and space between it and the optic disk lie next each other in the optic nerve; the discoloration of the temporal half of the disk proves that they are situated in this part of the nerve. Now these fibres which end around the nerve and in the macula run in the optic nerve next the sheath, while those which supply the anterior part of the retina run in the centre of the optic nerve. This is a settled anatomical fact. Hence the central scotomata occurring in diseases of the optic nerve are due to an isolated lesion of the bundles of fibres next the sheath, which would naturally and easily result from an inflammation of the sheath. This pathological condition is not an uncommon find in microscopic examinations of optic nerves. The shape of the scotoma, a horizontal oval, Leber thinks is due to a special participation of the fibres of the fasciculus cruciatus which supply the corresponding part of the outer half of the retina. These fibres, as demonstrated by Liebreich and Michel, pass in a horizontal direction outwards, while the fibres of the other fasciculus run in an oblique direction upwards and outwards, curve round the region of the macula and then run in the horizontal meridian. An atrophy of these bundles of fibres would cause a marked discoloration of the outer half of the papilla. (See "Bericht der Wiener Augenklinik," 1866, pp. 125–132; "Graefe u. Saemisch," l. c. p. 834.)—B.]

Leber[1] has found that the appreciation of colors is more or less impaired in all cases of central scotoma, for in thirty-one cases in which he made an accurate investigation upon this point, it was deteriorated in all. In some instances, the color-blindness led to the detection of a scotoma, which was unapparent by the usual modes of examination. In the slighter cases, red could not be appreciated; in the severer, the appreciation of colors gradually diminished more and more from the red to the violet end of the spectrum, just as occurs in atrophy of the optic nerve. The treatment must consist in local depletion by the artificial leech, the use of stimulant foot-baths, perhaps also the Turkish bath, the internal administration of iodide of potassium, or of tonics if the patient is feeble and his constitution much shattered. The most stringent rules must also be enforced as to the mode of life, and the abstinence from tobacco, stimulants, and debauchery of every kind. The prognosis must be guarded, but even in the severer cases need not be absolutely bad, for the disease does not lead to complete blindness, if the field of vision remains unimpaired for some length of time (Von Graefe).

[1] "A. f. O.," xv. 2, 70.

3.—ATROPHY OF THE OPTIC

I shall here confine myself to a desc
symptoms presented by different for:
reserve the consideration of the caus
until we come to treat of the amblyo

Some observers have thought that
are usually ushered in by a well-mark
Great care is, however, required, not
the color of the disk as being of pa
already stated, the nasal side of the
the outer side, its edge being therefore
a physiological appearance. In the a
(congestion) in the cerebral circulat
seen, as also after prolonged straini.
think that, as a rule, it is met with
progressive atrophy of the optic n·
nature of the simple, progressive at
doubtful. Some observers believe
irritation in the interstitial cellular
disappearance of the conducting n
might be urged the symptoms which
of the disease, e. g., pains in the hea
amaurosis nor in tabes dorsalis does
cellular tissue of the nerves, in the o

The ophthalmoscopic symptoms w
the optic nerve are a pale, white or t
diminution in the calibre and numbe:
the expanse of the disk, attenuation o
arteries, and frequently a peculiar ex

In atrophy of the optic nerve (r
cerebral or cerebro-spinal amaurosis)
grayish-pink tint, but looks pale and
great as to cause the disk to resem:
there is frequently a bluish-white c
lustre. In the former case, the plane
white color is chiefly due to the
hypertrophy and thickening of the
The bluish-white reflex is, on the o
tubules between the meshes of the la
of the latter peculiarly distinct. In
the nerve. Very frequently these tv
shallow excavation, with the details
disposed, the other portion being co
show (Von Graefe).

' Besides being pale and discolored
and peculiar clearness of tint, so tha
traced passing into the substance of
the disk may be somewhat irregular
defined, and the choroidal ring appe
papilla may also seem to be somewh:

¹ *Vide* Von Graefe's " Lectures on

should be attached to this symptom, which is, moreover, often due to causes situated in the refraction of the eye. The bluish, or bluish-green tint is often met with in cases of spinal amaurosis, of which indeed some authors consider it almost pathognomonic.[1]

The retinal vessels are generally diminished in size, and often considerably so. The little bloodvessels upon the disk are attenuated or have disappeared, and this of course also tends still more to blanch the papilla. The retinal arteries are often so narrow, as to resemble minute threads, being hardly traceable upon the retina at some little distance from the disk, but their principal trunks can generally be easily recognized upon the papilla. The retinal veins are mostly also somewhat diminished in calibre, but to a less extent than the arteries. We, however, sometimes meet with cases of chronic, complete amaurosis with well-marked symptoms of nerve atrophy, and yet the principal retinal vessels retain their normal diameter. The most marked attenuation of the vessel is seen in cases of atrophy consequent upon retinitis or choroido-retinitis.

Whilst the above are the symptoms presented by progressive atrophy of the optic nerve, the form of atrophy which is consecutive upon optic neuritis retains for a long time special characteristic peculiarities, which generally enable us to distinguish it from the former kind, and also from that which ensues upon retinitis pigmentosa, etc. Finally, however, these distinctive characteristics gradually fade away, and it assumes the appearance of progressive cerebral atrophy. In the earlier stage, it is chiefly distinguished from the latter by the fact that the papilla remains slightly swollen, having a dull and opaque, grayish-white, faintly clouded appearance. Its outline, moreover, is not sharply defined, but uneven and indistinct, passing over gradually and almost insensibly into the faintly clouded retina, so that the disk appears surrounded by a slight halo. The retinal veins also remain somewhat dilated, veiled, and tortuous. Sometimes, we may distinctly follow the atrophic changes in one portion of the papilla, whilst the other still retains the peculiar characters of neuritis. These appearances are well illustrated in Liebreich's "Atlas," Plate XI., Figs. 8 and 9.

I must here call attention to the fact that Mr. Wordsworth, Mr. Hutchinson, and some other observers, consider that a peculiar and characteristic form of atrophy of the optic nerve is met with in tobacco amaurosis.

Mr. Hutchinson, in a paper on "Tobacco Amaurosis" read before the Roy. Med. and Chir. Society,[2] says: "The cases which form the subject of this paper are recognized by the loss of vascular supply to the optic nerve itself. There is not usually much diminution in the size of the vessels which supply the retina, and often these remain of good size when the nerve itself is as white as paper. The first stage (one which is usually very transitory, and perhaps often altogether omitted) is one of congestion, during which the disk looks too red. Then follows pallor of the outer half of the nerve disk, that part which is nearest to the yellow spot. During these stages the patient complains merely of dimness of vision. Everything seems in a fog to him,

[1] Mauthner calls attention to the blue or bluish-green discoloration of the papilla, which was first described by Jäger, but does not consider that it is pathognomonic of atrophy of the nerve except other symptoms (e. g., attenuation of the retinal vessels) of the latter affection are also present. Where this is not the case, he still considers the prognosis hopeful as regards the sight, for not only may the degree of vision remain stationary, but even undergo wonderful improvement. He points out, moreover, that these changes in color of the disk are best seen in the erect mode of examination and binocular illumination, as with Helmholtz's or Jäger's ophthalmoscope. ("Lehrbuch der Ophthalmoscopie," p. 294.)

[2] "Transactions of the Roy. Med. and Chir. Society," 1867, p. 411.

but he has no pain in the eyes, nor any photophobia or photopsie. In a
later stage, the whole of the optic disk has become pale, even to blue-milk
whiteness; and later still there is proof, not only of anæmia of the nerve, but
of advanced atrophy. The stages generally occupy from four months to a
year. In many cases, the patient becomes at length absolutely blind; but in
others, the disease, having advanced to a certain point, is arrested. There is
from first to last no evidence of disease of any structure in the eyeball,
excepting the optic nerve, and even after years of absolute blindness, the
retina, choroid, etc., remain healthy and their blood supply good. Almost
always both eyes are affected, and progress almost *pari passu.* Sleepiness, a
little giddiness, and a little headache are usually the only constitutional
symptoms which attend it, and these disappear at a later stage and the
patient regains his usual health. As there is no tendency to fatal complications, opportunities for post-mortem examination of the brain are hardly
ever obtained."

In cases of lateral hemiopia, we may also in rare instances meet with a
partial atrophy of the disk with excavation, which corresponds to that half
of the optic nerve which is supplied by the fibres from the affected optic
nerve. But a long time elapses before symptoms of such atrophy begin to
show themselves; indeed, hemiopia may exist for a very long period without
the slightest trace of atrophy being recognizable.

4.—EXCAVATION OF THE OPTIC NERVE.

There are three forms of excavation or cupping of the optic nerve, viz.,
1. *The congenital physiological excavation.* 2. *The excavation from atrophy of
the optic nerve.* 3. *The glaucomatous or pressure excavation.*
In the *congenital physiological excavation,* we find that the cupping is
generally limited to the central portion of the optic disk; that it is mostly
very small and shallow, and that it may continue throughout life without
undergoing any changes. In some cases, the cup is not situated in the
centre of the disk, but slightly towards the outer (temporal) side. Sometimes the excavation is well marked and easily recognizable, the central
portion of the optic disk presenting a peculiar white, glistening appearance,
of varying size and form. This central glistening spot may be oval, circular,
or longitudinal, and its size is generally very inconsiderable in comparison
with that of the optic disk; it is surrounded by a reddish zone, which may
even be almost of the same color as the background of the eye. The width
of this zone varies with the extent of the excavation; if the latter be small,
the zone will be very considerable; but if it be large, the zone will be
narrow, and limited to the periphery of the disk. The edges of the cup are
generally slightly sloping, and never abrupt or steep, the excavation passing
gradually over into the darker zone, without there being any sharply defined
margin. But if the excavation is conical, or funnel-shaped the edges are
more abrupt, and the margin more defined. We find that the retinal vessels
also undergo peculiar changes in their course from the periphery towards the
centre of the disk, for when they arrive at the margin of the excavation,
instead of passing straight on, they describe a more or less acute curve as
they dip down into it. This curve may be very slight and gradual if the
cup is shallow, but if it is deep and extensive, the curve may be abrupt,
giving rise to a displacement of the vessels. In the expanse of the excavation, the vessels generally assume a slightly darker shade; sometimes they,
however, appear of a lighter, more rosy hue, and seem to be enveloped by a
delicate veil.

s easy to determine that an excavation is purely physio-
ı may prove to be one of amblyopia without ophthalmo-
the excavation; or there may be added to a physiological
n atrophic or a pressure excavation, or there may be a
ı of the optic nerve present.—B.]

s was first pointed out by H. Müller, the surface of the
w a physiological depression and elevation. The outer
is slightly excavated, whereas the nasal half is elevated,
of the papilla present most marked and striking differ-
easily be mistaken for pathological appearances by a
In such a case, we find that the cup has no sharply
l that in its expanse, the peculiar stippling due to the
ery observable, which is not the case in the other half.
cavated portion is pale and whitish, being in strong con-
ted part, which appears abnormally red and vascular.
disk also differs, for at the temporal side it is sharply
eral ring very apparent, whereas at the nasal side it is
or less hidden. The retinal vessels can be seen to mount
of the disk over the edge of the elevation, at which point
bent, sometimes to such a degree that their continuity

from atrophy of the optic nerve, we also meet with well-
aracteristic symptoms. The retinal vessels will be found
in calibre, the arteries small and thread-like, perhaps
he veins may at first retain their normal size, or be even
; in the course of the disease they also diminish greatly
olor of the disk is likewise changed; instead of the rosy-
which it presents in the normal eye, it assumes a more or
r bluish-white color, which may be limited to a portion
d to its whole expanse, lending it a peculiar glistening,
r-of-pearl appearance. The bluish-gray color of the optic
already stated, is often met with in spinal amaurosis;
iered almost characteristic of this affection. The atrophic
;h perhaps extensive on the surface, is generally very
t being gradual and sloping, not abrupt; consequently
on arriving at the edge of the cup from the periphery of
w any marked displacement, but only describe a more or
ometimes, this curve is so slight that it is hardly per-
those rare cases in which the excavation is tolerably
not abrupt, and for this reason there is no marked dis-
ssels at its edge; and on moving the convex lens of the
and fro, so as to make it act as a prism, the bottom of
not move as a whole, but only certain portions of the
a slight displacement; and this parallax is very different
guishable from, that met with in the glaucomatous cup.
n interruption of the overfilled veins at the edge of the
s so very characteristic in the glaucomatous form, is also

or pressure excavation (Plate VI., Figs. 15 and 16) is
following typical symptoms: The cup is not partial and
ral portion of the optic disk as in the physiological form,
e to the edge of the disk, its diameter equalling that of
lamina cribrosa being stretched and pushed backwards.
ay not yet have attained a considerable depth, the edge

is always abrupt and precipitous, thus differing greatly from the atrophic excavation, in which the descent is gradual and sloping. The edges may also overhang the cup, which has undermined the margin of the papilla. The disk is surrounded by a light, yellowish-white ring, which is due to the reflection of light from the anterior laminæ of the scleral ring, the choroid being thinned and atrophied at this point. This zone varies in width according to the depth of the excavation; the deeper and more advanced the latter, the broader and more marked will be the ring. The color of the disk is also much changed. Instead of the yellowish-pink appearance of the normal disk, the central, brightly shining, stippled portion is surrounded by a deep bluish-gray or bluish-green shadow, which gradually increases in darkness towards the periphery of the disk, where it may assume the appearance of a dark well-defined rim. On slightly moving the mirror or the object lens, this shadow will vary in intensity, more particularly in the central portion. On account of this peculiar shading of the disk, the latter looks, at the first glance, rather arched forward than hollowed and excavated. The course of the retinal vessels at the edge of the cup is also very peculiar. They do not pass, as in the normal eye, straight over the margin of the disk on to the retina without showing any curve or displacement; but if we trace their course from the retina, we find that when they arrive at the margin of the excavation, the dilated veins increase somewhat in size, and, making a more or less abrupt curve, descend into the cup; at the point of curvature the veins also appear somewhat darker in color. If the excavation is deep, the veins seem to curl round over the edge, and are considerably displaced, so that the prolongations of the veins on the optic disk deviate so considerably from those at the retinal edge of the cup, that they do not appear to belong to the same vessel. Their continuity seems interrupted, and this displacement of the two portions may equal the whole, or even more, of the diameter of the vessel. The extent and suddenness of this displacement vary with the depth of the cup. In the disk, the vessels appear indistinct and faded, and diminished in calibre; sometimes they may almost completely disappear, so that they can only be traced with difficulty. If the object lens be moved, so as to give it the action of a prism, a very marked parallax will appear; the whole bottom of the excavation shifts its position, and the broad scleral ring may seem to move over it, as if a frame were moved over a picture, the different portions of the excavation, however, shifting their individual positions but very slightly. The degree of the parallax also varies according to the depth of the excavation. It is particularly well seen, stereoscopically, with the binocular ophthalmoscope. The peculiarity of this parallax distinguishes, in a marked manner, the glaucomatous excavation from that met with in atrophy of the optic nerve; for in the latter case, as has been already pointed out, although certain portions of the excavation may shift their position, the bottom of the cup does not move as a whole. The displacement of the vessels in the glaucomatous excavation will also enable us to distinguish between this and the physiological form. In the former, the displacement is more or less abrupt, and occurs at the edge of the disk; whereas in the partial or physiological cup, the displacement or curvature is not abrupt, but slight and gradual, and does not occur at the edge of the disk, but within its area, at a greater or less distance from the margin, according to the extent of the excavation. Should a glaucomatous cup supervene upon a physiological one, we may at the outset of the disease sometimes observe the two existing together, the vessels showing the double displacement—the one at the edge of the physiological excavation and within the area of the papilla, the other more abrup and marked, and situated' at the edge of the optic disk. But at a later period the appearances of the physiological cup are lost, the latter becoming involved in the glaucomatous excavation.

In the majority of cases it is not difficult to distinguish the glaucomatous excavation from the others, even before it has reached any considerable depth; the extent of the cup, the abrupt and precipitous edges, the peculiar displacement of the vessels at its margin, and the spontaneous or easily producible arterial pulsation, will be found the surest guides. Where symptoms of atrophy of the optic nerve accompany the formation of a glaucomatous excavation, there may be some difficulty in ascertaining which is the primary affection, more particularly in those cases in which atrophy of the optic nerve, dependent upon cerebral amaurosis, has become complicated with inflammatory glaucoma. In such, a comparison of the two eyes and a careful and searching examination into the history of the case, will generally clear up the difficulty. But we must remember that, in glaucomatous excavation, the optic nerve often undergoes atrophic changes and becomes very white.

At the commencement of the glaucomatous excavation, the cupping may be partial, being confined to one portion of the optic disk; but it will already show the typical symptoms of the pressure excavation. The optic disk is perhaps completely surrounded by a broad scleral zone, the veins become somewhat dilated and abruptly displaced at the edge of the cupped portion, and there is a bluish shadow at the periphery of the latter, which is gradually shaded off to a lighter color towards the centre.

Von Graefe has pointed out the very interesting and important fact, that a glaucomatous excavation may become shallower after the operation of iridectomy, thus proving that the cup depends upon an increase in the intra-ocular tension. The best cases to illustrate this fact are those in which acute symptoms have supervened upon chronic glaucoma. In such cases, the excavation becomes more shallow and saucer-like, the ends of the vessels less abruptly displaced, and their interruptions disappear, so that the continuation of the vessel from the retina on to the disk can be distinctly traced, although it may be somewhat curved. We may also notice that vessels which were slightly curved at the edge of the disk, become straight again.

5.—PIGMENTATION OF THE OPTIC NERVE. [HEMORRHAGE INTO THE OPTIC NERVE.—B.]

When describing the normal appearances presented by the fundus oculí, I mentioned that we frequently meet with a more or less marked and extensive deposit of pigment at the edge of the optic disk, and that this is quite physiological, and has no pathological signification. Sometimes this deposit is but slight, and forms a narrow crescent at one part of the margin of the disk, just along the choroidal ring; in other cases it is more considerable in size, and may embrace a large portion of the edge of the optic nerve entrance.

In very rare instances, a considerable amount of pigment has been observed to be deposited in the expanse of the disk. Thus Liebreich[1] has published a case in which, after a severe accident, there ensued, in both eyes, atrophy of the optic nerve, with marked pigment deposit within the disk. This was especially the case in the left eye, in which the whole of the disk, except the very centre and a portion at the temporal side, was occupied

---

[1] "Annales d'oculistique," lii. 31.

b dense black pigment. Liebreich supposes that the black coloration of the disk was due to pigment cells, which had become developed in the connective tissue which replaces the nerve fibres in atrophy of the optic nerve. Knapp[1] also reports cases of extensive pigmentation of the optic disk, which had occurred after an accident, but considers that it is the result of hemorrhagic effusion within the sheath of the optic nerve, which afterwards undergoes pigment degeneration, the same thing, in fact, as we so often find occurring in blood-effusion in the retina. Another instance is recorded by Hirschberg,[2] in which a large deposit of pigment occurred in the optic disk, in an eye which had received a severe blow from a piece of iron.

Hemorrhages into the medullary sheath of the optic nerve fibres are rare, but hemorrhages between the sheaths are more frequent. These are generally bilateral, and come from an extravasation of blood at the base of the brain. The ophthalmoscopic signs are very vague, unless the blood is extravasated upon the papillæ. There may be a slight cloudiness of the retina near the disk, and possibly a hyperæmia of the veins. The pigment which results from these hemorrhages may show itself in the papilla itself as well as in the connective-tissue ring around it. Injuries, whether contusions or perforating wounds, are very liable to cause hemorrhages upon the papilla, which leave behind masses of pigment. The optic nerve may also become pigmented from melanotic infiltration. (See "Graefe und Saemisch's Hdb.," v. S. 906–909.)—B.]

Mauthner[3] has once observed, in a perfectly healthy eye, a minute brightly-glistening speck at the margin of the disk, which was evidently a cholesterine crystal; it is less rarely met with after certain morbid changes in the optic nerve, e. g., neuritis. Dr. Tweedie, of University College Hospital, has recently had under his care a case of optic neuritis, in the course of which five brilliantly-glistening specks of cholesterine crystals were formed on the disk. Subsequently four of them disappeared.

6.—TUMORS OF THE OPTIC NERVE, ETC.

Tumors of the optic nerve are of rare occurrence, and difficult to diagnose with the ophthalmoscope. [They may occur in the papilla as granuloma; or in the intra-orbital part of the nerve; or in the intra-cranial part of the nerve. Sometimes stratified concretions from the vitreous lamina of the choroid grow over into the papilla. In the orbit we meet with primary tumors of the nerve or inner sheath, which are myxomata, or myxo-sarcomata, or glio-sarcomata, or in rare instances neuromata. All these tumors start either from the inner sheath of the nerve or from the neuroglia. The nerve fibres are either lost in the tumor or they are pushed aside by the growth. When the tumor springs from the orbital tissue or the external sheath, the optic nerve, more or less atrophied, passes through the growth. The myxomata or myxo-sarcomata may grow to the size of a hen's egg, are very gelatinous, and may contain cysts. They grow somewhat slowly, the exophthalmos which results is usually in the direction of the axis of the eye, and the motility of the eyeball may not be markedly impeded. Diplopia may, however, be present even from the beginning. Vision may be very defective, or even entirely lost early in the course of the disease, from papillitis or from simple atrophy of the optic nerve. There is usually no pain until the growth has reached a considerable size, though there may be severe headache. The

---

[1] "A. f. O.," xvi. 1, 252.   [2] "Kl. Monats.," Oct. 1869, S. 824.   [3] Op. cit., p. 269.

growth, however, may be so rapid as to compress the eyeball, cause perforation of the cornea, and phthisis bulbi may be the result. An early extirpation of the tumor may prevent its recurrence.

True neuroma is very rare. A case is reported by Perls, which occurred in a child, was as large as a pigeon's egg, was covered by both sheaths, and consisted of gray medullary nerve fibres and nucleated cells. It was removed with the eyeball, and there was no return.

Sarcoma usually springs from the orbital tissue and involves the optic nerve secondarily, or the nerve becomes the seat of secondary deposits after a choroidal sarcoma. Here the growth is mainly along the inter-vaginal space. In cases of glio-sarcoma of the retina, deposits are very often found in the medullary sheath of the nerve fibres themselves.

Tumors involving the *intra-cranial* portion of the optic nerve are not very uncommon. Gummata of the brain or meninges not unfrequently involve the optic nerves and chiasm, and the latter may be the seat of cheesy tuberculous masses or of melanotic growths.

Knapp has reported a case of carcinoma of the sheath of the optic nerve.

A very marked hyperplasia of the chiasm and optic nerve has been described by Michel in a patient suffering from elephantiasis.

For detailed accounts of cases of tumor of the optic nerve, see "Arch. f. Ophth.," xix. 2, xix. 3; "Kl. Mon. f. Aug.," 1874, S. 439; "Graefe u. Saemisch," v. S. 912, 914; "Arch. of Ophthal.," iv. 3 and 4; v. 3 and 4; vi. 1 and 2, 3 and 4.—B.]

Von Graefe[1] records a case in which there was a large retro-ocular orbital tumor, causing a protrusion of the eye to the extent of nine lines. The sight was completely lost. With the ophthalmoscope, the retinal veins were found to be dilated and tortuous, but the arteries attenuated. At the inner half of the disk (to which it was confined) was noticed a peculiar steep and abrupt elevation. The latter projected about one line above the perfectly level outer half of the disk, and hung slightly over the inner edge. Within this elevated portion, the substance of the disk was of an opaque, grayish-red tint, and the retinal vessels were completely hidden. On microscopic examination by Drs. Recklinghausen and Schweigger, it was found to be a tumor (myxoma) of the optic nerve. In another case of orbital tumor reported by Dr. Jacobson,[2] the ophthalmoscope also revealed a striking projection of a portion of the optic disk, in which the retinal vessels were lost. The whole appearance of the disk, the variations in color of different portions of it, as well as the course of the retinal vessels, were most peculiar. This was also found to be a myxo-sarcomatous tumor of the optic nerve.

[7.—INJURIES OF THE OPTIC NERVE.

The optic nerve may be injured as it enters the eye, in the orbit, in the optic foramen, or at the base of the skull. The nerve may be simply contused; or it may be torn in the orbit, either by a perforating instrument or by a shot wound; or by a fracture of the sphenoid bone, especially of the clinoid process. If the nerve is injured anteriorly to the point of entrance of the central retinal artery, the ophthalmoscopic appearances are similar to those of embolus. If the seat of the injury is posterior to the entrance of the central retinal artery, either in the orbit or in the skull, the ophthalmoscope at first shows nothing; but after some weeks the papilla begins to grow pale, at first on the temporal side, but later the whole disk grows white

[1] "A. f. O.," x. 1, 194.   [2] Ibid., x. 2, 55.

and atrophic. Loss of vision is, of course, present from the beginning, though this may be partially recovered from, if the nerve was not divided.—B.]

A very extraordinary case of injury of the optic nerve, with rupture of the central vessels, has been described by Dr. Hermann Pagenstecher.[1] The injury occurred in a girl, aged twelve, who was hit on the right eye with the sharp point of an iron rod, which entered the orbit just below its upper margin, causing a wound of rather more than an inch in length. The lids were much swollen, the eyeball slightly prominent, its movement upward somewhat impaired, but no direct injury of the globe could be detected. The pupil was dilated and immovable, and the sight completely lost, there being not the faintest perception of even strong sunlight. The ophthalmoscope revealed a most peculiar condition, of which I can here only give the briefest outline. The optic disk was completely hidden by a brightly glistening white effusion, which extended in a broad zone over the retina, measuring about four times the diameter of a normal optic papilla ; no trace of any retinal vessel was evident on this patch, with the exception of one vessel running upwards (reverse image). In the course of a few days the effusion became slowly absorbed, the optic disk reappeared, the vessels showing, however, very peculiar interruptions on and near its expanse, and gradually the collateral circulation became established. Very extensive pigment deposits were formed in the choroid, and subsequently on the optic disk.

8.—OPAQUE OPTIC NERVE FIBRES.

Amongst the physiological peculiarities of the retina which are sometimes met with is one which, if it be at all fully developed, may easily be mistaken for an exudation into the retina. It is a well-known fact that, in the human subject, the nerve tubules of the optic nerve lose their medullary sheath at the cribriform plate, passing on to the most anterior portion of the papilla, and thence to the retina, denuded of their sheath, i. e., simply in the form of transparent axis cylinders. In certain animals, however, especially rabbits, the sheath is continued on to the retina. Now, this sometimes also happens in the human subject (as was first pointed out by Virchow), the optic nerve fibres retaining their medullary sheath for a short distance on to the retina, so that the latter, instead of being transparent, will at such points show a marked white opacity. The ophthalmoscopic diagnosis of opaque nerve fibres is by no means difficult, and a little care and reflection should guard any observer from mistaking these appearances for morbid changes in the retina. We notice in such cases that the optic nerve, instead of being sharply and clearly defined and surrounded by transparent retina, shows at certain points peculiar white, striated, tongue-like projections, which extend a little way into the retina. These patches terminate in an irregular manner, their outline showing faint "feathery" striæ. It is a fact of much diagnostic importance that the retina in the immediate vicinity of these ches is perfectly healthy and transparent, there being not the faintest of haziness of the retina due to serous infiltration ; whereas, in exudate to the retina, the contiguous portions always show a certain degree of

tinal vessels may be partly or completely hidden in these white which is especially the case if the latter are considerable in size. find that the vessels pass from the centre of the disk up to the edge of the opacity, become hidden by this, and reappear at its periphery, being thence distributed in a normal manner over the retina. These opacities vary much in size and number. In some cases, there are only two or three small patches; in others, there is one large, irregular white figure which surrounds the greater portion or even the whole of the disk, and extends, perhaps, for a considerable distance on to the retina. (For a beautiful illustration of such a condition, *vide* Liebreich's "Atlas," Plate XII., Figs. 1 and 2.) Sometimes the little white patches may even show themselves on the retina at some little distance from the disk, not being in contact with it, but separated from it by a portion of normal retina.[1] The opacity due to thickening of the optic nerve fibres may be particularly distinguished from an inflammatory exudation into the retina and optic nerve by the following symptoms:

1st. The optic disk itself is perfectly normal both in color and transparancy, and the vessels within its expanse are also quite healthy in appearance. In retinitis, especially when the morbid products are so close to the optic nerve, the disk is always more or less hyperæmic, indistinct, opaque, and perhaps somewhat swollen; the veins on its surface are dilated and perhaps tortuous, the arteries generally somewhat attenuated, and both sets of vessels perhaps slightly veiled. 2d. The opacities caused by thickened nerve fibres terminate, as has been already stated, in a peculiar manner, like the fine divisions of a tongue of flame. They end abruptly in the healthy retina, and only here and there can a faint trace of thickened nerve fibre be followed for a very short distance. 3d. The retina is perfectly normal, both in color and transparency, quite up to the opaque spot, the retinal vessels are also absolutely normal; whereas, in retinitis accompanied with inflammatory deposits in the retina, the condition is quite different, for then we find that the retina is more or less opaque and cloudy within a certain area around the exudations, this cloudiness gradually shading off into the normal retina. The vessels are also changed, the veins being dark, tortuous, and dilated, the arteries attenuated, and there are generally also extravasations of blood scattered about on, and between the vessels. 4th. If the eye is otherwise healthy, the sight and field of vision are perfect. If the opacity is extensive, the "blind spot," corresponding to the area of the disk, will be enlarged.

Mauthner[2] narrates a very interesting and peculiar case, in which there was a bifurcation of the optic nerve fibres, which appeared to be collected into two bundles, the one passing upwards, the other downwards, the retinal vessels taking the same course, whilst on the inner and outer portion of the disk there were no vessels. The fibres were devoid of their sheath, and hence their tint was not brilliantly white, but their situation and course were very marked and distinct, on account of the close super-imposition of the individual fibres, which rendered the upper and lower margin of the papilla quite lost and indistinct. [Von Jäger has also described a case of this kind in his "Ophthal. Hand-Atlas," Pl. VI., Fig. 33.

Another very rare anomaly is coloboma of the sheath of the optic nerve. This is usually accompanied by a fissure or defect in the choroid, but Nieden has recently reported four cases in which the coloboma was confined to the sheath of the nerve. The four cases referred to three patients, one having the anomaly in both eyes. The nystagmus present began in very early life. (See "Archives of Ophthal.," viii. 4, pp. 501–514.)—B.]

---

[1] This fact has been verified by dissection by Recklinghausen. *Vide* Virchow's "Archiv," vol. x. 164.

[2] Virchow's "Archiv," vol. x. 267.

CHAPTER XIII.

AMBLYOPIC AFFECTIONS.

UNDER the vague term "amaurosis" were formerly included all kinds of intra-ocular diseases that were not distinguishable with the naked eye; but since the discovery of the ophthalmoscope has revealed the true nature of the diseases of the inner tunics of the eye and of the optic nerve, we are able to confine the term "amaurosis" to very narrow limits. Indeed, it is of great practical importance, that a definite understanding should be arrived at, as to what diseases are to be included in the group of "amblyopic affections." Thus only can we remedy the confusion which still exists, from the fact that some writers apply the name amaurosis indiscriminately to all cases of total blindness dependent upon deep-seated intra-ocular affections, whilst others give to it a more limited signification, and confine it to the loss of sight dependent upon intra-cranial disease. I think, therefore, that Von Graefe's signification should be universally adopted. He excludes from the term "amblyopic affections" (amblyopia and amaurosis) all disturbances of sight dependent upon material, perceptible changes in the refractive media, in the internal tunics of the eye, on neuro-retinitis and embolism of the central artery of the retina.[1] It may be questioned whether we should exclude cases of optic neuritis from this group, as they are generally due to intra-cranial disease, and but too frequently pass over into consecutive atrophy of the optic nerve and retina, and more or less complete blindness. But even in these cases, I think it would be better and more definite to term such blindness, amaurosis from optic neuritis, just as we should speak of amaurosis (or amblyopia, as the case may be) from retinitis pigmentosa, from glaucoma or embolism of the central artery of the retina; in fact, that we should strictly confine the term amaurosis to cases of blindness from primary atrophy (degenerative atrophy) of the optic nerve, and that of amblyopia (in a special sense), to impairment of vision produced by irregularities in the circulation of the nervous system, which may lead in the end to primary atrophy of the optic nerve.

Amblyopic affections are also sometimes classified according to the degree of impairment of sight. Thus the term "amaurosis" is often confined to cases of absolute blindness, in which there is not the faintest perception of even very strong light; the name "amblyopia" embracing all degrees of impaired sight.

Liebreich[2] distinguishes three different forms: 1st. Amaurotic amblyopia, in which the sight is so much deteriorated that even large objects are only

---

[1] *Vide* Von Graefe's Lectures on "Amblyopic Affections," "Kl. M.," 1865. An able translation of these important and valuable Lectures by Mr. Z. Laurence will be found in the "Ophthalmic Review," ii. 282.

[2] "Nouveau Dictionnaire de Méd. et de Chir. Prat.," 785.

distinguishable with difficulty, or the patient is not able to guide himself. 2d. *Amaurosis;* in this condition even large objects can no longer be distinguished, there being no qualitative but only quantitative perception of light, which may exist either in the whole or only a part of the field of vision. 3d. *Absolute amaurosis*, where the patient has not the faintest power of distinguishing between light and darkness.

In examining the sight of cases of amaurosis and amblyopia, it is very important to ascertain the condition of the field of vision with the greatest accuracy. In these diseases, it does not suffice to examine the field by daylight, because slight contractions or interruptions may thus easily escape detection, which will become at once apparent if the field is tested by a more subdued light, for which purpose Von Graefe's graduated disk of light will be found the best. The mode and extent of the contraction or interruption of the field of vision, are of great importance in enabling us to form our prognosis as to the risk of a total loss of vision, or the chances of an improvement, or even a restoration of the sight.

In the following description of the different kinds of contraction and interruption of the visual field, and their bearing upon the prognosis as to the ultimate condition of the sight, etc., I have mainly followed the views of Von Graefe, as expressed in the above-mentioned lectures on amblyopic affections; indeed, he is the first writer who has attempted to lay down anything like definite rules with regard to the chief points that should influence our prognosis in this class of diseases. This, in fact, could only be done by one who had for many years closely watched the course of a vast number of cases, and carefully studied their minutest details. A mere hypothetical generalization, not founded upon absolute, sufficient, and closely scrutinized data, would be simply valueless.

Several different forms of contraction of the field of vision may be observed in amblyopic affections.

The contraction frequently commences at the temporal side of the field of vision (the nasal portion of the retina being the first to suffer), and from thence either passes on laterally towards the centre, or along the periphery in an upward and downward direction, extending finally towards the nasal side; and then, when the whole periphery of the field has become impaired, the contraction advances concentrically towards the axis of vision. The outlines of both these forms of contraction of the field are often very irregular and undulatory. The contraction of the field in cases of amaurosis generally commences at the temporal side, but this is not always the case, for it may begin at the nasal; whereas, in the contraction met with in glaucoma, it is a very characteristic feature that, as a rule, it commences at the nasal side (the outer portion of the retina becoming first impaired). We occasionally find that some time after the first eye has become affected (and perhaps even amaurotic), a gradually progressive contraction of the field shows itself in the second eye, commencing perhaps at a point quite symmetrical to that in which the contraction began in the eye originally affected. Such cases afford a most unfavorable prognosis, more especially if the central vision is greatly impaired, or already perhaps sunk below that of the eccentric portion of the retina, for these symptoms indicate but too surely a progressive atrophy of the optic nerve.

The contraction of the field may be equilateral in both eyes, *e. g.*, the right half of each field may be wanting, and the line of demarcation between this and the normal half of the field be quite sharply defined, and situated in the axis of vision. This is termed equilateral or homonymous hemiopia, on account of the corresponding halves (the right or left as the case may be) being affected. The nature of this condition is self-evident, when we remember the anatomical relations of the optic nerves to each other, and the fact that their fibres decussate at the optic commissure (chiasma) in such a manner that the right optic nerve supplies the right half of each retina (the

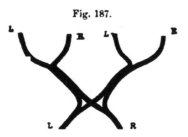

Fig. 187.

temporal side in the right eye, the nasal in the left), and the left optic nerve of the left half. A glance at Fig. 187 will explain the arrangement.

This figure represents the commissure of the optic nerves and their prolongation to the retina. R the right optic nerve. L the left optic nerve.

[The question of the course of the nerve fibres in the chiasm, and of their relation to each other, to the optic centres, and to the eyes, is the all important one in matters relating to defects in the field of vision due to intracranial lesions. During the last five or six years, investigations have been undertaken by numerous observers to settle this much vexed question. The view generally accepted, that there was a partial decussation of the fibres, as has been already described, has been rejected by Biesiadecki, Mandelstamm, and Michel, who claim, after careful experimentation and observation, that in man, as in the lower animals, the decussation of the nerve fibres in the chiasm is complete. According to these authors the nerve fibres take a curved course in the chiasm instead of a straight one, and their interweaving or interlacing is most intricate. This view has been most decidedly opposed by Gudden, and also in a short clinical paper by Mohr. Gudden, by experiments on animals, from which he has enucleated eyes, and from clinical observations and autopsies on patients, convinced himself that the old view of the partial decussation of the fibres was the correct one. Mohr's paper is a very interesting one, being based on clinical observation of an intracranial tumor with the results of the autopsy. From his observations he concluded that the nerve fibres which supply the macula lutea and its vicinity run along the tract and nerve of the same side, while fibres of less importance for central vision pass to the macula from the opposite tract. The important fibres destined for the macula lutea of the left eye come from the left optic tract, and with them come also from the left tract, fibres destined for the external half of the left retina, and finally some fibres which supply the more internal parts of the retina bordering on the macula. The nerve bundles destined for the macula of the right eye and the vicinity, as well as the fibres destined for the external half of the retina, run in the right optic tract. Mohr's case, which was one of typical hemiopia, seems to furnish positive proof of the semi-decussation of the fibres in the chiasm. Schwalbe, who writes the article on microscopic anatomy of the optic nerve in " Graefe und Saemisch's Handb. der Augenheilkunde," endorses the total decussation idea. The whole subject is still in an unsettled condition, but the majority of ophthalmologists still hold to the partial decussation theory as offering the most satisfactory explanation of the various symptoms relating to the field and acuity of vision. (For a full discussion, see "Graefe u. Saemisch's Handb.," i. S. 326–328; "Arch. f. Ophth.," xix. 2; xx. 2; xxi. 3; xxv. 1; xxv. 4; and exhaustively in "Graefe und Saemisch's Handb.," S. 929–950.)

Purtscher has recently published six cases of unilateral optic nerve atrophy, in which the results all agreed with the views of Gudden. In these cases the uncrossed, as well as the crossed bundles of fibres of the tracts were completely degenerated, except the small islands at the anterior border. In every case the atrophy was ascending, the optic nerve differing in this respect from all other peripheral nerves. (See "Archiv für Ophthalmologie," xxvi. 2.)

In this connection the investigations of Stilling into the ultimate anatomical connections of the optic nerves are of some interest. He found that diverging from the optic tract, a large number of fibres join the inner surface of the corpus geniculatum mediale, without, however, entering the gray substance of this ganglion. They run in a spiral course under the brachium conjunctivum posticum, and pass directly into the so-called loop. Between the lines of the latter, the optic nerve fibres can be followed as far as the lower olivary process. Besides these connections other bundles of fibres, diverging directly from the optic tract, run upon the inner surface of the corpus geniculatum mediale, and from here a part of these fibres pass directly to the nucleus of the oculomotorius, while others pass into the crus cerebelli. The optic nerve is the first nerve with which a certain connection with the cerebellum can be demonstrated. Participation of this organ in the act of vision is therefore proven, and many cases of disturbance of vision which had been attributed to affections of the cerebellum, are now thoroughly intelligible.—B.]

If, therefore, a tumor or an hemorrhagic effusion compresses the right optic nerve on the central side of the commissure in such a manner as completely to destroy its conductibility, the right half of each retina will be impaired, and consequently the left half of each field of vision be wanting. But if the compression is limited to the commissure, affecting only the crossed fibres, and leaving the lateral ones unimpaired, the appearance will be different, for then the nasal half of each retina will be affected, and the temporal half of each field be wanting. In such cases, however, the hemiopia is not so sharply defined as in the equilateral form, for there is generally a more or less broad line of transition, in which the defective portion of the field passes over gradually into the healthy part. The seat of the disease may not, however, be confined to the commissure, but be situated principally in front of, or behind the latter. This may be suspected if other symptoms coexist with the hemiopia, such as paralysis of other nerves, hemiplegia, impairment of the mental functions, etc. It will be seen, hereafter, that the prognosis is less favorable in the temporal than in the equilateral hemiopia. It is extremely rare to meet with hemiopia of the upper or lower halves of the field, and the real nature of such cases is at present quite unexplained.

If the cause of the compression is situated at the distal end of the optic nerve, i. e., after the crossing of the fibres in the commissure, of course the corresponding eye is alone affected.

In addition to the contraction of the field of vision, we often meet with interruptions in its continuity, which appear in the form of dark irregular clouds or spots before the patient's eyes. These "scotomata" (as they are called) may be situated in or near the centre of the field, or at its periphery. On examining the field in cases of scotomata, we find that within a certain area there is a more or less considerable gap, in which the object becomes indistinct, or even lost. If the scotoma is situated in the axis of vision, it of course produces great impairment of sight, and the patient often squints in a certain direction, in order that the rays from the object may fall upon a more sensitive (in this case eccentric) portion of the retina. Whereas, if the interruption occurs at the periphery of the field, and is only inconsiderable in size, it is generally altogether overlooked by the patient.

These scotomata generally make their appearance very suddenly; sometimes, however, a few weeks elapse before they become fully developed. They are not unfrequently met with after exhausting general diseases, or after great mental emotions, and are accompanied, perhaps, by cutaneous insensibility to pain. The circumscribed central scotomata are also sometimes due to disturbance in the circulation and impairment of the nutrition of the optic nerve; or, as has been previously stated, to retro-ocular neuritis (vide p. 570). I have already mentioned that Leber has found the appreciation of colors more or less impaired in all cases of circumscribed central scotoma, and his researches upon this point have led him to divide the affection into the following four classes, according to the state of appreciation of colors and of the field of vision:[1] 1. The central scotoma is not apparent by the usual mode of examination, but only by testing the appreciation of colors, the periphery of the visual field having a normal appreciation of colors. 2. The scotoma is also recognizable without testing the appreciation of colors: the latter is, however, only abnormal within the scotoma, being unaffected throughout the periphery. 3. The appreciation of colors is completely lost, or greatly impaired, in the scotoma, the periphery showing a greater degree of impairment; but the eccentric acuteness of vision is perfectly unaffected. In such cases, the scotoma is generally also recognizable by the ordinary modes of examination, but the opposite may occur. 4. The transition into atrophy of the optic nerve is formed by those cases in which, besides the symptoms enumerated, there is indistinctness of peripheral vision. We cannot, however, sharply define these four classes from each other, for one may gradually pass over into the other. The third class, in which the periphery of the field also shows a slight impairment of the appreciation of colors, is, according to Leber, to be regarded on the whole as the more severe and advanced form of the disease, for there often already exists partial discoloration of the disk, or, where this is absent, more or less cloudiness of the retina, so that we but rarely obtain a negative result from an ophthalmoscopic examination. Hence the prognosis as to a restoration ad integrum is less favorable, and some of these cases resist all treatment. In amblyopia potatorum the impairment of the sense of color, although it may only reach a slight degree, sometimes not only affects the centre of the field, but also extends in an irregular manner over the greater part of the periphery. We sometimes meet with very peculiar and characteristic cases in which the scotoma is surrounded by a circular zone, which is perfectly or almost perfectly normal, whilst at the periphery there is again marked color-blindness.

In cases of peripheral anæsthesia of the retina, we often meet with the interesting phenomenon that the phosphenes continue to exist in portions of the retina which are quite insensitive to light, and this is of prognostic importance, as it does not occur in amaurosis. The sight is generally very considerably affected, and may finally become quite lost, so that the patient cannot distinguish between light and dark.

In cerebral amaurosis, the pupil is generally somewhat dilated and sluggish, or immovable and large, if the eye is quite blind. If the pupil is dilated to its fullest extent, so that the narrow rim of iris is hardly discernible, we must assume that there coexists an irritation of the sympathetic fibres, causing a contraction of the dilatator pupillæ. If one eye only is affected, we often find that its pupil is dilated and immovable under the stimulus of light when the other eye is closed, but that it at once contracts

[1] "A. f. O.," xv. 3, 71.

consentaneously with the pupil of its fellow, when the latter is uncovered. This fact may prove of use in detecting the simulation of blindness in one eye by the dilatation of the pupil by atropine, when of course this consentaneous action could not occur. Great importance cannot, however, be attached in cases of amaurosis to the behavior of the pupil, for we sometimes find that, even in complete blindness, it retains its activity. In spinal amaurosis, the pupil is unusually and perhaps irregularly contracted (oval), and acts but very sluggishly and imperfectly upon the application of atropine. The great contraction is due to the paralysis of the sympathetic fibres. [See an article on "Lesions of the Optic Nerve and Pupil in certain Affections of the Spinal Cord," in "Amer. Journ. Med. Sciences," July, 1875.—B.]

The ophthalmoscopic symptoms of cerebral and cerebro-spinal amaurosis consist in certain changes in the appearance of the optic nerve, indicative of its progressive atrophy. Care must, however, be taken not to mistake simple anæmia, or blanching of the disk, for incipient atrophy. The small nutritive vessels, which are distributed upon the expanse of the disk, disappear, and this partly produces the white color; whilst the vessels distributed over the retina may retain their normal calibre, even when the optic nerve is quite atrophied, but generally they soon become attenuated. The symptoms of atrophy of the optic nerve have already been fully described (p. 572).

According to the researches of Leber, color-blindness is almost a constant symptom of atrophy of the optic nerve, whether this be primary, and dependent upon cerebral or spinal lesions, or secondary, and consequent upon optic neuritis; and it may appear at any stage and in any degree of the disease. In thirty-six cases of atrophy of the optic nerve, he found color-blindness completely absent in three cases, in five it was only slight, but in the remaining twenty-seven cases it was very marked. Such patients are at first generally unable to distinguish red, but, as the disease advances, the appreciation of other colors is gradually lost, blue being, as a rule, recognised the longest. This condition closely resembles the color-blindness which manifests itself in perfectly normal eyes, when the illumination is diminished. He has also observed color-blindness in atrophy of the optic nerve consequent upon glaucomatous excavation.

We have now to turn our attention to the various causes which may produce cerebral and cerebro-spinal amaurosis. But this subject is far too extensive for the scope of this work, and I must therefore confine myself to giving a mere outline of the principal causes, and must refer the reader for fuller information to special works and articles upon this subject. Amongst these I would especially recommend those of Von Graefe, Hughlings Jackson, Ogle, Galezowski, etc.

It must, however, be candidly confessed that we cannot diagnose the special cerebral cause, or localize its seat, simply from the ophthalmoscopic symptoms presented by the optic nerve. In order to aid and guide us in arriving at a conclusion as to the cause and its situation, other local and general symptoms must be searched for. But, even with their aid, we often fail to determine these points with anything approaching certainty, and may find, on post-mortem examination, that we have been quite mistaken. Indeed we sometimes meet with cases of simple progressive atrophy of the optic nerve, leading to blindness, in which it is quite impossible to detect any special cause, either cerebral, spinal, or constitutional. On the other hand, the trunk of the optic nerve may be seriously implicated in the intra-cranial disease, without the sight being in the least affected.[1]

[1] "A. f. O.," xii. 2, p. 111.

[It should be carefully borne in mind that it is possible to have marked intra-cranial disease without any sign of atrophy of the optic nerve visible with the ophthalmoscope; and that, on the other hand, there may be a purely local atrophy in the optic nerve without any intra-cranial lesion.—B.]

Still, the ophthalmoscope proves of immense use to the physician in the practice of his art, and may often lead him to the discovery of diseases which he would, without it, have passed over or misinterpreted.

As I have already mentioned, the various affections of the brain which may produce optic neuritis, I shall now only consider those which may give rise to progressive atrophy of the optic nerve.

Meningitis of the base of the brain is a very frequent cause of disease of the optic nerve. The symptoms of acute meningitis are generally so marked and characteristic that the diagnosis is not difficult, but it is different with the chronic form, the course of which is often very insidious, and its symptoms masked and indistinct. But its presence may be suspected, if there are febrile attacks accompanied by violent and recurrent paroxysms of headache, severe vomiting and retching, unconsciousness and sensitiveness of the cranium to palpation. Moreover, as the inflammation of the meninges is generally somewhat diffuse, we find that other cerebral nerves become affected, being either paralyzed or in a state of irritation. Thus, we sometimes find that some of the muscles of the eye are paralyzed, whilst others are in a state of spasmodic contraction (Von Graefe). The inflammation of the meninges may extend from the membranes to the cortical substance of the brain, perhaps to a considerable depth, reaching, according to L. Meyer,[1] even to the optic thalami.

With regard to the headaches which may occur in cases of amblyopia, we must be on our guard not to attribute them always to some cerebral affection; for, as Von Graefe has pointed out, they are often only due to the failing sight, and are produced by the intent endeavor of the patient still thoroughly to realize the visual impressions. On account of this there occur disturbances of sensibility akin in nature to those which are met with in double vision, circles of diffusion upon the retina, etc. If the headache be simply due to this cause, cessation from work will rapidly cure it; for it can be easily understood that its intensity may be materially increased by any cause that produces congestion of the brain or the eye, such as stooping, etc.

Acute meningitis, more especially the tubercular form, generally gives rise to optic neuritis, and this often ensues rapidly upon the outbreak of the cerebral affection; whereas, in the chronic form, the optic nerve often remains altogether, or for a long time, unaffected, and then it undergoes progressive atrophy, its nutrition becoming impaired by the chronic congestion of the brain and meninges.

Chronic periostitis of the base of the brain may also produce amaurosis.

Tumors within the brain may cause progressive atrophy of the optic nerve, either by the latter becoming directly implicated in the morbid process and its nervous elements destroyed, or by its being compressed, stretched, or pushed aside by the tumor, so that its conductibility and its nutrition are greatly interfered with; but the impairment of nutrition may also be due to pressure upon the bloodvessels of the optic nerve. Although sarcomatous and carcinomatous tumors are the most frequent morbid growths, we must include other neoplasms, such as masses of tubercle, syphilitic gummata, glioma, etc. Such morbid growths may be situated at the base of the brain or within its substance. Their diagnosis is very uncertain and obscure, except

[1] L. Meyer, "Centralblatt für die med. Wissensch.," Nos. 8, 9, 10, 1867.

other general or local symptoms coexist, which may aid us in determining the probable nature and seat of the cerebral disease. Thus in equilateral hemiopia (say of the left half of the visual field) we should suspect that a tumor or hemorrhagic effusion is pressing upon the right optic nerve.

[Atrophy of the optic nerves from direct pressure of the tumor is comparatively uncommon, as only a small proportion of the intra-cranial tumors are situated in this vicinity. Compression by exostoses, cheesy tuberculous masses or gummy neoplasms in the vicinity of the chiasm are the most common.

Hydrocephalus internus also causes atrophy by pressure on the chiasm.

The symptom known as hemianopsia, hemiopia, or hemiopsia, is of two varieties: 1st, a permanent defect of half the visual field of both eyes from pressure on the tract or chiasm, or from functional disturbance of the optic centres in one cerebral hemisphere; and, 2d, transient attacks of half-sided blindness without organic lesion, and called amaurosis partialis fugax, or flittering scotoma. The hemiopia generally affects one of the lateral halves of the visual field in both eyes; a superior or inferior hemianopsia is very rare. The hemiopia is either lateral, affecting the external half of one field and the internal half of the other; or it is temporal, affecting the temporal halves in both fields. A nasal hemiopia only exists, according to Leber, as a symmetrical disease of both optic nerves. In lateral hemiopia central vision is generally very good. In temporal hemiopia the dividing line is not a sharply defined perpendicular through the point of fixation. In pure hemiopia the color-sense is normal in the unaffected half of the visual field. Permanent superior or inferior hemiopia of both eyes is very rare, and the simplest explanation is that the optic nerves have been compressed at the base of the skull from above, or from below by some pathological product. Still it might be explained by a symmetrical primary lesion in both optic nerves.

In lateral hemiopia of central origin there is for a long time a normal fundus, as a descending atrophy requires time to reach the optic disk. It may be inferred from Gudden's experiments that central atrophy of the brain may extend peripherally to the optic tracts and nerves. If the lesion is in the chiasm, discoloration of the optic disk will occur sooner, though it may be preceded by the signs of neuritis.

Lateral hemiopia often appears suddenly with signs of cerebral apoplexy, and the cause is here an apoplectic clot, or an embolus, or a tumor in the opposite hemisphere. Tumors at the base in the region of the chiasm are common, such as sarcoma of the sella turcica or of chiasm, tubercle, and gummata. The locality of the tumor can only be determined from all the accompanying symptoms, and not always then.—B.]

If the temporal half of each field is impaired, the crossed fasciculi of the nerves are involved, and the seat of the disease is at the commissure. In such cases the impairment of vision is often very rapid, the sight being perhaps utterly destroyed within a few days. The contraction of the visual field begins at the periphery of the temporal side and extends up to or beyond the centre, so that finally only a slight glimmer of light may be left on the nasal side. If the cerebral tumor is very slow in its development, the brain substance and the nerves may gradually accommodate themselves to its growth, and there may only periodically arise some compression of the vessels at the base of the brain, which, setting up disturbance in the intra-cranial circulation, will give rise to ephemeral hemiplegia, ischæmia, and fainting or epileptoid fits. But symptoms of paralysis of the cerebral nerves may supervene if the tumor pervades, irritates, or presses upon the nerve substance, or if the vessels become compressed and the nutrition of the nerve impaired.[1]

[Wilbrand, in a paper upon what he calls "psychic blindness," localizes the central visual centre in the cortex of the occipital lobe of each cerebral hemisphere. Symptoms of this psychic blindness in pathological conditions of the cortex of the occipital lobe are only of value when a partial disease of one visual sphere is present; for, in extensive disease of both occipital lobes, bilateral cerebral amaurosis appears; while in unilateral functional disturbance of one visual sphere, the homonymous retinal halves of both eyes are completely blind. The condition of affairs is different in cases of partial disease of one visual sphere, which are distinguished by the appearance of an incomplete lateral hemianopsia of the opposite side.

Ferrier's investigations into affections of vision from cerebral disease have led him to the recognition of a distinct visual centre. He found in the monkey, that it included not only the angular gyrus, but the occipital lobe. A portion only of one visual centre would in time suffice for vision with both eyes. It would appear as if the hemispheres had a double relation with the eyes. The connection of the angular gyri was mainly crossed; hence lesions here and in the corresponding medullary fibres caused crossed amaurosis in amblyopia. Where there was a unilateral lesion of the angular gyrus and occipital lobe together, but not of each singly, hemiopia occurred and lasted for some time.—B.]

Tumors in the Cerebellum nearly always produce blindness (generally from optic neuritis) by setting up a general disturbance (Hughlings Jackson), whereas abscess of the cerebellum, as a rule, does not do so, on account of its limited extent and effect.

Cerebral hemorrhage may be suspected if the amaurosis comes on very suddenly; this sudden equilateral hemiopia of the left side would make us suspect hemorrhage in the right hemisphere. Such equilateral contractions of the field often remain behind in persons who have been affected with an apoplectic fit. Loss of the right side of the field is more irksome than that of the left, more especially in reading, as the patient cannot read so easily and rapidly on account of his not being able to foresee the words (Von Graefe). In slight degrees of cerebral hemorrhage, the sight is often quite unaffected. Hemiopia may, however, be also produced by temporary affections of the nerve trunk, e. g., syphilis.

Senile softening of the brain is not, as a rule, accompanied by amaurosis, but, of course, the atrophic changes in the brain may extend to the optic nerves, the nutrition of the latter becoming impaired on account perhaps of the disease of the vessels.

Epilepsy may produce amaurosis when it is due to some disease of the brain, for instance, meningitis, for epilepsy must be looked upon as a symptom and not as a disease.

In diseases of the spinal cord, more especially chronic myelitis and locomotor ataxy, amaurosis, from progressive atrophy of the optic nerves, is not unfrequently met with. But it hardly ever makes its appearance in locomotor ataxy until a late period of the disease of the spine, long after the impairment of the mobility and sensibility of the lower limbs, and the paralytic affections of the muscles of the eye, the latter often being amongst the first symptoms of the spinal disease. In some very rare instances, the atrophy of the optic nerves has preceded by a long period (several years) the first symptoms of spinal disease (Von Graefe). This late occurrence of

---

[1] "Kl. Monatsbl.," 1865, p. 259.

amaurosis is explained by the fact that the degeneration ascends from the vertebral canal to the cavity of the cranium. Amblyopia often occurs at the commencement of the spinal affection, and a careful examination as to the true nature of the impairment of vision should be made, for it may only be due to a loss of the power of accommodation from paralysis of the ciliary muscle, and be not at all dependent upon any disease of the optic nerve. A want of care in the examination as to the true cause of such amblyopiæ, has led to much confusion amongst writers upon this subject. In cases in which the atrophy of the optic nerve is dependent upon locomotor ataxy, the former may remain stationary for a few weeks and then again progress (Von Graefe).

[The most common cause of amaurosis in spinal disease is gray degeneration of the posterior columns, but it occurs also in myelitis of the lateral columns. According to Von Graefe, thirty per cent. of cases of progressive atrophy of the optic nerve is due to spinal disease. An interesting variety of optic nerve atrophy is described by Charcot, accompanied by atrophy of one-half of the body and contraction of the extremities. ("Comptes rendus Soc. de biol.," iv. p. 191.)—B.]

The affection of the optic nerve in diseases of the spine is probably due to a lesion of the great sympathetic, through its communication with the anterior roots of the spinal nerves.

[On this point see an article by the Editor, in "Amer. Journ. Med. Sciences," July, 1875.—B.]

In some cases simple atrophy of the optic nerve exists for a long time without any appreciable cause, or the appearance of any symptoms indicative of a cerebral or spinal lesions; and, even after death, nothing is perhaps found except atrophy of the optic nerves or atrophy of those parts of the brain which are continuous with the optic nerve. In some of these cases, however, insanity may supervene. And this brings us to a very important point, viz., the great use the ophthalmoscope is likely to prove to the alienist in establishing the study of insanity upon a more positive basis.[1] In England, we are almost entirely indebted to Dr. Allbutt for our knowledge of this subject, and I would refer the reader to his valuable and interesting paper, entitled "On the state of the Optic Nerves and Retinæ as seen in the Insane," read before the Roy. Med.-Chir. Society, February 25, 1868. In this, he mentions that in general paralysis of the insane, atrophy of the optic nerve is constantly found, and is commonly accompanied by atrophy of the olfactory nerves. It is not distinctly seen till the end of the first stage, as it slowly travels down from the optic centres, and it is in relation with the state of the $p_u pi_l$, which is contracted in the early stage and dilated in the fatty atrophic stage.

In mania, the ophthalmoscope often reveals symptomatic changes. In dementia, organic disease and affection of the eye generally occur together.

In idiots, atrophy of the optic nerve is of frequent occurrence. Out of twelve cases, it was found of a marked character in five; one was changing, and two were noted as doubtful.

We have now to consider the *prognosis* which may be made in cases of amaurosis or amblyopia, as to whether the impairment of vision will improve, remain stationary, or the sight become permanently lost. In framing our

---

[1] For further information, I would particularly recommend Dr. Leber's very interesting paper "On Gray Degeneration of the Optic Nerve," "A. f. O.," xiv. 2, 177; also Dr. Westphal's important papers in the "Archiv .für Psychiatrie und Nervenkrankheiten." [Also the "West Riding Lunatic Asylum Reports," first four years.—B.]

prognosis, we must be especially guided by the mode of attack, the condition of the field of vision, and the appearances presented by the optic nerve. The nature of the primary disease which has caused the affection of the eye must naturally also be taken into anxious consideration; for the prognosis will, of course, be materially influenced by the fact, that the intra-cranial affection is of a kind that permits of resolution or amelioration through the absorption of morbid products, or hemorrhagic effusions, or the amendment of irregularities in the circulation.

If atrophy of the optic nerve has already set in, the prognosis as to the arrest of the disease must be very guarded, as in such cases there is always a great tendency to progression, and termination in absolute blindness. But this is not necessarily always the case, and it would be committing a grave error to irrevocably condemn an eye, simply because the optic nerve shows symptoms of commencing atrophy. The state of the field of vision is our best guide in such cases.

[Gray degeneration of the optic nerve, in connection with spinal symptoms, is hopelessly incurable.—B.]

If the loss of sight has occurred with great suddenness and rapidity, the prognosis need not necessarily be bad, for we occasionally meet with cases in which great improvement, or complete restoration, of sight takes place after its sudden loss. Sudden equilateral hemiopia is generally due to hemorrhagic effusions (apoplexies), which is seldom the case in double central scotomata. Von Graefe[1] considers that the prognosis of sudden amaurosis is better in children than in adults. He also states that the best prognosis is furnished by those cases in which the sudden loss of sight is the result of mental shock; also if the phosphenes continue to exist in the blind retina, and complete darkness proves beneficial. This form of anæsthesia is often associated with cutaneous insensibility to pain, and is perhaps referable to vaso-motor action.

The prognosis is also inclined to be favorable if the disease has remained stationary for some length of time, for although the dangerous forms of amaurosis likewise halt in their progress, yet this interruption does not extend beyond a few weeks or months, when they again progress. The former cases often depend upon a combination of deleterious causes, such as alcohol, tobacco, dissipation of every kind, overwork of the eyes and brain, or irregularities in the digestive organs or the uterine system.

The prognosis is bad, if the atrophy of the optic nerve is of slow development, and manifests a persistent, though perhaps tardy progress.

When the atrophy of the nerve cannot be traced to any particular cause, but appears to be a disease *per se*, the prognosis is generally also very unfavorable.

In those cases in which the condition of the visual field is quite normal (even after the affection has existed for several months), and the acuity of vision has not sunk considerably (only to one-sixth or one-tenth), we may decidedly regard the disease as not being due to progressive atrophy. The impairment of vision may not, however, undergo much improvement.

With regard to the prognosis afforded by the different forms of contraction and interruption of the visual field, we may briefly state, that it is more favorable when it is equilateral; with a sharply defined line of demarcation, than when it is concentric, or its edges (in the lateral form) are undefined and irregular. Indeed, patients affected with equilateral hemiopia never become absolutely blind, except the disease extends to the commissure, or

---

[1] " Kl. Monatsbl.," 1865, 149.

some other cerebral affection supervenes.[1] Such patients often enjoy excellent central vision, being able to read the finest print, and the affection frequently remains unaltered for a very long time. I have cases still under supervision in which equilateral hemiopia has existed for some years, and the patients are still able to read perfectly, nor has the condition of the eye changed, nor have any other symptoms shown themselves.

The most dangerous cases are those in which irregular contractions of the field of vision occur either simultaneously in both eyes, or in quick succession. Also those, in which the condition of the one eye being already very bad (the degree of its central vision being perhaps even less than the eccentric), the second eye becomes affected in an exactly similar manner, the contraction of its visual field commencing at a point symmetrical to that at which it began in the first eye.

Central scotomata never indicate progressive atrophy, if the periphery of the visual field is normal. But if they have existed unaltered for several weeks, and the optic nerve begins to show symptoms of commencing atrophy, a restitution *ad integrum* can no longer be expected. If the central portion of the retina maintains its superiority of vision over the outlying parts (so that the patient can see through the scotoma), the prognosis is always better than when the reverse obtains. If the peripheral portion of the field of vision beyond the scotoma is impaired, progressive atrophy is to be feared, which is not the case when this part of the field is normal, for this shows that the power of conductibility in the part of the retina affected with the scotoma is perfectly retained (Von Graefe).

We cannot form our prognosis of the case simply from the appearances presented by the optic nerve, for, as Von Graefe remarks, it is impossible to tell from these alone whether the atrophy be progressive or stationary. In conjunction with the appearance of the optic nerve, we must therefore be guided by the condition of the field of vision, and the mode in which the attack occurred. Even the absence of atrophic symptoms in the nerve does not exclude the most unfavorable result. In cases of amblyopia due to disturbances in the circulation, or to alcohol, or in that form which is sometimes met with in very nervous females and in children, the presence of symptoms of atrophy of the optic nerve are always of material consequence, as they greatly cloud the prognosis.

Treatment.—This must of course be specially directed against the primary cause of the affection of the eye. In those cases of simple progressive atrophy, in which we fail to detect any appreciable organic or functional cause, we must be extremely upon our guard not to submit the patient to a very active course of treatment, more especially of a lowering or depressing kind; for great mischief is thus often produced, and the progress of the disease hastened, instead of being arrested or retarded. The best treatment for such cases consists in the administration of tonics, especially the tincture of the muriate of iron, or a combination of steel with quinine or strychnine. The lactate or sulphate of zinc may also be given in gradually increasing doses, commencing with two or three grains daily, and augmenting this gradually until

[1] Von Graefe says: "Total blindness in cases of unilateral brain disease can only ensue (1) when the other hemisphere likewise becomes the seat of disease; (2) when fresh effusions in the hemisphere originally affected occasion diffuse cerebral disease, chiefly through anæmia cerebri; (3) when a basilar affection supervenes, directly affecting the trunks of the optic nerves; (4) when some encroachment on the space of the cerebral cavity results in compression of the sinus cavernosus with consequent venous incarceration of the papilla; (5) when propagated encephalo-meningitis leads to neuritis descendens." ("Kl. Monatsbl.," 1865, 220; "Ophth. Review," ii. 359.)

the patient takes eight or ten grains a day. The diet should be nutritious but light, and the effect of stimulants be closely watched. The patient's course of life should be carefully regulated, a sufficiency of sleep be insisted on, and all amusements and employment that may prove injurious to his eyes or general health be strictly forbidden. The use of tobacco must also be absolutely given up.

If there is any evidence of the existence of chronic meningitis, irregularities in the circulation (more especially the cerebral), or a suppression of customary discharges, such as the menstrual, or the exhalations from the skin, more particularly the feet, a derivative course of treatment must be employed. Leeches should be applied behind the ears, or the artificial leech to the temple, and a seton may be inserted at the nape of the neck, which often affords great and speedy relief to the severe and persistent headache. The bichloride of mercury should be given in small doses, in combination perhaps with the iodide and bromide of potassium, more especially if any syphilitic taint is suspected. The sudden suppression of the normal exhalations from the skin is not an unfrequent cause of amblyopic affections, more especially after long exposure to cold and wet. Thus persons who have stood for many hours in the water (sportsmen, fishermen, etc.) are sometimes affected with amblyopia, on account of the suppression of the exhalations from the feet. In such cases, hot, stimulating pediluvia, together with diaphoretics and diuretics, should be prescribed. Von Graefe also advocates the Roman or Turkish bath, as especially exciting the action of the skin, which will also prove of benefit in the different forms of congestive amblyopia.[1]

If the affection of the eye is due to some sudden fright or shock to the nervous system, tonics should also be prescribed.

In the amaurosis due to locomotor ataxy, innumerable remedies have been tried. Dr. Althaus[2] states that he has derived much benefit in cases of locomotor ataxy from the administration of small doses of nitrate of silver. He gives it together with the hypophosphite of soda, and he never goes beyond the dose of half a grain of the nitrate of silver. It should be employed for from four to six weeks consecutively, and then discontinued for a fortnight or three weeks, a slight aperient mineral water being given in the meanwhile. Then the use of the remedy may be again commenced, and continued for a month or so. The gums should be examined from time to time, as the peculiar dusky discoloration of the skin, which the long-continued use of nitrate of silver produces, first appears in the mucous membranes.

If there is any reason for supposing that syphilis is the cause, a prompt and long-continued use of mercurials and iodide of potassium is indicated. The use of the constant current has been highly recommended by many observers, but no rules have been laid down for its application, and the majority of

An important and interesting fact in connection with this subject has been noticed . . . . Having found that persons affected with fulness and congestion of the . . . . much benefited by the Turkish bath, he thought that the readiest . . . . the effect of the latter upon the cerebral circulation would be by . . . . upon the bloodvessels of the retina. Mr. Wordsworth therefore . . . . . eyes with the ophthalmoscope just prior to his entering the . . . . had remained in the hottest chamber (196° F.) for a quarter . . . . a decided and marked paleness of the optic nerve, and a . . . . the retinal vessels. The same effect was noticed in four per- . . . . negro, an East Indian, an Englishman, and a German), ... F., who were examined at the same time by Mr. Words-

. . . . teria, and Atary," 1866.

ophthalmic surgeons have little faith in its efficacy. [The internal administration of strychnia has seemed to do good in some cases, but the manner in which it acts has never been satisfactorily explained.—B.]

The treatment of amaurosis by subcutaneous injections of strychnine is described at p. 604.

If central scotomata have been developed during a protracted enfeebling general illness, such as typhoid or scarlet fever, diphtheria, childbed, etc., tonics and generous diet, with stimulants, are the best remedies; and, subsequently, when the sight is beginning to improve, much benefit is often derived from methodically practising the sight (even the eccentric) with strong convex lenses, as is done in cases of amblyopia from non-use. An improvement upon the ordinary single convex lens is recommended by Von Graefe, viz., a combination of two biconvex lenses (the one six inches, the other four) set in a tube or ring at a distance of one inch from each other. We thus gain a relatively considerable magnifying power with only slight spherical aberration. The eye should at first be only practised for a very short time (about two or three minutes), and with print that can be pretty easily deciphered.

If there is any disturbance in the functions of the liver or digestive organs, mild aperient mineral waters should be prescribed, such as the Pullna, Karlsbad, or Kissingen.

1.—AMBLYOPIA.

This affection is often due to passive congestion of the brain, the eye, or other organs, such as the liver, uterus, etc., or to disturbances of the nervous functions.

We must admit that the term passive congestion is very vague, and that we do not know with any certainty the mode in which the sight becomes affected, and whether this is due to a retardation of the blood-supply and a consequent insufficiency of its aëration, or whether it is loaded with noxious ingredients, such as alcohol, nicotine, lead, etc., which exert a toxic influence, and thus impair the functions of the nervous system.

For practical purposes, we must, however, draw a line of demarcation between the amblyopia which is due to simple irregularities in the circulation or nervous function, and that which depends upon some blood-poisoning, if this term may be accepted.

The insufficiency of blood-supply which gives rise to the *anæmic amblyopia* may be due to some excessive discharge from the uterus, to the debility consequent upon very severe illnesses, to a prolonged and very exhausting confinement, or to over-suckling. Copious hemorrhages (*e. g.*, after confinement) may likewise produce it. Cases are also recorded in which vomiting of blood (probably dependent upon an ulcer of the stomach) has produced amaurosis.[1] In these cases, the loss of sight had come on rapidly (leading to complete blindness in the course of a few days), affected both eyes, and was incurable. The ophthalmoscopic appearances were either negative, or were those of anæmia of the optic nerve and retina, leading subsequently to atrophy. When the loss of blood is very considerable, the function of the optic nerve is probably impaired by the anæmia of the brain and the insufficient excitation of the retina. But it is remarkable (as Von Graefe has pointed out) that the sight does not necessarily return with a restoration of the blood-supply and a restitution of the other functions. This is prob-

[1] O'Reilly, "Lancet," 1862; Von Graefe, "A. f. O.," vii. 2, 143.

ably owing to the fact, that the temporary deficiency in the blood-supply had caused permanent changes in the nutrition of the more delicate nerve structures.

[The amaurosis does not usually occur at the time of the loss of blood, but several days afterwards, and the cause cannot be found solely in the resulting anæmia, for the patients have often recovered from the loss of blood before the blindness has made its appearance. The amaurosis is probably due to a peripheral affection, to a disturbance of function of the optic nerves, the seat of which is at the base of the skull. If the amblyopia is partial, the prognosis is better than it is in the amaurosis. The treatment should consist of tonics, wine, good food, and strychnine injections.—B.]

Temporary or "transitory" amaurosis is sometimes met with in severe acute diseases, which are accompanied by blood-poisoning or great poverty of the blood, such as scarlet and typhus fever. [Intermittent fever is also a cause of amaurosis, which is sometimes intermittent and sometimes permanent. The amaurosis affects both eyes, and when it is of the intermittent type appears with the beginning of the chill, lasts through the hot stages, and disappears with the sweating stage. The ophthalmoscopic signs are negative. The permanent form of amaurosis from intermittent fever is much more rare, may not be complete, and may affect one or both eyes. Jacobi reports a case where neuritis optica was seen with the ophthalmoscope, and some few cases have been reported where atrophy of the nerve was the result. (See "American Journal of the Medical Sciences," April, 1877, and "St. Louis Courier of Medicine," May, 1880.)—B.] The blindness comes on very suddenly, and may be so complete that all perception of light is lost; this lasts from twenty to sixty hours, and then the sight returns. One peculiar and very important feature is, that even although all perception of light is lost, the pupil reacts perfectly to the stimulus of light. The ophthalmoscope, moreover, reveals nothing abnormal in the appearance of the fundus oculi, except occasionally a slight dilatation and tortuosity of the retinal veins. Such cases of transitory amaurosis have been reported, amongst others, by Ebert,[1] Henoch,[2] and Leber.[3] It is probable that they depend upon some disturbance of the cerebral circulation or upon an acute and temporary œdema of that portion of the brain which is situated between the corpora quadrigemina and the seat of the perception of light. Now, it is of course of the greatest importance to have, if possible, some guide as to the prognosis which may be made with regard to the restoration of sight. Von Graefe[4] lays the greatest stress on the behavior of the pupil, as being the most important point in the prognosis, for if it retains its activity when all perception of light is lost, the prognosis is favorable.[5] As he justly points out, the negative result of the ophthalmoscopic examination is no guide as to the prognosis, for we meet with cases of sudden blindness in severe acute diseases in which no changes in the fundus are visible for several weeks, and then symptoms of atrophy of the optic nerve supervene. In such instances, the seat of the disease is evidently situated in the retro-ocular portion of the optic nerve, so that the disk and retina remain for a time unchanged. But, of course, the pupil cannot react upon the stimulus of light, for this depends upon the stimulus being uninterruptedly conducted from the retina along the optic nerve to the corpora quadrigemina, thence to be reflected to the

---

[1] " Berliner klinische Wochenschrift," 1868, S. 21.   [3] Ibid., p. 96.
[2] Ibid., 1869, p. 395.   [4] Ibid., 1868, p. 22.
[5] Leber, however, reports a case of complete amaurosis from meningitis in which the pupils remained active, but the sight did not return. But this case does not belong to same category as the transitory amaurosis. Ib., 1869, p. 897.

third nerve and its ciliary branches; whereas if the pupil remains active, it shows that the cause of the blindness is not situated within this chain or circle of conductibility, but between the corpora quadrigemina and that portion of the brain in which the perception of light is localized. In fact, as Von Graefe says, " the negative result of the ophthalmoscopic examination exculpates the retina and the intra-ocular end of the optic nerve from being the cause of blindness; and the preservation of the activity of the pupil not only exculpates these, but also the whole optic nerve and the corpora quadrigemina." Hence, if the action of the pupil on the stimulus of light remains intact in cases of sudden blindness, the prognosis as to the restoration of sight is favorable.

The amblyopia which is met with in diabetes is sometimes due to paralysis of the accommodation, or to retinitis, somewhat akin in its nature to that met with in Bright's disease, and only rarely to anæmia. In *cholera*, we might expect that there would be great amblyopia on account of the poverty of the blood, but this is not so.

[Bresgen considers the characteristic symptoms in diabetic amblyopia to be a pericentric scotoma, within the limits of which the form-sense or perception is at first distinguished, with, at the same time, partial diminution of the color-sense, which afterwards may become total; and finally, diminution of the light-perception, while the peripheral parts of the retina performed their normal functions unimpaired.

Real diabetic affections of the optic nerve are of three kinds: 1. Simple amblyopia with a free field; 2. Atrophy; 3. Hemiopia. The retina is generally affected also in these cases. (See "Graefe u. Saemisch," v. 8. 894-899.)—B.]

Congestive amblyopia may be due to over-fulness of the system and congestion of the eye, brain, or other organs. It is not unfrequently met with in cases of suppression of customary discharges, deficiency or absence of the catamenia, and insufficient action of the skin or kidneys. Mr. Lawson[1] narrates a case in which suppression of the menses produced, within a few days, complete amaurosis in one eye, and great impairment of vision in the other. Under the use of iodide of potassium, and with the reappearance of the catamenia, the sight was restored.

A very interesting and extraordinary case is also reported by Mr. Lawson,[2] in which amaurosis repeatedly occurred during the period of gestation. [Cases of amaurosis during the period of gestation have also been reported by Dr. Loring and the Editor.—B.]

The real nature of amblyopia which is observed in certain cases of so-called blood-poisoning is at present quite obscure. It is generally supposed to be due to some disturbance in the circulation, producing what is termed passive congestion of the brain. But this explanation is indefinite and unsatisfactory, for, as Von Graefe says,[3] " Whether there is a real inundation of the nervous centre with venous blood, whether the current and change of the blood is only too slow, or whether the visual function is affected from the blood being overloaded with alcoholic and narcotic substances, are so many questions suggested by the term 'passive cerebral congestion.' This term, therefore, only serves to designate a condition where, failing all evidence of active congestion, the functional, or, as the case may be, also the nutritional existence of the cerebral centre of the optic nerve is interfered with by circulatory influences of the aforesaid order."

---

[1] " Med. Times and Gazette," 1868.   [2] " R. L. O. H. Rep.," iv. 65.
[3] " Ophth. Review," ii. p. 840.

This toxic influence may be especially produced by alcohol, tobacco, lead, and quinine.

The amblyopia met with in drunkards (amblyopia potatorum) generally commences with the appearance of a mist or cloud before the eyes, which more or less surrounds and shrouds the object, rendering it hazy and indistinct. In some cases the impairment of vision becomes very considerable, so that only the largest print can be deciphered, but if progressive atrophy of the optic nerve sets in, the sight may be completely lost. The visual field may remain normal, or become more or less contracted. The affection may exist for a very long time without causing any organic changes in the optic nerve or retina, excepting those of hyperæmia, and a certain loss of transparency of the disk. In other cases, if the disease progresses or the cause persists, atrophy of the optic nerve supervenes, and this always materially clouds the prognosis; for although we may, even in such cases, sometimes succeed in securing a great improvement of sight and an arrest of the atrophic degeneration, yet the vision is but seldom restored *ad integrum*. In cases of simple amblyopia, without any central scotoma or contraction of the field of vision, Leber has found that the appreciation of colors is not at all, or only very slightly, impaired.

[Romiée regards a weakening of the accommodation as the first manifestation of chronic alcoholism in the eye. This paresis of accommodation is sometimes the only sign of the influence of alcohol upon the eyes. The diminution of vision to one-sixth or below, occurring within a limited period of time and simultaneously in both eyes, he regards as pathognomonic of alcoholic amblyopia. He recognizes the existence of color-scotomata, which, however, he thinks are rarely extensive. The nature of the affection he considers to be a diffuse interstitial sclerosis of the neuroglia of the nerve-fibres, originating in the nerve centres.

In the few cases of this kind hitherto examined microscopically, the nerve fibres were the seat of fatty degeneration, and the connective-tissue framework was hypertrophied. The amblyopia may be acute or chronic, the latter being the more frequent. It occurs much oftener in men than in women. Scotomata are not always demonstrable in this disease, but in some cases central color-scotomata are very pronounced. With repeated attacks of alcoholic amblyopia, the tendency to atrophy becomes more certain. The disease is always bilateral, and in severe cases the patients often complain of persistent colored after-images.—B.]

In many of these cases, we cannot detect any abnormal appearances with the ophthalmoscope, and must therefore regard the impairment of sight as due to a functional, and not to an organic, lesion. In other cases there is some hyperæmia of the retina and optic nerve, with, perhaps, a certain degree of passive congestion, together with a diminution in the transparency of the disk, and subsequently symptoms of atrophy of the optic nerve may make their appearance. But I must here again warn the reader against too readily assuming the existence of hyperæmia and congestion of the optic nerve and retina, simply because the disk may seem to him to be slightly too red, or the veins somewhat large. It has been already stated that the appearances of the optic disk and of the retinal circulation vary very greatly within a perfectly physiological standard, and that it often requires an experienced and careful observer to determine whether or not some marked peculiarity in the appearance of these structures is physiological or pathological. In judging of these conditions, we must take into special consideration the age, the habits, the complexion, etc., of the patient.

The prognosis will depend chiefly upon the condition of the optic nerve, the length of time which the disease has existed, and the fact whether or not the patient is willing entirely to give up any habits which may have caused it.

The effect of tobacco in producing amblyopia and amaurosis was originally pointed out by Mackenzie; more lately Critchett, Wadsworth, Hutchinson, and Sichel have, amongst others, paid much attention to this subject, and believe that it gives rise to a peculiar and distinctive form of loss of sight, which they have therefore termed "tobacco amaurosis." It is supposed to produce a peculiar form of atrophy of the optic nerve, the symptoms of which are so special as to be considered characteristic of tobacco amaurosis (vide article on "Atrophy of the Optic Nerve"). One argument which has been brought forward to lend special weight to the theory that tobacco may produce amaurosis is, that simple progressive atrophy of the optic nerve occurs far more frequently amongst men than women. Whilst readily conceding this, I must also call attention to the fact that the causes which may produce amaurosis obtain far more among men than women. Thus the former are, as a rule, exposed to far greater corporeal and mental labor, to greater vicissitudes, and to greater indulgence in free living of every kind. Moreover, in all probability, the amaurosis is far more due to a combination of such deleterious influences than to the prevalence of one special one, e. g., tobacco. At least, in by far the greater number of cases of amaurosis which I have met with in heavy smokers, the patients readily admitted their free indulgence in other excesses. I fully admit the fact, that the excessive use of tobacco (but most frequently together with other causes) may produce considerable impairment of vision, and finally, if the habits of the patient be not entirely changed, and the use of tobacco, stimulants, etc., given up, even atrophy of the optic nerves. But I cannot, from my own experience, accede to the doctrine that there is anything peculiar in the form of atrophy of the optic nerve which would at once enable one to diagnose the nature of the disease, as depending upon excessive smoking. For the three peculiarities particularly insisted on, viz., the premonitory hyperæmia of the disk, the blanching of the latter first at the outer side, and the diminution in size or even disappearance of the nutritive vessels of the optic nerve, whilst the retinal vessels for a very long time retain their normal calibre, are met with in other forms of atrophy of the optic nerve, and are therefore not at all distinctive of tobacco amaurosis. Indeed, it is impossible to understand why tobacco alone should produce these peculiar changes. I believe that in the commencement of the amblyopia of smokers and drunkards the disturbance of sight is at first only functional, the retina being, so to say, "blunted," and its sensibility impaired, so that it does not react with normal acuteness. This impairment of its function is probably chiefly due to some irregularity in the circulation of the nervous centres, although it is also probable that in many cases (especially of tobacco amaurosis) there is some depressing influence exerted directly upon the nervous system. The truth of this hypothesis is proved by the fact that at first the optic nerve and the retina are quite healthy or only somewhat hyperæmic, and that great and rapid improvement takes place when the patient relinquishes smoking, drinking, etc., and is subjected to a tonic course of treatment, together, perhaps, with local depletion. But if the cause persists, if the patient continues his indulgence in smoking, drinking, etc., combined, perhaps, with severe mental or corporeal exertion, then the disease does not remain confined to mere functional derangement, but generally passes over into an organic lesion. The optic disk begins to show symptoms of atrophic degeneration, and the latter may gradually but steadily advance until the sight is greatly impaired or even quite lost (Von Graefe).

[The visual disturbance and ophthalmoscopic result, central scotomata, and discoloration of the optic disk are all like those in alcoholic amblyopia. Its course is slowly progressive. With these symptoms is very apt to be united a chronic conjunctival irritation with scarcely any secretion, occurring especially in those who work in tobacco.—B.]

The absorption of *lead* into the system will produce amaurosis. I have only met with one case in which the loss of sight could be distinctly traced to lead-poisoning. This was in a young woman, who some time ago came under my care at Moorfields. She had been a worker in lead, and had suffered from severe lead-poisoning. She was completely blind, and both optic nerves showed marked symptoms of atrophy consecutive upon optic neuritis. Mr. Hutchinson[1] has observed similar instances, in which lead-poisoning had given rise to optic neuritis, followed by atrophy of the optic nerves. [In these cases the amaurosis is generally very complete, but transient, but in rare instances the amaurosis lasts for weeks and even months. (See " Archives of Ophthalmology," viii. 4, and ix. 1.)—B.] Very generally, however, the only symptoms revealed by the ophthalmoscope are congestion and hyperæmia of the optic nerve and retina, the veins especially being somewhat dilated and tortuous. The sight and field of vision are even in such cases often considerably impaired. It must be mentioned that albuminuria is sometimes met with in lead-poisoning, and that consequently albuminuric retinitis may occur (Ollivier, Desmarres).

[The hyaline degeneration of vessels in saturnine amblyopia involves the smaller arteries and arterioles of the optic nerve trunk and retina, as far forward as the ora serrata, the nature of the disease being an endarteritis obliterans. This ends in obliteration of the calibre of arteries and capillaries, their walls being changed into a homogeneous solid mass, the original form of the vessel being in places retained, while in others there is a marked knobbed appearance. In the arteries the characteristic arrangement of the nuclei of the muscular coat end suddenly in places, and the calibre of the vessels become at most doubled. In place of the middle coat there is sometimes a very delicate membrane. The loss of elasticity of the vascular wall, and its transformation into a rigid tube, the narrowing of the calibre and the resulting increased resistance to the blood-current, leads ultimately to thrombosis of the vessels. These thrombi may be numerous and may undergo hyaline degeneration, or may soften. There is in these cases marked œdema of the external layers of the retina, which pushes aside the connective-tissue framework, and forms spaces filled with a serous fluid. There may be numerous capillary hemorrhages in the retina, and in the granule layers irregular, glistening, hyaline scales, besides more or less extensive deposits of fibrin coagula. (See " Virchow's Archiv," lxxxvi. 2.)

The amaurosis is almost always bilateral, though it may be in different degrees. It may be sudden and complete, coming on at the end of an attack of colic, and this form can be cured. But the most common variety is the slowly progressive, with central scotoma, and with other defects in the field. may be no other signs of lead-poisoning present.—B.]

. . . . ne in large doses has been in rare instances observed to produce . . . . , probably by causing great congestion of the cerebral circulation . . . . benefit was derived from the use of the artificial leech. [S . . . . . er. Med. Assoc.," 1879; " Archives of Ophthalmology," x. 1 a . . . . e Monatsblätter für Augenheilkunde," Beiträge, 1881.—B.] . . . . blyopia.—In the article upon retinitis albuminurica, it v . . . . , very sudden and complete blindness sometimes occurs

[1] " R. L. O. H. Rep.," vi. 1, and vii. 1.

Bright's disease, and is due to uræmic blood-poisoning. The sight may be lost within a very few hours, together with the appearance of symptoms of uræmic blood-poisoning, such as great pain in the head, epileptoid fits, etc.[1] Then, on the subsidence of these symptoms, the sight is also restored. This impairment of vision must be carefully distinguished from that dependent upon retinitis albuminurica.

[Uræmic amaurosis occurs in scarlatina, variola, and measles, in pregnancy, and in the lying-in woman. It may not be complete, and is always transient. It may complicate a retinitis albuminuriea in the pregnant woman. The reaction of the pupil is a favorable sign—if this is absent or very sluggish, the prognosis is unfavorable.—B.]

Amblyopia is sometimes due to reflex irritation originating in one of the branches of the fifth nerve, or in other parts of the nervous system. Thus severe and prolonged dental neuralgia may produce impairment of vision, which mostly disappears with the removal of the carious teeth. The ophthalmoscopic examination generally only affords negative results.[2] In a case of abscess of the antrum from a carious tooth, narrated by Dr. James Salter, the eye was considerably protruded and blind—the ophthalmoscope revealing extreme anæmia of the optic nerve (atrophy?). The sight was not improved by the removal of the tooth. In a case of herpes frontalis. accompanied by great pain, recorded by Mr. Bowman, the optic nerve was atrophied.[3]

[Under this head may also be considered sympathetic neurosis in one eye from irritation of ciliary nerves in the other eye, accompanied by limitation of accommodation, lachrymation, and retinal hyperæsthesia. Also the amaurosis occurring after injury to the frontal nerve. Most of the cases of hysterical amaurosis and of the blindness occurring in hystero-epilepsy belong in this category. It is probable also that the cases of blindness occurring with the presence of intestinal worms, so often reported, are examples of reflex amaurosis.—B.]

When one eye is excluded for any length of time from binocular vision, its sight generally begins to fail from non-use of the eye. This condition is termed *amblyopia ex anopsia*, and is especially met with in cases in which, on account of the presence of some opacity of the cornea or lens, or of strabismus accompanied with diplopia, the acuteness of vision of one eye is considerably greater than that of the other, so that the difference in the distinctness of the two retinal images proves very confusing to the patient, and, in order to remedy this, he unconsciously suppresses the recognition of the less distinct image. This *active* suppression of the one image by the mind must be distinguished from its *passive* suppression, caused by a dense opacity of the cornea or lens. the presence of which prevents any image being formed upon the retina. The active suppression of the retinal image is far more injurious to the sight than the passive. But both are especially so in children, for in them we often find that after a strabismus has existed for some time (six or twelve months), the sight of the squinting eye may be so much impaired that only large print can be deciphered with it, and yet in all other respects it appears perfectly normal. Moreover, if the squint is operated upon, and the eye then practised separately with strong convex glasses, the sight may be rapidly restored, if the impairment of vision has

---

[1] A case of this uræmic amaurosis followed afterwards by retinitis albuminurica is recorded by Von Graefe, "A. f. O.," vi. 2, 277.

[2] Cases of amblyopia, accompanying dental neuralgia, have been recorded by Mr. Hutchinson, "R. L. O. H. Rep.," vol. iv. 381; also by De Wecker, "Ann. d'oculistique," 1866.

[3] "R. L. O. H. Rep.," v. 1, p. 7.

not reached too high a degree. This proves that the defect of sight is not congenital, as has been sometimes supposed, but is due to the exclusion of the eye from binocular vision, and consequent disuse of the retina. Besides, if the squint is alternating, so that each eye is used in turn, the sight of both remains perfectly good. The rare cases of non-alternating strabismus, in which the sight of the squinting eye still retains its normal acuteness, is probably due to the absence of binocular vision, in consequence of which there is no diplopia, and of course no active suppression of the double image. This subject, however, is more fully explained in the article upon "Strabismus." In children, even the passive exclusion of the eye (*e. g.*, from cataract) leads to amblyopia far sooner than in adults, in whom complete cataract may exist for very many years (Von Graefe has recorded such a case in which a cataract had existed for sixty years), and yet, when it has been successfully removed by operation, the patient can see perfectly. In children, however, this is not the case, and the sensibility of the retina is apt permanently to suffer; hence the rule, that in children cataract, as well as strabismus, should be operated upon soon after its appearance.

Sudden and severe blows upon the eye may produce complete and instantaneous blindness, apparently from paralysis of the retina (*commotio retinæ*). [Traumatic anæsthesia of the retina is perhaps a better name.—B.] The same has been observed after a stroke of lightning.[1] The ophthalmoscope generally reveals no symptoms at all commensurate with the degree of blindness; perhaps there is only some hyperæmia of the retina and optic nerve, or a few scattered blood extravasations. In other cases nothing abnormal is observed, and the loss of sight is probably due to some disturbance or derangement in the retinal elements, which are, however, invisible with the ophthalmoscope.[2] But De Wecker mentions a case in which atrophy of the optic nerve subsequently supervened. The sight in these cases of paralysis of the retina often becomes perfectly restored, even although all perception of light may at first have been lost. [Well-marked cases of amblyopia due to poisoning by opium and morph¹ne have been reported; also a case of osmic acid amaurosis, by Noyes. One case has been reported of total amaurosis from a snake-bite ("Annales d'oeulistique," 1875, p. 90). Chrysophanic acid is another rare cause of amblyopia, which has recently been noted.—B.]

The treatment of the different forms of amblyopia must vary with the cause of the affection. Thus, in cases where the latter is evidently due to great debility, consequent, perhaps, upon severe illness, hyperlactation, etc., tonics, a generous diet, plenty of exercise in the open air, sea bathing, etc., must constitute the chief remedial agents. Whereas in the congestive amblyopia, great attention must be paid to the free action of the various eliminative organs, more especially the liver, skin, and kidneys. For this purpose saline mineral waters, diuretics, hot stimulating pediluvia, and the hot-air or Turkish bath, will prove of special advantage. In Germany, the prolonged use of the decoction of Zitmann is a favorite remedy, but this mode of treatment is accompanied by so much inconvenience, that but few English patients will submit to it. In the congestive amblyopia, I have often derived the greatest benefit from the repeated use of the artificial leech. In some cases, even its first application was followed by the most marked and surprising improvement in the sight. Hence, I would particularly insist upon the necessity of always giving the artificial leech a trial in cases of

[1] *Vide* also Saemisch, "Kl. Monatsbl.," 1864, S. 22.
[2] *Vide* also Schirmer, Ibid., 1866, 261.

amblyopia or amaurosis, in which there is evidence or suspicion of congestion, or of irregularities in the circulation; for this remedy is at present far too much neglected in England. The blood should be drawn rapidly, so that the glass cylinder becomes filled in three or four minutes. One or two cylinders full from each temple (if both are affected) will generally suffice. The operation may be repeated at intervals of five or six days, but if there is no improvement of sight after it has been performed two or three times, it should not be repeated. After each application of the artificial leech, the patient should be kept in a darkened room for about twenty-four hours, as the operation is generally followed by a good deal of reaction in the intraocular circulation.

We must also insist upon the patient leading a most regular life and abstaining from excesses of every kind, and in the amblyopia potatorum the allowance of spirituous liquors must be cut down to a minimum. If the nervous system is enfeebled, tonics must be administered in considerable doses, more especially steel, either alone or in combination with quinine or strychnine. The tinct. ferri muriat. (from fifteen to thirty drops or more, two or three times daily) often proves of much benefit. In the amblyopia of drunkards, Galezowski recommends large doses of bromide of potassium, and a collyrium of calabarine. [In amblyopia potatorum, the artificial leech is sometimes very useful and should always be employed.—B.]

In order to alleviate the extreme restlessness and nervous irritability of such patients, digitalis or hyoscyamus should be prescribed, and morphia should be administered at night to relieve the great and very trying sleeplessness, or the subcutaneous injection of morphia may be employed with advantage.

In tobacco amaurosis, the greatest stress must be laid upon the *absolute necessity* of the patient's entirely giving up the use of tobacco. Only in this way can we hope to cure or arrest the disease. Moreover, it is generally more easy for a great smoker to break himself at once and altogether of the habit, than to limit himself to one or two cigars or pipes a day, for then the temptation of exceeding this amount is constantly presented to him. At the same time tonics (particularly the tincture of steel, alone or in combination with strychnia) should be prescribed. By pursuing this course of treatment, we may generally succeed in rapidly curing the amblyopia if it be still only functional, or of arresting it and perhaps greatly improving the sight, if the optic nerve is only slightly atrophied.

In the impairment of vision from lead-poisoning, many remedies have been recommended, of which the most reliable is probably opium. This has been found to shorten the course of the constitutional disease, to diminish the frequency of paralytic affections, and to prevent relapses. The subcutaneous injection of morphia has been employed by Dr. Haase[1] with much benefit in amblyopia saturnina. As a rule, such cases afford a favorable prognosis, if symptoms of neuritis or atrophy of the optic nerve have not supervened. The patient must, however, be warned not again to expose himself to the risk of renewed lead-poisoning, otherwise a relapse may occur. [The first thing is to remove the patient from the influence of the lead, and to give such medicines as will eliminate the poison from the system through the bowels and kidney. Large doses of iodide of potassium and hypodermic injections of strychnia are also advisable.—B.]

The amblyopia due to disuse of the eye is best treated by methodically exercising the sight in reading, etc., with the aid of a strong convex lens, or

----

[1] "Klin. Monatsbl.," 1867, 225.

still better, Von Graefe's combination of two lenses set in a small tube. The eye should be practised frequently during the day, but only for the space of two or three minutes at a time. [If the amblyopia is due to the squint, this should be corrected.—B.]

In the loss of sight dependent upon paralysis (commotio) of the retina, the artificial leech, and blisters, should be applied, and the subcutaneous injection of strychnine tried.

I must now refer to two modes of treatment of amaurosis and amblyopia which have more recently come in vogue, and attracted much attention, viz., the subcutaneous injection of strychnine and galvanism by means of the constant (continuous) current.

Strychnine injections have recently assumed much prominence in the treatment of amaurosis and amblyopia, which is chiefly owing to the able and extensive researches of Nagel,[1] who has tried their effect in very numerous cases. They have sometimes proved beneficial, even in cases of progressive white atrophy of the optic nerve, frequently, however, only temporarily arresting the progress of the disease; they have also been useful in cases of atrophy following optic neuritis. But the greatest benefit has been derived in cases of amaurosis and amblyopia without organic ophthalmoscopic changes, such cases as occur from anæmia, copious hemorrhage (hæmatemesis, bleeding after confinement, etc.), severe blows on the eye, or from flashes of lightning; also in anæsthesia of the retina, hemeralopia, and amblyopia dependent upon an excessive use of tobacco or stimulants. I have tried this mode of treatment pretty largely, and have occasionally derived much benefit from its use in these forms of amblyopia. I have sometimes even seen some benefit accruing from it in cases of atrophy of the optic nerve. It appears but of little if any good in diseases accompanied by changes in the retina and choroid. Woinow[2] states, moreover, that it proves useless if there is a loss of the perception of colors. If the treatment is likely to prove beneficial, the improvement in sight generally manifests itself early, after the first two or three injections. At first one-fortieth of a grain should be injected once daily in the temple or arm, the dose being gradually increased to one-twentieth or one-fifteenth. According to Nagel, it is sometimes advantageous to interrupt the injections for a day or two, especially if any signs of a constitutional effect show themselves, such as twitching in the limbs, formication, pain in the head, dizziness, etc. Woinow generally injects one-fiftieth of a grain every two or four days, and daily gives one-sixteenth of a grain of extract of nux vomica internally as a pill. [The use of strychnia, both hypodermically and internally, has become very extensive in the United States for almost all kinds of amblyopia and amaurosis. It certainly does good in a great variety of cases, but it is not possible to lay down any rules which may indicate the limits of its usefulness. Though beneficial in some cases of amblyopia potatorum and nicotiana, it proves useless in others. Some cases of chronic degeneration of retina and choroid improve markedly under its use, while others show no change. Its effect may not be demonstrated until after several weeks in some cases, and this is contrary to the idea formerly held. It is well to begin with a daily dose of one-thirty-sixth or one-thirtieth of a grain, and rapidly increase it to toleration; then hold it at this point for some time before diminishing the dose. It is advisable to employ it in all cases of amblyopia, but not as a specific.—B.]

---

[1] "Die Behandlung der Amaurosen und Amblyopillen mit Strychnin," von Dr. Albrecht Nagel. Tübingen, 1871. Vide also an article on this subject by Prof. Horner in the "Correspondenz-Blatt für schweizer Aertze," Sept. 1, 1872.

[2] "A. f. O.," xviii. 2, 38.

As to the treatment of these diseases by the constant current, it must be confessed that this is not at present placed upon a firm basis, and I think that it has not received that attention from oculists which it deserves. At all events, it is most advisable that more extensive experiments should be made with it, if only for the purpose of testing the curative powers claimed for this agent by some observers, especially Benedikt,[1] Erb,[2] and Driver.[3] In cases of atrophy of the optic nerve, the positive pole of the constant battery should be applied to the back of the neck, and the negative to the closed eyelids, being moved gently over and around them; each sitting should not last more than one to three minutes; the number of cells employed may range from four to ten or fourteen, according to the nature of the case and sensitiveness of the eye and of the patient. The operation should not produce dizziness at the time, or headache afterwards. It is better to have a short sitting every day than a prolonged one at longer intervals. I have found Foveaux's (Weiss') constant battery one of the most convenient. [The younger the patient the greater is the probability of success, and the more recent the amaurosis the more likely is it to be benefited by treatment. The greater the amount of vision retained, the better hope is there of benefit. There seems to be a definite connection between the size of the large vessels and the probability of improvement under treatment.—B.]

2.—HEMERALOPIA [NIGHT-BLINDNESS].

This disease is especially characterized by the fact that, although the patient may be able to see very well during bright daylight, his sight rapidly deteriorates towards dusk, and still more so at nightfall; hence the term night-blindness. When the illumination is sufficient, a more or less dense gray or purple cloud surrounds and renders all objects indistinct and hazy, and also impairs the power of distinguishing colors. Thus, according to Förster,[4] certain colors, especially white, yellow, and green, can be more readily distinguished than blue, violet, or red. The pupil is wide and sluggish on the admission of light, but reacts normally on irritation of the branches of the fifth, e. g., on instillation of the tincture of opium. In retinitis pigmentosa, the pupil is, on the contrary, contracted. In severe cases the impairment of sight may be so great, that even large objects cannot be distinguished when the light is much diminished. It is, however, an error to suppose that the dimness of sight is due to the setting of the sun, and that it is thus linked to a certain time of the day. Identically the same symptoms appear if the illumination is artificially diminished, by placing the patient in a darkened room. This fact was most satisfactorily proved by Förster, with his ingenious photometer. The dimness of vision is only due to an impairment of the sensibility (torpor) of the retina, so that the patient requires the full stimulus of bright daylight, or artificial light, in order to see distinctly. This impairment of the sensibility of the retina may either be due to an insufficiency of blood-supply, to the impoverished condition of the blood, or to the nerve elements of the retina having been over-stimulated by prolonged exposure to extremely bright light. Very frequently, the hemeralopia is a result of a combination of these causes. [The functional disturbance does not always involve all parts of the retina alike, but there may be a number of scotomata. Both eyes are always affected, and the

[1] "Electrotherapie," by Benedikt.
[2] Ib., ii. 2.
[3] Knapp's "Archives," ii. 1.
[4] "Ueber Hemeralopie," Breslau, 1857.

patients are often annoyed by after-images. The color-perception is markedly dull by low illumination, and phosphenes can with difficulty be excited. Conjunctivitis is a not uncommon complication.—B.]

It appears, however, to be true that in the early morning, after a sound and refreshing sleep, the sensibility of the retina is greater than at a subsequent period of the day, so that the patient is then able to see even by a somewhat diminished illumination.

It is of great consequence to distinguish between simple hemeralopia, and that condition of night-blindness which accompanies retinitis pigmentosa. The former is simply functional and curable, the latter depends upon organic changes in the retina, and at a later period in the optic nerve, and incurable. Inattention to, or ignorance of, these facts has led to great confusion in the writings of some authors.

Hemeralopia may be caused by prolonged exposure to extremely bright light, such as the rays of the sun in tropical climates, or the glare of a vast expanse of brightly glistening snow. The ill-effects of such exposure make themselves especially felt, if the individual is in a condition of great debility or exhaustion, as after severe illness or long deprivation of food. Thus, we not unfrequently find hemeralopia existing among sailors returning from the tropics, who have been kept for a length of time without sufficient food, and have, perhaps, been suffering from scurvy. I have several times had four or five sailors from one vessel under my care at Moorfields, for hemeralopia. Their story was always the same. They had just landed from their vessel, after a long exposure to a tropical sun and a scanty allowance of food, and they had generally been suffering from great debility, or from scurvy. The hemeralopia had diminished somewhat on their reaching a more temperate zone, and rapidly disappeared on their arrival in England, under the administration of tonics and the enjoyment of a generous diet. In none of these cases was I able to discover anything peculiar with the ophthalmoscope; the retinal veins were, perhaps, slightly dilated, but I could not trace any diminution in the calibre of the arteries. Indeed, in almost all cases of this form of hemeralopia, the ophthalmoscopic examination yields a negative result. In several of these patients there were distinctly noticed those peculiar, silvery-gray, scaly patches of thickened epithelium at the outer portion of the ocular conjunctiva near the cornea, to which particular attention has been called by Bitot.[1] He considers these patches pathognomonic of hemeralopia, and states that they disappear consentaneously with the disappearance of night-blindness. I have, however, found them absent in several cases of hemeralopia, and they are evidently quite unconnected with this disease, and only due to a thickening and desiccation of the conjunctival epithelium from exposure to intense heat, which sets up a state of chronic congestion or inflammation of the conjunctiva. The appearance of these patches at the outer part of the cornea, is due to this portion of the ocular conjunctiva being most exposed, on account of the palpebral aperture at this point.

Hemeralopia has also been observed to break out epidemically in gaols, camps, etc. I need hardly point out that in such cases a careful examination should always be instituted, in order to guard against "malingering." According to Alfred von Graefe, the accommodative power of the eye is often somewhat impaired, there being also a certain degree of insufficiency of the internal recti muscles. [Hemeralopia is said to be by no means a rare complication in diseases of the liver. It appears ordinarily in attacks of varying duration, in chronic hepatic affections, especially in cirrhosis. It does not

[1] "Gazette hebdomadaire," 1868.

seem to be produced by icterus, but by a special alteration of the blood resulting from interference with the hepatic functions. Its occurrence is of grave significance. (See "Archives générales de médecine, Avril, 1881.)—B.]

The treatment must be chiefly directed to strengthening the general health by tonics and a generous diet. Amongst the former, quinine, steel, and cod-liver oil are the best; indeed, cod-liver oil is considered by Despouts as a specific for hemeralopia. At the same time, the patient must be carefully guarded against bright light. His room should be darkened, and he should only be allowed to go out when there is no sun, and even then wear eye-protectors. If the attack of hemeralopia is severe, it may be even necessary to insist upon keeping him in perfect darkness for several days, and he should then be gradually accustomed to a greater and greater amount of light. Blisters and local depletion have been strongly recommended by some authors, but they are generally contra-indicated by the debility and feeble condition of the patient. But if there are marked symptoms of congestion and hyperæmia of the retina and optic nerve, the effect of the artificial leech should be tried.

In *snow-blindness* the impairment of vision is also chiefly due to diminution of the sensibility of the retina from the great and prolonged glare, but it may likewise perhaps be owing to the effect of the great rarefaction of the atmosphere in high mountain ranges, which may not only produce inflammation of the conjunctiva, with extravasations of blood into its tissue, but also perhaps hemorrhagic effusions into the choroid and retina.

Closely allied to the above form of amblyopia, is the anæsthesia of the retina which occurs in consequence of prolonged exposure to extremely bright light (Ueberblendung der Netzhaut). Instances of this kind are met with amongst persons who have been long exposed to strong sunlight, or have greatly tried their eyes by excessive use of the microscope, etc., more especially by artificial light. They are often seized with a sudden dimness of sight, and notice (more especially if the illumination is but moderate) a more or less dense dark cloud or disk, which appears suspended before their eyes, and veils the central portion of an object or of the field of vision, leaving the periphery, perhaps, quite clear. The density and extent of the cloud, and the consequent degree of amblyopia, as also its duration, are subject to considerable variation. Thus, the cloud may only be observed for a few minutes after the exposure, or it may last for days and weeks, or even longer. The treatment should principally consist in guarding the patient against all use of the eyes and exposure to bright light. Indeed, if the case is severe, it may be necessary to insist upon his being kept in the dark for some length of time. The artificial leech is also often of much benefit. Cod-liver oil and steel should be prescribed internally.

[Nyctalopia or day-blindness is that condition in which the vision is markedly diminished during ordinary daylight, but is quite normal in a dim light. It is only a particular form of retinal hyperæsthesia. This must be distinguished from the modified day-blindness occurring in albinism, coloboma iridis, mydriasis, and partial cataract. It is said to be caused by long exposure to glistening surfaces, brilliantly illuminated by the sun: hence snow-blindness is a variety of nyctalopia.—B.]

In all the above forms of amblyopia the suboutaneous injection of strychnine should be tried.

[Congenital color-blindness is that defect wh
to distinguish colors without any disturbance i
eye. The degree and kind of this defect may
methods have been recommended for discoveri
the ability of the patient to discriminate bet
Maxwell's colored disks, which were formerly u
testing was tedious and lengthy. Methods b
Landolt, Herschel and Rose, and by Stilling, the
testing by successive or by simultaneous contrast
results have been obtained with the spectrosc
sunlight. The most useful and practical test of
gren, and which has been so thoroughly practis
by Dr. Jeffries, of Boston. It consists in throw
before the patient a large number of colored
and requiring him to pick out and lay aside
all the worsteds of the same color, or of differ
Thomson's instrument for the detection of col
flat sticks about two feet in length and one
hinge at one end, and connected together by a b
these, and concealed from view, are forty white
from one to forty engraved upon them, attach
hooks. To the eyes of these buttons are atta
wool. The test-skeins are three; light-green
These skeins are shown to the persons exam
directed to select from the stick the colors whic
stick the colors are arranged alternately to m
those confusion-tints which experience shows t
by the color-blind. (See "Trans. Amer. Op
formerly supposed that the examination of color
a sound basis for the theory of color-blindness
and endorsed by Helmholtz. But the rece
("Sitzungsber. d. Wien. Akad.," Bd. lxix., 18
this is not always possible. As is well known, c
or total, the first being much the more freque
that in which green is confounded with variou
and is called green-blindness, or red-green-blir
not be absolute for these two colors, for the per
weakened, and bright tints of red may be recog
for all shades of red. Red-green-blindness is
Daltonism. Green-blindness is distinguished fr
that the patient confounds pure green and its
white or gray. Blindness for blue and yellow i
by Stilling, which were examined by the spectr
the spectrum for blue-green, green, and violet
called red, and blue was called green.

Pflüger thinks that the most significant fact a
theory is that the divisions of color-blindness
blindness, cannot consistently be carried out.
upon the different chromatic systems, comes to

no right to consider the colors which are wanting in the different forms of dyschromatopsia as the fundamental colors of the normal system.

Total color-blindness is an exceedingly rare anomaly. Very few cases have been reported, and in these red appeared as black, and orange as gray. The spectrum was markedly shortened at both ends. (For a complete account of the theory of color-blindness, the reader is referred to the exhaustive articles of Holmgren, in the "Nordiskt. med. Arkiv.," vi. Heft 3; and in the "Upsala Läkaref. Förhandl.," 1874, Heft 2 and 3; and of J. Stilling in the "Klin. Monatsbl. Ausserordentl. Beiträge," Heft i. and ii. 1875. See also Dr. Jeffries' "Monograph on Color-Blindness.") Congenital color-blindness is frequently hereditary, affecting several generations of the same family. The hereditary form comes oftener from the mother's side than the father's. The male sex is much oftener affected than the female, though in some families only the latter were found color-blind. Recent researches place the proportion of from three to five per cent. of the males of all countries as color-blind in a greater or less degree.

It is almost without exception bilateral, and there is reason for believing that it is commoner in the lower classes than among the better educated. The importance can scarcely be overestimated of carefully testing all persons employed in occupations which render a good perception of color indispensable, as in sailors, and the employés on railroads. This whole subject has been most thoroughly investigated and admirably discussed by Dr. B. Joy Jeffries, in his book on " Color-Blindness: its Dangers and its Detection." The colored plates in the latest edition of Stilling's book have been regarded by some as the quickest, simplest, and most trustworthy means of detecting color-blindness. Macé and Nicota prefer the method of examination by colored glasses, because by both bright and moderate illumination, the normal limits of the visual field are nowhere reduced by the interposition of glasses. For the quantitative determination of the color-sense, Weber's tablets are perhaps the best for the purpose. The importance of a compulsory examination of all railway and steamboat employés as to color-blindness, as well as to acuteness of vision, has been fully brought forward by many writers, notably by Drs. Jeffries and Thomson in the United States, and the Editor would refer to Dr. Jeffries' monographs, and to an article by Dr. Thomson in "The Medical News" for Jan. 14, 1882.—B.]

Professor Maxwell[1] mentions the interesting fact that if a color-blind person looks at red or green through a red glass, the green will appear darker, but the red be nearly as bright as before; whereas if he uses a green glass, the red will appear darker, but the green hardly altered. He has thus been able to make color-blind people distinguish the colors of a Turkey carpet, and suggests that if such a patient wore a pair of spectacles with one eye red and the other green, he might in time be able intuitively to form a judgment of red and green things.

It is generally held that the inability to distinguish a certain color, e. g., red) is due to an insensibility of those nerve fibres of the retina which are sensitive to red. This view, has, however, been lately strongly opposed by Max Schultze, who considers that in such cases it probably depends upon an excessive development of the yellow pigment in the region of the macula lutea, which has the effect of diminishing the intensity of the red rays.[2] In connection with this subject it is of interest that, during santonin intoxica-

---

[1] " Philosophical Transactions," 1860.

[2] *Vide* Max Schultze's brochure " Ueber dem Gelben Fleck," etc., 1866; also his work, " Zur Anatomie und Physiologie der Retina," 1866

tion everything acquires a yellow or greenish-yellow tint, but violet and red become indistinct. For further information upon this subject, I would refer the reader to articles by Rose and Hübner, "A. f. O.," vii. 272, and xiii. 2. Niemetchek, on the other hand, does not believe that the seat of appreciation of color resides in the bulbs of the retina, for they may be destroyed and yet it may exist; nor can it be in the optic nerve.[1] He has observed that in persons in whom the sense of appreciation of color is very pronounced, the region of the frontal bone between the orbits is greatly developed; the reverse being the case in those in whom this sense is deficient. He therefore supposes that this sense is a cerebral function, and especially of the inner and inferior convolutions of the anterior lobes. In Mr. John Dalton, this part of the brain was found to be very little developed. This hypothesis is, moreover, strengthened by the fact that subjective appearances of color arise, or color-blindness, if morbid processes occur in this region of the cerebrum.

Steffan holds that there is in the central nervous organs a special centre for the color-sense, which is a double one, corresponding to the double centre for the sense of space in the gray cortex of both occipital lobes. If an apoplectic clot can destroy at the same time both these color-centres, they must be very near the median line, and probably very near the space-centres. This theory goes far towards placing the cause of congenital color-blindness in the brain. But neither the cerebral nor the retinal theory of congenital color-blindness can alone be the correct one, for the cause of such defect may lie as well in the conducting fibres of the optic nerve as in the retina or in the cerebral color-centres.

Color-blindness (especially dichromatic vision) is, as a rule, congenital, and even hereditary; but the interesting and important fact has been observed by Benedikt, Schelske, etc., that it is met with in atrophy of the optic nerve, and, according to Galezowski,[2] in various other diseases. Dr. Argyll Robertson[3] has seen it in a case of spinal disease, in which there also existed myosis. Dr. Chisolm,[4] of Baltimore (U. S. A.), has observed achromatic vision in a case of optic neuritis. But the most important researches are those to which I have already referred, just published by Leber,[5] who has examined a great number of patients suffering from various eye affections, as to the presence of color-blindness. He has found color-blindness an almost constant symptom in atrophy of the optic nerve, whether this was primary or secondary upon optic neuritis; also more or less in all cases of circumscribed central scotoma. I have already entered more fully into these affections, and the results of his experiments, at pp. 571, 587. In syphilitic retinitis, color-blindness is sometimes present, and in other cases not; the same is the case in detachment of the retina. In the later stages of choroido-retinitis, accompanied by atrophy of the retina and optic nerve, color-blindness not unfrequently occurs. Color-blindness may also be acquired without, however, any impairment of sight. Thus it has been observed during pregnancy, and sometimes in consequence of some cerebral disturbances. Lawson[6] has observed a case in which it was produced by over-use of the eyes, in constantly looking at different colors for the purpose of sorting them. [It is also sometimes a symptom of certain functional (hysterical) disorders of the nervous system. Von Hasner has described a new disease which he calls chromatophobia. He regards this disease as a symptom of increased irritability of the light-perceiving apparatus, and as a species of retinal photo-

[1] " Prager Vierteljahrschrift," 1868, iv. 284.
[2] " Chromatoscopie Rétinienne," 1868.   [3] " Edin. Med. Journal," Feb. 1869.
[4] " R. L. O. H. Rep.," vi. 214.   [5] " A. f. O.," xv. 8.
[6] " Diseases of the Eye," p. 187.

phobia. There is generally an increased irritability, and an aversion to certain colors, which may eventually lead to reflex symptoms. In all his cases, the color-sense was normal, and there was no ophthalmoscopic evidence of any lesion.—B.]

4.—SIMULATION OF AMAUROSIS.

We occasionally meet with cases of simulated blindness, more especially amongst nervous, hysterical females, or persons who wish to shirk their duties, as soldiers, prisoners, etc. In sharp and clever individuals it is sometimes very difficult to convict them of deceit. Absolute blindness of both eyes is but seldom simulated, except, perhaps, in those cases in which so considerable a degree of amblyopia really exists, that the patient is unable to gain his livelihood, and therefore pretends to be absolutely blind, in order to excite the commiseration and assistance of the charitable. In such cases, the behavior of the pupil under the stimulus of light is the best guide; for if a patient declares that he is so blind that he cannot distinguish between light and dark, and the pupils yet contract under the stimulus of light, we may generally insist upon its being a case of simulation. Such patients, however, sometimes dilate the pupils artificially with atropine, and this may be suspected if they are dilated *ad maximum*, for in the mydriasis due to amaurosis (except the branches of the fifth nerve supplying the dilatator pupillæ are irritated), the pupil is but moderately dilated. If the action of atropine is suspected, but a conviction appears impossible, paracentesis should, if practicable, be performed, and the aqueous humor applied to some other eye to see if it will produce dilatation of the pupil. Where the atropine has only been applied to one eye, the detection is far more simple, for not only will the pupil be dilated *ad maximum*, but it will not act consentaneously with that of the other eye, with the movements of the eyes, or during the act of accommodation (*vide* the article "Mydriasis," p. 290). But h re are several other methods of detecting the simulation of monocular amaurosis. One of the best of these is Von Graefe's test with prismatic glasses. Thus, if a patient complains that he is absolutely blind in one eye, and the examination of this eye is concluded, that of the other (both eyes, however, being open) should be proceeded with, and a prism of 10° or 15° be held with its base upwards or downwards before the healthy eye. The patient should then be casually asked (so as not to arouse his suspicion that we suppose him to be deceiving), whether this improves the sight or not. If he says that it causes diplopia, the simulation is proved, for if he was absolutely blind in one eye diplopia could not be produced, whereas this would not exclude a considerable degree of amblyopia. The prism should be turned in different directions, in order that we may ascertain if the double images correspond to the position of the prism.

Dr. Von Welz[1] places before one eye a prism of 10° or 15°, with its base turned horizontally outwards or inwards. If a corrective squint arises, or if, on removal of the prism, there is any change in the position of the optic axes, it proves at once that the patient enjoys binocular vision.

Mr. Zachariah Laurence[2] employed the stereoscope for the purpose of detecting simulation of monocular amaurosis. The slide used for this purpose has two different words or figures (e. g., a circle and a quadrant) upon it, so

---

[1] "Congrès Ophthalmologique," 1866; Compte-rendu.
[2] "Handy-Book of Ophthalmic Surgery," 17.

CHAPTER XIV.

THE ANOMALIES OF REFRACTION AND ACCOMMODATION OF THE EYE.

1.—THE REFRACTION AND ACCOMMODATION OF THE EYE.

THE affections of the refraction and accommodation of the eye are daily assuming more importance, and are engaging more and more the attention of some of our most able and scientific ophthalmologists. For it is now known that certain forms of asthenopia and amblyopia, which had in former times set all remedies at defiance, are not due, as was generally supposed, to serious lesions of the inner tunics of the eyeball, but are in reality dependent upon some anomaly of the refraction of the eye, or a peculiar asymmetry of the organ (astigmatism). Since the discovery of these important facts, a considerable group of cases has been found to be amenable to treatment; cases which had formerly sorely puzzled the oculist, and were by him but too often deemed incurable.

The greater the strides which have been made in the investigation of the affections of refraction and accommodation, the more evident has it become how essential it is that they should be thoroughly and carefully studied, and scientifically treated. I would therefore impress upon the student the fact that, after he has made himself conversant with the theoretical portion of the subject, it is only by a practical and oft-repeated examination of a considerable number of cases, that he can acquire the requisite facility in the examination of the state of refraction and of the range of accommodation, or in the choice of spectacles. To those who may consider these subjects as somewhat abstruse and difficult, I would reply, that the difficulties lie only on the surface, and that a little perseverance and practice will soon enable them to unravel the knotty points.

Before we enter upon the subject of the refraction and accommodation of the eye, we must very briefly consider the properties of optical lenses. For

Fig. 188.

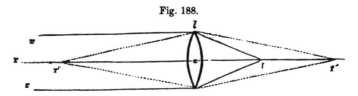

spectacles, the spherical biconvex and biconcave lenses are almost solely used, and I shall therefore confine myself to their description. In the article upon "Astigmatism," the properties of cylindrical lenses will be explained.

The biconvex lens is formed by the apposition of a segment of two spheres,

the radii of curvature of the two surfaces being equal). Such
also termed *converging* lenses, as they possess the power of
of light, passing through them, towards the axis. The line
the centre of the lens (Fig. 188, c) is termed the axis, and
through it (axial ray) is not deflected.

(1) If parallel rays (from a luminous object at an infini
upon a biconvex lens, they are united at a certain point
and this point is called the *principal focus* (or simply the f
The distance of this point from the optical centre of the le
the radius of the curvature of the lens), is termed the fo
lens. Thus, if in Fig. 188 *l* is a biconvex lens of six inch
rays (r r) will be united at *f*, six inches behind the lens. (
is now brought closer to the lens to *r'*, so that the rays er
assume a divergent direction, they will be brought to a foc
some distance behind the principal focus (*f*) of the lens. (
is situated at twice the focal length of the lens, the rays
united at a point placed twice the focal length behind the

Fig. 189.

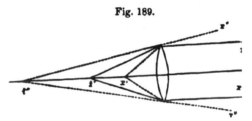

the distance of the object and of its focus from the lens v
(4) If the object be placed at the principal anterior foca
inches in front of the lens (Fig. 189, *f'*), the rays will emer
parallel to its axis r r. (5) If the object is placed *inside* th
(Fig. 189, *r'*) the rays from it will be so divergent that the
able to render them even parallel, and they will therefore
still somewhat divergent. This divergence will of course be
they entered the lens, and if the rays (*r'' r''*) are prolonged t
at which they would cut each other, this point would lie at *f*
further from the lens than the object *r'*. The focus (*f''*)
therefore imaginary, and situated on the same side of the le
(6) If convergent rays (rendered so by some other lens) fa
they will be brought to a focus on the other side of the lens,
nearer than the principal focus.

It has been shown above, that the further the object, from
rays fall upon the lens, is removed from the latter, the nea

[1] As the term infinite distance will necessarily be of frequent o
pages, it will be well to explain its signification at the outset. We
to be at a finite distance, as long as rays emanating from it fall in a
upon the eye. Of course rays, even from a very distant object, do
but this divergence (which naturally decreases in extent the furthe
moved) is already so slight when the object is placed at a distance of
feet, that the rays from it impinge, to all intents and purposes, par
We therefore consider rays coming from an object situated further
as parallel, and as emanating from an object at an *infinite* distance.
a nearer object are divergent in proportion to its proximity, and
coming from a *finite* distance.

of such rays approach the principal focus of the lens; whereas the closer
the object is brought (provided that it remains further off than the principal
focus) the more will its focus recede from the lens. On account of this
dependence of these two points (the position of the object and its focus)
upon each other, they are termed *conjugate foci*. Moreover, if the position
of the object and its focus were changed, so that the object were placed at *f'*
(Fig. 188), the rays from it would be brought to a focus on the other side of
the lens at *r'*, the point where the object was situated before; hence *f'* and *r'*
are *conjugate foci*. Again, if the object be placed at *f*, its rays will emerge
parallel from the lens.

Hitherto, we have only spoken of the refraction of rays which are parallel
to the axis of the lens, and whose focus is situated upon the axis. We must
now consider the focus of rays, the axes of which pass through the centre of
the lens, but which are inclined to the axis. Such are termed *secondary axes*.
The inclination must not, however, be too considerable, otherwise the rays
will not be brought to an exact focus, on account of the great spherical
aberration which occurs. Thus in Fig. 190, let *A B* be the principal axis
of a lens, *r* a luminous point situated on this axis, and *f* the focus at which

Fig. 190.

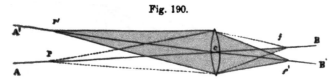

the rays from *r* are united. Now let *r'* be another luminous point situated
at the same distance from the lens as *r*, but not at the principal axis, but at
a certain inclination towards it. The secondary axis *A' B'* will pass straight
through the centre (*c*) of the lens without undergoing any deflection, and the
rays from *r'* will be brought to a focus at *f'*, which will be situated on the
secondary axis *A' B'*, at the same distance behind the lens as *f*. Just as *f* is
the conjugate focus of *r*, will *f'* be the conjugate focus of *r'*.

We shall now be able to understand the manner in which a biconvex
lens forms an image of any luminous object situated in front of it. Let
A B C (Fig. 191) be an object situated in front of the lens. The rays

Fig. 191.

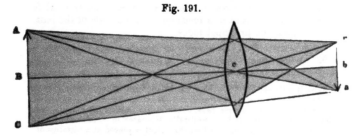

emanating from *A* will be focussed at a point *a*, situated on the secondary
axis, drawn from *A* through the centre *c* of the lens; *a* is consequently the
image of *A;* in the same manner, *c* is the image of *C*, and the rays from *B*,
situated on the principal axis of the lens, are united at *b*, likewise placed on
this axis, hence *b* is the image of *B*. A reverse and smaller image of the
object *A B C* is therefore formed behind the lens at *a b c*. The rays which

the radii of cu...
also termed co...
of light, passin...
the centre of t...
through it (ax...

(1) If para...
upon a bicon...
and this point...
The distance...
the radius of...
lens. Thus, i...
rays (r r) wil...
is now broug...
assume a div...
some distance...
is situated a...
united at a ...

... are not deflected; and a b c are the
... B and o b is also conjugate, for,
... verted and enlarged image would be

... by the lens will depend upon the dis-
... If the latter is placed at an infinite
... will be formed behind the lens at its
... approximated so as to lie at double
... image will be situated at double the
... the same size as the object. (3) If
... yet further than the anterior focus,
... away from the lens and be larger than
... at the anterior focus, no real image
... from the lens in a parallel direction.
... focal length, the rays will still issue in
... and the latter will act as a magnifying
... and situated behind the lens, but will
... in front of the lens, i. e., on the same side
... again this. If A B be an object situated

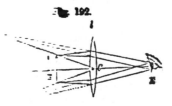

Fig. 192.

... or focus F, the rays from A will still diverge
... lens, and in such a direction as if they came
... will diverge as if they came from b. If the
... of the lens, it will see, instead of the object
... a b.

... lens will be greater according to the short-
... four-inch lens magnifies more than a five-inch,
six-inch lens. In order therefore to give the cor-
... demonstrate at once that a six-inch lens mag-
... designate the magnifying power of a lens by
... which are one, the denominators, the focal
... fourth is stronger than one-fifth, the latter
... former. Moreover, this way of expressing the
... correct, as indicating its power of refraction, for
... rays of light impinging upon it more than a

the dista...
(4) If th...
inches in...
parallel...
(Fig. 18...
able to...
still son...
they en...
at whi...
furthe...
theref...
(6) If...
they ...
neare...
It ...
rays ...

1 ...
pag...
to l...
upo...
but ...
mo...
feet ...
W...
us ...
n ...
co ...

... biconvex lens, they are united into a real focus
... ment, however, with a biconcave or "diverging"
... parallel rays, but renders them divergent. Thus
... (r r) fall upon a concave lens, they will be
... a direction as if they had proceeded from f, in
... wards of the divergent rays r' r' would cut one
... called the negative virtual focus of the lens, and
... situated upon the same side as the object. The

distance of this point for parallel rays from the lens gives the focal distance of the latter. Thus a concave lens of ten inches focus renders parallel rays so divergent, as if they came from a distance of ten inches in front of the lens. (2) If the object is brought closer to the lens, so that the rays emanating from it will diverge, they will be rendered still more divergent by the

Fig. 198.

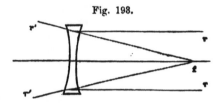

concave lens, and their focus will lie closer to the lens than its principal imaginary focus.

We have now to consider the manner in which the eye receives upon the retina a clear and sharply defined image of an object placed in front of it.

We may regard the eye as a camera-obscura, upon the screen (retina) of which is formed a diminished and inverted image of the object. The impression of the object will be formed upon the bacillar layer (rods and cones) of the retina, be conveyed thence through the fibres of the optic nerve to the brain, be there received, and then projected back again in an inverted direction outwards to the object. The most sensitive portion of the retina being situated at the yellow spot, this point is always directed towards any object at which we are looking. The sensibility of the retina, which diminishes rapidly from the yellow spot towards the periphery, may be excited by the undulations of rays of light, or by mechanical means. The former excitation occurs when rays, emanating from a luminous object, impinge upon the retina; the latter, when the eyeball is slightly pressed by the point of the finger, which will produce the appearance of luminous rings (phosphenes) situated apparently in a direction opposite to that of the pressure. Thus, if the outer portion of the sclerotic be pressed upon, the luminous rings will appear at the nasal side, and *vice versâ*.

The refractive power of the normal, emmetropic eye is such, that rays which emanate from a distant object and impinge in a parallel direction upon the cornea are brought to an exact focus upon the retina, and the eye receives a distinct image of such an object. [In this state there is total relaxation of the accommodation, the eye being adjusted for far distant objects.—B.] The dioptric system of the eye which causes this refraction of the rays of light, consists of certain media, which, taken conjointly, act as a biconvex lens. These refractive media are the cornea, aqueous humor, crystalline lens, and vitreous humor. On account of the slight thickness of the cornea, the parallelism of its two surfaces, and the fact that the refracting power of the cornea and aqueous humor are nearly equal, we may assume that the two form only one refracting surface. The index of the refraction of the vitreous humor is almost the same as that of the aqueous. But the refraction of the cornea and of the aqueous and vitreous humors would not suffice to bring parallel rays to a focus upon the retina in an emmetropic eye, for the focus would lie considerably behind it, and the lens is required to render the rays sufficiently convergent. The axis of the dioptric system is called the *optic axis*, the anterior extremity of which corresponds to the centre or apex of the cornea, and the posterior extremity to a point situated between the yellow spot and the entrance of the optic nerve. By the term *visual line*, is meant the line of direction drawn straight from the object (through the nodal point) to its image formed at the yellow spot. It was formerly supposed that the optic axis and visual line were identical, but this is not so, for according to Helmholtz,[1] the visual line outside the eye lies somewhat above and to the inner side of the optic axis, and its posterior extremity on the retina consequently lies a little to the outer and lower side of the axis. This fact will be found of practical importance with regard to the question of real and apparent strabismus.

If we now apply to the eye the principles laid down above as to the properties of biconvex lenses, we can easily understand the mode in which the reverse image of an object is formed upon the retina. Thus, if A B C (Fig. 194) be an object placed at the proper distance from the eye, a distinct inverted image of it will be formed upon the retina at a b c. Let B b be the

Fig. 194.

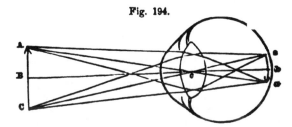

axial ray passing through the nodal point to the retina. Through this nodal point draw a straight line from A to a. This line A a will be a secondary optic axis, and all the rays emanating from A will be focussed upon the retina at a. The straight line C c, passing through the nodal point, will be another secondary optic axis, and all the rays from C will be united upon the retina at c. Hence a b c will be the inverted diminished image of A B C.

Now the question, whether or not the rays from the object will be brought to a focus upon the retina, and the latter thus receive a clearly defined image, will depend upon the situation of the object, and the distance for which the dioptric system of the eye is accommodated. The same principles as were laid down with respect to biconvex lenses apply to this case. Thus, if an eye is adjusted for parallel rays, these will be brought to a focus upon the retina. If the object is now brought nearer to the eye, so that its rays become divergent, they will no longer be united upon the retina, but behind it. The eye will consequently not receive a clearly defined image, but the latter will be blurred and indistinct, on account of the "circles of diffusion" formed upon the retina. As the focus of the rays lies behind the retina, each luminous point from the object is no longer presented by a point upon the retina, but by a circle (the section of each conical pencil of rays), and as these circles o e lap each other, the image is rendered in istinct. These are called "circles of diffusion," and take the form of the pupil, consequently their size diminishes with that of the pupil, and *vice versâ*.

For the more exact calculation of the passage of rays of light through the eye, Listing constructed a diagrammatic eye (Fig. 195) having six cardinal points, corresponding to those of optical lenses and situated on the optic axis.

---

[1] Helmholtz' "Handbuch der Physiologischen Optik," p. 70.

1. The focus F (Fig. 195) situated upon the retina, in which rays falling parallel upon the cornea would be united ; 2. The anterior focus F', at which rays coming from the retina, and whose course is parallel in the vitreous humor, would be brought to a focus; 3. The two "principal points" $H H'$, which lie on the optic axis in the anterior chamber close behind the cornea (in Fig. 195 these two points lie somewhat too far from the cornea); 4. The

Fig. 195.

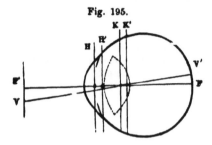

two "nodal points" $K K'$, in which the lines of direction cut each other, and which lie near the posterior surface of the lens.

On account of the extremely small distance (less than a quarter of a millimetre) between the two principal points and the two nodal points, this diagrammatic eye may be simplified, and these four cardinal points be reduced to two, viz., a principal point situated in the anterior chamber, and a nodal point, situated somewhat in front of the posterior surface of the lens. The two focal points remain the same. For the method of calculating the course of the rays of light, according to the cardinal points, I must refer the reader to Helmholtz, "Handbuch der Physiologischen Optik," and Donders' work on the "Anomalies of Accommodation and Refraction."

A glance at Fig. 195 will also explain the relative positions of the optic axis ($F F'$) and of the visual line ($V V'$). The latter is an imaginary line drawn from the yellow spot to the object point. They were formerly supposed to be identical, but Helmholtz has found that this is not the case, but that in front of the eye the visual line lies inwards and generally somewhat upwards of the optic axis, its posterior (retinal) extremity consequently lying to the outer side of the optic axis and slightly below it. Thus in Fig. 195 (which represents a horizontal section of the diagrammatic eye, the upper side of the figure being the temporal, the lower the nasal side) $V V'$ is the visual line, and $F F'$ the optic axis. At the cornea, the former lies to the inner side; at the retina, to the outer side of the optic axis. At the nodal point K they cross each other.

In the normal or emmetropic eye, the visual line impinges upon the cornea slightly to the inner side of the optic axis, forming with it an angle of about 5°. But Donders has shown that in the hypermetropic eye it lies still more to the inner side, so as to form an angle of 8° or 9°, whereas in myopia the visual line may correspond to the optic axis, or even lie to the outer side of it. These differences in the relation between the optic axis and visual line often give rise to an apparent strabismus.

The Visual Angle.—The apparent size of an object depends upon the size of its retinal image. If, for instance, the eye is adjusted for the object $A B$ (Fig. 196) and the lines of direction, $A A'$ and $B B'$, are drawn through the nodal point k, the angle $A k B$ will be the visual angle under which the object is seen, and this angle will equal the angle $A' k B'$. The visual angle stands in direct relation to the size of the object, for the larger the latter is, the greater will be the visual angle and consequently the image, and vice versâ. Moreover, the visual angle will also increase in size according to the proximity of the object, and diminished as the latter is further removed from the eye. If, however, the size of the object increases in due proportion with its distance, it will be seen under the same visual angle. Thus $A B$ (Fig. 196) and $a\, b$ are seen under the same visual angle, although the former is considerably further from the eye than $a\, b$. From this it will be easily understood, that the mere fact of a patient being able to read the

Fig. 196.

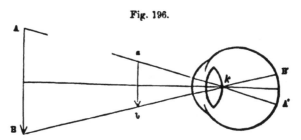

smallest print does not exclude a certain degree of amblyopia. In deciding upon this point, we must always take into consideration the distance at which he can read it, and the state of refraction and accommodation.

The smallest visual angle under which an object can be distinctly seen by the eye is one of five minutes. Hence this has been taken as the standard for determining the acuteness of vision, and the test-types of Snellen and Giraud Teulon have been devised upon this principle, as has been already stated (p. 37), each type being seen under an angle of five minutes at the distance in feet corresponding to its number. Thus No. 1 is seen at an angle of five minutes at one foot, No. 2 at two feet, etc.

We have now to turn our attention to the consideration of the subject of refraction and accommodation.

By the term "accommodation" is meant the power which every normal eye possesses of adjusting itself almost imperceptibly and unconsciously for different distances; at one moment, looking at something but a few inches from the eye; at the next, regarding some far distant object, or taking in at a glance the vast expanse of miles of scenery. [The limits of the accommodation are the far and the near points. The far point depends for its position on the refraction of the eye, and the near point depends upon the accommodation.—B.]

In a normal eye the whole apparatus of accommodation is so beautifully balanced, nad its functions are performed with such ease and accuracy, that, although in reality a voluntary act, its duties are from early childhood fulfilled intuitively, unconsciously. No wonder, then, that this power of adjustment of the eye to different distances has been a favorite study with some of the most eminent physiologists and natural philosophers.

That such a power is essentially necessary will become at once apparent by a consideration of the following fact, and a glance at Fig. 197.

It has been already stated that the emmetropic eye in a state of rest is adjusted for parallel rays $a\, a$ (Fig. 197), so that these are brought to a focus upon the retina b, without any effort of the accommodation. But if the object is now brought to *c* (twelve inches[1] from the eye), the rays will be very divergent, and will be focussed behind the retina at *d*, unless the eye can increase its power of refraction sufficiently to unite them upon the retina. If not, circles of diffusion will be formed upon the latter, and the object consequently appear blurred and indistinct. If the accommodation of the eye

Fig. 197.

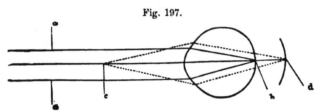

is paralyzed, rays from the object *c*, twelve inches in front of the eye, would be brought to a focus upon the retina by the aid of a biconvex lens of twelve inches focus, which would render the rays parallel and thus enable the eye to focus them upon the retina.

It is very necessary to carefully distinguish between the meaning of the terms refraction and accommodation, as they signify two perfectly different things. By refraction, is understood the passive power which every eye possesses, when in a state of rest—*i. e.*, adjusted for its far point—of bringing certain rays to a focus upon the retina without any active effort or participation of the muscular apparatus of accommodation. This power of refraction is due to the form of the eye and to its different refracting media.

We have just seen (Fig. 197) that the state of refraction of the normal eye is such that, when it is in a state of rest, parallel rays are brought to a focus upon the retina without any effort of the accommodation. Its furthest point of distinct vision lies at an infinite distance. Donders terms this condition emmetropia. He says,[2] " the refraction of the media of the eye at rest can be called normal in reference to the situation of the retina, only when the parallel incidcn: rays unite on the layer of rods and bulbs. Then, in fact, the limit lies precisely at the measure; then there exists emmetropia (from ἐμμετρος, modum tenens, and ὠψ, oculus). Such an eye we term emmetropic.   •

" This name expresses perfectly what we mean. The eye cannot be called a *normal* eye, for it may very easily be abnormal or morbid, and nevertheless it may be emmetropic. Neither is the expression *normally constructed eye* quite correct, for the structure of an emmetropic eye may, in many respects, be abnormal, and emmetropia may exist with difference of structure. Here the word emmetropia appears alone to express with precision and accuracy the condition alluded to."

The state of refraction may deviate in two ways from the emmetropic condition.

1. The principal focus of the eye, when adjusted for its far point, lies in front of the retina (Fig. 198), so that parallel rays are not brought to a focus upon the later, but in front of it at *f*, and circles of diffusion, *b b*, will be

---

I may remind the reader of the signification of the following symbols *A*, means range of accommodation; *r*, far point; *p*, near point; *x* (= 0), infinite distance; *'*, foot; *''*, inch; *'''*, line.

[2] Donders, " On the Anomalies of Accommodation and Refraction of the Eye," p. 81, " New Sydenham Society," 1864.

ved by a case of Von Graefe's, in which all the recti and obliqui
both eyes were paralyzed, so that the eyeballs were completely
and yet the power of accommodation was perfect.

length, however, been definitely settled, chiefly by the experi-
ramer and Helmholtz (conducted independently of each other),
essary change in the refraction of the eye during accommodation
alteration in the form of the crystalline lens. Helmholtz found,
f his ophthalmometer, that the lens did not change its position
ommodation for near objects, but this was brought about by a
he curvature of the anterior and posterior surfaces of the lens,
ne more convex (the lens itself thicker from before backwards),
lens acquires a higher power of refraction, and consequently a
istance, by which means rays from even very near objects are
a focus upon the retina. He found, with the ophthalmometer,
undergoes the following changes during accommodation for near

upil diminishes in size. 2. The pupillary edge of the iris moves
3. The peripheral portion of the iris moves backwards. 4. The
rface of the lens becomes more convex (arched), and its vertex
ards. 5. The posterior surface of the lens also becomes slightly
1, but does not perceptibly change its position. The lens, there-
es thicker in the centre.[1]
olume of the lens must remain the same, he thinks that we may,
ssume that the transverse diameter of the lens becomes diminished.
om calculation, that these changes in the lens are quite sufficient
mmodative purposes.[2]
illustrates the changes which the eye undergoes during accom-

Becker has found that in albinotic eyes the space between the ciliary pro-
e edge of the lens becomes increased in size during accommodation for
He thinks it probable that the volume of the ciliary processes varies in
onditions of the accommodation, and supposes that this is due to the differ-
lood-supply to the iris, which, he thinks, varies with the dilatation and
f the pupil.
s made numerous experiments and observations as to the accommodation,
r this purpose the eyes of persons upon whom iridectomy had been per-
found that the ciliary processes move forward and become somewhat
g accommodation for near objects; and that after the instillation of atropine
emarkably retracted; whereas, after the use of the Calabar bean they move
le his "Mechanism der Accommodation des Menschlichen Auges,"
). In the experiments as to the mechanism of the accommodation, which
r Hensen and Völckers upon dogs, it was found that during the action of
uscle, the choroid and retina are shifted forward. This fact would explain
e of the accommodative phosphenes of Czermak, and is moreover, as they
great practical interest and importance in diseases of these tissues. For if
sannot be immaterial in affections of the choroid and retina, whether the
on is employed or not, and the beneficial effect of atropine in such diseases
r be due to its paralyzing the power of accommodation, and thus obviating
t of the choroid and retina. The experiments of these observers lead them,
s, to agree with Helmholtz's theory of accommodation. (Hensen and
xperimental-Untersuchung über den Mechanism der Accommodation."

und, with the ophthalmometer, that the position of the reflection images
produced by the cornea and the anterior and posterior surfaces of the lens,
uange during accommodation for near objects. While the reflex image
es remains unchanged, that from the anterior surface of the lens approaches
mage and diminishes in size; the image from the posterior surface of
diminishes very slightly in size, but undergoes no appreciable change of

modation. The anterior portion of the eye is divided into two equal parts. The one half, F, shows the position of the parts when the eye is adjusted for distance, the other, N, when it is accommodated for near objects. When the eye is in a state of rest, the iris forms a curve (a) in the vicinity of Schlemm's

Fig. 200.

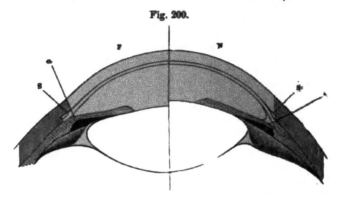

canal (s); but when accommodated for near objects, the fibres of the iris suffer contraction, the periphery of the iris becomes straightened (b), and the anterior chamber lengthened, so that its diminution in depth is compensated for by the advance of the anterior surface of the lens.

The question now arises, in what manner is this change in the form of the lens produced? There can be no doubt now that it is entirely due to the action of the ciliary muscle. Cramer, Donders, Helmholtz, Müller, as well as many other observers, considered that whilst the ciliary muscle played the most important part in the mechanism of the accommodation, it was materially assisted by the iris. Indeed, it was impossible to determine with accuracy, even after the most careful dissections and most elaborate investigations, the relative amount of importance of the iris and ciliary muscle. This question has now, however, been definitely set at rest by a case which occurred in Von Graefe's clinique, in which, together with a total absence of the iris (the latter was removed after an accident) the power of accommodation remained perfect. Moreover, on the application of a strong solution of atropine it became completely paralyzed.

[The process of accommodation is as follows: The lens, being elastic, tends to approach a spherical shape. The zonula, or suspensory ligament, which is attached to the ciliary processes and to the equator of the lens, is also elastic, and when the ciliary muscle is at rest, it is kept on the stretch, and the lens is thus flattened. When the ciliary muscle contracts, the zonula is at once relaxed, the lens is released, and assumes a greater convexity by reason of its own elasticity. It is probable that both the radiating and circular fibres of the ciliary muscle act simultaneously to relax the zonula.

Emmert holds that, owing to the intimate connection existing between the ciliary processes and the zonule of Zinn, the latter is always on the stretch, and never relaxed. The older the eye, the more does the anterior part of the ciliary processes seem to project beyond the ciliary body toward the lens. Assuming that the condition of rest of the ciliary muscle is when we look into distance, and the condition of activity is when we look at near objects, it is also deemed just to assume that for near vision the radial and meridional fibres assist the circular fibres, and that therefore the entire ciliary body approximates the edge of the lens. But Emmert holds that the lines of direction or diagonals of the various groups of fibres of the ciliary muscle never coincide with the line of direction of the resultant force. Actual observation shows that the ring muscle tends to draw the ciliary body, with its processes, towards the lens; while the radial muscle tends to draw it in the direction of its tendon towards the apex of the cornea. It is therefore scarcely intelligible that they tend simultaneously to effect the same purpose; and the simultaneous activity of the various groups of muscular fibres cannot, therefore, from a mechanical standpoint, be defended. With this conception of the existing relations, it will be conceded that contraction of the ring muscle, with simultaneous relaxation of the radial muscle, is necessary for near vision; and contraction of the radial muscle, with simultaneous relaxation of the ring muscle, is necessary for distant vision. It is also probable that the oculomotorius must be regarded as the motor nerve of the ring muscle, and the sympathetic as the motor nerve of the radial muscle. This anatomical explanation applies as well for myopic and hypermetropic eyes as for emmetropic eyes. It is also probable that the meridional fibres perform a similar function to that of the radiating fibres. Emmert's first conclusion is that irritation of the ciliary nerves causes an artificial accommodation, and that the choroid is drawn forward by the contraction of the ciliary muscle. (See "Archiv für Augenheilkunde," x. 4.)—B.]

2.—NEGATIVE ACCOMMODATION.

Some ophthalmologists of eminence, more especially Von Graefe and Weber, have thought that when the emmetropic eye is in a state of rest, it is not quite adjusted for its furthest point of distinct vision, but can become so by a slight alteration in its accommodation, which may be called the *negative* accommodation, in contradistinction to the *positive*, which enables it to adjust itself for near objects. Von Graefe has thought that, by the aid chiefly of the external muscles of the eyeball which exert a slight pressure upon the eye, and thus somewhat flatten the cornea, the refraction of the eye is slightly diminished, and the far point removed still further from the eye, than when the eye is in a state of absolute rest. Coccius likewise believes that the action of the external muscles of the eye, as well as the increased intra-ocular tension, may somewhat flatten the lens, and thus produce a certain amount of negative accommodation. Henke,[1] however, thinks that both the positive and the negative accommodation are produced by the action of the ciliary muscle; the former being due to the action of its circular fibres, the latter to that of its radial fibres.

The chief argument against the theory that the eye accommodates itself actively for distant objects is furnished by the action of a strong solution of atropine, which completely paralyzes the power of accommodation, but does not interfere with the distant vision of an emmetropic eye, and does not change the position of its far point.

[This is not, strictly speaking, correct, for, according to more recent and accurate investigations, atropia will produce a diminution of refraction varying from one-eightieth to one-fiftieth.—B.]

[1] "A. f. O.," vi. 2, 53.

od method for testing the range of accom-
ring whether the eye is emmetropic, myopic,

ten inches focus is placed before the eye.[1]
No. 1 of Snellen, and his far and near point
point (p') thus found, stand in such relation
(p), that the rays coming from r' are re-
ıe from r, those from p' being also refracted
ith convex six, r' (in the emmetropic eye)
r rays from an object at six inches distance
:endered parallel by it, and would, conse-
ı if they came from an infinite distance (the
oint (p') would lie at about two and two-
ver, with the age of the patient.
is, therefore, easily found by the formula

distance from the eye (about one-half inch)

point (r') lies at six inches, the near point

$$. \frac{1}{6} = \frac{1}{6}.$$

ıg by the following examples:
with convex six, $r' = 5''$, $p' = 3''$. The eye
not adjusted for the normal far point (six
e rays from which impinge in a divergent

$$. -\frac{1}{5} = \frac{1}{7\frac{1}{2}}.$$

ient require for infinite distance? By means
ıe changed this eye into a very myopic one,
ve should have to place a concave glass of
x, in order to enable it to see at a distance;
.er parallel rays as divergent as if they came
·der to find the proper concave glass for dis-
ım convex six. Hence the proper glass will

$$= \frac{1}{30}.$$

convex six, $r' = 8$, $p' = 3''$. The eye is,
far point lies beyond the normal far point

$$= \frac{1}{4\frac{1}{5}}, \text{ for } \frac{1}{A} = \frac{1}{3} - \frac{1}{8} = \frac{1}{4\frac{1}{5}}.$$

f the *absolute* range of accommodation which
eparately. Donders[2] has, however, pointed
other kinds of ranges, viz., the *binocular* and
the accommodation from the furthest point

ler that the patient may really command his far
pproximated so much that the minimum of the
ı any influence, and amblyopia is therefore ex-

ıs, with explanatory diagrams of this subject, will

r_2 to the nearest point p_2 when both eyes are tried together. The formula is:

$$\frac{1}{A_2} = \frac{1}{P_2} - \frac{1}{R_2}.$$

Although a certain connection exists between the accommodation and the convergence of the visual lines, yet this connection is not absolute and definite, for we find that the position of the visual lines may be changed, yet the accommodation remain the same; for if a prism of moderate strength be placed with its base outwards before one eye, the convergence of the visual lines will be greatly increased to overcome the diplopia, and yet the object can be distinctly seen at the same distance with both eyes. Again, the accommodation may be altered, and yet the state of convergence remain the same, for if we place weak concave or convex lenses before the eyes, an object can still be distinctly seen at a definite distance. This proves that the accommodation may be modified without any change of the convergence of the visual lines. These experiments show that there exists a certain independence between the convergence and the accommodation, and the range of accommodation over which we have control at a given convergence of the visual lines is termed the *relative* range, and is found by the formula $\frac{1}{A_1} = \frac{1}{P_1} - \frac{1}{R_1}.$ It consists, moreover, of two parts, the *positive* and the *negative*, the positive being the part which is disposable for a distance closer than the point of convergence, whereas the negative is the portion which is required to see an object lying beyond the point of convergence of the visual lines. Now the relation between these two parts of the relative range of accommodation is of much practical importance, for it is found that in order that the eyes may be employed comfortably for some length of time at near objects (reading, etc.), it is absolutely necessary that the positive part of the accommodation should bear a certain proportion to the negative (it should at the very least be equal to one-half).

The best objects for testing the range of accommodation are Snellen's test-types, or Von Graefe's wire optometer. But as the latter requires some exactitude and intelligence on the part of the patient, I find it more practical, especially with hospital patients, to use the test-types. If, whilst they are reading No. 1, we move the type a few times alternately nearer to and further from the eye, the nearest and furthest point of distinct vision can be readily ascertained. Von Graefe's optometer consists of a small square steel frame, across which a number of delicate parallel, vertical wires are stretched. This frame may be attached to a brass rod (graduated in inches and feet) upon which it is movable; or it may be fastened to a graduated tape. One end of the rod, or the bobbin of the tape, is placed against the forehead of the patient, and the frame moved to the nearest point at which the individual wires still look clearly and sharply defined; the distance of this point from the eye is read off from the graduated scale, and put down as the near point (p). The frame is then removed to the greatest distance at which the individual wires still appear sharply defined, and this is noted as the far point (r). The distance between p and r gives the range of accommodation. The wires only appear sharply defined when the eye accommodates itself perfectly for them; directly there is the slightest deviation from this perfect accommodation (the frame being too far from or too near to the eye), the wires seem indistinct, thickened, or as if surrounded by a halo; or colored double images of them may even appear in the transparent intervals. With the test-types the examination is still easier, the nearest point at which No. 1 (Snellen) can be distinctly and comfortably read is measured and noted as the near point, and then the furthest point (in an emmetropic eye No. 1 of Snellen should be read up to one foot, No. **xx** up to twenty feet) is measured and noted.

4.—MYOPIA.

It has been already shown that in myopia, parallel rays (emanating from an object at an infinite distance) are brought to a focus in front of the retina, and that only sufficiently divergent rays are united upon the latter. This is either due to the antero-posterior axis of the eyeball being too long, or to the refracting power of the eye being too high. In order somewhat to improve their sight for distant objects, short-sighted persons nip their eyelids slightly together. They in this way diminish the size of the circles of diffusion by narrowing the palpebral aperture, and also render the eye slightly less myopic by the pressure which is thus exerted upon the eyeball.

The anterior chamber is generally somewhat deeper, and the pupil somewhat larger in the myopic than in the emmetropic eye. If the myopia is considerable in degree, the eyeball appears abnormally large and prominent, the lids are widely apart, and the lateral movements of the eye somewhat curtailed. The increase in the length of the eyeball, and the sub-ovoid shape of its posterior portion can be easily recognized when the eye is turned far inwards towards the nose, the little hollow which exists in the emmetropic eye between the outer canthus and the globe having disappeared.

Myopia is frequently congenital, and often hereditary, and its existence may also be sometimes traced back through several generations, increasing perhaps somewhat in degree in each successive generation. It may also occur in several members of the same family.

The most frequent cause of myopia is an abnormal increase in the length of the eyeball in its antero-posterior axis. This extension occurs chiefly at the posterior portion of the globe, and may give rise to a more or less considerable ovoid bulging (posterior staphyloma), which is accompanied by thinning and atrophy of the choroid and sclerotic (*vide* the article on "Sclerectasia Posterior," p. 354). But even if this should not be present, the ophthalmoscope often reveals a hyperæmic and congested condition of the optic nerve and retina, especially if the eyes have been much overworked by artificial light.

It is also supposed by some, that long-continued work at near objects may produce myopia. For persons thus employed, continually accommodate for a very near point, their crystalline lens has, therefore, constantly to assume a more convex form, and, after a time, it may not be able quite to regain its original form, even when the necessity for adjusting itself for near objects no longer exists. The eye has in fact become somewhat myopic.

The production and increase of myopia by continuous use of the eyes at near objects, appear to find their explanation chiefly in the fact that the inner tunics of the eyeball become congested. The near approach of the object necessitates a strong convergence of the visual lines, which causes an accumulation of blood in, and congestion of, the inner tunics of the eyeball, these conditions being increased still more by the stooping position generally indulged in during such employment. We can easily understand that this congestion and augmentation in the pressure of the ocular fluids must, if long continued, necessarily lead to an extension of the tunics at the posterior pole, and thus give rise to sclerectasia posterior.

If the distention of the sclera is once established, it is easily intelligible how this may be increased by intra-ocular hyperæmia and a state of irritation.

Though in the majority of cases the primary cause of the myopia lies in a congenital weakness of the posterior part of the sclera, yet it may certainly be acquired. Myopia is often developed in children after measles or scarlet fever.—B.]

The seeds of short-sightedness are frequently sown in childhood, either through a premature over-exertion of the eyes at near objects, or through some affection of the refractive media (the cornea or lens). The cornea may, for instance, be clouded, and then the patient often brings the object very close to the eye, in order to obtain larger and more distinct retinal images, and thus myopia may be soon induced. The same thing may occur when the lens is somewhat opaque; thus it is well known that lamellar cataract frequently becomes complicated with short sight.

There can be no doubt that the degree of myopia is often greatly increased during childhood by long-continued study, more especially by insufficient illumination and a faulty construction of the tables or desks at which the pupils read and write. An insufficient illumination necessitates a close approximation of the object, which gives rise to straining of the accommodation and congestion of the eyes. A faulty construction of the tables, or of the distance between the latter and the seats, is also injurious by forcing the children to stoop. An interesting and valuable monograph has been written by Dr. Cohn[1] upon this subject. He examined the eyes of ten thousand and sixty school children, and could distinctly trace the increase in the proportion of the myopia according to the construction of the desks and the lighting of the school-rooms. But the valuable and interesting researches of Dobrowolsky[2] have shown that the rapid increase of myopia is often due to spasm of the ciliary muscle which gives rise to marked symptoms of asthenopia. Amongst the most prominent symptoms are: difficulty to continue work at near objects for any length of time, photophobia, lachrymation, pain in and around the eye, flushing of the eyeball, a contracted pupil, hyperæmia of the optic disk and fulness of the retinal vessels, and especially marked fluctuations in the state of refraction at different times of examination. This spasm of the ciliary muscle occurs much more frequently in the lower and medium degrees of myopia than in the higher, and more especially in young persons much engaged in reading, sewing, or other fine work. We must not, however, confound this condition with the apparent myopia occasionally observed in hypermetropic individuals which is entirely due to spasm of the ciliary muscle. The treatment must consist chiefly in paralysing the ciliary muscle by the methodical use of atropine, either applied in substance or in a strong solution (gr. iv ad f ʒj) two or three times daily, to be continued until the accommodation is quite relaxed and the muscle completely paralysed, or even somewhat longer. Sometimes the spasm yields in a few hours, in other cases not for several days. If the symptoms of hyperæmia of the fundus do not yield, and the myopia does not diminish after the atropine has been employed for several days, the artificial leech should be employed. The relaxation of the ciliary muscle generally produces a marked diminution in the degree of myopia.

[Dr. Just, of Zittau, has made a careful examination of the eyes of twelve hundred and twenty-nine scholars in the two high schools of Zittau, in which

---

[1] Dr. Cohn, " Untersuchung der Augen von zehn Tousend und sechzig Schulkindern." Leipsic, 1867. Vide also a paper by Dr. Erismann, "A. f. O," xvii. i. 1.

[2] " Kl. Monatsbl.," 1868; vide also more recent papers on the same subject by Dr Hosch, Basel, 1871, and Professor Schiess-Gemuseus, Basel, 1872.

of which the hygienic conditions of light, space, and arrangement of furniture leave nothing to be desired. He found that myopia was as frequent in the new schools of Zittau, as in other educational institutions of the same kind, and, hence, he concludes that it does not chiefly result from insufficient illumination of the school-rooms, but rather from the great and ever increasing demands on the industry of the pupils at home, forcing prolonged labor on their eyes during the evening hours, frequently by insufficient artificial light. (See "Arch. of Ophthal.," x. 1.)

The investigation into the condition of the eyes of the public-school children of Philadelphia, by Dr. Risley and his associates, has been very thorough. Dr. Risley found that myopia, commencing in the primary classes with a low percentage, steadily increases as the pupils pass to the highest grade in our public-school system; the percentage of increase is very much lower in the schools of Philadelphia than in the schools of Europe; the myopic eye presents a higher percentage of disease than eyes with emmetropic or hypermetropic refraction; and the percentage of disease is much higher when astigmatism is also present. The increase in myopia, is from eyes with already existing anomalies of refraction. While there is an evident and close relation between the increase of myopia and school-life, nevertheless the educational methods are responsible to only a limited degree. (See "Phil. Med. Times," July 30, 1881.)—B.]

It was formerly supposed that increased convexity of the cornea was the cause of myopia, but this is erroneous, for Donders has found that the cornea is, as a rule, less convex in myopic persons than the emmetropic. Increase of the curvature of the cornea (as in conical cornea) may, however give rise to myopia. We sometimes also find that persons suffering from incipient cataract become somewhat myopic, and see better at a distance with concave glasses. The real explanation of this fact is still uncertain, but it may perhaps be due to a slight swelling (?) of the lens, and a consequent increase in its power of refraction.

The diagnosis of myopia is generally a matter of no difficulty. The far point of distinct vision is more or less approximated to the eye, in consequence of which distant objects cannot be clearly distinguished, and a suitable concave lens is required to render them distinctly perceptible. We must be on our guard, however, not at once to pronounce a person short-sighted because he holds small objects (such as small print) very close to the eye, or because he cannot see well at a distance, for we shall hereafter point out that this may also occur in hypermetropia, in which case convex and not concave glasses are required to remedy this defect.

Together with the myopia, there is frequently present more or less amblyopia or weakness of sight. This is especially the case if there is a considerable degree of sclerotico-choroiditis posterior, and appears to be chiefly due to the stretching of the inner tunics of the eye, more especially of the light-conducting elements of the retina. The impairment of sight may also be due to opacities in the vitreous humor or the lens. Myopic eyes are often very irritable, so that prolonged use in reading or writing causes them to become red, hot, and very painful. This may be partly due to irritability and congestion of the inner tunics, or it may be caused by a weakness of the internal recti muscles, which are not sufficiently strong to maintain the requisite degree of conve g nce. If this insufficiency is developed to a considerable degree, it gives rise to marked symptoms of asthenopia and fatigue of the eyes (vide the article on "Muscular Asthenopia"). We may easily distinguish simple myopia from that complicated with amblyopia, by the fact that the former can be completely corrected by suitable concave

with the mirror, without any convex lens before it), we are at once struck by the fact, that we can see the details of the fundus at some distance from the eye. If we regard one of the retinal vessels or the optic disk, and move our head slightly to one side, we notice that the image moves *in the contrary direction;* if we move to the right, it moves to the left, and *vice versâ,* so that we obtain a reverse image of the background of the eye.

Fig. 201 will at once explain the reason of this. Let *a* be a very short-sighted eye ($m=\frac{1}{2}$), and *b* the eye of the observer; *a* being in a state of rest is adjusted for its far point (*c*), which lies four inches in front of the eye. The rays from the fundus, therefore, pass out of the eye in a strongly convergent direction upon the eye of the observer. If the latter be myopic (accommodated for divergent rays when his eye is in a state of rest), they may be united upon his retina (*b*) without the aid of any correcting lens behind the ophthalmoscope. But if his eye is emmetropic he will, if adjusted for his far point, require a suitable convex lens behind the mirror, in order to render the divergent rays parallel. If he, however, accommodates himself for a sufficiently near point, he will be able to unite the divergent rays upon his retina without any correcting lens. The reversed image of the eye represented in Fig. 201 (the myopia of which $=\frac{1}{2}$) will be seen at a distance of

Fig. 201.

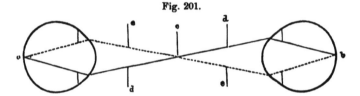

about seven to eight inches, because as the rays from it cross at *c*, the upper ray *e*, becomes the lower ray after they have crossed, and the lower ray *d*, becomes the upper.

II. In order to examine a myopic eye in the erect image, it will be necessary to place a suitable concave lens behind the mirror, so as to obtain a distinct image of the fundus; the greater the myopia the stronger must this concave glass be, and the nearer must the observer approach to the eye. The strength of this correcting concave lens will also enable us approximately to estimate the degree of the myopia,[1] which will be always somewhat less than the strength of the correcting lens. For instance, let us suppose that the eye of the observer is emmetropic, and not using its power of accommodation, and the patient's myopia $=\frac{1}{6}$ (*i. e.,* the rays emanating from a luminous point in the fundus will be brought to a focus six inches in front of its nodal point). Now if the examining eye is placed two inches in front of the optic centre of the patient's eye, the rays from the latter would impinge in so divergent a direction upon the eye of the observer, that they would be brought to a focus four inches behind it, and a concave glass of four inches focus would unite them upon his retina. Hence, if we add the distance between

---

[1] For a very full and valuable explanation of the determination of the state of refraction by the aid of the ophthalmoscope, I must refer the reader to Mauthner's ' Lehrbuch der Ophthalmoscopie." [And to an article by Dr. Edward G. Loring in the "Am. Journ. Med. Sci.," April, 1870, p. 323.—H.] [See also Snellen and Landolt's article "Ophthalmoscopie," in Graefe und Saemisch's " Hdb. der Augenheilk.," iii. S. 98–173, and the most admirably clear and concise monograph of Dr E. G. Loring, "The Determination of the Refraction of the Eye with the Ophthalmoscope," New York, 1876.—B.]

the optic centres of the observer's and patient's eyes (two inches) to the focal length of the correcting lens (four inches), we obtain the degree of myopia, viz., ¼.

["If the observer is a myope with relaxed accommodation, his myopia must be corrected by a concave glass before he can see the fundus of an emmetropic eye distinctly. If he cannot relax his accommodation, he is so much the more myopic for near vision, and this must also be accounted for in determining the result. If the eye examined is myopic, the degree of his own myopia must be subtracted from the glass which renders the fundus of the examined eye distinct, and the distance of the nodal point must also be taken into consideration." (Loring, "The Determination of the Refraction of the Eye with the Ophthalmoscope," 1876.—B.]

The field of vision will appear smaller, and the image nearer the eye of the observer than in the emmetropic eye. The image is also less bright in color and less illuminated, but apparently larger, for we cannot, as in the emmetropic eye (the size of the pupil being equal), overlook the whole expanse of the optic disk at a glance, but only a portion of it. In the indirect mode of examination, the image of the disk will be less than that of the emmetropic eye, on account of its being formed nearer to the object lens.

["For an emmetropic observer whose eye is at rest, the myopia in a given case will equal the weakest concave glass through which the fundus is seen distinctly, plus the distance of the glass from the nodal point of the observed eye." (Loring, loc. cit., p. 23.)

Weiss describes a new ophthalmoscopic symptom in myopic eyes, in the form of a curved white streak or line, situated at a varying distance in front of the plane of the retina, and veiling the retinal vessels in both the upright and the inverted image. This streak seems to surround the inner margin of the papilla, and the ends are somewhat removed from the border of the papilla. The greater the degree of the myopia, the further appears the streak from the margin of the papilla, and the further in front of the retinal plane does it seem to lie. Weiss thinks that it is connected with the changes which the vitreous and its central canal undergo in myopic eyes, under the form of detachment of the vitreous. It is possible that this change consists in the membrane which lines the central canal being torn away from its attachment to the hyaloid membrane, and becoming folded. The appearance of the streak on the inner side of the papilla only, is explained by the wall of the central canal at the funnel-shaped dilatation having a different inclination on this side, from the one it has on the outer side. (See "Med.-Chir. Centralblatt," Nov. 12 and 19, 1880.)—B.]

Myopia may run a very variable course. In some cases its progress is marked and rapid, in others slow and insidious; in the most favorable cases it remains stationary at the adult age. It is generally, however, somewhat progressive, especially between the ages of fifteen and twenty-five, and often remarkably so in hereditary myopia, or if the patients employ their eyes a great deal in reading, sewing, etc. A moderate degree of stationary or but slowly progressive myopia causes but little annoyance to the patient; but it is very different if its degree is very considerable and its progress marked and rapid, for in the latter case it is almost always accompanied by symptoms of irritation and inflammation of the inner tunics of the eyeball, giving rise to redness, heat, and ciliary neuralgia during prolonged work at near objects.

It is of consequence, both in the prognosis and treatment of myopia, carefully to watch its progress, and accurately to ascertain and note the degree of myopia at the commencement, so that we may hereafter be able to determine whether the disease has remained stationary or progressed, and, in the latter case, to know the extent and rate of such progress.

The popular idea that myopia diminishes with old age is not quite correct, although it is true that distant vision is somewhat improved by the diminution in the size of the pupil. Moreover, the senile changes (sclerosis) in the lens may slightly diminish the myopia.

[In speaking of progressive myopia, Javal considers that the variations of accommodation for near work, occurring in myopes, are not the cause of myopia, but rather a cause of its increase, and that it is necessary to distinguish between the production of myopia and its increase. There are certain eyes which elongate when their accommodation is called into play, and these eyes, predisposed to myopia, must be spared every effort of this kind. So far from prescribing concave glasses for reading for persons with such eyes, we should give them convex glasses. If the myopia has reached one or two dioptries, we must use glasses more or less strong, without ever going above three dioptrics. Instead of correcting the eye for infinity, correct it for a distance of twenty-five to thirty-three centimetres, by convex glasses when the myopia is not above three dioptrics, by concave glasses when it is above four or five dioptrics. (See "Annales d'oculistique," Juli–Août, 1880.)—B.]

With regard to the *prognosis* of short sight, it may be stated that there is nothing to be feared from a slight stationary myopia; but it is very different when the latter is high in degree, progressive, and associated with considerable sclerotico-choroiditis posterior, for then it is always a source of danger to the eye. There is a popular fallacy that short-sighted eyes are particularly strong, and even some medical men participate in it. But this is quite erroneous, indeed a myopic eye must be looked upon as unsound, more especially if the disease is extensive and progressive. In such cases care must, therefore, be taken that the patient avoids all employment or amusement that may hasten the progress of the myopia, or give rise to irritation and straining of the eye.

It is of much consequence in myopia that the spectacles should be selected with accuracy and care, for if they are unsuitable, more especially if they are too strong, they may prove very injurious to the eye.

The proper strength is rapidly and easily found in the following manner:

The degree of the myopia must in the first place be ascertained with exactitude by trying the furthest distance at which the patient can read No. 1. If he can do so up to ten inches from the eye, his far point (r) lies at ten inches, and his myopia = $\frac{1}{10}$; for a concave lens of ten inches focus would enable him to see at an infinite distance, as it would give to parallel rays a divergence as if they came from a point ten inches in front of the lens (the patient's far point). The position of r, therefore, always affords us a clue to the number of the concave lens required; but although No. 10 would be theoretically the proper glass, we find practically that it would be somewhat too strong. The reason of this is, that the convergence of the visual lines at ten inches prevents the eye from exactly accommodating itself for its far point, the latter being only attainable when we look at distant objects with parallel visual lines. Hence concave eleven or twelve would be the glass really suitable. Whether a given lens is accurately suited to the patient's sight, can be easily determined in the following manner: Let us return to the case above referred to of myopia = $\frac{1}{10}$. With concave ten the patient is able to read No. xx of Snellen at twenty feet, hence his V = 1. In order to determine whether No. 10 is exactly the right glass, we alternately place before it weak concave and convex glasses and try their effect. If weak concave glasses improve the sight, the original lens (No. 10) is too weak; if, on the other hand, weak convex glasses improve it, it is too strong. If neither concave nor convex glasses render any improvement, the original lens suits

exactly. The proper glass can be easily found by a very s
for if the myopia $= \frac{1}{10}$, and convex fifty improves the sig
vex forty making it worse, the original glass is somewhat t
must deduct $\frac{1}{40}$ from it. The proper glass will be $\frac{1}{12\frac{1}{2}}$, for,

We try concave thirteen and find that neither concave
render any improvement.

If the sight with the original lens ($\frac{1}{10}$) was most improve
of concave fifty, it was too weak, and a concave lens of about
will be required, for $\frac{1}{10} + \frac{1}{50} = \frac{1}{8\frac{1}{3}}$.

As a general rule, the weakest glass which neutralizes t
given.

If a myope desires to have spectacles to enable him to
about two feet (for reading music, etc.), the proper gl
found by the following calculation: If his myopia $= \frac{1}{17}$
see distinctly at twenty-four inches, the formula will be —.
and concave twenty-four will be the proper glass.

The degree of the patient's range of accommodation
the choice of spectacles, and the question as to whether
allowed their use for reading, writing, etc.

The range of accommodation may be tested in the
scribed, by finding the nearest and furthest point at whi
read with ease, and then deducting the latter from the for
the formula $\frac{1}{A} = \frac{1}{P} - \frac{1}{R}$.

The following plan, recommended by Donders, is, bowe
it allows the patient really to accommodate for his far poi
having been neutralized by the proper concave glasses, so
can read No. xx at twenty feet, the position of his near
glasses) is now found; if it lies at five inches, his range of
$= \frac{1}{5}$, for as r $= \infty$, and p 5", $\frac{1}{A} = \frac{1}{5} - \frac{1}{\infty} =$

In determining the degree of myopia, each eye should
separately, for the degree generally varies somewhat (ofter
the two eyes. The question as to what glasses should be
is any marked difference in the two eyes, either in the deg
in the refraction itself (the one eye being perhaps myopic
metropic), will be considered hereafter.

There is no harm in permitting myopic persons to wea
distance as just neutralize their myopia, especially if th
sight is but moderate. If the patient is young, the myo
range of accommodation good, he may even be permitt
glasses in reading and writing, as in such cases the myop
tendency to increase. But if the myopia is consideral
accommodation diminished, and the acuteness of vision im
should not be quite neutralized. The patient may, howeve
concave eye-glass before his spectacles when he desires to
very distinctly.[1]

[1] In very high degrees of myopia, I have found Steinheil's glass
distant objects, as it acts like a Galilean telescope. It consists of
glass, the base of which is convex, and the opposite surface concav
inch in length, and can be readily carried in the waistcoat pocket.

: purpose of reading music, I think it best to give patients spec-
ted for a distance of two or three feet, for if the myopia is consid-
d they use glasses which completely reutralize it for distance, the
e music is inconveniently diminished, and thus becomes somewhat
and difficult to decipher.

v come to the question whether myopic persons should wear glasses
;, sewing, writing, etc., and the answer to this must depend upon
rcumstances.

the myopia is but slight in degree (less than $\frac{1}{14}$), they may be dis-
th—or, if the employment is not continued for any length of time,
ce glasses may even be worn, but the type must be held at a greater
)therwise the eye becomes fatigued, and the accommodation strained.
find that it is less trying and more comfortable for such patients to
out their glasses.

nyopia is considerable in degree, so that the print has to be held
: to the eye, glasses should be prescribed which will remove the far
bout fourteen to sixteen inches, for this will prevent the necessity of
which causes an increased flow of blood to the eye, and an increase
sion of the intra-ocular fluids. This congestion of the eye greatly
promote the development of sclerotico-choroiditis posterior, intra-
norrhage, and detachment of the retina, which are so apt to occur
iort-sighted persons. For these reasons we should direct myopes
ith their heads well thrown back, and to write at a sloping desk.
unction must also be given against the habit of reading in the
t position, either in bed or on a couch, as this produces great con-
the eyes.

: strong convergence of the visual lines which takes place when the
, to be held close to the eye, is also a source of great danger, for it
accompanied by an increased tension of the eyeball and of the
lation. The latter is an associated action, not arising from the
n of the convergence, but existing within the eye itself, and may,
tly, easily give rise to an increase of the myopia. But besides
iressure of the muscles upon the eyeball is greater when the visual
onvergent than when they are parallel, and this increase of pressure
l to give rise to the development of posterior staphyloma, and to
progress. The increase in the tension of the eyeball is particularly
hen the internal recti muscles are weak, and thus render the con-
of the visual lines more difficult.

we afford such very short-sighted persons the use of glasses which
em to read and write at a distance of fourteen or sixteen inches
eye, we do away with the necessity of a considerable convergence
ual lines, the stooping position, and the evils to which these give

patient must be warned not to bring the type close to him when
)comes a little tired, for this would strain and fatigue the accom-
; but the book should then be laid aside for a few minutes, and the
d.

les may also be used for near objects in those cases in which the
accompanied by muscular asthenopia (depending upon an insuf-
: weakness of the internal recti muscles), which manifests itself as
e patient has worked at near objects for a short time.

the use of spectacles for near objects may be permitted with ad-
l the above forms of myopia, it must be forbidden if the range of
lation is very limited, and if the patient suffer from such a degree

of amblyopia (generally depending upon sclerotico-choroi
that they are unable to read No. 2 or 3 of Snellen's types.
diminish the size of the letters, and, in order to see them unde
angle, the patient will bring the object very close to the eye, v
the accommodation to be greatly strained, the intra-ocular t
creased, and serious mischief will but too surely ensue. Sp
not, therefore, be permitted for near objects when marked an

If the myopia is very considerable, we generally find that
employed for near objects; the convergence of the visual lii
fore annulled. Donders says, with reference to this point, "
me to be often a desirable condition : in strong myopia binocula
value, and the tension which would be required for it canu
than injurious. Now, in such cases, for reading no spectacl
the first place, because the acuteness of vision has usuall;
creased, and the diminution of concave glasses is now trou
second place, because, with the retrocession of r, injurious e
gence and at binocular vision might be excited. In any cas
should be so weak as to avoid these results."

[In the case of myopes who have strained their eyes for ɛ
and the use of atropia relieve the spasm of accommodation
recession of the far-point. But our best efforts should be d
avoiding the development of myopia. All near work shoul
during twilight or by any dim light. An erect position of tl
insured while reading, and in writing by the use of a desk
steeply inclined surface. If a high degree of myopia appeai
it should influence the choice of an occupation. All school-ı
properly lighted and furnished, and close work should, if n
quently interrupted.—B.]

5.—PRESBYOPIA.

The first symptom of presbyopia is that small objects |
needlework, etc.) cannot be seen with such ease, or at so shı
before. In order to see minute objects more distinctly, the ɪ
to remove them further from the eye, or even to seek a brigl
diminish the circles of diffusion upon the retina by narrowiɪ
pupil. But as the retinal images of these fine objects ▬▬
account of the distance at which they are held, he will ▪
commensurate difficulty in clearly distinguishing them; tl
stance,] will get indistinct and confused, and the eyes beooɪ
painfu .

In simple presbyopia, the far point is at a normal distanɪ
parallel rays are united upon the retina, and neither conɪ
glasses (even after the instillation of atropine) at all improv
The eye is neither myopic nor hypermetropic. There is, in ɪ
of refraction, but only a narrowing of the range of accoı
near point is removed too far from the eye, and hence the
curately distinguishing small objects.

Amblyopia sometimes coexists with presbyopia, and may ▪
for it, as the amblyopic patient likewise cannot see very sı
tinctly, and convex glasses also improve his sight. But in aı
(uncomplicated with amblyopia) we should be able to resı
acuity of vision and range of accommodation by the prope

With its aid the patient should be able to read No. 1 at eight inches; hence if he can only decipher No. 2 or No. 4, or is obliged to hold the print closer, he is also amblyopic.

Donders has found that in the emmetropic eye the near point gradually recedes, even from an early age, further and further from the eye. This recession commences about the age of ten, and progresses regularly with increasing years. At forty it lies at about eight inches, at fifty at eleven to twelve inches, and so on. In the emmetropic eye, no inconvenience is generally experienced from the recession till about the age of forty or forty-five. This change in the position of the near point is met with in all eyes, the emmetropic, hypermetropic, and myopic.

But the far point also begins in the normal eye to recede somewhat about the age of fifty, so that the eye then becomes slightly hypermetropic (distant vision being improved by convex glasses). At seventy or eighty years of age, the hypermetropia may $= \frac{1}{24}$, i. e., the patient can see distinctly at a distance with a convex glass of twenty-four inches focus. This hypermetropia, which is at first only acquired, may afterwards become absolute; so that the patient is not only unable to accommodate for divergent, but even for parallel rays.

The recession of the near point from the eye, and the consequent narrowing of the range of accommodation, are far more due to a change in those parts within the eye which are passively changed during the act of accommodation, than to an alteration in those which, through their activity, bring about the latter. For the ciliary muscle, the active agent of accommodation, is generally normal, although it may, later in life, undergo senile changes; whereas the passively changed organ of accommodation, the crystalline lens, gradually becomes more and more firm with advancing years, and in consequence of this increased firmness, the same amount of muscular action cannot produce the same change in the form of the lens as heretofore.

[This hardening begins at a very early age, affecting first the nucleus of the lens and spreading to the periphery. Later in life this hardening may be recognized by the stronger reflection of light from the lens when focussed upon by oblique illumination. True presbyopia is therefore a senile change and is accompanied by other senile changes, such as loss of transparency in the media of the eye, shallowness of the anterior chamber, atrophy of the muscle of accommodation, etc. Premature presbyopia may occur with marasmus, after prostrating disease, with incipient cataract, and also with the development of glaucoma. (See "Schweigger," l. c., pp. 25–28.)—B.]

At first, of course, no inconvenience is experienced from this gradual recession of the near point; we do not, in fact, notice it until the distance is so considerable that we cannot easily distinguish small objects. When are we, then, to consider an eye presbyopic? Donders thinks this should be done as soon as the near point has receded further than eight inches from the eye; for as soon as this is the case, patients generally begin to complain that continued work at small objects has become irksome and fatiguing. We, however, sometimes meet with persons with very strong sight, who can read and write for hours without experiencing any inconvenience, even although their near point may be eleven to twelve inches from the eye. But these cases are exceptional. Let us, therefore, with Donders, consider presbyopia to begin when the near point is removed further than eight inches from the eye.

The degree of presbyopia (Pr) may be easily found if we decide upon a definite distance (e. g., eight inches) as the commencement of presbyopia, for we have then simply to deduct the presbyopic near point (p') from this. Thus, if p' lies at sixteen inches, the presbyopia $= \frac{1}{16}$, for $\frac{1}{8} - \frac{1}{16} = \frac{1}{16}$. Hence convex sixteen will neutralize the presbyopia and bring the near point again to eight inches.

It will perhaps have already struck the reader, that if presbyopia is assumed to commence when the near point has receded further than eight inches from the eye, not only the emmetropic, but also the myopic and hypermetropic, eye may suffer from presbyopia; for if a person has a myopia $= \frac{1}{12}$, and his near point lies at twelve inches, he is also presbyopic. This cannot, of course, occur when the myopia is higher in degree than $\frac{1}{8}$. In hypermetropia the same thing may take place, for if, with the convex glass which neutralizes the hypermetropia, the near point lies at twelve inches, there is also presbyopia.

The range of accommodation is found by the formula $\frac{1}{A} = \frac{1}{P} - \frac{1}{R}$. If $p = 10''$, and $r = \infty$, $\frac{1}{A} = \frac{1}{10}$, for $\frac{1}{10} - \frac{1}{\infty} = \frac{1}{10}$.

There can be no question as to the advisability and necessity of permitting old-sighted persons the use of spectacles. They should be furnished with them as soon as they are in the slightest degree annoyed or inconvenienced by the presbyopia. Some medical men think that presbyopic patients should do without spectacles as long as possible, for fear that the eye should, even at an early period, get so used to them as to find them indispensable. This is, however, an error, for if such persons are permitted to work without glasses, we observe that the presbyopia soon rapidly increases.

The proper strength of the glasses may be readily calculated. If p (the near point) lies sixteen inches from the eye, $Pr = \frac{1}{8} - \frac{1}{16} = \frac{1}{16}$. A convex glass of sixteen inches focus will bring the near point back again to eight inches from the eye. We must generally, however, give somewhat weaker glasses, because, on account of the greater convergence of the visual lines, the near point will through these glasses (convex sixteen) be in reality brought nearer than eight inches. Late in life, when there is some diminution in the acuteness of vision, the near point may sometimes be brought even to six or seven inches, and it should be approximated the closer, the greater the range of accommodation.

If no hypermetropia exists, the weakest glasses with which No. 1 of Snellen can be distinctly and easily read at about twelve inches distance, may generally be given. But I have often found that if the person is much employed in reading and writing, and has always been accustomed to hold his book at a considerable distance, he will be at first much inconvenienced if his near point is brought to ten or twelve inches. We shall, therefore, have to give him glasses which will bring it only to about sixteen inches. With these he will be able to work with ease for a considerable length of time. They may afterwards be gradually changed for rather stronger ones.

In choosing spectacles for old-sighted persons, we must also be particularly guided by the range of their power of accommodation. If this is good, we may give them glasses which bring their near point to eight inches, but if it is much diminished, weaker glasses should be chosen, so that it may lie at ten to twelve inches from the eye. [The choice of glasses should never be left to the patient, as he is almost certain to choose those which are too strong, for the sake of their great magnifying power.—B.]

6.—HYPERMETROPIA.

It has already been stated that in hypermetropia the refractive power of the eye is so low, or its optic axis so short, that when the eye is in a state of rest parallel rays are not united upon the retina, but behind it, and only convergent rays are brought to a focus upon the latter. We must therefore give to parallel rays emanating from distant objects, a convergent direction by means of a convex glass, and the reader will now comprehend how it is that a hypermetropic eye requires convex glasses for seeing distant objects. The patient may require perhaps even a stronger pair for near objects. The consequence of this low refractive power of the eye is, that whereas the normal eye unites parallel rays upon its retina, without any accommodative effort, the hypermetropic eye has already, in order to do so, to exert its accommodation more or less considerably, according to the amount of hypermetropia. This exertion increases, of course, in direct ratio with the proximity of the object. If the degree of hypermetropia is moderate, and the power of accommodation good, no particular annoyance is perhaps experienced, even in reading or writing. But in *absolute* hypermetropia the patient will not be able to see well at any point.

It will be found that hypermetropia generally depends upon a peculiar construction of the eye. It is smaller and flatter than the emmetropic eye, and although all its dimensions are less than in the latter, this is more particularly and markedly the case in the antero-posterior axis. The eye does not appear to fill out the palpebral aperture properly, but a little space may be observed between the outer canthus and the eyeball. Upon directing the eye to be turned very much inwards, it will also be seen that the posterior portion of the eyeball is flatter and more compressed than in the emmetropic eye. Donders considers that the hypermetropic is generally an imperfectly developed eye, that the expansion of the retina is less, and that there is a smaller optic nerve with a less number of fibres. He thinks, moreover, that in hypermetropia there often exists a typical form of face, chiefly dependent upon the shallowness of the orbit, which lends a peculiar flatness to the physiognomy. The hypermetropic construction of the eyeball is congenital, and often hereditary.

[In the hypermetropic eye, the line of vision deviates inward from the corneal centre more than in emmetropia. It may develop during the growth of the body, but it is acquired comparatively seldom; aphakia being the most frequent cause of acquired hypermetropia. Hypermetropia may also be caused by the retina being pushed forward by exudations beneath it, or by a flattening of the eyeball posteriorly by orbital tumors. ("Schweigger," l. c.—B.)]

The ophthalmoscope also enables us to diagnose a hypermetropic eye, but in this case just the reverse obtains to what was seen in the myopic eye.

I. The fundus may also in this case be seen in the erect image at a considerable distance, but we obtain an erect image of it (and not, as in myopia,

Fig. 202.

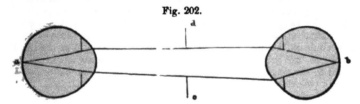

a reverse image), for if we regard the optic nerve or one of the retinal vessels, and move our head to one side, we find that the image *moves in the same direction*. For an explanation of this, let us glance at Fig. 202.

Let *a* be the hypermetropic eye, *b* the eye of the observer; *a* is adjusted for its far point (convergent rays), and the rays reflected from its back.

41

ground will, consequently, emanate from it in a divergent direction, as if they came from a point behind the retina, and they must, therefore, also fall in a divergent direction upon the eye of the observer. If the latter is myopic (adjusted for divergent rays), the rays will be united upon his retina without the aid of any correcting lens behind the ophthalmoscope. But if his eye is emmetropic (adjusted, when in a state of rest, for parallel rays), he will either have to place a convex lens behind the mirror, or have to accommodate for a nearer point. The strongest convex lens with which the details of the fundus can still be seen in the erect image, affords us a relative estimate of the degree of existing hypermetropia. Thus if the hypermetropia $= \frac{1}{8}$, the rays emanating from a luminous point on the retina will diverge as if they came from a point six inches behind the nodal point, appearing to the eye of the observer (placed two inches in front of that of the patient) as if they came from eight inches behind the nodal point of the eye under examination, and he will hence require a convex glass of eight inches focus to see the details of the fundus distinctly. The distance of the two eyes (two inches) from each other must be subtracted from the required lens (eight inches), in order to find the degree of hypermetropia, six inches; and the latter will always be greater than the focal distance of the lens.

The image of the observed eye will be erect, for c and d retain their relative positions.

II. On going closer, but still examining in the erect image, the field of vision appears much enlarged, and the image removed further from the eye; its size is considerably diminished, whereas the intensity of its light and color is much increased. If the hypermetropia is high in degree, we can overlook at a glance not only the whole optic entrance, but also a considerable portion of the fundus around it. In the indirect mode of examination, the size of the optic disk will appear much larger than in the emmetropic eye, which is due to its image being formed further from the object lens. If our eye is emmetropic, we must, in order to gain a distinct image, either place a strong convex lens behind the mirror, or else we must accommodate for a nearer point.

The ophthalmoscopic diagnosis of hypermetropia is frequently of much service, especially in young children affected with strabismus, the state of whose refraction we wish to ascertain, but who are too young to read. Again, in spasm of the ciliary muscle dependent upon hypermetropia, the latter may be so completely masked that the patient can only see at a distance with slightly concave glasses, and not at all with convex ones. We hence, perhaps, believe it to be a case of myopia, but on ophthalmoscopic examination we find that the refraction is markedly hypermetropic. In such cases the patient should, however, look at some distant object, or into vacant space, so that his accommodation may be quite relaxed. We may notice in such patients how the ophthalmoscopic appearances vary when the accommodation is relaxed, and when it is called into action by their regarding some near object. [In general terms, the hypermetropia in an observed eye is always equal to the glass used in the ophthalmoscope, minus the distance from the nodal point of the eye examined, supposing that the observer is emmetropic. If he is not, his own error of refraction must be taken into account or corrected by the proper glass.—B.]

We must distinguish various forms of hypermetropia, and in our classification of these we shall follow Donders' system, which is the most practical.

We may, in the first place, divide hypermetropia into two primary classes, the original and the acquired.

Owing to the senile changes in the lens which appear with advancing age, the far point begins to recede somewhat from the eye at the age of forty or forty-five. At sixty, the eye is generally already so hypermetropic that distant vision is markedly improved by convex glasses. At seventy or eighty years the hypermetropia often $= \frac{1}{7}$. This is termed acquired hypermetropia. The latter will, of course, be very considerable when the crystalline lens is absent (as after extraction of cataract).

Original hypermetropia may be divided into the manifest (Hm) and latent (Hl) form.

In order to determine the presence of hypermetropia, the patient is directed to read No. xx (Snellen) at twenty feet. Let us suppose that he can do so with ease; we then find the strongest convex glass with which he can still see the same number clearly and distinctly, and this gives us the degree of manifest hypermetropia. If convex twenty is the lens (convex eighteen making the sight worse), Hm $= \frac{1}{7}$. Each eye should be tried separately, as the degree of hypermetropia may vary. The range of accommodation with this glass is then tried.

But although convex twenty may be the strongest glass with which he can see at a distance, the degree of hypermetropia may in reality be very much higher than $\frac{1}{7}$. The fact being, that the patient has been so accustomed to exert his accommodation (even when regarding distant objects), that he cannot relax it all at once, even when there is no occasion for it, the malconstruction of the eye being compensated for by a convex lens. To find the real degree of hypermetropia, we must, therefore, paralyze his accommodation by a strong solution of atropine (four grains to one fluidounce).[1] This should be allowed to act for two or three hours. At the end of this time we again examine the patient, and now, perhaps, find that he cannot see No. xx at all at twenty feet without glasses, or even with convex twenty. To do so distinctly he, perhaps, requires convex eight; and this difference in the power of the glasses required before and after the paralysis of the ciliary muscle, shows us to what an extent he exerted his accommodation before the application of the atropine. But this great difference only exists in young persons with a good range of accommodation. The atropine should be only applied to one eye at a time; its effect goes off in about six or seven days. But as its effect proves very disagreeable and confusing to the sight it should only be applied in those cases in which it is of importance to know precisely the degree of latent hypermetropia. Its action may, if necessary, be neutralized by the extract of Calabar bean, which will, however, have to be repeated several times, as its effect is much more transitory.

A slight degree of hypermetropia is often unnoticed until the age of twenty-five or thirty, when symptoms of asthenopia show themselves if the patient is obliged to work much at near objects. If we try the sight for distance, we find that he can read No. xx at twenty feet, and also with a weak convex glass (thirty or forty). Or, perhaps, if only momentarily held before the eye it makes the sight worse, as the patient cannot at once relax his accommodation, but after looking through it for a few minutes he sees better. To make sure of the degree of Hl, the accommodation must be paralyzed with atropine. [After complete paralysis of accommodation from atropia, the latent hypermetropia returns, even when the patient wears continuously the proper correcting convex glasses.—B.]

---

[1] Dr. Berlin advises that in those cases of hypermetropia in which it is unadvisable to employ atropine, the degree of latent hypermetropia may be estimated by employing two abducting prisms (6° before each eye), so that the patient's visual lines may be parallel, and his accommodation consequently relaxed. ("Kl. Monatsbl.," Jan. 1869.)

Donders divides manifest hypermetropia into three classes, the *facultative*, the *relative*, and the *absolute*.

In *facultative* hypermetropia the patient can see well (with parallel optic axes) at an infinite distance, with or without convex glasses. He can also see to read small print with ease without glasses, so that he experiences no fatigue during work. Presbyopia, however, sets in unusually early, and then symptoms of asthenopia supervene.

In *relative* hypermetropia, the eye may also be able to accommodate itself either for parallel or for divergent rays, and see well both at a distance and near at hand, but it can only do so by converging the visual lines for a nearer point than that at which the object is situated; by acquiring, in fact, a periodic convergent squint. It is not of very frequent occurrence in childhood, but is more often met with after the age of puberty and in early manhood. The sight is always more or less affected, and the patient has a difficulty in finding the exact distance at which he can see best.

In *absolute hypermetropia* vision is indistinct, both for infinite distance and for near objects; for the patient cannot unite the rays upon the retina even with the strongest effort of accommodation, or with the strongest convergence of the visual lines. The focus of both divergent and parallel rays remains situated behind the retina. It is not often met with in youthful individuals, as they generally possess a sufficiently strong power of accommodation to overcome it. In a superficial examination, such a patient might be mistaken for a person suffering from myopia with amblyopia, for he will not be able to see distinctly at a distance without glasses, which may be erroneously attributed to myopia, nor will he be able to read very fine print, and this may be supposed to be due to amblyopia.

If the hypermetropia is considerable in degree, the patients often see better when the print is held very close to the eye, than when it is ten or twelve inches off. This is partly due to diminution in the size of the circles of diffusion, on account of the contraction of the pupil. Moreover, the circles of diffusion increase comparatively less in magnitude than the size of the retinal image, as the object is approximated (Von Graefe).

A hypermetropic eye may at a certain age become presbyopic. If with the glasses which neutralize the hypermetropia, the near point lies at twelve or fourteen inches, presbyopia coexists, and a stronger pair of glasses will be required for reading.

The range of accommodation is best found by neutralizing the patient's hypermetropia by means of the proper convex lens, and then finding where his near point lies with this glass.

In high degrees of hypermetropia the acuteness of vision is generally somewhat diminished. This, according to Donders, is partly due to the structure of the eye, for as the nodal point lies far back, the retinal images will be correspondingly small; hence convex glasses improve the sight, by advancing the nodal point, and increasing the size of the retinal image. It may also be due to astigmatism, or to the smaller number of nerve fibres in the optic nerve and retina.

Hypermetropia is a very frequent cause of asthenopia (seu hebetudo visus, impaired vision, etc.); this condition being distinguished by the following symptoms: The patient cannot look at near objects (in reading, writing, sewing, etc.) for any length of time without the eyes becoming fatigued. The print becomes indistinct, the letters run one into another, there is pain in and around the eye, and the latter may become red and watery, and feel hot and uncomfortable; yet the eye looks quite healthy, the refracting media are clear, vision is good, the convergence of the visual lines perfect, and the mobility of the eye unimpaired. Neither does the ophthalmoscope reveal anything abnormal, except perhaps slight hyperæmia of the optic nerve and retina. The symptoms of asthenopia quickly vanish when the work is laid aside, to reappear, however, when it is resumed. It was indeed a great boon when Donders discovered that most of these cases of asthenopia depended upon hypermetropia, and could be cured by the proper use of spectacles. If we wish permanently to cure such cases we must afford the patient the aid of glasses, and thus prevent all undue straining of the accommodation.

This accommodative form of asthenopia must be distinguished from the muscular, which depends upon weakness of the internal recti muscles, and from the retinal asthenopia. The latter is generally due to hyperæsthesia and irritability of the retina, accompanied by hyperæmia of the optic nerve and retina. It mostly occurs in feeble, nervous, and excitable persons, especially females.

Let us now consider how hypermetropic persons are to be suited with glasses.

Theoretically, it would appear right to neutralize the hypermetropia by a convex lens, and thus change the eye into an emmetropic one; this lens forming, so to speak, an integral part of the eye. But in practice we find that this does not answer.

In facultative hypermetropia, there will be no occasion to prescribe glasses for distance, as the patient can see well without them. Moreover, there is the disadvantage, that after convex spectacles have been worn for some time for distance, the power of seeing distinctly without them is lost, which is of course very inconvenient. For this reason they should never be ordered, except in cases of absolute or relative hypermetropia of a considerable degree. If there are symptoms of asthenopia, glasses should be given for reading, etc., which are somewhat stronger than those which correct the manifest hypermetropia. If these are found too strong and trying to the eye, they must be exchanged for weaker ones, and the strength be gradually increased until the asthenopia has disappeared.

In relative and absolute hypermetropia spectacles should also be worn for distance, as we find that in such instances distant vision is not distinct. In such cases, I generally commence with the glasses which neutralize the manifest hypermetropia, and in young persons order them to be worn both for near and distant objects. If they prove too strong for distance, a weaker pair must be prescribed, and their strength gradually increased. If they do not relieve the asthenopia, or if presbyopia coexist, a stronger pair must be given for reading, writing, and sewing.

In using the spectacles for reading, sewing, etc., it is always advisable to interrupt the work for a few minutes at the end of half an hour or an hour. This rests the eye, which is then able to resume the employment with renewed vigor and ease. If the asthenopia does not quite disappear under the use of glasses, we must examine the power of convergence, for together with the hypermetropia there may exist insufficiency of the internal recti muscles, and the asthenopia be partly due to this. If the accommodation has been greatly fatigued by prolonged work at near objects without the aid of glasses, or if there is a spasm of the ciliary muscle, the accommodation should be placed in a condition of complete rest, by being paralyzed by a strong solution of atropine; and this paralysis should be maintained for several weeks.

Donders has shown that convergent strabismus very frequently depends upon hypermetropia. A person suffering from the latter is always obliged to accommodate more or less, in order to see with distinctness. Even at a

a direction contrary to that of the observer's head; while in hypermetropia it moves in the same direction." (Loring, l. c., p. 47.)

The refraction of an eye may also be made out by means of the inverted image. In a myopic eye the inverted image must be smaller than in an emmetropic eye, since the nearer an image is formed behind a lens the smaller it will be; provided the same lens is used with each, and is held at or within its focal length from the eye. In a hypermetropic eye the image will be larger than in an emmetropic eye. In a myopic eye the size of the image increases as the lens is removed from the eye, while in hypermetropia it decreases as the lens recedes. (Loring, l. c., p. 50 and 51.)—B.]

7.—ASTIGMATISM.

We have seen that the anomalies of refraction resolve themselves into two, viz., myopia and hypermetropia. But the state of refraction may vary in the different meridians of the same eye; thus, it may be emmetropic in the vertical meridian, but myopic or hypermetropic in the horizontal, or *vice versâ*. Or differences in the degree or even in the form of emmetropia may exist in the various meridians. This asymmetry has been termed astigmatism (ɑ, privative, and στιγμα, a point), which signifies that rays emanating from a point are not reunited at a point. This peculiar defect[1] was first observed by Thomas Young (1793), who considered it due to some inequality in the structure of the lens; whereas, Wharton Jones thought its seat was in the cornea. Donders has shown that it is of frequent occurrence, and that many cases of congenital amblyopia are due to it, and may be cured by proper cylindrical glasses.

But even in the normal eye, the cornea does not refract equally in all its meridians, for the focal distance of the dioptric system is generally shorter in the vertical meridian than in the horizontal. On this account, fine vertical lines can be seen up to a further distance than horizontal lines, but the latter can be seen closer than the vertical lines. For this experiment, horizontal and vertical lines may be drawn upon a page, or Von Graefe's wire optometer may be used.

If the stripes or lines are arranged crosswise, we are unable to distinguish both the horizontal and vertical lines with equal clearness and distinctness at one and the same distance; thus, if we can see the vertical line clearly and sharply defined, we must approach the horizontal line nearer to the eye, in order to gain an equally distinct image of it, and *vice versâ*. These facts prove that the vertical meridian has a shorter focal distance than the horizontal, and for this reason horizontal lines are seen distinctly at a shorter distance than vertical ones. For, as the rays which are refracted in the vertical meridian are united in a point sooner than those in the horizontal plane, these latter give rise to circles of diffusion upon the retina in the form of small horizontal lines which do not confuse the images of horizontal lines, but interfere with those of vertical lines.

As it is of much consequence in the study of astigmatism that the reader should thoroughly understand these preliminary facts, I give the following extract and explanatory wood-cuts from Donders' work. After speaking of the fact that a vertical stripe can be seen further off, and a horizontal stripe at a closer distance, he continues: "These experiments prove that the points of the refracting meridians are not symmetrically arranged around one axis.

---

[1] For a most interesting historical account of this subject, see Donders' work, p. 589.

The asymmetry is of such a nature that the focal distance is shorter in the vertical meridian than in the horizontal. In order, namely, to see a vertical stripe acutely, the rays, which in a horizontal plane diverge from each point of the line, must be brought to a focus upon the retina; it is not necessary that those diverging in a vertical plane should also previously converge into one point, as the diffusion-images still existing in a vertical direction cover one another on the vertical stripe. On the other hand, in order to see a horizontal stripe acutely, it is necessary only that the rays of light diverging in a vertical plane should unite in one point upon the retina. Now horizontal lines are acutely seen, as I have remarked, at a shorter distance than vertical ones; consequently rays situated in a vertical plane, which are refracted in the vertical meridian of the eye, are more speedily brought to a focus than those of equal divergence situated in a horizontal plane, and the vertical meridian, therefore, has a shorter focal distance than the horizontal.

"The correctness of this view appears further from the form of the diffusion-images of a point of light. In accurate accommodation the diffusion-spot is very small, and nearly round, while a nearer point appears extended in breadth, and a more remote one seems to be extended in height. The signification of this phenomenon must be clearly understood, and appears, therefore, to demand more particular explanation.

"Let us suppose the total deviation of light in the eye to be produced by a single convex refracting surface, with the shortest radius of curvature in the vertical, and the longest in the horizontal meridian. These two are then the principal meridians. Through a central round opening (Fig. 203, *v v h h*)

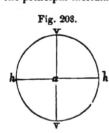

Fig. 203.

let a cone of rays proceeding from a point situated in the prolongation of the axis of vision, fall upon this surface; of this cone, let us consider only the rays situated in the vertical plane *v v*, and the rays situated in the horizontal plane *h h*, whereof respectively the points *v v* and *h h* are the most external. After the refraction, both approach the visual axis (which perpendicular to the plane of the drawing passes through *a*); *v v* does so, however, more rapidly than *h h*. Before union, they therefore lie in the ellipse *A*, as in Fig. 204, and where *v v* meet in one point *B*, *h h* have not yet come to a focus. Thereupon we now find in succession *v v* already intersected, *h h* approached to one another, *C*, *D*, *E*; further, *h h* united in one point, and *v v* after intersection more widely separated, *F*; finally, both intersected, *G*. The focus of *v v* therefore lies most anteriorly, that of *h h* most posteriorly in the axis. The

Fig. 204.

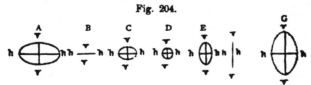

space between the two points, where rays of different meridians intersect, may be called the focal interval (*intervalle focal*, or Brennstrecke of Sturm). From the above figures, it is now evident what successive forms the section of the cone of light will exhibit. In the middle of the focal interval *D*, it will be nearly round, and anteriorly through oblate ellipses, *C*, with increasing eccentricity, it will pass into a horizontal line *B*; posteriorly through prolate ellipses, *E*, it will come to form a vertical line *F*, while before the focal interval a larger oblate ellipse, *A*, and behind it a larger prolate ellipse, *G*, will be found."

The position of these figures with regard to the focal interval is shown in Fig. 205. In the cone of light emanating from *L* are depicted the rays which impinge upon the vertical meridian *V V* and upon the horizontal meridian

Fig. 205.

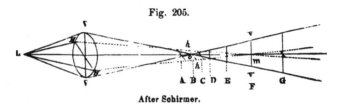

After Schirmer.

H H. The former are united in *m*, the latter in *m*, so that *o m* is the focal interval.

In Fig. 205, the letters *A, B, C, D, E, F*, and *G* correspond to the same letters in Fig. 204. The rays which lie in the plane of the vertical meridian *V V* (in Fig. 205) are brought to a focus at *o*, where the rays which lie in the plane of the horizontal meridian *H H*, are not yet united, but form the horizontal line *h h* (the *anterior* focal line). The rays *H H* are united further back at *m*, where the vertical rays form the vertical line *v v* (the *posterior* focal line). The distance between these two focal lines forms the focal interval. The anterior focal line *h h* corresponds to the position of the meridian of the lowest refractive power, whereas the posterior focal line *v v*, to that of the meridian of highest refraction. Generally, the astigmatic patient endeavors unconsciously so to regulate his accommodation that the middle portion of the focal interval falls upon the retina; in this way only a small round circle of diffusion *D* (Fig. 204) is formed, and the object is more distinctly seen than it would be at the anterior or posterior extremity of the focal interval. In case the anterior extremity of the focal interval falls upon the retina, and if this should be the focus of the vertical meridian, a circular flame appears of a horizontal luminous line. The reverse will of course occur if the posterior extremity of the focal line (if this corresponds to the focus of the horizontal meridian) falls upon the retina, for then the flame will appear as a vertical, luminous line. Hence, horizontal and vertical stripes will be sharply and distinctly seen when the diffusion-images of all the points of the stripe form respectively horizontal and vertical lines, which cover one another in the stripe; and this will be the case when the beginning and the end of the focal interval correspond respectively to the percipient surface of the retina (Donders).

Although we have hitherto assumed that the principal axes of curvature correspond with the vertical and horizontal meridians, it must be mentioned that they may deviate considerably from these. Also, that instead of the minimum of curvature corresponding with the horizontal meridian, and the maximum with the vertical, the reverse may even obtain, and the maximum curvature coincide with the horizontal meridian.

The aberration which is due to a difference in the focal distance of the two principal meridians, is called *regular* astigmatism, and depends upon the curvature of the cornea; whereas the aberration which is due to a difference in the refraction in one and the same meridian, is called *irregular* astigmatism, and is generally caused by a peculiarity in the structure of the crystalline lens, and cannot be corrected by cylindrical glasses. It often gives rise to monocular polyopia. The two forms sometimes coexist. The degree of regular astigmatism met with in normal eyes is generally too slight to cause any impairment of vision ; but when it is more considerable, the sight is indistinct. This amblyopia is due to circles of diffusion being formed upon the retina, which cross and overlap each other. The greater the difference in the refraction of the principal meridians, the more considerable will be the circles of diffusion and consequent indistinctness of vision. If the astigmatism is at all high in degree, the acuteness of vision is much impaired, both for near and distant objects. If the eye is myopic or hypermetropic, we find that we cannot with any spherical lens produce a very decided improvement, or raise the acuteness of vision to the normal standard.

The diagnosis of astigmatism may generally be made without much difficulty ; but it is necessary to follow a settled line of examination, otherwise the beginner will fall into great confusion, and waste a large amount of time. Numerous modes of discovering the presence of astigmatism, and of estimating its degree are in use ; but the following are the simplest and most practical.

In the first place, we must carefully examine the acuteness of vision, and ascertain which number of Snellen's types the patient can see at a distance of twenty feet. If the acuteness of vision is below the normal standard (if he cannot read No. xx), we must try whether it can be raised to this by concave or convex spherical lenses. If we fail in doing so, we must suspect the presence of astigmatism, and next proceed to determine the situation of the two principal meridians (*i. e.*, the maximum and minimum of curvature). This may be done by directing the patient to look at a small, distant point of light (varying from two to four millimetres in diameter, and seen through a small opening in a large black screen). The patient should be placed at a distance of from twelve to sixteen feet, and directed to look at the luminous point. The latter will not appear round if the eye is astigmatic, but will be elongated in a certain direction, according to the fact whether the light is nearer or further off than the point for which the eye is accommodated. Thus, if the maximum of curvature coincides with the vertical meridian, the luminous line will be horizontal if the eye is accommodated for a further point, and vertical if it is adjusted for a nearer point. Weak concave and convex lenses are then placed alternately before the eye (the latter being thus changed into a myopic or hypermetropic one), and the anterior and posterior focal line brought alternately upon the retina. The direction of this line will depend of course upon the direction of the principal meridian.

A better test-object is, however, formed by a series of straight lines, which cross each other in the centre of a circle. For this purpose, I have found Dr. Green's[1] test-objects the best, and use them in preference to any others. He employs three figures, which can be arranged in such a manner as to amplify and check the results obtained. I have, however, found that one of the diagrams (Fig. 206) is sufficient. It consists of a circle, traversed by a set of twelve triple lines, corresponding to the figures on a watch dial ; the figures being placed at the extremity of the sets of lines, as in Javal's optometer (Fig. 207). Each line is equal in thickness to the lines employed

---

[1] *Vide* Dr. Green's paper on "The Detection and Measurement of Astigmatism," in the "American Journal of the Medical Sciences," January, 1867. More recently Dr. Green has devised a still more complete set of tests for astigmatism, as well as some ingenious color-tests for the same purpose (*vide* "The Transactions of the American Ophthalmological Society," 1869). [Dr. Green has still more recently devised some additional tests for astigmatism, which will be found in the "Trans. Amer. Ophthal. Soc.," 1878.—B.]

by Snellen in the construction of No. **xx** of his test-types, and is designed to be distinctly seen at a distance of about twenty feet. The circle is about twelve and one-half inches in diameter. Snellen uses a semicircle of straight lines.

This test-circle is to be placed at the distance of twenty feet, and if the patient can see all the lines distinctly and sharply defined (any existing myopia or hypermetropia being corrected by suitable spherical lenses), he is not astigmatic. But if only the line in one meridian appears clear and sharply defined, whilst the others are indistinct, the presence of astigmatism

Fig. 206.

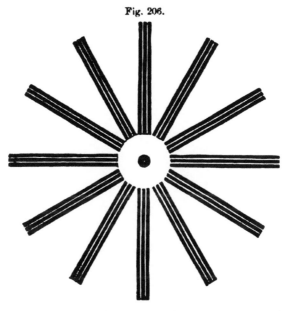

is proved, and the direction of the distinct line corresponds to the meridian of the highest refraction. If we now wish to discover the degree and nature of the astigmatism, and are only supplied with spherical lenses, we try the weakest concave or the strongest convex lens which, placed in a stenopæic apparatus,[1] enables the patient to see all the radiating lines with equal distinctness. If a concave lens is required, it is a case of myopic astigmatism; whereas it is hypermetropic if a convex lens is required. Dr. Pray has devised some very useful test-letters, which are composed of stripes running at different angles, by which the presence of astigmatism may be readily discovered.[2] (Knapp's "Archives," i. p. 17.)

If we possess a trial case of cylindrical lenses, the weakest concave or

---

[1] The stenopæic apparatus employed for this purpose consists of a small cylinder open at one end, so as to fit closely to the eye, the other end being furnished with a small slit, which can be readily narrowed and widened. The effect of this slit (which should be set to a width of about one and one-half or two millimetres) is of course to admit only rays in a certain direction, excluding all the others. The box of the cylinder should be made to unscrew, in order that spherical lenses may be placed in it.

[2] Mr. Brudenell Carter has had Dr. Pray's original sheet photographically reduced to one-fourth of its size. It is sold by the Autotype Fine Art Company, 86 Rathbone Place, W.

manner that they can be used singly or together, thus allowing of most varied combinations. After the degree of astigmatism has been determined, the state of the refraction of the eye must be ascertained, and the same apparatus may be used for this purpose. After the examination of the one eye has been finished, that of the other should be proceeded with, the series of cylindrical lenses being turned over to the other side. The principal objection to this instrument is, that on account of the patient being conscious of the close proximity of the object, he may not relax his accommodation completely, and is hence not in reality accommodated for his far point, and we may therefore fall into error as to the degree of his astigmatism. This error is to a great extent avoided if we test him with the radiating lines at a distance, and completely so if in a case of hypermetropia the accommodation is paralyzed.

Dr. Thomson[1] has devised a practical test for ametropia which will be also found very useful in detecting astigmatism; it is based upon the experiment of Scheiner. He has shown that whenever the visual axis is too long (myopia), or too short (hypermetropia), a point of light used as a test-object will appear double to the eye of the observer when it is examined through two small perforations in an opaque screen. In myopia, the double images are homonymous; in hypermetropia, crossed. The patient is placed five metres from a small point of light, having before his eye an opaque screen with two

Fig. 208.

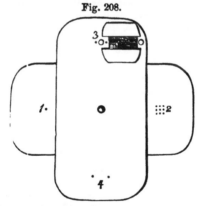

perforations in it, each one-half millimetre in diameter, and placed four millimetres apart. A piece of ruby glass is placed over one of the holes, so that he can readily distinguish between the two images.

[Dr. Thomson's optometer, which may readily be made with a visiting-card and a pin, consists of four screens of thin metal or cardboard perforated as follows:

No. 1. One hole, 1 millimetre diameter.
" 2. Nine holes, ½ " "
" 3. Two holes, 8 millimetres apart, ½ millimetre diameter.
" 4. " " 4 " " ½ " "

The patient should be placed in a darkened room, at not less than sixteen feet from a lighted candle, and should look through No. 1, and, at the same time, move the screen quickly before his eye. If the length of the axis of

[1] "Transactions of the American Ophthalmological Society," 1870, p. 28 [and "Am. Journ. of Med. Sci.," Jan. 1870, p 76, and Oct. 1870, p. 414. Also "Gross' Surg.," 6th ed., vol. ii. p. 237.—H.]

the eye be normal, and the refraction hence emmetropic, the point of light will remain stationary; should the eye be ametropic, the light will move with each movement of the screen. With No. 2, the light will appear single to an emmetropic eye, multiplied to an ametropic. With No. 3, the light which enters the two perforations will appear to the observer, when placed near his eye, to come from two large circles at the screen, which overlap each other at their inner borders. In this overlapping space only will the test-light appear double to an ametropic eye; and care must be exercised that the patient uses both apertures, and that his attention is fixed upon the overlapping space. This screen is provided with a slide of ruby-colored glass which can be pushed over either perforation, and thus color red the light which passes through it. To an ametropic eye, the light point in the overlapping space will appear as two lights. On sliding the red glass over the perforation on the right side, the light on the right appears crimson, and thus indicates that the axis of the eye is too long. To an hypermetropic eye, the left-hand light would become colored, indicating the axis to be too short.

With No. 4, we can determine, without test-glasses, the degree of optical defect, by estimating the apparent distance apart of the two lights as they appear to an ametropic eye. There is a measured and fixed quantity, four millimetres, in the screen, and the patient should be placed at a fixed distance, sixteen feet, from a small point of light, when the degree of the defect, and the proper glasses for its correction, can be ascertained by the measurement of the distance between the two lights. Where the single point of light appears double, approach to it a second light, until of the four points which the patient then perceives, the right-hand one of the fixed, and the left-hand one of the moving lights, are superimposed, and he then sees but three. By measuring the distance between the two lights, we are able to ascertain the optical defect by reference to the table below.

Distance of Lights Apart.	Degree of Ametropia.	Distance of Lights Apart.	Degree of Ametropia.
¼ inch	=	5 inches	=
1 "	=	6 "	=
1½ "	=	7 "	=
2 "	=	8 . "	=
3 "	=	9 "	=
4 "	=	10 "	=

A blackened disk, ten inches in diameter, having white lines one inch apart painted on its face, attached to a spring candlestick by a pivot, having

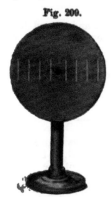

Fig. 209.

in its centre an opening one-fourth inch in diameter, through which the light of a candle may be transmitted, affords a very useful instrument. Let the patient regard this point of light, and when it appears double, he can determine the number of white lines between the lights, and hence the distance, since the lines are one inch apart. By rotating the disk and changing the position of the screen, in cases of astigmatism, any meridian of the eye can be examined.

The following diagram (Fig. 210) of an emmetropic eye indicates the path of the light admitted through each opening, and the position of each image which is thus formed. When the eye is emmetropic, the two images are superimposed and appear as one; when hypermetropic or myopic, two images are formed upon the retina. The dotted line represents the path of the red ray which falls upon one side of the retina in hypermetropia, and upon the other in myopia; a fact which enables these defects to be instantly distinguished.—H.]

[In 1878, Dr. Thomson, of Philadelphia, presented to the American Ophthalmological Society an instrument, called an ametrometer, for the rapid diagnosis of errors of refraction, a full description of which will be found in the "Transactions" for that year, pages 455 to 461. It consists of a thimble which can be attached to a common gas-burner, to which is attached a graduated half-circle. Connected with this is a horizontal bar, the end of which is a pointer, which can be placed at any part of the graduated half-circle by elevating or depressing the other end of the bar. Upon this bar slides a small box which is connected with a gas-jet, and at the upper end of the

Fig. 210.

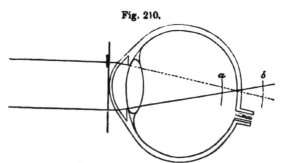

Diagram showing Hypermetropia at *a*, Myopia at *b*.

thimble and at right angles is a fixed gas-jet, the two jets being connected by a flexible rubber tube. These two jets may be placed in contact or at any distance from each other up to thirty centimetres, the length of the bar, and at any possible angle with the bar by the pivotal action of the latter. The description of the method of using is too long to transcribe, but the instrument is applicable for the determination of the kind and degree of simple ametropia, and also for that of astigmatism. The bar is divided into spaces of two and one-half centimetres with a half space between on one side, and into English inches and half inches on the other. Each space of two and one-half centimetres will indicate an ametropia of one dioptric, and each inch one-thirty-sixth of the old system. Dr. Thomson has since added a fifth disk of thin brass, one and one-half inch in diameter, having in its centre ten perforations, one-half of a millimetre each in diameter and one-half of a millimetre apart, arranged in the form of a cross. A scratch across the face of the disk, in a line with the stem, enables it to be placed at any angle in the trial frames. The test-object should be a small bright point of light at a distance of not less than sixteen feet from the patient, whose accommodation should be entirely paralyzed. For the clinical correction of astigmatism, the meridians of greatest and least ametropia must be carefully ascertained by the circular opening advised by Donders and Dr. Green's radiating lines. The disk may then be placed in the trial frames, with the stem of the cross corresponding to one of these, and by passing a card in front of each part of the cross, the refraction of each meridian may be separately ascertained. ("Trans. Amer. Ophthal. Soc.," 1873.)—B.]

[Javal and Schiötz have invented a new practical ophthalmometer for the determination of errors of refraction, and claim for it the following advantages: 1. It suppresses the error of collimation by replacing the heliometric plates of other instruments by a bi-refracting crystal. 2. It does away with all calculations and admits of reading off the refraction of each meridian immediately in dioptrics. 3. It diminishes the number of readings for each position, in increasing the precision of the instrument sufficiently to admit of limiting the examination in all security to a single reading. 4. In examining for astigmatism alone, the meridians of maximum and minimum curvature are found immediately by its aid, which reduces enormously the amount of labor in a given case. 5. It does away with the necessity of a special room, by permitting the work to be done by daylight. 6. The instrument is sufficiently small to admit of its being placed on any table. (See "Annales d'oculistique," Juli–Août, 1881.)—B.]

Donders has distinguished three forms of astigmatism, viz.: I. Simple astigmatism; II. Compound astigmatism; III. Mixed astigmatism.

I. Simple Astigmatism.—The state of refraction of the one principal meridian is emmetropic, whereas that of the other is either myopic or hypermetropic. If we, in such a case, turn the slit of the stenopæic apparatus in the direction of the normal meridian, the acuteness of vision will be perfect, whereas a certain concave or convex spherical lens will be required if the slit is turned in the direction of the other meridian.

Simple astigmatism is divided into: 1. Simple myopic astigmatism (Am), in which myopia exists in the one principal meridian, and emmetropia in the other. 2. Simple Hypermetropic Astigmatism (Ah). In this there is hypermetropia in the one principal meridian, and emmetropia in the other.

II. Compound Astigmatism.—In this form, myopia or hypermetropia exists in both principal meridians, but it varies in degree. If the stenopæic slit be used in such cases, it will be found that a different concave or convex lens will be required in each of the principal meridians, in order to render the acuteness of vision normal.

We must here also distinguish two forms: 1. Compound Myopic Astigmatism (M + Am). Myopia exists in both principal meridians. 2. Compound Hypermetropic Astigmatism (H + Ah). Hypermetropia exists in both principal meridians.

III. Mixed Astigmatism.—This is a rare form, in which the one principal meridian is myopic, the other hypermetropic. We must here also distinguish: 1. Mixed astigmatism, with predominant myopia (Amh). 2. Mixed astigmatism, with predominant hypermetropia (Ahm).

Knapp and Schweigger have pointed out that the ophthalmoscope also furnishes us with a valuable and easy diagnostic symptom of regular astigmatism. On examining in the direct method an eye affected with astigmatism, it will be found that the optic disk, instead of being round, appears elongated in one direction, and that the latter corresponds exactly to the meridian of greatest curvature. For as the focal distance is shorter in this meridian than in the other, the image must also be more magnified in this direction. If we now examine the same eye in the inverted image, the optic disk will appear elongated in the opposite direction; thus, if in the erect image the disk appears oval in the vertical direction, in the inverted it will appear oval in the horizontal direction, and this at once proves the existence of regular astigmatism, and shows also that the vertical meridian is of greater curvature, and consequently, has a less focal distance than the horizontal. The comparative examination in the erect and inverted image, therefore, furnishes us with a most valuable aid to diagnosis, which will often spare us the necessity of a long and intricate subjective examination.

["   the inverted image of an astigmatic eye the recession of the lens causes a variation in the size and shape of the optic disk. If the long diameter of the oval contracts when the lens is moved from the eye so as to become equal to the short, and thus make a circle, then the astigmatism is hypermetropic. If, on the contrary, the short diameter expands so as to become equal, at the focal distance of the lens, to the long, and thus make a circle, the astigmatism is myopic." (Loring, l. c., p. 55.)—B.]

In examining, in the erect image, an eye affected with hypermetropic astigmatism, it will also be found that in order to see with equal distinctness the vessels running in different directions, the state of accommodation of the observer's eye has to undergo a change.

Mr. Bowman "has been sometimes led to the discovery of regular astigmatism of the cornea, and the direction of the chief meridians by using the mirror of the ophthalmoscope much in the same way as for slight degrees of conical cornea. The observation is more easy if the optic disk is in the line of sight and the pupil large. The mirror is to be held at two feet distance, and its inclination rapidly varied, so as to throw the light on the eye at small angles to the perpendicular, and from opposite sides in succession, in successive meridians. The area of the pupil then exhibits a somewhat linear shadow in some meridians rather than in others."[1]

Mr. Couper has lately shown[2] that cases of mixed astigmatism may be readily diagnosed with the ophthalmoscopic mirror alone; an inverted or an erect image becoming alternately visible according as the observer views the fundus through the meridian of the greatest or of the least curvature. Mr. Couper has kindly furnished me with a brief outline of some of his observations; and I can, from my own experience, recommend his mode of examination as very practical and useful. For this examination he employs a concave mirror of silvered glass of about thirty inches focus, which enables him to illuminate the fundus at a maximum distance of about five feet. A concave mirror of six or eight inches focus scatters the rays too much to permit of an adequate illumination at even half this distance. A twofold object is served by commencing the examination from an extreme distance of five feet. 1. Very small degrees of myopia can be recognized by the inverted aerial image, which is thus placed beyond the observer's near point. 2. The meridian planes of maximum and minimum curvature are sometimes clearly revealed by the distortion which the image undergoes when viewed from a distance. It is best to have the accommodation paralyzed with atropine, and the surgeon should then recede to a sufficient distance to make sure of gaining an inverted image, and next direct the patient to follow with the eye under observation gentle movements of the forefinger, in a horizontal and vertical direction, and then notice in which direction and at what distance he gains the inverted or the erect image.

Mr. Couper lays special stress upon the fact, that in this mode of examination the observer may—by taking strict account of the adjustment of his own eye—gain a much more definite result than the mere existence of asymmetry of the media. For instance, if the observer, with his eye adjusted for parallel rays, obtains at a minimum distance a clear image of the linear details of the fundus in one particular direction, and if, being emmetropic, he cannot, by any adjustment of which his eye is capable, obtain a clear image of those details running at a right angle to the former, he knows that he has before him a case of simple myopic astigmatism. Whereas, if he gets a clear image of certain details when his eye is accommodated for parallel rays, and can then, by exerting his accommodation, render this

---

[1] Donders, p. 490. [2] "Med. Times and Gazette," Jan. 30, 1869.

image dim, and at the same time gain a distinct view of linear details lying at a right angle to those first seen, he knows that he has to deal with simple hypermetropic astigmatism. Again, if no part of the image be distinct at the minimum distance except he exerts a certain amount of accommodation, and if, moreover, he is obliged to exert a different degree of accommodation in order to see in succession linear details placed at a right angle to each other, it proves that it is a case of compound hypermetropic astigmatism. Mr. Couper has also found that it is possible to diagnose astigmatism by means of the change of form which the inverted image of the optic disk undergoes, when the distance of the object lens from the eye is varied. This test is founded on an observation of Mr. Jonathan Hutchinson's regarding certain contrasted peculiarities of the inverted image in myopia and hypermetropia. In hypermetropia the size of the disk appears to diminish as the object lens is moved further from the eye of the patient; whereas in myopia it is enlarged. Now Mr. Couper has observed that in simple hypermetropic astigmatism the image of the disk contracts, as the lens recedes from the eye, in the diameter corresponding to the plane of minimum curvature, and undergoes little or no change in the size in the opposite diameter; whereas in simple myopic astigmatism, its image is enlarged in the diameter of maximum curvature, and remains unchanged in the opposite diameter. [The determination of astigmatism with the ophthalmoscope is a much more difficult matter, and the results less accurate than in cases of simple refractive anomaly. We know from Schweigger that in an astigmatic eye, seen with the erect image, the optic disk is elongated in the direction of the meridian of greatest refraction, while with the inverted image, it is in the meridian of least refraction. The glass that does away with the distortion is the measure of the degree of astigmatism. The test-point for examination in these cases is the light streak seen on the centre of curvature of the vessels. This streak loses its brilliancy and clearness of definition the moment the vessel is out of focus. This gives the direction of one of the principal meridians, and it is known that the other is at right angles to it. The refraction of each meridian is now to be determined separately, and the difference between the two will be the degree of astigmatism present. (Loring, loc. cit., pp. 34–41.) —B.]

Astigmatism is generally congenital and often hereditary; it may, however, also be acquired. [A certain degree of meridional asymmetry exists in all eyes, and cannot be regarded as abnormal, unless the acuteness of vision suffers thereby.—B.] The congenital astigmatism is mostly regular and dependent upon asymmetry of the cornea. In the majority of cases it is present in both eyes, although perhaps in varying degree. Donders has found that abnormal astigmatism occurs far more frequently in hypermetropic eyes than others; indeed, he even thinks that out of six hypermetropic eyes one suffers from abnormal astigmatism. The amblyopia which often exists in hypermetropia, and which cannot be remedied by spherical convex lenses, is mostly due to astigmatism. We often find that persons unconsciously correct a certain amount of astigmatism by holding their head on one side, and thus looking slantingly through their spectacles.

Acquired astigmatism is mostly caused by inflammatory changes in the cornea, which lead to consecutive flattening of the cornea, and leave behind them opacities and cicatrices; it may also be caused by irregularity in the position of the edges of the incision after the operation of extraction of tract. We occasionally find that if iridectomy, or iridodesis, is performed areas of opacity of the cornea, a considerable degree of amblyopia persists after the operation, although the pupil is now brought opposite to a transparent portion of the cornea. On examination, we then observe that in many of these cases this weakness of sight is due to astigmatism, and that vision is greatly improved by a cylindrical lens. Acquired astigmatism may also be caused by dislocation of the crystalline lens, more particularly if it is obliquely displaced in the area of the pupil.

The best examples of pure regular astigmatism are furnished by successful cataract operations, for then any irregular astigmatism which may have been caused by the lens, will, of course, have been removed.

The disturbance of vision produced by even a slight degree of astigmatism is often very great and annoying, as the form and shape of minute objects (such as small letters) are so changed, that they cannot be seen with distinctness, but look blurred and confused. This is due to the fact that certain portions of a letter are yet quite distinct, whilst others are faint or unapparent. Thus the vertical lines of the letter H may appear quite dark and clear, whilst the horizontal connecting line is almost invisible. This also gives a peculiar tremulousness and uncertainty to the outline of the object. On account of the coexistence of irregular astigmatism, the patient may also be affected with monocular diplopia or polyopia.

Regular astigmatism may be remedied by the use of cylindrical lenses, which enable us to correct the anomaly of refraction in each of the principal meridians.

A cylindrical lens is the segment of a cylinder, and refracts those rays of light the strongest which strike it in a plane at right angles to the axis of cylindrical curvature; whereas the rays which pass through its axis suffer no deviation at all. In this, therefore, the cylindrical lens differs from the spherical, which refracts the rays in all planes of the segment.

Now, if in a case of simple astigmatism the one principal meridian is normal, so that rays passing through it are united exactly upon the retina, and the other principal meridian is myopic or hypermetropic, and the rays passing through it are brought to a focus before or behind the retina, we should correct this anomaly of refraction by means of a cylindrical lens whose axis corresponds to the normal meridian. The effect of this would be that the rays which pass through its axis would undergo no refraction, whereas those that pass in a plane at right angles to the axis would undergo the necessary refraction, and thus neutralize the anomaly which obtains in this meridian.

A convex cylindrical lens should be placed in such a direction that its axis lies in the plane of the highest refracting meridian, in order that it may give to the rays which undergo the smallest degree of deflection such an increased amount of convergence as if they passed through the meridian of the greatest refraction.

The reverse obtains in the case of concave cylindrical lenses, for here the axis must correspond to the meridian of least refraction, so that the focal length of the meridian of greatest curvature may be increased, and made equal to that of the meridian of least refraction. A glance at Fig. 205, p. 649, will readily explain this.

I will now illustrate the choice of cylindrical lenses by some examples.

I. *Simple Astigmatism.*—The state of refraction of the one principal meridian is emmetropic, whereas that of the other is either myopic or hypermetropic.

1. *Simple Myopic Astigmatism* (Am).—Let us suppose that there is emmetropia in the principal horizontal meridian (the far point lying at an infinite distance, *i. e.*, $R = \infty$), but that in the principal vertical meridian there is myopia $= \frac{1}{8}$, then $Am = \frac{1}{8} - \frac{1}{\infty} = \frac{1}{8}$.

In order to correct this, a concave cylindrical lens of eight inches focus will be required, its axis corresponding to the horizontal meridian, so that the rays of light may here pass without undergoing any refraction, and only those which pass at a right angle to the axis (vertically) be refracted, so as to neutralize the myopia which exists in the principal vertical meridian. To be quite accurate, the lens should be slightly stronger (seven and one-half inches focus), for one-half an inch should be deducted from the strength of the concave lens, on account of the distance of the latter from the nodal point. In hypermetropia, on the other hand, this distance of about one-half an inch must be added to the number of the convex lens. In slight degrees of myopia or hypermetropia (below $\frac{1}{15}$ or $\frac{1}{10}$) we may, however, omit this distance in the calculation.

2. *Simple Hypermetropic Astigmatism* (Ah).—In the horizontal meridian let there be hypermetropia $= \frac{1}{10}$, in the vertical emmetropia, then Ah $= \frac{1}{10} - \frac{1}{\infty} = \frac{1}{10}$, and the patient will require a convex cylindrical lens of ten inches focus with its axis placed vertically.

II. *Compound Astigmatism.*—In this form it will be remembered, that myopia or hypermetropia exists in both the principal meridians, but that it varies in degree.

It will be found very much to facilitate the understanding of these cases of compound astigmatism, if we consider the eye to be affected with simple myopia or hypermetropia, but that there exists besides a maximum degree of this anomaly of refraction in one of the principal meridians. We have, therefore, a certain degree of myopia or hypermetropia common to the whole eye, besides a certain, special degree in one of the principal meridians.

1. *Compound Myopic Astigmatism* (M + Am).—Myopia exists in both meridians, but to a higher degree in the one than in the other.

In the principal vertical meridian let M $= \frac{1}{30}$.

In the principal horizontal meridian let M $= \frac{1}{15}$. We then have myopia $= \frac{1}{30}$ and Am $= \frac{1}{15} - \frac{1}{30} = \frac{1}{30}$, to be written as M $= \frac{1}{30} +$ Am $\frac{1}{30}$.

In such a case, a spherico-cylindrical lens is required, the one surface of which has a spherical, the other a cylindrical curvature, and its action is that of a plano-cylindrical lens combined with a plano-spherical lens, and it may be expressed by the formula for each of the refracting surfaces, united by a sign of combination.

The case which we have supposed, would therefore be corrected by

$$-\frac{1}{30} \, \text{s} \subset -\frac{1}{30} \, \text{c}.$$

For the spherical and cylindrical surface would require to have a negative focal distance of thirty inches, and the axis of the cylindrical surface would have to be placed horizontally.

2. *Compound Hypermetropic Astigmatism* (H + Ah).—Hypermetropia exists in both principal meridians, but more in the one than in the other.

In the vertical meridian let H $= \frac{1}{18}$. In the horizontal meridian let H $= \frac{1}{12}$. We have then H $= \frac{1}{18}$, and moreover Ah $= \frac{1}{12} - \frac{1}{18} = \frac{1}{36}$, and we write H $\frac{1}{18} +$ Ah $\frac{1}{36}$. Hence a positive spherico-cylindrical lens will be required, and it will be corrected by $\frac{1}{18} \, \text{s} \subset \frac{1}{36} \, \text{c}$, the axis of the cylindrical surface being placed vertically.

III. *Mixed Astigmatism.*—In this form, in which myopia exists in the one principal meridian, and hypermetropia in the other, we must make use of bi-cylindrical glasses. These consist of two cylindrical surfaces of curvature, the axes of which are perpendicular to one another, the one surface is concave, the other convex. In consequence of this, the effect of such lenses is to render parallel incident rays divergent in the plane of one axis, and convergent in that of the other. The axis of the concave surface must be placed in the direction of the hypermetropic meridian, and the axis of the convex surface in the direction of the myopic meridian. Their action may be expressed by the formula for each of the two planes, united by a sign of a right angle $\lfloor$.

1. *Mixed Astigmatism, with predominant myopia* (Amh).

In the vertical meridian let $M = \frac{1}{10}$. In the horizontal meridian let $H = \frac{1}{20}$. Therefore $Amh = M \frac{1}{10} + H \frac{1}{20} = \frac{1}{6\frac{2}{3}}$, and is corrected by $\frac{1}{20} c \lceil -\frac{1}{10} c$.

The axis of the convex surface to be placed vertically, that of the concave horizontally.

2. *Mixed Astigmatism with predominant hypermetropia* (Ahm).

In the vertical meridian let $M = \frac{1}{18}$. In the horizontal meridian let $H = \frac{1}{12}$. Therefore $Ahm = H \frac{1}{12} + M \frac{1}{18} = \frac{1}{7\frac{1}{5}}$, and is corrected by $\frac{1}{12} c \lceil -\frac{1}{18} c$.

The axis of the convex surface to be placed vertically, that of the concave surface horizontally.

These examples illustrate the method to be adopted in finding glasses to correct the astigmatism and the ametropia. But in many cases it is not advisable completely to neutralize the anomaly of refraction, both on account of the difference in the size of the retinal images which will occur if the lenses are strong, and also on account of the disturbance in the combined action of the ciliary muscle and the internal recti muscles. It is often desirable that the astigmatism should be wholly corrected, but that only a certain portion of the myopia or hypermetropia should be neutralized.

After the operation of extraction of cataract, the sight is often materially improved by cylindrical lenses, even although before the opacity of the lens the sight had been perfectly normal. Such cases can only be explained on the supposition that a certain degree of corneal astigmatism had been neutralized (compensated for) by some lenticular astigmatism, so that, when the lens is absent, the ill-effects from the corneal astigmatism make themselves felt. This condition must of course be distinguished from the acquired astigmatism due to a faulty cicatrization of the section. In all cases of extraction, in which the sight is not as good as might be expected from the general appearance of the eye, the presence of astigmatism should be looked for, and the effect of cylindrical lenses tried.

It is of great consequence that the axes of the surfaces of curvature of the cylindrical glasses should be situated in the principal meridians of the eye, for even a very slight deviation will give rise to considerable indistinctness of vision. In order to insure the exact adaptation of the glasses to the eye, the lenses should be set in round frames, which permit of their being readily rotated in any direction. When the proper position of the axis is found, the screw should be tightened, and the lens thus firmly fixed in the desired position. The clumsy and awkward appearance of the circular frames may be greatly diminished by making them of a smaller diameter, or by having the glasses ground down into oval ones, and then reset into oval frames. But this requires great exactitude and nicety.

Irregular astigmatism may be divided into two classes, the normal or physiological, and the abnormal or pathological.

Normal irregular astigmatism is due to irregularities in the structure and density of the crystalline lens, so that an aberration of the rays occurs as they traverse the different sectors, in consequence of which there is an imperfect coincidence, even after accommodation, of the images of the different sectors; and there is also the astigmatism proper to the image of each sector in itself. The normal irregular astigmatism is of course wanting in eyes in which the lens has been removed. The chief symptom of this form of irregular astigmatism is polyopia, but the acuteness of vision is not affected. Whenever the latter is diminished, we must regard it as abnormal irregular astigmatism.

Abnormal irregular astigmatism may depend upon some defect in the curvature of the cornea, or some irregularity in the structure or position of the lens. The irregularity in the curvature of the cornea may be due to thinning of the latter after keratitis, to conical cornea, or to a faulty union of the section in extraction of cataract. The defect of the lens may be owing to changes in its structure, *e. g.*, commencing cataract, or to displacement of the lens, so that its edge lies partially in the area of the pupil, which may also give rise to this form of astigmatism. On account of these irregularities in the cornea or lens, the refraction of luminous rays is much distorted; for not only do the rays in a certain diameter undergo irregular refraction, but even perhaps individual rays in the same diameter. The retina, therefore, receives a very confused and blurred image, and hence there is always a considerable degree of impairment of vision, the objects, moreover, looking more or less crooked and distorted (metamorphopsia). Monocular diplopia or polyopia is often also present. Amongst the objective symptoms of irregular astigmatism may be mentioned irregularity of the corneal reflections, the surface of the iris appearing perhaps also somewhat wavy. With the oblique illumination, changes in the curvature of the cornea or of the position of the lens are easily recognized. On examining the fundus with the ophthalmoscope, the optic disk and retinal vessels will appear distorted and irregular, and there will be a more or less well-marked parallax.

Whilst the irregular astigmatism cannot be corrected by cylindrical glasses, it is often susceptible of improvement by stenopæic spectacles, which render the image less distorted and confused, by excluding a large portion of the irregularly refracted rays. If regular astigmatism coexist with the irregular, it will generally be advantageous to correct this by proper cylindrical lenses.

8.—APHAKIA (ABSENCE OF THE CRYSTALLINE LENS).

This condition may be due to an operation for cataract, to absorption of the lens after traumatic cataract, or dislocation of the lens into the vitreous humor; it may also be congenital. The state of refraction is, of course, greatly altered by the absence of the lens. Thus, an emmetropic eye becomes strongly hypermetropic; a hypermetropic eye still more so; whereas a myopic eye will become less short-sighted, or, if the degree of myopia was very great, it may even become emmetropic. The power of accommodation is completely absent in aphakia. This has been now incontrovertibly proved by Donders' numerous and most exact experiments.

The acuteness of vision, even after the most successful operations for cataract, and with the aid of the most suitable glasses, does not usually reach the normal standard. In old persons, this is frequently due to certain senile changes which take place in all eyes, and often considerably deteriorate the sight. But we must not forget that the insufficient aid furnished by spherical glasses may be due to astigmatism, and we should, therefore, always try the effect of cylindrical glasses in such cases. Another not unfrequent cause is to be found in the presence of secondary cataract, or even in the wrinkling of the transparent capsule, which may produce considerable distortion and confusion of the retinal image.

Patients who have been operated upon for cataract require very strong convex glasses to neutralize the acquired hypermetropia. The strength of these glasses will vary according to the degree of the hypermetropia, i. e., the length of the optic axis; for the shorter the latter is, the stronger will the lens require to be. Two sets of glasses will be wanted, one for distant objects, and one for reading, sewing, etc. For the former purpose, the number generally ranges from four inches to five inches focus; for the latter, from two inches to two and a half inches focus. But as this varies considerably, different numbers must be tried until the best is found, and it must be remembered that in these lenses of high power, a slight difference may exert a very considerable effect upon the sight. In order to remedy the great spherical and chromatic aberration of light which is produced in these lenses from the difference in the thickness at the centre and at the periphery, such spectacles are generally set in a broad horn or tortoise-shell frame, which leaves only the more central portion of the glass exposed. If the patient is astigmatic, he will require a sphero-cylindrical glass, which, if made in the ordinary manner, will be very heavy and clumsy. To remedy this defect, Dr. Loring[1] has had the lenses made in the following manner: "A simple cylindric glass of the required strength is first set in the spectacle frame in the usual way, the axis of the glass, of course, running in the required direction. A thin plano-convex glass is then ground, and, taking advantage of the fact that lenses can be cemented by Canada balsam, this is firmly fixed by its plane surface to the back or plane surface of the cylindric glass." The weight of the two combined lenses when nicely made is only one-fourth of the ordinary cataract-glasses.

9.—PARALYSIS, SPASM, AND ATONY OF THE CILIARY MUSCLE.

Diminution or loss of accommodation from paralysis or atony of the ciliary muscle is occasionally met with after severe illness, the whole muscular system being greatly debilitated. In such cases, it is not unfrequently mistaken for amblyopia dependent upon general debility. It is also often met with after diphtheria, and appears to depend less upon general constitutional weakness, than upon some special and peculiar cause, the exact nature of which is undetermined. [A cold is often regarded as a cause, and often no cause can be found. Many cases are due to brain disease.—B.]

The symptoms of paralysis of the accommodation are very marked in emmetropic eyes. The patients find that they cannot accurately distinguish near objects, so that they are quite unable to read, write, or sew; but at a distance they can see distinctly. The far point has undergone no change in

---

[1] "Transactions of the Ophthalmological Society," 1871, p. 108.

position, but the near point has receded further from the eye. If we test the sight with a convex lens of six inches focus, we find, perhaps, that the near point has receded to five or five and one-half inches from the eye, and that the far point lies at six inches (the focal distance of the lens), hence that the power of accommodation is almost entirely lost. The position of the near point will, of course, vary with the degree of paralysis; if this is but slight (paresis), the near point may be but little removed from the eye, and the disturbance of vision but inconsiderable. If there is complete paralysis, the patients cannot generally distinguish any print smaller than No. 14 or 16 of Jäger, but can easily read the finest type with strong convex lenses. The sight is much less affected in short-sighted persons, for if the myopia $= \frac{1}{12}$ or $\frac{1}{14}$, they are still able to read at their far point (twelve or fourteen inches), as only the near point undergoes a change, and the far point lies sufficiently close to the eye to permit of small objects being seen distinctly. In hypermetropic patients it is, however, quite different, for in them both the near and distant sight is impaired, just as after the instillation of atropine. In incomplete paralysis, the symptoms often resemble those of asthenopia, and the true nature of the affection may be easily overlooked, if the range of the accommodation is not examined. Together with the paralysis of the accommodation, there is almost always paralysis of the constrictor pupillæ, and consequent dilatation of the pupil, as both muscles are supplied by the third nerve; and frequently other muscles of the eye supplied by this nerve, are also affected. In trying the sight, attention should be paid to this dilatation of the pupil, and the consequent presence of circles of diffusion upon the retina, and the patient should be directed to read through a small stenopæic opening. [Paralysis of accommodation also occurs without participation of the sphincter of the iris, and here the annoyance to vision is not so great, because the circles of dispersion are not so great. Micropsia is often complained of in these cases.—B.]

The treatment of cases of paralysis of the ciliary muscle must depend upon the cause. If the patient has been suffering from diphtheria or any debilitating disease, tonics must be our chief remedy. In the rheumatic form (due to exposure to cold or draught) or the syphilitic, iodide and bromide of potassium are of much use, as also a suppurating blister behind the corresponding ear. I have often found the most marked and speedy benefit from the latter remedy, so that a patient, who before could only decipher letters of 14 or 16 Jäger, was able, within twenty-four or forty-eight hours after the application of the blister, to read the finest print. I have also used the solution of the extract of Calabar bean with excellent results. I employ it of a strength sufficient to cause considerable contraction of the ciliary muscle and constrictor pupillæ, without, however, over-straining, and thus fatiguing these muscles. I then allow the effect to pass off entirely, and after a few days' rest, the extract is reapplied, so that the muscles may be periodically stimulated. The action of Calabar bean, and its peculiar effect upon the pupil, were fully investigated, in 1862, by Dr. Fraser,[1] in his valuable graduation thesis for the University of Edinburgh, on the "Characters, Action, and Therapeutic Uses of the Ordeal Bean of Calabar." And in 1863, Dr. Argyll Robertson discovered its effect upon the accommodation.[2]

[1] Further investigations on the physiological action of Calabar bean are contained in a more recent paper by Dr. Fraser, in the "Transactions of the Royal Society of Edinburgh," vol. 24.

[2] Shortly after this discovery of Dr. Argyll Robertson, I had the opportunity of carefully studying the effect of Calabar bean upon a case of paralysis of the ciliary muscle; a full account of which will be found in the "Med. Times and Gazette," May

On the application of a minute quantity of a strong solution (one drop equalling four grains of the bean) to the inside of the lower eyelid, a little irritation and redness are produced, but these pass off very rapidly. Within five or ten minutes the pupil begins to contract, and at nearly the same time the spasm of the ciliary muscle commences. The contraction of the pupil reaches its maximum degree (about one line in diameter) in from thirty to forty-five minutes. After two or three hours it gradually dilates again, but does not regain its normal size till after the lapse of two or three days, when it may even become larger than before. Even during its greatest contraction, the pupil is still under the influence of light. [A better preparation of the Calabar bean is the sulphate of eserine, solutions of two and four grains to the fluidounce of distilled water being used. It is not well, however, to use this drug for any lengthy period or very frequently, for it is apt to produce conjunctivitis and even iritis, besides occasioning considerable pain by the spasm of the muscle.—B.]

The spasm of the accommodation commences about the same time as the contraction of the pupil, and both the near and far point become greatly approximated to the eye, which becomes, in fact, strongly myopic. The far point in the emmetropic eye may be brought to five or six inches from the eye, and the near point to three or three and one-half inches. The effect upon the accommodation passes off much sooner than that upon the pupil, for three or four hours generally suffice to restore the state of refraction and accommodation to its normal condition.

That the spasm of accommodation is due to the action of the drug upon the muscle of accommodation, and not upon the iris, was incontrovertibly proved by Von Graefe[1], who tried its effects in a case of complete absence of the iris, and found that the action upon the accommodation took place at about the same time, and in exactly the same manner, as in eyes in which the iris was present. This action of the Calabar bean is, therefore, exerted upon the ciliary muscle, and is completely independent of its effects upon the iris.

The effect of Calabar bean in counteracting the action of atropine, has also been proved by many experiments. The weaker solutions of atropine are easily overcome by a strong solution of Calabar bean. But the complete paralysis of the accommodation by a strong solution of atropine (four grains to the fluidounce), is only temporarily overcome even by a very strong solution of Calabar bean, one drop equalling four grains; the pupil becomes smaller, and the state of refraction increased, but the action of atropine reasserts itself in the course of a few hours. In such cases, we must repeat the application of the Calabar bean when necessary, until the effect of the atropine upon the accommodation has disappeared.[2] [The hopes placed on Calabar bean have not been realized. The prognosis is generally favorable, but we should rely mainly upon a tonic course of treatment. In some cases, the galvanic current and faradic current have proved useful in restoring the muscle to its proper tone.—B]

Great fatigue of the ciliary muscle through over-exertion at near objects, may give rise to very severe symptoms of asthenopia, and this is best treated by the use of strong convex glasses (six to ten inches focus), for reading, etc. After they have been used for some time, the accommodation should be gradually exercised by employing weaker glasses, the distance of the object

---

[1] "A. f. O.," ix. 3, 118.

[2] Instead of the extract, the more elegant preparation of the gelatine disks may be employed. But these do not answer so well when we wish to stimulate the partially paralyzed muscle, as we cannot regulate the strength so exactly as in the solution.

remaining the same. The accommodation may also be rested by the application of a strong solution of atropine continued for some little time.

Spasm of the ciliary muscle (apparent myopia) is not of such unfrequent occurrence as is often supposed. We have already seen that it may accompany myopia and astigmatism; but it is most frequently observed in youthful hypermetropes who have strained their eyes much in reading, sewing, etc., without using convex glasses; this continued tension of the accommodation producing a spasmodic contraction of the ciliary muscle, or apparent myopia. Such patients complain chiefly of two sets of symptoms, viz., those of marked asthenopia during reading and fine work, and also that they are short-sighted. Dobrowolsky[1] states that the following are the principal symptoms of apparent myopia: The pupil is generally small, the shape of the eye is often decidedly hypermetropic, the anterior chamber shallow, and the iris arched forwards from the increased curvature of the lens, the optic disk and retina are hyperæmic, and there is not unfrequently a posterior staphyloma. There may be also a convergent squint, and there are marked variations in the state of refraction, the patient sometimes preferring one glass, sometimes another. On examining the sight of such patients, I have often found a great difference between the position of the far point in reading small print, and the degree of apparent myopia. Thus, for instance, the patient may not be able to read No. 1 further off than eight inches from the eye, and we suspect a myopia $= \frac{1}{8}$; but on trying him for distance, we discover our mistake; he can only read, perhaps, Snellen 50 at twenty feet, but a very weak concave lens (fifty or forty) enables him to read No. 20 $\left(V = \frac{20}{xx} \right)$. This fact should at once arouse our suspicions that we have to deal in reality with a case of apparent myopia, due to spasm of the ciliary muscle. If we now examine him with the ophthalmoscope, we find, when he is looking vacantly into the far distance, that the refraction is highly hypermetropic.

Liebreich[2] considers that spasm of the ciliary muscle is sometimes due to insufficiency of the internal recti, the excessive effort therefore required to maintain the necessary degree of convergence for reading, etc., being accompanied by excessive contraction of the ciliary muscle; in such cases he recommends the use of abducting prisms. The treatment of apparent myopia must consist chiefly in the methodical and prolonged use of a strong solution of atropine (gr. iv ad f$\mathfrak{z}$j) three or four times daily; sometimes it must be continued for several weeks before the spasm is overcome, and the ciliary muscle completely paralyzed. The effect of the atropine is often markedly accelerated by the application of the artificial leech, which also proves very useful in diminishing the symptoms of hyperæmia, or irritation of the optic nerve and retina. When the ciliary muscle is completely paralyzed, we can ascertain the exact degree of hypermetropia, and it is best to give the patient the proper convex glasses at once, so that he may wear them and get accustomed to them during the time the muscle is recovering from the effect of the atropine; for if we do not do this, we shall find that the spasm is apt to recur after the atropine has been left off for some time. If patients will not submit to the prolonged application of atropine, I generally give them strong convex glasses for reading, and try to persuade them to wear weak convex glasses (e. g., + 40) for distance. The effect of the latter is gradually to diminish the spasm of the muscle, so that after they have been worn for some time, a patient, who before could not perhaps decipher No. 50 of Snellen at twenty feet without a weak concave lens, may be able to see No. 20 without

[1] "Kl. Monatsbl.," 1868, p. 141.   [2] "A. f. O.," viii. 1, 259.

any glasses. But as they render distant objects indistinct for a length of time, but few patients will submit to this inconvenience. Where the patient will neither submit to the use of atropine nor of weak convex glasses for distance, I prescribe strong convex glasses for reading, and permit him the occasional and short use of the weakest concave glasses which make $V = \dfrac{20}{xx}$.

In doing this we must warn him strictly, that the concave glasses should only be used for a short time occasionally, as at the theatre, etc. Nagel has found benefit from the subcutaneous injection of strychnine in spasm of the ciliary muscle.[1] If the internal recti are weak, we may combine the use of convex glasses for reading, with the use of a prism (base inwards).

10.—SPECTACLES.

The spectacles which are generally used for the purpose of correcting some optical defect in the eye are either spherical or cylindrical lenses, or a combination of both. The properties of such lenses have been already sufficiently explained, and I shall, therefore, now only add a few remarks as to the different kinds of spectacles and their construction.

From the perusal of the different anomalies of refraction and accommodation, the reader will have been sufficiently impressed with the importance of the proper and scientific selection of spectacles. I have no hesitation in saying that the empirical, haphazard plan of selection generally employed by opticians, is but too frequently attended by the worst consequences; and that eyes are often permanently injured, which might, by skilful treatment, have been preserved for years. For this reason I must strongly urge upon medical men the necessity of not only examining the state of the eye, and ascertaining the exact nature of the affection of refraction or accommodation, but of going even a step further than this, and determining with care and accuracy the number of the required lens. For this purpose they must possess a case of trial-glasses,[2] containing a complete assortment of concave and convex lenses, glasses of corresponding number being kept by the optician. Written directions as to the focal distance of the required glass, and whether it is for distance or for reading, are to be sent to the optician.

The strength of any given convex lens may be easily ascertained by finding the distance at which the image of a distant object (a candle, the bars of a window frame, etc.), is distinctly formed on a sheet of white paper or the wall. The distance of this distinct image from the lens, gives the focal length of the latter. But if we have a set of trial glasses at hand, a

---

[1] "Kl. Monatsbl.," 1871, 391.

[2] Such trial cases are made by Messrs. Paetz and Flohr, of Berlin, and contain complete sets of concave and convex lenses, prismatic and tinted glasses, and a clip spectacle frame for holding the lenses. These lenses are defined in Prussian inches, which are almost identical with the English; whereas the French are considerably more. As the arrangement of the lenses in these trial cases is, however, made without any system, so that whilst there are very many and but slight gradations in the weaker glasses, those in the stronger are not sufficiently numerous, the difference in the refraction of the higher numbers is very great. Thus, whilst the difference in the refraction between the convex sixty and fifty is only one three-hundredth, that between three and one-fourth and three is one-thirty-ninth. To remedy these defects, as well as to simplify the trial cases, and greatly diminish the number of lenses, Zehender has proposed a new combination scale of glasses (vide "Klin. Monatsbl.," 1866). At the meeting of the International Ophthalmological Congress held last year in London, a large number of members agreed to substitute the use of the metre measure for that of inches in the determination of the strength of lenses, in order that their number may be the same in all countries, and for other practical reasons.

more simple and ready mode is to find the concave lens which completely neutralizes the convex one, and this at once gives us the number of the latter.

The complete neutralization of the convex lens by the concave is known by the fact that if the two are placed in close apposition, we can read as well through them as without any glass before the eye. Another test is, that if we regard a vertical line (e. g., the vertical bar of a window) through them, it remains perfectly immovable when the glasses are moved to and fro before the eye; whereas the line will distinctly move, if the two glasses do not neutralize one another, the more so, the greater the difference between them. If the object moves in the contrary direction to that in which the lenses are moved, it proves that the convex lens is the stronger of the two; whereas, if it moves in the same direction, the concave is the stronger. The strength of concave lenses may be tried in the same way.

Care should be taken that the spectacles fit accurately; that the glasses are on the same level, so that one is not higher than the other; that they are sufficiently close to the eyes; and that the centre of each glass is exactly opposite the centre of the pupil. The last point should be particularly observed in the selection of glasses which fit on the nose by means of a spring (pince-nez), for we find that, on account of their oval shape, these generally are not accurately centred. If they do not fit properly, so that their centre corresponds to the centre of the pupil, they act as prisms, and give rise to diplopia or a corresponding squint, and the latter may even become permanent, if their use is persisted in. Concave glasses should be quite close to the eye, otherwise they will diminish the size and distinctness of the retinal image. As the rays which impinge upon a concave lens are rendered divergent by it, it follows that the further the glass is removed from the eye, the fewer peripheral rays will enter the latter, in consequence of which the retinal image is diminished in size and intensity.[1] The reverse obtains in the case of convex glasses, for as they render the rays which impinge upon them more convergent, a greater number of peripheral rays will enter, the further (up to a certain point, of course) the convex glass is removed from it, the retinal image becoming at the same time larger and brighter.

Single eyeglasses should not, as a rule, be permitted, as they often lead to weakness of the other eye from non-use.

Besides the spherical and cylindrical spectacles, we must also consider the following kinds:

The periscopic glasses consist of concavo-convex, and convexo-concave lenses (so-called positive and negative menisci), and consequently have only a very slight spherical aberration. On this account, when the concave surface is turned towards the eye, there is less irregular refraction at the edge of the glass, so that the regularity of the images is much less impaired. In consequence of this, the observer can look more obliquely through them, as was first shown by Wollaston, who on this account termed them periscopic. Their chief disadvantages are that they reflect the light more, and are also more heavy and expensive than spherical lenses.

Spectacle glasses are sometimes required to have a different focus in the upper and lower part (pantoscopic spectacles). This is more especially the case if presbyopia coexists with myopia or hypermetropia. Thus, Franklin,

---

[1] It has already been stated that concave glasses diminish the retinal image by moving the nodal point further back, thus diminishing the angle of vision; whereas, convex glasses enlarge the retinal image, as they move the nodal point forwards, and thus increase the size of the angle of vision.

who was presbyopic and also slightly myopic, employed glasses, the lower half of which was convex, to neutralize the presbyopia, and the upper half concave to neutralize the myopia. In Paris such glasses are termed *verres à double foyer*, and are constructed by grinding in the upper part of the spectacle-glass, the surface which is turned from the eye, with another radius. Such spectacles must be placed at a proper height before the eyes, so that in looking at near objects the rays only fall upon the eye through the lower part; whereas, those from distant objects must only fall upon the upper part. This form of spectacle is found very useful by miniature painters, lecturers, etc.

Prismatic spectacles are sometimes employed either for the purpose of exercising and thus strengthening certain of the muscles of the eyeball, or to relieve them. The action of prisms has been already explained in the introduction (p. 47), and the use of prismatic spectacles will be found described in the article upon "Muscular Asthenopia." The prisms are generally turned with their base inwards (to relieve the internal recti muscles), and may either be used alone or in combination with convex or concave lenses. In the latter case, they are ground in such a manner as to combine the effect of a prism with that of a spherical lens. By turning the base of the prism inwards, the rays will be deflected somewhat to the inner side of the yellow spot, the eye will consequently move slightly outwards so as to bring the rays again upon the yellow spot; there will consequently be a less convergence of the visual lines, the effect being the same as if the object were placed somewhat further off, but it is seen under the same visual angle, and the divergence of the rays is also the same.

Closely allied to the prismatic glasses, are the decentred lenses of Giraud Teulon. They are constructed in such a manner, that the eccentric portions of two convex lenses are used instead of the centre, so that they must thus acquire a slightly prismatic action. Thus in convex lenses the centre should lie a little to the inner side of the visual lines, whereas in concave glasses the reverse obtains, and the centre should lie a little to the outer side of the visual lines.

Dr. Scheffler proposes to substitute for the common spherical lenses, glasses which are cut out from the periphery of a large lens, in such a manner as to act as decentred lenses. The advantage which he claims for them is, that with them the convergence of the visual lines undergoes an alteration in harmony with the change in the accommodation, which is not the case when the common spherical lenses are used. His work "Die Theorie der Augenfehler und der Brille," in which this subject is fully treated, has been translated into English by Mr. R. B. Carter.

[Stenopæic glasses often improve vision markedly in cases of cloudy cornea or lens, and they are most applicable for near objects. They have been recommended in cases of high degrees of myopia combined with loss of distinct vision, where, in connection with weak concave glasses, they improve the vision by lessening the size of the circles of dispersion without affecting that of the retinal images.—B.]

Eye-protectors are found of much service to guard the eye against very bright light, dust, or cold winds. The best are the medium blue curved eye-protectors. They are curved somewhat like a watch glass, so as to fit closely, except at the temporal side, where they permit a sufficient amount of air to enter and come in contact with the eye, to maintain the evaporation of the conjunctival moisture. They are greatly to be preferred to the goggles with wire or silk sides, or the glass spectacles with large glass side-pieces, for these keep the eye much too hot and close. The goggles are useful if the patient is exposed to the atmosphere very soon after a severe operation, when the eye is still inflamed and very susceptible to cold, but for all other purposes the curved glasses are to be preferred. Messrs. Salom (of 137 Regent Street) have lately introduced an excellent modification of the goggles, by adding thin gauze side-pieces to the curved blue eye-protectors, which render them quite as efficient as the goggles, and much lighter, as well as less unsightly and conspicuous.

The sense of dazzling of which many (more especially myopic) patients complain when they are exposed to bright sun or gaslight, is most effectually relieved by cobalt-blue glasses. It was formerly supposed that the red rays of the solar spectrum were the most trying to the eye, and consequently green glasses (which exclude the red rays) were much in vogue. But it is now a well-known fact, that it is not the red but the orange rays which are irritating to the retina, and as blue excludes the orange rays this is the proper color for such spectacles. Moreover, the blue color, on account of its more eccentric position in the solar spectrum, makes a less impression upon the retina. Smoke-glasses are not so good, and they more or less subdue and diminish the whole volume of light and color, and thus render the image somewhat indistinct.

It is often very desirable to combine the blue tint with the use of convex or concave spherical lenses; in the weaker glasses this can be very effectually done, but in the higher numbers it is difficult, for the varying thickness of the glass causes a considerable difference in the tint in the centre and at the edges of the lens. In such cases it will be well to adopt Mr. Laurence's suggestion, viz., to join a very thin piece of plain tinted glass with Canada balsam, to the back of a colorless spherical lens.

Besides the colored eye-protectors, which are used in order to diminish the bright glare of light, or to keep off the cold wind, dust, etc., there are those which are employed by workmen in order to protect the eye during their work against injury from pieces of stone, chips of steel, etc. The best are those made of thick plate glass, with wire or gauze sides, for they are sufficiently strong to resist the force of any, excepting a very large projectile. The chief objections to these are their expense and their weight. To obviate these defects, Dr. Cohn[1] has recommended the use of spectacles made of mica instead of glass. If the mica is of good quality, it is quite as transparent as glass, but lends a faint gray tint to objects, which does not, however, in the least diminish the acuity of vision, but rather tempers the light. They are made in the shape of the large curved eye-protectors, and should fit close to the eye, leaving only the temporal side somewhat open. They are much lighter and cheaper than the glass spectacles, and do not break on falling down.

11.—DIFFERENCE IN THE REFRACTION OF THE TWO EYES.

Differences in the refraction of the two eyes are not of unfrequent occurrence, and generally consist in differences in the degree of the myopia or hypermetropia in the two eyes; or, again, one eye may be emmetropic, the other myopic or hypermetropic; or myopia may exist in one eye, and hypermetropia in the other. [Unilateral astigmatism may also occur, but usually with myopic astigmatism in one eye there is myopia in the other, or with hypermetropic astigmatism in one eye there is hypermetropia in the other.— B.] Absence of the lens (aphakia) in one eye, gives rise of course to a very great difference in the state of refraction of the two eyes. In the majority of

[1] " Berliner Klinische Wochenschrift," February 24, 1868.

cases, the refraction of the two eyes is very nearly alike. Sometimes, however, we find considerable differences in the degree of myopia or hypermetropia. The practical question is, what kind of glasses are we to give to such patients? It might appear proper to furnish each eye with the glass suitable to its own state of refraction, but in practice we find that this does not generally answer, for the patients, as a rule, complain that such spectacles render their vision confused and indistinct, on account of the difference in the size of the two retinal images. It is best, therefore, to furnish both eyes with the glass which suits the least ametropic (hypermetropic or myopic) eye. If it is very desirable that the patient should enjoy the greatest possible acuteness of vision, we may give two different glasses, so as completely to neutralize the difference in the state of refraction, and the patient must try whether he is able to see distinctly and comfortably with them. Sometimes a little practice will enable him to do so, and then their use may be allowed. If this is not the case, we may partially neutralize the difference, and thus diminish the size of the circles of diffusion. Thus if the myopia of the one eye $= \frac{1}{14}$, and that of the other one-sixth, we may prescribe concave fifteen for the former, and concave nine or ten for the latter. It has also been advised that when the sight of the two eyes (which differ considerably in the degree of their myopia) is equally good, the glass which lies midway between the two degrees of myopia should be given for both. If, for instance, the one eye requires concave four and the other concave eight, it would be advisable to prescribe concave six for both eyes. But such glasses prove unsuitable, as they suit neither eye, being too strong for the one, and too weak for the other.

If there is a difference in the refraction of the two eyes—the one being myopic, the other hypermetropic—it is also often difficult to suit them with glasses which shall neutralize each anomaly. This is owing to the difference in the size of the retinal images which will be produced, for the convex lens will enlarge, the concave lens diminish, the size of the retinal image, and this may prove a source of considerable confusion. In all cases of difference in the refraction of the two eyes, the patient should try the glasses for some little time, so as, if possible, to become accustomed to them, before we decide definitely as to the kind of glasses which we shall prescribe.

[In nearly all cases of difference of refraction with good vision in both eyes, it can be demonstrated that only that eye is used for near vision, which receives distinct retinal images with the least effort of accommodation. Still a normal binocular vision *may* exist in spite of the dissimilarity of the retinal images, the circles of dispersion in one eye being overlooked. If one eye be hypermetropic and the other emmetropic or myopic, the former is usually amblyopic.

If there is a difference of refraction, and at the same time there exists the mutual visual act and binocular fixation, the first thing to determine is which eye possesses the better vision and also the least error of refraction. The proper lens is then chosen for this eye, and *generally* the same lens may be prescribed for the other eye. Sometimes, however, the best results are gained by providing each eye with its best correcting lens. If the eye with the best vision has also the greatest error of refraction, it is better to give the other eye a proportionately weak lens. ("Schweigger," loc. cit., pp. 74-76.)—B.]

CHAPTER XV.

AFFECTIONS OF THE MUSCLES OF THE EYE.[1]

1.—ACTIONS OF THE MUSCLES OF THE EYE.

In order properly to understand the physiological action of the different muscles of the eyeball, we must consider the eye as a sphere, the centre of which being fixed, its movements can only be rotations around a fixed axis, and hence there can be no change of locality.[2] But for the purpose of accurately determining these rotations, it does not suffice to ascertain the change of position which *one* point upon the surface of the sphere may undergo, but we must take into consideration the position of a *second* point, which must not, however, stand in the relation of a pole to the first. If we take the centre of the cornea for the one point, and the vertical meridian (the greatest circle standing perpendicular to the equator of the eye) as the second, we shall be easily able to determine the rotations which the eye undergoes, by watching in which direction the centre of the cornea moves, and what kind of inclination the vertical meridian undergoes.

For the purpose of discovering the inclination of the vertical meridian in the different positions of the eye, Donders devised the following ingenious experiment. Having vertically suspended a colored thread, he looked at it until its image was impressed upon his retina (this image was of course in the vertical meridian of the eye), he next moved his head in the different directions in which he desired to ascertain the inclinations of the vertical meridian, and then measured the angle which the image upon his retina formed with a line held vertically before his eye. As the position of the retinal image of course agreed with that of the vertical meridian, he was

---

[1] For further information upon the diseases of the muscles of the eye, I must refer the reader to Von Graefe's articles in the "A. f. O.," vols. i. and iii., and to his work entitled "Symptominlehreder Augenmuskellähmungen;" to Alf. von Graefe's "Motilitätsstörungen des Auges;" and also to my articles in the "R. L. O. H. Rep.," vols. ii. and iii.; and in the "Med. Times and Gazette," 1865. [Graefe und Saemisch's "Handbuch der Augenheilk.," vi. 1.—B.]

[2] It is, however, not quite correct to consider the eye as a sphere (globe) and its centre of motion as situated in the centre of the visual axis, for it is in reality placed somewhat behind it, as was shown by numerous measurements made by Donders and Doyer. They found, moreover, that the exact position of the centre of motion (turning point) varies with the state of refraction of the eye. On this subject Donders says: "1. In the emmetropic eye, the centre of motion is situated at a considerable distance (one and seventy-seven one-hundredths millimetre) behind the middle of the visual axis. 2. In myopic individuals the centre of motion is situated more deeply in the eye, but also further from the posterior surface, and indeed so that in the eyes of such persons the relation between the parts of the visual axis situated before and behind the centre of motion is nearly the same as in the emmetropic eye. 3. In the hypermetropic eye the centre of motion is situated not so deeply, but relatively closer to the posterior surface of the eye."—"Anomalies of Refraction and Accommodation," p. 182.

enabled in this way readily to ascertain the direction of the vertical meridian in every movement of the eyeball.

I must here point out that from habit we see objects vertical and not slanting, even although the vertical meridian should be inclined.

Based upon these experiments, Donders laid down the following rules as to the position of the vertical meridian in the different movements of the eye:

1. In looking in the horizontal meridian plane, straightforwards, to the right or to the left, the vertical meridian suffers no inclination, but remains vertical.

2. In looking in the vertical meridian plane, straightforwards, upwards or downwards, the vertical meridian also remains vertical.

3. In looking diagonally upwards to the left, the vertical meridians of both eyes are inclined[1] to the left and parallel (that of the left eye slanting outwards, that of the right inwards).

4. In looking diagonally downwards to the left, the vertical meridians of both eyes are inclined to the right and parallel (that of the left eye inwards, that of the right outwards).

5. In looking diagonally upwards to the right, the vertical meridians of both eyes are inclined to the right and parallel (that of the right eye outwards, that of the left inwards).

6. In looking diagonally downwards to the right, the vertical meridians of both eyes are inclined to the left and parallel (that of the right eye inwards, that of the left eye outwards).[2]

For the sake of simplicity, we may consider the muscles which move the eyeball as consisting of three pairs. The two muscles of each pair act in an antagonistic way to each other, but each pair has a common traction-plane, and hence, also, a common axis of turning, around which the one muscle describes a positive, the other a negative rotation. Now, although these three pairs of muscles would be capable of placing the eyeball in every kind of position, we find that only a small portion of all the possible positions really occurs; for Donders has demonstrated, that as every position of the eye is given by the direction of the visual line with regard to the head, and by the simultaneous rotation (inclination of the meridian planes to the visual plane), so a given direction of the visual line is always associated with a definite degree of rotation (Donders' law). This, of course, considerably curtails the number of the positions of the eye, and substitutes a physiological certainty for the unlimited mechanical possibility (Von Graefe).[3]

In order to ascertain the direction in which a muscle acts, we must draw through it a straight line, which shall unite the middle of its origin with the middle of its insertion. A plane laid through this line and the turning-point of the eye, is termed the *plane of the muscle* (*muscle-plane*), and a line standing perpendicularly upon this plane in the turning-point is called the *axis of turning*. Now, we shall find it of the greatest importance in the paralyses of the different muscles of the eyeball, to know in which positions of the eye certain muscles act most upon the height of the cornea, and in which positions most upon the vertical meridian. We shall find that the effect upon the height of the cornea is the greater, the more the muscle-plane coincides with the vertical meridian plane, and the more the axis of turning

---

[1] The *upper* end of the vertical meridian line is the one always described.

[2] These rules have been translated from Alfred von Graefe's excellent work, "Klinische Analyse der Motilitäts-störungen des Auges."

[3] "Symptomenlehre der Augenmuskellähmungen," p. 81.

approaches the horizontal diameter. On the other hand, the power over the vertical meridian will be least in this position, but will increase in proportion as the eye is turned in the opposite direction, for the axis of turning then approaches more and more the position of the optic axis.

1. The axis of turning of the first pair (rect. ext. and int.) is vertical, and coincides with the vertical diameter of the eyeball.

2. The axis of turning of the second pair (rect. sup. and infer.) lies also in the horizontal meridian, and is directed from before and inwards to behind and outwards, in such a manner that it forms with the optic axis an angle of about 70°.

3. The axis of turning of the third pair (oblique sup. and infer.) lies also in the horizontal meridian, and is directed from before and outwards to behind and inwards, in such a manner that it forms an angle of about 35° with the optic axis,

Let us now consider the action of the different muscles upon the position of the eyeball and the direction of the vertical meridian.

[Fig. 211.

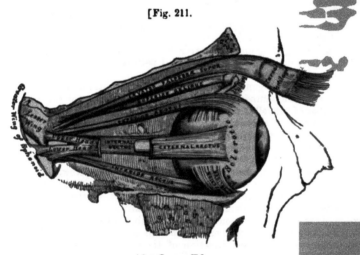

After Gray.—H.]

The superior rectus muscle arises from the portion of bone just in front of the optic foramen, and runs obliquely over the globe to be inserted into the sclerotic, about three lines from the cornea. But its course is so oblique, that the internal portion of its insertion lies almost one line nearer the cornea than its external portion. Its action is to move the eye upwards and slightly inwards, inclining the vertical meridian inwards. [Fig. 211.—H.]

The inferior rectus also arises from the optic foramen, and its tendon is inserted about three lines from the lower edge of the cornea, but somewhat (about half a line) to the inner side of a supposed vertical line drawn through the centre of the cornea. It moves the eye downwards and inwards, and inclines the vertical meridian outwards.

The superior and inferior recti exert most influence upon the height of the cornea, when the eye is turned outwards, as the muscle-plane then coincides more and more with the vertical meridian plane, and the axis of turning approaches the horizontal diameter. These muscles act most upon the inclination of the vertical meridian, when the eye is turned inwards, as the axis of turning then approaches more and more the optic axis.

The external rectus arises from the common tendon, and runs along the outer side of the eyeball to be inserted about three lines from the external edge of the cornea. It moves the eye directly outwards, without producing any inclination of the vertical meridian.

The internal rectus is the strongest of the ocular muscles, and nearly four lines in width; it arises from the common tendon, and is inserted into the sclerotic about two and a half lines from the inner edge of the cornea. It moves the eye directly inwards, and does not incline the vertical meridian.

The superior oblique arises just in front of the inner portion of the optic foramen, and runs along towards the inner angle of the eye, where its tendon passes through the trochlea, and then, bending outwards and backwards, it spreads out like a fan to be inserted into the upper, outer, and posterior quadrant of the eyeball, by a tendon three lines in length, the convexity of which looks backwards. The action of the superior oblique is to roll the eye downwards and outwards, and to incline the vertical meridian inwards.

The inferior oblique arises from a depression in the orbital edge of the superior maxillary bone, slightly towards the outer side of the lachrymal sac, and passes along the floor of the orbit in an outward, downward, and backward direction, until it has passed beneath the inferior rectus (to which it is connected by fibro-cellular tissue), when it curves upwards and backwards, and passes to the inner side of the external rectus, to be inserted by a short tendon close to the insertion of the superior oblique. The inferior oblique rolls the eye upwards and outwards, and inclines the vertical meridian outwards. The two oblique muscles act most upon the height of the cornea when the eye is moved inwards, as their muscle-plane then coincides more and more with the vertical meridian plane; whereas, they act most upon inclination of the vertical meridian when the eye is turned outwards, for then the axis of turning approaches more and more the optic axis.

Having described the action of the individual muscles, we must now pass on to the consideration of the movements of the eye which are produced by the combined action of several muscles. In so doing, we have to consider the following eight different movements of the eye:[1]

1. The movement vertically upwards, in which the vertical meridian remains vertical, is brought about by the action of the superior rectus and inferior oblique. The superior rectus alone draws the cornea upwards and inwards, and inclines the vertical meridian inwards, hence some other muscle (inferior oblique), whose action is to draw the cornea upwards and outwards and incline the vertical meridian outwards, must associate itself with the superior rectus, in order to counterbalance its action.

[1] In order to comprehend the various combined movements of the eye, we must assume a "primary position" of the eye, starting from which the visual line (Blicklinie) may be moved directly upwards or downwards, or directly to the right or to the left, without the occurrence of any rotatory turning or movement, i. e., without any inclination of the vertical meridian towards the visual line. This primary position corresponds very closely to that of the eyes when (the head being erect) they are fixed upon some object on the horizon lying in the median plane of the head. According to Helmholtz, the law regulating the movements of the normal eyes directed parallel may therefore be expressed as follows: "If the visual line passes from the primary position into any other position, the rotatory movement of the eyeball in this secondary position is of such a kind as if it (the eyeball) had been turned round a fixed axis lying perpendicular to the first and second direction of the visual line." (Listing's law.) "Physiologischen Optik," p. 466.

2. In moving the eye diagonally upwards and inwards, the vertical meridian being inclined inwards, the superior rectus is chiefly associated with the internal rectus. But as the latter has no effect upon the vertical meridian, the superior rectus would incline it too much inwards, and hence disturb its parallelism with the vertical meridian of the other eye (which is inclined outwards). Some other muscle, whose action is to incline the vertical meridian outwards, must, therefore, be called into play, in order to check the action of the superior rectus. We shall again find in the inferior oblique the muscle required; moreover, on account of its having least influence on the vertical meridian when the eye is turned upwards and inwards, it will not over-correct the action of the superior rectus, but only limit it.

3. In moving the eye diagonally upwards and outwards, the vertical meridian being inclined outwards, the superior rectus acts in conjunction with the external rectus. But as the latter has no influence on the position of the vertical meridian, and as the superior rectus turns it inwards, we must call into requisition some other muscle, which shall not only counterbalance the effect of the superior rectus upon the vertical meridian, but shall even more than correct it, and incline the latter outwards. The inferior oblique will be able to do this, for the eye is now in the position (upwards and outwards) in which the inferior oblique acts most upon the vertical meridian.

4. The movement vertically downwards, the vertical meridian remaining vertical, is produced by the combined action of the inferior rectus and superior oblique. The action of the inferior rectus alone, would be to draw the eye downwards and inwards, and to incline the vertical meridian outwards, hence it must be associated with the superior oblique, whose action is to move the eye downwards and outwards, and to incline the vertical meridian inwards, and thus to counterbalance the inferior rectus.

5. In the movement diagonally downwards and inwards, the vertical meridian being inclined outwards, the inferior rectus is associated with the internal rectus, and the superior oblique is required to limit the effect of the inferior rectus upon the vertical meridian, and to preserve the parallelism of the meridians.

6. In the movement diagonally downwards and outwards, the vertical meridian being inclined inwards, the inferior rectus is associated with the external rectus, and the superior oblique is called into play, not only to counterbalance the effect of the inferior rectus upon the vertical meridian, but to over-correct this, and incline the latter inwards.

7. The movement directly outwards is produced by the action of the external rectus.

8. The movement directly inwards is produced by the action of the internal rectus.

The following tabular arrangement will enable the reader to remember more easily the manner in which the different movements of the eye are produced:

Movement	Is produced by the action of the
Upwards	Superior rectus and inferior oblique.
Downwards	Inferior rectus and superior oblique.
Inwards	Internal rectus.
Outwards	External rectus.
Upwards and inwards .	Superior rectus, internal rectus, and inferior oblique.
Upwards and outwards .	Superior rectus, external rectus, and inferior oblique.
Downwards and inwards .	Inferior rectus, internal rectus, and superior oblique.
Downwards and outwards	Inferior rectus, external rectus, and superior oblique.

The effect of the recti muscles is to draw the eye *into* the orbit, that of the oblique muscles is to draw it out.

The nerves supplying the muscles of the eye are the third, fourth, and sixth.

The third nerve supplies the superior, inferior, and internal rectus, the inferior oblique, the levator palpebræ superioris, the constrictor pupillæ, and the ciliary muscle.

The fourth nerve supplies the superior oblique.

The sixth nerve supplies the external rectus.

There are two different kinds of binocular movements, viz., the associated and the accommodative [or converging.—B.]. In the former, the visual lines remain parallel, whereas in the accommodative movements they converge towards each other, and meet in the object. When the muscles of both eyes are quite at rest, the angle formed by the visual lines of the two eyes is called the muscular mesoropter; and the convergence of the visual lines is such, that their prolongation would meet at a point varying from eight to twelve feet in front of the eyes. I must here mention the fact, that in looking downwards there is always an increased tendency to convergence, whereas in looking upwards, there is a greater tendency to divergence. Hence a convergent squint becomes more marked when the patient looks downwards, and divergent squint when he looks upwards.

We have now briefly to consider the symptoms, diagnosis, and treatment of the paralytic affections of the different muscles of the eye, and I shall commence with the simplest and easiest form of paralysis, viz., that of the external rectus muscle.

To prevent needless repetition, and to avoid the chance of any symptom being overlooked, it is always best to follow a certain routine in examining patients supposed to be affected with strabismus, or paralysis of one or more of the muscles of the eye. Such an examination is best begun, by directing the patient (who should hold his head quite straight and immovable) to follow with his eyes some object, such as a pen or ruler, held at a distance of a few feet, and moved in all directions.* Any abnormality in the movement of either eye will thus become at once apparent. We next cover one eye (say the right) with our hand, the patient the while keeping his eyes steadily fixed upon the object, and we then observe whether the left eye remains immovable, or makes a movement in order to bring its visual line to bear upon the object. In the latter case, we know at once that this eye had before deviated from the object; thus, if it moves downwards, it before stood too high, and *vice versâ.*

2.—PARALYSIS OF THE EXTERNAL RECTUS MUSCLE (OF THE LEFT EYE.)

If the object (a lighted candle) is held in the horizontal meridian plane about four or five feet in front of the patient, we find that both visual lines are steadily fixed upon it, for upon the closure of either eye the other makes no movement. The object is then successively moved to the right of the patient, then upwards and downwards, and still both eyes follow it accurately. But when it is moved somewhat to the left side of the median line, we find that the left eye lags behind, thus giving rise to a convergent squint, which increases in proportion as the object is moved further to the left. As the paralysis of a muscle only shows itself when the eye is moved in a direction which calls into action the muscle in question, the paralysis of the left external rectus does not become manifest until the eye has to be moved in a direction to the left of the median line.

In a recent case of complete paralysis of the external rectus, it will be found that when the healthy eye is closed, and the object moved slightly into the left half of the field of vision, the left eye will attempt to follow it, not, however, in a straight, horizontal direction, but by a zigzag, rotatory movement, brought about by the action of the superior and inferior oblique.

[This is by no means always so, for in many cases of recent paralysis, there is absolutely no motion beyond the median line. In the cases where an oscillatory motion or zigzag action is observed in the affected eye, the external rectus is not completely paralyzed, but only partially so. There can be no motion where there is complete paralysis of a motor nerve.—B.]

A third symptom is that the secondary deviation is considerably greater than the primary.[1] This is a symptom of great importance in distinguishing the paralytic from the common concomitant squint. The deviation of the squinting eye is termed the *primary* deviation. Now if the healthy eye is covered, the other will move in a certain direction to adjust its visual line upon the object, which movement will be accompanied by an associated movement of the healthy covered eye, which thus becomes the squinting eye, and this movement of the healthy eye is termed the *secondary* deviation.

To render this more intelligible, let us presume that in our supposed case of paralysis of the left external rectus, the object is moved somewhat to the left side of the patient. At a certain point, a slight degree (say one line) of convergent squint of the left eye will appear owing to the inability of this eye to follow the object. If we now cover the right eye with our hand, the left will make an outward movement of one line in order to direct its visual line upon the object, but the right eye will simultaneously make an associated movement inwards of perhaps two and a half or three lines. This secondary deviation (two and a half or three lines) is therefore considerably greater than the primary (one line). The reason of this is easily explained. As the external rectus of the left eye is insufficiently innervated, it demands a greater impulse of the will to bring about this movement of one line, than if the innervation were normal. But this increased impulse also affects the associated, healthy internal rectus of the right eye, and thus produces a greater amount of movement in this eye. Hence, it is an invariable rule in all cases of paralysis, that the secondary deviation considerably exceeds the primary, whereas in the common concomitant squint the two are exactly equal.

The linear measurement of a squint may be made as follows: We note a spot upon the lower eyelid, which would correspond to an imaginary

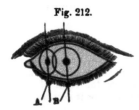

Fig. 212.

vertical line drawn through the centre of the pupil of the squinting eye, when the other eye is fixed upon an object held at from eight to twelve inches distance. The normal eye is then closed, and the squinting eye directed upon the object, and the spot on the lower lid which now corresponds to a vertical line drawn through the centre of the pupil is again noted, and the distance between the first and second spot gives the linear size of the squint. These spots may be at first marked with a dot of ink upon the lower lid, but a little practice will soon enable us quickly and accurately to estimate the distance between

[1] To watch the position of the eye excluded from participation in the act of vision, a slip of slightly frosted glass should be placed before the one eye, instead of covering it with the hand; for whilst the glass prevents the patient from seeing, it does not prevent our observing the position of the eye.

them. This proceeding is illustrated in Fig. 212. *A* represents the mark corresponding to the centre of the pupil when the eye is squinting, *B* the mark corresponding to the centre of the pupil when the eye is fixed upon the object. The distance between *A* and *B* gives the size of the squint.

It is, however, still more convenient to employ Mr. Laurence's strabismometer (Fig. 213), which consists of any ivory plate (*P*) moulded to the conformation of the lower eyelid. Its border is graduated in such a manner, that while the centre is designated 0, Paris lines and half lines are marked off on each side of 0. The handle (*H*) is attached to the plate. The plate is applied to the border of the lower eyelid of the squinting eye, and the size of the squint can be read with great ease and accuracy.[1]

[Dr. Galezowski's[2] binocular strabismometer consists of a graduated horizontal bar, upon which slide, in the sulcus of a screw, two needles; these, when placed opposite the centre of each corresponding cornea, indicate, by means of the scale on the bar, the degree of deviation.

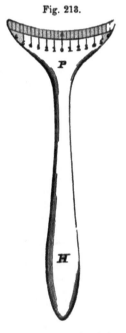

Fig. 213.

The transverse bar is held on a level with the eyelids, the handle of the instrument upwards, and the fork of the bar against the root of the nose. By turning the little buttons at the extremities of the bar, the needles are moved until each is found opposite the centre of the cornea, as is shown in Fig. 214. The graduation of the transverse bar enables us to determine the degree of deviation with ease and precision. Thus, with this ingenious and simple little instrument, we can measure with exactitude the degree of deviation as well as the precise result obtained by tenotomy.—H.]

Another symptom which is at once characteristic of a paralytic affection, is the erroneous projection of the visual field. For instance, if we close the right eye and tell the patient to strike quickly with his finger (if he does it slowly, he will have time to correct his mistake) at an object held somewhat towards the left median line, he will miss hitting it by going too much to the left side of it. The reason of this is, that the insufficiently innervated external rectus requires to make a contraction far exceeding the extent of the required movement, and far greater than would be necessary if the innervation were normal. In consequence of this, the patient overestimates the amount of movememt and believes the object to lie further to the side of the affected muscle than it really does, and consequently strikes too much to the left. If the paralytic affection is not too complicated, the patients in time learn to correct these errors of projection. The dizziness which they often complain of is not necessarily due to a cerebral lesion, but is generally owing to the confusion which arises from the diplopia, and the erroneous projection of the visual field.

[Von Graefe's method is more complicated but somewhat more exact. By its means he is enabled to determine the degree of the squint and the relations

---

[1] Meyer and Galezowski have more lately devised binocular strabismometers, which are, however, more expensive and less handy.

[2] ["Medical Times and Gaz.," 1869, i. 401.—H.]

of the squinting eye to its collective motion in the horizontal plane, and he also makes the measurements directly upon the scleral curvature, all starting from the external commissure of the lids. (See Graefe u. Saemisch's "Handb. d. Aug.," vi. 1, S. 98.)—B.].

[Fig. 214.]

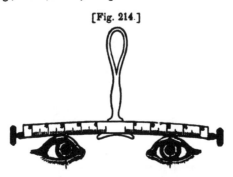

The manner of examining the position of double images, and the action and uses of prismatic glasses, have been explained in the introductory chapter, p. 46.

In a case of paralysis of the external rectus, the diplopia will appear when the object is moved into the left half of the visual field, but will be absent in the right half. The distance between the double images will increase the further the object is moved to the left. The double images show only lateral differences, being parallel, of the same height, and homonymous. It is, however, an interesting fact, that although the external rectus has no direct influence upon the vertical meridian, it yet, by assisting in the external diagonal positions of the eyeball, helps in preserving the parallelism of the vertical meridians of the two eyes. For instance, if the patient be directed to look at an object held diagonally upwards to the left, the right eye will be moved into the necessary position, by the combined action of the superior rectus, inferior oblique, and the internal rectus, its vertical meridian being inclined to the left. The left eye requires, in order to be moved upward and outwards, the combined action of the superior rectus, the inferior oblique, and the external rectus. But as the latter is paralyzed, the left eye will remain almost straight, and its vertical meridian vertical (instead of being inclined towards the left); the parallelism of the vertical meridians is therefore destroyed, and they converge at the top, whilst the double images appear to the patient to diverge at the top. But as in conformity with the laws of normal vision, the image which falls in the slanting meridian of the healthy right eye appears straight to the patient, the image of the affected eye will necessarily appear slanting.

Hence, in the diagonal positions to the left, viz., upwards and outwards, and downwards and outwards, the double images will show not only a difference in inclination, but also in height. As the external rectus is engaged, together with the superior rectus and inferior oblique, in bringing about the movement f the eye diagonally upwards and outwards, its paralysis must impair this, nd also affect the position of the vertical meridian, which, instead of being allel with that of the right eye, and inclined to the left, will be nearly cal, and consequently the two vertical meridians will converge at the top, ouble images appearing to the patient to diverge. A glance at Fig. 215 eadily explain this.

In Fig. 215, I represents the healthy right eye, whose vertical meridian $A B$ is vertical, and whose horizontal meridian $C D$ is horizontal, the image $a b$ falls in the vertical meridian.   II is the left eye affected with paralysis of the external rectus, in the position upwards and outwards the vertical meridian $A' B'$ is not parallel to that of the right eye, but converges towards it ($A'' B''$).   The image $a' b'$ will consequently not fall in the vertical meridian, but in the upper and outer ($A'' D''$), and the inner and lower ($C'' B''$)

Fig. 215.

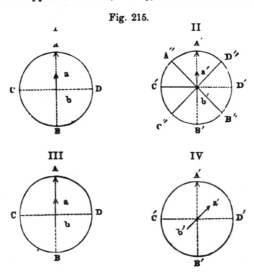

quadrants of the retina.   The double image will, therefore, appear to the patient to be turned towards the left, and to diverge at the top from that of the right eye (III and IV, $a b$ and $a' b'$).

I must here again call attention to the fact that the inclinations of the vertical meridians are merely relative, so that, although in reality the image of the healthy eye may be the one which is inclined, it generally appears to the patient to be straight, and the image of the affected eye is the one which seems to be slanting, although its vertical meridian may remain vertical.

We also meet with a curious phenomenon in this movement (upwards and outwards), viz., a difference in the height of the double images, without any

Fig. 216.

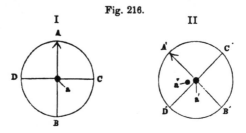

difference in the height of the cornea.   This apparent anomaly is easily explained by a glance at Fig. 216.   In I the rays from the object will fall on the yellow spot *a*, but in the left eye (II), on account of the convergence of the eyes and the inclination inwards of the vertical meridian (*a' a''*), the rays will not fall upon *a'*, but on *a''*, a point in the inner and upper quadrant of the retina, and hence the double image will lie to the left side, and below the object. Whereas, in the diagonal position downwards and outwards, the double image will lie to the left and above the object, and be inclined towards the right.

The position of the head is also characteristic, for the patient carries it turned slightly to the left, in order to avoid the diplopia, by bringing all objects as much as possible into the right half of the field of vision.

The *prognosis* is generally favorable if the paralysis of the external rectus muscle is acute, not too considerable in extent, and not dependent upon a cerebral lesion. Such cases are often completely cured, or very greatly relieved. Sometimes, however, secondary contraction of the internal rectus of the same eye supervenes, on account of the diminished force opposed to the action of the latter muscle. In this way, a permanent convergent squint of this eye may be produced. But if the affected eye enjoys the better sight of the two, and is only suffering from a partial paralysis of the external rectus, the patient may use it, in spite of the effort required, in preference to the other, which will squint considerably inwards, and perhaps permanently so.

In paralysis of the external rectus, a prism would have to be applied with its base to the temple, so that the rays may be refracted outwards; for, on account of the convergence of the visual line, the rays from the object will fall on the inner side of the yellow spot. Prismatic glasses may be used for two purposes: 1, simply to free the patient from the annoyance of diplopia; 2, for the purpose of slightly exercising the paralyzed muscle, and so gradually strengthening it. In the former case, we prescribe the number of prism which completely neutralizes the diplopia at a certain distance. Whereas, if we desire to exercise the affected muscle, we order a prism which only approximates the double images; this proves very confusing to the patient, and he endeavors, if possible, to fuse them into one by a voluntary exertion of the paralyzed muscle. In doing this, care must be taken that the prism is not too weak; at first, one should be selected which nearly fuses the double images, and then, as the muscle becomes stronger, a gradually weaker prism may be prescribed.[1]

3.—PARALYSIS OF THE THIRD NERVE.

The third is the principal motor nerve of the eyeball; it divides in the orbit into two branches, an upper and a lower. The former supplies the superior rectus and the levator palpebræ superioris, the latter, the internal rectus, inferior rectus, inferior oblique, sphincter, pupillæ, and ciliary muscle. According to Volkmann and Fäsebeck, the third also sends a small branchlet to the superior oblique and external rectus.

[1] This certain amount of power, which a partially paralyzed muscle generally possesses of still acting in order to unite the double images, is termed by Von Graefe "the power of fusion," and the extent of the field through which the muscle can thus extend single vision is termed "the range of fusion." He points out, moreover, that the extent of this power of fusion is of importance with regard to the diagnosis of the cause of the paralytic affection; for in cerebro-spinal paralysis the range of fusion is extremely small. In several cases of incipient dementia he has seen it almost entirely lost. ("Symptomenlehre der Augenmuskellähmungen," p. 36.)

The paralysis of the third nerve may vary in degree and extent, and may be complete or partial. 1. All the muscles supplied by it may be more or less implicated; they may be all completely or all partially paralyzed; or, again, some may be completely paralyzed, whilst the rest are only partially affected. 2. One or more muscles may be completely or partially paralyzed, the rest being unaffected.

Before describing the symptoms presented by the isolated paralyses of the individual muscles supplied by the third nerve, it will be well to glance at those which are caused by a paralysis of all branches of the nerve.

Let us, therefore, suppose the existence of a complete paralysis of the third nerve of the left eye. The following would be the symptoms present in such a case: The upper eyelid hangs down over the eye; upon lifting it and moving an object in different directions, we find that the eye fails to follow it in the upward, inward, and downward direction. It can still, however, move outwards by the action of the external rectus, and somewhat downwards and outwards by aid of the superior oblique. Generally, secondary contraction of the external rectus soon supervenes, and a marked divergent squint arises, accompanied by crossed diplopia.

If we move the object over to the right of the patient, a divergent squint arises (with crossed diplopia), which increases in proportion as the object is moved further in this direction. Upon moving the object upwards, the right eye will follow it, but the left will lag behind, the rays from the object will therefore fall upon a portion of the retina below the yellow spot, and the double image be projected above that of the right eye. If the object is moved downwards, the reverse will of course obtain, and the image of the left eye be projected beneath that of the right.

On account of the paralysis of the branch to the sphincter pupillæ, the pupil will be somewhat dilated (about two or two and one-half lines in diameter), and immovable. The paralysis of this branch may, however, precede that of general paralysis of the third nerve. Upon the application of atropine, the pupil dilates to its fullest extent. Finally, as the ciliary muscle is paralyzed, the eye will have lost its power of accommodation.

If the healthy eye is closed, and the patient directed to walk straight up to a certain object, he becomes giddy and faint, and reels in his gait; which is owing to the illusion which exists in his mind between the real and imaginary position of the object. There is generally some protrusion of the eyeball, on account of the paralysis of the three recti muscles, whose office it is to pull the eye into the orbit.[1] There is also marked ptosis, but the latter is not so excessive as when the orbicularis palpebrarum is also paralyzed. By relaxing the orbicularis and contracting the frontalis, the upper eyelid can still be somewhat lifted. Although we but seldom meet with a complete, isolated paralysis of the individual muscles supplied by the third nerve, it will be well briefly to consider the symptoms which paralysis of these different muscles would present.

4.—PARALYSIS OF THE INTERNAL RECTUS OF THE LEFT EYE.

When an object is moved from the left to the right side, both eyes will be fixed upon it nearly up to the middle line, but when it is carried over to

---

[1] H, Müller discovered in the inferior orbital fissure a reddish-gray mass, consisting of bundles of unstriped muscular fibre with elastic tendons, analogous to the orbital membrane of the mammalia. He supposed that its action is to protrude the eyeball; it is supplied by fibres from the sympathetic, and irritation of the latter in the neck has been found to cause protrusion of the eye, perhaps through the action of this muscle.

the right, the left eye will lag more and more behind, thus giving rise to a divergent squint. If the paralysis is complete, and the patient endeavors to move his left eye inwards, a vicarious, rotatory, zigzag movement inwards will be produced by the action of the superior and inferior rectus.   As the squint is divergent, the diplopia is crossed, and the lateral distance between the double images will increase in proportion as the object is carried over to the right, but there will be no difference in the height and straightness of the images in looking vertically upwards or downwards. But in the diagonal positions inwards, there will not only be a difference in the height of the double images, but the one will slant considerably.   In the oblique position of the object upwards and inwards, the double images will diverge at the top, that of the left eye being inclined to the right ; whereas, in the diagonal position downwards and inwards, the double images appear to converge at the top, that of the left eye being inclined towards the left.

In the diagonal positions inwards, there will also be a difference in the height of the images, even although there is no difference in the height of the cornea. The reason of this has been already explained in the description of paralysis of the external rectus muscle.

The line which divides the portion of the field in which the patient sees double from that in which single vision exists, does not run vertically from above downwards, but obliquely left to right ; lying to the left side of the vertical line above the horizontal line, and to the right side of it below the horizontal line.   This is explained by the fact that the divergence is much greater when the eyes look upwards, than when they look down.

The patient's head is turned towards the right, so as to avoid diplopia, by bringing objects as much as possible into the left half of the visual field.

6.—PARALYSIS OF THE SUPERIOR RECTUS OF THE LEFT EYE.

This muscle moves the eye upwards and inwards, and inclines the vertical meridian inwards.

The inefficiency of the paralyzed superior rectus will not be apparent in the movements of the eye below the horizontal diameter, but only in those above the latter.   The diplopia will consequently be also only apparent in the upper half of the field.   When the object is moved above the horizontal line, the left eye will lag behind, and this deviation will increase in proportion the higher the object is moved.   At the same time there will also be a divergent squint, for, on account of the paralysis of the superior rectus, the inferior oblique will move the eye somewhat outwards. If the right eye is covered, and the patient directed to look with the left at an object held slightly in the upper half of the visual field, the left eye will move upwards and inwards (the degree depending upon the amount of paralysis), showing that it had before deviated downwards and outwards. The covered eye will at the same time make a considerably greater associated movement upwards and outwards. The patient, in endeavoring to strike an object, will aim too high. He will carry his head thrown back, so as to bring all objects as much as possible in the lower half of the field.

The diplopia manifests itself in the upper half of the visual field. The double images show lateral differences, are crossed, different in height, and not parallel.

As the cornea deviates downwards and outwards, the rays from an object held above the horizontal meridian line fall upon the outer and lower portion of the retina, and will consequently be projected upwards and inwards;

the double image of the affected eye (*pseudo-image*) lying above and to the right of the image of the right eye.

As the action of the superior rectus upon the height of the eye increases as the latter is moved outwards (to the left), the inefficiency of the paralyzed muscle in raising the cornea, will also be most evident in this direction. The difference in the height of the double images, therefore, increases as the eye is turned outwards, and diminishes as it is turned inwards. On the other hand, the inclination of the vertical meridian will be most apparent when the eye is turned inwards, and least so when it is turned outwards (to the left). On account of the paralysis of the superior rectus, the vertical meridians are not parallel, but that of the left eye is turned outwards by the unopposed action of the inferior oblique. Hence the pseudo-image would appear to converge towards the image of the right eye, but the double images are crossed, and hence they diverge at the top, the pseudo-image being inclined towards the right.[1]

6. –PARALYSIS OF THE INFERIOR RECTUS OF THE LEFT EYE.

The symptoms arising in a paralysis of this muscle are just the reverse of those in paralysis of the superior rectus. The want of movement and consequent diplopia are only apparent when the object is held below the horizontal meridian line. The pseudo-image lies *below* that of the right eye, and towards its right. The double images increase in height when the eyes are moved to the left, and in inclination when they are moved to the right. The double images are crossed and the pseudo-image inclined towards that of the right eye (*i. e.*, inclined towards the left).

7.—PARALYSIS OF THE INFERIOR OBLIQUE OF THE LEFT EYE.

As it is extremely doubtful whether an isolated paralysis of this muscle ever occurs, I shall not describe the symptoms which would be presented by such an affection, but simply state that they would be just the reverse of those met with in paralysis of the superior oblique, and from a knowledge of which these symptoms could easily be constructed. [Dr. Noyes, of New York, has described a well-authenticated instance of traumatic paralysis of the right inferior oblique muscle in his own person. It differs somewhat from the description of the symptoms of paralysis of this muscle as given by Alf. von Graefe, in that the images were crossed. The cause of the paralysis was a fracture through the malar bone across the origin of the inferior oblique muscle, and Noyes thinks it possible that only those fibres going to the outer side of its insertion were impaired, and that in this way the adductive power was impaired. (See "Trans. Amer. Oph. Soc.," 1879.)—B.]

8.—PARALYSIS OF THE SUPERIOR OBLIQUE OF THE LEFT EYE, ETC.

The paralysis of the superior oblique illustrates, better than that of any other of the ocular muscles, the correctness of the rules laid down as to the action of the different muscles, and the nature of the diplopia presented by their paralysis. Indeed, the deviation of the visual line is so extremely

---

[1] As patients often find it difficult to estimate accurately the obliquity of a small object, such as the flame of a lighted candle, it is better to use as an object a white staff, or a roll of paper about twelve inches in length.

... in cases of paralysis of the superior oblique, that ...
... detection, and we must, therefore, place our chief re...
... of the double images to assist us in determining the ...

A person affected with paralysis of the left superior obli...
... that objects (the floor, steps, etc.) in the lower half of th...
... and irregular in outline. Above the horizontal me...
visual lines are fixed upon the object and no diplopia exists.
... held in the horizontal median line or a very little below it,
deviation of the left eye in an upward and inward direction is n...
becomes more and more marked the further the object is mo...
lower half of the field, more especially towards the right. If th...
is closed, the left makes a well-marked movement downwards an...
and there will be an erroneous projection of the visual field i...
direction. Upon closing the healthy right eye, and testing the ...
the left, we might at first suppose it to be unimpaired in all dire...
on closer examination we find that downwards and inwards (tow...
nose there is a distinct want of mobility. Instead of following the ...
sweep of the object from below to the inner side, the visual line mo...
diagonal spring upwards and inwards. The double images are homony...
and show a difference both in height and laterally, and the one slants.
Diplopia is confined to the lower half of the visual field, and is absent ir
upper. On account of the convergent squint which arises below the
mental line, the diplopia is homonymous, and as the left eye remains a
same time too high, its image will appear beneath that of the right
The lateral difference between the double images increases the mor
further the object is moved downwards, as the convergence of the visual
then becomes greater, on account of the unopposed action of the in
rectus. The difference in the height of the double images increase
more, the further the object is moved over to the right, and diminishe
is moved over to the left. This is owing to the fact, that the su
oblique exerts the greatest influence upon the height of the eyeball wh
eye is moved downwards and inwards, and hence its loss of power up
height of the cornea will also be felt the most in this direction. On th
hand, the inclination of the double images will be greatest when the
is moved over to the left, and least when it is carried over to the
for the superior oblique exerts most influence on the position of the v
meridian, when the eye is moved downwards and outwards. On acco
the paralysis of the superior oblique, the inferior rectus will exercise
sway over the vertical meridian in all the movements of the eye
the horizontal median line, and incline it outwards. The parallelism
vertical meridians will, therefore, be destroyed, and they will diverge
up, the double images appearing to converge; for, on account of the ab
upwards of the vertical meridian of the left eye, the image of the
will not fall in the vertical meridian, but upon the upper and inner
corner and outer quadrants of the retina, and the pseudo-image will,
appear to the patient to be inclined towards the right, and to co
towards the image of the right eye. A glance at Fig. 215, p. 681
render this intelligible, it being remembered, however, that the v
meridian is turned outwards in paralysis of the superior oblique, and in
that of the external rectus.

When the object is carried very far down into the lower half of the
... phenomenon is observed, viz., that the pseudo-image appears
... of the right eye, even although the left cornea still remains highe
... This is due to the extreme inclination of the vertical mer

base of the skull, and this must be especially suspected if several muscles of one or both eyes are affected, or if some other nerves (such as the facial or some branches of the fifth) are also implicated. We find that the causes situated at the base of the brain generally produce paralysis by a direct compression of the nerves which lie at this situation. Amongst such causes we must especially enumerate syphilitic and rheumatic ostitis and periostitis, exostoses, syphilitic tophi, tubercular deposits, effusions of blood, and tumors of various kinds. In cases of tumor or aneurism, the progress of the paralysis is generally slow, whereas the reverse is the case in inflammatory exudations.

[Pagenstecher says that in epidemics of diphtheria, paralyses of the extrinsic muscles of the eyes are not uncommon, and are noticeable for the rapidity with which they appear and disappear, and for the fact that they only occur in the stage of convalescence. They are also said to occur in the course of and after febrile infectious diseases.—B.]

The cause may, however, be situated in the brain itself, and we then generally find that the patient shows some derangement of the intellectual functions. His memory fails him, and he experiences a difficulty in arranging his ideas, or in giving expression to them. These derangements are often very transitory, and may vary greatly in extent, from a slight impairment of memory to a state bordering on idiocy. Ptosis is not unfrequently a symptom of a cerebral affection, whereas lagophthalmos is only exceptionally so. Amongst the various lesions within the brain which may produce paralysis of the muscles of the eye, must be mentioned softening of the brain, effusions of blood, tubercular deposits, aneurisms, impermeability of some of the cerebral bloodvessels, tumors situated within the brain, hydrocephalus, etc. The nature of the diplopia aids us to a certain extent in localizing the cause of the paralysis, for in paralysis due to a cerebral lesion we observe that there is a great difficulty in the fusion of the double images. It is found very difficult, or almost impossible, to unite them, even with the more carefully selected prism, the patient being unable to fuse them by a voluntary effort, even although they are brought very close together. [A diagnosis of the nature and seat of the cause of paralysis of central origin can only be made from an accurate knowledge of the origin and course of the various motor nerves going to the ocular muscles. It should be remembered that the third, fourth, and sixth nerves all rise in the vicinity of the floor of the fourth ventricle and aqueduct of Sylvius, the nucleus of origin of the third being the most anterior, close behind it that of the fourth, and in the region of the posterior third of the pons lies that of the sixth. Furthermore there is a complete decussation of the fibres of the fourth nerves, and probably a partial decussation of the fibres of the third nerves; while the sixth nerves are not crossed. Hence any abnormal growth or diseased process in the region of origin of the fourth or sixth would cause homonymous paralysis of the sixth and crossed paralysis of the fourth nerves.

Among the causes not mentioned above, must be mentioned hyperæmia of the brain and its membranes, on the authority of Niemeyer; disseminate sclerosis of the brain, and degeneration of the posterior columns of the cord.—B.]

The *prognosis* of the different kinds of paralysis varies with the cause, the degree, and length of duration of the paralysis.

With regard to the *general* prognosis of paralytic affections of the muscles of the eye, it may be laid down as a rule that it is the more favorable, the more recent the affection. Again, a partial paralysis affords a more favorable which becomes so great when the eye is moved far downwards that a dislocation of the quadrants of the retina takes place, the rays from the object falling no longer upon the inner and upper quadrant of the retina, but upon the inner and lower, and they are hence projected upwards and to the left.

The double images in paralysis of the superior oblique are not at the same distance from the patient, but that of the affected eye is considerably nearer to him. This was, I believe, first noticed by Dr. Michaelis. It would appear to be due to the projection of the image upon a horizontal surface below the eye (e. g., the floor of the room), for this symptom disappears with an alteration of the surface of projection.[1]

The line which divides the field of single from that of double vision does not run horizontally, but obliquely downwards from the right to the left. The patient carries his head turned downwards and to the right, so as to bring the objects as much as possible into the upper and left portion of the field, as the diplopia arises sooner in the right half. Prisms must be turned with their base downwards and outwards.

After a paralysis of the superior oblique has existed for some time, secondary contraction of the inferior oblique often supervenes. The diplopia then extends into the upper half of the visual field, but here becomes crossed, the pseudo-image, however, being still beneath that of the right eye. This is due to the cornea being moved abnormally upwards and outwards, on account of the contraction of the inferior oblique. The increase in the height of the double images will augment towards the right, and diminish towards the left; the reverse obtaining with regard to the inclination of the double images.

Having considered the various symptoms presented by the paralytic affections of the different muscles of the eye, we must now turn our attention to the causes, prognosis, and treatment.

We may distinguish peripheral and cerebral causes. Amongst the former, cold and rheumatism are the most frequent. In such cases the affection is rapidly developed, and is generally accompanied by more or less severe rheumatic pains in the corresponding side of the face and head. Very frequently there is no difficulty in tracing the cause to a cold which the patient has caught from a sudden exposure to a great change in temperature, or to a draught of cold wind. This is soon followed by pain in and around the orbit, accompanied by a slight degree of diplopia. The pathological changes in such cases generally consist in a rheumatic inflammation of the nerve sheath.

The causes may be situated in the orbit. Amongst these we must enumerate effusions of blood, all the different forms of orbital tumor, abscess of the orbit, exophthalmic goitre, etc.

The most frequent cause is, however, syphilis. According to Von Graefe, about one-third of the paralytic affections of the muscles of the eye are due to it. In many cases it is, however, impossible to determine with any degree of accuracy the exact seat of the cause; we must be satisfied with the fact that the patient has suffered from syphilis, and we frequently find that a rapid recovery ensues under proper anti-syphilitic treatment.

Syphilitic nodes or exostoses may be situated in the orbit, or at the base of the brain, and cause the paralysis by direct pressure upon the nerve. Syphilitic neuromata may also produce it.

Paralysis of the ocular muscles is often due to some cause situated at the

---

[1] Vide Von Graefe's "Symptomenlehre der Augenmuskellähmungen," p. 145.

base of the skull, and this must be especially suspected if several muscles of one or both eyes are affected, or if some other nerves (such as the facial or some branches of the fifth) are also implicated. We find that the causes situated at the base of the brain generally produce paralysis by a direct compression of the nerves which lie at this situation. Amongst such causes we must especially enumerate syphilitic and rheumatic ostitis and periostitis, exostoses, syphilitic tophi, tubercular deposits, effusions of blood, and tumors of various kinds. In cases of tumor or aneurism, the progress of the paralysis is generally slow, whereas the reverse is the case in inflammatory exudations.

[Pagenstecher says that in epidemics of diphtheria, paralyses of the extrinsic muscles of the eyes are not uncommon, and are noticeable for the rapidity with which they appear and disappear, and for the fact that they only occur in the stage of convalescence. They are also said to occur in the course of and after febrile infectious diseases.—B.]

The cause may, however, be situated in the brain itself, and we then generally find that the patient shows some derangement of the intellectual functions. His memory fails him, and he experiences a difficulty in arranging his ideas, or in giving expression to them. These derangements are often very transitory, and may vary greatly in extent, from a slight impairment of memory to a state bordering on idiocy. Ptosis is not unfrequently a symptom of a cerebral affection, whereas lagophthalmos is only exceptionally so. Amongst the various lesions within the brain which may produce paralysis of the muscles of the eye, must be mentioned softening of the brain, effusions of blood, tubercular deposits, aneurisms, impermeability of some of the cerebral bloodvessels, tumors situated within the brain, hydrocephalus, etc. The nature of the diplopia aids us to a certain extent in localizing the cause of the paralysis, for in paralysis due to a cerebral lesion we observe that there is a great difficulty in the fusion of the double images. It is found very difficult, or almost impossible, to unite them, even with the most carefully selected prism, the patient being unable to fuse them by a voluntary effort, even although they are brought very close together. [A diagnosis of the nature and seat of the cause of paralysis of central origin can only be made from an accurate knowledge of the origin and course of the various motor nerves going to the ocular muscles. It should be remembered that the third, fourth, and sixth nerves all rise in the vicinity of the floor of the fourth ventricle and aqueduct of Sylvius, the nucleus of origin of the third being the most anterior, close behind it that of the fourth, and in the region of the posterior third of the pons lies that of the sixth. Furthermore there is a complete decussation of the fibres of the fourth nerves, and probably a partial decussation of the fibres of the third nerves; while the sixth nerves are not crossed. Hence any abnormal growth or diseased process in the region of origin of the fourth or sixth would cause homonymous paralysis of the sixth and crossed paralysis of the fourth nerves.

Among the causes not mentioned above, must be mentioned hyperæmia of the brain and its membranes, on the authority of Niemeyer; disseminate sclerosis of the brain, and degeneration of the posterior columns of the cord.—B.]

The *prognosis* of the different kinds of paralysis varies with the cause, the degree, and length of duration of the paralysis.

With regard to the *general* prognosis of paralytic affections of the muscles of the eye, it may be laid down as a rule that it is the more favorable, the more recent the affection. Again, a partial paralysis affords a more favorable prognosis than if it is complete, even although the latter may be of much shorter duration. The character of the diplopia is also prognostically of importance, for the double images which only show a lateral difference and none in height are far more easily united when there is a difference in height. Slight cases of paralysis of the internal or external rectus may be spontaneously cured by the effort of the act of vision, which causes the fusion of the images.

The prognosis is generally very favorable in the rheumatic paralysis, especially if the patient applies soon after the outbreak of the disease. If the cause is situated within the orbit, the prognosis will principally depend upon the fact whether the cause can be removed or dispelled.

In the syphilitic form of paralysis, the prognosis leans towards the favorable side of the scale, but is greatly influenced by the seat and extent of the cause. If the paralysis is due to some cerebral lesion, it is, however, much more unfavorable, although a complete cure may arise if the primary affection is removed (as in absorption of exudations, etc.).

The treatment must also vary with the nature of the cause. In rheumatic paralysis, a free purge should be administered, and diaphoretics be prescribed, together with a good-sized blister behind the ear. I have found the greatest benefit from the latter remedy, as also from the use of iodide of potassium internally. When the inflammatory symptoms have subsided, and the nerves are regaining some power, faradization or galvanization should be applied. In syphilitic cases, the iodide and bromide of potassium are found of the greatest service; or mercurial inunction may be employed, if necessary. Zittmann's decoction is also very serviceable, as it acts not only as an antisyphilitic, but also as a diaphoretic. Its use, however, entails a good deal of inconvenience and discomfort.

To relieve the patient from the annoyance and confusion produced by the diplopia, the affected eye should be excluded from the visual act by a shade or a piece of frosted glass (if spectacles are used). This exclusion also obviates the tendency of the patient to carry his head turned to one side.

Prismatic glasses may likewise be employed for the purpose of fusing the double images, and their strength, as well as the direction in which their base is to be turned, will depend upon the muscle affected, and the degree of deviation. In paralysis of the internal rectus, the base should be turned inwards; in that of the external rectus, outwards. If the double images show both a difference sideways and in height, we may divide the prisms, placing one with its base laterally, and the other with its base turned upwards or downwards as the case may be; or we may divide these two prisms between the two eyes. In accordance with the fact, that the eye can readily overcome lateral differences in the double images, whereas it cannot correct any but the very slightest difference in height, we often find that if we correct the latter by a prism, the lateral differences are at once corrected by an effort of one of the horizontal muscles of the eye. This fact is of much importance in those cases in which we operate for the sake of curing diplopia. I have already stated, when speaking of paralysis of the external rectus, that when we desire to use prisms therapeutically, the double images should not be fused into one, but only approximated, in order that the paralyzed muscle may be stimulated to an effort to unite them.

Electricity (both faradization and galvanization) is often found of great service in the treatment of paralysis of the muscles of the eye, especially if the cause is peripheral. The negative pole of the instrument is applied to the closed eyelid in a situation corresponding to the affected muscle, the

44

positive being placed on the temple or the back of the neck; the sitting should not extend beyond two or three minutes. In galvanization, from six to fourteen cells should be employed, according to the point of application and the degree of effect we desire. Hitherto, it has generally been supposed that electricity acts beneficially by a direct excitation of the paralyzed motor nerves, but according to Benedikt[1] this is not so, for he states that its effect is due to a reflex excitation of the fifth nerve. He found, moreover, that in most cases a curative action was only produced when the excitation was relatively weak, and when no trace of muscular contraction was produced by the electricity. The proper measure for the strength of the current is the sensitiveness of the fifth nerve. If the latter is extremely sensitive, the battery may have to be reduced to three or four cells; if, on the other hand, the fifth is very insensible, it may have to be raised to twelve or fifteen. The current should be sufficiently intense to produce a slight sensation in the parts excited, but the excitation should only continue for about half a minute at each sitting. In paralysis of the external rectus, Benedikt applies the positive pole to the forehead, and the negative over the neighborhood of the cheek bone. In mydriasis, the latter should be applied to the same place, but the positive to the closed eyelid. In ptosis, the positive may be either on the forehead, or may be applied by means of a short catheter-like reophore to the mucous membrane of the cheek, while the negative is drawn over the lid. For all the other branches of the third nerve, the positive pole is applied as above. In order to act upon the internal rectus or inferior oblique, the negative pole should be drawn over the skin of the side of the nose, near the inner angle of the eye; and in order to act upon the inferior rectus, over the lower margin of the orbit. Benedikt found that in the greater number of cases the improvement takes place instantaneously, as shown by increased mobility of the eye, and a diminution of the field in which diplopia arises; and when this is not the case, a longer continuance and increased strength of the excitation are not indicated. When the paralysis has been unaffected by fourteen days of treatment, he has not seen any benefit arise from its longer continuance. Not unfrequently, however, faradization succeeds after galvanization has failed, and *vice versâ*. Dr. Althaus[2] therefore recommends that if the one has not produced any effect after some time (*e. g.*, ten to fourteen days), the other should be tried. Mr. Brudenell Carter[3] advises the combination of faradization of the paralyzed muscle with tenotomy of the contracted opponent. The lids are to be held apart by a speculum and the current applied to that part of the conjunctiva which corresponds to the paralyzed muscle. But this is very painful, and should only be tried, I think, in very obstinate cases.

Paralytic affections of the muscles of the eye may run the following different courses: 1. The paralysis may be completely cured, which is most likely to occur when the affection is recent, and due to some peripheral cause. 2. The cure may be incomplete, the muscle being only partially restored to its former power. 3. The paralysis may remain complete; but this condition generally soon leads to the next (4) state, viz., to a secondary contraction of the opponent muscle. Thus in paralysis of the left external rectus, the diplopia may extend more and more into the right half of the

---

[1] *Vide* a very interesting paper by Dr. Moritz Benedikt, "On Electro-Therapeutical and Physiological Researches on Paralysis of the Ocular Muscles." "A. f. O.," x. 1, translated in "Ophthalmic Review," vol. ii. p. 143.

[2] *Vide* Dr. Althaus' excellent "Treatise on Medical Electricity," p. 495.

[3] "Lancet," December, 1868.

visual field, and a decided convergent squint of the left eye be apparent, even when the object is held in the right half of the field.   The opponent muscle may in time contract so much as to drag the eye almost immovably to its own side.

When all other remedies have failed to effect a cure, it may be necessary to have recourse to operative interference, and the nature of this will depend upon the degree of paralysis which remains behind.   Thus, if only a slight degree of paralysis of the external rectus remains, so that the want of mobility outwards amounts to about one line or one and a half lines, division of the opponent muscle (internal rectus) will be indicated.   But when the mobility exceeds this degree, and amounts to two or three lines, this operation will not suffice, and we must combine with it the operation of bringing forward the insertion of the paralyzed muscle (the latter operation is generally termed that of "readjustment"), so as to increase its power over the mobility of the eyeball.   This operation should not be deferred too long, for after a time the paralyzed muscle may undergo fatty degeneration, which renders it unfit for the requisite degree of contraction, even if its innervation were completely, or in great part restored ; and it also favors secondary contraction of the opponent.   The method of performing the operation of readjustment will be considered together with that of strabismus.

[In extreme cases of secondary contraction of the antagonistic muscle, it does not suffice to divide the latter and advance the paralyzed muscle; but it becomes necessary to divide the coördinating muscle of the other eye: the internal rectus if the paralyzed muscle is the external rectus, and the external rectus if the paralyzed muscle is the internal rectus.

The defect is a much more difficult one to remedy when the superior or inferior rectus is the muscle affected, owing to the oblique direction of their insertions, and the difficulty of producing the exactly desired effect, without overdoing or underdoing it.—B.]

9.—SPASMODIC AFFECTIONS OF THE MUSCLES OF THE EYE. NYSTAGMUS, ETC.

The symptoms of nystagmus consist in a peculiar, restless movement or oscillation of the eyeballs.   This oscillation is generally horizontal, but occasionally rotatory, the eyeballs oscillating round the axis of the oblique muscles.   In very rare instances, the nystagmus may be vertical.   I have seen two such cases.   In one, the eye was affected with convergent squint, and made a constant upward and downward movement, which was not arrested or even improved by tenotomy of the internal rectus.   The other occurred in a man affected with choroido-retinitis, and here both eyes showed a well-marked vertical nystagmus.   Zehender[1] has also met with one case.   I lately saw a very curious form of nystagmus in a patient of Mr. James Adams, where the oscillations only occurred when he looked below the horizontal meridian, the eyes being quite steady exactly in the horizontal meridian and in all the movements above it.   The oscillation may be periodical, and its degree is often very variable at different times, being markedly increased by any nervous excitement, and by the effort of accommodation. To remedy the indistinctness of vision produced by the unsteadiness of the eyes, the patients often make a contrary movement of the head ; or they hold the print in a slanting or vertical, instead of a horizontal position, so

---

[1] " Kl. Monatsbl.," 1870, 112.

that the lines run vertically instead of horizontally. The reason of this is easily intelligible, for they can then see the individual lines chiefly by the aid of the superior or inferior recti, and the circles of diffusion caused by the oscillation of the eye will then extend the letters vertically, instead of horizontally; the length of the letters will consequently be considerably more increased than their breadth, which is less confusing to the sight, as their lateral separation will be preserved. Whereas, when they are extended horizontally, one letter runs into the other, its outline is blurred and confused, and the power of distinguishing them much impaired.

Although there may be considerable oscillation of the eyeballs, the movements of the eyes are unaffected and perfect in all directions, and the two eyes may act perfectly together, but binocular vision is often disturbed, and the sight of the two eyes frequently very different. The oscillation sometimes diminishes greatly, or is even arrested when the eyes are moved very far outwards or inwards, or in one of the diagonal positions downwards (Böhm).[1]

Nystagmus generally appears in early infancy, and is especially met with in cases in which a considerable degree of exertion of the ocular muscles is required for distinct vision; the object having, perhaps, to be held very close to the eye, either on account of some anomaly of the refraction, or some opacity in the refracting media. Thus the affection is often met with in infants together with opacities of the cornea or of the lens, in cases of strabismus, in albinos, etc.

[Nystagmus is almost always bilateral, and the movements associated ones. The degree of the nystagmus with respect to the rapidity and amplitude of the excursive movements is not always constant, and here a psychic causation is of undeniable influence. In certain cases of horizontal nystagmus, the movements may be caused to cease by strongly converging the eyes. In the majority of cases the nystagmus occurs at a period in early life when, in addition to the causes above enumerated, there is an abnormal disposition of the muscle in addition. Although nystagmus is apt to be connected with various forms of congenital amblyopia, it does not, by any means, occur in all; and though its hereditary propagation is well recognized, the occurrence of an actual congenital nystagmus has not yet been proven. There is a peculiar variety of nystagmus, occurring in minors, which is still but imperfectly understood. It is acquired in adult or declining years by men who have worked for a long time in coal mines. Diminution of the acuity of vision is, as a rule, not present. The nystagmus is of a periodic character, the paroxysms being favored by a dim illumination. It appears especially when the eyes are turned in a certain direction. Darkness plays an important *role* in the development of this anomaly, in rendering the vision and fixation very difficult, for there is an almost constant effort to recognize distinctly certain objects in the darkness. It was formerly supposed that the position of the miners, lying down, kneeling, or crouching, with the eyes elevated, had some influence in producing the nystagmus, but this is now doubted. The form and direction of the movements are less variable in this variety of nystagmus than in the former variety. Warlomont defines this variety of nystagmus as a myopathy of both elevators of the eyeball and of the internal rectus, intimately connected with anæmia and paralysis of accommodation.

Another kind of nystagmus is due to disease of the central nervous system. Though a periodic oscillatory motion of the eyes occurs in a variety of brain diseases, the constant typical nystagmus is a very common symptom

[1] Böhm, "Der Nystagmus."

of insular sclerosis of the central nervous system. A similar trembling motion is also seen in the arms and legs in this disease. The nystagmus is usually bilateral. (See "Arch. f. Ophth.," xxiii. 3, p. 241-254; "Graefe u. Saemisch, Handb.," vi. 1, s. 223-241.)—B.]

The disease may diminish, or even disappear, as the patient grows older, but it generally remains permanent, varying, perhaps, somewhat with the state of health; any debility or nervous excitement increasing its intensity. If strabismus coexists, this should be cured by an operation, and in some cases the nystagmus is also considerably diminished by the tenotomy. In others it must, however, be confessed, that either no benefit, or only a very temporary one, results. Hence I do not consider it advisable to perform tenotomy of any of the ocular muscles for the chance of curing the nystagmus, except there is also strabismus. Any anomaly of refraction should be corrected by suitable lenses, and benefit is sometimes experienced from the use of blue eye-protectors, to diminish the intensity and glare of the light.

Spasmodic affections of the ocular muscles are extremely rare. Clonic spasms are sometimes met with in children affected with chorea or basilar meningitis; also in cases of lead-poisoning, and in some of the affections of the brain and spinal cord. Tonic spasms of the ocular muscles are occasionally observed in epilepsy.

[The abnormal deviation of the eyes in certain cerebral diseases, called by Prevost "conjugate deviation," and the observations of Longet upon the same subject, look to the existence of a special centre for associated movements; and as the associated .relation of the muscles is a certain form of coördination, these cases may be regarded as spasm of coördination. (See "Graefe und Saemisch, Handb.," vi. 1, s. 221.)

The subject of conjugate deviation of the eyes in bulbar lesions of the encephalon has been very carefully studied by Quioc, who draws the following conclusions: 1. The abducens nerve furnishes an anastomosis, formed of the peripheral fibres, which passes obliquely across the medulla oblongata from the nucleus of the sixth nerve to the trunk of the third nerve on the opposite side. 2. Every lesion, involving either the nucleus or the trunk of the sixth nerve and the anastomotic branch which passes to the third nerve of the opposite side, causes a conjugate deviation of the eyes. 3. The conjugate deviation of the eyes in paralysis of the external rectus and conjugate inaction of the opposite internal rectus, and occurring on the side of the paralyzed muscles, is due to a lesion in the posterior part of the bulbar region, in a territory comprising the nucleus of the sixth nerve and a peripheral zone. 4. There may also occur a conjugate deviation of the eyes on the opposite side from the lesion, when the latter is situated in the cerebellum, or in that portion of the fasciculi of the cerebral peduncle which extends between the tubercula quadrigemina and the nucleus of the abducens. 5. The conjugate deviation of the eyes occurs on the same side as the lesion when the latter is located in the hemispheres, the peduncle of Megnert, or the protuberance, provided in the latter case the region of the bulbar protuberance is not involved. (See "Lyon médical," Juli 3, 10, 17, and 24, 1881. See also a paper by Leichtenstern in the "Deutsche med. Wochenschrift," October 29, 1881.)—B.]

Spasm of the orbicularis palpebrarum is described in the article upon the "Diseases of the Eyelids."

[Abadie reports some cases of what he calls *ocular vertigo*, in which the vertigo was the main symptom, accompanied by a severe pain in the back of the neck, an inability to elevate the pupils more than two or three millimetres above the horizontal plane, and a feeling as if the patients were falling backward. The vertigo increased almost to syncope when the patients attempted to look upward, and the pain in the spine and the sense of constriction in the root of the nose increased also. Under the influence of small doses of belladonna, there was a marked amelioration of all the symptoms. See "Le Progrès méd.," Dec. 31, 1881, and Jan. 6, 1882.—B.]

10.—STRABISMUS.

We have now to turn our attention to the consideration of the various forms of squint and their treatment. The surgeon should thoroughly master the theoretical portion of this subject before he attempts to operate for the cure of this affection; for although the operation for squint is not per se a difficult one, we yet meet with many cases which require very great exactitude and nicety, not only in the preliminary examination, but also in the mode of operation. Still more difficult and intricate are those cases in which we operate less for the cure of the deformity, which is, perhaps, hardly observable, than for the purpose of freeing the patient from the great and constant annoyance of diplopia. These demand a thorough knowledge of the individual actions of the muscles of the eyeball, an intimate acquaintance with the various forms of diplopia, and considerable manual dexterity in the performance of the operation, the extent and character of which should be accurately determined upon beforehand. Such cases, indeed, often form some of the most difficult problems in ophthalmic surgery, and can be only successfully treated by those who have mastered the theory of this and kindred subjects. A want of such knowledge brought the operation for squint into almost complete disrepute, and we are chiefly indebted to Von Graefe for having extricated it from the obloquy with which it had, not undeservedly, been visited, and for having rendered it one of the most successful operations in surgery. He has achieved this success not so much by improving the mode of operation, as by his elaborate researches into the physiology and symptomatology of the various forms of squint, which have enabled him to lay down exact data for their successful treatment.

Symptomatically we mean by the term "squint," an inability to bring both visual lines to bear simultaneously upon one point, the one always deviating in a certain direction from the object. If the squinting eye deviates inwards, it is called convergent squint, if outwards, divergent squint; if it squint upwards, strabismus sursumvergens, if downwards, strabismus deorsumvergens.

The name strabismus was formerly indiscriminately applied to all abnormal deviations of the visual lines, whatever their cause; whether they were due to paralysis or spasm of one or more of the muscles of the eyeball, or whether some tumor, etc., of the orbit prevented the free movement of the eye in certain directions.

We now, however, limit the term strabismus (or strabismus concomitans of Von Graefe, a name we shall adopt) to that group of cases which presents the following well-defined and constant symptoms:

1. The visual line of one eye being fixed upon one object, that of the other always deviates from the latter at a certain angle, and in a certain direction. In convergent squint it deviates to the inner, in divergent squint to the outer · of the object. In order to determine which is the squinting eye, the ient should be directed to look steadily at an object (a lighted candle or uplifted finger) held in the horizontal median line, at the distance of a · feet. Then, alternately covering each eye with our hand, we note

whether the uncovered eye remains steadily fixed upon the object, or has to change its position before it can bring its visual line to bear upon it. In the former case, it is the one generally used for fixation; in the latter, it deviates from the object. We may, however, fail to detect the deviation in this manner, if it is so very slight as to be almost objectively inappreciable, in which case we must call the diplopia to our aid, as it enables us to detect the most minute deviations of the visual lines. But the concomitant squint is generally very evident.

If we cover the healthy eye with one hand, the other will move in a certain direction in order to fix the object (in convergent squint it will move outwards, in divergent inwards), the healthy, covered eye making at the same time an *associated* movement (which has been designated the *secondary* deviation), becoming now, in fact, the squinting eye.

I have already (p. 679) explained the method of measuring the linear extent of the deviation with Laurence's strabismometer. I need only add that the degree of strabismus should be tested both for near and distant objects, as it is often far more considerable during a strong effort of accommodation, as in reading small type, than when the eye is looking at a distant object.

We sometimes find that there is not only a lateral deviation, but also a slight difference in the height of the two eyes. It is important in such a case, to determine whether (in a case of convergent squint) this is due to the upper fibres of the internal rectus being more contracted than the middle or lower fibres, or whether it is owing to the superior rectus being also affected, for upon this will hinge the question of operating upon more than one muscle.

The associated movement, which the healthy eye makes when it is covered and the squinting eye fixes the object, will enable us to determine this, for if the internal rectus is alone at fault, the associated movement of the healthy eye will be only lateral, without any deviation in height; whereas, if the superior rectus is also implicated, the healthy eye will make not only an inward, but also a downward movement, corresponding to the outward and downward movement of the other eye. In the former case, we shall almost always succeed in curing the inward and slightly upward deviation by a tenotomy of the internal rectus alone, more particularly if we freely divide the upper portion of the tendon. In the latter case, we shall have not only to operate upon the internal, but also upon the superior rectus.

2. The primary and secondary deviations are quite equal in extent. The meaning of these terms has been already fully explained at page 677. Let us suppose that the left eye squints inward to the extent of two lines. Now, if the right is covered, the left will have to move outwards to the extent of two lines in order to fix the object, and the covered eye will make at the same time an associated movement inwards of two lines, this secondary deviation being, therefore, exactly equal-to the primary.

3. The extent of movement of the two eyes is quite normal and equal, the arc of mobility being exactly of the same extent in both eyes, and only a little shifted towards the side of the shortened muscle. Thus, in a convergent squint it is shifted slightly inwards, but what is gained in this direction is lost in the movement outwards. This increase in the mobility towards the side of the shortened muscle, is, however, very slight when compared with the degree of the squint. On account of this complete accompaniment of the squinting eye in all the movements of the healthy one, it has been called strabismus concomitans. If we hold an object in the horizontal median line, and then move it to the right and left, the visual line of the

squinting eye will exactly accompany that of the healthy eye in all its movements, deviating from it, however, always at the same angle, except, indeed, at the extreme portions of the field of vision.

In order to note accurately, and to keep an easy and diagrammatic record of the extreme lateral movements of each eye inwards and outwards, Mr. Bowman has for some time adopted the following simple and practical method: He notes the extreme range inwards, by marking the position of the pupil on extreme inversion, compared with that of the lower punctum; and the extreme range outwards, by marking the position of the outer edge of the cornea, on extreme eversion, compared with that of the external canthus.

The following figures illustrate this method, the patient being supposed to face the observer:

Fig. 217 shows R the right outer canthus, and L the left outer canthus, crossed by a vertical line a, or b, or c, which indicates by its position the extent to which the outer edge of the cornea approaches the canthus, or even goes beyond it, on *extreme eversion* of the eye. And Fig. 218, in like manner,

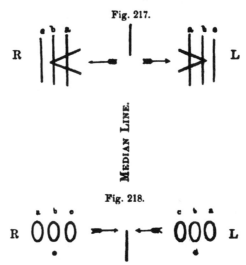

Fig. 217.

MEDIAN LINE.

Fig. 218.

exhibits for R the right eye, and for L the left eye, the position which the pupil, O, takes with regard to the punctum, . ,when the eye is moved inwards to the extreme degree. It may fail to reach it, as at a a, or be over it, as at b b, or pass more or less inwards beyond it, as at c c.

In taking the relation of the pupil to the punctum if the eye is much inverted, the observer should, as it were, face the pupil in its inverted position, otherwise the interval between it and the punctum is not so correctly estimated. Or the parts may be viewed from above, the surgeon raising the upper lid, and standing behind the patient, who sits on a chair. But a little practice soon renders this unnecessary.

If the outer edge of the cornea, in extreme eversion, passes under cover of the canthus, its actual position can be readily enough marked by noting how much of the iris is hidden from view.

A diagrammatic record should be kept of the range of mobility, in order that we may hereafter be able to estimate the effect of the operation upon the lateral movements of the eye.

The accommodative movements of the eye should also be accurately tested, for they are extremely important, as will be shown hereafter, in determining the mode and extent of the operation. On bringing the object nearer and nearer to the eyes, the visual line of the healthy eye will remain fixed upon it, converging the more the nearer the object is approximated : the position of the squinting eye (convergent strabismus) may, at the same time, undergo the following changes:

1. It may retain its original position, sustaining only a few oscillating, irregular, lateral movements.

2. It may remain completely stationary, so that the angle of squinting will diminish the more, the nearer the object is brought, until, at a certain point (if the squint be not excessive), its visual line will also be fixed upon the object, and there will no longer be any squint. If, however, the object is approximated still closer, a divergent squint will arise; for, whilst the healthy eye converges still more, the other retains its position, and now deviates (passively) outwards.

3. It retains its position up to a certain point, and then, as the healthy eye moves inwards to follow the object, it makes an *associated* movement outwards.

4. It deviates suddenly and spasmodically inwards, when the object is approximated very closely.

[*Alfred von Graefe* denominates concomitant strabismus as muscular or myopathic squint, and asserts that the excess of contraction which gives rise to the abnormal position, when the squint is permanent, is only passive. In strabismus, the squinting position is that of rest, and the excess of tension of the rectus internus is a purely physical condition of the muscle, independent of any innervation. ("Graefe u. Saemisch, Handb.," vi. 1.)

V. Hasner holds somewhat similar views, and looks upon strabismus as an abnormality in the primary binocular position, laying great stress on the anatomical equilibrium. ("Beiträge zur Phys. u. Path. des Auges.")

Hansen, of Copenhagen, differs from both Von Graefe and Hasner. The real cause of squinting, he thinks, is the abnormal situation of the range of accommodation. When strabismus does not appear in a person who is hypermetropic, this is due among other things to the range of the relative accommodation being sufficiently great to make it independent of convergence. He regards it as established that in strabismus the innervation to convergence is equally strong in both eyes, and that the conditions in squinting are fully explained by "considering them to consist of an active shortening of the muscle, brought about by increased innervation to convergence." In the normal eye the convergence for a fixed point "fulfils the demands of binocular vision," while in the squinting eye "the convergence satisfies the want of accommodation and puts aside the demands of binocular vision." As the result of his consideration upon the subject, he states the following: " Every hypermetropic squint depends upon the relation between accommodation and convergence. Convergence is partly an immediate expression for the accommodation used in the moment of fixation, partly an expression for the unconscious innervation to convergence arising from accommodation, and lasting during its state of rest." (See a very interesting paper by Hansen in "Trans. Fifth Internat. Ophthal. Congress," New York, 1876.)—B.]

Concomitant squint may be either monolateral or alternating. In the former case, the squint is always confined (when both eyes are open) to one and the same eye. If the healthy eye be covered, the other will move in order to fix the object, but directly the former is again uncovered, it will at once resume its squinting position. In alternating squint it is different, for sometimes the one eye deviates, sometimes the other. If we, in this case, cover the healthy eye, the other will make a movement in order to adjust its visual line upon the object, and will retain its position when we uncover the sound eye. The latter has now, in fact, become the squinting one. If we then cover the other, the squint will alternate again. It appears almost, or quite, immaterial to the patient which eye he uses. In such cases, there is generally no difference in the sight of the two eyes; whereas, in monolateral strabismus the vision of the squinting eye is almost always affected, on account of the suppression of the double image, sometimes, indeed, very considerably.

The active negation of the double image by the brain soon leads to a more or less considerable deterioration in the sight of this eye. We occasionally find, however, that the vision of the squinting eye remains good, although the strabismus is not alternating. Indeed, I have seen cases (exceptional, I grant) in which the patients could read the very finest print with it, never having, as far as they could remember, suffered from diplopia. Here binocular vision had most likely never existed, and hence the absence of diplopia and the call for the suppression of the double image.

It was at one time proposed to cure squint by closing the healthy eye, and thus necessitating the fixation of the other upon the object. The error of such treatment is, however, self-evident, as the squint is merely transferred to the excluded eye; for just the same thing occurs, as when we place our hand over the healthy eye in order to estimate the primary and secondary deviation. The vision of the squinting eye is exercised, but the disease remains uncured. But this proceeding often proves very valuable in practice, for by it we may render a monolateral squint alternating, and preserve the sight of both eyes. If, for instance, a child squints (seeing perfectly with both eyes), and the operation has to be postponed for some reason, we may preserve the sight of the squinting eye by the periodical exclusion of the other. In this way, we may not only maintain the alternating character of the strabismus, and the sight of both eyes, but we may even change a monolateral into an alternating squint.

The question as to whether binocular vision exists or not in a case of strabismus, is of much importance in the prognosis. For if it does not exist, we cannot expect a perfect, but only an approximative, cure, for there will not be any diplopia, and the perfect cure of squint depends upon the fusion of the double images. Hence, the presence of binocular vision should always be ascertained before the prognosis of a strabismus operation is made. Its presence is of course proved at once by the existence of binocular diplopia. The sight of each eye may be good, and there may be no deviation of the visual lines when both are open, and yet both may not be used at the same time. The existence of binocular vision is easily proved by the aid of prisms. Each eye should, however, be first examined separately, and its acuity of vision, range of accommodation, and state of refraction be accurately ascertained; notice being also taken as to whether the visual line is adjusted upon the object, or whether the eye "fixes" the latter with an eccentric portion of the retina, and not with the yellow spot. In the former case it is termed "central," in the latter "eccentric fixation." The patient is next directed to look with both eyes at a lighted candle situated at a distance of four or six feet, and a prism, with its base outwards, is then placed before one eye (let us suppose the left). One of the following three things will then occur: 1, diplopia; 2, a *corrective squint* if the prism is not too strong, for the left eye will endeavor to overcome the annoyance of the diplopia by squinting inwards, and thus fusing the double images; 3, the prism may have no effect, producing neither diplopia nor a corrective squint. This proves the absence of binocular vision, and that the prism has been held before the eye which is not used. For if we place it (still with its base outwards) before the other eye, this will move inwards in order to bring the deflected rays again upon the yellow spot, which is, of course, accompanied by an associated movement outwards of the eye which is excluded from binocular vision.

Binocular vision is frequently only lost in certain portions of the retina, more especially in those which, though not identical with, are constantly excited simultaneously with the central portion of the retina of the other eye.

Thus in convergent squint we find that, in the squinting eye, the portion of the retina which lies internal to the yellow spot is the first to suffer a loss of binocular vision, for it is directed towards the object, and is therefore (though not identical with it) constantly excited simultaneously with the central portion of the retina of the other eye, which is fixed upon the object. The reverse occurs in divergent squint, for there the external portion of the retina is the first to fail. At first, this loss of binocular vision only extends horizontally, so that if we turn a prism with its base upwards or downwards (or place it even in a diagonal position), we at once produce double images, which show not only a difference in height, but also, if there is any squint, a lateral difference. We may thus determine, with the greatest nicety, which part of the retina has lost the power of binocular vision. Sometimes it extends over the whole retina, so that we fail to produce diplopia even with the strongest prisms turned in any direction; in other cases, this loss of binocular vision is tolerably circumscribed, being confined to a very small portion of the retina. In convergent strabismus, for instance, only a small portion of the retina internal to the yellow spot may have suffered; so that on placing a prism, with its base towards the nose, before this eye, and deflecting the rays still more inwards, double images are at once produced, although the deflected rays now impinge upon a more eccentric, and naturally less sensitive portion of the retina. Occasionally, we may in such a case also produce diplopia, if we, by means of a prism, bring the rays nearer to the macula lutea. Thus, a sudden alteration of the position of the visual line of the affected eye, may at once give rise to diplopia; as, for instance, after the operation for squint, or in cases of paralysis or spasm of the other muscles of the eyeball.

Von Graefe has found that binocular vision is absent in about ninety per cent. of cases of concomitant squint; that we can produce diplopia by prisms in about twenty-five per cent.; and that after the operation, binocular vision is found to exist in about fifty per cent. The reason why binocular vision is so frequently absent in concomitant squint is, that on account of the annoyance and confusion produced by the diplopia, the patient soon acquires the habit of mentally suppressing the retinal image of the squinting eye. This active suppression of the pseudo-image is mostly accompanied by considerable amblyopia, and the latter is especially apt to increase very rapidly in children, so that, perhaps, within a few months after the first appearance of the squint, the child may hardly be able to decipher large letters (No. 16 or 20 of Jäger) with the squinting eye. This being so, the operation should never be unnecessarily deferred. The question is often debated, as to whether a child of two or three years of age should be operated upon for squint, or whether it is not better to postpone the operation until it is much older. My opinion is very strongly opposed to the latter practice, and is urgently in favor of the operation being performed as soon as possible, whilst binocular vision still exists, and the sight of the squinting eye is good. If it is, however, absolutely necessary to postpone the operation, the vision of the squinting eye should be very frequently practised, and each eye alternately used for reading, etc.

The amblyopia due to the suppression of the retinal image is often greatly improved by the operation, and especially by practising the sight afterwards with a strong convex lens, or by Von Graefe's arrangement of two lenses placed in a short tube. The improvement produced by the operation varies with the degree of amblyopia, and is greatest when the patient can still read moderate-sized print (from No. 4 to 14 Jäger), when the sight is improved by convex glasses, and when the fixation is central and the visual field good.

The sudden and very marked improvement of sight which occasionally takes place directly after the division of the tendon, is probably due to the relief of the compression exercised by the contracted muscle upon the sclerotic, and through it upon the retina. It is difficult otherwise to explain this very sudden and striking improvement of vision.

[The theory of *amblyopia ex anopsia*, or from disuse, which has been so generally accepted. has been questioned energetically by Schweigger, Alfred von Graefe, and others. The former believes that the amblyopia in squint is congenital. He thinks that a real amblyopia resulting from squint is true only in a partial sense, viz., as a regional amblyopia, not identical with scotoma, but in the sense that over the locality upon which the image falls when the eye squints, there is either a dulness of perception or a habitual negation of vision. We know that some patients can recover the function of the squinting eye, and combine it with its fellow, and that to other persons this is impossible; and the impossibility may lie either in the incurability of the impaired sight, for which no ophthalmoscopic lesion can be discovered, or because of mental incapacity to coördinate and combine both eyes. (See Schweigger's "Handbuch der Augenheilkunde," 4th edition, 1880. Noyes' "Treatise on Diseases of the Eye," 1881, pp. 107 and 108.)

According to Javal, the amblyopia of divergent squint resists all amelioration by exercise. When, however, the squint is due simply to insufficiency of the interni, optical treatment gives excellent results. If glasses do not give binocular vision, then stereoscopic exercises must be undertaken. The amblyopia of convergent squint is incurable when there is fixation by a peripherical part of the retina. When the fixation is uncertain, isolated exercises may produce considerable amelioration. When the amblyopia is slight, it is certain that the squint has lasted a long while, and here Javal prefers to close the good eye for a certain time, followed by the temporary use of glasses correcting the total hypermetropia, which sometimes gives brilliant results. (See "Bull. gén. de thérapeutique," Dec. 30, 1880.)—B.]

We must now briefly consider the different forms of strabismus, and the various causes that may give rise to them. Before doing so, I must, however, again call attention to the fact that we occasionally meet with cases of *apparent strabismus*. In such there is an undoubted and well-marked deviation (either convergent or divergent) of the optic axes, and yet both eyes are steadily fixed upon the object, and neither moves in the slightest degree when the other is closed. Hence the squint is not real, but only apparent. Donders has called particular attention to this fact, and has furnished us with the explanation.

I have already mentioned (p. 619) that, according to Helmholtz, the optic axis and the visual line (an imaginary line drawn from the yellow spot to the object-point) do not correspond, but that the latter impinges upon the cornea slightly to the inner side of the optic axis, forming with it an angle of about 5°. It will, therefore, be at once apparent, that if the visual lines are parallel, the optic axes must necessarily be slightly divergent, and such is indeed the case in the normal eye; but this divergence is so very slight, and we are so accustomed to it, that it escapes our observation. In some cases, the visual line may change its position with respect to the optic axis, and if this deviation be at all considerable, an apparent squint will arise. In myopia, for instance, the visual line, instead of lying to the inner side of the optic axis, may correspond to the latter, or even lie to the outer side of it; and in the latter case, there will consequently be an apparent convergent squint; for whilst the visual lines meet in the object-point, the optic axes must necessarily cross on this side of it. In hypermetropic eyes, the reverse may obtain; the visual line may lie more than normally to the inner side of the optic axis, forming with it, perhaps, if the hypermetropia be excessive, an angle of 8° or even 9°, instead of one of 5°. If such eyes look at a distant object, they will appear to be affected with a divergent squint, for whilst the visual lines are fixed upon the object, the optic axes will diverge from it. This explanation of Donders is not only exceedingly interesting, but is also of much use to us in practice, for it will guard us against an erroneous diagnosis and treatment of such cases.[1] Some of the cases of so-called incongruence of the retinæ were probably really cases of apparent strabismus.[2]

(1) CONVERGENT STRABISMUS.

Convergent squint is in the vast majority of cases due to hypermetropia. According to Donders,[3] the latter is present in about seventy-five per cent. of the cases of convergent strabismus. De Wecker places it even at a higher figure (eighty-five per cent.). The presence of hypermetropia is often overlooked, because it is either latent, or because the patients are very young, and do not know how to read. The ophthalmoscope would, however, in such cases, at once enable us to detect the true state of refraction.

[While hypermetropia is certainly the most frequent cause of convergent squint, there are statistics of very many cases which show that essential muscular defects are also influential in its production. Hence Donders' views must be modified.—B.]

It will be remembered that we understand by the term "hypermetropia," that condition of the eye in which its refracting power is too low, or the optic axis (antero-posterior axis) too short, so that rays which impinge parallel upon the eye (emanating from distant objects) are not brought to a

[1] From these facts the reader will see how necessary it is that the terms "optic axis" and "visual line" should no longer be used as being identical in signification; for this is not only incorrect, but must lead to constant confusion and misapprehension.

[2] We occasionally meet with cases in which the double images do not at all agree in character with the position of the visual lines. Thus, after an operation for convergent strabismus, we may find that, even although a considerable degree of convergent squint is left, the diplopia is not homonymous, but crossed. This incongruence of the retinæ occurs, almost without exception, only in cases in which the disturbance in the binocular vision dates from early childhood (before the eighth year), which leads in all probability to a faulty development of the appreciation of the identity of the two retinal impressions; a faculty which appears to be purely psychical, and chiefly developed in childhood. (*Vide* Von Graefe's "Symptomenlehre der Augenmuskellahmungen," p. 60; also Nagel, "Das Sehen Mit Zwei Augen, und die Lehre von der Identischen Netzhautstellen," 1861; and Alfred von Graefe, "A. f. O.," xi. 2.

[3] *Vide* Donders' article on "The Pathogeny of Squint," "A. f. O.," ix. 1, 99; also an able translation of this by Dr. Wright, of Dublin.

focus upon the retina, when the eye is in a state of rest, as occurs in the normal eye, but more or less behind it, according to the amount of hypermetropia present. The effect of this low refractive condition is that, whilst the normal eye unites rays from distant objects upon the retina without any accommodative effort, the hypermetropic eye has already, in order so to do, to exert its power of accommodation more or less considerably. This exertion must increase, of course, in a direct ratio with the approximation of the object to the eye; for if the accommodation has already to be brought into play to unite parallel rays upon the retina, how much more must this be the case when the object is closely approximated, and the rays from it impinge in a very divergent direction upon the eye? Now, in order to increase the power of accommodation, one eye often squints inwards, for the following reason: Because, together with the increase in the convergence of the visual lines, there is also an increase in the power of accommodation. We can easily prove the truth of this statement, by placing a prism (with its base outwards) before a hypermetropic eye; for the latter, in looking at distant objects, will then squint inwards, in order to avoid diplopia, and this convergence of the visual lines will now enable it to unite parallel rays (from distant objects) upon the retina, whereas, when its visual lines were parallel, it could only unite convergent rays. Again, on placing a concave lens before a normal eye, we change it into a hypermetropic one, for parallel rays are now united behind the retina, and it will require either a convex glass or an effort of the accommodation, to bring these rays once more to a focus on the retina. If this concave glass be but weak, an increased effort of the accommodation will neutralize its effect, and overcome this artificial hypermetropia. If, however, the concave lens be too strong for this, the eye often overcomes its effect by squinting inwards, and thus increasing its power of accommodation. This shows, therefore, apart from other consequences, the danger of giving a short-sighted person too strong a glass, for we may thus induce a convergent squint. Now, the same thing often occurs in hypermetropia—the one eye squints inwards in order to increase the power of accommodation. At first this squint is but periodic, appearing only when the patient is intently regarding some object. As soon as he looks at any object, near or distant, the one eye may move inwards. Frequently, however, the squint only occurs when he is looking at near objects, as in reading, writing, etc. This squint has, therefore, been termed periodic squint; and hypermetropia is by far the most frequent cause of it. It is even surprising that squint is not more common amongst the hypermetropic. This form of periodic strabismus is often met with in young children, frequently showing itself first about the fourth or fifth year, when they are learning to spell, etc. In such cases we may fail (on only cursorily glancing at the eyes) to detect the slightest squint; if we, however, direct the patient to look fixedly at something—as in reading, etc.—one eye directly squints inwards, this deviation, however, disappearing again as soon as the object is removed. Sometimes this periodic squint shows itself whenever the person is looking intently at any object, be it near or distant; in other cases, however, it only occurs when the eyes are looking at near objects, the squint disappearing as soon as they regard distant objects. The strabismus may, also, be frequently corrected by placing suitable convex glasses before the eyes, so as to neutralize the hypermetropia. If the latter is not neutralised by the constant use of lenses, the squint will generally soon become permanent, acquiring symptoms of concomitant squint. As hypermetropia is often ... frequently exists in several members of the same family, ... also causes strabismus, the popular idea that a squint may be produced by imitation, has gained considerable credence, even in the profession. I have often had occasion to examine such cases of squint occurring in different members of the same family, and have almost invariably found that both patients, the supposed imitator and the imitated, have been hypermetropic; a common cause had produced the same affection.

The reason why the majority of hypermetropic persons do not squint, is evidently due to the fact, as pointed out by Donders, that they prefer to sacrifice a certain degree of distinctness and sharpness of vision in order to avoid diplopia. This is often proved by the fact, that if we cover the one eye of a hypermetropic patient with our hand, it will soon deviate inwards when the other is used for reading, etc. But it is otherwise when the images of the two eyes are very different as regards distinctness, as, for instance, if the degree of hypermetropia is much greater in one eye than in the other, or if there is some opacity in the refracting media of one eye. In such cases, a convergent squint easily becomes developed. The same occurs if the internal recti muscles are very strong. A great difference between the position of the visual line and the optic axis (the two forming a considerable angle) seems also in hypermetropic eyes to predispose to strabismus (Donders).

Convergent squint is most frequently met with in the moderate degrees of hypermetropia (from one-fortieth to one-tenth), being generally absent in the high degrees. This is evidently due to the fact, that when the hypermetropia is very considerable in degree, the accommodation is sufficient (even when the visual lines are abnormally converged) to produce a perfect retinal image, and the patient therefore accustoms himself to gain correct ideas from imperfect representation, rather than improve these by a maximum of effort (Donders).

Impaired vision of the one eye is a frequent cause of strabismus, as we can often notice in cases of opacity of the cornea or of the lens, or of some affection of the deeper structures of the eye; the distinctness of the retinal image of the affected eye being consequently impaired. This difference in the sharpness and intensity of the retinal images of the two eyes is often very confusing and annoying to the patient, and, in order to escape from this annoyance, he involuntarily squints with the affected eye, so that the rays from the object may impinge upon a more peripheral (and, therefore, less sensitive) portion of the retina; and the image of this eye be consequently so much weakened in intensity as not to prove any longer of annoyance. The direction in which this deviation may take place, is generally determined by the relative strength of the different muscles. If one proves preëminently strong, the eye will squint in the direction of this muscle. The latter will contract more and more, and the squint will soon assume all the characters of concomitant strabismus. The image of the squinting eye will be gradually suppressed, and then amblyopia from non-use of the eye will be superadded to the weakness of sight caused by the original affection (opacities in the refracting media, etc.). It must, however, be admitted, as has been pointed out by Pagenstecher, that in very many of these cases of impaired vision hypermetropia coexists, and must, therefore, be regarded as the true cause of the squint. Donders thinks that the inflammation which causes the corneal opacity, may extend to some of the muscles, and at first bring on a spasmodic and then an organic contraction of the muscular tissues. Convergent squint may also arise as a secondary affection, after paralysis, or wounds and injuries of the opponent muscle. Marked instances of this secondary form of squint are but too often furnished by excessive operations for strabismus; the extent of the operation having either been too great for the requirements of the case, or the muscle having been divided instead of the tendon. Spasmodic contraction of the internal rectus may also produce convergent squint, but this does not, strictly speaking, belong to our present subject.

[Cases of intermittent convergent squint have been reported in which it was supposed that the periodicity of the affection pointed to a malarial origin. Samelsohn reports such a case in a girl, six years of age, in which the squint was of a strictly tertian character. There was slight corneal opacity in both eyes, and a hypermetropia of 1.25 D. On the intervening days there was never the slightest degree of squint. Three years later the squint had lost its strictly intermittent type. Long-continued treatment with quinine and arsenic had produced no effect upon the periodicity of the early squint.—B.]

Von Graefe[1] has pointed out, that in rare instances myopia may be the cause of convergent squint. This occurs only in cases in which the myopia is moderate in extent, and in which the eyes are much used for very near work. After a time, the internal recti become contracted from this constant and excessive use, and cannot be relaxed when the patient looks at a distant object, the external recti being too weak to overcome the action of the internal recti. Consequently a convergent squint arises, which is at first periodic, but may in time become permanent, and appear as soon as the patient looks at any object which is not very close to him.

This squint is not met with in cases of very considerable myopia, because in these the necessary convergence of the visual lines can generally not be maintained on account of the close proximity of the object, and therefore the patient only uses one eye. This form of strabismus mostly becomes developed in early manhood, more especially amongst students or literary men who are not in the habit of wearing glasses.

(2) DIVERGENT STRABISMUS, ETC.

Just as hypermetropia is by far the most frequent cause of convergent squint, myopia is the most frequent cause of divergent strabismus. The latter may be constant or absolute, the one visual line always diverging from the object, and this divergence existing for all distances, so that both eyes cannot be brought to converge upon the object at any distance. The divergence, however, sometimes diminishes somewhat when near objects are regarded. Absolute divergence is especially met with in cases in which the sight of one eye is greatly impaired (amaurosis, mature cataract, etc.), in paralysis of the internal rectus muscle, or in cases in which the latter has been too freely divided in an operation for convergent squint.

The principal cause why myopic eyes are so subject to divergent strabismus is to be sought in the elongation of the antero-posterior axis of the eyeball in myopia. On account of the ellipsoidal shape of the globe, its range of mobility is diminished, and it cannot be moved so freely inwards or outwards. The outward limitation of mobility does not matter much, as it only comes into account in the extreme lateral movements of the eye, and the inconvenience arising from it can easily be remedied by a turn of the head.

We find, however, that it is very different if there is a considerable curtailment of the inward movement, as the necessary degree of convergence for a very near point can then only be maintained with great difficulty and exertion. The internal recti muscles are much strained and fatigued, symp-

[1] "A. f. O.," x. 1, 156.

toms of asthenopia appear, and then, to relieve these and the strong muscular effort, one eye is allowed to deviate outwards; when the work can be continued without difficulty. This is one form of periodic or relative divergent strabismus, and the same thing occurs, as Donders has pointed out, whenever the degree of myopia is so extreme that the object has to be approximated so closely to the eye, that the visual lines cannot possibly be brought to converge upon it. Relative divergence may be due simply to the elongation of the eyeball, together with great myopia, the internal recti being healthy; or to weakness of the internal recti, without the presence of myopia; but in most instances these two causes coexist. The tendency to divergent squint is also increased by the small angle which the visual line forms with the optic axis in cases of myopia. We likewise find that divergent squint may only appear when the myopic patient is looking at any object beyond his far point, and which he does not see distinctly; or that it occurs when he is looking vacantly before him without fixedly regarding any object. On account of the indistinctness of the object, there is no effort at binocular vision, and the one eye will follow its natural muscular impulse, and deviate outwards, if the external rectus is relatively stronger than the internal; but if the patient is furnished with suitable concave glasses for distance, so that he can see the objects clearly and distinctly, the desire to maintain binocular vision will overcome the divergence; the same occurring if he is looking at any object within his range of accommodation. When one eye is blind, or there is a great difference in the refraction of the two eyes, divergent strabismus frequently occurs; for as there is no impulse to maintain binocular vision, the internal rectus gradually diminishes in strength, and the external rectus perhaps undergoes secondary contraction. The relative form of divergent squint, dependent upon insufficiency of the internal recti, is a subject of such great importance, and one which demands such careful and special examination and treatment, that I shall treat of it separately under the name of "Muscular Asthenopia."

We must now pass on to the treatment of strabismus. The nature of concomitant squint is totally different from that of the paralytic. In the latter, the innervation of one or more of the muscles of the eyeball is impaired; whereas, concomitant squint is due to a change—an increased degree of tension—in the muscle in the direction of which the squint occurs. But its innervation is normal, as is at once proved by the perfect mobility of the eyeball in this direction, and by the fact, that the secondary deviation exactly equals the primary, and does not exceed it as in cases of paralysis. Practically, we may regard the affected muscle as shortened. We often meet with fixed forms of squint, for paralytic and spasmodic affections of the muscles of the eye may give rise to concomitant squint, leaving behind them but very slight traces of the original affection. But just as paralysis may be the cause of concomitant squint, so may the latter, if it be excessive in degree and of long standing, produce changes in the opponent muscle. Let us, for instance, suppose that there is an excessive convergent squint of the one eye; if the latter is not frequently exercised, and made to fix its visual line upon the object either by an artificial or natural alteration, the non-use of the external rectus will gradually induce atrophy of this muscle. The internal rectus will at the same time become somewhat hypertrophied, and the mobility of the eye outwards will be more or less curtailed. These changes in the structure of the muscles are best prevented by the frequent separate exercising of the squinting eye.

In slight cases of strabismus, it may be advantageous to exercise the weaker muscle by frequent and systematic "orthopædic" exercise; so that it may be gradually strengthened, and enabled to overcome the excessive action of its opponent in the direction in which the eye is deviated. Such exercises are, however, only indicated when the squinting eye possesses a fair degree of sight; when binocular vision exists; and when there is intolerance of diplopia, so that when the double images are brought sufficiently close together, they are fused into one by a voluntary muscular effort. These exercises may be performed by the aid of prisms, the double images being approximated so closely to each other, that they can be readily united As the strength of the muscle increases, that of the prism must be diminished, for thus the distance between the images will be increased, and the muscle more exerted. Javal[1] has introduced a very ingenious stereoscopic arrangement for these orthopædic exercises. The latter consist in the fusion of two large dots (one in each half of the stereoscope), and subsequently of letters and words, gradually diminishing in size. But both the prismatic and stereoscopic exercises demand very great patience and exactitude, and hence most patients infinitely prefer the more speedy cure by operation. These exercises, however, often prove very useful in perfecting the results of an operation. The sight of the squinting eye should also be often practised by itself.

Absolute concomitant squint can be cured only by an operation. De Wecker[2] is, however, of opinion that hypermetropic convergent strabismus not infrequently undergoes a spontaneous cure later in life.

The object of the operation is to weaken the muscle in whose direction the squint occurs, so that its influence upon the movements and position of the eyeball may be diminished. This is effected by carefully dividing the tendon as closely as possible to its insertion; the muscle will then recede slightly, and acquire a new insertion somewhat further back. This recession is, however, accompanied by a certain diminution of power, for the further back the insertion lies, the less power can the muscle exercise upon the movements of the eyeball. As we wish to weaken the muscle, but at the same time to preserve as much of the lateral mobility as possible, we must carefully regulate and adapt the amount and nature of the operation to the requirements of each individual case, and we shall see hereafter how its effects may always be estimated to a nicety. The success depends less upon manual dexterity than upon a thorough knowledge of the theoretical part of the subject.

After the tenotomy and retrocession of the muscle, the eyeball will incline passively to the side of the opponent to about the same extent as the muscle receded on the sclerotic. The diminution in the lateral mobility towards the side of the operated muscle, will, however, exceed the extent of this retrocession. If, for instance, the muscle has receded two lines, the loss of mobility will be from two to three lines, and this would impair the results of the operation considerably (particularly with regard to the accommodative movements) if it was not for the fact, that the mobility of the squinting eye is pathologically increased towards the side of the shortened muscle. Hence the mobility will be in reality but slightly diminished by the operation, or it may even remain equal to that of the other eye.

The question, whether one or both eyes are to be operated on, does not hinge upon the fact whether both eyes squint or not, but depends solely upon the extent of the strabismus. It is quite erroneous to confine the

[1] "Annales d'oculistique," 1868, p. 76; also 1867, p. 5.
[2] "Kl. Monatsbl.," 1871, 458.

operation to one eye, merely because the squint is monolateral, and to perform the double operation only in cases of alternating strabismus.

If the squint measures from two to two and one-half lines we may generally correct it by a single operation; by incising the subconjunctival tissue somewhat freely, and by using a larger hook, we may even obtain an effect of two and one-half or three lines. This is particularly the case in children. If the deviation exceeds two and one-half or three lines, we must always divide the operation between the two eyes.

Let us suppose, for instance, that a patient is affected with a convergent squint of the right eye of about four and one-half lines. To correct this by one operation, we should have to divide the tendon of the internal rectus muscle of this eye to such an extent that the muscle might recede four and one-half lines. This would be, however, accompanied by a diminution in the mobility inwards of about five and one-half lines; and even supposing that the pathological increase in the mobility in this direction had been previously about one line, we should still have a deficiency of about four and one-half lines after the operation. The associated movements towards the left side of the patient would, therefore, be greatly impeded; and this want of mobility inwards would make itself particularly felt during the accommodative movements, for it would prevent the proper convergence of the visual lines during reading, etc., as the visual line of the right eye would deviate slightly outwards from the object, and this divergent squint would soon increase in extent and become permanent. In order to obviate this, we must divide the operation between the two eyes. Let us suppose that the tenotomy of the right internal rectus has corrected two and one-half lines of the deviation, there will, consequently, still remain an inward squint of this eye of about two lines. On covering the left eye with our hand, and telling the patient to look at the object with the right, the latter will have to make an outward movement of two lines, and this will be accompanied by an inward, associated movement of the left eye of the same extent. We must now calculate the extent of the operation which will be necessary to correct the secondary squint of the left eye, just as if the latter was primarily affected with a convergent squint of two lines. Let us now assume that the left internal rectus has been divided, and that we have obtained an effect of two lines; the eye will consequently incline outwards to this extent, a divergent squint of two lines being in fact produced; and it will, therefore, require an extra exertion of the internal rectus to bring the visual line of the left eye to bear again upon the object. Now, this inward movement of two lines will be accompanied by an associated outward movement of the right eye to the same extent; hence the convergent squint which had remained after the first operation will be completely corrected. If binocular vision exists, the double images will now be so very closely approximated, that a very slight muscular effort will be able to unite them permanently, and the cure of the squint will be perfect.

The operation is always to be performed in such a manner, that the greater amount of correction is apportioned to the squinting eye, as the mobility is pathologically increased in the direction of the shortened muscle.

I shall confine my description to three operations, viz., Von Graefe's, the subconjunctival operation of Mr. Critchett, and Liebreich's modification of Von Graefe's operation.

I may mention, however, that the old operation, in which the conjunctiva and subconjunctival tissue were widely incised, the capsule of Tenon lacerated, and the muscle itself, and not its tendon, divided, should never be performed. Its effect is generally most unhappy, and it brought the operation for strabismus into great disrepute.

The principle of Von Graefe's operation consists in a very careful division of the tendon close to its insertion, with the smallest possible amount of laceration of the subconjunctival tissue, and the tendinous processes of the capsule of Tenon. We diminish the power of the muscle by giving it a more backward insertion; but we, at the same time, preserve its length intact. Our object is only to weaken the muscle, and not to render it more or less impotent. Before proceeding to consider this method of operating, I would, however, dwell for a moment upon the anatomical relations of the muscles of the eye with the ocular sheath. Commencing at the optic foramen and loosely embracing the optic nerve, the sheath expands, and passes on to the eyeball, which it encloses like a capsule. It is loosely connected with the sclerotic by connective tissue—so loosely, indeed, as to allow of the free rotation of the globe within it. At the equator of the eyeball, it is pierced by the tendons of the oblique muscles, and, more anteriorly, by the tendons of the four recti muscles, with which it becomes blended; being finally lost on, rather than inserted into, the sclerotic, close to the cornea. The posterior portion of the sheath, up to the passage of the tendons, has been called the capsule of Bonnet; the anterior portion, from the passage of the tendons to its insertion in the sclerotic, having been designated the capsule of Tenon. On piercing the capsule, the tendons of the recti muscles become connected with it by slight cellular processes, sent forth from the capsule. These processes prevent the too great retraction of the muscle after the division of its tendon, which would be followed by a great loss of power. It is, therefore, of much consequence that these connecting processes should not be severed by the tendon being divided too far back, or be lacerated by rude and careless manipulations with the strabismus hook. Von Graefe has, moreover, pointed out that the result may be unfavorable, even although the tendon has been divided anterior to these fibres, as the sheath of the tendon becomes thickened from the point at which it passes through the capsule, and this thickening extends nearly up to its insertion. If the tendon is, therefore, not divided sufficiently close to its insertion, it is apt to retract within this thickened sheath, and this retraction will in many cases prevent its reunion with the sclerotic. In the old operation, the muscle was divided far back, frequently even posterior to its passage through the eyeball, and it was consequently often rendered so powerless that the eyeball could not be moved in this direction; its opponent acquired a corresponding preponderance of power, giving but too frequently rise to a secondary squint in the opposite direction. Hence the popular dread of the operation, "lest the eye should go the other way." But such an unfortunate result is not to be feared if the surgeon performs the operation with care and circumspection, and is thoroughly conversant with the theoretical part of the subject. It is an important rule, never to do too much, for nothing is so difficult as to retrace one's steps and to patch up a fault which has been committed. It is far easier subsequently to increase the effect of the operation than to diminish it. I know of no surgical operation which is so safe and so sure in its cure as that for strabismus when properly performed. Let us now pass on to the description of Von Graefe's operation.

As it is sometimes very painful, the patient should be placed under chloroform or methelyne. [In the United States, sulphuric ether is the anæsthetic generally employed, and very recently the bromide of ethyl has been recommended.—B.] The eyelids are to be kept apart by the spring speculum, or, if this proves not sufficiently strong, by the broad silver elevators. An assistant should evert the eye with a pair of forceps (I am supposing that the internal rectus of the right eye is to be operated on), taking care to do so in the horizontal direction, without rotating the eyeball on its axis; otherwise the horizontal position of the internal rectus will be changed. The operator should then seize, with a pair of finely pointed forceps [Fig. 219],

[Fig. 219.]

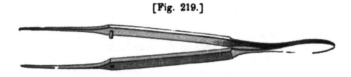

a small but deep fold of the conjunctiva and subconjunctival tissue close to the edge of the cornea, and about midway between the centre and lower edge of the insertion of the internal rectus. He next snips this fold with the scissors (which should be bent on the flat, and blunt-pointed [Fig. 220]),

[Fig. 220.]

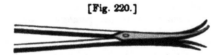

and, burrowing beneath the subconjunctival tissue in a downward and inward direction, makes a funnel-shaped opening beneath the subconjunctival tissue, this being, however, done, very carefully, so as not to divide it to too great an extent. If the subconjunctival tissue is thick and strong, it will be better first to take up a small fold of the conjunctiva only, to open this, and then, seizing the subconjunctival tissue, to divide the latter. The squint-hook, which should be bent at a right-angle, and have a slightly bulbous point (vide Fig. 221), is then to be passed through the opening to the lower edge of the tendon. Its point being pressed somewhat firmly against the sclerotic, the hook is to be turned on the point and slid upwards beneath the tendon, as close to its insertion as possible, and the whole expanse of the tendon caught up. The operator must be careful not to direct the point of the hook upwards and outwards, otherwise it may perforate the fibres of the tendon, and only a portion of the latter be caught up; the direction of the point should, therefore, be rather upwards and inwards. When the tendon has been secured on the hook, the conjunctiva which covers its upper portion may be gently pushed off with the points of the scissors, so as to expose the tendon, which is then to be carefully snipped through with the scissors as closely as possible to its insertion. When it has been completely cut through, the conjunctiva is to be slightly elevated on the point of the hook, and a smaller hook passed upwards and downwards to ascertain whether the lateral expansions of the tendon have been divided. Should a few fibres remain, they must be divided, and the surgeon should again ascertain whether any others are still present. He should never omit to satisfy himself upon this point, for sometimes the lateral expansions are considerable,

Fig. 221.

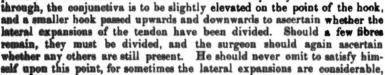

the tendon spreading out like a fan, and although a few fibres only might remain undivided, they would suffice to spoil the effect of the operation.

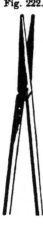

Fig. 222.

I have lately adopted a slight modification of Von Graefe's operation, and perform it more subconjunctivally. I use a pair of straight blunt-pointed scissors [Fig. 222], and, instead of pushing off the conjunctiva from the hook so as to expose the tendon caught up by the latter, I divide the tendon subconjunctivally, quite close to its insertion. In this way, the advantages of Von Graefe's and the subconjunctival operation are combined. On account of the smaller size of the hook, and the situation of the incision (which is between the centre and lower edge of the tendon), the subconjunctival tissue is stretched and incised to a much less extent than in the subconjunctival operation. Again, the position and direction of the conjunctival wound are such that a suture can be at once applied, if necessary; whereas in the subconjunctival operation the incision would have to be considerably enlarged upwards, before any effect could be produced by a suture upon the two cut edges of the tendon. But where the degree of strabismus is so considerable that it is certain no suture will be required, the subconjunctival operation may be employed; and also if we have no assistant at hand to roll the eye in the opposite direction.

If it is found, on the first introduction of the hook, that this slides up to the edge of the cornea without having caught up the tendon, it is certain that we have either not divided the subconjunctival tissue at all, or that the hook has been passed between it and the conjunctiva. If the former is the case, we must open the subconjunctival tissue, and then, on reintroducing the hook, we shall have no difficulty in finding the tendon. The opening in the conjunctiva and subconjunctival tissue should be but small, and the excursions with the hook limited, otherwise the subconjunctival tissue and the lateral processes of the capsule of Tenon will be extensively lacerated, which may be followed by too great a recession of the muscle.

The after-treatment is very simple. The eye, after having been well washed and cleansed of any blood coagula, is to be kept constantly moist with cold-water dressing during the day of operation, so as to prevent any extensive effusion of blood under the conjunctiva. No button of granulations will form on the stump of the tendon, if the latter has been divided close to its insertion, and if the opening in the conjunctiva has been made near the upper or lower edge of the tendon, so as not to leave the latter exposed.

The effect upon the squint which follows immediately upon the operation will not be the permanent one. We may, indeed, distinguish three stages in the effect produced by the operation: 1st. The period immediately following the operation; 2d. After three or four days have elapsed; 3d. After the interval of a few months—this being the permanent effect. During the first stage, the effect will be considerable, for the eye can now only be moved in the direction of the divided muscle by the indirect connection of the latter with the sclerotic by the lateral processes of the capsule of Tenon. As soon as the divided end of the tendon becomes reunited with the sclerotic, which generally occurs within three or four days, the effect will diminish, for the muscle now again exerts a direct influence upon the eyeball. This is the second stage. But we find that a further alteration in the position generally shows itself a few weeks or months after the operation, the effect being then again somewhat increased. This is due to the action of the opponent muscle, which, on account of its antagonist having been weakened, can now exert a greater influence upon the position of the eyeball.

A clue to the permanent result of the operation is furnished by the position of the operated eye during the accommodative movements of the eyes, when they are directed upon some near object. It is, therefore, of great consequence always to test the position of the eyes during accommodation immediately after the operation, as soon as the effect of the anæsthetic has gone off. We have already seen that the position of the squinting eye (convergent strabismus) may vary when the object is approximated closely to the eyes; for whilst the visual line of the healthy eye remains fixed upon the object, converging the more the nearer the latter is brought, the position of the squinting eye may undergo the following changes: 1st. It may retain its original position, sustaining only a few oscillating, irregular, lateral movements. 2d. It may remain completely stationary, so that the angle of squinting will diminish the more the nearer the object is brought, until at a certain point (if the squint be not excessive), its visual line will also be fixed upon the object, and there will no longer be any squint. If, however, the object is approximated still closer, a divergent squint will arise; for whilst the healthy eye coverges still more, the other retains its position, and now deviates (passively) outwards. 3d. It retains its position up to a certain point, and then, as the healthy eye moves inwards to follow the object, it makes an associated movement outwards. 4th. It deviates suddenly and spasmodically inwards when the object is very closely approximated.

We should, therefore, soon after the operation, when the effect of the anæsthetic has passed off,[1] ascertain whether both visual lines can be steadily fixed upon the object, when it is brought to a distance of from four to six inches from the eyes (their state of refraction being normal). If the eyes are very short-sighted, the distance should be still less. The final result of the operation may be predicted from the position which the operated eye now assumes. If it remains stationary when the object is brought up to within eight inches from the eye, so that a passive divergence will arise on its being approximated still closer, we must expect a certain amount of divergence in the course of a few months. But this will be still more the case, if the eye, instead of simply remaining stationary, makes an associated movement outwards. It is necessary to test this at short distances (four or six inches), for the eye might be able momentarily to fix its visual line upon the object, although quite incapable of maintaining this position for any length of time. In both the above cases, the effect of the operation is to be diminished by a conjunctival suture, and particularly so in the latter instance. The effect of the suture will vary with its position, and with the amount of the conjunctiva embraced in it. Its effects will be considerable if it be inserted in a diagonal direction from downwards and inwards to upwards and outwards, so that the inner and outer lips of the wound are united. By giving it this direction, we also prevent any sinking of the caruncle. The suture diminishes the effect of the operation by readvancing the tendon, which is closely connected with the conjunctiva and subconjunctival tissue; the divided ends will consequently be more closely approximated, and the retraction of the muscle diminished. The suture may remain in for from twenty-four to thirty-six hours. Sutures should not be applied in all cases, as is recommended by

[1] For some time past I have often employed methelyne in place of chloroform in strabismus operations, iridectomies, etc.; its chief advantages over chloroform are that its effect is not only much quicker, but also passes off again much sooner. If it be well given, I like it even for extraction of cataract.

some authors; for this is quite erroneous, they being only indicated if the effect of the tenotomy is too considerable.

The fourth position which the operated eye may assume during accommodation, viz., making a sudden spasmodic movement inwards, must make us fear that there will be a relapse—that in the course of a few months the inward squint will again show itself; for this convergent squint, which at first only showed itself during accommodation for near objects, will gradually extend also to greater distances. In such cases, the operation is said to have been only of temporary benefit; but on examination we mostly find that the patient is hypermetropic, and that suitable glasses generally correct the squint.

The extent of the operation must be regulated according to the degree of the squint.

In very slight degrees of strabismus (one line to one and one-half lines) a partial tenotomy was formerly often practised, the tendon not being completely divided, but a few of the upper or lower fibres (as the case might be) being left standing. But this does not answer, as the power of the muscle is but slightly, if at all, impaired. In such cases we should, therefore, make a complete tenotomy, and, if necessary, insert a suture. The conjunctival opening should be small and the hook but of moderate size. The accommodative movements must be accurately tested immediately after the operation; for if there is the slightest tendency to divergence when the object is brought up to eight or six inches from the eye, a suture should be inserted. In a squint of two or two and one-half lines, the cellular tissue may be somewhat more freely incised, and a larger hook employed. In children we find that the effect is generally more considerable, for the muscle is not hypertrophied and the surrounding cellular tissue is very elastic; we may, therefore, in them easily attain an effect of two and one-half or three lines by a single operation.

If the squint exceeds two and one-half or three lines, we must always operate upon both eyes. We should perform a free tenotomy in the squinting eye and a very careful one in the other, limiting the effect in the latter by a suture. In this we must be guided by the amount of squint left after the affected eye has been operated upon. As a general rule, I do not think it advisable to operate upon both eyes at the same time, except the squint is very considerable, exceeding four and one-half or five lines; for if both muscles have been divided at the same time, we cannot accurately test the accommodative movements directly after the operation, and we thus lose the only clue to the permanent effect. It is, therefore, far safer to operate first upon the affected eye, and then, after a few days have elapsed, and the divided tendon has again reunited with the sclerotic, to ascertain how much of the squint is still left. The amount still remaining will guide us as to the extent of the operation necessary upon the healthy eye. If, after having operated upon the latter, we find that the effect somewhat exceeds our wishes, we can always diminish it by a suture. It certainly is far more brilliant to operate upon both eyes at the same time, and thus rid the patient at once of the squint, but, then we run the risk of the unpleasant contingency of the eye subsequently "going the other way." It should always be remembered that the cure is to be permanent, and not temporary. In some exceptional cases, however, the risk must be run—if, for instance, the time of the patient limited, or a second visit impossible. If the squint exceeds five lines, we may, particularly in adults, operate safely upon both eyes at the same time. may be occasionally necessary to operate not only upon both eyes, but n to repeat the operation upon the squinting eye, before we can cure the n. This generally occurs only in cases of excessive squint, or if the nus existed for a long time, and the muscle has become hypertrophied. This second operation upon the affected eye requires considerable care, for the effect of the correction will exceed the extent of the retraction, as the influence of the muscle upon the eyeball diminishes in proportion to the backward position of its insertion.

But in severe cases, it is still better to operate first upon the squinting eye, and to increase the effect as much as possible by making the patient look over to the opposite side for some days after the operation, so that the cut edges of the tendon may be stretched apart and widely separated. The effect of this will be that the union will take place further back than would have occurred if the eye had maintained a median position. If the internal rectus of the right eye has been divided, and we desire to increase the effect of the operation, the patient should be directed to look, as far as possible, towards his right side. The easiest way of attaining this is, by making the patient wear spectacles, the left half of each glass being covered with a piece of court-plaster, for he will in this way be obliged to look to the right. They should be worn during the first three or four days after the operation. Or two pieces of card may be fixed over the left half of the eyes, by means of a tape passing over the forehead. By this means we shall obtain a very considerable effect by the operation, and the amount of squint still remaining must then be treated by an operation upon the other eye.[1]

Von Graefe points out the fact that, occasionally, though rarely, we meet with cases in which the operation is followed by no effect, either upon the position or mobility of the eyeball, and yet no lateral fibres of the tendon have remained undivided. In such cases, there is a second connection of the muscle with the sclerotic further back, near the equator of the eye; in one instance, indeed, he found it even posterior to the equator.

If the operation for squint be carefully performed, there is no fear of any but the slightest sinking of the caruncle. A little sinking will occasionally occur, whatever mode of operation be employed; indeed, I know of no method which can guarantee a *perfect* immunity from it. Von Graefe thinks that the sinking does not depend so much upon the gaping of the conjunctival wound and retraction of its inner lip, as upon the cicatrization of the connective tissue situated between the muscle and conjunctiva, by which the movable caruncle is retracted. The further back this cicatrization extends, the more will the caruncle sink. Hence the danger of incising the tendon too freely, and of any considerable sweeping about with the hook, and consequent extensive laceration of the subconjunctival tissue.

Mr. Critchett's subconjunctival operation is to be performed as follows: The patient having been placed under the influence of an anæsthetic, and the

---

[1] In cases of very considerable squint (both internal and external) Von Graefe advises that the effect of the operation should be increased by the insertion of a suture on that side of the eye which is opposite the tenotomy. Thus, if the internal rectus has been divided, a curved needle, armed with a strong silk thread, is to be inserted in the ocular conjunctiva, near the outer canthus, and pushed towards the cornea, beneath the conjunctiva, to an extent of four or five lines, and then removed. In this way a broad fold of conjunctiva will be included within the loop of silk, which is to be tightly drawn together and firmly knotted. This will cause the eye to roll outwards, and considerably limit the movement inwards. The suture is to remain in for two and one-half or three days. I have treated many cases in this way with marked success. In some severe cases (especially of divergent squint) I have inserted a strong suture passed for two or three lines beneath the conjunctiva, close to the edge of the cornea, opposite to the muscle which is to be divided, and then, after the tenotomy, rolling the eye to the opposite side, and keeping it fixed in this position by means of the suture, so that the divided ends of the tendon are widely stretched apart. This suture is to be retained for two or three days.

eyelids kept apart by the stop-speculum, he seizes a small fold of the conjunctiva and subconjunctival tissue at the lower edge of the insertion of the
rectus muscle, and with a pair of blunt-pointed straight scissors,
makes a small incision at this point through these structures.
The lower edge of the tendon, close to its insertion, is now exposed. A blunt hook (Fig. 223) is next to be passed through
the opening in the subconjunctival tissue beneath the tendon, so
as to catch up the latter, and render it tense. The points of the
scissors (but slightly opened) are then to be introduced into the
aperture, and one point passed along the hook behind the tendon,
the other in front of the tendon between it and the conjunctiva,
and the tendon is then to be divided close to its insertion by successive snips of the scissors. A small counter-puncture may be
made at the upper edge of the tendon, to permit of the escape of
any effused blood, and thus prevent its diffusion beneath the
conjunctiva (Bowman).

Fig. 223.

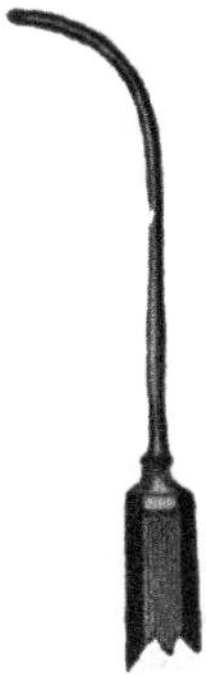

[In this operation the tendon, owing to the cutting action of the
scissors, is apt to slip off the hook before it has been completely
divided. To remedy this, Dr. Theobald[1] has devised the "crochet
hook" (Fig. 224). With the exception of the crochet point, it is similar to
Von Graefe's strabismus hook. The tendon being secured by it, it is not
necessary to force the point up against the conjunctiva, as is ordinarily done,

Fig. 224.

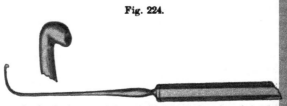

a. Crochet hook, natural size.   *b.* Magnified view of crochet point.

so as to throw the tendon into the angle of the hook, while it is being divided,
but simply to hold the handle at right angles to the muscle.—H.]

Mr. Liebreich[2] has lately introduced a modification of the operation of
strabismus, based upon a different view of the anatomical relations of the
conjunctiva, subconjunctival tissue, and the capsule of Tenon to the muscles
of the eye. He considers the capsule of Tenon as divided into two portions—
an anterior and a posterior—the division being formed at the point where
the recti muscles pierce it from without inwards; the capsule being at this
point so closely connected with the muscles as to render any displacement
between the two impossible. The posterior half of the capsule, with its
smooth, firm, inner surface, forms a cup, in which the eyeball moves as freely
as the head of a joint in the socket. The close connection between the
muscles and the posterior half of the capsule is increased by sheath-like processes, which run backwards from the outer surface of the capsule towards
the orbit, and which are, for a certain distance, closely connected with the
muscles. But there are no sheath-like processes between the inner portion
of the posterior capsule and the sclerotic. The anterior half of the capsule
of Tenon adheres to the upper surface of the muscle, and is intimately con-

[1 "Amer. Journ. of Med. Sci.," April, 1872, p. 406.—H.]
[2 "A. f. O.," xii. 2, 298; also "British Medical Journal," Dec. 15, 1866.

ueeted with it. But Liebreich denies the presence of sheath-like processes derived from the capsule, where they pierce the latter, and accompanying the muscles as far as their insertion. He states, moreover, that "the caruncle, together with the semilunar fold, rests upon a band-like ligament, which passes from the capsule of Tenon towards the edge of the orbit. Now, when the internal rectus is contracted, and the eye rolled inwards, this band is rendered tense; and the caruncle, which is fixed to it, is consequently drawn in towards the inner edge of the orbit. But the outer edge of the caruncle, together with the semilunar fold, and an adjoining portion of conjunctiva are drawn backwards into a furrow." This intimate connection between the muscle, capsule, and caruncle, is the reason of the sinking of the caruncle and semilunar fold, which is occasionally observed after an extensive division of the internal rectus. To obviate these disadvantages, and yet to obtain a considerable effect, Liebreich operates in the following manner:

"If the internal rectus is to be divided, I raise with a pair of forceps a fold of conjunctiva at the lower edge of the insertion of the muscle; and, incising this with scissors, enter the points of the latter at the opening between the conjunctiva and the capsule of Tenon. I then carefully separate these two tissues from each other as far as the semilunar fold, also separating the latter, as well as the caruncle, from the parts lying behind. When this portion of the capsule, which is of much importance in the tenotomy, has been completely separated from the conjunctiva, I divide the insertion of the tendon from the sclerotic in the usual manner, and extend the vertical cut, which is made simultaneously with the tenotomy, upwards and downwards—the more so if a very considerable effect is desired. The wound in the conjunctiva is then closed with a suture.

"The same mode of operating is to be pursued in dividing the external rectus; and the separation of the conjunctiva is to be continued as far as that portion of the external angle which is drawn sharply back when the eye is turned outwards.

"The following are the advantages of my proceeding:

"1. It affords the operator a greater scope in apportioning and dividing the effect of the operation between the two eyes.

"2. The sinking back of the caruncle is avoided, as well as every trace of a cicatrix, which not unfrequently occurs in the common tenotomy.

"3. There is no need for more than two operations on the same individual, and therefore of more than one on the same eye."

I have performed Liebreich's operation in numerous instances with success, and should prefer it to any other in those cases in which it is desirable to gain a very considerable effect, and yet confine the operation to one eye. For I have not found that we are able by any other operation to obtain so considerable an effect with so slight a loss of mobility, and so very little (if any) sinking of the caruncle; yet the inadmissibility of chloroform and the insertion of the sutures have prevented my practising this operation extensively. If an anæsthetic is given, we cannot estimate with exactitude the degree of effect which we are producing by the free incisions in the capsule; and but few patients are willing to submit to a lengthened and very painful operation, unless an anæsthetic is administered. The removal of the sutures a day or two after the operation is frequently attended with a good deal of difficulty in children and nervous, hysterical women, for although the proceeding is quite painless, yet it is often regarded by the patient and his friends as a second operation. Where it is absolutely necessary for the success of the operation to insert a suture, I never hesitate to do so, but in Von Graefe's operation this is the exception, whereas in Liebreich's it is the rule.

[Dr. Noyes, of Detroit, operates for the cure of squint by making the tenotomy on the antagonistic, or what he calls the elongated tendon. The shortening necessary to correct the squint is made by lapping the ends of the divided tendon, and maintaining them in position by two sutures passed through the conjunctiva and lapped ends of the tendon, above and below, and tied lightly. He considers the operation applicable in all cases. It is practically an advancement of one muscle without the tenotomy of the antagonist. ("Trans. Amer. Ophth. Soc.," 1874, p. 273.)—B.]

I must now describe the method in which certain special forms of strabismus should be treated. The question sometimes arises, whether the periodic squint which is caused by hypermetropia should be operated on, or whether it is to be corrected by the use of suitable convex glasses. If it is but slight in extent, glasses may suffice, but if it is considerable, and the internal rectus is very strong, tenotomy should be performed; for by dividing the internal rectus, we diminish its power, and a greater exertion of this muscle will consequently be demanded, in order to bring the visual line to bear again upon the object. This extra exertion will be accompanied by an increased power of accommodation, as was the case before, when the eye squinted. But we shall now have an increased power of accommodation with a normal position of the visual lines.

On examining such cases of periodic squint with prisms, we generally find that the internal recti muscles are abnormally strong, this preponderance in strength extending throughout the whole field of vision, so that the correct position of the visual lines, which may occur when convex glasses are interposed, is frequently forced. A carefully performed tenotomy of the internal rectus muscle is, consequently, productive of very favorable results. By advising an operation for this form of periodic squint, I do not propose to set aside the use of convex glasses for the treatment of the hypermetropia; I only think it beneficial to balance the strength of the muscles of the eyeball, and to restore their normal equilibrium, for this will be accompanied by increased facility and comfort in the use of the eyes, particularly for prolonged work at near objects. Whether or not both eyes will require to be operated on, will depend upon the amount of the squint, and the relative strength of the internal recti muscles.

I believe that the best treatment for this form of periodic squint consists in a careful tenotomy of the internal rectus, with subsequent neutralization of the hypermetropia by means of convex glasses. In some cases, the question may, however, arise, whether, by operating upon the periodic squint, we may not only free the patient from the deformity, but also obviate the necessity for spectacles; for, after the operation, the increased exertion of the accommodation in reading, etc., will be unaccompanied by a squint. This question arises chiefly with ladies, who desire not only to be freed from the squint, but also from the necessity of wearing spectacles.

Dr. John Green[1] strongly recommends, in the periodic convergent hypermetropic strabismus in young children, the periodic instillation of atropine until the accommodation is completely paralyzed, which leads to the speedy abandonment of the habit of squinting, and then giving them suitable convex glasses.

The periodic squint which occurs in the short-sighted generally only shows itself when the object is removed beyond the range of accommodation. As this squint disappears as soon as the myopia is neutralized by the proper

---

[1] "Transactions of the American Ophthalmological Society," 1870 and 1871.

concave glasses, it might appear unnecessary to have recourse to an operation, but we yet find that this greatly facilitates the continued use of the eyes for near objects.   On excluding the affected eye from the act of vision by shading it with our hand, we observe that it then moves inwards, even although the object is held within its range of accommodation; its fixation was, therefore, forced.   On testing such cases with prismatic glasses, the internal rectus muscle is generally found to be abnormally strong.   It is, therefore, necessary to weaken it, and thus restore the equilibrium, so that the strength of the different muscles of the eyeball may be evenly balanced. But great care must be taken that we do not produce too great an effect, and render convergence of the visual lines for near objects impossible.   Hence the power of convergence for a very near point (three or four inches) must always be carefully and accurately tested, and if it is found that it is only produced with difficulty, the effect of the operation must be at once diminished by a conjunctival suture.   In order that we may not be misled by the temporary insufficiency of the divided muscle, which afterwards partly disappears again, Von Graefe recommends that the point of fixation (both for near and distant objects) should not lie in the median line, but towards the temporal side of the operated eye; for in this position, the temporary insufficiency of the internal rectus will come less into play, and the temporary result will correspond more closely to the permanent.

In slight cases of this form of periodic squint, it may suffice to give the patient concave glasses, so that he may be able to hold the object (book, etc.) at a greater distance.   Or, again, we may combine the concave glasses with abducting prisms.

Operation for the cure of Diplopia.—We are sometimes called upon to operate for the cure of diplopia, the deviation of the visual line being, at the same time, perhaps, hardly perceptible.   These form the most difficult and intricate cases, for here less depends upon mere manual dexterity than upon a complete mastery of the theoretical portion of the subject, and a thorough knowledge of the actions of the muscles of the eyeball, and their effect upon the position of the vertical meridian, etc.   Having already explained these subjects, I shall only mention the chief points to b considered in the treatment.   We must, in the first place, ascertain in what directions prisms have to be turned in order to fuse the double images, and whether any active tendency exists to unite the images if they are closely approximated.   We find that certain kinds of double images are far more difficult to unite than others.   It is quite impossible to fuse images which are of a different height, except, indeed, this difference be of the very slightest, equalling a prism of $1°-2°$.   Crossed double images, again, are more difficult to unite than homonymous.   If the double images show a difference in height, we must first endeavor to remedy this by an operation, and then, when this is cured, the patient may be able to fuse them if they are sufficiently close to each other.   Should they be crossed, we must change them into homonymous, and approximate them close to each other, so that they may be easily united.

Secondary Strabismus after Paralysis of the Opponent Muscle.—Our treatment must vary with the amount of immobility in the direction of the paralyzed muscle.   Let us assume that, after a paralysis of the abductor, the immobility outwards amounts to from one to one and one-half line, but that there is no deviation inwards, so that the diplopia only extends up to the middle line, or but slightly into the opposite half of the field of vision. In such cases, a simple tenotomy of the internal rectus will generally suffice. If the immobility exceeds one or one and one-half line, ranging between this and two or two and one-half lines, a simple tenotomy will not suffice, and we must then bring forward the insertion of the paralyzed muscle (operation of "readjustment"), and combine with this a tenotomy of the opponent and a suture. If the want of mobility in the direction of the paralyzed muscle exceeds two and one-half lines, we must bring forward the paralyzed muscle, and, at the same time, divide its opponent. Our object in bringing forward the insertion of the paralyzed muscle is to afford it an increased amount of power over the eyeball; for the more anterior its insertion the greater its power. This operation of readjustment, as it is called, is also to be performed in those cases of secondary strabismus which sometimes follow tenotomy of the opponent muscle. I also do it in cases of considerable divergent strabismus, where tenotomy of the two external recti would prove insufficient.

I now generally perform the operation of readjustment in the following manner: Let us suppose that the insertion of the internal rectus is to be brought forward accompanied by tenotomy of the external rectus. I commence by making, with the blunt-pointed strabismus scissors, a vertical incision in the conjunctiva about one and one-half or two lines from the inner edge of the cornea and extending somewhat beyond its upper and lower margin; this incision must not be made too close to the cornea, otherwise the portion of conjunctiva left standing next the cornea will not be sufficiently wide to admit of strong, firm sutures being passed through it. In the next place, all the parts covering the inner side of the globe (conjunctiva, subconjunctival tissue, capsule of Tenon, and the internal rectus muscle) are to be dissected off with the scissors quite close to the sclerotic. This dissection should reach to the equator of the eyeball, and when the flap thus formed, containing the muscle and portion of capsule appertaining to it, has been rendered freely movable, it is to be pulled well forward with a pair of forceps, and if there appears to be rather too much conjunctiva, a portion of this is to be snipped off, but care must be taken not to cut away too much, or any portion of the muscle. I next pass five curved needles through the flap of conjunctiva left standing at the edge of the cornea; the three central needles are very small and carry fine silk, the two lateral ones are larger and armed with very strong silk. The central suture is to be opposite the centre of the cornea, and the next two nearer the upper and lower margin of the cornea, and the two strong lateral ones are to lie above and below the cornea, and embrace a good-sized piece of conjunctiva; for these two sutures are of special importance, as the chief pull upon the muscle, etc., is to be made by them, and they thus take off most of the strain from the smaller central sutures, which are otherwise very apt to give way. The sutures are then to be passed (very far back) through the flap raised at the inner side of the eye, and at points exactly opposite to those in the corneal flap, and firmly tied. I tied the lateral first, and then the central ones, for in this way we greatly diminish the strain upon the latter, and there is less chance of their breaking. I next proceed to the division of the external rectus, but before doing so, I pass a curved needle, carrying a strong silk thread, beneath a broad portion of the conjunctiva, midway between the insertion of the external rectus and the cornea, but I do not tie the suture until the tendon has been divided, otherwise it puckers up the conjunctiva and renders the tenotomy more difficult. The eyeball is finally rolled far inwards by means of this suture, the ends of which are to be firmly fixed by strips of plaster to the bridge of the nose. [Various modifications of this operation have been proposed, all differing merely in the quantity of tissue included in the sutures, and the points at which the needles are introduced through the muscle to be advanced. In Agnew's operation, the lateral sutures are passed beneath the conjunctiva as far as the vertical meridian of the cornea, and then brought out and tied. The conjunctiva is dissected up from the muscle as far as the caruncle, and made to cover it after it is advanced. A more recent method of performing this operation, which possesses some advantages, is that proposed by Dr. Prince, of Jacksonville, Ill., and a description of which will be found in the St. Louis "Medical and Surgical Journal" for June, 1881; and in Noyes' "Treatise on Diseases of the Eye," p. 116.—B.]

In bringing forward the internal rectus, some operators draw forth the muscle somewhat and pass the stitches through it. Schweigger recommends a flat tenotomy hook to be passed beneath the insertion of the muscle, and then behind the hook a suture, with a needle at each end; the tendon is next divided, and the muscle can then be easily drawn forward by the suture. As there is generally considerable reaction after this operation, cold compresses should be applied for the first day or two. The suture by which the eyeball is pulled in should be removed at the end of forty-eight or seventy-two hours, but those which keep the internal rectus in position should be allowed to remain for eight or ten days, if possible.

11.—MUSCULAR ASTHENOPIA (INSUFFICIENCY OF THE INTERNAL RECTI MUSCLES)[1]—[LATENT DIVERGENT SQUINT.—B.]

This affection is of common occurrence, and is characterized by very marked symptoms of asthenopia, which sometimes prove so irksome and harassing to the patient as to incapacitate him from reading, etc. Such patients complain that after they have been working or reading for a certain length of time, the eyes become hot and uncomfortable, the print grows dim, the letters become confused and run into, or overlap each other. This is generally preceded by a feeling of tension and weight in the eyes and over the brow, and some patients distinctly feel how the one eye becomes unsteady and wavering in its fixation, and then moves gradually outwards. They often also anticipate these symptoms by closing one eye. After resting for a short time, reading may be resumed, to be, however, again interrupted by the same train of symptoms.

[The pain in these cases is often through the temple or forehead, or even at the vertex. Many cases of obstinate headache, which have resisted all treatment, originate in disorders of the ocular muscles, and disappear when these disorders are corrected. The assertion has been made that chorea, epilepsy, and other functional nervous disorders, are caused by conditions of muscular asthenopia; but this is extremely doubtful, and it is much more probable in the case of chorea it gives rise itself to debility and irregular action of the ocular muscles as one of its manifestations. The statement that chorea can be cured by relieving the ocular trouble, whether the latter is a refractive or muscular error, has not been substantiated by the Editor in a single case out of a large number examined and treated. (See on this subject, "A Treatise on Diseases of the Eye," by Henry D. Noyes, 1881, p. 88.)—B.]

On examining the eyes, we find that they look normal, that the acuity of vision and range of accommodation are good, but that there is, as a rule, a

---

[1] For fuller information upon this subject, I would refer the reader to Von Graefe's articles, "A. f. O.," viii. 2, and "Kl. Monatsbl.," 1869, p. 225.

considerable degree of myopia. If we direct the patient to l
with both eyes at an object (a pencil, or our finger), and gradua
mate this to the eye, we find that when the object is brought
inches from the patient, the one eye becomes unsteady and wa
fixation, and then either gradually and slowly, or suddenly an
cally, deviates outwards. The same deviation occurs (even pe
object is some feet distant) when we cover one eye with our h
of ground glass, so as to exclude it from participation in bino
Such a deviation will likewise manifest itself if a prism is held
upwards or downwards so as to produce diplopia, for the do
cannot be fused into one, as the eyes are unable to unite do
which show any but the very slightest difference in height. Th
more delicate test than that of covering one eye with our han
enable us to detect degrees of deviation of the visual lines w
slight to be appreciated by the eye. But in many instances
asthenopia we find that, although a prism with its base turned
downwards does not produce divergence at a distance, yet t
rectus is able to overcome a prism of 10°, 14°, 18°, for distance.
(facultative divergence), as Von Graefe points out, is much incr
patient is ordered to wear an abducting prism for a day or tw
final trial is made.

We find that the normal eye is generally able to overcom
from 20° to 30° with its base turned outwards, and one of 6° o
base turned inwards. This is owing to the fact that the exter
much stronger and more exercised than the external. But very
can overcome more than a prism of 1° or 2° with its base turn
or downwards. In consequence of this, diplopia will, therefore l
the visual impulse will be annulled, and the eye yiel

Fig. 225.   ponderating influence of the strongest muscle. In th
the muscles are equally balanced, and the double ima,
show a difference in height, standing straight one abo
But if either the internal or external rectus consideri
the normal standard of strength, the double images
show a difference in height, but also a lateral differe
internal rectus is insufficient, the eye will move outw
prism is held with its base upwards or downwards, an
consequently, be not only a difference in the height o
images, but they will also be crossed, on account of t
squint. We may then easily express the degree of
by the degree of the prism (base turned inwards) whic
to bring the double images one above the other. I
the presence of insufficiency of the internal recti mus
not be gui ed by the position of the binocular ne
youthful myopes may be able to converge for even t
half inches, and yet there may be a considerable di
the lateral equilibrium of the eyes. Hence Von G
upon the importance of carefully estimating the lateral
of the muscles at the distance at which the patient ge
or writes, this being best done in the following man
is drawn on a piece of paper, and is bisected by a very fine
(Fig. 225). This paper is placed at the usual distance of readin,
and the patient is directed to regard the dot with both eyes. A

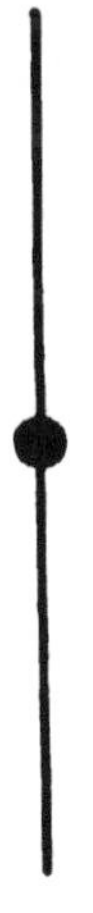

1 " Kl. Monatsbl.," 1869, p. 247.

(with its base upwards) is then to be placed in front of one eye. This will at once produce diplopia, and the image of the eye before which the prism is held will be beneath that of the other eye. If the eyes are normal, the double images will only show a difference in height, but not any lateral difference; they will lie straight above one another. But if the internal rectus is insufficient, the eye moves outwards, and consequently the double images will not only show a difference in height, but also a lateral difference, and they will be crossed. We next try what prism (with its base inwards) is required to neutralize the effect of this deviation, and bring the images straight above each other. In order to ascertain whether the images are crossed or homonymous, we place a slip of red glass before the other eye, and this will enable us at once to distinguish which image belongs to the right and which to the left eye. Von Graefe points out that if the line is not very thin and the dot sufficiently large, the patient may bring the linear double images into one, which of course entirely deceives us as to the dynamic equilibrium of the muscles. We may know, however, that this endeavor at fusion of the double images has occurred, if the slightest lateral turn of the vertical prism does not at once produce a corresponding horizontal deviation of the double images. We must next test the degree of the disturbance in the lateral equilibrium a little further off, and finally at a distance, a lighted candle forming the best object. Von Graefe, however, strongly insists upon the fact that the absence of dynamic divergence for distance (or even the presence of a certain degree of dynamic convergence) does not contra-indicate the necessity for an operation.[1]

We must next ascertain the power of abduction (facultative divergence) for distance, i. e., we must find the strongest prism (with its base turned inwards) which the patient can overcome by a voluntary exertion of the external rectus, when the object is placed at a distance of eight or ten feet. In testing this, the object must not be held in the horizontal visual plane, but about 20° below it. A prism of 18° (with its base turned inwards) should be placed before one eye, and the candle be then gradually removed from the eye, until homonymous double images appear; the furthest point at which single vision can be maintained for a few minutes being noted, for a mere momentary fusion should not suffice. If the power of abduction is very slight compared with the disturbance of the lateral equilibrium at a short distance, an abducting prism (the strength divided between the two eyes) should be worn in spectacles for a few days, which will soon greatly increase the power of abduction. In these experiments great care must be taken that the prisms are held quite horizontal, for any difference in height renders their voluntary fusion extremely difficult, or even impossible. Von Graefe points out the importance of detecting and correcting the little differences in the height of the double images which sometimes exist in these cases, and which should always be suspected if the power of abduction is very small, for it will be found that when these differences in height are equalized by a suitable prism, the power of abduction is generally often very greatly increased. We must also be upon our guard that the patient does not suppress (exclude) the one image, for in this way he may apparently overcome excessively strong prisms, and his single vision may altogether mislead us as to the necessity and extent of an operation. Hence it is of much importance to ascertain in all cases whether or not the patient excludes. If the one eye is not excluded, we find that each remains steadily fixed upon the object when the other is covered.

[1] "Kl. Monatsbl.," 1869, 250.

Having ascertained the strength of the external recti muscles of each eye, we may next test that of the internal recti, by finding the strongest prism which they can overcome by voluntary convergence.

[Latent insufficiency is not always unmasked by Von Graefe's test. The accommodation is undisturbed, and if there be spasm, the full measure of error of the motor muscles will not appear. This criticism holds for many cases of emmetropia, and still more for hypermetropia. This test applies only to errors of adduction and abduction. There are cases in which the weakness obtains only in the vicinity of the eye, and not for remote distances, but it may concern remote as well as near vision. In testing for muscular errors, it is important to eliminate the accommodation, by moderately darkening the room and testing with a lighted candle at some distance, say twenty feet. Let the patient fix this, and then put a red glass over one eye, say the patient's right; the flame may remain single. Then put over the other eye a prism of 5°, base upwards. Two flames will be seen; if the red, which belongs to the right eye, stand directly above the white, there may be equilibrium; but if it go to the left, we have insufficiency of adduction; if it go to the right, we have insufficiency of abduction. But if the lights stand vertically, move the candle several feet to the right or to the left; or bid the patient turn his head far to the right and then to the left, still fixing the flame; in these lateral positions, want of perpendicularity may be detected, and thus the faulty muscle be found out. The next step is to measure the capacity of the muscle at twenty feet; first for abduction by holding before one eye a prism of 5° axis, horizontal, and base inwards. At first two flames will be seen, which quickly merge into one; if they do not, weak externi may be suspected. If, on the contrary, the abductive power prove to be greater than 8°, some error of adduction is usually indicated, and we then proceed to test for this by prisms with base outwards, and increase the strength of these until the patient is no longer able to fuse the images. In connection with these tests, proper regard must be had to the state of refraction, and when an error is present, the correcting glasses must invariably be used for myopic cases; and for hyperopic cases, the test is to be taken both with and without them. (See Noyes' "Treatise on Diseases of the Eye," pages 89 et seq.)—B.]

Insufficiency of the internal recti is most frequently met with in cases of considerable myopia. The reason of this can be readily understood, if we remember that a person with a myopia of ⅕ would have to hold any small object (a book, etc.) at a distance of about five inches. This, however, necessitates a considerable degree of convergence of the visual lines, and great exertion of the internal recti muscles. After a time the latter become fatigued, symptoms of asthenopia arise, and if the work is persisted in, one eye deviates outwards. But a temporary insufficiency of the internal recti may also be produced by severe constitutional diseases, which greatly weaken the system (such as fevers, diphtheria, etc.), but it disappears when the patient has regained his strength. It may also coexist with hypermetropia, and its presence should always be suspected if the symptoms of asthenopia persist in spite of the use of convex lenses.

[According to Hansen (l. c., p. 121 et seq.) latent divergence is not dependent upon a muscular anomaly, but upon different kinds of anomalies of innervation. He considers that convergence of the act of vision is regulated by, 1, the consciousness of the approximate distance of the object; 2, by accommodation; and, 3, by the tendency of fusion, or of bringing the macula lutea of both eyes to bear upon the same object. A purely latent divergence is dependent on some disturbance in the central apparatus.

Relative insufficiency is the most frequent form, and is only found in myopes. Next in frequency, and quite different from the relative form, is the latent divergence which occurs in emmetropia, or in hypermetropia and minor degrees of myopia. The third and least frequent form is the divergence depending on the want of fusion, and betrays itself by diplopia, which occurs at the ordinary working distance.—B.]

The disease may be treated in various ways, according as our purpose is merely to alleviate the asthenopia, or to cure it. It may be alleviated by the use of concave glasses for reading and working, so that the patient can hold the object at a distance of twelve or fourteen inches, and thus require a much less degree of convergence. Moreover, the use of prisms with their base turned inwards will relieve the internal recti, but the fear is that, from want of sufficient exercise, those muscles should, after a time, become still weaker. This mode of using prisms is only indicated in the slighter cases of insufficiency, or if there is only a very limited power of abduction for distance, so that there is a risk of producing convergent squint by a tenotomy of the external rectus. These prisms may often be advantageously combined with concave glasses.

Again, the internal recti may be strengthened by frequent exercises with prisms (base turned outwards). The object (a lighted candle, white wand, etc.) is to be placed at a distance of six or eight feet, and a prism with its base outwards should be held before one eye. Crossed diplopia will be produced, and in order to overcome this the patient will voluntarily squint inwards. The strength of the prisms will be gradually increased, but should not be too strong at first, otherwise the internal rectus will be weakened by over-exertion. If the patient is short-sighted, he should wear concave glasses when he is looking at the object. This plan of treatment, however, requires much patience and accuracy, and generally soon proves irksome to the patient. Galvanization of the internal rectus may also be tried.

The best mode of treatment consists in the division of the external rectus, for we thus indirectly strengthen the internal rectus, which will have a less resistance to overcome. In a myopia of $\frac{1}{4}$, our chief object must be to enable the patient to converge easily, and for some time, for a distance of about four and one-half inches, as he will hold the print or his work at about five and one-half or six inches. But besides this, the operation has the great and important advantage of materially arresting the progress of the myopia (Von Graefe). For this progress is much accelerated by the continued effort of convergence which a patient affected with insufficiency of the internal recti is obliged to make.

[According to Alfred von Graefe, the question of an operation should be considered only under the following circumstances: " 1. When the muscular trouble is undoubtedly the source of the asthenopic symptoms and their consequences, and when the pathological conditions cannot be overcome by the ordinary means at our command. 2. When the symptoms disappear with the change from latent to manifest divergence, but at the expense of binocular single vision; while the fitness of both eyes seems to indicate the maintenance of the latter as important and practicable. 3. When there is reason for believing that forced use of the internal muscles produces an involuntary increase of the accommodation, a certain variety of spasm of accommodation, which causes the degree of myopia connected with the insufficiency to appear greater than it really is." ("Graefe und Saemisch," l. c., vi. 1, S. 199.)—B.]

But great care and circumspection are required in accurately apportioning the extent of the operation to the degree of the disturbance in the lateral equilibrium; for if the effect of the tenotomy is excessive, a convergent

—will be produced for distance, which
... rectus be then divided to remedy
... for reading, etc., will be reproduced.
... results, the preliminary examination as
... must be very carefully made, and the
... apportioned to this, and the after-treat-
... to. Thus Von Graefe lays it down
... of from 15°–18° can be overcome for
... a simple tenotomy should be performed.
... than 14°, the effect of the operation must
... application of a conjunctival suture; the
... and being tied the tighter, the greater
... rule, the operation is not to be recommended
... can be overcome. But if, in a case where
... it is very desirable to divide the operation
... gain a very symmetrical effect, a very broad
... three lines) of conjunctiva towards the outer
... the suture, and the latter very firmly tied. If
... a prism of 18°, the operation should, as a rule,
... eyes: but if from some reason this is not desir-
... may be increased by applying a subcon-
... (inner) side of the eyeball as recommended
... squint (p. 713, note), and thus rolling the eye

... recovered from the effects of the anæsthetic we
... of the operation, and ascertain whether or not
... lateral equilibrium for distance. In order, how-
... by a temporary insufficiency of the operated
... the object (which is to be about 10 feet off) in the
... to the side of the healthy eye, and as much below
... A prism with its base turned downwards is to be
... the double images should lie straight above one
... lateral equilibrium, which should exist directly
... Only in certain instances (according to Von Graefe)
... exceptions to this rule. Thus, if the case is just on the
... for an operation (i. e., if the abduction power = a
... very slight divergence of a prism of 1° or 2° may be
... convergence of 3° must be considered excessive, and
... by a suture. If the effect of the operation is to be
... may be released or removed; if it is to be diminished,
... applied, or made to include more conjunctiva, or drawn

... a proper examination in this position will prevent any
... and diplopia in the median line, it does not guard as
... of diplopia towards the temporal side. Hence we
... the defect of the absolute mobility of the eye towards the side
... muscle, and such a defect should not exceed two and one-half
... if the power of abduction equalled a prism of 14°; or one
... if the latter was but slight (Von Graefe).
... after the operation there is generally some increase in
... there may be in the median line a dynamic convergence
... that a prism of 8°–16°, the homonymous diplopia commenc-
... or four feet. But this need not alarm us if we have accu-
... lateral equilibrium and the extent of the want of mobility

directly after the operation. This increase in the effect is chiefly due to
the tension of the conjunctiva by the blood effusion. If the increase is,
however, too considerable, the effect of the tenotomy must be limited by a
fresh suture.

The suture should remain in for about two days. If, at the end of the
first week, the effect of the operation is found to be considerably too great,
the wound in the conjunctiva must be reopened, the slight adhesions formed
by the tendon gently separated with the squint-hook and a suture applied.
If, on the other hand, some increase of the defect is desired, the patient
should be supplied with a pair of strabismus spectacles, which are so constructed that the half of each glass which corresponds to the operated eye is
covered with court-plaster or paper, so that he is obliged to look considerably
to the other side, which of course puts the divided muscle more on the
stretch, and thus increases the effect of the tenotomy. Von Graefe, on the
other hand, does not deem it advisable that the patient should be directed to
look towards the affected side during the first few days, for the purpose of
diminishing the effect; this is only indicated at the end of the second or
third week.

If it is subsequently, at the expiration of a few weeks, found desirable to
increase the effect, the patient should be furnished for distance with proper
concave glasses, combined with adducting prisms (the base turned outwards)
so as to practise and strengthen the internal recti muscles.

[Abadie advises partial tenotomy of the external rectus muscle in cases
of pure muscular asthenopia without consecutive permanent strabismus, the
object being simply to weaken the muscle and not to displace it backward.
He opens the conjunctiva in the usual way, slides the strabismus hook under
the tendon, and carefully wipes away any blood that flows, however little.
Then, with a pair of sharp-pointed scissors, he divides the tendons by little
cuts, commencing at the side of the free border of the hook, and stopping
when near the centre of the tendon. He then divides the tendon on the other
side of the hook, leaving a few median fibres adherent to the sclera. These
suffice to prevent the displacement of the muscle backward. By this method
he has succeeded in removing the asthenopic symptoms in cases where
prismatic glasses had failed. This partial tenotomy has the advantage of
being a method of treatment applicable to any case as soon as the insufficiency of the internal recti muscles becomes manifest, and thus the progress
of the myopia may be combated most efficaciously. (See "Annales d'oculistique," Mai-Juin, 1880.)—B.]

In settling the question as to which eye should be selected for operation,
we must be chiefly guided by the fact whether or not one and the same eye
always deviates outwards when the object is approximated, which will become especially apparent if the object is held above the horizontal meridian.
If so, this should be selected. If the deviation alternates, we must try the
power of abduction for distance, and operate upon the eye which has the
greatest power of facultative divergence. If here, again, the power is equally
balanced, the eye should be selected whose acuity of vision is the worst
(Von Graefe). If the facultative divergence is so great that a stronger
prism than 18° or 20° can be overcome, it will be necessary to divide the
operation between the two eyes. But this demands the greatest care, and
should never be done at one sitting. First one eye must be operated upon,
and then, after two or three weeks, when the final result of the tenotomy is
apparent, the operation must be performed upon the other; special care
and attention being paid to the preliminary and subsequent examinations
as to the power of abduction, etc.

When the insufficiency is but inconsiderable, and the power of abduction very slight, we must give the patient (if myopic) concave spectacles for reading, combined with the proper abducting prisms (base turned inwards); abducting prisms being worn for distance, so as to exercise and strengthen the internal recti muscles.

[For a most careful and elaborate consideration of this whole subject, the reader is referred to the paper by Alfred von Graefe, in Graefe und Saemisch's "Handbuch der Gesammten Augenheilkunde," Bd. vi. Part i. S. 183–187.—B.]

CHAPTER XVI.

THE USE OF THE OPHTHALMOSCOPE.

IT was formerly supposed that the black appearance of the pupil is due to the fact that all the light which enters the eye is absorbed by the choroid, and consequently that none is reflected towards the observer. This, however, is not the case, for a considerable portion is diffusely reflected, and may be caught up by the observer's eye if this is placed in the direction of the emerging rays. In such a case, the pupil no longer appears black, but is luminous, having a bright red glow. Cumming, in 1846, pointed out that all normal eyes are luminous, more especially if the pupil is dilated; but that it is necessary, in order to obtain this luminosity, that the eye of the observer should be placed parallel to the incident rays, that is, as nearly as possible in the direct line between the source of light and the eye observed. But in the ordinary mode of examination this is next to impossible, as the observer's head must be placed between the light and the patient's eye, and will, therefore, cut off the rays passing to the latter. Moreover, even if some of the reflected rays could be caught up, they would only afford the appearance of a bright red glow, or, at the best, but a very confused and indistinct image of the fundus, owing to the insufficiency of the illumination and to the direction of the emerging rays. For in consequence of the optical condition of the eye, the incident rays, if the eye is accommodated for the object, are so reflected that they emerge again in exactly the same direction as they entered, and would, therefore, be brought to a focus at the point whence they originally emanated, that is at the source of light. The object

Fig. 226.

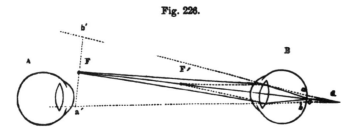

and its retinal image are, in fact, in the position of conjugate foci. The pupil of the patient's eye will therefore appear black if it is accommodated for the pupil of the observer, as the latter will then only see the reflection of his own pupil.

A glance at Fig. 226 will readily explain this. If F is the object, and c its image formed upon the retina, rays reflected from c will be brought to a focus at F, so that whichever of these two points is the radiant-point, the other will be the focal point. Now, if we place our eye at F, the luminous rays emanating from our pupil (which is black) will be insufficient to illuminate the fundus of the patient, and hence his pupil will also appear black.

But in certain conditions of the eye, a considerable amount of reflection may be obtained, as, for instance, in the eyes of albinos, and in cases in which the retina is bulged forward by morbid products. It is a well-known fact that the pupil of the albino is markedly luminous. This is not caused, as if often supposed, by a greater reflection of the rays which enter the pupil, on account of the deficiency of the pigment in the choroid, but is due to the great amount of light which passes through the iris and sclerotic. The truth of this statement was proved by Donders, who placed before an albinotic eye a small screen, having a circular aperture for the pupil, but covering the iris and sclerotic in such a manner that no light could pass through them. It was then found that the pupil lost its luminosity, and at once acquired the usual darkness of other eyes.

Again, if the position of the retina is altered, it being bulged forward by a tumor behind it (amaurotic cat's eye) or by fluid, more light will be reflected, and the fundus will appear luminous. Moreover, on account of the more anterior position of the retina, the emerging rays will be divergent, and hence easily brought to a focus upon the retina of the observer.

Brücke, in 1844–47, made a series of interesting experiments with regard to the luminosity of the eye, and showed that if the eye under examination is neither accommodated for the light nor for the pupil of the observer, but for some other nearer point, a portion of the light reflected from its background may be caught up by the observer, and the pupil will then appear red and luminous. This is shown in the preceding figure (Fig. 226). If F is a luminous point for which the eye under observation (B) is accommodated, the rays emanating from F will be brought to a focus upon the retina at c, at which point a clear and distinct image of F will be formed. This being so, the rays reflected from c will unite at F, for F and c are conjugate foci. If the eye of the observer (A) be placed beside F, it will receive no luminous rays from B, and will hence see the pupil of the latter black. Now, if whilst the eye, B, remains accommodated for the luminous point, F, the latter is brought nearer to the eye, to F', the rays emanating from it will no longer be brought to a focus on the retina at c, but behind it at d, and a circle of diffusion, a b, will be formed upon the retina. As the eye is accommodated for the distance, F, the rays emanating from the points of the circle of diffusion, a b, will be brought to a focus at a' b', and there form an enlarged and inverted image of a b. Hence the eye of the observer, placed at A, will receive a portion of this reflected light, and therefore the pupil of B will appear more or less luminous.

We shall see, hereafter, that Helmholtz turned this experience of Brücke's to a practical use, and constructed his simplest ophthalmoscope upon this principle. Before entering upon this, I must state that Helmholtz, in 1851, devised an apparatus by which the observer was enabled to place his eye in the direct line of the emerging rays, and thus gain a view of the fundus. The accompanying figure and description of this instrument are from Mr. Carter's admirable translation of Zander's work on the ophthalmoscope—a work I cannot too warmly recommend to all who wish to gain a thorough knowledge of the theory of the ophthalmoscope, its use in practice, and the different morbid changes of the fundus which may be recognized with it. The student will also derive great benefit from the perusal of Mr. Hulke's and Mr. Wilson's excellent works on the ophthalmoscope, which, though shorter and less exhaustive, yet contain a great amount of information, conveyed in a very clear and concise manner.

"Under certain conditions, however, we may see the fundus of the human eye shine with a reddish lustre. Such conditions are shown in Fig. 227, where F is a luminous point, and S a polished plate of glass, which reflects the light $a\,b$ falling upon it, into the observed eye B, in a direction as if it came from a point F' lying as far behind the plate S as the actual point F lies before it. Disregarding the loss of light caused by irregular reflection and other circumstances, the rays $a\,d$ and $b\,c$, reflected from S, enter the observed eye, and become united at e. The emerging rays in their exit from B, must take precisely the same course as in their entrance; they proceed, therefore, in the converging cone $c\,b\,a\,d$ to the plate of glass, by which they are partly reflected back to F, while the remainder proceed in an unaltered direction forwards to unite in a focus at F' and then again to become divergent. If now the eye of the observer be placed so as to intercept them from their union, as at A', it receives from e convergent rays that, made more convergent by its own refraction, are united before they reach its retina, upon which, after crossing, they form only the dispersion circle $a'\,\beta'$. The eye of A' would certainly, therefore, receive no image, but only the sensation of light—it would see the eye B illuminated, and the same would happen if it were so placed as to intercept the diverging rays behind the point F'.

"After this principle was announced by Von Erlach, Professor H. Helmholtz, then of Königsberg, and since of Heidelbe g [and now Professor of Physics in the University of Berlin.—B.], was the first to discover the reason why the retina was not distinctly seen, and to find the means of rendering it visible. The problem was threefold: the observed eye must be sufficiently illuminated; the eye of the observer must be placed in the direction of the emerging rays, and these must themselves be changed from their convergence, and rendered divergent or parallel. The solution of the main difficulty was obtained when, in a darkened chamber, the light of a lamp was allowed to fall on a well-polished plate of glass in such a manner that the rays reflected therefrom entered the eye to be observed. The observer placed himself on the other side of the glass plate, and made the convergent rays divergent by a concave lens. Thus in Fig. 227 we place the concave glass c before the eye of the observer A, and convert the convergent pencil $b\,g\,f\,a$, coming through S, into the divergent pencil $g\,i\,k\,f$, so that the eye A may form upon its retina e' a clear image of the point e.

"The combination of such an illuminating apparatus with suitable lenses forms an instrument by which it is possible clearly to see and examine the details of the background of the eye of another person. To this instrument Helmholtz gave the name of eye-mirror, or ophthalmoscope."

In order to obtain a better illumination, Helmholtz afterwards employed three plates of glass instead of a single slip. A still greater advance was made when Helmholtz utilized Brücke's experiment above referred to, and employed a strong convex lens, held before the patient's eye, to converge the rays reflected from a large circle of diffusion formed upon the retina. In this way an enlarged and inverted image of the fundus was formed between the lens and the observer. This constitutes the "examination of the actual inverted image."

Helmholtz placed the flame of a candle before the eye under observation, and a screen behind the flame, so that the observer's eye could be brought close to the source of light, and thus catch the rays after they had been united by the convex lens, and formed an image of the fundus. This point of union lies at the focal distance of the lens. This mode of examination was, however, troublesome and inconvenient, and hence Ruete had recourse to a concave mirror having a central aperture for the observer's eye, and he

Fig. 227.

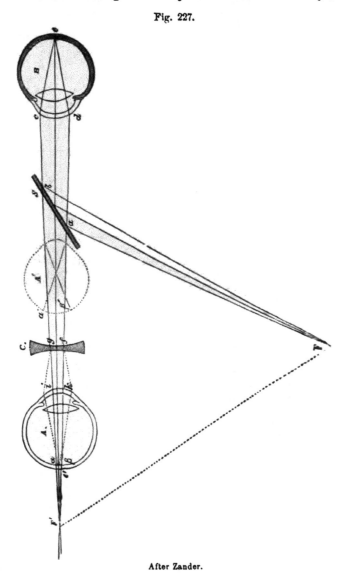

After Zander.

thus still more increased the illuminating power. Since then different forms of mirror have completely superseded the plates of polished glass.

The following description and illustration from Zander clearly explain the action of the concave mirror in the inverted examination, *i. e.*, the use of a convex lens placed a short distance from the eye under observation, so as to converge the rays emanating from the circle of diffusion formed upon its retina. The patient is to accommodate for an infinite distance, so that the rays issue parallel from this eye.

"*Examination of the actual Inverted Image.*—In Fig. 228, *F* is again the flame, *S* the mirror, *L* the convex lens, and *B* the eye observed. The rays *a e b f*, proceeding convergent from the mirror, and rendered more convergent

Fig. 228.

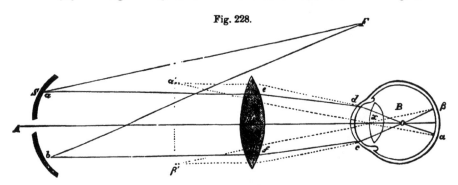

by their passage through the lens, strike the cornea of *B* in *c* and *d*. Rendered still more convergent by the dioptric apparatus of *B*, they intersect at some point in front of the retina, for example at *o*, and form on the retina the dispersion circle *a β*. On account of the passive state of accommodation of the eye, the rays proceeding from it will follow courses parallel to the lines of direction *a x* and *β x*, and after their refraction by the lens *L* will unite to form at *a′ β′* an actual inverted image of *a β*."[1] In this mode of examination it will be observed that the aerial image of the fundus is situated between the observer and the convex lens, and that it is inverted and enlarged. If we desire to increase the size of the image, a somewhat weaker object-lens (three and one-half or four inches focus) should be employed, for as this renders the rays less convergent, the image will be proportionately enlarged, but will at the same time lie somewhat further from the eye; this is, however, accompanied by the disadvantage that the field of vision is much diminished in size. Hence the best plan is to use first a lens of two or two and one-fourth inches focus, so as to gain a view of the whole fundus, and then to change this for a weaker lens if we desire to examine any special part of the background with particular care and minuteness. The size of the image may also be considerably magnified by placing a convex lens of eight or ten inches focus in the little clip behind the mirror. In this case the observer must, however, approach somewhat closer to the patient.

"*In the examination of the virtual erect image* the mirror alone is used, without the aid of an object lens, the observer approaching very closely to the patient's eye. He will thus obtain an erect, geometrical image of the fundus, the image being apparently situated behind the patient's eye, as in Fig. 229.[2] *E* is the examined eye, and *E′* the position of the examiner's

---

[1] Carter's translation of Zander, p. 20.
[2] This figure and its explanation are from Mr. Hulke's able work on the "Ophthalmoscope."

eye; *r r* are divergent rays from *F*, a flame, incident on the concave speculum *A B*, which reflects them convergingly as *r′ r′* to *E*, about two inches distant, upon the fundus of which they form the circle of dispersion *d d′*. The rays

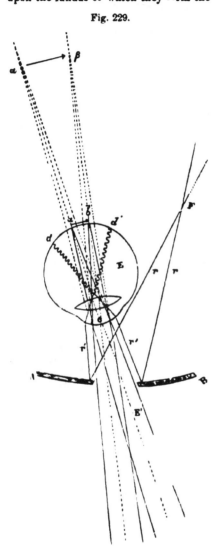

Fig. 229.

reflected from any point *a b* within the circle, after leaving *E*, assume a direction parallel to the prolongations of the lines *a o b c* (which pass through *a*, the optical centre of *E*) and reach the observer's eye at *E′*, on the retina of which they form an inverted image of *a b*, which is mentally projected as the *enlarged, erect, geometrical image a β*." It will be explained hereafter that it is generally necessary to make use of an ocular lens behind the mirror, in order to gain a clear and distinct image of the fundus. The nature and strength of this lens depend upon the state of refraction of the eye of the observer and that of the patient.

I must now pass on to a brief description of the different forms of ophthalmoscope which are in most frequent use. For a full and accurate description of the various kinds of ophthalmoscope which have been invented, I must refer the reader to Mr. Carter's translation of Zander.

Ophthalmoscopes may be divided into four different classes:

1. The portable or hand ophthalmoscopes. Of these I shall notice those of Liebreich, Coccius, and Zehender [and Loring.—H.], [and Knapp.—B.].

2. The fixed or stand ophthalmoscopes, such as Liebreich's, and its excellent modification by Smith and Beck.

3. T e binocular ophthalmoscopes of Giraud-Teulon, and of Laurence and Heisch.

4. The aut-ophthalmoscope.

All ophthalmoscopes may also be divided into two principal classes, the *homo-centric* and the *hetero-centric*. In the *homo-centric* the mirror is concave, and its focus, calculated from its surface, is fixed and definite; whereas in the *hetero-centric* the mirror is plane or convex, and the focus is negative, situated behind the mirror, and can be altered according to the strength of the biconvex lens which is fixed beside the mirror.

1.—THE PORTABLE OR HAND OPHTHALMOSCOPES.

(1) THE OPHTHALMOSCOPE OF LIEBREICH.

As has been already mentioned above, Ruete was the first to employ a concave perforated mirror (which was, however, fixed) as a substitute for the slips of glass of Helmholtz, and this principle has formed the base for the numerous modifications at present in use. Of all the different forms of concave mirror, I think Liebreich's (Fig. 230) the most handy and useful. It consists of a concave metal mirror, about one and one-fourth inches in diameter, and eight inches focal length. Its centre is perforated by a small aperture, about one line in diameter, the edges of which are exceedingly thin. The bronze back of the speculum around this opening is bevelled off towards the edge, so that the latter may be as thin as possible, in order that the peripheral rays of the cone of light, which passes through the aperture, may not be intercepted and cut off by a thick broad edge, which would give the opening the character of a short canal. Behind the speculum, which is fixed upon a short handle, is a small clip for holding a convex or concave lens.

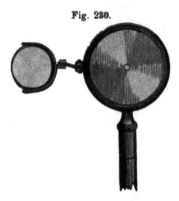

Fig. 230.

(2) THE OPHTHALMOSCOPE OF COCCIUS.

This instrument consists of a plane mirror combined with a lateral biconvex collecting lens. Its chief advantages over the concave mirror are: that the observer's eye is placed within the cone of reflected light, instead of being behind it; that the focal distance of the mirror can be altered according as the lens at the side is approximated or placed further from the speculum, or as the power of the lens is changed; the light can be more concentrated upon one point of the retina; and the corneal reflex is far less. These advantages over the concave mirror are especially marked in the examination in the direct image. With the concave mirror, only a cone of light corresponding in size to that of the pupil is admitted into the eye, and as the size of this cone diminishes with the approximation of the mirror, it follows that in the direct examination the illumination of the fundus is but slight. Moreover, on account of the very close proximity in which the mirror has to be brought to the patient's eye, much of the light from the lamp is often intercepted, whereas this is obviated by the collecting lens in Coccius' instrument. The latter is, therefore, to be much preferred to the concave mirror for the direct method of examination. For the indirect method the advantages are less marked, but even for this I prefer it, for reasons which I shall mention hereafter.

Coccius' ophthalmoscope (Fig. 231), as made at present, consists of a plane metal mirror, having a small central aperture. Behind the mirror is a hinged clip to hold a convex or concave lens. A lateral biconvex lens of five or seven inches focal length is held in a large clip mounted on a jointed bracket, which is so connected with the neck of the handle that it permits of the lens being moved to either side of the mirror.

Fig. 231.   [Fig. 232.]

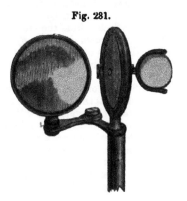

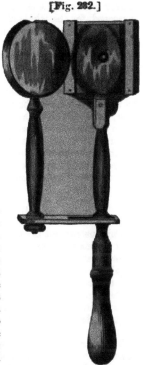

The original form of Coccius' ophthalmoscope [Fig. 232] differed from that which I have described above, and which is at present in general use, both in being square in shape, and in being made of glass instead of metal. The square mirror was inconvenient, and could not be steadied so well against the orbit as the circular. But the great disadvantage of the glass mirror was (as Helmholtz pointed out) that the aperture could not be bevelled down to so fine an edge as the metal one, in consequence of which more or less of a canal existed, which intercepted many of the peripheral rays, and produced considerable diffraction.

The mode of using Coccius' ophthalmoscope is as follows: The collecting lens is to be turned towards the flame, which should be somewhat more than twice the distance of the focal length of the lens from the observer. The mirror is then to be set somewhat slanting to the lens and the eye of the patient. If the mirror is properly adjusted for the lens and the flame, we shall obtain, if we throw the image of the flame upon the palm of our hand or the cheek of the patient, a bright circle of light, with a small dark central spot, which corresponds to the opening in the speculum. The dark spot is then to be thrown into the pupil of the eye under examination, the surgeon placing the mirror close to his own eye, and looking through the aperture into the patient's eye, which should afford a bright luminous reflex. For the indirect mode of examination a biconvex lens of from two to three inches focus is to be held before the eye under observation. I, moreover, also use a convex lens of eight or ten inches focus behind the mirror, in order still more to magnify the image. If the direct examination is employed, a concave lens will generally be required behind the speculum. At first this instrument may be somewhat more difficult to use than the concave mirror, on account of our having to regulate the position of the collecting lens with respect to the flame and the mirror; but a little practice and perseverance will very soon overcome this difficulty.

This consists in the combination of a slightly convex mirror with a bi-convex collecting lens. The illumination of the retinal image is thus greatly increased, for the whole of the cone of light reflected from the mirror can be collected into a narrower section, and can be thrown into the eye without the peripheral rays being intercepted by the edge of the pupil; more light can also be diffused over the fundus, and it can be more strongly concentrated upon one point.

This ophthalmoscope is, in fact, a modification of that of Coccius, and it very closely resembles the present form. Indeed, at the first glance, they may be readily mistaken for each other. On closer observation it will be, however, noticed, that Zehender's mirror is convex, whereas that of Coccius is quite plain. Moreover, on looking into Zehender's, we get a smaller image of our face than is the case with that of Coccius. It is certainly the better ophthalmoscope for the direct examination, but I prefer Coccius' for the indirect mode of observation. Indeed, the latter answers so well for both purposes, that for the general surgeon it will amply suffice.

[(4) The Ophthalmoscope of Loring.

This instrument is extremely useful for the direct method of examination, as it avoids a constant change of lens behind the mirror, and expedites the determination of errors of refraction. It is so constructed[1] as to contain the requisite convex and concave glasses in three cylinders placed behind the mirror, and their rotation enables the surgeon to rapidly obtain the proper lens for his examination. Each cylinder is pierced for eight glasses, forming in the aggregate a series of lenses extending with but comparatively slight differences in focal value, from convex $\frac{1}{70}$ to $\frac{1}{3}$ and from concave $\frac{1}{70}$ to $\frac{1}{2}$.

The manner in which the glasses are divided among the cylinders will be readily understood from the accompanying figures (Fig. 233). The first cylinder is made up entirely of convex glasses, by means of which all ordinary degrees of hypermetropia can with sufficient exactness be determined. One hole (0) is left vacant to represent emmetropia, without the necessity of removing the cylinder, and for examination by the inverted image without an eye-piece; should, however, the latter be desired, the observer has a large selection at his command. The second cylinder contains the concaves of moderate focal power, and the third is composed of the high numbers, both positive and negative. These strong numbers are designed for the determination of the highest degrees of errors of refraction and for the measurement of the inequalities of the fundus, such as excavations and elevations of the optic nerve, projections of tumors, retinal detachments, membranes in the vitreous, etc.

The mirror, being contained in a separate case, is made detachable from the rest of the instrument, which can then be used as an optometer, the patient himself revolving the cylinder till the suitable glass is obtained.

Besides the common concave mirror, Dr. Loring has had another constructed, which was originally designed for a stenopæic slit to be used with the instrument when employed as an optometer for the determination of

[1] "Amer. Journal of Med. Sci.," April, 1870, p. 340.

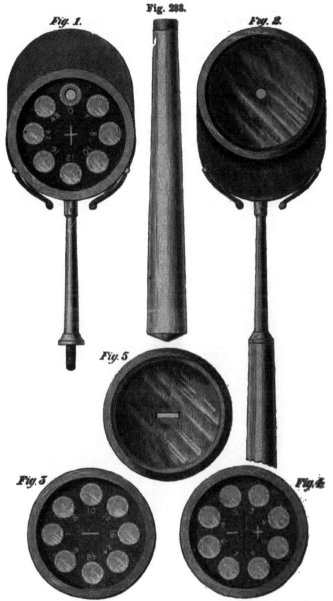

Fig. 233.

Fig. 1.   Fig. 2.

Fig. 5

Fig. 3   Fig. 4.

Fig. 1. Back of Loring's ophthalmoscope with cylinder in position. *Fig.* 2. Front view of instrument. *Figs.* 3 and 4. Remaining cylinders detached. *Fig.* 5. Astigmatic optometer and mirror.

astigmatism. It consisted of a thin plate with a slit in it, whose length was equal to the diameter of the perforations in the cylinder. This was mounted like the mirror, and made to fit in the mirror cell in which it revolved, so as to allow the slit to correspond with any given meridian of the cornea. The meridian once determined, the patient turned the cylinder till the suitable glass was obtained. This plate was subsequently made with a polished surface in front, and then was made to serve also as a mirror for determining, by means of the ophthalmoscope, the amount of astigmatism in the principal meridians of the eye.—H.]

[The modification of the Rekoss system adopted by Knapp consists of two undetachable, revolving disks, one containing concave and the other convex glasses. These are placed upon each other so that they rotate past each other, and thus the strength of each glass can be diminished by adding the different glasses of the other disk. This, however, necessitates considerable calculation to determine the actual value of the glass used. The advantage of this instrument is that it is in one piece, and has no detached cylinders. ("Trans. Amer. Ophthal. Soc.," 1873.)

De Wecker's modification consists in a revolving disk with twenty-four convex and concave glasses, which can be set in motion by a cog-wheel apparatus. The disadvantage consists in the very small size of the inserted glasses. ("Kl. Monatsbl. f. Augenheilk.," 1873.)

[Fig. 284.]

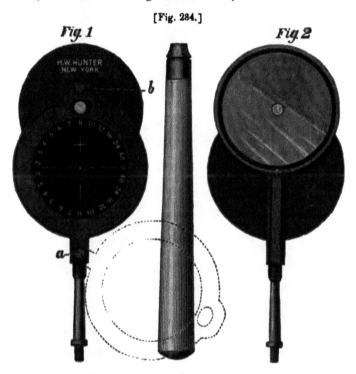

Loring's first modification of his original instrument consists in replacing the detachable disks by a single stationary one, one inch and a half in diameter, in which the glasses are arranged in two concentric circles. The glasses consist of twelve convex and twelve concave, the weaker ones being arranged in the outer circle, and the stronger ones in the inner circle. The outer or inner circle can be rapidly brought into position by sliding the disk upwards or downwards on the hand, without removing it from the eye. ("Amer. Journ. Med. Sciences," Jan. 1874.)

Knapp has also adopted an instrument similar to De Wecker's. Both these instruments have the glasses covered by a piece of metal to prevent scratching and soiling. ("Arch. of Ophthal.," iii. No. 2; Ib. iv. No. 1.)

Loring's instrument has also been provided with a cover in the shape of a thin flat ring, which swings round on a pivot, and, when closed, is held in position by sliding under the edge of a second pivot. Fig. 234. (See "Determination of the Refraction of the Eye with the Ophthalmoscope," New York, 1876.)

The instrument recommended by Mr. C. J. Oldham consists in a similar modification of the original instrument with the disks, and has no advantage over those already mentioned. ("Trans. of Fourth Ophth. Congress," London, 1872.)

At the Fifth International Ophthalmological Congress held in New York, in 1876, Dr. Loring presented an ophthalmoscope for determining refraction, in which the glasses were numbered according to the metric system, the glasses being dioptrics or fractions of a dioptric. This admits of application to his instrument with twenty-five perforations, by having the disk contain a regular series of whole numbers, and adding a clip behind the mirror, provided with two glasses, + and — .5, or half a dioptric.

The metric ophthalmoscope of Knapp contains thirty-two glasses, running from 0.5 dioptric to 18 dioptrics, positive and negative.

A modification of Loring's last instrument by Dr. Wadsworth, of Boston, consists in an additional mirror for use in the upright image. It is very small, circular, and has a diameter of fifteen millimetres. It rotates from right to left, and admits of an inclination of 20°; but necessitates the use of two mirrors for the instrument. Loring has himself modified this in two ways, as follows: he first cut off a lateral segment of the ordinary circular, concave mirror, and swung this on two vertical pins, or by a hinge from the mirror-case. A second modification consists in cutting off both sides of the ordinary mirror, so that a circle is changed to a parallelogram. This is swung on two pivots, and admits of an inclination of 25°. It tilts both ways, and can be used for either the upright or inverted method of examination.

The latest modification of the ophthalmoscope adopted by Dr. Loring, and in some respects the best, is a successful attempt to combine two essential points, viz.: first, that the glasses should have a diameter of not less than six millimetres; and, secondly, to have a sufficiently large number of glasses. This is done by a single disk and the segment of a disk, the latter being the quadrant of a circle (see Fig. 235).

The single disk contains sixteen glasses on the metric system, the plus being numbered in *white*, and the minus in *red*.[1] The first row of numbers, or that just beneath the glass, shows the *real* value of the glass; the second, or inner row, shows the result of the combinations when the quadrant is in position. The quadrant rotates immediately over the disk and around the same centre, and contains four glasses — .5 — 16. and + .5 + 16.

When not in use, the quadrant is beneath its cover. The instrument then represents a simple ophthalmoscope with sixteen perforations, the series run-

---

[1] To designate the figures in *red*, numerals have been used. In the instrument the bright scarlet figures produced by actual pigment, are even more vivid and brilliant than the white, especially under gaslight.

ning with an interval of 1. D, and extending from 1. to 7. plus, and from 1. to 8. minus.

This is ample for all ordinary work, as the interval of 1. D is as close as even an expert usually desires, and can, with a little experience, be used for even very minute discrepancies. For if in a given case the fundus is seen distinctly with 1. D and a little to spare, while 2. D blurs the picture, we know at once that the refraction must be between the two, or 1.5 D. If, however, for any reason we wish to prove this conclusion, we can bring up 0.5 D. From this glass we get successive half-dioptrics from 1. to 8. plus, and from 1. to 9. minus. In this way we have, so to speak, a fine and coarse adjustment, as in the microscope.

If the higher numbers are desired, these are obtained by combination with those of the quadrant. These progress regularly up to 16. D, every dioptric being marked upon the disk; above this, up to + 23. D and − 24. D, we have to simply add the glass which comes beneath the 16. D, turning always in the same direction. By the various combinations a total series of sixty-five glasses can be obtained.

Beginning with 0, and revolving always from left to right, we obtain ·			Beginning with 0, and revolving always from *right* to *left*, we obtain :		
PLUS			MINUS		
	0			1	
	1			2	
	2			3	
	3			4	
	4			5	
	5			6	
	6			7	
	7	Bring up + 16		8	Bring up − 16
+ 16 − 8 =	8		− 16 + 7 =	9	
" − 7 =	9		" + 6 =	10	
" − 6 =	10		" + 5 =	11	
" − 5 =	11		" + 4 =	12	
" − 4 =	12		" + 3 =	13	
" − 3 =	13		" + 2 =	14	
" − 2 =	14		" + 1 =	15	
" − 1 =	15		" + 0 =	16	
" 0 =	16		" − 1 =	17	
" + 1 =	17		" − 2 =	18	
" + 2 =	18		" − 3 =	19	
" + 3 =	19		" − 4 =	20	
" + 4 =	20		" − 5 =	21	
" + 5 =	21		" − 6 =	22	
" + 6 =	22		" − 7 =	23	
" + 7 =	23		" − 8 =	24	

Thus, with the superposition of a *single* glass (+ 16. or − 16.), and with an uninterrupted rotation, a series is obtained of successive dioptrics from 1. to 23. plus, and from 1. to 24. minus.

With the use of the 0.5 we can obtain in addition the following series with an interval of half a dioptric:

+ 0.	− 0.5
+ 0.5	− 1.
+ 1.	− 1.5
+ 1.5	− 2.
+ 2.	− 2.5
+ 2.5	− 3.
+ 3.	− 3.5
+ 3.5	− 4.
+ 4.	− 4.5

By a simple displacement of the quadrant, the instrument becomes a single-disk ophthalmoscope. (See "Trans. Fifth Internat. Ophthal. Con-

Fig. 235.

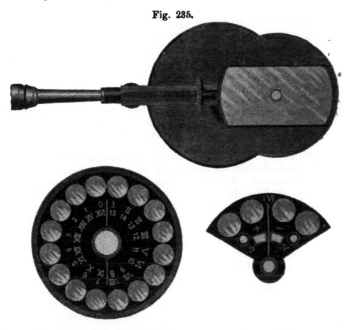

gress," 1876, and "Trans. Amer. Ophth. Soc.," 1878.) (These various modifications made by Dr. Loring of his original instrument can all be obtained of Mr. H. W. Hunter, 1132 Broadway, N. Y.) [Dr. H. D. Noyes has described in his own "Treatise on Diseases of the Eye," 1881, pp. 28 and 29, an ophthalmoscope with certain modifications, based upon Loring's latest model, devised for the purpose of putting at command, in rapid succession, the full series of glasses which may be required. The mechanism by which this is effected is by cog-wheels, and there are two disks carrying lenses. The mirror, besides swinging in the trunnions, may be rotated in a circular direction, and thus assume any angle. The front disk is moved by the lowest wheel, and the back disk by the upper and exposed wheel. There is a spring clip on the back of the instrument which will carry a cylindric glass. It gives command of a complete set of spherical glasses, both positive and negative, seventy-six in number. In other particulars the instrument is copied after Loring's latest model.

Parent has joined the army of modifiers of the ophthalmoscope by modifying his own instrument. He has added a ring, of a diameter of thirty-eight millimetres, upon which is fixed eccentrically a disk containing ten concave cylindrical glasses, ranging from D 0.5 to D 6. The zero of this wheel has the shape of a triangular sector, which admits of the reading of the spherical glasses placed beneath. For the determination of myopia and hypermetropia without astigmatism, the cylinders are placed with their axes vertical. The combination of three disks, rotating in a concentric manner, makes a necessarily heavy and clumsy instrument.—B.]

2.—THE FIXED OR DEMONSTRATING OPHTHALMOSCOPE OF LIEBREICH.

This instrument is constructed upon the principle of the concave mirror as it is employed in the indirect mode of examination, and is so arranged that the whole apparatus (mirror and object-lens) is fixed to a table, thus allowing the surgeon free use of his hands, and when it is properly adjusted, enabling even an unskilled observer to see the details of the fundus.

The instrument consists of two tubes, moving one over the other. That nearest to the surgeon has a small oblong portion cut out of its side, in order to admit the light to the concave mirror, which is attached to its extremity. Behind the speculum, there is a small clip for an ocular lens. The other tube carries, at its free end, a biconvex object-lens of from two to two and one-half inches focus, which is to be placed about two and one-half inches from the patient's eye. The two tubes are movable, one upon the other, by a rack and pinion, so that the mirror and the object-lens may be adjusted to any required distance. The whole apparatus is supported on an upright stem, and may be fixed by a clamp to the corner of a table. This stem is also supplied with a movable rest to receive the patient's chin, and thus to steady his head, which purpose is likewise assisted by a small arc, supported by a rod adjusted to the upper end of the stem, the arc receiving the patient's forehead. Two small black shades are adjusted to the tubes, so as to cut off the light of the lamp from the eyes of the patient and the observer. The lamp is to be placed a few inches from the instrument, and nearly opposite to the opening in the tube containing the mirror, so that its rays may fall direct upon the latter. The patient is to be seated at the other end of the apparatus, having the eye under examination on a level with the object-lens, and about two and one-half inches from it. Before illuminating his eye, it will be best to throw the light upon the palm of our hand, upon which it should form a bright circle of light having a small central dark spot; if this is obtained, the instrument is properly adjusted, and the light should be thrown into the patient's pupil, which should be widely dilated by atropine. If the reflection is not round, but jagged or faint, there is some fault in the adjustment of the lamp, mirror, or object-lens, which must be corrected before the examination is commenced. If the reflections of the lamp on the retina confuse the image, the object-lens should be slightly turned, so as to separate the two reflections and remove them from the centre of the field of view.

This instrument is especially useful for demonstration to a class; or for the purpose of drawing the appearances of the fundus, as it leaves both hands of the surgeon at liberty. For common examination it is too tedious and inconvenient, as we are completely dependent upon the patient, for the slightest movement of his eye will throw the object out of view, whereas with the hand ophthalmoscope we are chiefly dependent upon our own dexterity.

A very excellent modification of Liebreich's instrument has been made by Messrs. Smith and Beck, as suggested by Mr. Kilburn. It is more easily adjustable, and its position with regard to the patient and observer can be more readily changed. Instead of being screwed on to the edge of the table, this instrument is fixed upon a small board supplied with rollers, which enables its position to be changed with great facility, and quite independently of the patient. Moreover, the standard carries a paraffin lamp, so that the position of the ophthalmoscope towards the light always remains the same, even although the former may be moved nearer to, or further from, the patient. This arrangement saves a great deal of time and trouble, and obviates the constant change of position between the lamp and the ophthalmoscope, necessitated by any movement of the latter. The rest which supports the patient's chin, instead of being attached to the instrument, is independent of it, and is supported on a separate standard. This permits the position of the instrument to be changed without affecting that of the patient.

Dr. Lionel Beale has devised a very ingenious ophthalmoscope, which can be used without darkening the room, and which will be found especially useful in the light wards of a hospital, and in the physician's consulting-room. I have been able to see the details of the fundus perfectly with it by broad daylight.

Dr. Beale has obtained this result by enclosing the reflector and lens in a tube, to the side of which is adapted a small paraffin lamp, with a large plano-convex lens. The illumination is so strong that it is not necessary for the tube to fit at all accurately to the margin of the orbit, and, indeed, the instrument can be used quite successfully even if two or three inches of daylight intervene. The reflector is fixed in the tube at the proper angle, and the lens is made to incline a little, so as to remove the reflections upon the retina out of the field of vision. With this instrument the optic disk is at once brought into view without any difficulty, and as the lamp moves with the mirror and lens, experienced persons can use the apparatus successfully almost upon the first trial. The instrument weighs nearly a pound, but it can be made very much lighter. The lamp is the same as that which Dr. Beale has adapted to the hand microscope he used for the demonstration of objects in his lectures. For making ophthalmoscopic drawings, the instrument can be fixed to a pillar and stand. The artist can work in daylight with very little effort, while the patient can retain the eye fixed in the proper position without exertion.

The instrument has been made by Mr. Hawkesly, of Blenheimstreet, Bond Street, who is now engaged in simplifying the arrangements, as much as possible, and in carrying out some improvements and reducing the weight of the metal-work. Mr. Hawksley thinks the cost will be less than two guineas.

Mr. Brudenell Carter's new demonstrating ophthalmoscope is by far one of the best. "The apparatus requires the use of a table, which should be four feet long, and which need not be more than eighteen inches wide; or it may be arranged across one end of an ordinary dining-table. The person whose eye is to be observed should be seated comfortably, as shown at A in Fig. 236, with his chin supported by a chin-rest, which can be fixed at any desired height, and which should render the plane of the face vertical. The mirror (M), of thirteen inches focal length and four inches diameter, should then be arranged with its central aperture about the same height as the eye to be examined, and should be placed opposite the face at the other side of the table, about forty inches from the chin-rest. The flame of the lamp (F) should be placed at the same height, distant about thirteen inches in a direct line from the centre of the mirror, and about eight inches to the right or left of a line drawn from the mirror to the chin-rest. The screen (s) should cut off all direct lamplight from the patient; and the stand (G), which carries a square of blue glass, should be interposed between the flame and the mirror, but close to the former, and with the glass at such an angle that it shall not reflect light to the patient. The lens, of eight inches focal length and four inches diameter, roughly set to the height of the eye by the screw at B, is then placed about eight inches from the patient, with its long double hands

(H) turned towards the observer, who first so disposes the mirror and lens as to throw a circle of light about the size of a shilling upon the eye of the patient, and then seats himself behind the mirror to complete the adjustments required for a perfect view of the fundus oculi. Whilst looking

Fig. 236.

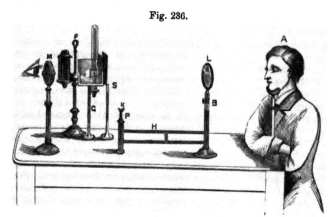

through the aperture he may impress slight movements upon the mirror, turning it either upon the vertical axis of its stem, or upon the horizontal axis on which it swings in its gimbal. By means of the handle (H) with its terminal pillar (P), he may move the lens nearer to or further from the patient, or across the table in such a manner as to transfer the light even from one eye to the other. By causing the pillar (P) to move in an arc he may render the plane of the lens oblique, so as to displace reflected images, and, by the fine adjustment governed by the screw (K), he may regulate the height of the lens with exactness. So complete is the mastery over all parts of the apparatus that a very little practice renders it possible to follow all slight movements of the eye as readily as with a hand ophthalmoscope, while the resulting image is about four times as large as any that an ordinary hand ophthalmoscope will afford. The large mirror and the position of the lamp combine to furnish a very powerful illumination, and the absorption

Fig. 237.

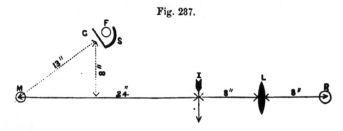

of yellow rays by the blue glass renders the light so little irritating that it has scarcely any tendency to produce contraction of the pupil, and the use of atropine is therefore in most cases unnecessary. The arrangement of the apparatus is shown in ground-plan in Fig. 237, where M shows the position of the mirror, R that of the chin-rest, F that of the flame, with its screen S, and its blue glass G; L shows the lens, and I the position of the inverted image."

3.—BINOCULAR OPHTHALMOSCOPES, ETC.

We are indebted for this valuable and ingenious instrument to **Dr. Giraud-**Teulon, who was the first to solve the difficult problem how it was possible to gain a binocular view of the details of the fundus, and thus give a stereoscopic effect to the image.

The annexed diagram (Fig. 238) will explain its mode of action. Let O

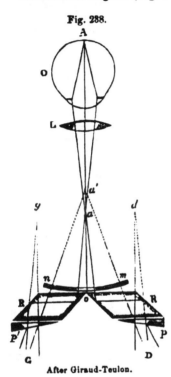

Fig. 238.

After Giraud-Teulon.

be the eye of the patient, L the objectlens, and m n, the concave mirror, having a central aperture. Behind the mirror are two rhombs (R R) of crown glass, ground so as to afford a double refraction at an angle of 45°. These rhombs are in contact at the edge o, thus equally dividing the aperture of the mirror. The effect of this arrangement is that each pencil of rays, diverging from the actual image (a) of the background of the eye, after falling upon the mirror, is divided into two—a right and left half—and is then reflected by the opposite sides of the rhombs in such a manner that it will emerge parallel to its original direction, and give rise to two inverted images d and g. The one (d) belonging to the right eye, the other (g) to the left. In order to cause these two images to become united, two decentred lenses are adjusted behind the rhombs. The two images d and g are consequently united at a′, and the observer thus gains one stereoscopic view of the details of the fundus.

The disadvantage of this ophthalmoscope, as originally constructed, was, that as the rhombs were adjusted for a certain fixed distance, it only suited persons whose eyes were a corresponding width apart from each other; for if they were either nearer or further apart than the ocular openings, the surgeon either found that one eye was altogether excluded from participation in the visual act, or that he saw double. This difficulty has now been removed by a division of one of the rhombs into two parts, the outer of which is movable, and thus allows of the instrument being adapted to all eyes.

The mode of using this instrument differs somewhat from that of the ordinary monocular ophthalmoscope. Before attempting to use it, the observer should accurately adjust it for his eyes, so that when he is looking with both eyes at an object, he receives a single, clearly defined image. The readiest mode of adjusting the instrument is, to pull out to its furthest extent the screw at the end, which governs the position of the movable half of the prism, and then to look through the ocular openings at the flame of the lamp placed at a distance of from twelve to eighteen inches. If the observer only sees one image of the flame, he must alternately close each eye, and notice whether the image remains apparent on the closure of either eye; if so, the instrument is properly adjusted. But if the image disappears when one eye is shut, it shows at once that the observer was only looking through one ocular opening, and that the position of the rhomb must be changed. If two images are seen, the screw must be gently pushed in (or out, as the case may be) until they are brought closer and closer together, and are at last fused into one clear and well-defined image, which must remain apparent on the closure of either eye. The lamp is then to be placed directly behind the patient, so that its rays may pass over his head to the observer, who is seated straight before him. Before the examination is commenced, the surgeon should again convince himself of the proper adjustment of the instrument, by throwing the light into the pupil and noticing whether or not he sees one image of it, and whether this remains apparent when either eye is closed. At first, it is better to dilate the pupil with atropine, as this greatly facilitates the examination, for even to an accomplished ophthalmoscopist the binocular ophthalmoscope will prove somewhat strange at the commencement, and will require to be used a few times before he becomes thoroughly familiar with it. In the more recent form of Giraud-Teulon's instrument, the mirror admits of a lateral movement, so that the lamp may be placed at the side of the patient. I, however, much prefer the illumination from above; still, this is not always convenient, and therefore it is necessary that the mirror should have a lateral movement, more especially for the direct examination, which it renders more easy.

A very excellent form of binocular ophthalmoscope has been invented by Messrs. Laurence and Heisch. [Fig. 239.] It consists of a set of prisms arranged so as to divide the rays into two. The two central prisms are fixed, but the two lateral ones are movable in such a manner that they not only allow of a lateral movement, but their inclination can also be changed, so that the angle of divergence of the rays from the median line can

[Fig. 239.]

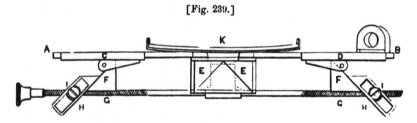

be altered as may be necessary. On account of this arrangement, the decentred lenses of Giraud-Teulon are unnecessary, and, instead of these, convex spherical lenses may be employed, and the image be thus considerably enlarged.

"The instrument[1] consists of a horizontal metallic plate [A B] one and one-half centimetre wide and ten centimetres long, with a central perforation. Behind this plate the central prisms [E E] are fixed, and the lateral ones [F F] slide in movable settings, furnished with an index and graduated scale, by which their distance apart can be read off at a glance. Their inclination is regulated by a screw [G G] that acts upon both of them at once. The mirror [K] turns upon a pin on the upper part of the plate, and the

[1] *Vide* Carter's translation of Zander, p. 61.

instrument is completed by a movable wooden handle. Th
tions are constructed of aluminium bronze, and the total   is
reduced to two ounces and fifty grains. The case, as fitted   Messrs.
Murray and Heath, contains also

[Fig. 240.]

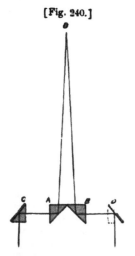

and two pairs of oculars, and is made of a shape
and size convenient for the pocket."

[The optical action of the instrument is represented in Fig. 240. "O A and O B are the extreme outer rays of a pencil proceeding from a
point (O) of the inverted image formed by the
ordinary object-lens; the ray O B is reflected by
the prism B to the prism D, and hence to the observer's right eye placed behind D. Similarly,
the ray O A is reflected to the observer's left
He then sees two images of the fundus oculi.
inclining the ocular prisms (D and C) inw
by the mechanism described at Fig. 237, the two
images are fused into one.

"The manner of using this instrument differs
but little from that of using the ordinary ophthalmoscope, excepting that the light is placed above
the head of the patient, and in the same vertical
plane as that of the eye to be examined. (Fig.
241.) The observer holds the instrument horizontally, with the ocular prisms opposite his eyes,
and reflects the light into the eye of the patient by tilting the mirror on i
hinge; in all other respects it is used as an ordinary ophthalmoscope."—H.]

Fig. 241.

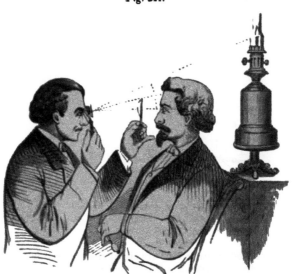

This ophthalmoscope possesses, certainly, several advantages over that of
Giraud-Teulon. In the first place, it is much lighter, which is very con-

venient if numerous cases have to be examined, for then a heavy instrument proves irksome and fatiguing. Again, on account of the alteration which can be made in the inclination of the prisms, the strain upon the internal recti muscles, in maintaining a forced convergence in order to unite the double images is done away with. But this instrument is rather more apt to get out of order than that of Giraud-Teulon, if it be carelessly handled, as is apt to be the case in a class, where it is used by many different persons.

[Coccius has constructed a modification of Giraud-Teulon's instrument, as follows: Immediately behind the mirror of six inches focus, and in front of the prism apparatus, is a convex lens of twelve inches focal length, which imparts greater distinctness to the image, and, at the same time, admits of a greater magnifying power. The latter is obtained by a small opera-glass adapted for near objects, which is connected with the mirror and prism apparatus. ("Trans. Fourth Ophthal. Congress," London, 1876.)

Schweigger employed two mirrors, separated from each other by the same distance as exists between the two eyes, each mirror turning upon a horizontal and a vertical axis. This instrument is not applicable for the examination in the inverted image. ("Graefe und Saemisch's Hdb. der Augenheilk.," iii.)—B.]

The great advantage of the binocular ophthalmoscope consists in its affording us a stereoscopic view of the details of the fundus, so that they are brought into relief. We are thus enabled to judge of the real thickness of the retina, and can readily determine whether this is abnormally increased or diminished. The slightest degrees of detachment of the retina are also easily recognized. The optic disk shows itself in its reality, and we can detect at a glance whether its surface is level, arched forward, or excavated; whereas, with the monocular ophthalmoscope, slight changes in the level of the disk are often very difficult to determine with certainty, even by an accomplished ophthalmoscopist. Again, we can ascertain with facility the exact position of extravasations of blood, exudations of lymph, or collec-

Fig. 242.

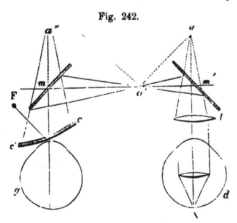

tions of pigment, and whether they are situated in the retina or the choroid, or perhaps in both these tissues. These points in the differential diagnosis are often of much importance in framing the prognosis.

[An ophthalmoscope for two observers was first attempted by De Wecker and Roger in 1870. Sichel has since constructed one which admits of useful application (see "Graefe und Saemisch," l. c., iii. S. 161). Burke's instrument is also adapted to this purpose. All instruments for two observers divide the rays of light coming from the object into two parts; the images are, therefore, of a lower degree of illumination, and hence more indistinct.—B.]

Various forms of *aut-ophthalmoscopes*, by which the surgeon could examine his own eye, have been devised, the first who succeeded in constructing such an instrument being Coccius; since then Heymann, Giraud-Teulon, and Zehender have invented different kinds of aut-ophthalmoscopes. The best and simplest of these is, I think, Giraud-Teulon's. Its action is explained by the accompanying diagram (Fig. 242), copied from Giraud-Teulon's article in the French translation of Mackenzie. The instrument consists of two plane mirrors m m', inclined to one another at an angle of 90°, and placed in front of the observer. A concave mirror (c d) is held obliquely before the left eye (g), so that the rays from a flame (F) are reflected on to m, and thence on to m', which will reflect them into the right eye (d). A double convex lens l is placed between d and m', by which an inverted aerial image of A is formed, which is situated in reality at a' between the two mirrors, but which will appear to g to be situated beyond the mirror m at d'. In fact the rays emanating from d, instead of passing straight on, are bent twice at a right angle, and brought back to g, without having undergone any change in their relative positions.

4.—THE EXAMINATION WITH THE OPHTHALMOSCOPE.

In the selection of a portable monocular ophthalmoscope, our choice for the examination of the inverted image lies, I think, between the instruments of Coccius and Liebreich. The latter, on account of its being somewhat easier to use, is the one most generally employed. But as certain difficulties in the use of the ophthalmoscope have always to be overcome by beginners, I think it just as well that they should commence at once with the best instrument, even although the difficulty of the examination be thereby somewhat enhanced. I have for many years used Coccius' instrument for the inverted image, in preference to any other, as it possesses certain decided advantages over the concave mirror. Thus, on account of the lateral collecting lens, we can alter the focal length of the mirror and the intensity of the illumination to any desired extent, and we can also more fully concentrate the pencil of light upon any given portion of the fundus which we wish to submit to special examination. The corneal reflex is also much less, and this is of great importance if the pupil is very small, as is frequently the case in elderly people, in whom, with the concave mirror, we can often obtain, on account of the great corneal reflex, but a very imperfect view of the fundus without artificial dilatation of the pupil.

Coccius' ophthalmoscope is also decidedly better than Liebreich's for the examination of the erect image, although it is for this purpose somewhat inferior to Zehender's. But to persons who desire to have only *one* ophthalmoscope, which shall serve them for all purposes, I should recommend that of Coccius, as fulfilling this desideratum better than any other. [Any of the modern ophthalmoscopes are better for all purposes of examination than the instruments first invented. The introduction of the principle of the Rekoss disk, or of any apparatus at the back of the mirror for holding the necessary glasses, is an absolute necessity in the practice of modern ophthalmology. All the modern instruments in use are good, but special preference should be given to Dr. Loring's.—B.]

For conducting an ophthalmoscopic examination, a darkened room and a bright, steady-burning lamp are essentially necessary. In arranging a room for this purpose in a public institution, care must be taken that a bright stream of daylight does not enter directly in front of the patient, as this produces great reflection, weakens the illumination of the fundus, and renders the examination far more difficult, and needlessly trying to the eyes of the surgeon.

The best gas-lamp for ophthalmoscopic purposes is that employed at Moorfields, which has an Argand porcelain burner, perforated by a number of small apertures, and closed underneath by a very fine wire gauze, so as to regulate the draught, and thus steady the flame. The burner should not be too small, but should give a full round flame, as this affords a much better illumination than if the flame is long and thin. It is attached to a bracket, which admits of a universal movement in all directions. In the consulting room, a standard upright burner, connected with a gas-pipe by means of an elastic tube, will be, however, perhaps more convenient. Or a good, bright-burning moderator lamp may be employed. The lamp or burner is to be covered only by a chimney, and not a globe. In order to decrease the intensity of the light, and thus to diminish the contraction of the pupil, a blue chimney may be employed, or what is still better, a blue object-lens, as suggested by Mr. Carter, which is made by cementing a plane, light-blue glass (A tint) between two plano-convex lenses of the required power.

It is best for the beginner to have the pupil widely dilated by atropine, as this greatly facilitates the examination; but when he has acquired some dexterity in the use of the ophthalmoscope, he must learn to examine with an undilated pupil, for the use of atropine proves very inconvenient to patients. It should, therefore, only be employed exceptionally, and when it is absolutely necessary, as for instance when the pupil is very small, and the periphery of the fundus has to be examined for a suspected slight detachment of the retina, or morbid changes in the outlying portions of the choroid and retina. The examination in the region of the yellow spot is also very difficult, on account of the great reflection of the light, and the great contraction of the pupil when this part of the eye is illuminated. If atropia is used, only a weak solution should be employed, otherwise the dilatation of the pupil will not only last some time, but there will also be much inconvenience from the paralysis of the accommodation, which will, perhaps, prevent the patient from using his eyes for reading and writing for several days. For the purpose of simply dilating the pupil for ophthalmoscopy, a drop of a solution of one grain of atropine to ten or twelve fluidounces of water will suffice to produce the requisite degree of dilatation in about an hour, and it will continue from twelve to thirty hours. The atropinized gelatine disks will be found very convenient, as the patient can himself place one in the eye, before his visit to the surgeon.

[By far the best explanation of the principles of the ophthalmoscopic diagnosis of refraction has been offered by Dr. Loring, and it is, therefore, here given in his own words:

"Ophthalmoscopic diagnosis of the refraction of an eye can only be done accurately when the accommodation is at rest. As a preliminary to such an examination the observer must have a thorough knowledge of the state of his own refraction and accommodation. Generally, sufficient relaxation can be obtained in emmetropia by making the patient look at a distance, or into vacancy. This is much easier for a myope than for a hypermetrope, as he has only to look at some point beyond his far point. In the observer the ability to relax the accommodation varies very much, from the power to

diagnosticated by simple inspection of the corneal reflex. This reflex, as also the movement of the light and shadow on the cornea when the mirror is turned on its axis, depends, in low degrees of ametropia, almost entirely on the distance of the observer from the observed eye. These appearances will vary according as a concave or a plane mirror is used. This method of inspection affords no means of distinguishing between axile ametropia and ametropia of curvature. In a myopic eye the *bright portion* of the corneal crescent is situated at the periphery, on the side from which the light comes, and increases in extent in proportion to the degree of myopia. In a hypermetropic eye the *shadow* occupies this position, and diminishes in extent in proportion to the degree of hypermetropia present. In simple myopic astigmatism, the illuminated portion will assume the form of a crescent, or of a triangle with its apex toward the summit of the cornea, and will be large in proportion to the degree in which myopia is present. The movement of the shadow upon the astigmatic meridian corresponds to the movement of the mirror. In compound myopic astigmatism, in both meridians the shadow will move in the same direction as the mirror, but the illuminated portion of the pupil will be relatively larger in the more myopic meridian. In simple hypermetropic astigmatism, the shadow will, in both meridians, move in a direction contrary to the movements of the mirror. In the hypermetropic meridian it will be well at the periphery, and will be more pronounced in proportion to the amount of hypermetropia present. In compound hypermetropic astigmatism, the shadow will be deeper and smaller in that meridian in which the hypermetropia is the most marked. (See "Royal London Ophthalmic Hospital Reports," August, 1880.)—B.]

5.—THE EXAMINATION OF THE ACTUAL INVERTED IMAGE.

The patient is to be seated on a chair, and the lamp should be placed beside, and somewhat behind him, at the side corresponding to the eye which is to be examined. The surgeon then seats himself directly opposite to the patient, and, holding the mirror in his right hand, places it close before his eye, so that its upper edge rests against the superior margin of the orbit. Then, turning the mirror slightly towards the lamp, he throws the reflection of the flame into the eye, the pupil of which will be brightly illuminated. This movement of the mirror must be very slight, and simply made by rotating the hands a very little between the fingers, otherwise the reflection will be thrown considerably above or to the side of the patient's head. The beginner always finds some difficulty in acquiring these slight movements of the mirror, as also the power of moving his own head in different directions, and yet constantly keeping the eye well illuminated. When the fundus is thoroughly lighted up, the rim of the biconvex object-lens is to be taken lightly between the forefinger and thumb of the left hand, and held about two inches from the eye under examination. The ring finger is to be placed against the upper edge of the orbit, in order to steady the hand, and this leaves the little finger free for lifting the upper lid if necessary. [Fig. 243.] The object-lens should be held at such a distance from the eye, that its focal length coincides with the pupil. A two-inch lens should, therefore, be held a little less less than two inches from the cornea, and a three-inch lens a little less than three inches. At first, some difficulty is always experienced in keeping the eye illuminated during the adjustment of the object-lens, as the observer's attention is apt to be entirely directed to it, and he forgets all about the illumination. Indeed, one of the chief difficulties that the be-

ginner has to overcome, is that of learning to work both hands readily together.

When the fundus is well illuminated, we should first endeavor to gain a
view of the optic disk, and the patient should therefore be directed to look
at the ear of the observer which is on the opposite side to the eye under examination, so that the optic axis of the latter may be turned somewhat
inwards.   Thus, if the right eye is to be examined, the patient should look
towards the surgeon's right ear, and *vice versâ*; for as the entrance of the
optic nerve is not situated in the optic axis (centre of the retina), but towards
its nasal side, it is necessary that the patient should look inwards, in order
that the disk may be brought directly opposite to the observer's eye.   To
gain this position, the patient may also be directed to look at the uplifted
little finger of the hand holding the ophthalmoscope.   In this case its handle
may be held horizontally, and the left hand used for holding the mirror
when the left eye is under examination.   It is still more convenient to have

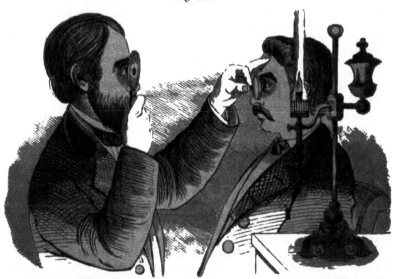

Fig. 248.

a screen or board, divided into differently numbered compartments, placed
at some distance behind the surgeon.   The patient is then directed to look
at a certain figure upon the board, according to the part of the fundus which
we desire to examine.   The object should always be placed at some distance,
in order that the patient's accommodation may be relaxed to the utmost.
The entrance of the optic nerve is readily recognized by its presenting a
whitish reflex, instead of the red glare reflected from the fundus.   As soon
as this white reflex is obtained, the object-lens should be adjusted, and we
shall then have no difficulty in finding the optic nerve entrance, which appears in the form of a circular pinkish-white disk, on whose expanse are
noticed numerous bloodvessels, which diverge from it to be distributed to
different portions of the retina.   If the disk is not in view, it may also be
easily found by tracing some of the retinal vessels up to the point towards
which they converge—*i. e.*, the optic nerve entrance.   The disk having been

found, the observer should very carefully study its color, the appearance of its surface and margin, and the course of the bloodvessels upon it, in order that these different points may be well impressed upon his memory. In the next place, passing from the disk, the different portions of the fundus should be successively examined, and the appearance and mode of distribution of the retinal vessels, and the difference between them and those of the choroid be carefully studied. The beginner should at first always examine a considerable number of healthy eyes, and study very attentively the physiological appearances of the fundus, and the various peculiarities which may occur within normal limits. And then, when he has become thoroughly conversant with these diversities, he should pass on to the examination of the pathological conditions. The examination of the rabbit's eye, also, affords excellent practice; and in the Albino rabbit, the distribution of the choroidal and retinal vessels can be most beautifully seen. As the opportunity of examining a considerable number of human eyes is not always to be had, the following instrument, made by Nachet, of Paris, will be found extremely useful for practising ophthalmoscopy, and for studying many of the morbid appearances of the fundus. It consists of an artificial eye, or dummy, made of brass, and fitted in front with a lens in the situation of the cornea. This lens is covered with a black metal cap, having a central aperture corresponding to the pupil. There are two of these caps, the one having a very small central opening corresponding to the normal size of the pupil; the other a large aperture, like a widely dilated pupil. By changing the lens, we may convert the eye into a hypermetropic, myopic, or astigmatic one. The posterior half of the eye opens, so as to admit of the insertion of a papier maché cup or disk, colored to represent the appearance of a healthy fundus, or of some pathological condition, as, for instance, retinitis pigmentosa, excavation of the optic nerve, posterior staphyloma, etc. In the box containing the instrument there is a series of these colored disks, illustrating many of the morbid ophthalmoscopic appearances of the fundus. The eye is fixed upon a standard for placing it upon a table. It is termed Perrin's artificial eye.

I have already mentioned, that if we desire to increase the size of the image in the indirect mode of examination, we must employ a weaker object-lens, e. g., of three or four inches focus, which must be held somewhat further from the eye. In order to magnify the image still more, Coccius[1] has devised a compound object-lens which consists of two convex lenses (one of which has a focal length of two, the other of two and a quarter inches), inserted in the extremities of a brass tube, composed of two portions, each of which is two and a quarter inches in length, and made to slide, one within the other. The effect of this is, that parallel rays reflected from an emmetropic eye will be united within the tube into an actual inverted image, the rays from which will then pass through the second lens, which will afford a magnified virtual image of the actual image within the tube. The disadvantages of this compound object-lens are, that it is expensive, and very cumbersome, proving very fatiguing. if many patients have to be examined in succession. I find, moreover, that we may gain almost as great an enlargement, by using an ordinary object-lens of four inches focus, and a convex lens of eight inches focus behind the mirror.

[1] Mr. R. B. Carter has given an excellent description of this apparatus and its mode of action in the "Lancet," March 18, 1866.

6.—THE EXAMINATION OF THE VIRTUAL ERECT IMAGE.

It has already been stated, that in this mode of examination the observer must go very close to the patient's eye. The lamp must therefore be placed on the side corresponding to the eye under examination, and the surgeon will find it most convenient to examine with his right eye the corresponding eye of the patient, and *vice versâ*. For the examination of the erect image, the ophthalmoscope of Coccius or Zehender will be found preferable to that of Liebreich. Not only is the illumination better, and the corneal reflex considerably less, but it is also easier, on account of the lateral collecting lens, to maintain a good illumination of the eye, and to keep the optic axis of the observer's eye in a line corresponding to that of the patient, which is often difficult, if the mirror has to be considerably turned in order to catch the rays from the lamp. If the surgeon is not much accustomed to this mode of examination, and the pupil is small, the latter should be dilated with atropine, for this will increase the size of the field of vision, and facilitate the lighting up of the fundus. If the observer and the patient are both emmetropic, and their accommodation is suspended (*i. e.*, if they are accommodated for their far point, in this case for parallel rays), the surgeon will receive a clearly defined and distinct image of the details of the fundus. The beginner, however, generally finds considerable difficulty in completely relaxing his accommodation, more especially as his close approximation to the patient leads him involuntarily to accommodate for a point considerably nearer than his far point, *i. e.*, he is accommodated for more or less divergent rays. This will render the image indistinct, and necessitate the use of a concave ocular lens, in order to give the requisite degree of divergence to the parallel rays emanating from the patient's eye. In certain conditions of the refraction either of the patient's or surgeon's eye, a concave ocular lens is absolutely necessary to render the image of the fundus distinct. Thus, if the patient's eye is emmetropic, but that of the surgeon myopic, the rays from the former will be parallel, and be consequently brought to a focus in front of his retina, and a concave lens will be required to give them the necessary degree of divergence. The strength of this lens should be such as to neutralize his myopia for distance. A still stronger concave lens will be required, if the eyes of the surgeon and patient are both myopic, for then the rays will impinge in a convergent direction upon the surgeon's eye. But if the surgeon is myopic, and the patient hypermetropic, the former may be able to see the fundus distinctly without the aid of a concave lens, for the following reason: the focus of the dioptric system of the eye under examination, will in this case lie behind the retina, and the eye will therefore be adjusted for more or less convergent rays. The emerging rays will consequently be divergent, and will be readily united upon the observer's retina, if his myopia is not too considerable in degree. The same will occur if the surgeon is hypermetropic or emmetropic, but then he will have to use his power of accommodation, in order to bring the divergent rays to a focus upon his retina. If, on the other hand, the observer is hypermetropic, he may also be able to examine a myopic or emmetropic eye (if the myopia is not too great) without the aid of a concave lens, for he will be able to unite convergent rays upon his retina, and also parallel rays by an effort of the accommodation. The cases containing the portable ophthalmoscopes are supplied with a series of concave ocular lenses, varying in focal length from four to ten or twelve inches, and fitting into the clip behind the mirror. The surgeon should select the strength of the lens according to the state of the refraction of his own and the patient's eye.

The chief advantage of the erect image is, that we obtain a much larger image, so that the minute details of the fundus can be studied with much greater accuracy. This mode of examination is therefore of much importance in solving any doubts which may exist with the reverse image, as to the exact nature or situation of any morbid appearances. But the field of vision is more limited, and the examination somewhat more difficult. Moreover, it is not always convenient or agreeable to examine all patients in such close proximity. The latter may be one reason why this mode of examination is far too much neglected in England in favor of the inverted image. As a rule, it is best to obtain a general view of the appearances of the fundus in the inverted image, and then, if we desire to examine any particular point with greater minuteness and accuracy, to have recourse to the direct method.

[The degree of enlargement produced by the upright image, and the method of ascertaining it, does not admit of an explanation within the space of a few lines. The first thing necessary to determine the size of a retinal image is to know the distance at which the object is seen, for the relative size of the images of an object on the retina stand in the same proportion to each other as the corresponding distances of the object in front of the nodal point of the eye. The distance from the latter to the retina of the human eye is a known quantity (six and seven-tenths Paris lines). The magnifying power of a glass for an object seen at its focus is obtained by dividing some arbitrary distance assumed as a standard by the focal length of the glass. A standard of eight inches has been assumed, and dividing this by the focal length of the dioptric system of the eye, the magnifying power of the latter is found to be fourteen and one-third. Hence the retina of an emmetropic eye is seen to be enlarged by the upright method of examination fourteen and one-third diameters. (Loring's "Determination of the Refraction of the Eye with the Ophthalmoscope," 1876.) From observations made by Mauthner, we now know that the image of a myopic eye seen in the upright image with the error of refraction corrected is larger than the image of an emmetropic eye, while the image of a hypermetropic eye is smaller. With the inverted image, the reverse is the case. (Mauthner's "Lehrbuch der Ophthalmoscopie," 1867.)—B.]

7.—THE OPHTHALMOSCOPIC APPEARANCES OF HEALTHY EYES
(Plate I., Figs. 1 and 2).

Before commencing any ophthalmoscopic examination of the fundus, the condition of the cornea, iris, pupil, and crystalline lens should be examined by the oblique illumination. This having been done, the same structures should be viewed by transmitted light, i. e., the surgeon should examine the eye by the direct method (without the interposition of a convex lens between the mirror and the patient's eye), but the mirror should be held at some distance (fourteen to eighteen inches) from the eye under examination. In this way no opacity of the refracting media can escape detection, which is not unfrequently the case if these modes of examination are neglected, and the fundus only examined with the inverted image. We can also in this way readily ascertain the state of refraction of the eye.

The examination of the refracting media in a healthy condition, of course, affords a negative result. Sometimes small flakes of mucus may be noticed on the cornea, giving it a somewhat irregular appearance. They disappear on closure of the lids.

It has been already stated (p. 427) that certain physiological changes occur in the lens in advancing age, and we must be upon our guard not to mistake these for commencing cataract. The lens-substance becomes thickened and consolidated, and the nucleus assumes a yellowish tint, which is especially apparent by reflected light. Indeed this opacity is sometimes so considerable, that it may be mistaken for a tolerably advanced cataract, but on examining the lens by transmitted light (with the mirror only) it will be found perfectly transparent, and the details of the fundus quite distinct.

On the other hand, the healthy appearances presented by the fundus oculi deserve and demand the closest and most attentive study, in order that the many diversities which they may present may not be mistaken for morbid phenomena. It is only by an intimate knowledge of the many physiological peculiarities which may exist in a perfectly normal eye, that we can avoid committing grave errors in diagnosis. Beginners are but too apt to hurry over the examination of healthy eyes with a careless, "Oh, there is nothing the matter; the fundus is quite healthy," craving only after the most marked pathological changes, such as large posterior staphylomata, very deep excavations of the optic nerve, and huge patches of atrophied choroid; and completely overlooking the minuter shades of difference between a healthy and morbid condition of the fundus, a knowledge of which proves of the greatest importance in practice.

On looking at No. 1 of the ophthalmoscopic plates, the reader will be at once struck by the marked difference in the appearances presented by Figs. 1 and 2, and yet both illustrate a perfectly healthy fundus.

In Fig. 1 (which is taken from a person with black hair and a dark-brown iris) the optic nerve entrance appears circular, and of a yellowish-white tint. The bloodvessels emerge somewhat to the left of the centre of the disk, which is here of a deeper white. The paler vessels are the retinal arteries, the darker ones the veins. They pass over the disk to the retina, where they course and divide in different directions, chiefly upwards, downwards, and towards the left. At some little distance to the right of, and slightly below, the disk, is noticed a large dark-red spot, with a small white dot in the centre. This is the macula lutea, or yellow spot, with its [fovea] centralis. It will be observed that the vessels course round the yellow spot, leaving it free. The fine gray film in the region of the disk and the yellow spot is due to the reflex yielded by the retina; it is only observable in dark eyes, and is consequently altogether absent in Fig. 2. The fundus of the eye is of a rich dark-red tint, and only the retinal vessels are apparent, those of the choroid being hidden by the density of the pigment in the epithelial layer and stroma of the choroid.

[An explanation of the glittering ring or halo seen round the macula lutea with the inverted image was first given by Dr. Loring in 1871, whose words are as follows: "This region of the fundus bears in its formation a strong resemblance to a shallow cup, of which the rim is represented by a convex and the bowl by a concave surface. If we look upon these curved surfaces as mirrors, they would each have their foci, one lying behind and the other front, according to their respective degrees of curvature. And if light should be thrown perpendicularly against such a combination of curves, the ... of the outside rim or convex surface would, from well-known optical ... appear illuminated, while the inside or concave surface would appear ... or less in shadow. Thus, we should have the effect of a darker centre, surrounded by an illuminated edge." From these considerations, which were illustrated by practical experiments upon eye-phantoms, he is of the opinion that the halo round the macula "is the product of reflection and refraction from the combination of curved surfaces which enter into the construction of this portion of the retina, and that the principal sources of light from which these reflections are produced are the images of the ophthalmoscope and lamp situated in the media of the eye." (See "Trans. Amer. Ophthal. Society," 1871, and "Report of the Fifth Internat. Ophthal. Congress," 1876.)—B.]

In Fig. 2 (taken from the eye of a person with very light hair and a blue iris) the appearances are quite different. The disk is of a more rosy tint, the retinal vessels, although very distinct, are less markedly so than on the darker background of Fig. 1. The region of the yellow spot is of a bright red color, and the foramen centrale appears in the form of a little light circle. But the greatest difference is noticed in the pale, brilliantly red color of the fundus, and the distinctness with which the finest branches of the choroidal vessels can be traced. The ciliary arteries enter in the region of the yellow spot, and, running towards the periphery, ramify in various directions, and partly pass over directly into the larger branches of the vasa vorticosa, situated at the equator of the eye.

The red color of the background of the eye, as seen with the ophthalmoscope, is due to the reflection of the light from the bloodvessels of the retina and choroid, more especially the latter. As the retina is very translucent, but little light is reflected by it, and the sclerotic can only be seen through the choroid, and will therefore be the more apparent the less pigment there is in the latter. The appearance presented by the fundus will, therefore, vary greatly according to the degree of pigmentation of the choroid. If its epithelial layer and stroma are darkly pigmented, the vessels of the choroid may be completely hidden, even at the periphery of the fundus; but if the epithelial layer contains but little pigment, and the stroma is, on the other hand, richly pigmented, the choroidal vessels will appear like bright red bands or ribbons, divided by dark islets or intervals, the so-called intravascular spaces. These vessels are chiefly situated in the stroma of the choroid, for they are less covered by the pigment than those of the venæ vorticosæ, which lie deeper (nearer the sclerotic), or the smaller vessels (Schweigger). The intra-vascular spaces are of a longitudinal shape near the equator of the eye, and more oval or circular in the vicinity of the disk. If the stroma is light, and the epithelium but moderately pigmented, the epithelial cells may be well seen with a considerable magnifying power, as has been shown by Liebreich, and may be recognized as small circumscribed dots uniformly studded over the fundus, giving it a markedly granular appearance. In eyes in which the pigmentation of the choroid is but very slight, the choroidal vessels may be most beautifully traced to their smallest divisions, as also the large stems of the venæ vorticosæ as they perforate the sclerotic. The red color of the background is also influenced by age and the illumination. It is of a brighter tint in young persons than in older individuals. If the illumination is strong, the brightness will be uniform; if it is weak, it will decrease from the disk towards the periphery of the fundus.

The retina is extremely translucent, and reflects but little light. On this account it is not visible in light eyes, but becomes so when the fundus is dark, appearing like a thin gray film or halo over the background. In very dark eyes, such as those of negroes, the retina is very distinctly apparent, showing a gray striated appearance, especially in the vicinity of the disk. These striæ are not, Schweigger thinks, due to the nerve fibres, but to the peculiar arrangement of the connective tissue.

8.—THE OPTIC DISK.

The normal disk is subject to numerous and sometimes marked differences in shape, color, and size. An exact knowledge of all the peculiarities which come within the normal and physiological standard is absolutely necessary to prevent the surgeon from falling into errors in diagnosis, and mistaking some perfectly physiological appearances as being of pathological import.

The entrance of the optic nerve is generally round, but not perfectly circular; it is often oval, having the long diameter vertical. This oval appearance is particularly striking in cases of astigmatism. The disk is generally of a transparent, grayish-pink tint, with a slight admixture of blue. This tint varies in appearance with the pigmentation of the choroid; thus in dark eyes the disk appears white and glistening, whereas in very light eyes it assumes a more rosy hue. The admixture of the color of the optic nerve entrance is made up from three sources: the white is due to the reflection from the connective tissue of the lamina cribrosa, the red to the blood in the capillaries on its expanse, and the bluish-gray to the nerve tubules lying in the meshes of the cribriform tissue. The outline of the disk appears sharply defined, but on closer observation we notice that it may be divided into an internal gray ring, the real boundary of the nerve; outside this is the white line of the sclerotic ring, which varies somewhat in size, being broadest and most apparent at the outer side of the disk. External to the scleral zone, is the dark-gray line of the opening in the choroid. This choroidal ring is somewhat irregular in shape and color, being most marked at the outer side, at which there is often a well-defined deposit of pigment molecules, assuming the appearance of a broad black crescent, which is frequently mistaken by beginners for some pathological change.

The retinal vessels generally emerge from the central portion of the disk, or somewhat to the inner side of it. If the division of the central artery takes place after its passage through the lamina cribrosa, the division of the main trunk into the different branches can be distinctly observed; whereas, if the division occurs before the passage of the trunk through the lamina cribrosa, the main branches pierce the disk in an isolated manner, so that their point of division from the trunk cannot be distinguished. The number, mode of division, and course of the retinal vessels vary very considerably, being constant only in this, that the principal branches run upwards and downwards. As a rule, no main branch runs inwards, but only a considerable number of small vessels; whereas towards the outer side only a few very small, short twigs are sent. The most frequent arrangement is, that an artery and two veins pass upwards, and the same downwards; but sometimes there are two arteries and two veins. The arteries may be readily distinguished from the veins by being lighter in color, smaller, and straighter in their course. Moreover, along the centre of the vessels is noticed a bright stheak. Various opinions have been advanced as to the cause of this central white stripe. Von Trigt and Jaeger originally explained it thus: That the rays of light which fall perpendicularly upon the cylindrical walls of the vessels are reflected in a perpendicular direction; whereas the rays which fall external to the centre of the vessel are reflected laterally, and hence cause the sides to appear dark. This explains the reason why the white stripe varies in position according to that of the visual line of the observer, for if we look at the side instead of the centre of the vessel, the light stripe will also shift to the side. More recently, Jaeger has given us this opinion, and believes that the column of blood within the vessels and not the walls of the latter produce the reflection.[1] Loring, on the other hand, believes,[2] "that the light striking the wall nearest the observer passes through this on account of its transparency, without being reflected to any appreciable degree, traverses the contents of the vessel, and is then reflected back slightly from the opposite wall, but principally from the subjacent tissues." This view has been again opposed more recently by Schneller,[3] who maintains that the light streak is due to the reflection of light from the anterior wall of the artery. [Schneller's views have been carefully reviewed in a later paper by Loring, who does not consider them tenable, either from a mathematical or physiological point of view. His own explanation has been accepted by Giraud-Teulon, who has also adduced some additional experiments of his own in support of it. (See "Trans. Amer. Ophthal. Soc.," 1873.) Parent's idea of the phenomenon is that the reflection from the vessels is caused by the column of blood itself, in this agreeing with Jaeger. He thinks the posterior wall of a vessel acts like a concave cylindrical mirror; the reflected rays following the meridian parallel to the axis might return to the eye of the observer if the absorbent power of the blood were less considerable; but the rays which fall upon the wall of the vessel perpendicular to its axis cannot be reflected outside of this; hence these rays cannot contribute to the formation of a reflex, for they are extinguished in the interior of the vessel, and absorbed by the column of blood. He also speaks of a general reflection from the suface of the retina, which is sometimes so intense as to interfere materially with an ophthalmoscopic examination. This he regards as due to the internal limiting membrane, which, especially in children, is really a vitreous membrane and gives off a reflex, resembling that from glass. Parent's views will probably be rejected by most authorities.—B.] The retinal veins are of a darker tint, larger, and more undulating than the arteries. On account of the greater tenuity of the walls of the veins, and of the blood-tension being less in them than in the arteries, they are somewhat flattened and not cylindrical in form. Hence the reflection of light is very slight, and the central bright streak hardly observable. Even on the normal disk the sheath of the vessels is sometimes apparent, giving rise to a double contoured white stripe at the edge of the principal vessels, arteries, and veins. This is generally confined to the disk and its immediate vicinity (Mauthner). The blood supply of the most anterior part of the optic nerve is maintained not only by the small twigs given off to it from the central vessels of the retina by the vessels of the external and internal sheath, but also by a series of branchlets emanating from a vascular circle, which is situated close to the edge of the optic nerve, and which is formed by three or four of the short posterior ciliary arteries.[4] Leber, moreover, has found that numerous arteries and some veins also pass directly from the choroid to the optic nerve, anastomosing there with the network of vessels which surrounds the nerve fibres.[5]

[1] "Ophthalmoskopischen Hand-Atlas," 1869, S. 82.

[2] "Trans. of American Ophthalmological Society," 1870, p. 122; also Knapp's "Archives," ii. 1, 199.

[3] "A. f. O.," xviii. 1, 118.

[4] Vide Jäger, "Ueber die Einstellungen des Dioptrischen Apparatus in Menschlichen Auge," S. 55; also Leber, "A. f. O.," xi. 1, 5.

[5] Galezowski's opinion that the minuter vessels of the disk, through which the latter obtains its reddish tint, are not branches of the central vessels of the retina, but of the vessels of the pia mater and brain, is disproved by Leber, "A. f. O.," xviii. 2, 25; vide also Dr. Wolfring's article, ib., p. 10.

9.—THE OPHTHALMOSCOPIC EXAMINATION OF DISEASED EYES.

THE REFRACTING MEDIA.

Before commencing any ophthalmoscopic examination of the fundus, the refracting media should always be examined by the oblique illumination and by transmitted light (*vide* p. 755). By making this a constant rule, the beginner will avoid falling into many errors in diagnosis which might otherwise occur, such as mistaking opacities of the cornea, the capsule, or the lens for some deeper-seated lesion. In making an examination of the lens or the vitreous humor, the pupil should be widely dilated, although an expert observer will often be able, even with an undilated pupil, to detect opacities which are situated at the margin of the lens, or the periphery of the vitreous humor, by making the patient look very far in the opposite direction, which will enable the surgeon to look quite behind the iris. The color of opacities in the refracting media will vary according to the amount of illumination, and the fact whether they are examined by reflected or transmitted light. In the former case, they will appear in their true colors, the fundus being in the shade, so that they will look like gray or whitish opacities situated upon a dark background. It is different, however, when the fundus is lighted up with the ophthalmoscope, for then the opacities will appear like dark specks, of varying size and form, upon a bright red background, for their surfaces can reflect but little light, and they are thus seen in shadow. On this account, very small opacities are best seen by a weak illumination, for in consequence of their very slight reflection, they become invisible if the illumination is too bright. It is of much importance to be able rightly to estimate the depth at which any opacity in the refracting media is situated. There cannot be the slightest difficulty about this when the opacity is in the cornea, the capsule, or the anterior portion of the lens, for with the oblique illumination we shall be able to ascertain the position of the opacity in relation to the pupil. Indeed, for opacities in the anterior half of the eyeball the oblique illumination is of most service, but for those in the posterior half the ophthalmoscope should be used. But it is best to avail ourselves of both modes of examination. When the opacity is situated in the vitreous humor, it is more difficult to ascertain its exact depth. The two following methods of examination will, however, enable us to decide this: If, for instance, the observer (using the direct method) looks in such a direction that his visual line passes through the turning-point of the patient's eye, it will be found that this point and the corneal reflection of the mirror will alone remain stationary when the eye is moved in different directions. Any opacity which is situated in front of this point will move in the same direction as the cornea, whereas any opacity situated behind the turning-point will move in a direction opposite to that of the cornea. The further the opacity is from the turning-point of the eye, the greater will its excursion be. Now the turning-point corresponds as nearly as possible to the posterior pole of the crystalline lens. If there should consequently be an opacity situated at this spot (posterior polar cataract), it will remain stationary during the various movements of the eye. If the opacity is situated in front of the posterior pole, it will move in the same direction as the cornea: if the latter moves upwards, the opacity will do the same; the reverse will occur if the opacity is situated behind the turning-point, for then it will move downwards as the cornea moves up, and vice versa.

It is more difficult to determine the exact position of the object when it lies very close to the retina. This is best done by the surgeon making a slight movement with the object-lens (in the examination with the reverse image), his own and the patient's eye being at the same time kept stationary. The nearer that the object is to the observer, the more marked will be its movement in the same direction as the lens. To illustrate this, Liebreich[1] cites the following example: If we suppose that a filiform opacity were to extend from the posterior pole of the lens to the centre of the retina, it would appear like a point when seen from in front. If we were then to move the convex lens from right to left, the anterior extremity of the opacity would pass to the corresponding side, in front of its posterior extremity, so that the opacity would no longer appear like a point, but a line. The depth of opacities in the vitreous is, however, best determined by the aid of the binocular ophthalmoscope.

Opacities of the cornea are best seen with the oblique illumination, and appear like small gray or white spots, and their situation and extent can thus be ascertained with the greatest nicety. This method of examination will also be found useful in the detection and removal of foreign bodies from the cornea. In the direct mode of examination with the ophthalmoscope, small opacities or facets in the cornea lend a peculiar mottled or marbled appearance to the fundus, as if little dark spots or streaks are studded over its red expanse. We may thus also readily detect changes in the curvature of the cornea, and diagnose the earliest stage of conical cornea, for the conical portion yields a bright reflection, like a transparent bead or drop of water, with its base half in shadow; the situation of the latter varying with the movements of the mirror.

The appearances presented by different forms of cataract, etc., both by reflected and transmitted light, have already been described at length in the chapter upon the "Diseases of the Lens."

---

[1] French translation of Mackenzie's "Treatise on the Diseases of the Eye," p. 31.

CHAPTER XVII

DISEASES OF THE ORBIT.

1.—INFLAMMATION OF THE CELLULAR TISSUE OF THE ORBIT (CELLULITIS ORBITÆ).

THE symptoms and course of this disease are generally of a very acute and severe inflammatory character. The eyelids become rapidly swollen, red, and hot, the palpebral and ocular conjunctiva much injected, and there is mostly great serous chemosis, surrounding the cornea in the form of a thick, dusky-red mound, the edges of which may even overlap and partially hide the cornea. The patient complains of intense, intermittent pain in and around the eye, and extending over the corresponding side of the forehead. There is also, generally, marked febrile constitutional disturbance; and if the inflammation should extend from the orbit to the brain, severe cerebral symptoms will supervene. The eyeball soon becomes protruded. At the outset of the disease, this protrusion is not very marked, and may only become evident when the two eyes are compared; but when the inflammatory swelling of the orbital cellular tissue increases, and still more when pus is formed, the exophthalmos rapidly augments, perhaps even to such a degree that the dusky, swollen lids can no longer be closed over the eyeball, but the latter projects more or less between them. If the pus collects chiefly at the bottom of the orbit, the protrusion is uniform and straightforward in the axis of the eyeball, and not in one particular direction, as is generally the case in the exophthalmos accompanying periostitis of the orbit. The movements of the eyeball are also uniformly impaired, and not especially so in one direction. If the patient attempts to move the eye, or it is touched, more especially if it is slightly pushed back into the orbit, intense pain is produced. But this is not the case if the point of the little finger be gently passed along and somewhat beneath the edge of the orbit, and we do not find a special point, where its touch excites great pain, as is the case in periostitis. The formation of pus is generally accompanied by well-marked rigors.

From the exposure of the protruded eyeball to the atmosphere, the secretions on the surface of the conjunctiva and the chemotic swelling become dried in the form of hard, dark crusts. The surface of the cornea may also become roughened and clouded, from desiccation of its epithelium and its exposure to mechanical irritants. The sight is often much impaired by the stretching of, or pressure exerted upon, the optic nerve, and the retinal veins are generally more or less engorged and tortuous; there being, perhaps, at the same time a serous infiltration of the disk and the retina in its vicinity. The field of vision is also somewhat contracted, often considerably so. If the exophthalmos lasts for any length of time, optic neuritis may supervene upon the congestion and engorgement of the optic nerve, followed, perhaps, by consecutive atrophy of the latter. [Sometimes the nutrition of the eyeball is so interfered with by the compression of the infiltrated orbital tissues, that the cornea becomes opaque, sloughs, and then the suppurative process extends to the eyeball.—B.]

If the pus be formed in sufficient quantity, it makes its way forward from the bottom of the orbit, and may cause distinct fluctuation behind the conjunctiva or the lids; and it perforates either through the lid or through the conjunctiva, and in the latter case, it will appear to come from within the eye. But the inflammation and suppuration may also invade the eyeball, and panophthalmitis be set up; pus will appear in the anterior chamber, the pain will be still more increased in severity, and will only be ameliorated when the cornea gives way, and the lens and the humors of the eye are evacuated. Sometimes the swelling of the eyelids is so tense and great that all sense of fluctuation is lost.

Although the severity of the inflammatory symptoms met with in orbital cellulitis varies considerably in degree, the disease generally runs a more or less acute course. But, according to Mackenzie,[1] the latter may, in very rare instances, be extremely chronic. Not until a very long time, perhaps many months, has elapsed, does matter accumulate in the orbit, and then the eye gradually protrudes, the lids become somewhat swollen and red, the pus makes its way to the surface, the skin gives way, and a sinus may be left, often proving extremely obstinate in the treatment. [Sometimes, although all the inflammatory symptoms may be well marked, no pus is formed, in spite of hot applications and free incisions. The tissue cuts like brawn, and there is very little hemorrhage. These are the most unfavorable cases, for the process of resolution is slow, and the great pressure frequently destroys the eye.—B.]

In framing our prognosis, we must always remember that cellulitis not unfrequently becomes complicated with periostitis, leading subsequently to caries or necrosis. That, moreover, the inflammation may extend backwards along the periosteum to the membranes of the brain, producing meningitis or abscess of the brain. If caries or necrosis of the walls of the orbit has taken place, the pus may make its way through this aperture into the cranium or antrum of Highmore, etc. Moreover, the patient's general health, already perhaps undermined by a long and very serious illness, may give way beneath the acute and protracted sufferings produced by the disease, if the latter is improperly allowed to run its course, and is not arrested and relieved by a timely evacuation of the pus.

[The prognosis in most cases must be regarded as bad, as far as the integrity of the eye is concerned, and rapid suppuration is to be favored.—B.]

Amongst the most frequent causes of inflammation of the cellular tissue of the orbit, are contused or incised wounds of, and the lodgement of foreign bodies in, the orbit. The disease may also be caused by sudden changes of temperature, and exposure to cold and wet; and it may occur secondarily in severe constitutional diseases, such as pyæmia, puerperal fever, etc. It may also be due to the extension of the inflammation from neighboring parts, as in erysipelas of the head and face, severe inflammation of the lachrymal sac, or operations performed upon the latter, more especially its destruction by the galvano-caustic apparatus or very strong caustics; or it may ensue upon panophthalmitis, or operations upon the eye or eyelids.

[The connection between orbital cellulitis and erysipelas of the face has been very clearly presented by Leber. In this form of inflammation, thrombo-phlebitis of the numerous small orbital veins plays an important

---

[1] "Diseases of the Eye," p. 299.

part. The erysipelatous poison or mycosis enters a small vein, causes an infecting thrombosis and phlebitis, which extends through the veins with great rapidity, and produces in their vicinity suppuration and the formation of an abscess. In the same way the thrombo-phlebitis may extend to the cavity of the skull. When both orbits are affected, the cellulitis breaks out simultaneously, as when the erysipelas occupies the entire face or middle frontal region; or else by the anastomosis of the frontal and supra-orbital veins of both sides in the centre of the forehead, the thrombo-phlebitis outside the skull is communicated from one side to the other. (See "Archiv für Ophthalmologie," xxvi. 3.)

It has been known to be caused by an iridectomy, the inflammation beginning in the capsule of Tenon, close to the wound, and rapidly involving the orbital tissue. (See "Amer. Journ. Med. Sciences," July, 1878.—B.]

The treatment should be chiefly directed to subduing and arresting the inflammatory symptoms. If the disease is due to an injury, the treatment suitable to its special character (vide "Injuries of the Orbit") must be adopted, and cold compresses and leeches should be applied. But if suppuration has already set in, these applications should be changed for hot poppy fomentations or hot poultices, and a free incision with a bistoury should be made at an early period, in order that the pus may be evacuated. If much doubt exists as to the true nature of the disease, a small exploratory incision should be made, and if pus is found to ooze out, the incision should be sufficiently enlarged to permit of its free and ready escape. If possible, the opening should be made through the conjunctiva, and not through the eyelids; but if the abscess points directly beneath the latter, the incision must be made at this spot.

In making the incision through the conjunctiva, the upper lid should be raised with the finger, and a scalpel, or the point of a cataract-knife, passed through the conjunctiva above the upper edge of the eyeball into the orbit. Care should be taken that the globe is not injured, and to avoid this, the edge of the knife should be directed somewhat upwards. Warm poultices are then to be applied, and the edges of the wound are to be kept open by daily passing a probe between them. If the track of the wound is deep and long, and fear is entertained that it may not heal from the bottom, a small dossil of lint should be inserted as a tent, and changed every day. The sinus should also be syringed out once or twice a day with a mild astringent lotion (zinc. sulph. gr. iv, ad aq. dest. f℥ij). If the healing of the sinus prove obstinate and protracted, a careful examination must be made as to the presence of carious or necrosed portions of bone. In the latter case, time should be allowed for the loosening or detachment of the spicula of bone, and the incision should then be sufficiently enlarged, and the fragments of bone removed with a pair of forceps.

If panophthalmitis coexist with the abscess in the orbit, and there is pus in the anterior chamber, paracentesis should be performed, and the pus evacuated.

The patient's health should be sustained by a generous diet and tonics, care being at the same time taken that the bowels are kept well open, and febrile symptoms alleviated by maintaining a free action of the kidneys and the skin.

When the pus has been evacuated, the protrusion of the eye will gradually diminish, and the latter reassume its normal position. If the eye has otherwise escaped all injury, and the impairment of vision was simply due to stretching of the optic nerve and stasis in the retinal circulation, the sight will rapidly improve. Sometimes, however, a curtailment of the movements of the eye in certain directions may remain behind.

We meet with two forms of periostitis of the orbit, the *acute* and the *chronic*.

In *acute* periostitis, the inflammatory symptoms are often very severe and pronounced. The patient complains of great pain in and around the eye, and the constitutional symptoms may also be very severe. The eyelids, more especially the upper one, become swollen, red, hot, and painful, but the swelling and redness are, as a rule, not so extreme, and do not advance with such rapidity as in cellulitis of the orbit; moreover, in periostitis, the swelling of the two lids is not alike in degree, but one is generally more swollen than the other. The ocular conjunctiva and subconjunctival tissue are injected, and there is more or less serous chemosis. The eyeball becomes somewhat protruded, even perhaps to such a degree (if much pus is formed) that the eyelids cannot be closed. The protrusion is not, however, straightforward, as is generally the case in abscess of the orbit, but towards one side; the movements of the eyeball are therefore not curtailed equally in all directions, but more in certain directions than in others. This is due to the fact that the periostitis is chiefly and specially confined to one wall or one portion of the orbit. Thus, if the inner and upper wall of the orbit are affected, the eyeball would protrude downwards and outwards, and the movements would be especially curtailed in the upward and inward direction. If the tip of the little finger is passed along the upper or lower edge of the orbit, and pushed somewhat back into the cavity, we are often able to detect a point where its pressure causes severe pain, and where there is distinct swelling, thus indicating the seat of the disease. Sometimes, the patients can themselves localize the situation of the periostitis with much exactitude. In the course of acute periostitis, the cellular tissue generally also becomes extensively inflamed, a great amount of pus may be formed, the eye be very considerably protruded, and its movements greatly, or even completely, impaired. The disease then assumes a mixed type of periostitis and abscess of the orbit. The periostitis is generally accompanied from the outset by a certain degree of inflammation of the bone itself.

In *chronic* periostitis, the inflammatory symptoms are far less pronounced, and the disease is more protracted and insidious in its course. The swelling and redness of the eyelids, the injection of the conjunctiva, the chemosis, and the protrusion of the eye, are generally far less severe than in the acute form. Pain is experienced in and around the eye, which mostly increases in severity towards night, and is markedly augmented by pressure upon the edge of the orbit, or by pressing the eye backwards in a certain direction. Sometimes, decided swelling of the orbit can be detected at one point. A certain amount of suppuration generally takes place, and if pus is formed in considerable quantity, it will, of course, cause great protrusion of the eye. As a rule, however, the suppuration is limited, and the pus is apt to accumulate between the periosteum and the bone, and lift up the former. The periosteum often becomes greatly swollen and thickened, giving rise perhaps to little nodules or tuberosities. These may subsequently again diminish in size, and finally only leave a somewhat thickened condition of the periosteum, or they may undergo ossification, and thus give rise to exostoses. If the bone becomes involved, caries and often necrosis will result, and the inflammation or the pus may extend through the aperture in the orbit to the cavity of the cranium, or into the frontal sinus. Indeed, the great danger of the disease is, that the inflammation should extend from the orbit back to the membranes of the brain, and set up fatal meningitis, or that an abscess should be formed in the brain.

Periostitis is sometimes met with in infants, and is indeed far more common amongst young persons than in adults. The most frequent causes of acute periostitis are penetrating wounds of the orbit with sharp cutting instruments; or severe contusion of its edge from blows, or blunt instruments; and the lodgement of foreign bodies within the orbit. It may also be secondary, the inflammation extending from the periosteum of some of the neighboring cavities, *e. g.*, frontal sinus, maxillary space, etc. Exposure to damp and cold and to sudden changes of temperature may also give rise to it. As already stated, it may likewise appear in the course of inflammation of the cellular tissue of the orbit. Chronic periostitis is most frequently due to syphilis. [See a paper by the Editor in the "Trans. of the New York Academy of Medicine" for 1881.

Periostitis may also be caused by the presence of intra-orbital tumors.—B.]

The general plan of treatment resembles very closely that recommended for inflammation of the cellular tissue of the orbit, and if the presence of pus is suspected, it should be evacuated as early as possible. Where the disease is due to syphilis, the iodide and bromide of potassium, in combination with some preparation of mercury, should be administered, or the mercurial bath should be employed. Care should be taken not to enfeeble the patient's health, but to fortify it as much as possible by tonics and a generous diet.

3.—CARIES AND NECROSIS OF THE ORBIT.

At the commencement of a carious affection of the bones of the orbit, there is generally a certain degree of œdematous swelling of the eyelids, which are also somewhat red and perhaps painful. The conjunctiva and subconjunctival tissue are injected, and the eye is irritable and watery. The œdema of the eyelids is often very considerable, particularly in children of a scrofulous diathesis. Soon, a spot is noticed where the eyelid assumes a more dusky-

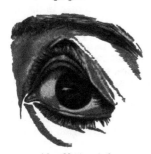

[Fig. 244.

After Mackenzie.]

red tint; here the abscess points, the skin gives way, and through this small perforation a thin, scanty, muco-purulent or "stringy" discharge oozes out. On passing a probe through this aperture, we find that it leads to a portion of bare, roughened bone. The edges of the opening generally become somewhat everted, swollen, and ulcerated, and covered perhaps with fleshy granulations. A portion of the bone, as a rule, becomes necrosed, and small fragments are exfoliated. After this condition has lasted for more or less considerable length of time, the sinus closes up, and the aperture heals; but during the process of cicatrization, the integuments become adherent to the periosteum, and thus an eversion of the lid, perhaps of very considerable extent, may be produced, causing a great exposure of the eyeball (lagophthalmos) with all its deleterious consequences. [Fig. 244.]

The course of the disease is often most protracted, especially in persons of feeble health, and of a scrofulous or syphilitic diathesis, in whom relapses are very apt to occur. The disease improves, the sinus and external aperture appear to be healing kindly, when a relapse takes place, fresh symptoms of inflammation supervene, the discharge again increases in quantity, and fresh portions of bone are perhaps exfoliated.

Caries and necrosis may occur in different portions of the orbit; thus, the bottom of the latter may be the seat of the disease, as is often the case after periostitis of this portion of the cavity. In rarer instances, it may

[Fig. 245.

Fig. 246.

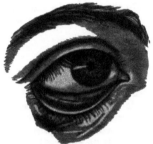

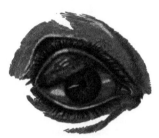

After Mackenzie.

After Mackenzie.]

supervene upon inflammation of the cellular tissue of the orbit, accompanied by periostitis. Sometimes the caries is confined to the margin of the orbit, or it occurs just within the cavity near the edge. In such cases, the upper or lower lid, according to circumstances, may become extensively involved in the cicatrix, and a very considerable ectropium result [Figs. 245 and 246]. These cases of caries and necrosis of the margin of the orbit are generally the result of a blow or fall upon this part, and are frequently met with in children, more particularly those of a scrofulous diathesis. Syphilis is a frequent cause of caries of the orbit, and the disease of the bone may in such cases be due to an extension of the affection from the nasal fossæ. [See a paper by the Editor in the "Trans. of the New York Academy of Medicine" for 1881.—B.]

The principles of treatment should resemble those recommended for periostitis. The pus should be evacuated as early as possible, the fistulous sinus be washed out frequently with warm water or mild astringent injections, and a small tent of lint should be introduced, in order to cause the sinus to heal from the bottom. If a loose sequestrum of bone is detached with the probe, the external opening should be somewhat enlarged, and the fragment be carefully removed with forceps. The treatment of the lagophthalmos and ectropium consequent upon the caries, is fully described in the articles upon these subjects.

[Occasionally a carious process is developed in the lachrymal or ethmoid bones, which gives rise to an uncommon pathological condition, a prelachrymal abscess. A swelling slowly develops at the inner canthus, above the internal canthal ligament, lying in the hollow of the lachrymal bone and side of the nose, immediately beneath the upper margin of the orbit, and involving the inner end of the upper lid. When the skin is cut through here, there is seen a distinct cyst-wall which bulges, but an attempt to dissect out the cyst fails, for it is found closely united with the periosteum of the lachrymal or ethmoid bones. After being opened, its cavity is found smooth and communicating at the bottom with a hole in the bones. A probe passed through this enters the ethmoidal cells, and dead bone is discovered. This

49

prelachrymal abscess resembles somewhat abscess of the lachrymal sac, but has no connection with the lachrymal passages, and causes no epiphora. The caries does not admit of operative interference, on account of its proximity to important cavities, and the most that can be hoped for is that a careful syringing of some astringent or some caustic, like a weak solution of argentic nitrate, for a protracted period; or the introduction of a drainage-tube of flexible silver through the hole into the superior nasal meatus, may eventually put an end to the caries, and admit of the cavity filling by granulations from the bottom. These cases are usually the result of a blow at the inner angle of the orbit, as from a foil in fencing. (See a paper by the Editor, in "Amer. Journ. Med. Sci.," July, 1880.)—B.]

4.—INFLAMMATION OF THE CAPSULE OF TENON.

The fibrous capsule which envelops the eyeball (capsule of Tenon) is occasionally subject to inflammation. This disease is particularly distinguished by the appearance of a more or less marked chemosis round the cornea, there being at the same time considerable conjunctival and subconjunctival injection. On closer examination, we find that there is no apparent cause for this chemosis, for the cornea, iris, and deeper tunics of the eye are unaffected, and the sight and the field of vision are also good. The eyelids are likewise somewhat red and swollen. The eyeball is, moreover, slightly protruded, although perhaps to so inconsiderable a degree that it might escape observation unless the state of the two eyes is compared. There is, at the same time, a certain impairment of the movements of the eyeball, which is especially evident in the extreme movements in different directions, when diplopia will also arise. The pain in and around the eye may be somewhat severe, but it never reaches the same intensity as in cellulitis or periostitis of the orbit. The progress of the disease is generally slow, eight or ten weeks perhaps elapsing before it is cured.

It is generally of rheumatic origin, being due to a draught of cold air, as, for instance, in railway travelling, etc., or to sudden changes of temperature. It is also seen in cases of irido-choroiditis supervening upon operations, especially those for cataract. According to De Wecker, it may also follow the operation for strabismus, if the sclerotic has been much exposed, or the capsule of Tenon too freely incised.

If the inflammatory symptoms are severe, a few leeches should be applied to the temple, and warm poppy fomentations be prescribed, together with the compound belladonna ointment. If the inflammation is due to traumatism, as, for instance, in the operation for strabismus, ice compresses should be applied.

5.—EXOPHTHALMIC GOITRE (GRAVES' DISEASE, MORBUS BASEDOWII, ETC.).

This is a very interesting and peculiar disease, the true nature and cause of which are at present unknown. Amongst the first symptoms are, generally, great palpitation and acceleration of the action of the heart, the pulse perhaps reaching one hundred and twenty or one hundred and fifty beats in the minute. There is at the same time much nervous excitement and dyspnœa. Sometimes there are, moreover, symptoms of gastric derangement, such as frequent and obstinate retching and vomiting, or diarrhœa. It is now, perbaps, also noticed that the eyes have a peculiar and somewhat staring look, which is partly due to a retraction of the upper eyelid, leaving the eyeball much uncovered, and giving an expression of astonishment to the patient. Moreover, as Von Graefe has pointed out, the upper lid does not quite follow the movements of the eyeball when the person looks upwards or downwards, but remains somewhat too elevated. This is quite independent of the exophthalmos, and generally appears during the stage of progression, and may disappear without any diminution in the protrusion of the eye. This retraction is probably due to irritation of the unstriped muscular fibres of the upper lid which are supplied by the sympathetic, and is relieved by the subcutaneous injection of morphia. Stellwag[1] has lately called attention to the fact, that the normal, involuntary nictitation takes place very imperfectly, and at unusually long intervals. The lids can, however, be easily and perfectly closed by a voluntary effort. The cardiac symptoms may have lasted perhaps some little time before those of bronchocele and exophthalmos present themselves. The latter symptoms generally appear about the same time, but do not necessarily bear any absolute relation to each other, and need not coexist; for, according to Praël,[2] in exceptional instances, the bronchocele may be absent. There is, moreover, nothing peculiar in this form of bronchocele, excepting that the veins are generally much dilated, even perhaps to such a degree that the disease might be termed "bronchocele aneurysmatica;" and often a distinct diastolic murmur can be heard in them. According to Virchow,[3] there is, at the commencement, only a simple swelling of the thyroid gland, the disease becoming gradually developed into a true bronchocele. Degenerative changes, of a gelatinous or cystoid nature, may then occur, or nodulated, fibroid indurations be formed. As all these changes occur also in common bronchocele, Virchow thinks it probable that the affection of the thyroid is of a *secondary* nature.

At the commencement, the cardiac affection seems simply to consist in the greatly increased action and violent palpitations of the heart, but after a time dilatation and hypertrophy, more especially of the left ventricle, ensue. There is often a marked bellows murmur, without, perhaps, any valvular affection, and the murmur may extend into the aorta and carotid. The pulsation in the carotid is sometimes quite evident at a little distance from the patient. The aorta and larger arteries have occasionally been found to have undergone atheromatous changes.

The exophthalmos may become so considerable, that the eyelids cannot be closed over the cornea, but the latter, and a more or less considerable portion of the sclerotic, protrude between them. The protrusion of the eye is not generally straightforward, in the direction of the optic axis, but towards one side, frequently the nasal. On account of the constant exposure of the uncovered cornea to the influence of external irritants, its epithelial covering becomes roughened and thick, ulcers are formed, which, extending in circumference and depth, may lead to extensive perforation of the cornea, and even to subsequent atrophy of the eyeball. The eyelids at the same time become inflamed, the ocular conjunctiva injected, and perhaps œdematous, and of a dusky-red color from constant exposure to the atmosphere and irritants. The suppuration which may occur in this disease is not, however, of neuro-paralytic origin, but Von Graefe thinks it is due to a paralysis of the "trophic" fibres of the fifth nerve, as was shown in Meissner's experiments.

Cases of suppuration of the cornea are not, however, of frequent occurrence,

[1] " Wiener medezinische Jahrschrift," xvii., 1869.
. [2] " A. f. O.," iii. 2, 209.   [3] " Krankheiten Geschwülste," iii. 1, 76.

and I have only met with a single instance of the kind, where a young woman affected with exophthalmic goitre had lost both eyes from suppuration of the cornea; and the eyeballs, although shrunken, were still very prominent. According to Von Graefe, it occurs more frequently amongst men than women; thus out of fourteen cases in which suppuration took place, it occurred ten times in men and four times in women.[1]

The exophthalmos is due to hypertrophy of the adipose cellular tissue of the orbit, and to a hyperæmic swelling of this tissue, which may at first be diminished by pressure, and rapidly disappears after death.[2] [This has been proven by Snellen, who, while examining such an eye with the stethoscope, heard a distinct vascular murmur. Such murmurs occur only in places where the blood-channels dilate, and in connection with the exophthalmos, they probably indicate a distention of the orbital vessels.—B.] Recklinghausen has also observed fatty degeneration of the muscles of the eyeball. Dr. Wright[3] found, besides the strong dilatation of the veins, a small quantity of half-coagulated blood extravasated over the eyeball.

The true cause of the disease and the nature of the connection between the affection of the heart, the thyroid gland, and the eye are at present unknown. It was supposed by some authors, that the pressure of the enlarged thyroid upon the cervical bloodvessels caused the protrusion of the eye. In opposition to this view it may, however, be urged that we often meet with very large bronchoceles without any exophthalmos; and, on the other hand, as has been shown by Praël, the latter may exist without any enlargement of the thyroid gland. Others have supposed that the symptoms are due to anæmia, and Mackenzie speaks of the disease as "Anæmic Exophthalmos." But it is impossible that anæmia could be the direct cause of such a condition, and it could, therefore, as Virchow points out, only act in so far, that the morbid condition of the blood exerts a deleterious influence upon the nerves.

It is, however, far more probable that the affection is due to an irritation or neurosis of the sympathetic nerve, producing hypertrophy of the adipose tissue of the orbit and dilatation of the veins. There is, moreover, another fact which would argue in favor of this view of irritation of the sympathetic, viz., the retraction of the upper lid; for H. Müller discovered unstriped muscular fibres in the upper lid, which are supplied by branches of the sympathetic. Any irritation of these nervelets would cause an elevation of the lid; whereas, if this irritability were allayed, the retraction would disappear. Now the latter, as has already been mentioned, may be observed to occur after the subcutaneous injection of morphia. The anatomical conditions of the sympathetic have, however, been found to vary considerably. Thus some observers (Wright, Moore, Trousseau, etc.) found the cervical ganglia of the sympathetic enlarged, hard, and firm; and on microscopical examination they were seen to be filled with a granular substance, like a lymphatic gland in the first stage of tuberculosis. The trunk of the sympathetic, as well as the branches going to the inferior thyroid and vertebral arteries, were found to be enlarged; whereas Recklinghausen,[4] on the contrary, observed that the trunk and the ganglia of the sympathetic were diminished in size, as if atrophic, without, however, presenting any histological changes. One fact, which argues rather against the assumption that the disease is due to irritation of the sympathetic, is the condition of the pupil; for the latter was only in some cases dilated.

---

[1] "Berliner klin. Wochenschr.," 1867, 649.   [2] Virchow, l. c., 76.

[3] "Med. Times and Gazette," Nov. 1865.   [4] Virchow, loc. cit., p. 80.

Virchow, in speaking of the functional disturbances, also calls attention to the fact, that together with the disappearance of the bronchocele in consequence of small doses of iodine, marked acceleration of the pulse, and palpitation of the heart may be observed. Now as the same thing has been occasionally noticed when spontaneous diminution of the bronchocele has taken place, the question arises whether these symptoms may not be due to an admixture of soluble goitre-material with the blood.

The disease occurs most frequently in women, especially during the time of puberty, or during confinement. It is also observed to be paired with disturbances of the uterine functions, particularly chlorosis, suppression of the catamenia, etc.; it may also supervene upon severe constitutional diseases. According to Von Graefe, it is not only more rare amongst men, but in them it occurs at a later period, and with greater severity. It has been caused by severe bodily labor, or mental shocks, fright, great depression, etc.

The course of the disease is mostly very slow and protracted, and relapses are very apt to occur, more especially if there still exists great disturbance in the action of the heart. Amongst men, the prognosis should be very guarded, as the disease assumes a much more severe character, and is more frequently complicated with serious affections of the cornea. On account of the impediment produced in the intra-ocular circulation by the exophthalmos, the retinal veins are sometimes dilated and tortuous, but otherwise there are no changes in the fundus, and the function of the retina is generally unimpaired. Hypermetropia may arise on account of the flattening of the eye. [Death may follow upon an increase of all the symptoms, sometimes speedily, with great cerebral disturbance, or it may ensue slowly from gradual failure of all the powers. Sometimes a complete recovery takes place rapidly, though the progress in either direction is usually slow.—B.]

With regard to treatment, the most benefit seems to be derived from the administration of tonics, more especially the preparations of quinine, together with a generous diet, plenty of open-air exercise, and, if necessary, a change of air and a prolonged residence in the country. Both Von Graefe and Trousseau[1] consider that preparations of steel are contra-indicated, more especially when there is much excitation of the vascular system. Trousseau strongly recommends the use of digitalis, which is to be freely given until the pulse sinks to seventy or sixty beats a minute, when the dose is to be considerably diminished or the remedy suspended. He also advocates bleeding to diminish the danger of asphyxia from the pressure of the congested thyroid, and to alleviate the violent palpitations of the heart. He has likewise found benefit from hydropathy, and the continuous application of cold compresses on the thyroid and over the region of the heart. On the other hand, he is opposed to the use of iodine in cases of exophthalmic goitre, although he admits that, in rare and exceptional instances, it may temporarily prove beneficial. I have often derived much benefit from the administration of quinine and steel, combined with large doses of digitalis, if there is great acceleration of the heart's action. Should the steel be not well borne, I only give quinine and digitalis. Dr. Cheadle,[2] in his recent paper on "Exophthalmic Goitre," states that he has employed iodine with advantage both internally and topically to the throat, and believes that it is probably most useful in those cases in which the goitre is large and exerts dangerous pressure. A firm compress bandage will often cause the exophthalmos to diminish considerably. [Tinct. veratri viridis has proven beneficial in some

---

[1] "Clinique médicale," 2d edit., vol. ii. 502.
[2] "St. George's Hospital Reports," 1869, vol. iv. 192.

cases, beginning with doses of one drop and gradually increasing; but this may cause diarrhœa, and should be combined with opium. Belladonna has also been given in some cases with benefit. If anæsthesia or infiltration of the cornea occur, atropine and the pressure bandage should be employed.—B.]

Galvanization of the sympathetic nerve has lately been strongly recommended, amongst others by Chvostek,[1] and Moritz Meyer.[2] The latter has found it very successful in curing the exophthalmos and the goitre, as well as in improving the general health; but on the other hand, it does not appear to exert any influence on the acceleration of the pulse or the palpitation of the heart. I have lately tried it, and in one case with marked benefit, as to the diminution of the exophthalmos. I generally apply the positive pole to the auriculo-maxillary fossa, and the other I move gently over the closed eyelids, and afterwards over the goitre. I employ about six to ten cells for the eye, and eight to fourteen for the goitre, applying the electricity for about one and one-half to two minutes to each part. We may besides this, galvanize the cervical ganglia of the sympathetic, applying one electrode to the auriculo-maxillary fossa, the other to the sixth or seventh cervical vertebra, or manubrium sterni. It may take about twenty to thirty sittings before any very marked improvement is noticed in the exophthalmos or goitre; and considering the little effect that other treatment has upon the disease, I think that galvanization should always have an extended trial.

The peculiar retraction of the upper eyelid may be, if necessary, alleviated by an operation upon the levator palpebræ, as has been advised by Von Graefe. He was formerly in the habit of recommending tarsoraphy for this elevation of the upper lid, but now prefers a partial tenotomy of the levator palpebræ superioris. The latter operation is to be performed as follows:[3] The horn spatula having been introduced beneath the upper lid, so as to put it well on the stretch, he makes a horizontal incision through the skin of the upper lid, extending nearly the whole length of the latter, and situated about one line above the upper edge of the tarsal cartilage. He then divides the orbicularis, or still better, excises a small horizontal portion of it, in order to gain a better view of the subjacent parts. A careful exposure of the tarso-orbital fascia will bring into view the vertical or oblique striation which indicates the tendon of the levator palpebræ, which here passes over into, and becomes blended with, the cartilage. With a very narrow knife, the point where they are blended is then to be incised at each side, so that only a narrow central bridge (of about one line in width) remains standing. Care must of course be taken not to perforate the conjunctiva. The result of the operation is an incomplete ptosis, which diminishes considerably during the first few weeks, the remainder just neutralising the retraction of the upper lid which before existed.

6.—TUMORS OF THE ORBIT.

It would be quite beyond the plan and scope of this work to enter at length into all the varieties of tumor that may be met with in the orbit, as well as the points of difference in their structure, diagnosis, and mode of de-

---

[1] " Weiner med. Presse," 1869.
[2] " Berliner klin. Wochenschrift," Sept. 23, 1872.
[3] Vide " Compte rendu du Congrès d'ophthalmologie," 1867; also " Kl. Monatsbl.," 1867, p. 372.

velopment; I shall, therefore, confine myself to a broad and practical division of this subject, and shall endeavor briefly to give the most characteristic and leading features presented by the principal varieties of tumor, as well as the different modes of treatment which are more especially indicated.

Tumors of the orbit may be developed primarily in the latter, or may commence within the eye or one of the neighboring cavities, and, gradually increasing in size, finally make their way into the orbit. As long as the tumor is confined within the eye, its progress may be slow and protracted; but when it has once perforated the ocular tunics, its growth, being no longer restrained by the firm sclerotic, is often very rapid, so that it may, within a short time, attain a very considerable size.

Tumors may be developed from any part of the orbit; they may spring from the bottom of the cavity, from its walls, or from its most anterior part close to the edge. As the morbid growth increases in size, the eyeball will be more and more protruded, and the direction of this protrusion will depend upon the principal situation of the tumor. The exophthalmos may finally become so great, that the eyeball is quite pushed out of the orbit upon the cheek. Together with the protrusion, the movements of the globe will be more or less impaired. The eyelids are generally swollen and œdematous, and the œdema may be so great that it is impossible to judge of the true nature of the tumor, or it may even obscure the presence of the latter. If the tumor is chiefly situated at the upper part of the orbit, a certain degree of ptosis is frequently present. The eyelids are, in other cases, greatly everted, their exposed conjunctival surface being swollen and fleshy in appearance. There is often also a very considerable degree of chemosis of a dirty, dusky-red tint. The sight may suffer from the optic nerve being stretched or pressed upon by the tumor, or from the impediment to the intraocular circulation. The efflux from the retinal veins is retarded, symptoms of inflammation of the optic nerve may supervene, and if the tumor be not removed, the optic nerve may undergo consecutive atrophy. But the sight may also be greatly impaired or even lost from inflammation or extensive ulceration of the cornea, dependent upon its constant exposure to the action of external irritants, when the eye is much protruded. Perforation or sloughing of the cornea may ensue, and, the contents of the globe escaping, the eye may gradually undergo atrophy.

In attempting the removal of any tumor of the orbit by operation, we should always take into anxious consideration its size, rate of progress, suspected nature, and situation; as well as the condition of the eye, and the general health of the patient. If there is still sight, we should always endeavor to remove the morbid growth, if possible, without sacrificing the eye. But in some cases, more especially of malignant tumors, it is quite impossible to remove the whole of the morbid growth without the removal of the eye; and in such instances, it is far wiser to sacrifice the latter, than to run the risk of leaving portions of tumor behind, to prove the ready source of a recurrence of the disease. We should, if possible, remove the tumor through the conjunctiva, but if this is not practicable, the incision must be carried through the skin of the lids. The incision should, in such a case, be always horizontal, and perhaps slightly curved, so as to correspond with the natural wrinkles of the skin, and thus avoid the formation of unsightly cicatrices.

[Schimemi speaks of the excision of the ophthalmic ganglion in a case where it became necessary to operate upon a sarcoma of the orbit. The immediate consequences of the operation were immobility of the lower lid, owing to marked recession of the eye; almost complete immobility of the eyeball, complete anæsthesia of the cornea, dilatation and immobility of the

pupil. The cornea ulcerated in one spot, but soon heale
days later a large corneal ulcer appeared, with hypopyon,
worse, until the edges of the lids were stitched togethe
heal. See " Annali di ottalmologia, ix. 2.)—B.]

In order to gain more room to work in, it may also be
the outer canthus. We should always endeavor to e
without any injury to the neighboring parts, and for t'
must not be too freely used, but the attachments of the
be loosened with the tip of the finger, the handle of a
point of a silver knife. In some tumors, it is necessa:
different portions, or to snip them off the walls of the pe
of blunt-pointed, curved scissors. The use of the chlo
cases of removal of malignant tumors, as well as those w
be feared, will be considered when speaking of these tur

(1) Fibrous Tumors.

The fibrous tumor is especially characterized by the f
closely resembles that of radiating fibrillar connective
being closely packed together. On section, such a tu:
and perhaps somewhat rough surface, traversed by bund
Its color is of a grayish-white or grayish-yellow tint. T
surrounded by a distinct sheath of thickened connectiv
trated by a small number of vessels. These tumors ma:
changes, and cysts may be formed, and in such a ca
diminished, and a certain degree of fluctuation may be
this is considerable, they may be easily mistaken for cy
may undergo osseous or calcareous changes, the bone
with in the form of small sequestra.

These tumors grow from the periosteum either by a b
or more pedicles. They are generally formed near th
and if they are stalked, they may be felt in the form of
scribed, movable growths. The consistence of the tu:
considerably. It is generally firm and hard, from the
densation of the radiating connective-tissue elements.
ever, it is softish and perhaps lobulated, or the surface
central portion, or that nearest to the point of origin f
may be firm and hard. The progress of the tumor is
and the firmer varieties do not, as a rule, acquire a ve
It is difficult, however, with the softer kinds, as they
magnitude. Thus Mooren[1] mentions a fibrous tumor
after a former operation, attained the size of a child's
the bones of the face and head. Mr. Critchett[2] narrate
of fibrous tumor of the orbit removed at two sittings.
recorded a case, in which he successfully removed a
(preserving the eye), and applied the chloride of zinc
plaster to the bottom of the orbit, the surface of the l
caustic paste was spread being turned outwards away fi
latter protected by the interposition of a thick layer of
ever, only just sufficed to save the eyeball from the ac

[1] Mooren, "Ophthalmiatrische Beobachtungen," p. 41.
[2] "Med. Times and Gazette," 1852, p. 465.

the outer surface of the globe was covered by a slight layer of eschar, the sclerotic remaining, however, uninjured.

If the fibrous tumors are small in size, and situated near the edge of the orbit, they can generally be removed without any danger; but if they are large, extend deeply into the orbit, and are widely attached to the periosteum, either by a broad base or by several pedicles, operative interference must be extensive, and may set up very considerable inflammation, extending perhaps to the periosteum of the orbit, and even to the brain. Or the operation may be followed by fatal erysipelas.[1]

(2) SARCOMATOUS (FIBRO-PLASTIC) TUMORS.

Sarcomatous tumors are particularly distinguished in their minute structure by the fact that they are composed of variously shaped, closely packed cells, and a scanty intercellular substance. These cells vary much in size and form, being stellate, circular, oblong, spindle-shaped, etc. If the cells contain pigment, it is termed melanotic sarcoma. The fibro-plastic variety shows marked spindle-shaped cells with a large ovoid nucleus and long, perhaps subdivided, filamentous extremities. On account of this peculiar shape of the cell and these long terminal projections, it was formerly supposed that the connective tissue was formed by a division of these cells. But this, as Virchow[2] points out, is erroneous, for it is the special characteristic of these tumors that their cells persist as cells, and do not become developed into connective tissue; for if this development took place, and a considerable formation of fibrillar intercellular substance really occurred, and if the cells were transformed into fibres, the tumor would simply be a fibroma and not sarcomatous. In fact, the fibro-plastic tumor is nothing but a spindle-shaped cell sarcoma. The malignant fibrous and recurrent fibroid tumors of Paget are also varieties of sarcoma. The amount of the fibrillar intercellular substance varies considerably in quantity. In some cases, it is firm and dense, in others, on account of the great development of the cells, it may have nearly disappeared; in the latter case, the tumor is very soft and becomes medullary. In rare instances the tumor also contains cysts, and is then termed "cysto-sarcoma."[3]

Sarcomatous tumors are not benign in character, but show a great tendency to infection of neighboring organs, commencing first in the homologous tissues, and then passing on to the heterologous. But they affect distant organs, and as the lymphatic glands frequently remain unaffected, it has been supposed that the infection is carried more by the blood than by the lymphatic vessels.

According to Virchow, sarcomatous tumors of the orbit "are generally developed from the adipose cellular tissue behind the eye, after a time pushing the eyeball out of the orbit, and appearing beneath the conjunctiva in the form of round, firm protrusions, finally assuming a fungoid character. Their commencement may often be traced to distinct traumatic causes. If no operation is performed, the eye is in the end destroyed by pressure or inflammation, and at the best becomes atrophied. Or again, the fungus may grow inwards, reach the dura mater, invade the cranium, and generally ends in metastases, amongst which those of the bones of the skull are the most remarkable. Most of the orbital sarcomata have rather a soft consistence, and belong to the melano-, myxo-, or gliosarcomata. They are generally multi-

---

[1] *Vide* Mackenzie, p. 327.   [2] " Krankheiten Geschwülste," ii. 1, 180.
[3] *Vide* " Kl. Monatsbl.," 1869, March, ii. 2.

cellular; but even those consisting of smaller cells may be operated upon with success."[1] Frequently the sarcomatous tumors, especially melanotic sarcoma, originate in the eyeball, and subsequently make their way into the orbit. In some cases the sight remains perfect for a long time, in others it becomes greatly impaired or entirely lost from optic neuritis, atrophy of the optic nerve, detachment of the retina, extension of the tumor into the optic nerve, etc.

The great danger of the disease is its extension into the neighboring cavities, the bony walls, which separate these from the orbit, being destroyed by caries or necrosis, or worn through by the pressure of the tumor. In such a case, the extension of the growth in an outward direction may be slow and protracted. The operator, thinking that he has only to deal with a moderate, sharply defined tumor, is surprised to find it extending far into neighboring cavities, in which it has perhaps reached a very considerable size (Stellwag). [In not a few instances the sarcomatous growth starts from the periosteum of the orbit, and grows very rapidly. It is not uncommon to find that these grow from both the orbital and intracranial sides of the roof of the orbit. Some authors have advocated the removal of the orbital plate of the frontal bone in these cases, and it has been done with success; but the danger of injury to the dura mater is certainly great, and seems a very serious thing to risk. Still, a radical and complete extirpation may in this way be possible.—B.]

But the tumor may be originally developed in some other cavity, as, for instance, the nasal fossa,[2] or antrum of Highmore,[3] and extend thence into the orbit. [Growths originating in this way are very serious cases. They are generally of very rapid growth, have widely extended ramifications, and are almost always complex in character, such as combinations of sarcoma with myxoma, adenoma, osteoma, enchondroma, or carcinoma. It is scarcely possible to remove these growths completely without an excision of the superior maxilla alone or of portions of other bones of the face; and the diseased process has frequently extended so far in all directions, that even such a severe surgical procedure as the above proves unsuccessful. (See "Trans. Fifth Internat. Ophth. Congress," 1876, pp. 58–62.)—B.]

These tumors are very apt to recur, and may have to be operated upon several times. Thus in a case narrated by Mr. Quinn, he operated three times.[4] If the sight is unaffected, we should endeavor to remove the tumor without sacrificing the eyeball, and in order that all remains of the morbid growth may be removed, the chloride of zinc paste, spread upon strips of lint, should be inserted into the wound, care being taken that the dry side of the lint is turned towards the eye, and the latter should still further be protected by the interposition of layers of charpie. That the caustic may be applied without injury to the eyeball or its muscles, was already shown in Zehender's case; Mr. Hulke[5] has more lately published a similar instance. The eyeball may generally be saved as long as the disease has not extended into the conical space (Muskeltrichter) enclosed by the four recti muscles (Von Graefe).[6]

But where the disease is extensive, the eyeball lost, or there is no doubt as to the malignant nature of the disease, the globe must be excised with the tumor, and the latter should be as thoroughly removed as possible; but the excision of the morbid growth with the knife and blunt-pointed, curved scissors alone, will not suffice in cases where the tumor is of a sarcomatous

[1] "Krankheiten Geschwülste," p. 349.   [3] Von Graefe, "A. f. O.," i. 1, 419.
[2] Pagenstecher, "Klinische Beobachtungen," 1861, i. 76.
[4] "Med. Times," 1854, No. 204.   [5] "R. L. O. H. Rep.," v. 4, 345.
[6] "A. f. O.," x. 1, 197.

or carcinomatous nature, and infiltrates more or less the neighboring structures; for then it cannot with certainty be completely removed, and remnants of tumor are sure to be left behind. The surgeon should endeavor to remove as much as possible of the morbid growth by chipping it away from the walls of the orbit, exploring beforehand with the finger the mass which he is about to excise. If the walls of the orbit are also affected, the periosteum, or even portions of the diseased bone, may be readily removed with the elevator. In order to check hemorrhage, and to destroy any remaining portions of the morbid growth which cannot be reached with the scissors, the hot iron should be applied to the wounded surface, and then, when all bleeding has ceased, the chloride of zinc paste, spread upon strips of lint, is to be applied to the wound. The chloride of zinc paste has been used extensively and most successfully at the Middlesex Hospital, where the following formula is generally employed: One part by weight of chloride of zinc is rubbed up with four parts of flour, to which sufficient laudanum is added to make a paste of the consistence of honey.

To many surgeons, the use of the hot iron and of an escharotic to the orbit will appear a most dangerous proceeding, on account of the thinness of the roof of the orbit, which divides it from the brain; but experience proves that this proceeding, if carefully and expertly performed, is not fraught with any particular risk, for the action of the hot iron is superficial, and that of the chloride of zinc can also be very well regulated. Moreover, it produces little or no constitutional disturbance, and only excites slight inflammation of the living tissues beyond the slough. The truth of these statements is sufficiently proved by the very remarkable cases in which this line of treatment has been pursued by Mr. de Morgan, Mr. Moore, Mr. Hulke, and Mr. Lawson, and which have been brought before the notice of the profession at different periods.

Mr. Hulke[1] reports a very interesting case of large fungating melanotic sarcoma which had become developed from a shrunken eyeball, filled the cavity of the orbit, and protruded between the eyelids, which was successfully extirpated with the aid of the actual cautery and chloride of zinc paste.

A very interesting and important case of recurrent fibroid tumor, which has been operated upon several times by Mr. Lawson, is recorded in the "R. L. O. H. Reports," vi. 3, 206. [See also "Trans. Fifth Internat. Ophthal. Congress," 1876, pp. 258 to 263; "Trans. Amer. Ophth. Soc.," 1879.—B.]

(8) FATTY TUMORS OF THE ORBIT. [LIPOMATA.—B.]

The fatty tumors are developed in the adipose cellular tissue of the orbit, either in its cavity or between the recti muscles, just beneath the conjunctiva. They generally occur in early life, and are sometimes perhaps congenital. They increase slowly in growth, are not accompanied by any symptoms of pain or inflammation, and vary much in size and consistence. The latter will depend upon the relative amount of the fatty material, and the firmness and quantity of the fibro-cellular tissue. They are often very elastic to the touch, and give rise to a sense of fluctuation, which may deceive us as to their true nature, and cause them, perhaps, to be mistaken for a cyst. No difficulty is generally experienced in their removal, which should, if possible, be done from within the eyelid. [They do not return.—B.]

[1] "R. L. O. H. Rep.," v. 3, 181.

(4) Osseous and Cartilaginous Tumors.

According to Mackenzie,[1] we may distinguish three forms of exostosis of the orbit: 1, the cellular; 2, the craggy, or semi-cartilaginous; 3, the ivory. The cellular exostosis is characterized by its being composed of an osseous crust, which surrounds rather a soft substance, traversed by numerous delicate bony partitions. Sometimes, it may contain hydatids. This form of exostosis springs from the periosteum, does not generally acquire a considerable size, and may remain quite stationary. The craggy or semi-cartilaginous exostosis generally consists in the centre of osseous laminæ, which are surrounded by cartilage, over which the periosteum may be imperfectly traced, but it has no complete shell. It may grow from the cancelli or from the periosteum.

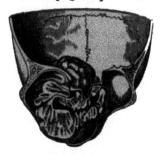

[Fig. 247.]

The ivory exostosis is the form most frequently met with in the orbit; it is excessively hard, and consists of perfectly developed, dense, and very firm bone tissue. According to Mackenzie, it originates in the diploë, presses the compact tissue of the bone before it, and forms a round, smooth, or somewhat nodulated tumor. [Fig. 247.] It, moreover, shows a disposition to extend into the cranium.

Exostosis frequently supervenes upon periostitis and ostitis, and may be due to a scrofulous or syphilitic diathesis, or be produced by injuries, such as falls or blows upon the orbit, or by fractures of the latter.

These osseous tumors are more or less hard to the touch, slow in their progress and growth, and generally accompanied by little or no pain or inflammatory symptoms. Sometimes, the pain may, however, be severe, more especially if symptoms of periostitis supervene in the course of the disease. The degree of exophthalmos and impairment of the movements of the eye will vary with the extent and situation of the exostosis. It is often quite impossible to determine the exact nature of the disease before operation, more especially when the tumor is situated deep in the orbit. Ivory exostosis is frequently developed from the frontal or ethmoid bone.

[According to Knapp, these bony tumors grow on the periphery only, converting the connective tissue over them into bone. Their bulk may spread out beyond the base, and their adhesion to the underlying bone is sometimes less firm than their consistence. Their periosteal covering may contain cysts, and thus render the diagnosis very difficult. Knapp advises, when they grow from the roof of the orbit, that they should be removed with their base by chisel and mallet, and by traction in various directions, thus leaving the dura mater exposed. (See "Trans. Fifth Internat. Ophth. Congress," 1876, p. 54.)

An interesting case of ivory exostosis of the bones of the orbit, in which the skull was examined after death, is reported by Carreras-Aragó. The tumor probably arose from the diploë of the frontal bone, near the orbital arch toward the external angle. It involved the entire upper margin of the orbit, filled the whole orbital cavity, involved all the walls of the orbit, and

---

[1] "Diseases of the Eye," 4th edition, p. 41.

penetrated the cavity of the skull by the optic foramen and sphenoidal fissure. It also extended into the nasal fossae, and filled the anterior cerebral fossae. Outside of the orbit, it extended into the zygomatic fossa. It was very dense and compact, without any medullary spaces or Haversian canals, and weighed about five hundred grammes. The growth probably began in ossification of the periosteum of the frontal sinuses, and perhaps also of the ethmoidal sinuses. The cerebral symptoms were intense convulsions, occurring with greater frequency and violence, and ending in imbecility which lasted till death. (See "La Crónica oftalmológica," Dic. 12, 1880. See also interesting cases reported by Drs. H. Sands and H. Knapp in the "Archives of Ophthalmology," ix. 4.)—B.]

In the early stage, the treatment should be directed to promote the absorption of the tumor, by the administration of iodide of potassium internally, the application of mercurial ointment over the brow, etc. The patient's general health must be attended to, and kept up by a generous diet and tonics, residence in the country or at the seaside, etc.

If the exostosis is small and remains stationary, it should not be interfered with by operation. But if it is increasing in size and is producing exophthalmos, etc., the surgeon should endeavor to remove it.

The tumor should be freely exposed by one or more incisions, carried through the integuments and between the fibres of the orbicularis, or, if necessary, by dissecting back the lids. In order to gain plenty of room, it may also be necessary to divide the commissure of the lids. The tumor, having been thus exposed, is to be stripped of its periosteum and carefully excised with a scalpel, assisted by cutting pliers and strong bone forceps. Great care must be taken not to injure the upper and inner wall of the orbit by a rough and thoughtless use of the instruments. The ivory exostoses are frequently so firm and hard, and so intimately and widely connected with the bone, that it is only possible to remove a certain portion of the morbid growth. Mr. Haynes Walton narrates a case in which he successfully removed a large ivory exostosis.[1] Two similar instances are recorded by Maisonneuve. [For these very dense tumors, the chisel and mallet are better than the saw, but a still better instrument is the dental lathe with drills of various sizes, the rapid revolution of which makes it possible to use lateral pressure.—B.]

Sometimes, however, the tumor is so excessively hard, and its attachment so extensive, that it resists all efforts made with the saw, cutting pliers, or mallet; little splinters of bone may be chipped off, but the great mass of the growth is impregnable, and the operation has to be abandoned. Such instances have been recorded by Mackenzie[2] and Knapp.[3] In Knapp's case, seven weeks after the operation, the first five having been passed very quietly and favorably, the patient was attacked with symptoms of meningitis, of which she died. On post-mortem examination, a general thickening of the cranium was discovered, together with a large exostosis, about the size of a goose's egg, springing from the frontal bone. In a subsequent case of ivory exostosis, Knapp succeeded in removing the tumor.[4]

[A very interesting case of large osteoma of the maxillary sinus and floor of the orbit is reported by Manz. The tumor was entirely removed, and the patient recovered with fair vision. ("Archives of Oph.," viii. 3, pp. 320–328.)—B.]

The true cartilaginous tumors (enchondroma) are only very rarely met

---

[1] "Surgical Diseases of the Eye," 286. [2] Loc. cit., 48.
[3] "A. f. O.," viii. 1, 289. [4] "Kl. Monatsbl.," 1865, 376.

with in the orbit.   Many of the cases which have been recorded under this name, were in reality instances of osteo-steatoma or osteo-sarcoma.   This mistake is the more easily made, as some of these tumors in the course of their development undergo cartilaginous changes before becoming ossified.

Although these cartilaginous tumors, as a rule, spring from the bone, they may also become developed from the softer tunics of the orbit.   They are most frequently met with in youthful individuals.   In a case of Von Graefe's,[1] it occurred in a child only seven months old, it being stated that the tumor had existed since the first month after birth.

(5) Cystic Tumors of the Orbit.

Cysts may occur at various parts of the orbit, either deep in its cavity behind the eyeball, or near its upper or lower margin.   Whilst some of these cysts contain hydatids, others are developed from the follicles of the lids.   At first, their true nature may be readily recognizable, but when they attain a considerable size, the connection between the cyst and the follicle may become so attenuated, stretched, or even torn through, that their real mode of origin is often overlooked.   The consistence and contents of these follicular cysts are subject to considerable variations.   Thus in the atheromatous form, the contents are of a friable, cheesy, or curdy nature; whereas in the steatomatous, they rather resemble suet.

Other cysts spring from the glandular structures of the conjunctiva, and may contain a yellow, serous, or rather viscid and albuminous fluid, like white of egg (the latter kind of cyst is termed hygroma).   They may be about the size of a pea or bean, and situated near the surface of the conjunctiva.   But they sometimes extend back into the orbit, attain a very considerable size, and then give rise to great exophthalmos.   In rare instances, the cysts contain a brown hemorrhagic fluid.

Some orbital cysts have been found to have hairs, etc., growing from their internal walls.   [See "Report of Fourth Internat. Ophthal. Congress," London, 1872, article on "Intra-orbital Dermoid Cysts."

The subject of the connection between congenital serous cyst of the orbit and coloboma of the eye, is one which of late has excited some attention.   The cysts here considered are of complete dermoid texture, presenting at the level of the plane of the fronto-orbital aperture, either at the internal or external angle.   In most of the cases they present a pedicle attaching them to the skeleton, a pedicle which is either full or hollow.   They are not perceived at first during a varying period, but about the age of puberty they grow and excite attention.   It is well known that an irregular closure of the ocular cleft in the fœtus may end in a pronounced ectasia of the cicatrix and its immediate vicinity; that is, of the floor—so called—of the eye.   Van Duyse found that, in one case of his own, one slightly microphthalmic eye presented a sclerectasia, caused by the expansion of a coloboma of the choroid and of the sheath of the optic nerve.   The other eye showed a still more pronounced degree of the same anomaly, it having remained rudimentary, in consequence of the development of the coloboma.   The latter had become encysted, and developed in filling the orbit and pushing before it the conjunctiva and lower lid.   (See "Annales d'oculistique," Sept.–Oct. 1881.)—B.]

Two kinds of hydatids are met with in the orbit, the echinococcus, and the

[1] "A. f. O.," i. 1, 415.

cysticercus. The former is much larger, and occurs in greater numbers than the cysticercus. Thus, echinococcus may acquire the size of a filbert, and be present in great quantities, causing an excessive protrusion of the eye. In a case of Lawrence's, quoted by Mackenzie,[1] half a teacupful of echinococci, varying in size from a pea to a filbert, were emptied from an orbital cyst. Mr. Bowman[2] operated upon a somewhat similar case, in which three hydatids came away a few days after the operation. Two were as big as large marbles, the third about half the size. In a case of Waldhauer's,[3] some of the hydatids, of which there was a great quantity, had acquired the size of a hazel-nut. The hydatid is enclosed in a capsule of thickened connective tissue, besides the proper cyst-wall. The cysticerci are much smaller in size than the echinococci, and their cyst-wall much slighter and thinner.

Cystic tumors of the orbit are generally slow in their progress, and may remain but small in size; if they, however, grow considerably, the eyeball will gradually be protruded. The development is generally unaccompanied by any pain, but when they are very large, and have caused great exophthalmos, the sufferings of the patient are often most intense, the pain extending perhaps over the corresponding side of the head and face. The tumor is not, however, tender to the touch. If the cyst is situated near the front of the orbit, so that it can be seen and felt, it will present a round or ovoid appearance [Fig. 248] of varying size, and is observed to be quite

[Fig. 248.

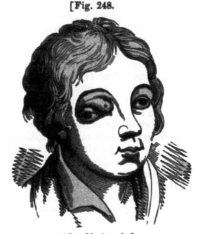

After Mackenzie.]

unconnected with the eyeball. When the cyst-wall is thin and soft, the tumor will be very elastic to the touch, and distinctly fluctuating. If firm pressure is applied, it may perhaps be made to recede into the orbit, reappearing, however, when the pressure is relaxed. If the cyst-wall is thick, or the integuments over the tumor are swollen, the latter will, on a superficial examination, feel somewhat firm, the fluctuation being only discovered on deeper pressure. When any doubt exists as to the nature of the tumor, an explanatory puncture or incision should be made, and then, if the cyst is

[1] Mackenzie, 1067. [2] Ib., 1068.
[3] " Kl. Monatsbl., 1865, p. 385.

found to be only moderate in extent, and not reaching very far back, and if its contents are dense, it should be excised, which is best done by dissecting it out with the aid of a spatula, or the end of the handle of a scalpel, assisted by the finger. If the contents are fluid, and the cyst is large, it will be better to empty it (if necessary, repeated several times) by an incision, and then to permit it to close by adhesive inflammation. Sometimes strips of lint are inserted, thus setting up suppurative inflammation; but this is dangerous if the cyst extends deeply into the orbit, as the inflammation might extend to the lining membranes of the brain. Injections of iodine have been recommended, but they are also accompanied by considerable risk.

I may state that at the commencement of the disease it is often extremely difficult, or even impossible, to diagnose with anything like certainty, whether the nature of the orbital tumor is benign or malignant. There are, however, certain points, which may assist us in our diagnosis. Thus, in malignant affections the general health of the patient mostly suffers considerably even at an early stage; whereas, in benign tumors this is not the case, the patient retaining good, and even blooming health, excepting indeed the tumor has attained a very considerable size, and produces great pain by pressing upon the eyeball or stretching the nerves.

The progress of a malignant tumor is also, as a rule, much more rapid than when it is benign. The rapidity of its growth will, however, vary according to circumstances. Thus, as long as it is confined to the posterior portion of the orbit, the pressure of the eyeball offers a certain degree of check to its development, and somewhat restrains its rapid growth. The same is the case in intra-ocular malignant tumors, whose progress may be comparatively very slow as long as they are confined by the external coats of the eye; but when these have once given way, and the tumor sprouts forth, its increase in size is always most marked and rapid. The pain is also much more intense and continuous in malignant tumors, but this symptom is not very reliable, for even in benign tumors it may be very severe, if the eye is much protruded.

Von Graefe[1] lays great importance upon the degree to which the muscles of the eye and their nerves are implicated, as a point of diagnosis between benign and malignant tumors of the orbit. Malignant growths, according to him, always cause a much greater and earlier impairment of the movements of the eye, so that the latter may be already almost immovable, whilst the exophthalmos is yet but slight in degree. In estimating the amount of immobility, we must, of course, take into consideration the mechanical effect of the tumor, and the change of position of the eyeball.

The skin and neighboring parts are more frequently affected in malignant tumors, so that the boundaries of the latter cannot be so exactly made out, and the skin is not so movable over them. Malignant growths of the orbit are also of more common occurrence in children than in adults. Thus Leber has found that in one-third of the cases of cancer of the eye and orbit, the patients were under ten years of age.

Whether or not the tumor springs from the eye or is continuous with it, may be estimated by the nature of the movements of the eyeball. If the movements take place round the turning-point of the protruded eye, it proves that the normal layer of connective tissue between the posterior hemisphere of the eyeball and the tumor still exists; whereas if the tumor and the globe are continuous, the movements will not be round the turning-point of the eye (Von Graefe).

Cancerous tumors of the orbit may be developed from the walls of the

----

[1] "A. f. O.," x. 1, 194.

latter, from the adipose cellular tissue, or may extend into the orbit from neighboring cavities or from the eyeball.

The medullary and melanotic cancer are far more frequently met with in the orbit than scirrhus.

Scirrhus of the orbit is generally due to some injury, or to prior inflammation. It may show itself in the form of one large scirrhous mass implicating the whole of the orbit, or in the form of small, circumscribed, hard tumors, which closely resemble exostoses in their appearance. Its growth is generally slow, and not accompanied by much or severe pain.

The following case of scirrhous tumor of the orbit is of rare importance and interest, as illustrating the great benefit to be derived from extirpation, followed by the application of the hot iron and chloride of zinc paste.

A woman, aged 48, upon her admission into the Middlesex Hospital under Mr. Lawson, January 30, 1866, had her left eye protruded to a full inch beyond its fellow by a hard, solid growth, which could be distinctly felt with the finger to be filling the orbit. The surface of the cornea was ulcerated, and the eye had only perception of light. The upper lid could not close over the globe. About four months before the admission a hard scirrhous tubercle was noticed in front of the ear, it was now about the size of a bean. Mr. Lawson excised the eyeball and the whole of the cancer down to the

Fig. 249.   Fig. 250.

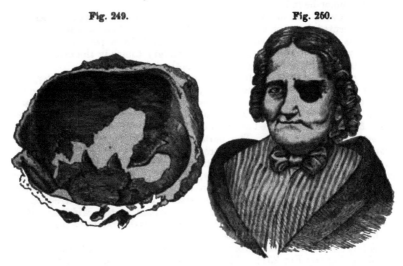

orbital walls, and then applied the actual cautery to arrest the bleeding. Strips of lint, covered with chloride of zinc paste, were then applied to the bottom of the orbit and around its walls. He next excised the tubercle on the face, and also applied to this, after all bleeding had ceased, the chloride of zinc paste. Large superficial sloughs were at first detached, and in about three months afterwards the whole bony orbit became completely detached, and Mr. Lawson pulled it away in one piece (Fig. 249).[1]

1 "Transactions of the Pathological Society," 1867, p. 283.

The exact size and appearance of the orbit after its removal are here very correctly represented. It is now in the museum of the Middlesex Hospital. The patient had a good deal of pain in the head and sickness during the separation of the bone from the neighboring tissues, but all these symptoms at once ceased after the orbit had come away.

Up to this date, June, 1873, nearly seven and one-half years after the operation, she is still perfectly well, and has had no recurrence of the disease. Her present appearance is well illustrated in Fig. 250.[1]

(7) MEDULLARY CANCER.

This is especially distinguished by its soft consistence, which greatly resembles that of rice, by the peculiar cauliflower excrescences, or the red, fleshy, fungous appearance (fungus hæmatodes) which it presents when protruding from the orbit. The form of the tumor may be tolerably circumscribed, and it may not be very adherent to the periosteum; or it may be closely connected with the latter, also invading and destroying the muscles of the eye, the periosteum, and, finally, the bones of the orbit, and then extending into the neighboring cavities. It may likewise extend along the optic nerve to the brain.

The tumor may grow with considerable rapidity, and attain an enormous size, and this is especially the case when it recurs, after the eyeball and the primary tumor have been extirpated.

The following case of Mr. de Morgan's graphically illustrates the appearances presented by such a tumor, as well as the mode of treatment which should be adopted, and which proved successful for a period of fourteen months, when the patient died from a secondary tumor in the cranium, the disease having travelled back along the optic nerve.

The patient,[2] James Vinall, was thirty-three years of age, healthy, and also of a healthy family, when he received, in August, 1863, a blow on the left eye. In two months the sight became impaired, and there was deep-seated pain in the orbit, and in February, 1864, he was quite blind in this eye. Mr. Woolcott detected an intra-ocular, cancerous growth, and removed the eye on the 20th April. The parts healed rapidly, and his health improved. In May, he had again severe darting pain at the back of the orbit, and shortly afterwards a tumor protruded between the lids. The morbid growth increased with great rapidity, and his health and strength failed greatly. In August, the tumor began to bleed, and hemorrhage recurred daily. In October, a piece, about the size of a large walnut, dropped off from the centre of the mass. He became a patient in the Middlesex Hospital, on November 3, 1864. Mr. de Morgan gives the following description of the tumor, and the operation performed upon it:

"A large, irregular tumor projected from the orbit, excavated in the centre, and sloughing (see Fig. 251). The margins of the lids could be traced over it, spread out and stretched to a remarkable degree. At the lower and outer part, the tumor involved the structure of the cheek. Its general surface was somewhat flattened and circular, and measured four inches across. It projected nearly four inches forward from the cheek on the outside, and about two inches and three-quarters from the nasal side. No alteration could be detected in the cranial bones; nor were any diseased glands to be felt.

[1] These woodcuts (which were kindly lent by Mr. Lawson to the author) are from photographs by Mr. Heisch.
[2] "Pathological Society's Transactions," 1866, 265.

The patient had never had any cerebral symptoms. He was in a wretched state of health from continued bleeding and offensive discharge, and from severe and constant pain. As, at two hospitals, the surgeons who saw him declined to operate, he was fully impressed with the hopelessness of his case, but he was anxious to have anything done to free him for a time from the pain and discharge. With this view I consented to operate, anticipating only a short reprieve from death, but hoping that I might be able by destroying the disease as it sprouted again, to give him some relief and comfort. The success which attended Mr. Moore's operation on the case of rodent

Fig. 251.

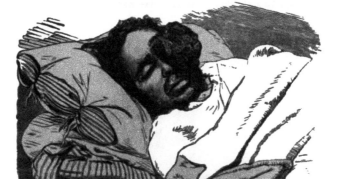

ulcer, brought before the British Medical Association, determined me to follow the same plan, and thus destroy the disease as effectually as I could. I removed the tumor on the 23d of November, 1864, by first cutting the mass from the orbit with strong curved scissors, and then removing all the parts to which the growth extended external to the lids themselves. The actual cautery was then freely applied over the whole surface of the orbit and parts around, and finally the whole was covered with a layer of cotton-wool, thickly coated with the chloride of zinc paste.

"There was very little hemorrhage, and he scarcely had pain after the operation. In a fortnight a large mass of charred tissue was thrown off, with some parts of the orbital bones. Portions of the bones of the orbit exfoliated from time to time, until much of the framework came away, exposing in one part the dura mater, and opening the nasal and maxillary cavities. Healthy granulations soon covered the whole surface. He rapidly gained health and strength. One or two little millet-seed looking excrescences remained at the inner part of the wall of the cavity, but they did not appear to grow: from time to time, however, they were touched with chloride of zinc, or nitrate of silver."

In September, 1865, he again applied, suffering from severe rheumatic pains in the right hip; he had lost flesh, and the pulse was up to 100. The excrescences on the inside of the orbit, having increased in size (one was as large as a small nut), were cut away by Mr. de Morgan, and the tissue around them destroyed by the chloride of zinc.

The microscopic examination of the tumor, made by Mr. Hulke, showed it to be medullary cancer. The optic nerve appeared healthy on section; but extending between the inner and outer sheath in the loose connective tissue, were small diffused patches of cancer elements, lying in the meshes of the healthy tissue.

Fig. 252 shows the patient's condition when he appeared before the Pathological Society, on February 6, 1866.[1] He was then apparently quite well.

Fig. 252.

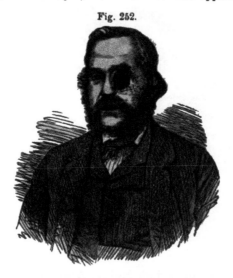

Although the patient appeared to be quite well in February, 1866, he died on July 11th, having lived one year and eight months after the operation. He had for some time suffered greatly from sciatica, which was soon followed by paraplegia. He had also vertical hemiopia of the remaining eye. On post-mortem examination, a large tumor was found in the middle fossa of the skull, growing apparently from the orbital foramen and sphenoidal fissure, the optic nerve as far as the commissure being involved in, and undistinguishable from it. Cancerous deposits were also found in the glands around the aorta, and adhering to the nerve trunks of the cauda equina. The orbit was empty, and free from any cancerous growth.

The return of the disease, and its fatal termination, were consequently only due to the fact that the optic nerve was involved in the cancerous affection. Mr. de Morgan therefore thinks that these facts justify the belief that, had the operation been done in the same manner at an earlier period, the patient might have remained well.

[1] This and the preceding cut are from photographs by Mr. Heisch, and have been kindly lent to the author by the Council of the Pathological Society.

(8) MELANOTIC CANCER.

Melanotic tumors of the orbit are, like those within the eye, often either of a sarcomatous or a mixed character, one portion of the morbid growth being of a sarcomatous nature, another carcinomatous. The character and progress of melanotic cancer have already been given in the articles upon " Tumors of the Choroid " (p. 375) and need not be entered upon here, as the disease does not differ essentially in its course and nature (excepting its color) from other cancerous affections of the orbit.

(9) EPITHELIAL CANCER.

Epithelial cancer of the orbit is also occasionally met with, originating in the skin of the temple, cheek, or nose, and extending into the orbit. Mr. Hulke[1] narrates a most interesting case of epithelial cancer of the orbit caused by a severe blow upon the cheek, in which the symptoms presented by the disease closely resembled those of carbuncular cellulitis.

[(10) Among the rare tumors of the orbit may be mentioned the *cylindroma*. These tumors are usually mixed, containing generally a large number of sarcomatous elements, but also more or less of the cylindroid arrangement of epithelial cells, which is the characteristic feature of these growths. An interesting case of this kind is reported by Sattler. (See the " Vierteljahrsch. f. prakt. Heilk.,''Bd. I.) They are malignant and tend to recur after removal.

There are a few cases on record of *congenital encephalocele*, which grow to an enormous size. One such case is reported by Raab. (See the " Wein. med. Wochensch.," May 11, 1876.)—B.]

7.—VASCULAR TUMORS OF THE ORBIT.

(1) CAVERNOUS TUMOR.

Only four instances of this very rare form of orbital tumor have been recorded, by Lebert,[2] De Ricci,[3] Von Graefe,[4] and De Wecker.[5]

These tumors do not present any specially characteristic features in their external appearance, excepting that they are prone to undergo marked spontaneous changes in size, which are dependent upon mechanical hyperæmia of the morbid growth. Thus, any straining or violent exertion, or stooping position of the head, may be followed by a striking increase in the size of the tumor. In Von Graefe's case, the mere pressure of the pillow in bed upon this side of the head and face gave rise to a temporary protrusion of the eye, accompanied by great congestion of the conjunctival and subconjunctival vessels.

The growth of these tumors is generally slow, more especially if they are situated deeply in the orbit, for then the pressure of the eyeball restrains their rapid development.

---

[1] " R. L. O. H. Rep.," v. 336.
[2] " Abhandlungen aus dem Gebiete der praktischen Chirurgie." Berlin, 1848, S. 88.
[3] " Dublin Quarterly Journal," 1865, November, p. 338.
[4] " A. f. O.," vii. 2, p. 12.
[5] De Wecker, " Maladies des Yeux," 2d edit., i. 798.

The cavernous tumor[1] is surrounded by a capsule of dense cellular tissue, which is only very loosely connected to the adipose tissue of the orbit, so that the tumor can be very readily and completely removed, with but a very slight amount of hemorrhage. On section, it is seen to be of a spongy nature, and to be traversed by delicate meshes of fibrillar connective tissue, dividing it into a vast number of little compartments. These interspaces contain blood, which can be readily squeezed out by a little pressure, and this causes a considerable diminution in the bulk of the tumor, which at the same time becomes of a pale grayish tint.

The erectile tumors (telangiectasis) which are met with in the orbit, almost invariably take their origin from the eyelids, and then, increasing in size, extend into the orbit. They are described in the article on "Tumors of the Eyelids."

[Pulsating tumors of the orbit with exophthalmos may be due to one or more of several causes: 1st. They may be due to true aneurism of the ophthalmic artery or one of its branches, though this is perhaps the most infrequent cause of all. 2d. The cause may be a false aneurism from rupture of an artery, the result of injury to the head or orbit. 3d. There may be no disease of any artery, but simply some cause of compression of the ophthalmic vein at its exit from the cavity, as by an aneurism of the internal carotid, or phlebitis of the cavernous sinus.—B.]

(2) ANEURISMS OF THE ORBIT.

Aneurism by anastomosis is of far less frequent occurrence in the orbit than was at one time supposed, and many of the cases which have been described

[Fig. 258.]

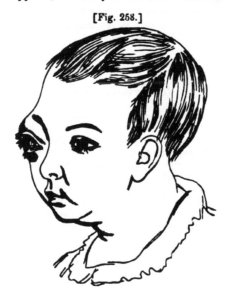

under this name, were evidently instances of diffuse aneurism. Aneurism by anastomosis is met with principally in young children, and is mostly con-

---

[1] Virchow, " Die Krankheiten Geschwülste," iii. 1, 358.

genital. The tumor commences in or near the skin, is connected with the subcutaneous tissue, and presents the appearance of an irregular nodulated growth, consisting of convolutions of dilated arteries; the vessels of the neighborhood participating in the increased action. [Fig. 253.] The origin of the tumor is neither sudden nor produced by direct violence, but is slow, and its increase in size is tardy and gradual. The size of the swelling is much increased by any position or exertion which causes congestion of the head, e. g., stooping, straining, coughing, etc. Although the tumor presents distinct signs of pulsation and thrilling, no effect (or only a very tardy one) is produced upon these symptoms, or upon the swelling, by compression of the carotid artery. Moreover, as was strongly insisted upon by Mr. John Bell, aneurism by anastomosis is not curable by ligature of vessels. The best treatment is that of subcutaneous ligature of the tumor, the ligature being either applied in a circular manner, so as to include the base of the tumor within a single loop, or else the figure-of-8 ligature should be employed. If the growth is of considerable size, and is divided into different nodulated portions, these may be operated upon successively by the ligature; or threads saturated with a solution of the perchloride of iron may be drawn through the tumor, so that they cross and recross each other in various directions. These modes of operating are far more safe than, and much to be preferred to, the injection of the perchloride of iron or other agents for the purpose of producing coagulation. Dr. Althaus' treatment by electrolysis might also be tried.

True aneurisms of the orbit are of rare occurrence, and do not attain any considerable bulk, on account of the small size of both the ophthalmic artery and the central artery of the retina. In a case recorded by Mr. Guthrie,[1] an aneurism of the ophthalmic artery of each side, about the size of a large nut, was discovered after death. The ophthalmic vein was greatly enlarged, and obstructed near its passage through the sphenoidal fissure by the great increase in size of the recti muscles, which had also acquired an almost cartilaginous hardness. Although the eyes were greatly protruded, the sight was hardly affected, and the exophthalmos was evidently as much due to the state of the muscles as to the dilatation of the vessels. There was an audible hissing noise in the head, which was attributed to aneurism. As the disease existed on both sides, Mr. Guthrie did not propose ligature of the carotid.

Cases of aneurism of the central artery of the retina have been observed by Von Graefe (senior), Schmidler, and A. Cooper. In Von Graefe's case the central artery of the retina was dilated to the size of a stalk of grass. Sous'[2] was in one case able to diagnose the affection with the ophthalmoscope. He observed, in a woman of sixty-four, a red ovoid tumor on the left optic disk, extending somewhat beyond its margin, and, after becoming suddenly narrower, passing over into one of the retinal arteries. It presented evident signs of pulsation, the dilatation being synchronous with the systole of the heart. The other retinal arteries were very narrow and threadlike, the veins somewhat dilated.

Diffuse or false aneurism of the orbit is of far more frequent occurrence. It may be either primary and traumatic, or consecutive in its origin. In the former case, the walls of the artery are torn or ruptured by a sudden blow or wound of the head or orbit, or a fall upon the head, and the effect

1 "Lectures on Operative Surgery," p. 158.
2 "Annales d'oculistique," 1865.

is immediate, blood is effused into the orbital cellular tissue, and a certain degree of exophthalmos may be produced. As the exophthalmos increases, the eyelids become swollen, red, and œdematous, the conjunctival and sub-conjunctival vessels congested, the movements of the eyeball diminished, and the sight perhaps more or less impaired. The bloodvessels around the eye are also sometimes dilated and tortuous. A bluish, elastic, soft tumor now makes its appearance at some point of the edge of the orbit, and shows distinct pulsations, which are evident both to the eye and touch, are synchronous with the systole of the heart, and accompanied by an audible thrill. If the ear is applied, a peculiar humming or whirring sound is heard, like the action of a steam-engine, threshing-machine, or humming-top, and this proves a source of the greatest distress and anxiety to the patient. This may extend over a considerable portion of the head. In a case narrated by Dr. Joseph Bell,[1] this whirring sound was audible to a bystander at the distance of a yard. There is often also intense pain in and around the orbit and over the corresponding side of the head. Compression of the carotid artery at once stops the pulsation, and pressure upon the tumor generally causes it distinctly to diminish in size. In some cases, the appearances of an aneurismal tumor do not come on till some length of time after the accident, and its increase is slow and gradual; in other instances, the symptoms super-vene immediately, or very rapidly upon the injury.

The consecutive diffuse aneurism of the orbit is frequently preceded by a true aneurism, accompanied by a fatty or atheromatous degeneration of the walls of the vessel, which thus become weakened. But the disease of the walls of the bloodvessels may also be alone present. Any sudden strain or exertion on the part of the patient causes the vessel to give way, and this is accompanied by a very marked and sudden pain through the head and eye, as if a pistol had been shot off, or something had given way within the head. The blood flows through the rent in the artery, and, becoming infiltrated in the surrounding cellular tissue, a cavity, communicating directly with the vessel, is formed. Symptoms of exophthalmos, together with pulsation and a bruit in the tumor, and other signs of aneurism supervene, the patient at the same time experiencing intense pain. Sometimes the disease may appear spontaneously, without the slightest apparent cause, and without any accident or violent exertion. It has been frequently met with in women during the time of pregnancy or childbirth. Compression of the carotid causes a con-siderable diminution or arrest of the pulsation and bruit, but is sometimes accompanied by severe pain and distressing symptoms of fulness in the head (Gioppi). Or these may be produced to a very marked degree by sudden relaxation of the pressure. whereas a gradual removal produces no pain.[2]

But all the symptoms of orbital aneurism may exist without the presence of any such affection within the orbit; the pulsating orbital tumor being simply due to some compression of the ophthalmic vein, which prevents the efflux of the blood from the orbit. The cause of this compression is fre-quently the presence of an aneurism of the ophthalmic artery near its origin, or of the internal carotid artery. Thus Mr. Nunneley, in his valuable and interesting paper on "Vascular Protrusion of the Eyeball,"[3] narrates, amongst other cases, that of a patient in whom he successfully tied the carotid, in 1859, for a pulsating tumor of the orbit. In 1864 she died, and on post-mortem examination the presence of a circumscribed aneurism of the ophthalmic artery was discovered, just at its origin, of the size of a hazel-

[1] "Edinburgh Medical Journal," 1861, p. 1064.
[2] Dr. Joseph Bell, l. c., p. 1065.
[3] "Med.-Chir. Trans," vol. 48, 1865, p. 29.

nut. The trunk and branches of the ophthalmic artery, continued forwards into the orbit, being of small size. The following case of Mr. Bowman's[1] is also of much interest, as showing how all the symptoms of orbital aneurism may be simulated without the existence of any such affection. The patient, a woman, aged forty, noticed severe pain in the left temple, very shortly after a blow from a fist on the left side of the head and temple. A fortnight afterwards, she felt a constant rushing sensation on the same side of the head, like the beat of a steam-engine, which increased with acceleration of the heart's action. On her admission into King's College Hospital, under Mr. Bowman, the eye was prominent and congested, the pupil dilated but active, distant sight was perfect, but she was unable to read. There was a loud sibilant bruit over the left side of the head, being synchronous with the beating of the heart; also distinct pulsation of the left eye, apparent to the touch, and a loud bruit could be heard when the stethoscope was placed on the closed eyelids. Mr. Bowman tied the common carotid, and the pulsation and bruit, hitherto felt and heard over the front of the eye, at once ceased. But the patient died eighteen days after the operation from phagedenic ulceration and hemorrhage from the wound. On post-mortem examination, no appearance of an aneurism could be discovered, and it is difficult, as Mr. Hulke says, in reporting the case, " to explain the aneurismal symptoms by the pathological appearances, which were those of phlebitis of the cavernous, transverse, circular, and petrosal sinuses. The internal carotid may have been partially compressed by the swollen walls of the cavernous sinus against the side of the body of the sphenoid bone, giving rise to the bruit, which would have a good conducting medium in the cranial bones. The plugging of the trunk of the ophthalmic vein, where it joins the cavernous sinus, by obstructing the return of blood from the orbit, accounts for the protrusion of the eyeball, and perhaps also for the pulsation which was felt when the finger was laid on it, because each diastole of the ophthalmic artery must have been attended by a general momentary increase of the whole quantity of blood in the orbit, because its exit through the ophthalmic vein was cut off, and t e resisting bony walls of the orbit could permit a distention in front only"

The operation of ligature of the common carotid has proved very successful in cases of aneurism or supposed aneurism of the orbit. Dr. Noyes,[2] of New York, has given a tabulated account of all cases of ligature of the carotid for pulsating tumors of the orbit, which had occurred up to 1869. He has collected forty-five cases, of which thirty-two were cured, two partially successful, four unsuccessful, and seven died.

Digital compression of the carotid has [been tried in nine cases and] proved successful in three cases, viz., in those of Gioppi,[3] Vanzetti,[4] and Freeman.[5] In a case of Szokalsky's,[6] digital compression was continued for fifty-six hours, together with ice-cold compresses and small doses of digitalis, but proved quite unavailing. Ligature of the common carotid was then performed with perfect success. Digital compression may be applied in such a manner as to press the common carotid directly back against the vertebral

[1] "R. L. O. H. Rep.," ii. p. 6.
[2] "New York Medical Journal," March, 1869. *Vide* also Dr. Morton's papers in "Amer. Journal of Med. Sciences," April, 1865, and July, 1870; also Zehender's article, "Kl. M.," 1869, 99.
[3] "Annales d'oculistique," Novembre et Décembre, 1858.
[4] "Annali univers. di med. e chir.," 1858, p. 148; *vide* also "Lancet," March 15, 1862.
[5] "American Journal of Med. Sciences," July, 1866.
[6] "Kl. Monatsbl.," 1864, 427.

column; but in this mode the jugular vein is very apt to be also compressed, which produces great congestion of the head. It is, therefore, better to raise the carotid somewhat, and compress it between the fingers. Relays of assistants should be ready to alternate in this duty. Sometimes, however, it cannot be borne for longer than four or five minutes at a time. The success of these cases should encourage us to give this method of treatment by digital compression a fair trial, before having recourse to ligature of the carotid, for this operation can always be performed if compression fails.

Two cases have been successfully treated by styptics;[1] and Dr. Holmes mentions an instance of traumatic aneurism cured by the administration of the extract of ergot, and tincture of green hellebore, together with complete rest and low diet.[2] Two cases in which electrolysis and injection of the perchloride of iron were tried, are narrated in Zander and Geissler.[3] The latter remedy is, however, excessively dangerous, for instantaneous death has been caused by it more than once.

[The difficulty of diagnosis in cases of orbital pulsating tumors is thus very great. In examining a case we must note the effect of: (1) compression of the common carotid on the same side; (2) steady pressure on the eyeball through the closed lids, whether on removing the pressure the former state is *slowly* or *quickly* reproduced; (3) the seat of greatest pulsation, whether the pulsation is strong or weak, the effect of posture, the presence of a bruit heard by the stethoscope or at a distance through the air, and the character of any sound heard by the patient in his own head; (4) pain and inflammatory symptoms and history of injury; pain is often severe in cases of traumatic aneurism with extravasation and orbital inflammation. (Nettleship.)

Harlan has reported two cases of vascular disease of the orbit, in one of which the cause was supposed to be aneurism by anastomosis in the orbit, which was probably congenital, or at least came on in early childhood. In the second case, which was of traumatic origin and was at first supposed to be orbital aneurism, Harlan seems later to have been somewhat doubtful of the diagnosis, and to have adopted Nunneley's idea of vascular protrusion. At the present day most ophthalmic surgeons seem inclined to agree with Nunneley, that in the great majority of such cases of protrusion of the eyeball, there is no disease whatever in the orbit, but that the symptoms depend on obstruction to the return of blood through the ophthalmic vein. Orbital aneurism is certainly a very rare disease, and its symptoms are often imitated by cases in which only the veins are affected. (See "Trans. Amer. Ophthal. Soc.," 1875.) Gruening has reported an interesting case of vascular protrusion of both eyes of traumatic origin, which he thought was probably due to an arterio-venous communication in the cavernous sinus.

There was double choked disk and total blindness. Compression of the left common carotid entirely stopped the bruit and headache. Ligation of the left common carotid five days after complete amaurosis set in, restored the vision completely in one eye, and very markedly improved it in the other. The entire absence of all cerebral symptoms is against the possibility of a true or diffuse aneurism of the left internal carotid within the skull, and all the symptoms pointed to an intra-cranial arterio-venous communication. (See "Arch. of Ophthal. and Otology," v. i. pp. 40–47.)

---

[1] Dr. Noyes has collected ("New York Med. Journal," March, 1869) six cases treated by injection of styptics, and in all with a successful result.—H.]

[2] "Amer. Journ. of Med. Sci.," July, 1864.

[3] "Die Verletzungen des Auges," 433.

In the "Archives of Ophthalmology," viii. 3, pp. 328 to 344, Nieden reports three cases of pulsating vascular tumor of the orbit cured by ligation of the common carotid. The first case he diagnosed as a rupture of the ophthalmic artery, free communication of the blood in the retro-orbital cellular tissue with the arterial current, and a cure eighteen months later by the formation of a thrombus. The second case was probably due to an impediment to the return of the blood by phlebitis behind the orbit. The third case he considered to be an aneurismal dilatation of the internal carotid, or a rupture of the artery in the cavernous sinus, with a direct communication between arterial and venous blood.

In the "Med.-Chirurg. Trans.," lviii. pp. 184–218, Rivington has published an interesting paper on pulsating tumor of the orbit, including autopsies on twelve cases, which contains most of the literature on the subject.

One of the latest communications on the subject is by Schlaefke, who reports a case of supposed traumatic rupture of the left internal carotid artery in the cavernous sinus, with the formation of an arterio-venous aneurism. The bruit and pulsation ceased immediately after ligation of the common carotid. The patient recovered, but died three months later from empyema and purulent pericarditis. At the autopsy, the left optic nerve was found atrophied, and the left cavernous sinus widened, and its walls very much thickened. All the orbital veins were enormously dilated, and their walls thickened. The left internal carotid in the cavernous sinus was dilated and connected by three openings. There was no change in the ophthalmic artery. Numerous thrombi in the orbital veins. The paper is a long and interesting one, but contains nothing new. (See "Archiv für Ophthalmologie," xxv. 4, pp. 112–162.)

Hirschberg reports a case of pulsating exophthalmos in the left eye of ten days' duration, occurring in a woman of thirty-five. The eye was immovable, the cornea anæsthetic, and vision was reduced one-half. There was a well-marked bruit, isochronous with the radial pulse. The fundus was normal. The patient had left facial paralysis and constant headache. Ten days later, complete blindness suddenly ensued. Injections of ergotin, subcutaneously, into the orbit, put a stop to the pulsations, but they returned two days later. The left common carotid was then tied, and the pulsations ceased permanently. Seventeen days later, the exophthalmos had disappeared, but the immobility, anæsthesia, and blindness remained. Four months later, some mobility had been regained in the eye, and the facial paralysis had nearly disappeared. There was atrophic excavation of the optic nerve, with remains of retinal hemorrhages. (See "Centralblatt für Praktische Augenheilkunde," July, 1880.)

Secondi reports an interesting case of pulsating exophthalmos, bilateral in character. The patient had fallen, striking his forehead a violent blow, and became unconscious. Consciousness was not regained for several hours, and the patient bled from the mouth, nose, and ears. There was ecchymosis of the conjunctiva and eyelids, marked exophthalmos, and severe pain in the head for fifteen days. Secondi diagnosticated a fracture of the base of the skull, with subsequent development of an arterio-venous aneurism. He assumed that the rupture of the left internal carotid artery in the corresponding venous sinus was caused by the fracture. (See "Annali di ottalmologia," x. 2.)

Another case of aneurism of the orbit cured by ligature of the common carotid artery is reported by Wolfe. The patient was a woman, æt. twenty-two, with a large nævus on the right temple, and another on the left breast. After a blow on the left eye, she began to suffer pain, with severe knocking in the head. When seen, there was a general dilatation of the orbital tissues, and a slight protrusion of the eyeball. There was no pulsation, but a slight bruit was audible in the orbit. Vision was not affected. Five months later, there was considerable protrusion of the eye, the lids were infiltrated, the conjunctiva was injected, and the eye pushed downwards and outwards, and markedly limited in its movements. A tumor of half the size of a walnut was seen near the inner canthus, soft and pulsating. The pulsation was visible at some distance, and the noise very audible. When the carotid artery of the same side was compressed, the bruit ceased and the tumor partially disappeared. The ophthalmoscope showed all the signs of choked disk, vision was very much impaired, the outer margin of the cornea was ulcerated, and the pupil sluggish. The carotid was ligated in the usual way, and pulsation in the orbit immediately ceased, the tumor was considerably diminished, and the eyeball retracted within the orbit. The ulceration of the cornea was arrested, and vision subsequently became normal. The retinal veins remained dilated and tortuous at the periphery. (See "Lancet," Dec. 3, 1881.)—B.]

8.—EFFUSION OF BLOOD INTO THE ORBIT.

The effusion of blood into the orbit is generally rapid, and can mostly be traced to some direct cause, such as a blow or fall upon the eye or head, incised or punctured wounds of the orbit, or the lodgement of a foreign body within the latter. In rarer instances, the hemorrhage may be due to violent exertion or straining, or may even be spontaneous in its origin. The eye generally becomes rapidly protruded, and its mobility curtailed. Frequently the protrusion, as well as the impairment of the mobility of the eyeball, occur chiefly in certain directions. The sight is more or less affected, and this is chiefly due to direct pressure upon the optic nerve by the effusion, but in cases of injuries to the head, it must be remembered that the affection of the sight may be dependent upon some cerebral lesion. Thus consecutive neuro-retinitis may become developed, being due to the inflammation of the meninges.[1] On account of the impairment of the mobility of the eye, there is also diplopia. The eyelids are often much swollen, contused, discolored, and perhaps studded with ecchymoses, which may also occur in the conjunctiva and subconjunctival tissue. Moreover, although the blood may be at first confined to the posterior portion of the orbit, it may press forward and become diffused beneath the conjunctiva, and thus produce considerable chemosis. In cases of orbital hemorrhage dependent upon fracture of the bones of the orbit, it has been supposed that the presence of ecchymoses in the eyelids is a guide to the diagnosis of the seat of the fracture. Velpeau especially insisted on the importance of this symptom. When ecchymosis of the lids exists alone, or precedes the subconjunctival effusion, it was supposed to be indicative of a fracture of the margin of the orbit; whereas subconjunctival effusion existing with other symptoms of fracture of the orbit, in which there was no ecchymosis of the eyelids, or this only came on subsequently, was supposed to be pathognomonic of the injury being situated deeper in, or at the bottom of the orbit. But absolute reliance cannot be placed upon these symptoms, for the bones of the orbit may be fractured, and yet there may not be the slightest effusion of blood either under the conjunctiva or into the eyelids. If there is a fracture of the inner or lower

[1] Vide Manz, "A. f. O.," xii. 1, 1.

wall of the orbit, emphysema of the latter may also be produced, and then the protrusion of the eye will be increased when the nose is blown.

The treatment must be chiefly directed to hastening the absorption of the blood. Cold compresses and a firm bandage will be found most serviceable. Only in those cases in which the effusion of the blood is very great, and causes extreme exophthalmos, with very severe suffering to the patient, is it advisable to make incisions, in order to permit of the escape of the blood. In the majority of cases, it is wiser to allow it to be absorbed.

9.—EMPHYSEMA OF THE ORBIT.

Emphysema of the orbit is generally accompanied by a similar condition of the eyelids. The affection may be produced by a rupture of the ethmoidal cells, by fracture of the frontal sinus, in which case the swelling may extend to the forehead and temple, or, as is most frequently the case, by a rupture of the lachrymal sac. The air is admitted into the cellular tissue of the orbit and eyelids, causing great protrusion of the eye and swelling of the lids, both subsiding considerably when gentle pressure is applied to the eyeball and lids. If the affection is due to a rupture of the lachrymal sac, the swelling may be immediately produced by the patient's forcibly blowing his nose. The emphysematous swelling is very elastic to the touch, and there are marked symptoms of crepitation. [It may occur from fracture of the lachrymal bone. (See "Amer. Journ. Med. Sci.," July, 1880, Art. IX. "Lesion of Bones of Orbit.")—B.]

[10.—HYPEROSTOSIS AND PERIOSTOSIS OF THE BONES OF THE ORBIT.

The bones of the orbit occasionally undergo hypertrophy, and the proliferation may affect either the bone substance itself or the periosteum. The two commonly coexist in the bones of the face. The excessive development of one or more of the bones of the orbit would of course produce the most singular changes in the shape of this cavity. According to Wagner, hyperostosis may affect only the external compact tissue or the medullary substance alone, or it may be met with in both at the same time. It seems, however, to involve mainly the external table of the bones. It is a mistake to suppose that inflammatory action is at the bottom of this proliferation in all cases, for cases have been known to occur in which a facial bone has continued to increase in size without any symptoms except those produced by its increase in bulk. As a result of the change in size and shape of the bones of one orbit, the two orbits do not occupy a corresponding position, but one of them is found to be on a higher plane than the other. Periostosis may result from long-continued subacute periostitis of traumatic origin. (See "Trans. Amer. Ophthal. Society," 1879, pp. 598–602.)—B.]

11.—PRESSURE UPON THE ORBIT FROM NEIGHBORING CAVITIES,

Dilatation of the cavities in the vicinity of the orbit will cause a contraction and malformation of the latter, accompanied by more or less considerable exophthalmos, curtailment of the mobility of the eyeball, and impairment of vision.

Diseases of the frontal sinus[1] may produce considerable dilatation of this cavity, which then encroaches upon the orbit, giving rise to a contraction and malformation of the latter, and consequent protrusion of the eyeball. Amongst such affections of the frontal sinus, must be enumerated acute and chronic inflammation of its lining membrane, giving rise to the formation of a purulent or muco-purulent discharge; in rarer instances, polypi, cystic tumors, and entozoa are met with; also, perhaps, exostosis. The latter is, however, according to Mackenzie, so extremely rare, that he is not aware of a single recorded case of exostosis of the frontal sinus, although he happens to have two specimens in his own collection.[2] Of these diseases of the frontal sinus, acute and chronic inflammation, terminating in abscess, are the most common.

The symptoms presented by abscess of the frontal sinus are often somewhat obscure, and may mislead even an experienced surgeon, for they may so closely simulate those presented by an intra-orbital tumor, that the true nature of the disease is not recognized until an exploratory incision has been made, or the abscess has perhaps burst through the upper lid, and a fistulous opening is found, leading into the frontal sinus. Again, if the swelling extends somewhat lower down, so that it is crossed by the tendo oculi, it may be mistaken for distention of the lachrymal sac. But we should be guarded against such a mistake, by the absence of epiphora and symptoms of inflammation, as well as by the hardness of the swelling, if it be due to distention of the wall of the sinus.

The disease generally presents the following symptoms: The patient experiences a feeling of fulness and uneasiness over the eyebrow, accompanied by a dull aching pain, which is sometimes increased by pressure upon this spot, or by any exertion or posture which causes an acceleration of the circulation. In the acute abscess, the muco-purulent discharge generally perforates the roof of the orbit, or makes its way into the nose at an early stage, before there has been time for the sinus to become much dilated. If the discharge has made its way into the orbit, the eyelid becomes red and swollen, the upper lid perhaps drooping a little, and a small elastic tumor appears at the inner and upper angle of the orbit. As the abscess increases in size, the eyeball is displaced in a downward and outward direction, becomes more and more protruded, and its mobility impaired, in consequence of which, diplopia manifests itself when the patient looks upwards. If the abscess is not opened, it will point and burst through the skin of the upper eyelid, generally near its inner angle, or perhaps lower down, just above the tendon of the orbicularis, when the fistulous opening which remains may be mistaken for inflammation of the lachrymal sac. But if a probe be passed into the opening, the sinus will be found to extend in an upward and backward direction, perhaps to a very considerable distance. Sometimes there are several fistulous openings. In a chronic abscess, the frontal sinus often becomes very considerably distended by the collection of mucus, and this produces great exophthalmos, and gives rise to a marked prominence over the eyebrow. The progress of the chronic abscess is often extremely slow and protracted, and accompanied by but little pain and discomfort, until symptoms of exophthalmos and diplopia supervene. Inflammation and abscess of the frontal sinus are, in the majority of cases, caused by blows or falls upon this part of the face, but they may arise spontaneously.

---

[1] *Vide* Mr. Hulke's articles on "Diseases of the Frontal Sinus," "R. L. O. H. Rep.," iii. 147.
[2] Mackenzie's "Diseases of the Eye," 4th edit., i. p. 59.

[Leber has made some observations upon empyema of the frontal sinus and the secondary symptoms in the eyes. The course of the disease is very chronic, and it may exist for many years before the anterior wall of the sinus becomes absorbed and a fluctuating tumor presents. The symptoms are a swelling of the upper and inner orbital margin, slight exophthalmos, sometimes diplopia from paresis of the trochlearis, and epiphora from compression of the lachrymal sac. (See "Archiv. für Ophthalmologie," xxvi. 3.)—B.]

As the symptoms are generally at the outset very obscure, the treatment can then be only directed to the alleviation of the pain or inflammation, by the application of warm poppy fomentations. But when the presence of matter is ascertained, a free incision should be made into the swelling just beneath the supra-orbital arch, and the pus be thoroughly evacuated, the finger or small piece of sponge being introduced into the cavity of the frontal sinus for this purpose. The point of the forefinger should then be inserted into the dilated sinus in order to ascertain its relation with the neighboring cavities, and also the condition of its lining membrane. The point of the little finger should next be introduced up the corresponding nostril as high as the floor of the dilated sinus, and a bistoury or trocar should be passed through the opening in the frontal sinus, and the lower wall of the latter, just over the tip of the finger introduced by the nostril, should be incised, so that a free communication may be established between the sinus and the nasal cavity. A stout seton, composed of several thick silk threads, is then to be passed through the aperture in the skin into the sinus and thence through the nostril; the free end, projecting through the latter, being tied to that which projects from the incision in the skin, so that a large and easily movable loop is formed, which should be freely moved by the patient two or three times a day, so as to keep the opening between the nasal cavity and the sinus permanently patent. It is, however, much better to employ an India-rubber drainage-tube, having holes cut at short intervals. This is to be fastened to a director, and the latter passed in the same manner as the seton, and the tube be then drawn through. Or it may be passed up the nostril into the sinus, and thence into the orbit and out by the external wound, the one end being fastened to the forehead by a strip of plaster, the other being left to project a little from the nostril. The cavity of the sinus should be washed out several times daily with water or an astringent lotion (Zinc. sulph. gr. j, Alumen. gr. iij, Aq. dest. f ℥j), this being injected through the tube; the latter is also to be moved a little once or twice daily. The patient is to be kept in bed for some days and closely watched. The seton should be worn for several weeks, or even longer, but should be removed if it gives rise to much irritation or to cerebral symptoms. When the communication with the nose has been established, the seton or tube should be removed, and the opening in the skin will then granulate and heal. I have seen several cases very successfully treated in this way by Mr. Bowman and Mr. Lawson. The following case of my own also illustrates well the symptoms of the disease:

R. S., aged 40, baker, perceived, about twelve years ago, that the right upper lid was swollen, and hung down over the eye. This swelling disappeared spontaneously in the course of a week, but recurred about every two years; and six months ago he noticed that, beside the tumefaction of the lid, there was a small swelling at the inner angle of the upper lid close to the root of the nose; and as it gradually increased in size, he applied for advice at King's College Hospital, on June 4, 1869. He then presented the following appearance: The right eye protrudes considerably, and is so much displaced dowards and outwards, that the upper edge of the cornea is below the level of the left lower lid (*vide* Fig. 254). The movements of the eyeball are greatly curtailed both upwards and inwards. The upper lid is considerably swollen, and at its inner angle is noticed an oval tolerably defined swelling, about the size of a large hazel-nut, which extends upwards to the eyebrow. But the nasal prominence on this side is only very slightly enlarged. The outline of the upper and lower margin of the orbit can be easily traced with the finger, and is found to be sharply defined and not at all swollen, or concealed by any tumor. The oval swelling, though firm and tense, is elastic, yields a distinct sense of fluctuation, and is slightly tender to the touch; the

Fig. 254.

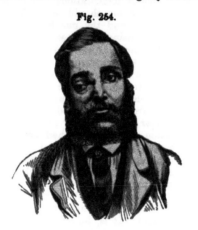

patient also experiences some dull pain, extending from the inner corner of the eye outwards over the orbit. The eye is somewhat injected and becomes irritable and watery on exposure to cold winds or bright light. But the sight and visual field are good, and the fundus oculi is quite normal, nor has the exophthalmos, and consequent stretching of the optic nerve, produced hyperæmia and œdema of the retina or optic nerve. I considered the case one of abscess of the frontal sinus, which had burst through the wall of the orbit, and strongly advised an operation, which was performed on June 16. A free incision was made over the most prominent part of the swelling; the skin and fibres of the orbicularis muscle were somewhat dissected back, and the point of the knife was then plunged into the tumor, the incision being enlarged to the size of the external wound. A large quantity of thick, greenish pus escaped, the eyeball gradually sinking back into its normal position. On passing the little finger through the incision in the direction of the frontal sinus, a large irregular opening was discovered leading into the latter and readily admitting the finger. A good deal of matter having been removed from the cavity of the distended sinus, the little finger of the other hand was passed up the right nostril, until its tip could be touched by that of the finger in the sinus, only a thin plate of bone intervening. This was then carefully punctured at the lowest part with a trocar. An India-rubber drainage-tube, having holes cut at short intervals, was fastened to a probe, and the latter passed up the nostril into the sinus, and thence out through the orbit by the external incision; the tube was then easily pulled through in the same direction, and its one extremity fastened to the forehead by a strip or two of plaster, the other being left to project a little from the nostril. In this way a free communication was maintained between the sinus and the nose, so that the former could be flushed out with water and astringent injections, and the discharge flow off through the nostril. The operation was followed by a certain degree of inflammatory reaction, swelling of the lids and cheek, etc., but these symptoms soon yielded to hot poppy fomentations

Fig. 255.

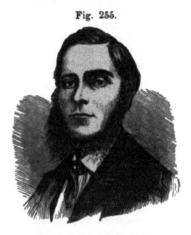

and poultices. The incision was kept open so as to permit the free exit of the discharge, and the drainage-tube was syringed out with lukewarm water several times a day, in order to keep it patent, being also slightly moved up and down twice daily. The patient recovered rapidly, and was made an out-patient on July 3, the tube still remaining in. The swelling had now almost entirely disappeared, the eyeball had resumed its natural position, and its range of mobility upwards and inwards was very greatly increased. The tube was allowed to remain in till September 23, when it was removed, as there had been no return of the swelling, and all discharge had ceased. The external wound now quickly closed; the eye having by this time regained its normal appearance (*vide* Fig. 255), and its mobility was perfect in all directions. He was seen last in the beginning of February, 1870, and was still perfectly well.

Enlargement of the maxillary sinus, the nasal cavity, and the cavity of the cranium may also cause pressure upon, and a contraction of, the cavity of the orbit, accompanied by protrusion of the eye and limitation of its movements. For interesting cases illustrative of these different conditions, I must refer the reader to Mackenzie's "Treatise on Diseases of the Eye." [See also an article by Knapp, in the "Trans. Fifth Internat. Ophthal. Congress," 1876, pp. 55 and 56.—B.]

12.—WOUNDS AND INJURIES OF THE ORBIT.

Incised and punctured wounds of the orbit should always be watched with care, for serious symptoms do not always arise directly after the injury, and may not manifest themselves till some time afterwards. The instrument which has inflicted the injury should be examined, in order that we may ascertain whether a portion of it has not been broken off, and perhaps remains lodged within the orbit. Even if the eyeball itself and the bones of the orbit have escaped direct injury, inflammation of the cellular tissue of the orbit and a more or less extensive formation of pus are very likely to occur.

Foreign bodies, more especially if they are small in size, such as shot,

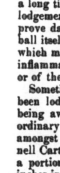

[Fig. 256.]

splinters of glass, steel, etc., may remain for a long time undetected within the orbit. The lodgement of a foreign body in the orbit may prove dangerous by direct injury to the eyeball itself, the optic nerve, or the orbital walls, which may be fractured. Or it may produce inflammation of the cellular tissue of the orbit, or of the periosteum, etc.

Sometimes, very large foreign bodies have been lodged in the orbit without the patient being aware of their presence. Very extraordinary cases of this kind have been recorded, amongst others by Nélaton,[1] and Mr. Brudenell Carter[2] [Fig. 256]. In the latter instance, a portion of hat-peg three and three-tenth inches in length had remained impacted in the orbit for from ten to twenty days without the patient's being aware of it. It was so successfully removed by Mr. Clarke, that the patient recovered without a single unfavorable symptom, the vision and movements of the eye being unimpaired.

Fractures of the walls of the orbit are extremely dangerous, more especially when the roof or upper portion of the inner wall is fractured, for the foreign body (frequently the stem of a pointed instrument, as the ferrule of an umbrella, etc.) may penetrate the cranium, or the splinters of the fractured bone may set up great irritation and inflammation of the brain and meninges. The severe character of the injury and the presence of cerebral symptoms, may not show themselves for a day or two after the accident.

If the fracture extends from the orbit into the ethmoidal or frontal cells, there is generally emphysema of the orbit and eyelids.

[Injuries to the superior orbital margin or its vicinity, which do not involve the roof of the orbit, are often borne very well, even when caries is the result; and this is true of pistol-shot wounds as of other injuries. The carious process is here very slow, and the sinus or fistula leading down to it, is generally very tortuous and long. The removal of the carious bone in the most thorough manner is, of course, at once indicated. Pistol balls have been found embedded in the orbital edge of the frontal bone without causing any grave symptoms. (See

[1] Zander and Geissler, loc. cit., 225.   [2] "Ophth. Rev.," No. 4, p. 837.

a paper by the Editor, in "Amer. Journ. of Med. Sciences," July, 1880, on Traumatic Lesions of the Bones of the Orbit.) Gunshot wounds of the orbit are not uncommon, and sometimes the ball may pass through the orbital walls transversely, destroying one or both eyes in its transit, usually the injury inflicted will depend both upon its penetration and direction; and is often fatal.

Dislocation of the malar bone from a violent fall upon the face, may cause extensive orbital hemorrhage and possibly diplopia from paralysis of the inferior oblique muscle. Anæsthesia of the infra-orbital nerve may last for a considerable period. A fracture of the orbit may occur from an injury to the head, without any of the ordinary symptoms of this lesion, and without at first any demonstrable ophthalmoscopic signs, until after a time the optic nerve may show signs of inflammation or atrophy. Other cases occur, in which an autopsy shows a line of fracture running through the optic foramen or roof of the orbit and uniting with a fracture at the base of the skull, together with more or less hemorrhage within the sheath of the optic nerve. (See "A Treatise on Diseases of the Eye" by Henry D. Noyes, 1881, p. 337 et seq.)—B.]

The treatment of injuries of the orbit must vary with their nature. In cases of incised and punctured wounds, we must endeavor to subdue the inflammatory reaction by cold compresses, leeches, etc., and an early evacuation of the pus. Foreign bodies should be removed as soon as possible, unless they are of so small a size that they would be found with difficulty, and their removal might cause more disturbance than their presence.

Before an operation is attempted for the removal of a foreign body, the size, nature, and position of the latter should be ascertained as accurately as possible by a careful examination. If the foreign body be considerable in size, and situated deeply in the orbit, so that it must be cut down upon, the outer canthus may have to be divided, in order that the upper or lower lid (as the case may be) can be turned up or down. The conjunctiva between the eyeball and the lid should be divided over the point where it is supposed that the foreign body is situated, and a probe or tip of the little finger be introduced to ascertain its exact position, so that it may be grasped and extracted with a pair of forceps. The incision should never be made through the skin of the eyelid, for the contraction consequent upon the cicatrization of the wound might give rise to subsequent ectropium. The lips of the incision at the outer canthus are then to be united by two or three fine sutures, or the twisted wire suture.

In fractures of the orbit the most absolute rest must be enforced, the patient should be placed upon low diet, and the use of stimulants should be forbidden. Cold compresses, and, if necessary, leeches, should be applied.

The eyeball may be dislocated and pushed out of the orbit by a foreign body, e. g., a piece of iron, the ferrule of an umbrella or stick, etc., being thrust into the socket. In such cases, the eye lies upon the cheek, protruding far beyond the lids, which cannot be closed over it. The optic nerve is, of course, greatly stretched, and vision more or less completely lost, but on the removal of the foreign body, and replacement of the eye, the sight may be perfectly restored. The foreign body should be immediately extracted, and the eye replaced. The latter is to be done by gently, yet firmly and steadily, pressing the eyeball back, which will cause it suddenly to spring back into the orbit, the sight being then generally at once restored. The eye should be retained in its position by a firm compress bandage.

13.—EXCISION OF THE EYEBALL.

The modern method of removing the eye was first devised by Bonnet and O'Ferral in 1841, independently of each other. Stoeber practised it in 1842, and Critchett first introduced it in London in 1851.

The principal advantages of this operation over the old one are, that the eye is removed from the ocular capsule without any injury to, or interference with, the cellular tissue of the orbit, or a division of the outer commissure of the eyelids; that the muscles are divided quite close to their insertion into the sclerotic, that nearly the whole of the conjunctiva is preserved, and that only a few bloodvessels are divided. Thus there is but a moderate amount of hemorrhage, and an excellent degree of mobility is preserved for the insertion of an artificial eye.

The operation is best performed in the following manner: The patient should lie on a couch, and a large sponge should be placed beneath the temple and cheek of the side corresponding to the eye about to be removed. so that the blood may not flow down his neck or over his clothes. An assistant should be ready with several smaller sponges, to wipe away the blood from the eye during the different steps of the operation. The patient having been brought thoroughly under the influence of an anæsthetic, and the eyelids held apart by the stop-speculum, the operator places himself behind the patient, and, fixing the eyeball steadily into a pair of forceps, divides the conjunctiva all round the cornea and quite close to the latter, with a pair of strong blunt-pointed scissors curved on the flat [Fig. 257]. He next incises the subconjunctival tissue at one point, and, passing a strabismus hook through this aperture, catches up one of the recti muscles, and divides it quite close to its insertion. The four recti muscles are to be thus divided in succession. When this has been done, the operator presses back the upper and lower eyelid, so as to make the eyeball spring forth through [Fig. 257.] the small opening in the conjunctiva and protrude between the eyelids. The cut end of the tendon of the external or internal rectus muscle being seized with the forceps, and the eyeball rolled to the corresponding side, the scissors (closed) are to be passed along the posterior surface of the globe until the optic nerve is reached, when the blades are to be opened and the nerve divided close to the sclerotic. The eyeball should now be lifted forward by the fingers, and any portions of conjunctiva or subconjunctival tissue which may adhere to the globe, as well as the insertion of the oblique muscles, are to be divided close to the sclerotic. This finishes the operation, and the eye will have been removed quite free from conjunctival or muscular tissue, and present a perfectly smooth and polished appearance.

As the operator stands behind the patient, it will be found most easy to divide the optic nerve of the right eye from the temporal side, the eye being at the same time rotated inwards the left optic nerve, on the contrary, is best divided from the nasal side. By so doing, the right hand can be used for either eye, and the operator is not obliged to alter his position.

The hemorrhage which ensues upon the division of the optic nerve and ophthalmic artery, is generally soon stopped by making a stream of cold water from a sponge (or, for want of this, from the narrow spout of a small jug) play upon the bottom of the orbit, and it will not be necessary to ligature any vessel. When the hemorrhage has stopped, the lips of the conjunctival aperture, through which the eye has been removed, may be brought together by a fine suture, passed through the four little lappets left in the interval of the recti muscles. The suture, which is best inserted with the long needle with a handle devised for this purpose by Mr. Hulke, may then be tied or twisted, so that the lips of the incision may be accurately brought together. It is still better, however, to wait with the tying of the suture for an hour or two, until all hemorrhage has ceased. Although the insertion of the suture brings the edges of the conjunctival wound very nicely together, it should not be employed in those cases in which the excised eye is acutely inflamed, as it prevents the exit of inflammatory exudations. When the operation is finished, a thick pledget of folded lint or a sponge should be pressed firmly for a few minutes against the lids, in order to stop the bleeding. Should this not arrest the hemorrhage, a compress of lint soaked in cold (or iced) water is to be tied very tightly over the eye. This is far less painful than keeping the lids open with a wire speculum for an hour or two, and packing the orbit with lint and small portions of sponge.

The after-treatment of cases of excision of the eye is generally very simple. A cold compress should be applied during the first few days, and the orbit syringed out with a little lukewarm water, to cleanse away the discharge. If the latter should continue for longer than a week or ten days, and the conjunctiva looks red and swollen, a mild astringent injection of sulphate of zinc or alum should be used two or three times daily. If symptoms of inflammation of the cellular tissue of the orbit should supervene, warm bread-and-water poultices or warm poppy fomentations should be applied, and the exit of pus be facilitated by a free incision into the conjunctiva: this should never be neglected if the lips of the wound have been closed by a suture. Should small granulations make their appearance on the conjunctival cicatrix, these should be at once snipped off with a pair of scissors.

When the eye is excised on account of the presence of an intra-ocular tumor, the optic nerve, instead of being divided close to the globe, must be cut as far back as we can reach, in order that all the diseased portion may, if possible, be removed. Or Von Graefe's preliminary division of the optic nerve may be performed, a description of which will be found in the article on "Glioma of the Retina" (p. 552). The extirpation of the eye together with the soft parts of the orbit, as in orbital tumors, is a more severe and protracted operation than the simple excision. The outer commissure of the lids must generall be divided, in order to give more room for the extirpation of the eye and the morbid contents of the orbit.

[For a discussion of the subject of "Optico-ciliary Neurotomy and Neurectomy," see the chapter on "Sympathetic Ophthalmia."—B.]

14.—THE APPLICATION OF ARTIFICIAL EYES
(PROTHESIS OCULI).

The use of an artificial eye should not be allowed until five or six weeks after the excision, when the cicatrix has become firmly united, and the parts are quiet and free from all irritation. If the eye has been removed on account of sympathetic irritation of the other, special care must be taken that no artificial eye is worn until all the sympathetic symptoms have permanently disappeared for some months, and the eye must be carefully watched for some time afterwards, lest the artificial eye might re-awaken them. Indeed, the wearing of an artificial eye for too long a time, so that it sets up great irritation, may even give rise to sympathetic disease.[1]

[1] *Vide* an interesting case of this kind recorded by Mr. Lawson, "R. L. O. H. Rep.," vi. 2, 128.

At first, a small eye should be worn for a short time each day, and then, when the parts have become accustomed to it and there is a complete absence of all symptoms of irritation, a larger one may be adopted and worn for a longer period, and at last the whole day, but it should *always be removed at night.* After the lapse of some months, the internal surface of the eye becomes rough, and as this is a ready source of irritation and discomfort a new one is required.

As the insertion and removal of the artificial eye require some little knack and practice, I subjoin the following concise and plain rules, which are given to the patients at the Royal London Ophthalmic Hospital.

Instructions for Persons wearing an Artificial Eye.—It should be taken out every night, and replaced in the morning.

To put the Eye in.—Place the left hand flat upon the forehead, with the fingers downwards, and with the two middle fingers raise the upper eyelid towards the eyebrow; then with the right hand, push the upper edge of the artificial eye beneath the upper eyelid, which may be allowed to drop upon the eye. The eye must now be supported with the middle fingers of the left hand, whilst the lower eyelid is raised over its lower edge with the right hand.

To take the Eye out.—The lower eyelids must be drawn downwards with the middle finger of the left hand, and then with the right hand the end of a small bodkin must be put beneath the lower edge of the artificial eye, which must be raised gently forward over the lower eyelid, when it will readily drop out; at this time care must be taken that the eye does not fall on the ground or other hard place, as it is very brittle, and might easily be broken by a fall.[1]

After it has been worn daily for six months, the polished surface of the artificial eye becomes rough; when this happens, it should be replaced by a new one; for unless this is done, uneasiness and inflammation may result.

[It is sometimes necessary to perform certain plastic operations upon the orbit, before an artificial eye can be introduced and worn. When the eye, orbit, and lids have been injured by extensive burning, whether by hot metals or fluids, the culs-de-sac become so contracted that an operation has to be done to make a place for the insertion of the eye. This also sometimes becomes necessary after severe orbital cellulitis.—B.]

---

[1] In order to avoid this accident, the patient should stoop over a cushion or handkerchief placed on a table, or over a bed.

EXPLANATION OF THE PLATES.

PLATE I.

Figs. 1 and 2.

The Normal Fundus Oculi (*vide p.* 755).

In Fig. 1 (which is taken from a person with black hair and a dark-brown iris) the optic nerve entrance appears circular, and of a yellowish-white tint. The bloodvessels emerge somewhat to the left of the centre of the disk, which is here of a deeper white. The paler vessels are the retinal arteries, the darker ones the veins. They pass over the disk to the retina, where they course and divide in different directions, chiefly upwards, downwards, and towards the left. At some little distance to the right of, and slightly below, the disk, is noticed a large dark-red spot, with a small white dot in the centre. This is the macula lutea, or yellow spot, with its fovea centralis. It will be observed that the vessels course round the yellow spot, leaving it free. The fine gray film in the region of the disk and the yellow spot is due to the reflex yielded by the retina; it is only observable in dark eyes, and is consequently altogether absent in Fig. 2. The fundus of the eye is of a rich dark-red tint, and only the retinal vessels are apparent, those of the choroid being hidden by the density of the pigment in the epithelial layer and stroma of the choroid.

In Fig. 2 (taken from the eye of a person with very light hair and a blue iris) the appearances are quite different. The disk is of a more rosy tint, the retinal vessels, although very distinct, are less markedly so than on the darker background of Fig. 1. The region of the yellow spot is of a bright red color, and the fovea centralis appears in the form of a little light circle. But the greatest difference is noticed in the pale, brilliantly red color of the fundus, and the distinctness with which the finest branches of the choroidal vessels can be traced. The ciliary arteries enter in the region of the yellow spot, and, running towards the periphery, ramify in various directions, and partly pass over directly into the larger branches of the venæ vorticosæ, situated at the equator of the eye.

Plate I.

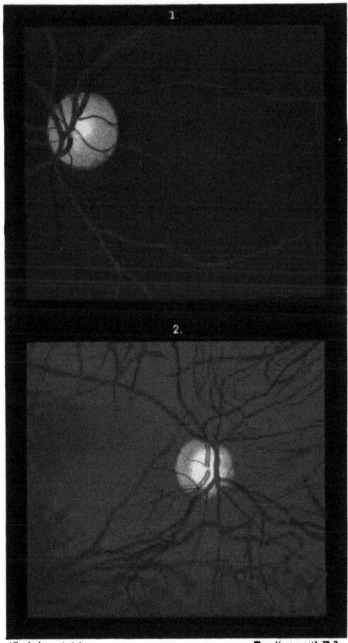

after Liebreich's Atlas

EXPLANATION OF THE PLATES.

PLATE I.

Figs. 1 and 2.

The Normal Fundus Oculi (*vide p.* 755).

n Fig. 1 (which is taken from a person with black hair and a dark-brown iris)
optic nerve entrance appears circular, and of a yellowish-white tint. The
odvessels emerge somewhat to the left of the centre of the disk, which is here
a deeper white. The paler vessels are the retinal arteries, the darker ones the
as. They pass over the disk to the retina, where they course and divide in
erent directions, chiefly upwards, downwards, and towards the left. At some
ue distance to the right of, and slightly below, the disk, is noticed a large dark-
red spot, with a small white dot in the centre. This is the macula lutea, or yellow
spot, with its fovea centralis. It will be observed that the vessels course round
the yellow spot, leaving it free. The fine gray film in the region of the disk and
the yellow spot is due to the reflex yielded by the retina; it is only observable in
dark eyes, and is consequently altogether absent in Fig. 2. The fundus of the eye
is of a rich dark-red tint, and only the retinal vessels are apparent, those of the
choroid being hidden by the density of the pigment in the epithelial layer and
stroma of the choroid.

In Fig. 2 (taken from the eye of a person with very light hair and a blue iris)
the appearances are quite different. The disk is of a more rosy tint, the retinal
vessels, although very distinct, are less markedly so than on the darker background
of Fig. 1. The region of the yellow spot is of a bright red color, and the fovea
centralis appears in the form of a little light circle. But the greatest difference is
iced in the pale, brilliantly red color of the fundus, and the distinctness with
the finest branches of the choroidal vessels can be traced. The ciliary arteries
the region of the yellow spot, and, running towards the periphery, ramify
ns directions, and partly pass over directly into the larger branches of the
ticosa, situated at the equator of the eye.

PLATE II.

Fig. 3.

Sclerotico-choroiditis Posterior (*Staphyloma Posticum*), p. 354.

This figure illustrates the appearances presented by an extensive sclerotico-choroiditis posterior. Towards the outer side of the disk is observed a large white figure, over which the retinal vessels appear to run a somewhat straighter course, and to be rather more numerous and distinct. The disk is oval, and its shortest diameter (in this case the horizontal) shows the direction in which the ectasia (bulging) is situated. In the vicinity of the disk and of the white figure, the choroid is observed to be somewhat thinned; on the left, the pigment in the epithelial layer is diminished, and hence the choroidal vessels are particularly marked. The intra-vascular spaces are here also peculiarly conspicuous and striking, which is due to the increase in the pigment of the stroma. Whereas, on the right side of the figure, the pigmentation of the epithelial layer conceals the subjacent tissue and the vessels.

Fig. 4.

Choroiditis Disseminata Syphilitica, with Secondary Atrophy of the Retina and Optic Nerve (p. 351).

In this figure we notice very numerous, irregular, circumscribed spots, of palish-pink or whitish tint, surrounded by a dark fringe of pigment; others, appearing simply as small black patches. In some of the larger spots, a choroidal vessel can be distinctly seen to pass over it. The optic disk is atrophied, and of a bluish tint. It is completely devoid of bloodvessels, excepting the two little twigs which can just be discerned running over its edge. But not a single retinal vessel can be seen over the whole fundus; and on account of this atrophy of the retina, the choroidal vessels appear with unusual distinctness.

PLATE II.

Fig. 3.

Sclerotico-choroiditis Posterior (Staphyloma Posticum), p. 354.

This figure illustrates the appearances presented by an extensive sclerotico-choroiditis posterior. Towards the outer side of the disk is observed a large white figure, over which the retinal vessels appear to run a somewhat straighter course, and to be rather more numerous and distinct. The disk is oval, and its shortest diameter (in this case the horizontal) shows the direction in which the ectasia (bulging) is situated. In the vicinity of the disk and of the white figure, the choroid is observed to be somewhat thinned; on the left, the pigment in the epithelial layer is diminished, and hence the choroidal vessels are particularly marked. The intra-vascular spaces are here also peculiarly conspicuous and striking, which is due to the increase in the pigment of the stroma. Whereas, on the right side of the figure, the pigmentation of the epithelial layer conceals the subjacent tissue and the vessels.

Fig. 4.

Choroiditis Disseminata Syphilitica, with Secondary Atrophy of the Retina and Optic Nerve (p. 351).

In this figure we notice very numerous, irregular, circumscribed spots, of palish-pink or whitish tint, surrounded by a dark fringe of pigment; others, appearing simply as small black patches. In some of the larger spots, a choroidal vessel can be distinctly seen to pass over it. The optic disk is atrophied, and of a bluish tint. It is completely devoid of bloodvessels, excepting the two little twigs which can just be discerned running over its edge. But not a single retinal vessel can be seen over the whole fundus; and on account of this atrophy of the retina, the choroidal vessels appear with unusual distinctness.

PLATE III.

Fig. 5.

Retinitis Pigmentosa (p. 527).

Numerous large, irregular, black figures are observed scattered about the fundus, being arranged at some points along the retinal vessels, which are extremely attenuated, and here and there quite unapparent. At other situations, the black patches show irregular prolongations, the extremities of which touch those of other spots. Hence they assume a certain similarity to bone corpuscles. The optic nerve is white and atrophied, and the retinal arteries are excessively small and attenuated.

Fig. 6.

Retinitis Albuminurica (p. 513).

This illustration is peculiarly characteristic of the ophthalmoscopic appearances presented by the retinitis met with in Bright's disease. At the disk, and its vicinity, is observed a delicate gray opacity, which is caused by a serous infiltration and proliferation of the connective tissue of the retina. Beyond this lies the white, glistening mound, which is due to sclerosis of the optic nerve fibres and fatty degeneration of the connective-tissue elements. The extreme margin of this white mound is broken up into small, irregular patches, which assume, in the region of the yellow spot (to the left of the disk), a peculiar stellate arrangement, looking as if they had been splashed in with a brush. The retinal arteries are much diminished, both in calibre and number. The veins are dilated and tortuous, and the vessel running upwards, is interrupted in its course by the infiltration, and, at the point of interruption, are noticed well-marked blood extravasations. These, as well as most of the other hemorrhages, show by their irregular outline and striated, feathery appearance, that they lie in the optic nerve layer of the retina.

Plate III.

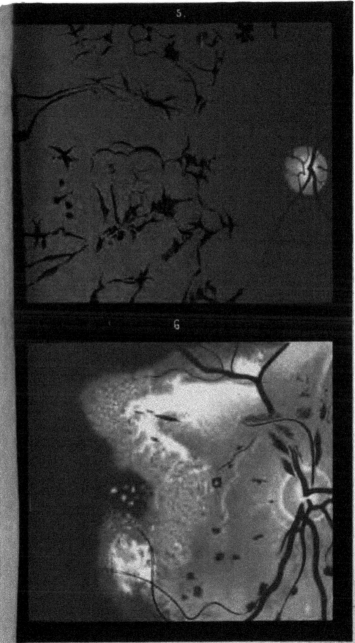

5.

6.

ter Liebreich's Atlas.   Thos Hunter Lith Phila.

PLATE IV.

Fig. 7.

Hemorrhagic Effusions into the Retina, Retinitis Apoplectica (p. 524).

In Fig. 7, numerous blood effusions of varying size and shape are noticed in the retina, being situated in different layers of the latter. But even between the larger patches, the retina is not free, for minute hemorrhagic spots are strewn about in all directions. The retinal arteries are here and there filled with blood coagula, but at other points they are quite bloodless, and changed into narrow white bands. In a few branches, the circulation is, however, unimpeded.

Fig. 8.

Embolism of the Central Artery of the Retina (p. 541).

Here we notice, in the region of the yellow spot, a well-marked, grayish-white opacity, which is due to a serous infiltration of the retina. In its centre is a conspicuous cherry-colored spot, which is not caused by a blood effusion. as might be supposed at the first glance, but is due to the fact that the retina is transparent at this point, and thus permits the choroid to shine through, which assumes a redder tinge in consequence of the contrast with the grayish-white opacity. The vessels running towards the yellow spot are particularly conspicuous on account of the blood coagula which they contain, and of the white opacity. The outline of the disk is slightly undefined and encircled by a faint opacity. The retinal veins show a distinct retardation in the circulation, and contain here and there blood coagula. The arteries are greatly diminished in size, and become quite indistinct at certain points of their course.

PLATE V.

Fig. 9.

Cysticercus in the Vitreous Humor (p. 502).

This figure illustrates the appearance presented by a cysticercus in the vitreous humor. The entozoon shows itself in the form of a well-defined, bluish-gray vesicle, which is so transparent, that in the central portion the red tint from the choroid can be distinctly seen to shine through. The neck is more opaque in tint than the rest of the entozoon, and it is studded with small white dots (chalky particles). At the head, two suckers can be recognized, the other two being placed posteriorly. The buccal extremity is directed upwards. The small, circular, gray spots which partly encircle the vesicle, are caused, according to Liebreich, by a peculiar opacity of the vitreous humor due to the suction of the entozoon, and are quite characteristic of the presence of a cysticercus.

Fig. 10.

Detachment of the Retina (p. 532).

Fig. 10 represents a case of old-standing and extensive detachment of the retina. The lower half of the retina (which shows a tolerable sharply-defined edge towards the left) bulges forwards into the vitreous humor, and is thrown into well-marked folds, and on this account, as well as of the color of the subjacent fluid, it shows a peculiar greenish-gray tint. The retinal vessels are undulating and tortuous, riding on the folds of the retina, and they assume a darker tint in consequence of the gray background.

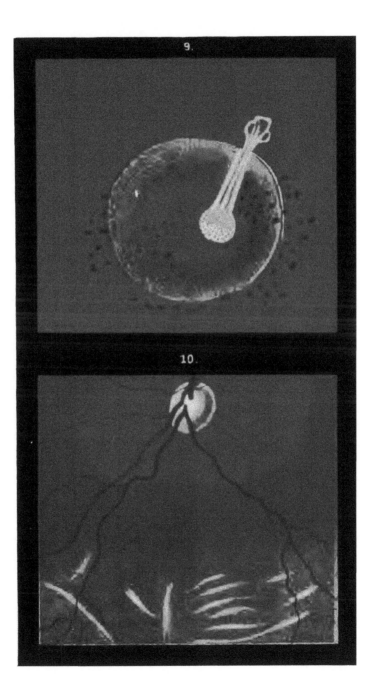

F
pat
peo
spi
of
The
tho
due

I
neu
vei
hie
tw
tin
a g
vei

B
les
In
at
sic

PLATE VI.

Figs. 11 and 12.

Atrophy of the Optic Nerve (p. 572).

Fig. 11 shows the appearances presented by atrophy of the optic nerve, in a patient affected with locomotor ataxy. The disk is slightly excavated, and of the peculiar bluish mottled tint, so frequently observed in the atrophy dependent upon spinal disease. The arteries are small and attenuated. Fig. 12 represents a case of white atrophy after meningitis. The disk is very white, and faintly cupped. The arteries are much diminished in calibre, and some of the veins (as some of those in Fig. 11) show a well-marked, white streak along their margin, which is due to sclerosis of the tunica adventitia.

Figs. 13 and 14.

Optic Neuritis (p. 556).

In Fig. 13 is represented the swollen and enlarged papilla consequent upon optic neuritis, the opacity of the disk being dense and markedly striated. The retinal veins are enlarged and tortuous, the arteries diminished in size, and, here and there, hidden by the exudation. Fig. 14 shows the condition of the same optic nerve two years later, when consecutive atrophy had supervened. The uniformly opaque tint of the disk, as well as its somewhat undefined margin, help to distinguish it at a glance from the progressive form of atrophy (Fig. 12). Moreover, although the veins are less dilated than in Fig. 13, they yet retain a certain degree of tortuosity.

Figs. 15 and 16.

Glaucomatous Excavation of the Optic Nerve (p. 575).

the two figures are observed different degrees of glaucomatous excavation. sent all the characteristic features of this disease, but in Fig. 15 they are ed than in Fig. 16, in which the cup is much deeper and more abrupt. ase, the disk is surrounded by a pale, light girdle, its color is much darker riphery than in the centre, and the retinal vessels are more or less con- bent or interrupted at the edge of the papilla.

pa
pe
sp
of
Tl
th
dι

nι
vι
h
tι
ti
a

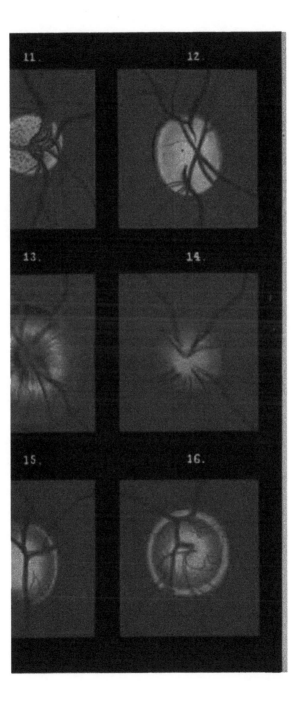

SELECTIONS FROM THE TEST-TYPES

OF

PROF. EDWARD JAEGER, OF VIENNA,

AND

DR. H. SNELLEN, OF UTRECHT.

TEST-TYPES,

CORRESPONDING TO THE SCHRIFT-SCALEN OF
EDWARD JAEGER, OF VIENNA.

No. 1.—*Diamond.*

A Fox being caught in a trap, was glad to compound for his neck by leaving his tail behind him; but upon coming abroad into the world, he began to be so sensible of the disgrace such a defect would bring upon him, that he almost wished he had died rather than come away without it. However, resolving to make the best of a bad matter, he called a meeting of the rest of the Foxes, and proposed that all should follow his example. "You have no notion," said he, "of the ease and comfort with which I now move about: I could never have believed it if I had not tried it myself; but really when one comes to reason upon it, a tail is such an ugly, inconvenient, unnecessary appendage, that the only wonder is that, as Foxes, we could have put up with it so long. I propose, therefore, my worthy brethren, that you all profit by the experience that I am most willing to afford you, and that all Foxes from this day forward cut off their tails." Upon this one of the oldest stepped forward, and said, "I rather think,

No. 2.—*Pearl.*

my friend, that you would not have advised us to part with our tails, if there were any chance of recovering your own." A Man who had been bitten by a Dog was going about asking who could cure him. One that met him said, 'Sir, if you would be cured, take a bit of bread and dip it in the blood of the wound, and give it to the dog that bit you." The man smiled, and said, "If I were to follow your advice, I should be bitten by all the dogs in the city." He who proclaims himself ready to buy up his enemies will never want a supply of them. A certain man had the good fortune to possess a Goose that laid him a Golden Egg every day. But dissatisfied with so slow an income, and thinking to seize the whole treasure at once, he killed the Goose, and cutting her open, found her—just what any other goose

No. 4.—*Minion.*

would be! Much wants more and loses all. A Dog made his bed in a Manger, and lay snarling and growling to keep the horses from their provender. "See," said one of them, "what a miserable cur! who neither can eat corn himself, nor will allow those to eat it who can." A Viper entering into a smith's shop began looking about for something to eat. At length, seeing a file, he went up to it, and commenced biting at it; but the File bade him leave him alone, saying, "You are likely to get little from me whose business it is to bite others." A Cat, grown feeble with age

No. 6.—*Bourgeois.*

and no longer able to hunt the Mice as she was wont to do, bethought herself how she might entice them within reach of her paw. Thinking that she might pass herself off for a bag, or for a dead cat at least, she suspended herself by the hind legs from a peg, in the hope that the Mice would no longer be afraid to come near her. An old Mouse, who was wise enough to keep his distance, whispered to a friend, "Many a

No. 8.—*Small Pica.*

bag have I seen in my day, but never one with a cat's head." "Hang there, good Madam," said the other, "as long as you please, but I would not trust myself within reach of you though you were stuffed with straw." Old birds are not to be caught with chaff. As a Cock was

scratching up the straw in a farm-yard, in search of food for the hens, he hit upon a Jewel that by some chance had found its way there. Ho! said he, you are a very fine thing, no doubt, to those who

prize you; but give me a barley-corn before all the pearls in the world. The Cock was a sensible Cock; but there are many silly people who despise what is precious only

because they cannot understand it. A Man who kept a Horse and an Ass was wont in his journeys

to spare the Horse, and put all the burden upon the Ass's

No. 16.—2-line Great Primer.

back. The Ass, who had been some while ailing, besought the Horse one day to relieve

No. 18.—Canon.

him of part of his load; For if, said he, you would take a portion,

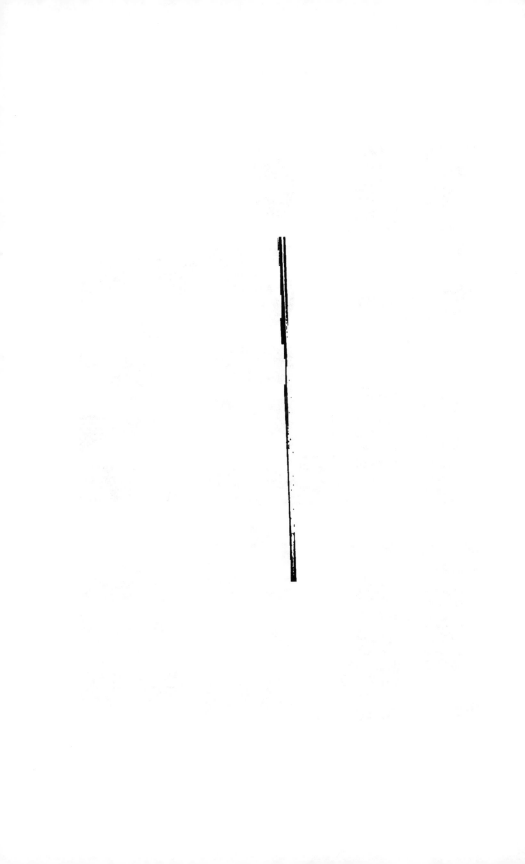

No. 19.—4-line Condensed.

I shall soon get well again; but if you

No. 20.—8-line Roman.

refuse to hel

I.

[illegible]

II.

F H K O S U Y A C E G L 2

III.

C E G L N P R T V Z B D 3

IV.

V Z B D F H K O S U Y A 4

V.

S U Y A C E G L N P R T 5

VI.

N P R T V Z B D F H K O 6

VII.

F H K O S U Y A C E G L 7

VIII.

C E G L N P R T V B D 8

X.

Z B D F H K O S U Y A 10

XII.

S U Y A C G N P R 12

XV.

P R B D H K O 15

XX.

Y A C E G L

XXX.

H K O

XL.

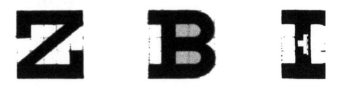

Z B I

L.

P R T

LXX.

G L

Snellen's Test-Types

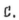 C C.

C.

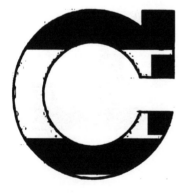

INDEX.

A TREATISE ON THE PRINCIPLES AND PRACTICE OF MED-ICINE. By Austin Flint, M. D. Professor of the Principles and Practice of Medicine and of Clinical Medicine in Bellevue Hospital Medical College. Designed for the use of Students and Practitioners. Fifth edition, thoroughly revised and much improved. In one large and closely-printed octavo volume of 1150 pages. Cloth, $5.50; leather, $6.50; very handsome half Russia, raised bands, $7.

Flint's Treatise is the work of an accomplished hospital physician, and is remarkable for its masterly descriptions of disease. It is a work on clinical medicine, embodying the experience of a lifetime. It has been carefully brought up to the present day, and the additions and alterations have been so great that it is virtually a new work, and not merely a new edition. In making these alterations, Flint openly confesses that he has not been too careful to maintain a character for consistency, but has endeavored to give his reader his views more matured, and, as he believes, more truthful views, careless of any discrepancy between them and those he formerly advanced. Flint is right; and only in this way could he produce a work worthy of being looked upon as a standard. — *Edinburgh Medical Journal*, June, 1882.

A HANDBOOK OF DIAGNOSIS AND TREATMENT OF DISEASES OF THE THROAT, NOSE, AND NASO-PHARYNX. Second edition. In one very handsome 12mo. volume of 294 pages, with 77 illustrations. Cloth, $1.75. *Just ready*.

In preparing a second edition of this work, the author has endeavored to include all recent advances in this department of surgery. Voluminous additions have thus been necessitated in all portions of the book, and the number of illustrations has been increased by the addition of many beautiful and accurate engravings.

A SYSTEM OF MIDWIFERY, · INCLUDING THE DISEASES OF PREGNANCY AND THE PUERPERAL STATE. By William Leishman, M. D., Regius Professor of Midwifery in the University of Glasgow, etc. Third American edition, specially revised by the Author, with additions by John S. Parry, M. D., Obstetrician to the Philadelphia Hospital. etc. In one large and very handsome octavo volume of 740 pages, with 205 illustrations. Cloth, $4.50; leather, $5.50; half Russia, $6.

The author is broad in his teachings, and discusses briefly the comparative anatomy of the pelvis and the mobility of the pelvic articulations The second chapter is devoted especially to the study of the pelvis, while in the third the female organs of generation are introduced. The structure and development of the ovum are admirably described, then follow chapters upon the various subjects embraced in the study of midwifery. The descriptions throughout the work are plain and pleasing It is sufficient to state that in this, the last edition of this well-known work, every recent advancement in this field has been brought forward —*Physician and Surgeon*, January, 1880.

THE PRINCIPLES AND PRACTICE OF GYNÆCOLOGY, for the use of Students and Practitioners of Medicine. By Thomas Addis Emmet, M. D., Surgeon to the Woman's Hospital, New York. Second edition, thoroughly revised. In one large and very handsome octavo volume of 879 pages, with 133 illustrations. Cloth, $5; leather, $6; very handsome half Russia, raised bands, $6.50.

In no country in the world has gynæcology received more attention than in America. It is, then, with a feeling of pleasure that we welcome a work on diseases of women from so eminent a gynæcologist as Dr. Emmet. The work is essentially clinical, and leaves a strong impress of the author's individuality. We can say that the work teems with original ideas, fresh and valuable methods of practice, and is written in a clear and elegant style, worthy of the literary reputation of the country of Longfellow and Oliver Wendell Holmes. —*British Medical Journal*, February 21, 1880.

A COMPLETE PRACTICAL TREATISE ON THE DISEASES OF CHILDREN. By J. Lewis Smith, M. D., Clinical Professor of Diseases of Children in the Bellevue Hospital Medical College, N. Y. Fifth edition, thoroughly revised and rewritten. In one handsome octavo volume of 836 pages, with illustrations. Cloth, $4.50; leather, $5.50; very handsome half Russia, raised bands, $6.

There is no book published on the subjects of which this one treats that is its equal in value to the physician. While he has said just enough to impart the information desired by general practitioners on such questions as etiology, pathology, prognosis, etc., he has devoted more attention to the diagnosis and treatment of the ailments which he so accurately describes, and such information is exactly what is wanted by the majority of "family physicians."—*Virginia Monthly*, February, 1882.

HENRY C. LEA'S SON & CO., PHILADELPHIA.

A PRACTICAL TREATISE ON DISEASES OF THE SKIN.

use of Students and Practitioners. By JAMES NEVINS HYDE. M.D., Profess
matology and Venereal Diseases in Rush Medical College. Chicago.   In one handso
volume of 570 pages, with 66 illustrations.   Cloth. $4.25 : leather. $5.25.   *Just re*

Prof Hyde has given to the profession a valuable and comprehensive work upon this special subject—exposing the etiology, symptomatology and treatment of diseases of the skin in a concise and thorough manner The book is a valuable one for the student and practitioner, containing all the latest progress made in der-

matology, and will, without doubt, answ pected by its author—to make the genera thoroughly informed in regard to the tre taneous diseases; and it will prove a valu reference to the specialist. — *New Orleans Surgical Journal.* April, 1883.

A SYSTEM OF SURGERY; Pathological. Diagnostic. Therape

Operative.   By SAMUEL D. GROSS. M.D., LL.D., D.C.L. Oxon., LLI
Emeritus Professor of Surgery in the Jefferson Medical College of Philadelphia.   Si
thoroughly revised and greatly enlarged and improved.   In two large and beautif
imperial octavo volumes containing 2382 closely-printed pages. with 1623 (
Leather, raised bands. $15: very handsome half Russia, raised bands. $16.   *Part*

We have purposely abstained from comment to estimate of the book before us   It has formerly been noticed more than once in our columns, and it is enough
now to remark that the present edition fully maintains
the reputation the work has acquired.   Though Prof

Gross' book is the resource of his college
several parts have been extended, elabor
pified, and it has become a complete an
book of reference alike for the student an
a home.—*The Londric Lancet*. January 11,

A PRACTICAL TREATISE ON IMPOTENCE. STERILIT

ALLIED DISORDERS OF THE MALE SEXUAL ORGANS. By S
GROSS. A M., M.D., Professor of the Principles of Surgery and of Clinical Surgery
Person Medical College of Philadelphia.   Second edition.   In one very handsome
one of 168 pages, with 10 illustrations.   Cloth. $1.50.   *Just ready.*

The wide circulation of a large edition of this work, the favorable comments which it h from the medical press, its translation into the Russian language and the fact that it has pro... subject, constitute an evidence that it has filled the void for which it w designed.

... men in treating these cases will describe the direc
... gives the treatment very perspicuous...
... — *The Liverpool Medico-Chirurgical J.*

THE PRACTICE OF SURGERY By THOMAS BRYANT, F.R.C

... Third American from the third and revis
... John H. Roberts, M.D.   In one
... Cloth. $6.50. Leath

... to make the surgery what follows the...
... diagnosis and treatment in any c...
... — *Cincinnati New Remedy*

THE EAR ITS ANATOMY PHYSIOLOGY AND DISEA

... Surgeon ...
... Philadelphia Hospital. Surgeon in ch...
... Cloth but some botany of the
... Cloth. $3.50 : very handsome half Ru

... references are ...
...

HENRY C. LEA'S SON & CO.'S

(LATE HENRY C. LEA)

CLASSIFIED CATALOGUE

OF

MEDICAL AND SURGICAL

PUBLICATIONS.

In asking the attention of the profession to the works advertised in the following pages, the publishers would state that no pains are spared to secure a continuance of the confidence earned for the publications of the house by their careful selection and accuracy and finish of execution.

The large number of inquiries received from the profession for a finer class of bindings than is usually placed on medical books has induced us to put certain of our standard publications in half Russia; and, that the growing taste may be encouraged, the prices have been fixed at so small an advance over the cost of sheep as to place it within the means of all to possess a library that shall have attractions as well for the eye as for the mind of the reading practitioner.

The printed prices are those at which books can generally be supplied by booksellers throughout the United States, who can readily procure for their customers any works not kept in stock. Where access to bookstores is not convenient, books will be sent by mail postpaid on receipt of the price, and as the limit of mailable weight has been removed, no difficulty will be experienced in obtaining through the post-office any work in this catalogue. No risks, however, are assumed either on the money or on the books, and no publications but our own are supplied, so that gentlemen will in most cases find it more convenient to deal with the nearest bookseller.

' A handsomely illustrated catalogue will be sent to any address on receipt of a three-cent stamp.

HENRY C. LEA'S SON & CO.

Nos. 706 and 708 Sansom St., Philadelphia, June, 1883.

PROSPECTUS FOR 1883.

A NEW WEEKLY MEDICAL JOURNAL.

SUBSCRIPTION RATES.

The Medical News	Five Dollars.
The American Journal of the Medical Sciences .	Five Dollars.

COMMUTATION RATES.

The Medical News	} Nine Dollars per
The American Journal of the Medical Sciences	} annum, in advance.

THE MEDICAL NEWS.

A National Weekly Periodical, of from 28 to 32 Quarto Pages, containing more Reading Matter than any other Weekly Medical Journal in America.

The unprecedented growth of the subscription list of THE MEDICAL NEWS during 1882 is gratifying to all concerned in its publication, not only as assuring its continued success, but as proving that they were not mistaken in supposing that the profession felt the need of and would generously support a weekly journal, national in the fullest sense of the word, devoted to the best interests of medical science, and conducted with the forethought to devise and energy and ability necessary to execute every available plan for enhancing its usefulness. Encouraged by this approbation, those in charge of THE NEWS will make during 1883 renewed efforts to strengthen in every way its hold upon the respect and esteem of the of the regular profession, it is the chosen vehicle for the conveyance of the most important intelligence from all parts of the country.

The general plan of THE NEWS affords ample space for the presentation of articles upon all branches of medical science. The opening pages are devoted to **Original Lectures** by the ablest teachers of the day, which are invariably revised by their authors before publication, thus insuring an authenticity and exactitude otherwise unattainable. In the department of **Original Articles**, THE NEWS will endeavor, as heretofore, to surpass its contemporaries in the intrinsic value of its contributions. Under the caption of **Hospital Notes** is laid open the vast and rich store of clinical information developed in the chief hospitals of the globe. The department of **Medical Progress** consists of condensations of articles of importance appearing in the leading medical, pharmaceutical and scientific journals of the world. The **Editorial Articles** are from the pens of a large and able EDITORIAL BOARD, and discuss living subjects in all departments of medical science in a thoughtful, independent and scholarly manner. Important subjects, requiring unusually elaborate consideration, are treated in **Special Articles**. The **Proceedings of Societies** in all parts of the country afford a means of imparting valuable information, for which due space is reserved. For the collection of **News Items**, and for **Correspondence**, THE NEWS enjoys an organization similar to that of a daily newspaper, and by mail and telegraph receives notice of all professional events of interest through special correspondents, located in the following cities:—In the United States: Portland, Boston, New York, Baltimore, Pittsburgh, Washington, Charleston, New Orleans, Cincinnati, Chicago, Detroit, Kansas City and San Francisco. In Canada: Montreal. In Great Britain: London and Edinburgh. In Continental Europe: Paris, Berlin, Vienna and Florence. In Asia: Yokohama, Canton, Hong Kong and Calcutta. In South America: Rio Janeiro and Valparaiso. In Cuba: Havana. Due attention will be paid to **New Publications**, **New Instruments** and **New Pharmaceutical Preparations**, and a column will be devoted to **Notes and Queries**. Space is reserved each week for accurate reports of all changes in the **Army and Navy Medical Service**.

THE MEDICAL NEWS appears in a double-columned quarto form, printed by the latest improved Hoe speed presses, on handsome paper, from a clear, easily read type, specially cast for its use.

It will thus be seen that THE MEDICAL NEWS employs all the approved methods of modern journalism in its efforts to render itself indispensable to the profession; and, in the anticipation of an unprecedented circulation, its subscription has been placed at the exceedingly low rate of $5 per annum, in advance. At this price it ranks as the cheapest medical periodical in this country, and when taken in connection with THE AMERICAN JOURNAL at NINE DOLLARS per annum, it is confidently asserted that a larger amount of material of the highest class is offered than can be obtained elsewhere, even at a much higher price.

THE AMERICAN JOURNAL of the MEDICAL SCIENCES,

Edited by I. MINIS HAYS, A. M., M. D.,

Is published Quarterly, on the first days of January, April, July and October, each Number containing over Three Hundred Octavo Pages, fully Illustrated.

Founded in 1820, THE AMERICAN JOURNAL entered with 1883 upon the sixty-fourth consecutive year of faithful and honorable service to the profession. Being the only periodical in the English language capable of presenting elaborate articles—the form in which the most important discoveries have always been communicated to the profession—THE AMERICAN JOURNAL cannot fail to be of the utmost value to physicians who would keep themselves *au courant* with the medical thought of the day. It may justly claim that it numbers among its contributors all the most distinguished members of the profession, that its history is identified with the advances of medical knowledge, and that its circulation is co-extensive with the use of the English language.

During 1883 THE JOURNAL will continue to present those features which have long proved so attractive to its readers.

The **Original Department** will consist of elaborate and richly illustrated articles from the pens of the most eminent members of the profession in all parts of the country.

The **Review Department** will maintain its well-earned reputation for discernment and impartiality, and will contain elaborate reviews of new works and topics of the day, and numerous analytical and bibliographical notices by competent writers.

Following these comes the **Quarterly Summary of Improvements and Discoveries in the Medical Sciences,** which, being a classified and arranged condensation of important articles appearing in the chief medical journals of the world, furnishes a compact digest of medical progress abroad and at home.

The subscription price of THE AMERICAN JOURNAL OF THE MEDICAL SCIENCES has never been raised during its long career. It is still sent free of postage for Five Dollars per annum in advance.

Taken together, the JOURNAL and NEWS combine the advantages of the elaborate preparation that can be devoted to a quarterly with the prompt conveyance of intelligence by the weekly; while, by special management, duplication of matter is rendered impossible.

It will thus be seen that for the very moderate sum of NINE DOLLARS in advance the subscriber will receive free of postage a weekly and a quarterly journal, both reflecting the latest advances of the medical sciences, and containing an equivalent of more than 4000 octavo pages, stored with the choicest material, original and selected, that can be furnished by the best medical minds of both hemispheres. It would be impossible to find elsewhere so large an amount of matter of the same value offered at so low a price.

Gentlemen desiring to avail themselves of the advantages thus offered will do well to forward their subscriptions at an early day, in order to insure the receipt of complete sets for 1883.

☞ The safest mode of remittance is by bank check or postal money order, drawn to the order of the undersigned; where these are not accessible, remittances for subscriptions may be made at the risk of the publishers by forwarding in *registered* letters. Address,

HENRY C. LEA'S SON & CO., Nos. 706 and 708 Sansom St., Philadelphia, Pa.

₊ Communications to both these periodicals are invited from gentlemen in all parts of the country. Original articles contributed exclusively to either periodical are liberally paid for upon publication. When necessary to elucidate the text, illustrations will be furnished without cost to the author.

All letters pertaining to the *Editorial Department* of THE MEDICAL NEWS and THE AMERICAN JOURNAL OF THE MEDICAL SCIENCES should be addressed to the EDITORIAL OFFICES, 1004 Walnut Street, Philadelphia.

All letters pertaining to the *Business Department* of these journals should be addressed *exclusively* to HENRY C. LEA'S SON & CO., 706 and 708 Sansom Street, Philadelphia.

MEDICAL LEXICON; A Dictionary of Medical Science: Containing a concise explanation of the various Subjects and Terms of Anatomy, Physiology, Pathology, Hygiene, Therapeutics, Pharmacology, Pharmacy, Surgery, Obstetrics, Medical Jurisprudence and Dentistry, Notices of Climate and of Mineral Waters, Formulæ for Officinal, Empirical and Dietetic Preparations, with the Accentuation and Etymology of the Terms, and the French and other Synonymes, so as to constitute a French as well as an English Medical Lexicon. A new edition, thoroughly revised, and very greatly modified and augmented. By RICHARD J. DUNGLISON, M.D. In one very large and handsome royal octavo volume of 1139 pages. Cloth, $6.50; leather, raised bands, $7.50; very handsome half Russia, raised bands, $8.

The object of the author, from the outset, has not been to make the work a mere lexicon or dictionary of terms, but to afford under each word a condensed view of its various medical relations, and thus to render the work an epitome of the existing condition of medical science. Starting with this view, the immense demand which has existed for the work has enabled him, in repeated revisions, to augment its completeness and usefulness until at length it has attained the position of a recognized and standard authority wherever the language is spoken. Special pains have been taken in the preparation of the present edition to maintain this enviable reputation. The additions to the vocabulary are more numerous than in any previous revision, and particular attention has been bestowed on the accentuation, which will be found marked on every word. The typographical arrangement has been greatly improved, rendering reference much more easy, and every care has been taken with the mechanical execution. The volume now contains the matter of at least four ordinary octavos.

A book of which every American ought to be proud. When the learned author of the work passed away, probably all of us feared lest the book should not maintain its place in the advancing science whose terms it defines. Fortunately, Dr. Richard J. Dunglison, having assisted his father in the revision of several editions of the work, and having been, therefore, trained in the methods and imbued with the spirit of the book, has been able to edit it as a work of the kind should be edited—to carry it on steadily, without jar or interruption, along the grooves of thought it has travelled during its lifetime. To show the magnitude of the task which Dr. Dunglison has assumed and carried through, it is only necessary to state that more than six thousand new subjects have been added in the present edition.—*Philadelphia Medical Times*, Jan. 3, 1874.

About the first book purchased by the medical student is the Medical Dictionary. The lexicon explanatory of technical terms is simply a *sine qua non*. In a science so extensive and with such collaterals as medicine, it is as much a necessity also to the practising physician. To meet the wants of students and most physicians the dictionary must be condensed while comprehensive, and practical while perspicacious. It was because Dunglison's met these indications that it became at once the dictionary of general use wherever medicine was studied in the English language. In no former revision have the alterations and additions been so great. The chief terms have been set in black letter, while the derivatives follow in small caps; an arrangement which greatly facilitates reference.—*Cincinnati Clinic*, Jan. 10, 1874.

As a standard work of reference Dunglison's work has been well known for about forty years, and needs no words of praise on our part to commend it to the members of the medical, and likewise of the pharmaceutical, profession. Both especially are in need of a work which gives clear and reliable information on the thousands of new facts and terms which they are liable to encounter in pursuing their daily vocations, but which they cannot be expected to be familiar with. That they before us fully supplies this want.—*American Journal of Pharmacy*, Feb. 1874.

Particular care has been devoted to derivation and accentuation of terms. With regard to the latter, indeed, the present edition may be considered a complete "Pronouncing Dictionary of Medical Science." It is perhaps the most reliable work published for the busy practitioner. It contains information upon every medical subject in a form for ready access, and withal is as admirable as it is practical.—*Southern Medical Record*, Feb. 1874.

A valuable dictionary of the terms employed in medicine and the allied sciences, and of the relations of the subjects treated under each head, it well deserves the authority and popularity it has obtained.—*British Medical Journal*, Oct. 24, 1874.

Few works of this class exhibit a grander monument of patient research and of scientific lore.—*London Lancet*, May 13, 1873.

Dunglison's Dictionary is incalculably valuable, and indispensable to every practitioner of medicine, pharmacist and dentist.—*Western Lancet*, March, 1874.

It has the rare merit that it certainly has no rival in the English language for accuracy and extent of references.—*London Medical Gazette*.

HOBLYN, RICHARD D., M. D.

A Dictionary of the Terms Used in Medicine and the Collateral Sciences. Revised, with numerous additions, by ISAAC HAYS, M. D., late editor of The American Journal of the Medical Sciences. In one large royal 12mo. volume of 520 double-columned pages. Cloth, $1.50; leather, $2.00.

It is the best book of definitions we have, and ought always to be upon the student's table.—*Southern Medical and Surgical Journal*.

RODWELL, G. F., F. R. A. S., F. C. S.,
Lecturer on Natural Science at Clifton College, England.

A Dictionary of Science: Comprising Astronomy, Chemistry, Dynamics, Electricity, Heat, Hydrodynamics, Hydrostatics, Light, Magnetism, Mechanics, Mensuration, Pneumatics, Sound and Statics. Contributed by J. T. Bottomley, M.A., F.C.S., William Crookes, F.R.S., F.C.S., Frederick Guthrie, B.A., Ph.D., R. A. Proctor, B.A., F.R.A.S., G. F. Rodwell, Editor, Charles Tomlinson, F.R.S., F.C.S., and Richard Wormell, M.A., B.Sc. Preceded by an Essay on the History of the Physical Sciences. In one handsome octavo volume of 702 pages, with 143 illustrations. Cloth, $5.00.

HARTSHORNE, HENRY, M. D.,

Lately Professor of Hygiene in the University of Pennsylvania.

A Conspectus of the Medical Sciences; Containing Handbooks on Anatomy, Physiology, Chemistry, Materia Medica, Practice of Medicine, Surgery and Obstetrics. Second edition, thoroughly revised and greatly improved. In one large royal 12mo. volume of 1028 pages, with 477 illustrations. Cloth, $4.25; leather, $5.00.

The object of this manual is to afford a convenient work of reference to students during the brief moments at their command while in attendance upon medical lectures. It is a favorable sign that it has been found necessary, in a short space of time, to issue a new and carefully revised edition. The illustrations are very numerous and unusually clear, and each part seems to have received its due share of attention. We can conceive such a work to be useful, not only to students, but to practitioners as well. It reflects credit upon the industry and energy of its able editor.—*Boston Medical and Surgical Journal,* Sept. 3, 1874.

We can say, with the strictest truth, that it is the best work of the kind with which we are acquainted. It embodies in a condensed form all recent contributions to practical medicine, and is therefore useful to every busy practitioner throughout our country, besides being admirably adapted to the use of students of medicine. The book is faithfully and ably executed.—*Charleston Medical Journal,* April, 1875.

The work is intended as an aid to the medical student, and as such appears to fulfil admirably its object by its excellent arrangement, the full compilation of facts, the perspicuity and terseness of language, and the clear and instructive illustrations.—*American Journal of Pharmacy,* July, 1874.

The volume will be found useful not only to students, but to many others who may desire to refresh their memories with the smallest possible expenditure of time.—*N. Y. Med. Journ.,* Sept. '74.

The work before us has many redeeming features not possessed by others, and is the best we have seen. Dr. Hartshorne exhibits much skill in condensation. It is well adapted to the physician in active practice who can give but limited time to familiarizing himself with the important changes that have been made since he attended lectures. The manual of physiology has also been improved, and gives the most comprehensive view of the latest advances in the science possible in the space devoted to the subject.—*Penins. Jl. of Med.* Sept. '74.

NEILL, JOHN, M. D., and SMITH, F. G., M. D.,

Late Surgeon to the Penna. Hospital.   *Prof. of the Institutes of Med. in the Univ. of Penna.*

An Analytical Compendium of the Various Branches of Medical Science, for the use and examination of Students. A new edition, revised and improved. In one very large royal 12mo. volume of 974 pages, with 374 woodcuts. Cloth, $4; strongly bound in leather, raised bands, $4.75.

LUDLOW, J. L., M. D.,

Consulting Physician to the Philadelphia Hospital, etc.

A Manual of Examinations upon Anatomy, Physiology, Surgery, Practice of Medicine, Obstetrics, Materia Medica, Chemistry, Pharmacy and Therapeutics. To which is added a Medical Formulary. Third edition, thoroughly revised, and greatly extended and enlarged. In one handsome royal 12mo. volume of 816 large pages, with 370 illustrations. Cloth, $3.25; leather, $3.75.

The arrangement of this volume in the form of question and answer renders it especially suitable for the office examination of students, and for those preparing for graduation.

WILSON, ERASMUS, F. R. S.

A System of Human Anatomy, General and Special. Edited by W. H. GOBRECHT, M. D., Professor of General and Surgical Anatomy in the Medical College of Ohio. In one large and handsome octavo volume of 616 pages, with 397 illustrations. Cloth, $4.00; leather, $5.00.

SMITH, H. H., M. D., and HORNER, WM. E., M. D.,

Emeritus Prof. of Surgery in the Univ. of Penna., etc.   *Late Prof. of Anat. in the Univ. of Penna.*

An Anatomical Atlas, Illustrative of the Structure of the Human Body. In one large imperial octavo volume of 200 pages, with 634 beautiful figures. Cloth, $4.50.

CLELAND, JOHN, M. D., F. R. S.,

Professor of Anatomy and Physiology in Queen's College, Galway.

A Directory for the Dissection of the Human Body. In one 12mo. volume of 178 pages. Cloth, $1.25.

BELLAMY, EDWARD, F. R. C. S.,

Senior Assistant-Surgeon to the Charing-Cross Hospital, London.

The Student's Guide to Surgical Anatomy: Being a Description of the most Important Surgical Regions of the Human Body, and intended as an Introduction to Operative Surgery. In one 12mo. volume of 300 pages, with 50 illustrations. Cloth, $2.25.

HARTSHORNE'S HANDBOOK OF ANATOMY AND PHYSIOLOGY. Second edition, revised. In one royal 12mo. volume of 310 pages, with 220 woodcuts. Cloth, $1.75.

SHARPEY AND QUAIN'S HUMAN ANATOMY. Revised by JOSEPH LEIDY, M. D., Prof. of Anat. in Univ. of Penna. In two octavo volumes of about 1300 pages, with 511 illustrations.

HORNER'S SPECIAL ANATOMY AND HISTOLOGY. Eighth edition, extensively revised and modified. In two octavo volumes of 1007 with 320 woodcuts. Cloth, $6.00.

HEATH'S PRACTICAL ANATOMY. From London edition, with additions by W. W. M. D. In one 12mo. volume of 578 pp. 247 woodcuts.

A System of Human Anatomy, Including Its Medical and Surgical Relations. For the use of Practitioners and Students of Medicine, with an Introductory Chapter on Histology. By E. O. Shakespeare, M. D., Ophthalmologist to the Philadelphia Hospital. In one large and handsome quarto volume of about 60 double-columned pages, with 380 illustrations on 109 lithographic plates, many of which are in colors, and about 250 engravings in the text. In six Sections, each in a portfolio. Section I. Histology (*Just Ready*). Section II. Bones and Joints (*Just Ready*). Section III. Muscles and Fasciæ (*Just Ready*). Section IV. Arteries, Veins and Lymphatics (*Just Ready*). Section V. Nervous System (*In Press*). Section VI. Organs of Sense, of Digestion and Genito-Urinary Organs (*In Press*). Price per Section, $3.50. *For sale by subscription only.*

EXTRACT FROM INTRODUCTION.

It is the design of this book to present the facts of human anatomy in the manner best suited to the requirements of the student and the practitioner of medicine. The author believes that such a book is needed, inasmuch as no treatise, so far as he knows, contains, in addition to the text descriptive of the subject, a systematic presentation of such anatomical facts as can be applied to practice.

A book which will be at once accurate in statement and concise in terms; which will be an acceptable expression of the present state of the science of anatomy; which will include nothing that can be made applicable to the medical art, and which will thus embrace all of surgical importance, while omitting nothing of value to clinical medicine, — would appear to have an excuse for existence in a country where most surgeons are general practitioners, and where there are few general practitioners who have no interest in surgery.

Among other matters, the book will be found to contain an elaborate description of the tissues; an account of the normal development of the body; a section on the nature and varieties of monstrosities; a section on the method of conducting post-mortem examinations; and a section on the study of the superficies of the body taken as a guide to the position of the deeper structures. These will appear in their appropriate places, duly subordinated to the design of presenting a text essentially anatomical.

A book like this is an ideal rarely realized. It will do, we have no doubt, what its accomplished author hopes: "make anatomy what unfortunately it rarely is—*an interesting study*." It has long been an opprobrium to America that our anatomical text-books were all foreign, but this work will remove the stigma. It is a mine of wealth in the information it gives. It differs from all preceding anatomies in its scope, and is, we believe, a vast improvement upon them all. The chief novelty about the book, and really one of the greatest needs in anatomy, is the extension of the text to cover not only anatomical descriptions, but the uses of anatomy in studying disease. This is done by stating the narrower topographical relations, and also the wider clinical relations, of the more remote parts, by giving a brief account of the uses of the various organs, and by quoting cases which illustrate the "localization of diseased action." The plates are beautiful specimens of work by one who long since won a deserved reputation as an artist.—*The Medical News,* October 21, 1882.

It is to be considered a study of applied anatomy in its widest sense—a systematic presentation of such anatomical facts as can be applied to the practice of medicine as well as of surgery. Our author is concise, accurate and practical in his statements, and succeeds admirably in infusing an interest into the study of what is generally considered a dry subject. The department of Histology is treated in a masterly manner, and the ground is travelled over by one thoroughly familiar with it. The illustrations are made with great care, and are simply superb. It would be impossible, except in a general way, to point out the excellence of the work of the author in the second Section—that devoted to the consideration of the Bones and Joints. There is as much of practical application of anatomical points to the every-day wants of the medical clinician as to those of the operating surgeon. In fact, few general practitioners will read the work without a feeling of surprised gratification that so many points, concerning which they may never have thought before, are so well presented for their consideration. It is a work which is destined to be the best of its kind in any language.—*Medical Record,* Nov. 25, '82.

The appearance of the book marks an epoch in medical literature. It is the first important work on human anatomy that has appeared in America; and, more than this, its scope is new and original. It is intended to be both descriptive and topographical, scientific and practical, so that while satisfy-

ing the anatomist it will be of value to the practising physician. Such a work is certainly novel, and it will bring the greatest honor to the author. The illustrations of this book are very fine. The figures of the parts, muscular attachments, etc., are printed either on the page or close beside, so that they are easily read. Dr. Allen's treatment of the joints is admirable, and the illustrations made from the author's dissections deserve the highest praise. They bear witness to his skill with the scalpel and to that of the artist with his pencil. They are well conceived and well executed, handsome artistically and clear anatomically. As the author points out, such a work as he has undertaken to produce is very much needed, and the result shows that he has brought to it a mind well prepared for the task by extensive reading, critical judgment and literary ability. We can cordially recommend the work to the profession, believing that it is suited not only to those of scientific tastes, but that it will be of use to the practising physician.—*Boston Medical and Surgical Journal,* Jan. 11, 1883.

It has fallen to the lot of the fortunate publishers to be able to bring out the best anatomy yet produced in America, and one which will prove much more useful to the general practitioner than the foreign works now accepted as standard. The descriptions are clear, tersely expressed and well up to date. The work, as a whole, shows a great amount of research, and reflects credit upon its author. Its pages teem with well-culled facts which cannot be found in the ordinary anatomical treatises. The lithographic plates are beautifully executed, and deserve unqualified praise. To the more advanced students in anatomy, as well as to the profession at large, it will prove a valuable companion, and one often referred to.—*New York Medical Journal and Obstetrical Review,* Nov., 1882.

The distinguishing feature of this work is that, while a thorough treatise on human anatomy, it is neither prepared from the standpoint of the anatomist without knowledge of or sympathy with clinical requirements, nor from the standpoint of the surgeon, who often disregards the wants of the student and physician. The purpose has been maintained throughout of adapting the work to the wants of the student, the surgeon, and the physician. The Sections are beautifully illustrated with plates of wonderful fidelity and beauty; the text is simple, concise, accurate and clear.—*Louisville Medical News,* Dec. 2, 1882.

GRAY, HENRY, F. R. S.,
Lecturer on Anatomy at St. George's Hospital, London.

Anatomy, Descriptive and Surgical. The Drawings by H. V. CARTER, M. D., and Dr. WESTMACOTT. The dissections jointly by the AUTHOR and Dr. CARTER. With an Introduction on General Anatomy and Development by T. HOLMES, M.A., Surgeon to St. George's Hospital. A new American from the eighth enlarged and improved London edition. To which is added the second American from the latest English edition of LANDMARKS, MEDICAL AND SURGICAL, by LUTHER HOLDEN, F. R. C. S, author of "Human Osteology," "A Manual of Dissections," etc. In one magnificent imperial octavo volume of 903 pages, with 523 large and elaborate engravings on wood. Cloth, $6.00; leather, raised bands, $7.00; half Russia, raised bands, $7.50.

The author has endeavored in this work to cover a more extended range of subjects than is customary in the ordinary text-books by giving not only the details necessary for the student, but also the application of those details to the practice of medicine and surgery, thus rendering it both a guide for the learner and an admirable work of reference for the active practitioner. The engravings form a special feature in the work, many of them being the size of nature, nearly all original, and having the names of the various parts printed on the body of the cut, in place of figures of reference with descriptions at the foot. They thus form a complete and splendid series, which will greatly assist the student in forming a clear idea of Anatomy, and will also serve to refresh the memory of those who may find in the exigencies of practice the necessity of recalling the details of the dissecting-room. Combining, as it does, a complete Atlas of Anatomy with a thorough treatise on systematic, descriptive and applied Anatomy, the work will be found of great service to all physicians who receive students in their offices, relieving both preceptor and pupil of much labor in laying the groundwork of a thorough medical education.

To the present edition has been appended the recent work by the distinguished anatomist, Mr. Luther Holden—"Landmarks, Medical and Surgical"—which gives in a clear, condensed and systematic way all the information by which the practitioner can determine from the external surface of the body the position of internal parts. Thus complete, the work, it is believed, will furnish all the assistance that can be rendered by type and illustration in anatomical study.

It is difficult to speak in moderate terms of this new edition of "Gray." It seems to be as nearly perfect as it is possible to make a book devoted to any branch of medical science. The addition of Holden's "Landmarks" will make it as indispensable to the practitioner of medicine and surgery as it has been heretofore to the student. As regards completeness, ease of reference, utility, beauty and cheapness, it has no rival. No student should enter a medical school without it; no physician can afford to have it absent from his library. —*St. Louis Clinical Record*, Sept. 1878.

ALSO FOR SALE SEPARATE—

HOLDEN, LUTHER, F. R. C. S.,
Surgeon to St. Bartholomew's and the Foundling Hospitals, London.

Landmarks, Medical and Surgical. Second American from the latest revised English edition, with additions by W. W. KEEN, M. D., Professor of Artistic Anatomy in the Pennsylvania Academy of the Fine Arts, formerly Lecturer on Anatomy in the Philadelphia School of Anatomy. In one handsome 12mo. volume of 148 pages. Cloth, $1.00.

This little book is all that can be desired within its scope, and its contents will be found simply invaluable to the young surgeon or physician, since they bring before him such data as he requires at every examination of a patient. It is written in language so clear and concise that one ought almost to learn it by heart. It teaches diagnosis by external examination, ocular and palpable, of the body, with such anatomical and physiological facts as directly bear on the subject. It is eminently the student's and young practitioner's book.—*Physician and Surgeon*, Nov. 1881.

To the student or young surgeon this is practically a most useful little book. We heartily recommend this work to all students and young practitioners, for whom it has been written, and who by its aid will readily be able to make thorough and intelligent examination, or in surgical operations to cut down upon any part with confidence.—*Medical and Surgical Reporter*, Sep. 3, 1881.

DALTON, JOHN C., M. D.,
Professor of Physiology in the College of Physicians and Surgeons, New York.

The Topographical Anatomy of the Brain. In one very handsome quarto volume of about 200 pages of descriptive text. Illustrated with forty-nine life-size photographic illustrations of Brain Sections, with a like number of outline explanatory plates, as well as many carefully-executed woodcuts through the text. *Preparing.*

ELLIS, GEORGE VINER,
Emeritus Professor of Anatomy in University College, London.

Demonstrations of Anatomy. Being a Guide to the Knowledge of the Human Body by Dissection. By GEORGE VINER ELLIS, Emeritus Professor of Anatomy in University College, London. From the eighth and revised London edition. In one very handsome octavo volume of 716 pages, with 249 illustrations. Cloth, $4.25; leather, $5.25.

Ellis' Demonstrations is the favorite text-book of the English student of anatomy. In passing through eight editions it has been so revised and adapted to the needs of the student that it would seem that it had almost reached perfection in this special line. The descriptions are clear, and the methods of pursuing anatomical investigations are given with such detail that the book is honestly entitled to its name.—*St. Louis Clinical Record*, June, 1879.

DALTON, JOHN C., M. D.,
Professor of Physiology in the College of Physicians and Surgeons, New York, etc.

A Treatise on Human Physiology. Designed for the use of Students and Practitioners of Medicine. Seventh edition, thoroughly revised and rewritten. In one very handsome octavo volume of 722 pages, with 252 beautiful engravings on wood. Cloth, $5.00; leather, $6.00; very handsome half Russia, raised bands, $6.50.

The reputation which this work has acquired as a compact and convenient summary of the most advanced condition of human physiology renders it only necessary to state that the Author has assiduously labored to render the present edition worthy a continuance of the marked favor accorded to previous issues, and that every care has been bestowed upon the typographical execution to make it, as heretofore, one of the handsomest productions of the American press.

The merits of Professor Dalton's text-book, his smooth and pleasing style, the remarkable clearness of his descriptions, which leave not a chapter obscure, his cautious judgment and the general correctness of his facts, are perfectly known. They have made his text-book the one most familiar to American students.—*Med. Record*, March 4, 1882.

Certainly no physiological work has ever issued from the press that presented its subject-matter in a clearer and more attractive light. Almost every page bears evidence of the exhaustive revision that has taken place. The material is placed in a more compact form, yet is delightful charm is retained, and no subject is thrown into obscurity. Altogether this edition is far in advance of any

previous one, and will tend to keep the professor posted as to the most recent additions to our physiological knowledge.—*Michigan Medical News*, April, 1882.

One can scarcely open a college catalogue that does not have mention of Dalton's Physiology as the recommended text or consultation-book. For American students we would unreservedly recommend the edition of Dr. Dalton's work now before us. Let it suffice to state that revisions have been made to such an extent as to bring the volume as fully up to the present state of physiological knowledge as it is practicable for any author of a book to do.—*Virginia Medical Monthly*, July, 1882.

FOSTER, MICHAEL, M. D., F. R. S.,
Professor of Physiology in Cambridge University, England.

Text-Book of Physiology. Second American from the latest English edition. Edited, with extensive notes and additions, by EDWARD T. REICHERT, M. D., late Demonstrator of Experimental Therapeutics in the University of Pennsylvania. In one handsome royal 12mo. volume of 999 pages, with 250 illust. Cloth, $3.25; leather, $3.75.

A more compact and scientific work on physiology has never been published, and we believe ourselves not to be mistaken in asserting that it has now been introduced into every medical college in which the English language is spoken. This work conforms to the latest researches into zoology and comparative anatomy, and takes into consideration the late discoveries in physiological chemistry and the experiments in localization of Ferrier and others. The arrangement followed is such as to render the whole subject lucid and well connected in its various parts.—*Chicago Medical Journal and Examiner*, August, 1882.

Dr. Michael Foster's *Manual of Physiology* has been translated from the German, with a preface, by Professor Kühne. Kühne points out in his

preface that the abundant material, in spite of the moderate size, is not condensed to systematic shortness, but the whole is related in a narrative style. Further on he writes: "To give to students and physicians a book which is not intended merely for reference, but which, by its lively style, invites the reader to go through it, is always useful, especially when the contents, including numerous matters in a state of active discussion in which physiology is now so rich, instruct with truth and calm impartiality, such the author has preserved throughout." The translation of it into German is a well-merited compliment, since Germany is the especial home of physiology, and its literature is abundantly rich in text-books, monographs and periodicals on physiology.—*American Med. Bi-Weekly*, June 12, 1882.

CARPENTER, WM. B., M. D., F. R. S., F. G. S., F. L. S.,
Registrar to the University of London, etc.

Principles of Human Physiology. Edited by HENRY POWER, M. B., Lond., F. R. C. S., Examiner in Natural Sciences, University of Oxford. A new American from the eighth revised and enlarged edition, with notes and additions by FRANCIS G. SMITH, M. D., late Professor of the Institutes of Medicine in the University of Pennsylvania. In one very large and handsome octavo volume of 1083 pages, with two plates and 373 illustrations. Cloth, $5.50; leather, $6.50; half Russia, $7.

Without departing materially from the judicious arrangement which the author originally chose, the latest researches in physiology have been introduced, and with a careful hand. The American editor has added what few paragraphs were necessary to bring the work up to the level of the science since the last English edition, and has thus rendered it a thoroughly complete compendium of physiology. Altogether there are few, if any, treatises on the subject so well calculated to attract and instruct a student as this one.—*Medical and Surgical Reporter*, Dec. 2, 1876.

The editors have, with their additions to the only work on physiology in our language that, in

the fullest sense of the word, is the production of a philosopher as well as a physiologist, brought it up fully to the standard of our knowledge of the subject at the present day. The additions by the American editor give to the work as it is a considerable value beyond that of the last English edition. We have been agreeably surprised to find the volume so complete in regard to the structure and functions of the nervous system in all its relations—a subject that in many respects is one of the most difficult of all, in the whole range of physiology, upon which to produce a full and satisfactory treatise of the class to which the one before us belongs.—*Jl. of Nerv. and Ment. Dis.*, Apr. '77.

FOWNES, GEORGE, Ph. D.

A Manual of Elementary Chemistry; Theoretical and Practical. Revised and corrected by HENRY WATTS, B. A., F. R. S., Editor of A DICTIONARY OF CHEMISTRY, etc. A new American from the twelfth and enlarged London edition. Edited by ROBERT BRIDGES, M. D. In one large royal 12mo. volume of 1031 pages, with 177 illustrations on wood and a colored plate. Cloth, $2.75; leather, $3.25.

The book opens with a treatise on Chemical Physics, including Heat, Light, Magnetism and Electricity. These subjects are treated clearly and briefly, but enough is given to enable the student to comprehend the facts and laws of Chemistry proper. It is the fashion of late years to omit these topics from works on chemistry, but their omission is not to be commended. As was required by the great advance in the science of Chemistry of late years, the chapter on the General Principles of Chemical Philosophy has been entirely rewritten. The latest views on Equivalents, Quantivalence, etc., are clearly and fully set forth. This last edition is a great improvement upon its predecessors, which is saying not a little of a book that has reached its twelfth edition.—*Ohio Medical Recorder*, Oct. 1878.

The student will value the clear and full expositions of *Physical Science*, and the *tabular form* of so many facts which are thus more readily retained in the memory. The medical practitioner will turn with pleasure to its copious index for the most recent facts in the somewhat hazy and nebulous domain of organic chemistry. In point of fulness the work is a *Modern Dictionary of Chemistry*. In its explanations it is a clear and able treatise, embracing many valuable tables from the standard works of Graham, Miller and Gmelin.—*Canada Medical Record*, Sept. 1878.

The work is too well known to American students to need any extended notice; suffice it to say that the revision by the English editor has been faithfully done, and that Professor Bridges has added some fresh and valuable matter, especially in the inorganic chemistry. The book has always been a favorite in this country, and in its new shape bids fair to retain all its former prestige.—*Boston Journal of Chemistry*, Aug. 1878.

When we state that, in our opinion, the present edition sustains in every respect the high reputation which its predecessors have acquired and enjoyed, we express therewith our full belief in its intrinsic value as a text-book and work of reference.—*American Journal of Pharmacy*, Aug. 1878.

ATTFIELD, JOHN, Ph. D.,
Professor of Practical Chemistry to the Pharmaceutical Society of Great Britain, etc.

Chemistry, General, Medical and Pharmaceutical; Including the Chemistry of the U. S. Pharmacopoeia. A Manual of the General Principles of the Science, and their Application to Medicine and Pharmacy. Eighth edition, specially revised by the Author. In one handsome royal 12mo. volume of 701 pages, with 87 illustrations. Cloth, $2.50; leather, $3.00.

We have repeatedly expressed our favorable opinion of this work, and on the appearance of a new edition of it little remains for us to say, except that we expect this eighth edition to be as indispensable to us as the seventh and previous editions have been. While the general plan and arrangement have been adhered to, new matter has been added covering the observations made since the former edition. The present differs from the preceding one chiefly in these alterations and in about ten pages of useful tables added in the appendix.—*American Journal of Pharmacy*, May, '79

Each of these editions has been a decided improvement on its predecessor, until now the present edition is as perfect as one could well expect a work of this kind to be. It possesses the advantage over other chemical works intended specially for medical students of being also quite complete as a *general* chemical text-book. It is even more particularly serviceable to pharmaceutical students and apothecaries, as it "includes the whole of the chemistry of the U. S Pharmacopoeia, of the British Pharmacopoeia and of the Pharmacopoeia of India"—*Virginia Medical Monthly*, May, 1879.

The author has bestowed arduous labor on the revision, and the extent of the information thus introduced may be estimated from the fact that the index contains three hundred new references relating to additional material —*Druggists' Circular and Chemical Gazette*, May, 1879.

This very popular and meritorious work has now reached its eighth edition, which fact speaks in the highest terms in commendation of its excellence. It has now become the principal text-book of chemistry in all the medical colleges in the United States. The present edition contains such alterations and additions as seemed necessary for the demonstration of the latest developments of chemical principles and the latest applications of chemistry to pharmacy It is scarcely necessary for us to say that it exhibits chemistry in its present advanced state.—*Cin. Med. News*, April, 1879.

The popularity which this work has enjoyed is owing to the original and clear disposition of the facts of the science, the accuracy of the details, and the omission of much which freights many treatises heavily without bringing corresponding instruction to the reader. Dr. Attfield writes for students, and primarily for medical students; he always has an eye to the pharmacopoeia and its officinal preparations, and he is continually putting the matter in the text so that it responds to the questions with which each section is provided. —*Medical and Surgical Reporter*, April 19, 1879

BLOXAM, CHARLES L.,
Late Professor of Chemistry in King's College, London

Chemistry, Inorganic and Organic. New edition. In one very handsome octavo volume of about 700 pages, with about 300 illustrations. *In press.*

REMSEN, IRA, M. D., Ph. D.,
Professor of Chemistry in the Johns Hopkins University, Baltimore.

* **Principles of Theoretical Chemistry,** with special reference to the Constitution of Chemical Compounds. New edition. In one handsome royal 12mo. volume of about 250 pages. *Preparing.*

Wöhler's Outlines of Organic Chemistry. Edited by RUDOLPH FITTIG, Ph. D., Nat. Sc. D., Professor of Chemistry in the University of Tübingen. Translated by IRA REMSEN, M. D., Ph. D., Professor of Physics and Chemistry in Williams College, Mass. In one 12mo. volume of 550 pages. Cloth, $3.

BOWMAN'S INTRODUCTION TO PRACTICAL   American from the sixth London edition. In

HOFFMANN, F. A.M., Ph.D., & POWER, F.B., Ph.D.,

P... A... ... ... New York.   *P... of Anal. Chem... in Phil. C... Pa...*

A Manual of Chemical Analysis, as applied to the Examination of Medicinal Chemicals and their Preparations. Being a Guide for the Determination of their Identity and Quality, and for the Detection of Impurities and Adulterations. For the use of Pharmacists, Physicians, Druggists and Manufacturing Chemists, and Pharmaceutical and Medical Students. Third edition, entirely rewritten and much enlarged. In one very handsome octavo volume of 621 pages, with 179 illustrations. Cloth, $4.25. *Just ...*

The first portion of this work, treating of operations and reagents, and giving a general account of the methods of chemical analysis, has been considerably enlarged and completed so that now it affords an efficient and explicit guide in the practical execution of chemical analysis. That on volumetric analysis has been correspondingly extended, and a new chapter on the separation and estimation of the alkaloids has been added. The second and main part of the work, containing the physical and chemical characteristics of medicinal chemicals and of the methods of establishing their identity, quality and purity, has been much enlarged and improved, new chemicals of recognized therapeutical value have been added, and new tables and many additional illustrations, introduced. The methods for the quantitative estimation of many chemicals have also received an increased share of attention. Especially is this true in regard to the identification and separation of those of poisonous properties. The labors and results of pharmacopoeial revisions both here and in Europe, as well as the kindred literature, have not been neglected; so that the work will be found to correspond with the most recent advances in chemical knowledge.

CLOWES, FRANK, D. Sc., London,

Senior Science-Master at the High School, Newcastle-under-Lyme, etc.

An Elementary Treatise on Practical Chemistry and Qualitative Inorganic Analysis. Specially adapted for use in the Laboratories of Schools and Colleges and by Beginners. Second American from the third and revised English edition. In one very handsome royal 12mo, volume of 372 pages, with 47 illustrations. Cloth, $2.50.

The one object of the author of the present work was to furnish one which was sufficiently elementary in the description of apparatus, chemicals, modes of experimentation, etc., so as to "reduce to a minimum the amount of assistance required from a teacher." It is a generally recognized fact that one of the most serious hindrances to the utility of a great many of the smaller textbooks is the too great condensation of the language employed, which renders it unintelligible to the primary student unless supplemented by copious verbal explanations from the teacher. The *Elementary Treatise* of Dr. Clowes, examined with reference to the above claims, is found to be a great improvement on other elementary works. A student who carefully reads this text will scarcely need the assistance of a tutor in following out any of the experiments described.—*Pro M... ... M... ... Ap... 1...*

GALLOWAY, ROBERT, F. C. S.,

Professor of Applied Chemistry in the Royal College of Science, Dublin, late.

A Manual of Qualitative Analysis. From the sixth London edition. In one handsome royal 12mo, volume, with illustrations. *Preparing.*

CLASSEN, ALEXANDER,

Professor in the Royal Polytechnic School, Aix-la-Chapelle.

Elementary Quantitative Analysis. Translated, with notes and additions, by Edgar F. Smith, Ph. D., Assistant Professor of Chemistry in the Towne Scientific School, University of Pennsylvania. In one handsome royal 12mo, volume of 324 pages, with 36 illustrations. Cloth, $2.00.

Classen's work has for some time been the laboratory companion of the student in most of the first-class schools of the continent of Europe, while it has been received with equal favor by practical chemists in France, Russia and Poland. Every line in the book has practical stamped upon it. Laboratory work alone can teach chemistry, and Classen's Manual is the best guide to it we have seen.—*St. Louis Chemical Record, Oct. 1878.*

It is probably the best manual of quantitative nature extant, inasmuch as its methods are the best. It teaches by examples, commencing with single determinations, followed by separations, and then advancing to the analysis of minerals, of such products as are met with in applied chemistry. It is an indispensable book for students of chemistry.—*Boston Journal of Chemistry, Oct. 1878.*

GREENE, WILLIAM H., M. D.,

Demonstrator of Chemistry in the Medical Department of the University of Pennsylvania.

A Manual of Medical Chemistry. For the use of Students. Based upon Bowman's Medical Chemistry. In one royal 12mo, volume of 310 pages, with 74 illustrations. Cloth, $1.75.

It is a concise manual of three hundred pages, giving an excellent summary of the best methods of analyzing the liquids and solids of the body, both for the estimation of their normal constituents and the recognition of compounds due to pathological conditions. The detection of poisons is treated with sufficient fulness for the purpose of the student or practitioner.—*Boston R. of Chem., June, '80.*

The author has availed himself of all the recent discoveries and advances in this important branch of medicine to bring his work fully up to the times. As a handbook for the busy practitioner who will necessarily be now and then called upon to make a chemical analysis, this little work will prove invaluable.—*Nashville Journal of Medicine and Surgery, June, 1880.*

The above little book is concise, practical, and thorough as the physician could desire. The methods of examination are simple, require but little apparatus, and are easily performed. The drawings are four and faithful. We recommend the book to our readers.—*Am. Practitioner, June, '80.*

H, EDWARD,

Late Professor of Materia Medica in the Philadelphia College of Pharmacy.

A Treatise on Pharmacy. Designed as a Text-book for the Student, and as a Guide for the Physician and Pharmaceutist. With many Formulæ and Prescriptions. Fourth edition, thoroughly revised, by THOMAS S. WIEGAND. In one handsome octavo volume of 985 pages, with 230 illustrations. Cloth, $5.50; leather, $6.50; half Russia, $7.00.

Perhaps one of the most important, if not the most important, book upon pharmacy which has appeared in the English language has emanated from the transatlantic press. "Parrish's Pharmacy" is a well-known work on this side of the water, and the fact shows us that a really useful work never becomes merely local in its fame. Thanks to the judicious editing of Mr. Wiegand, the posthumous edition of "Parrish" has been saved to the public with all the mature experience of its author, and perhaps none the worse for a dash of new blood.—*Lond. Pharm. Journal*, Oct. 17, 1874.

We have here an encyclopædia of pharmacy, of equal value as a text-book for the student and as a guide for the pharmacist and physician, which has reached its fourth edition A work which has gained such a hold upon the confidence of the profession stands in no need of the recommendation of the press. We have called the treatise an encyclopædia as the name most descriptive of its character—a work in which may be found all that the pharmacist or student of medicine need to know of pharmacy. On whatever point of pharmacy he may be seeking information, he will be fully instructed in this handbook, which is heartily recommended —*American Practitioner*, July, 1874

GRIFFITH, R. EGLESFIELD, M. D.

A Universal Formulary; Containing the Methods of Preparing and Administering Officinal and other Medicines. The whole adapted to Physicians and Pharmaceutists. Third edition, carefully revised and much enlarged, by JOHN M. MAISCH, Phar. D., Professor of Materia Medica in the Philadelphia College of Pharmacy. In one large and handsome octavo volume of 775 pages, with illustrations. Cloth, $4.50; leather, $5.50.

A more complete formulary than it is in its present form the pharmacist or physician could hardly desire. To the first some such work is indispensable, and it is hardly less essential to the practitioner who compounds his own medicines Much of what is contained in the introduction ought to be committed to memory by every student of medicine. As a help to physicians it will be found invaluable, and doubtless will make its way into libraries not already supplied with a standard work of the kind —*The American Practitioner*, July, 1874.

HERMANN, Dr. L.,

Professor of Physiology in the University of Zurich.

Experimental Pharmacology. A Handbook of Methods for Determining the Physiological Actions of Drugs. Translated, with the Author's permission, and with extensive additions, by ROBERT MEADE SMITH, M. D., Demonstrator of Physiology in the University of Pennsylvania. In one handsome 12mo. volume of 199 pages, with 32 illustrations. Cloth, $1.50. *Just ready.*

TRANSLATOR'S PREFACE.

The translation of Hermann's Manual of Pharmacology was undertaken to furnish the student with a work that would assist him in his studies of the physiological action of drugs, enabling him to make the experiments himself that would otherwise require the assistance of the instructor. The translator has attempted to elucidate the text with a careful selection of illustrations; and he trusts that his additions, which constitute nearly one-half of the entire volume, will render the work a more perfect guide to the student.

This work is a text-book for students for their guidance in the physiological laboratory. To the translation the editor has added many original paragraphs, and he has introduced numerous illustrations from the larger volumes of Sanderson, Foster, Bernard and others In size this work is much more handy than similar laboratory manuals, and must prove acceptable to the student in this department of study If only such books are added to the literature of this advancing branch of medical research, we shall ere long have no reason to regret that the laws of Great Britain have closed their physiological laboratories only to open our own —*N. C. Medical Journal*, Feb 1883.

MAISCH, JOHN M., Phar. D.,

Professor of Materia Medica and Botany in the Philadelphia College of Pharmacy.

A Manual of Organic Materia Medica; Being a Guide to Materia Medica of the Vegetable and Animal Kingdoms. For the use of Students, Druggists, Pharmacists and Physicians. In one handsome royal 12mo. volume of 451 pages, with 194 beautiful illustrations on wood. Cloth, $2.75.

A book evidently written for a purpose, and not simply for the purpose of writing a book It is comprehensive, inasmuch as it refers to all, or nearly all, that is of essential value in organic materia medica, clear and simple in its style, concise, since it would be difficult to find in it a superfluous word, and yet sufficiently explicit to satisfy the most critical The text is freely illustrated with woodcuts, which cannot fail to be valuable in familiarizing students with the physical, microscopic and macroscopic appearance of drugs The work is preceded by a table of contents, and completed with that without which no book should be considered complete, i. e., an index In fact, the little book is just what it pretends to be, and is worthy of unqualified commendation.—*Chicago Medical Journal and Examiner*, Aug. 1882.

The above manual, by a well-known authority in this department and one of the authors of the National Dispensatory, is a work for which students of pharmacy should be grateful The subject is one in which the beginner needs the guidance of a good classification in order to avoid the bewilderment which follows the attempt to grasp a subject having so many details. This condition the book fulfils, the classification adopted being a simple and practical one, the notice of each drug is brief and clear, non-essentials being omitted. It is fully illustrated by some two hundred woodcuts. —*Boston Med. and Surg. Journal*, Jan 19, 1882.

Professor Maisch, in the work before us, has in as concise a manner as seems consistent with clearness given us the origin, habitat, botanical description, chemical constituents and medicinal properties of the drugs of the vegetable kingdom This book is an admirable one indeed.— *Michigan Medical News*, April 10, 1882.

The National Dispensatory: Containing the Natural History, Chemistry, Pharmacy, Actions and Uses of Medicine, including those recognized in the Pharmacopœias of the United States, Great Britain and Germany, with numerous references to the French Codex. Third edition, thoroughly revised and greatly enlarged. In one magnificent imperial octavo volume of about 1600 pages, with several hundred fine engravings. *In press.*

The publishers have much pleasure in announcing to the Medical and Pharmaceutical Professions that a new edition of this important work is in press, and that it will appear in the shortest time consistent with the care requisite for printing a work of immense detail, where absolute accuracy is of such supreme importance. Besides its revision on the basis of the U. S. Pharmacopœia of 1880, it will include all the advances made in its department during the period elapsed since the preparation of that work. To this end all recent medical and pharmaceutical literature, both domestic and foreign, has been thoroughly sifted, and everything that is new and important has been introduced, together with the results of original investigations. The Therapeutical Index has been enlarged so that it contains about 8000 references, arranged under an alphabetical list of diseases, thus placing at the disposal of the practitioner, in the most convenient manner, the vast stores of therapeutical knowledge constantly needed in his daily practice. The work may therefore be justly regarded as a complete Encyclopædia of Materia Medica and Therapeutics up to 1883.

The exhaustion of two very large editions of THE NATIONAL DISPENSATORY since 1879 is the most conclusive testimony as to the necessity which demanded its preparation and to the admirable manner in which that duty has been performed. In this revision the authors have sought to add to its usefulness by including everything properly coming within its scope which can be of use to the physician or pharmacist and at the same time by the utmost conciseness and by the omission of all obsolete matter to prevent undue increase in the size of the volume. No care will be spared by the publishers to render its typographical execution worthy of its wide reputation and universal use as the standard authority.

A few notices of the previous edition are appended.

The authors have embraced the opportunity offered for a thorough revision of the whole work, striving to include within it all that might have been omitted in the former edition, and all that has newly appeared of sufficient importance during the time of its collaboration and the short interval elapsed since the previous publication. After having gone carefully through the volume, we must admit that the authors have labored faithfully and with success in maintaining the high character of their work as a compendium meeting the requirements of the day, to which one can safely turn in quest of the latest information concerning everything worthy of notice in connection with Pharmacy, Materia Medica and Therapeutics. —*Am. Jour. of Pharmacy,* Nov. 1879.

The authors have produced a work which for accuracy and comprehensiveness is unsurpassed by any work on the subject. There is no book in the English language which contains so much valuable information on the various articles of the materia medica. The authors have succeeded in producing a dispensatory which is not only *national*, but will be a lasting memorial of their learning.—*Edinburgh Med. Jour.,* Nov. 1879.

The National Dispensatory is beyond dispute the very best authority. It is throughout complete in all the necessary details, clear and lucid in its explanations, and replete with references to the most recent writings, where further particulars can be obtained if desired. Its value is greatly enhanced by the extensive indexes—a general index of materia medica, etc., and also an index of therapeutics. No practising physician can afford to be without The National Dispensatory.—*Canada Med. and Surg. Journ.,* Feb. 1880.

The first edition of this great work appeared only a few months ago, and that the publishers should find it necessary to issue a second edition in the same year is most conclusive evidence that the work has really supplied a want felt by the medical and pharmaceutical professions. The material embodied in the work is truly immense, as shown by the almost countless number of subjects treated. It is now, undoubtedly, the most perfect book of its kind in any language.—*Buffalo Medical and Surgical Journal,* Nov. 1879.

The work may be looked upon as a kind of international codex, available to the English-speaking community of all nations; emphatically, we would repeat, a book for the practitioner—one well calculated to give him hints as to treatment and most suggestive as to remedies.—*London Medical Times and Gazette.*

STILLÉ, ALFRED, M. D., LL. D.,

Professor of Theory and Practice of Med. and of Clinical Med. in the Univ. of Penna.

Therapeutics and Materia Medica. A Systematic Treatise on the Action and Uses of Medicinal Agents, including their Description and History. Fourth edition, revised and enlarged. In two large and handsome octavo volumes, containing 1900 pages. Cloth, $10.00; leather, $12.00; very handsome half Russia, raised bands, $15.00.

The rapid exhaustion of three editions and the universal favor with which the work has been received by the medical profession are sufficient proof of its excellence as a repertory of practical and useful information for the physician. The edition before us fully sustains this verdict.—*American Journal of Pharmacy,* Feb. 1875.

We can hardly admit that it has a rival in the multitude of its citations and the fulness of its research into clinical histories, and we must assign it a place in the physician's library; not, indeed, as fully representing the present state of knowledge in pharmacodynamics, but as by far the most complete treatise upon the clinical and practical side of the question.—*Boston Medical and Surgical Journal,* Nov. 4, 1874.

For all who desire a complete work on therapeutics and materia medica for reference in cases involving medico-legal questions, as well as for information concerning remedial agents, Dr. Stillé is par excellence the work.—*St. Louis Medical and Surgical Journal,* Dec. 1874.

specially revised by the Author. Enlarged and adapted to the U. S. Pharmacopœia by FRANK WOODBURY, M. D. In one very handsome 12mo. volume of 524 pages. Cloth, $2.25. *Just ready.*

Dr. Farquharson's Therapeutics is constructed upon a plan which brings before the reader all the essential points with reference to the properties of drugs. It impresses these upon him in such a way as to enable him to take a clear view of the actions of medicines and the disordered conditions in which they must prove useful. The double-columned pages—one side containing the recognized physiological action of the medicine, and the other the disease in which observers (who are nearly always mentioned) have obtained from it good results—make a very good arrangement. The early chapter containing rules for prescribing is excellent. We have much pleasure in once more drawing attention to this valuable and well-digested

book, and predict for it a continued successful career.—*Canada Medical and Surgical Journal*, Dec. 1882.

The general arrangement, the excellent manner in which the individual articles are presented, the eminently practical character together with the positiveness of expression in both the physiological and therapeutical indications of special remedies, and the fact that it is fully abreast with the most recent developments of scientific investigations, all tend to make this little volume peculiarly valuable. It is throughout complete in all the necessary details, clear and lucid in its explanations, and is not only a handy little volume, but may be regarded as an authority.—*The Southern Practitioner*, Dec. 1882.

GREEN, T. HENRY, M. D.,
Lecturer on Pathology and Morbid Anatomy at Charing-Cross Hospital Medical School, etc

Pathology and Morbid Anatomy. Fifth American from the sixth enlarged and revised English edition. In one very handsome octavo volume of about 350 pages, with about 150 fine engravings. *Preparing.*

COATS, JOSEPH, M. D., F. F. P. S.,
Pathologist to the Glasgow Western Infirmary.

A Treatise on Pathology. In one very handsome octavo volume of about 900 pages, with 339 beautiful illustrations. *In press.*

CORNIL, V.,   and   RANVIER, L.,
Prof. in the Faculty of Med. of Paris.   *Prof. in the College of France.*

A Manual of Pathological Histology. Translated, with notes and additions, by E. O. SHAKESPEARE, M. D., Pathologist and Ophthalmic Surgeon to Philadelphia Hospital, and by J. HENRY C. SIMES, M. D., Demonstrator of Pathological Histology in the University of Pennsylvania. In one very handsome octavo volume of 800 pages, with 360 illustrations. Cloth, $5.50; leather, $6.50; half Russia, raised bands, $7.

We have no hesitation in cordially recommending the translation of Cornil and Ranvier's "Pathological Histology" as the best work of the kind in any language, and as giving to its readers a trustworthy guide in obtaining a broad and solid basis for the appreciation of the practical bearings of pathological anatomy.—*American Journal of the Medical Sciences*, April, 1880.

One of the most complete volumes on pathological histology we have ever seen. The plan of study embraced within its pages is essentially practical. Normal tissues are discussed, and after their thorough demonstration we are able to compare any pathological change which has occurred in them. Thus side by side physiological and pathological anatomy go hand in hand, affording that best of all processes in demonstrations, comparison. The admirable arrangement of the work affords facility in the study of any part of the human economy.—*New Orleans Medical and Surgical Journal*, June, 1882.

This important work, in its American dress, is a

welcome offering to all students of the subjects which it treats. The great mass of material is arranged naturally and comprehensively. The classification of tumors is clear and full, so far as the subject admits of definition, and this one chapter is worth the price of the book. The illustrations are copious and well chosen. Without the slightest hesitation, the translators deserve honest thanks for placing this indispensable work in the hands of American students.—*Philadelphia Medical Times*, April 24, 1880.

Their book has been written in the laboratory beside the microscope. It bears the marks of personal knowledge and investigation upon every page. Its translation has made it the best work in pathology attainable in our language, one that every student certainly ought to have.—*Archives of Medicine*, April, 1880.

The best and most complete work ever issued on the subject from the press of any country.—*London Medical Press and Circular.*

SCHÄFER, EDWARD ALBERT, M. D.,
Assistant Professor of Physiology in University College, London.

A Course of Practical Histology. Being an introduction to the use of the Microscope. In one handsome royal 12mo. volume of 308 pages, with 40 illustrations. Cloth, $2.00.

It is a clear, practical guide for the student of histology, written by one who thoroughly understands not only his subject, but how to teach it. We are very much pleased with the book, which teaches the student simply how to use his instruments and conduct his studies without going further into the microscopic anatomy of the tissues and organs than is absolutely necessary. What we particularly praise in it is the way in which it takes the student by the hand, as it were, showing him what to do, and explaining simply but thoroughly how to do it.—*Boston Medical and Surgical Journal*, April 12, 1877.

This is a book which we do not hesitate to recommend to the profession. In these progressive times, when many physicians are taking up the study, this is a book that is needed, and might be appropriately named the study of microscopy and histology without a teacher.—*American Practitioner*, June, 1877.

GLUGE'S ATLAS OF PATHOLOGICAL HISTOLOGY. Translated, with notes and additions, by JOSEPH LEIDY, M. D. In one volume, very large imperial quarto, with 320 copper-plate figures, plain and colored, and descriptive letter. Cloth, $4.00.

HORNER'S SPECIAL ANATOMY AND TOLOGY. See page 5.

the use of Students and Practitioners of Medicine. Fifth edition, entirely rewritten and much improved. In one large and closely-printed octavo volume of 1150 pages. Cloth, $5.50; leather, $6.50; very handsome half Russia, raised bands, $7.

We cannot conclude this notice without expressing our admiration for this volume, which is certainly one of the standard text-books on medicine; and we may safely affirm that, taken altogether, it exhibits a fuller and wider acquaintance with recent pathological inquiry than any similar work with which we are acquainted, whilst at the same time it shows its author to be possessed of the rare faculties of clear exposition, thoughtful discrimination and sound judgment.—*London Lancet*, July 23, 1881.

In a word, we do not know of any similar work which is at once so elaborate and so concise, so full and yet so accurate, or which in every part leaves upon the mind the impression of its being the product of an author richly stored with the fruits of clinical observation, and an adept in the art of conveying them clearly and attractively to others.—*American Journal of Medical Sciences*, April, 1881.

Flint's Treatise is the work of an accomplished hospital physician, and is remarkable for its masterly descriptions of disease. It is a work on clinical medicine embodying the experience of a lifetime. It has been carefully brought up to the present day, and the additions and alterations have been so great that it is virtually a new work, and

not merely a new edition. In making these alterations, Flint openly confesses that he has not been too careful to maintain a character for consistency, but has endeavored to give his reader the more matured, and, as he believes, more truthful view, careless of any discrepancy between them and those he formerly advanced. Flint is right; only in this way could he produce a work worthy of being looked upon as a standard.—*Edinburgh Medical Journal*, June, 1881.

This work is so widely known and regarded as the best American text-book on the practice of medicine that it would seem hardly worth while to give this, the fifth edition, anything more than a passing notice. But even the most cursory examination shows that it is, practically, much more than a revised edition; it is, in fact, rather a new work throughout. This treatise will undoubtedly continue to hold the first place in the estimation of American physicians and students. No one of our medical writers approaches Professor Flint in clearness of diction, breadth of view, and, what is of transcendent importance, rational estimate of the value of remedial agents. It is thoroughly practical, therefore pre-eminently fitted for American readers.—*St. Louis Clin. Rec.*, Jan. '81.

HARTSHORNE, HENRY, M. D.,
Late Professor of Hygiene in the University of Pennsylvania.

Essentials of the Principles and Practice of Medicine. A Handy-book for Students and Practitioners. Fifth edition, thoroughly revised and rewritten. In one handsome royal 12mo. volume of 669 pages, with 144 illustrations. Cloth, $2.75; half bound, $3.00. *Just ready.*

The author of this book seems to have spared no pains to bring it up to the modern standpoint, for as we turn over its pages we find many subjects introduced which have only lately been brought before the profession. Certainly amongst books of its class it deserves and has obtained a good position. On the whole it is a careful and conscientious piece of work, and may be commended.—*London Lancet*, June 24, 1882.

Within the compass of 600 pages it treats of the history of medicine, general pathology, general symptomatology, and physical diagnosis (including laryngoscope, ophthalmoscope, etc.), general therapeutics, nosology, and special pathology and practice. With such a wide range, condensation is, of course, a necessity; but the author has endeavored to make up for this by copious references to original

papers, etc. We cannot but admit that there is a wonderful amount of information contained in the work, and that it is one of the best of its kind that we have seen.—*Glasgow Medical Journal*, Nov. 1881.

An indispensable book. No work ever exhibited a better average of actual practical treatment than this one; and probably no one writer in our day had a better opportunity than Dr. Hartshorne for condensing all the views of eminent practitioners into a 12mo. The numerous illustrations will be very useful to students especially. These essentials, as the name suggests, are not intended to supersede the text-books of Flint and Bartholow, but they are the most valuable in affording the means to see at a glance the whole literature of any disease, and the most valuable treatment.—*Cincinnati Medical Journal and Examiner*, April, 1882.

WOODBURY, FRANK, M. D.,
Physician to the German Hospital, Philadelphia; late Chief Assistant to the Medical Clinic in Jefferson College Hospital, etc.

A Handbook of the Principles and Practice of Medicine. For the use of Students and Practitioners. In one royal 12mo. volume, with illustrations. *Preparing.*

BRISTOWE, JOHN SYER, M. D., F. R. C. P.,
Physician and Joint Lecturer on Medicine at St. Thomas' Hospital.

A Treatise on the Practice of Medicine. Second American edition, revised by the Author. Edited, with additions, by JAMES H. HUTCHINSON, M.D., physician to the Pennsylvania Hospital. In one handsome octavo volume of 1085 pages, with illustrations. Cloth, $5.00; leather, $6.00; very handsome half Russia, raised bands, $6.50.

The second edition of this excellent work, like the first, has received the benefit of Dr. Hutchinson's annotations, by which the phases of disease which are peculiar to this country are indicated, and thus a treatise which was intended for British practitioners and students is made more practically useful on this side of the water. We see no reason to modify the high opinion previously expressed with regard to Dr. Bristowe's work, except by adding our appreciation of the careful labors of the author in following the latest growth of medical science.—*Boston Medical and Surgical Journal*, Feb. 1880.

His accuracy in the portraiture of disease, his care in stating subtle points of diagnosis, and the

faithfully given pathology of abnormal processes have seldom been surpassed. He embraces many diseases not usually considered to belong to theory and practice, as skin diseases, syphilis and insanity, but they will not be objected to by readers, as he has studied them conscientiously and drawn from the life.—*Medical and Surgical Reporter*, Dec. 27, 1879.

The reader will find every considerable subject connected with the practice of medicine ably presented, in a style at once clear, interesting and concise. The additions made by Dr. Hutchinson are appropriate and practical, and greatly add to its usefulness to American readers.—*Buffalo Medical and Surgical Journal*, March, 1880.

REYNOLDS, J. RUSSELL, M. D.,
Professor of the Principles and Practice of Medicine in University College, London.

A System of Medicine. With notes and additions by HENRY HARTSHORNE, A. M., M. D., late Professor of Hygiene in the University of Pennsylvania. In three large and handsome octavo volumes, containing 3056 double-columned pages, with 317 illustrations. Price per volume, cloth, $5.00; sheep, $6.00; very handsome half Russia, raised bands, $6.50. Per set, cloth, $15; sheep, $18; half Russia, $19.50. *Sold only by subscription.*

VOLUME I. Contains GENERAL DISEASES and DISEASES OF THE NERVOUS SYSTEM.
VOLUME II. Contains DISEASES OF RESPIRATORY and CIRCULATORY SYSTEMS.
VOLUME III. Contains DISEASES OF THE DIGESTIVE, BLOOD-GLANDULAR, URINARY, REPRODUCTIVE and CUTANEOUS SYSTEMS.

Reynolds' SYSTEM OF MEDICINE, recently completed, has acquired, since the first appearance of the first volume, the well-deserved reputation of being the work in which modern British medicine is presented in its fullest and most practical form. This could scarce be otherwise in view of the fact that it is the result of the collaboration of the leading minds of the profession, each subject being treated by some gentleman who is regarded as its highest authority—as, for instance, diseases of the bladder by Sir Henry Thompson, malposition of the uterus by Graily Hewitt, insanity by Henry Maudsley, consumption by J. Hughes Bennet, diseases of the spine by Charles Bland Radcliffe, pericarditis by Francis Sibson, alcoholism by Francis E. Anstie, renal affections by William Roberts, asthma by Hyde Salter, cerebral affections by H. Charlton Bastian, gout and rheumatism by Alfred Baring Garrod, constitutional syphilis by Jonathan Hutchinson, diseases of the stomach by Wilson Fox, diseases of the skin by Balmanno Squire, affections of the larynx by Morell Mackenzie, diseases of the rectum by Blizard Curling, diabetes by Lauder Brunton, intestinal diseases by John Syer Bristowe, catalepsy and somnambulism by Thomas King Chambers, apoplexy by J. Hughlings Jackson, angina pectoris by Professor Gairdner, emphysema of the lungs by Sir William Jenner, etc., etc. All the leading schools in Great Britain have contributed their best men, in generous rivalry, to build up this monument of medical science. That a work conceived in such a spirit and carried out under such auspices should prove an indispensable treasury of facts and experience, suited to the daily wants of the practitioner, was inevitable; and the success which it has enjoyed in England, and the reputation which it has acquired on this side of the Atlantic, have sealed it with the approbation of the two pre-eminently practical nations.

Its large size and high price having kept it beyond the reach of many practitioners in this country who desire to possess it, a demand has arisen for an edition at a price which shall render it accessible to all. To meet this demand the present edition has been undertaken. The five volumes and five thousand pages of the original have, by the use of a smaller type and double columns, been compressed into three volumes of over three thousand pages, clearly and handsomely printed, and offered at a price which renders it one of the cheapest works ever presented to the American profession.

But not only is the American edition more convenient and lower priced than the English; it is also better and more complete. Some years having elapsed since the appearance of a portion of the work, additions were required to bring up the subjects to the existing condition of science. Some diseases, also, which are comparatively unimportant in England, require more elaborate treatment to adapt the articles devoted to them to the wants of the American physician; and there are points on which the received practice in this country differs from that adopted abroad. The supplying of these deficiencies has been undertaken by HENRY HARTSHORNE, M. D., late Professor of Hygiene in the University of Pennsylvania, who has endeavored to render the work fully up to the day, and as useful to the American physician as it has proved to be to his English brethren. The number of illustrations has also been largely increased, and no effort spared to render the typographical execution unexceptionable in every respect.

There is no medical work which we have in times past more frequently and fully consulted when perplexed by doubts as to treatment, or by having unusual or apparently inexplicable symptoms presented to us, than "Reynolds' System of Medicine." It contains just that kind of information which the busy practitioner frequently finds himself in need of. In order that any deficiencies may be supplied, the publishers have committed the preparation of the book for the press to Dr. Henry Hartshorne, whose judicious notes distributed throughout the volume afford abundant evidence of the thoroughness of the revision to which he has subjected it.—*American Journal of the Medical Sciences,* Jan. 1880.

Certainly no work with which we are acquainted has ever been given to the English-reading profession which treats of so many diseases in a manner so concise and thorough, and withal so lucid and trustworthy. In that branch of medicine in which the rank and file of the profession are mainly interested, viz., the practical part, therapeutics, Reynolds, without intending any invidious comparison, stands pre-eminent. The therapeutics of the English correspond more closely than those of any other country with those of this country, and the American editor of Reynolds' has brought this branch up to the most advanced American standard.—*Michigan Medical News,* Feb. 15, 1880.

WATSON, THOMAS, M. D.,
Late Physician in Ordinary to the Queen.

Lectures on the Principles and Practice of Physic. Delivered at King's College, London. A new American from the fifth English edition, revised and enlarged. Edited, with additions, and 190 illustrations, by HENRY HARTSHORNE, A. M., M. D., late Professor of Hygiene in the University of Pennsylvania. In two large and handsome octavo volumes, containing 1840 pp. Cloth, $9.00; leather, $11.00.

and Surgery. Second edition. In one very handsome octavo volume of 292 pages, with 109 illustrations. Cloth, $2.50. *Just ready.*

FROM THE PREFACE TO THE SECOND EDITION,

In the present edition I have made many additions and improvements to render the work more useful to those for whom it is intended. At the same time, in response to what seems to me an increasing desire for scientific treatment, I have developed more fully the modern methods of ascertaining and expressing current strength, tension, resistance, etc. I have also entered more fully into the polar method, and into the action and uses of the magnet. Notwithstanding an increase in the number of lines to the page, and the condensation of the matter new and old, the work has been enlarged by the addition of thirty pages. Thus improved, I may be permitted to hope that the new edition will continue to enjoy the favor so largely bestowed on the first.

The second edition of this work following so soon upon the first would in itself appear to be a sufficient announcement; nevertheless, the text has been so considerably revised and condensed, and so much enlarged by the addition of new matter, that we cannot fail to recognize a vast improvement upon the former work. The author has prepared his work for students and practitioners—for those who have never acquainted themselves with the subject, or, having done so, find that after a time their knowledge needs refreshing. We think he has accomplished this object. The book is not too voluminous, but is thoroughly practical, simple, complete and comprehensible. It is, moreover, replete with numerous illustrations of instruments, appliances, etc, is printed on fine paper, and handsomely bound in cloth.—*Medical Record,* Nov. 18, 1882.

It is, fortunately, not such an interminable treatise as most electro-therapentists like to write. It is not burdened with a needlessly learned terminology, and is written more from the point of view of the physician than of the specialist. The second edition has been considerably increased over the first, and has been brought up to the most recent advances of the science. It can in every way be recommended to those who wish to read a lucid, manageable monograph on this form of therapeutics.—*Med. and Surg. Reporter,* Nov. 4, 1882.

A most excellent work, addressed by a practitioner to his fellow-practitioners, and therefore thoroughly practical. The work now before us has the exceptional merit of clearly pointing out where the benefits to be derived from electricity must come. It contains all and everything that the practitioner needs in order to understand intelligently the nature and laws of the agent he is making use of, and for its proper application in practice. In a condensed, practical form, it presents to the physician all that he would wish to

remember after perusing a whole library on medical electricity, including the results of the latest investigations. It is the book for the practitioner, and the necessity for a second edition proves that it has been appreciated by the profession.—*Physician and Surgeon,* Dec. 1882.

It is very evident that Dr. Bartholow was correct in his view that the profession desired a small, plain and complete work on the practical use of electricity. It is only about a year since the first edition of his book appeared. In preparing the second edition he has enlarged the book somewhat, and has added some new matter, but not much. In truth, the work was so complete for its purpose as it first appeared that no considerable alterations or additions would be possible. Every physician who owns a battery should possess and study this book.—*Columbus Medical Journal,* Jan. 1883.

The first edition of this work having been exhausted in less than a year, shows the great value in which it has been held by the profession. Only a work of unusually great merit could have met with such a rapid sale. It has been found to fill a want, notwithstanding having numerous competitors. It was the purpose of the author to prepare a work from the practitioner's rather than the merely scientific standpoint, and this he has certainly accomplished. — *Cincinnati Medical News,* Nov. 1882.

This work seems to be written for physicians and is easily intelligible to every practitioner. It is concisely written, and the author's diction is simple and always comprehensible. The edition is larger than the first, and well represents the science of medical electricity at the present time. Every physician must use electricity in his practice, and in doing so he can have no better guide and companion than this volume.—*Gaillard's Med. Journ.,* Nov. 1882.

RICHARDSON, B. W., M.A., M.D., LL.D., F.R.S., F.S.A.

Fellow of the Royal College of Physicians, London.

Preventive Medicine. In one octavo volume of about 500 pages. *In press.*

A CENTURY OF AMERICAN MEDICINE, 1776–1876. By Drs. E. H. CLARKE, H. J. BIGELOW, S. D. GROSS, T. G. THOMAS and J. S. BILLINGS. In one very handsome 12mo. volume of 370 pages. Cloth, $2.25.

This work appeared in the pages of the American Journal of the Medical Sciences during the year 1876. As a detailed account of the development of medical science in America, by gentlemen of the highest authority in their respective departments, the profession will no doubt welcome it in a form adapted for preservation and reference.

BARLOW'S MANUAL OF THE PRACTICE OF MEDICINE. With additions by D. F. CONDIE, M. D. 1 vol. 8vo., pp. 603. Cloth, $2.50.

STOKES' LECTURES ON FEVER. Edited by John William Moore, M. D., F. K. Q. C. P. In one octavo volume of 280 pages. Cloth, $2.00.

A TREATISE ON FEVER. By ROBERT D. LYONS, K. C. C. In one octavo volume of 354 pages. Cloth, $2.25.

LECTURES ON THE STUDY OF FEVER. By A. HUDSON, M. D., M. R. I. A. Physician to the

Meath Hospital. In one octavo volume of 308 pages. Cloth, $2.50.

LA ROCHE ON YELLOW FEVER, considered in its Historical, Pathological, Etiological and Therapeutical Relations. In two large and handsome octavo volumes of 1468 pp. Cloth, $7.00.

TODD'S CLINICAL LECTURES ON CERTAIN ACUTE DISEASES. In one octavo volume of 320 pages. Cloth, $2.50.

HOLLAND'S MEDICAL NOTES AND REFLECTIONS. 1 vol. 8vo., pp. 493. Cloth, $3.50.

A Handbook of Diagnosis and Treatment of Diseases of
Nose and Naso-Pharynx. Second edition. In one handsome royal 12mo. volume
of 294 pages, with 77 illustrations. Cloth, $1.75. *Just ready.*

BROWNE, LENNOX, F. R. C. S., Edin.,
Senior Surgeon to the Central London Throat and Ear Hospital, etc.

The Throat and its Diseases. Second American from the second English edition, thoroughly revised. With 100 typical illustrations in colors and 50 wood engravings,
designed and executed by the Author. In one very handsome imperial octavo volume of
about 350 pages. *Preparing.*

FLINT, AUSTIN, M. D.,
Professor of the Principles and Practice of Medicine in Bellevue Hospital Medical College, N. Y.

A Manual of Auscultation and Percussion; Of the Physical Diagnosis of
Diseases of the Lungs and Heart, and of Thoracic Aneurism. Third edition. In one handsome royal 12mo. volume of 240 pages. Cloth, $1.63. *Just ready.*

By the Same Author.
Physical Exploration of the Lungs by Means of Auscultation and
Percussion. Three lectures delivered before the Philadelphia County Medical Society,
1882-83. In one handsome small 12mo. volume of 83 pages. Cloth, $1.00. *Just ready.*

By the Same Author.
A Practical Treatise on the Physical Exploration of the Chest and
the Diagnosis of Diseases Affecting the Respiratory Organs. Second and
revised edition. In one handsome octavo volume of 591 pages. Cloth, $4.50.

By the Same Author.
Phthisis: Its Morbid Anatomy, Etiology, Symptomatic Events and
Complications, Fatality and Prognosis, Treatment and Physical Diag-
nosis; In a series of Clinical Studies. In one handsome octavo volume of 442 pages.
Cloth, $3.50.

By the Same Author.
A Practical Treatise on the Diagnosis, Pathology and Treatment of
Diseases of the Heart. Second revised and enlarged edition. In one octavo volume
of 550 pages, with a plate. Cloth, $4.

GROSS, S. D., M.D., LL.D., D.C.L., Oxon., LL.D., Cantab.

A Practical Treatise on Foreign Bodies in the Air-passages. In one
octavo volume of 452 pages, with 59 illustrations. Cloth, $2.75.

FULLER ON DISEASES OF THE LUNGS AND
AIR-PASSAGES. Their Pathology, Physical Diagnosis, Symptoms and Treatment. From the
second and revised English edition. In one
octavo volume of 475 pages. Cloth, $3.50.

SLADE ON DIPHTHERIA; Its Nature and Treatment, with an account of the History of its Prevalence in various Countries. Second and revised
edition. In one royal 12mo. volume, pp. 158.
Cloth, $1.25.

WILLIAMS ON PULMONARY CONSUMPTION;

Its Nature, Varieties and Treatment. With an
analysis of one thousand cases to exemplify its
duration. In one octavo volume of 300 pages.
Cloth, $2.50.

SMITH ON CONSUMPTION; Its Early and Remediable Stages. 1 vol. 8vo., pp. 253. $2.25.

LA ROCHE ON PNEUMONIA. 1 vol. 8vo. of 490
pages. Cloth, $3.00.

WALSHE ON THE DISEASES OF THE HEART
AND GREAT VESSELS. Third American edition. In 1 vol. 8vo., 416 pp. Cloth, $3.00.

HABERSHON, S. O., M. D.,
Senior Physician to and late Lect. on Principles and Practice of Med. at Guy's Hospital, London.

On the Diseases of the Abdomen; Comprising those of the Stomach, and
other parts of the Alimentary Canal, Œsophagus, Cæcum, Intestines and Peritoneum. Second
American from third enlarged and revised English edition. In one handsome octavo
volume of 554 pages, with illustrations. Cloth, $3.50.

This valuable treatise will be found a cyclopædia
of information, systematically arranged, on all diseases of the alimentary tract from the mouth to
the rectum. A fair proportion of each chapter is
devoted to symptoms, pathology and therapeutics.
The present edition is fuller than former ones in
many particulars, and has been thoroughly revised
and amended by the author. Several new chapters
have been added, bringing the work fully up to

the times, and making it a volume of interest to
the practitioner in every field of medicine and
surgery. Perverted nutrition is, in some form,
associated with all diseases we have to combat,
and we need all the light that can be obtained on
a subject so broad and general. Dr. Habershon's
work is one that every practitioner should read
and study for himself.—*N. Y. Medical Journal,*
April, 1879.

PAVY'S TREATISE ON THE FUNCTION OF DI-
GESTION; Its Disorders and their Treatment.
From the second London edition. In one octavo
volume of 238 pages. Cloth, $2.00.

CHAMBERS' MANUAL OF DIET AND REGIMEN
IN HEALTH AND SICKNESS. In one handsome octavo volume of 302 pp. Cloth, $2.75.

HAMILTON, ALLAN McLANE, M. D.,

Attending Physician at the Hospital for Epileptics and Paralytics, Blackwell's Island, N. Y., and at the Out-Patients' Department of the New York Hospital.

Nervous Diseases; Their Description and Treatment. Second edition, thoroughly revised and rewritten. In one handsome octavo volume of 598 pages, with 72 illustrations. Cloth, $4.

We are glad to welcome a second edition of so useful a work as this, in which Dr. Hamilton has succeeded in condensing into convenient limits the most important of the recent developments in regard to diseases of the nervous system. Of recent years nervous pathology has attained to such importance as to necessitate very careful description in special works, and among these this volume must take a high place. This volume is on the whole excellent, and is devoid of that spirit of plagiarism which we have unfortunately seen too much of in certain recent English works on nervous diseases. —*Edinburgh Medical Journal*, May, 1882.

When the first edition of this good book appeared we gave it our emphatic endorsement, and the present edition enhances our appreciation of the book and its author as a safe guide to students of clinical neurology. One of the best and most critical of English neurological journals, *Brain*, has characterized this book as the best of its kind in any language, which is a handsome endorsement from an exalted source. The improvements in the new edition, and the additions to it, will justify its purchase even by those who possess the old.—*Alienist and Neurologist*, April, 1882.

The book is made up of plain and practical descriptions of the chief disorders of the nervous system, with interesting discussions of pathological points and very sensible views as to treatment. It is a book which the general practitioner will find of great value.—*N. Y. Med. Jour.*, Sept. 1882.

The author's aim is to write a treatise on Nervous Diseases which is both concise and practical, while it is, at the same time, sufficiently comprehensive. We have pleasure in bearing testimony to the fact that his efforts have been crowned with success. The various diseases have been well described, the directions as to how to arrive at a correct diagnosis are very clear, and the hints in treatment are plain, practical and sound. Such a book should be considered a necessity in every medical library, as the ailments described are among the most common that come under observation in the everyday work of the general physician. To him, therefore, we recommend it with pleasure; in fact, we may go further and say that, all things considered, it is for his purpose the best work of the kind now available.—*Canada Jour. Med. Sciences*, April, 1882.

This work is well adapted to the wants of the general practitioner, for whom it seems to have been especially written. It is a thoroughly practical book, the careful study of which will render the diagnosis of nervous affections the more easy, and their treatment more successful. The book is very useful as a reference work to the busy practitioner, to whom we can recommend it.—*Medical and Surgical Reporter*, Jan. 21, 1882.

The most valuable, for the general purposes of the student and practitioner, of the host that has recently been published in the same field of professional literature.—*Amer. Practitioner*, May, 1882.

MITCHELL, S. WEIR, M. D.,

Physician to Orthopædic Hospital and the Infirmary for Diseases of the Nervous System, Phila., etc.

Lectures on Diseases of the Nervous System; Especially in Women. Second edition. In one very handsome 12mo. volume of about 250 pages. *Preparing.*

The life-long devotion of the Author to the subjects discussed in this volume has rendered it eminently desirable that the results of his labors should be embodied for the benefit of those who may experience the difficulties connected with the treatment of this class of disease. Many of these lectures are fresh studies of hysterical affections; others treat of the modifications his views have undergone in regard to certain forms of treatment; while throughout the whole work he has been careful to keep in view the practical lessons of his cases.

A few notices of the previous edition are appended:—

It is a record of a number of very remarkable cases, with acute analyses and discussions, clinical, physiological and therapeutical. It is a book to which the physician meeting with a new hysterical experience, or in doubt whether his new experience is hysterical, may well turn with a well-grounded hope of finding a parallelism; it will be a new experience, indeed, if no similar one is here recorded.—*Phila. Medical Times*, June 4, 1881.

The book throughout is not only intensely entertaining, but it contains a large amount of rare and valuable information. Dr. Mitchell has recorded not only the results of his most careful observation, but has added to the knowledge of the subjects treated by his original investigation and practical study. The book is one we can commend to all of our readers.—*Maryland Medical Journal*, May 1, 1881.

PLAYFAIR, W. S., M. D., F. R. C. P.

The Systematic Treatment of Nerve Prostration and Hysteria. In one handsome small 12mo. volume of 97 pages. Cloth, $1.00. *Just ready.*

TUKE, DANIEL HACK, M. D.,

Joint Author of The Manual of Psychological Medicine, etc.

Illustrations of the Influence of the Mind upon the Body in Health and Disease. Designed to illustrate the Action of the Imagination. New edition. In one handsome octavo volume. *Preparing.*

BLANDFORD, G. FIELDING, M. D., F. R. C. P.,

Lecturer on Psychological Medicine at the School of St. George's Hospital, London.

Insanity and its Treatment: Lectures on the Treatment, Medical and Legal, of Insane Patients. With a Summary of the Laws in force in the United States on the Continement of the Insane, by ISAAC RAY, M. D. In one very handsome octavo volume.

CLINICAL OBSERVATIONS ON FUNCTIONAL NERVOUS DISORDERS, by C. HANDFIELD JONES, | M. D. Second American edition. In one handsome octavo volume of 340 pages. Cloth, $3.25.

ASHHURST, JOHN, Jr., M. D.,

Professor of Clinical Surgery, Univ. of Penna., Surgeon to the Episcopal Hospital, Philadelphia.

The Principles and Practice of Surgery. Third edition, enlarged and revised. In one large and handsome octavo volume of 1060 pages, with 556 illustrations. Cloth, $6; leather, $7; very handsome half Russia, raised bands, $7.50. *Just ready.*

GIBNEY, V. P., M. D.

Orthopædic Surgery. For the use of Practitioners and Students. In one handsome octavo volume, profusely illustrated. *Preparing.*

ROBERTS, JOHN B., A. M., M. D.,

Lecturer on Anatomy and on Operative Surgery at the Philadelphia School of Anatomy.

The Principles and Practice of Surgery. For the use of Students and Practitioners of Medicine and Surgery. In one very handsome octavo volume of about 500 pages, with many illustrations. *Preparing.*

STIMSON, LEWIS A., B. A., M. D.,

Prof. of Pathol. Anat. at the Univ. of the City of New York, Surgeon and Curator to Bellevue Hosp.

A Manual of Operative Surgery. In one very handsome royal 12mo. volume of 477 pages, with 332 illustrations. Cloth, $2.50.

BRYANT, THOMAS, F. R. C. S.,
Surgeon to Guy's Hospital.

The Practice of Surgery. Third American from the third and revised English edition. Thoroughly revised and much improved, by JOHN B. ROBERTS, A. M., M. D. In one large and very handsome imperial octavo volume of 1009 pages, with 735 illustrations. Cloth, $6.50; leather, $7.50; very handsome half Russia, raised bands, $8.00.

Without freighting his book with multiplied details and wearying descriptions of allied methods of procedure, he is ample enough for reference on all the departments of surgery, not omitting such strict specialties as dental, ophthalmic, military, orthopaedic and gynaecological surgery. Some of these chapters are written by specialists in these respective branches, and all are amply sufficient for anyone not himself aiming at special practice. The labors of the American editor deserve unqualified praise. His additions to the author's text are numerous, judicious and germane. They add very distinctly to the value of the original treatise, and give a more equitable illustration of the part taken by American surgeons than the author was able to do.—*Medical and Surgical Reporter,* Feb. 12, 1881.

It is the best of all the one-volume works on surgery of recent date for the ordinary surgeon, containing enough of pathology, accurate description of surgical diseases and injuries, well-devised

plans of treatment, etc., to make the surgeon who follows the text successful in his diagnosis and treatment in any case in which success can be secured, according to the present state of the surgical art.—*Virginia Medical Monthly,* May, 1881.

It is a work especially adapted to the wants of students and practitioners. It affords instruction in sufficient detail for a full understanding of surgical principles and the treatment of surgical diseases. It embraces in its scope all the diseases that are recognized as belonging to surgery and all traumatic injuries. In discussing these it has seemed to be the aim of the author rather to present the student with practical information, and that alone, than to burden his memory with the views of different writers, however distinguished they might have been. In this edition the whole work has been carefully revised, much of it has been rewritten, and important additions have been made to almost every chapter.—*Cincinnati Medical News,* Jan. 1881.

ERICHSEN, JOHN E., F. R. S., F. R. C. S.,
Professor of Surgery in University College, London, etc.

The Science and Art of Surgery; Being a Treatise on Surgical Injuries, Diseases and Operations. Carefully revised by the Author from the seventh and enlarged English edition. In two large and beautiful octavo volumes of 1944 pages, illustrated by 862 engravings on wood. Cloth, $8.50; leather, $10.50; half Russia, raised bands, $11.50.

Of the many treatises on surgery which it has been our task to study, or our pleasure to read, there is none which in all points has satisfied us so well as the classic treatise of Erichsen. His polished, clear style, his freedom from prejudice and hobbies, his unsurpassed grasp of his subject and vast clinical experience, qualify him admirably to write a model text-book. When we wish, at the least cost of time, to learn the most of a topic in surgery, we turn, by preference, to his work. It is a pleasure, therefore, to see that the appreciation of it is general, and has led to the appearance of another edition.—*Medical and Surgical Reporter,* Feb. 2, 1878.

For the past twenty years Erichsen's Surgery has maintained its place as the leading text-book, not only in this country, but in Great Britain. That it is able to hold its ground is abundantly proven by the thoroughness with which the present edition has been revised, and by the large amount of valuable material that has been added. Aside from this, one hundred and fifty new illustrations have been inserted, including quite a number of microscopical appearances of pathological processes. So marked is this change for the better that the work almost appears as an entirely new one.—*Medical Record,* Feb. 23, 1878.

ESMARCH, Dr. FRIEDRICH,
Professor of Surgery at the University of Kiel, etc.

Early Aid in Injuries and Accidents. Five Ambulance Lectures. Translated by H. R. H. PRINCESS CHRISTIAN. In one handsome small 12mo. volume of 109 pages, with 24 illustrations. Cloth, 75 cents. *Just ready.*

The course of instruction is divided into five sections or lectures. The first, or introductory lecture, gives a brief account of the structure and organization of the human body, illustrated by clear, suitable diagrams. The second teaches how to give judicious help in ordinary injuries—contusions, wounds, haemorrhage and poisoned wounds. The third treats of first aid in cases of fracture and of dislocations, in sprains and in burns. Next, the methods of affording first treatment in cases of frost-bite, of drowning, of suffocation, of loss of consciousness and of poisoning are described, and the fifth lecture teaches how injured persons may be most safely and easily transported to their

homes, to a medical man, or to a hospital. The illustrations in the book are clear and good, and it will, we doubt not, command an extensive circulation.—*Medical Times and Gazette,* Nov. 4, 1882.

This little book contains much of the greatest usefulness, and, were it generally read and remembered, the confusion and disorder that generally attend injuries and accidents would be diminished and the injured not only rendered comfortable at once, but preserved from further injury. The clear and lucid style of the great German surgeon is readily recognized in all parts of the translation.—*Nashville Journal of Medicine and Surgery,* Feb. 1883.

DRUITT, ROBERT, M. R. C. S., etc.
The Principles and Practice of Modern Surgery. From the eighth London edition. In one octavo volume of 687 pages, with 432 illustrations. Cloth, $4.00; leather, $5.00.

SARGENT ON BANDAGING AND OTHER OPERATIONS OF MINOR SURGERY. New edition, with a Chapter on military surgery. One 12mo. volume of 383 pages, with 187 cuts. Cloth, $1.75.

MILLER'S PRINCIPLES OF SURGERY. Fourth American from the third Edinburgh edition. In one 8vo. vol. of 688 pages, with 340 illustrations. Cloth, $3.75.

MILLER'S PRACTICE OF SURGERY. Fourth and revised American from the last Edinburgh edition. In one large 8vo. vol. of 682 pages, with 364 illustrations. Cloth, $3.75.

PIRRIE'S PRINCIPLES AND PRACTICE OF SURGERY. Edited by JOHN NEILL, M. D. In one 8vo. vol. of 784 pp. with 316 illus. Cloth, $3.75.

COOPER'S LECTURES ON THE PRINCIPLES AND PRACTICE OF SURGERY. In one 8vo. of 767 pages. Cloth, $2.00.

SKEY'S OPERATIVE SURGERY. In one of 661 pages, with 81 woodcuts. Cloth, $

GIBSON'S INSTITUTES AND PRACTICE OF SURGERY. Eighth edition. In two of 965 pages, with 34 plates. Leather

HOLMES, TIMOTHY, M. A.,

Surgeon and Lecturer on Surgery at St. George's Hospital, London.

A System of Surgery; Theoretical and Practical. IN TREATISES BY VARIOUS AUTHORS. AMERICAN EDITION, THOROUGHLY REVISED AND RE-EDITED by JOHN H. PACKARD, M. D., Surgeon to the Episcopal and St. Joseph's Hospitals, Philadelphia, assisted by a corps of thirty-three of the most eminent American surgeons. In three large and very handsome imperial octave volumes, containing 3137 double-columned pages, with 979 illustrations on wood and 13 lithographic plates, beautifully colored. Price per volume, cloth, $6.00; leather, $7.00; half Russia, $7.50. Per set, cloth, $18.00; leather, $21.00; half Russia, $22.50. *Sold only by subscription.*

VOLUME I. contains GENERAL PATHOLOGY, MORBID PROCESSES, INJURIES IN GENERAL, COMPLICATIONS OF INJURIES AND INJURIES OF REGIONS.

VOLUME II. contains DISEASES OF ORGANS OF SPECIAL SENSE, CIRCULATORY SYSTEM, DIGESTIVE TRACT AND GENITO-URINARY ORGANS.

VOLUME III. contains DISEASES OF THE RESPIRATORY ORGANS, BONES, JOINTS AND MUSCLES, DISEASES OF THE NERVOUS SYSTEM, GUNSHOT WOUNDS, OPERATIVE AND MINOR SURGERY, AND MISCELLANEOUS SUBJECTS (including an essay on HOSPITALS).

This great work, issued some years since in England, has won such universal confidence wherever the language is spoken that its republication here, in a form more thoroughly adapted to the wants of the American practitioner, has seemed to be a duty owing to the profession. To accomplish this, each article has been placed in the hands of a gentleman specially competent to treat its subject, and no labor has been spared to bring each one up to the foremost level of the times, and to adapt it thoroughly to the practice of the country. In certain cases this has rendered necessary the substitution of an entirely new essay for the original, as in the case of the articles on Skin Diseases and on Diseases of the Absorbent System, where the views of the authors have been superseded by the advance of medical science, and new articles have therefore been prepared by Drs. Arthur Van Harlingen and S. C. Busey, respectively. So also in the case of Anaesthetics, in the use of which American practice differs from that of England, the original has been supplemented with a new essay by J. C. Reeve, M. D. The same careful and conscientious revision has been pursued throughout, leading to an increase of nearly one-fourth in matter, while the series of illustrations has been nearly trebled, and the whole is presented as a complete exponent of British and American Surgery, adapted to the daily needs of the working practitioner.

In order to bring it within the reach of every member of the profession, the five volumes of the original have been compressed into three by employing a double-columned royal octavo page, and in this improved form it is offered at less than one-half the price of the original. It is printed and bound to match in every detail with Reynolds' System of Medicine. The work will be sold by subscription only, and in due time every member of the profession will be called upon and offered an opportunity to subscribe.

The authors of the original English edition are men of the front rank in England, and Dr. Packard has been fortunate in securing as his American coadjutors such men as Bartholow, Hyde, Hunt, Conner, Stimson, Morton, Hodgen, Jewell and their colleagues. As a whole, the work will be solid and substantial, and a valuable addition to the library of any medical man. It is more widely and more useful than the English edition, and with its companion work—"Reynolds' System of Medicine"—will well represent the present state of our science. One who is familiar with those two works will be fairly well furnished head-wise and hand-wise.—*The Medical News,* Jan. 7, 1882.

This work is cyclopædic in character, and every subject is treated in an exhaustive manner. It is especially designed for a reference book, which every practising surgeon should have under hand in cases which require more than ordinary knowledge.—*Chicago Med. Journ. and Exam.,* Feb. 1882.

Great credit is due to the American editor and his co-laborers for revising and bringing within easy reach of American surgeons a work which has been received with such universal favor on the other side of the Atlantic as Holmes' System of Surgery. In the list of English contributors to the first volume we find the names of such well-known surgeons as Sir James Paget, Simon, Savory, Callender, Barclay, and others equally distinguished; while among the American writers we recognize men of no less celebrity. With regard to the mechanical execution of the work, neither pains nor money seem to have been spared by the publishers.—*Med. and Surg. Reporter,* Sept. 2, 1882.

In the revision of the work for the American edition not only has provision been made for a renegation of the advances made in our knowledge during the ten years since its first publication, but also for a presentation of the variations in practice which characterize American surgery and distinguish it from that of Great Britain. The work is one which we take pleasure in commending to the notice of our readers as an encyclopedia of surgical knowledge and practice.—*St. Louis Courier of Medicine,* Nov. 1881.

HOLMES, TIMOTHY, M. A.

Surgery, Its Principles and Practice. In one handsome octavo volume of 968 pages, with 411 illustrations. Cloth, $6.00; leather, $7.00; half Russia, $7.50.

Mr. Holmes is a surgeon of large and varied experience, and one of the best known, and perhaps the most brilliant writer upon surgical subjects in England. It is a book for students—and an admirable one—and for the busy general practitioner. It will give a student all the knowledge needed to pass a rigid examination. The book fairly justifies the high expectations that were formed of it. Its style is clear and forcible, even brilliant at times, and the conciseness needed to bring it within its proper limits has not impaired its force and distinctness.—*N. Y. Med. Record,* April 14, 1876.

It will be found a most excellent epitome of surgery by the general practitioner who has not the time to give attention to more minute and extended works, and to the medical student. In fact, we know of no one we can more cordially recommend. The author has succeeded well in giving a plain and practical account of each surgical injury and disease, and of the treatment which is most commonly adopted. It will no doubt become a popular work in the profession, and especially as a text-book.—*Cinn. Med. News,* April 1876.

STIMSON, LEWIS A., B. A., M. D.,

Professor of Pathological Anatomy at the University of the City of New York, Surgeon and Curator to Bellevue Hospital, Surgeon to the Presbyterian Hospital, New York, etc.

A Practical Treatise on Fractures. In one very handsome octavo volume of 598 pages, with 360 beautiful illustrations. Cloth, $4.75; leather, $5.75. *Just Ready.*

The author has given to the medical profession in this treatise on fractures what is likely to become a standard work on the subject It is certainly not surpassed by any work written in the English, or, for that matter, any other language Perfectly conversant with the American, English, French and German medical literature, the author tells us in a short, concise and comprehensive manner, all that is known about his subject. There is nothing scanty or superficial about it, as in most other treatises, on the contrary, everything is thorough. The chapters on repair of fractures and their treatment show him not only to be a profound student, but likewise a practical surgeon and pathologist. His mode of treatment of the different fractures is eminently sound and practical. We consider this

work one of the best on fractures; and it will be welcomed not only as a text-book, but also by the surgeon in full practice.—*N. O. Medical and Surgical Journal*, March, 1883

This practical treatise upon the subject of fractures of the various portions of the bony skeleton is a compendious exposition of the most recent as well as the best attested modes of treatment, but is not confined to this, as it also considers the pathology, etiology and mechanical principles involved in the different forms of fracture as well as the cause of delayed union, pseudo-arthrosis and other related topics. We have no criticism, but only commendation, for this excellent work.—*College and Clinical Record*, Jan. 15, 1883.

HAMILTON, FRANK H., M. D., LL. D.,

Surgeon to the Bellevue Hospital, New York.

A Practical Treatise on Fractures and Dislocations. Sixth edition, thoroughly revised and much improved. In one very handsome octavo volume of 909 pages, with 352 illustrations. Cloth, $5.50; leather, $6.50; half Russia, raised bands, $7.00.

The only complete work on its subject in the English tongue, and indeed it may now be said to be the only work of its kind in any tongue. It would require an exceedingly critical examination to detect in it any particulars in which it might be improved. The work is a monument to American surgery, and will long serve to keep green the memory of its venerable author.—*Michigan Medical News*, Nov. 10, 1881

Dr. Hamilton is the author of the best modern work in his own or any language on fractures and dislocations.—*Lond. Med. Times and Gaz.* Nov. 19, '81

This edition, besides being carefully revised, has in part been entirely rewritten—for instance, the chapter on fractures of the patella—and a chapter on general prognosis has been added. The work as a whole is one of the very few medical books of American origin that are everywhere accorded a standard character Its subject-matter unavoidably comes home to every general practitioner as a branch of our art in which he cannot afford to neglect the fullest and most practical information of such a character as it and it alone furnishes —*New York Medical Journal*, March, 1881.

WELLS, J. SOELBERG, F. R. C. S.,

Professor of Ophthalmology in King's College Hospital, London, etc.

A Treatise on Diseases of the Eye. Third American from the third London edition. Thoroughly revised, with copious additions, by CHARLES S. BULL, M. D., Surgeon and Pathologist to the New York Eye and Ear Infirmary. In one large and very handsome octavo volume of 883 pages, with 254 illustrations on wood, six colored plates, and selections from the Test-types of Jaeger and Snellen. Cloth, $5.00; leather, $6.00; half Russia, raised bands, $6.50.

NETTLESHIP, EDWARD, F. R. C. S.,

Ophthalmic Surg and Lect. on Ophth Surg at St Thomas' Hospital, London.

The Student's Guide to Diseases of the Eye. New edition. With a chapter on the Detection of Color-Blindness, by WILLIAM THOMSON, M. D., Ophthalmologist to the Jefferson Medical College. In one royal 12mo. volume of 416 pages, with 138 illustrations. Cloth, $2.00. *Just ready.*

This new edition of an excellent handbook embodies several improvements. A brief but clear introduction to the principles of geometrical optics, so far as they concern the ophthalmist, will be hailed by many a student whose preliminary scientific lessons are fading from his mind The advantage to all readers of having this fcount of physical principles thus readily at hand is manifest. We confidently recommended the first edition, we have only now to congratulate the author on his assured success—*The Practitioner*, Nov. 1882.

The second edition of Mr. Nettleship's excellent

little work contains many additions and improvements on the former one As it stands now the book forms one of the most complete, concise, and withal practical volumes in ophthalmology The principal additions that we recognize are an initiatory chapter on "Optical Outlines," which is evidently introduced to supply a decided want in the preliminary education of every medical student Operations are described stage after stage with great clearness as becomes one who is himself in the first line of operators.—*Australian Medical Journal*, Oct. 15, 1882

BROWNE, EDGAR A.,

Surgeon to the Liverpool Eye and Ear Infirmary and to the Dispensary for Skin Diseases.

How to Use the Ophthalmoscope. Being Elementary Instructions in Ophthalmoscopy, arranged for the use of Students. In one small royal 12mo. volume of 116 pages, with 35 illustrations. Cloth, $1.00.

LAWSON ON INJURIES TO THE EYE, ORBIT AND EYELIDS. Their Immediate and Remote Effects. In one octavo volume of 404 pages, with 92 illustrations. Cloth, $3.50.
LAURENCE AND MOON'S HANDY BOOK OF OPHTHALMIC SURGERY, for the use of Prac-

titioners Second edition In one octavo volume of 227 pages, with 66 illust. Cloth
CARTER'S PRACTICAL TREATISE ON ES OF THE EYE. Edited by JOHN Gi
In one handsome octavo volume.

BURNETT, CHARLES H., A. M., M. D.,

Aural Surg. to the Presb. Hosp., Surgeon-in-charge of the Infir. for Dis. of the Ear, Philadelphia.

The Ear, Its Anatomy, Physiology and Diseases. A Practical Treatise for the use of Medical Students and Practitioners. In one handsome octavo volume of 610 pages, with 87 illustrations. Cloth, $4.50; leather, $5.50; half Russia, raised bands, $6.00.

The medical profession will welcome this new work on otology, which presents clearly and concisely its present aspect, whilst clearly indicating the direction in which further researches can be most profitably carried on. Dr. Burnett has produced a work which, as a text-book, stands *facile princeps* in our language. To the specialist the work is of the highest value, and his sense of gratitude to Dr. Burnett will, we hope, be proportionate to the amount of benefit he can obtain from the careful study of the book and a constant reference to its trustworthy pages.—*Edinburgh Med. Journal, Oct. '78.*

As the title of the work indicates, this volume treats of the anatomy and physiology of the ear as well as of its diseases, and the author has taken special pains to make this difficult and complicated matter thoroughly clear and intelligible. Both student and practitioner can study this work with a great deal of benefit. It is profusely and beautifully illustrated.—*N. Y. Hosp. Gazette, Oct. 13, 1877.*

POLITZER, ADAM, M. D.,

Imperial-Royal Prof. of Aural Therap. in the Univ. of Vienna.

A Text-Book of the Ear and its Diseases. Translated, at the Author's request, by JAMES PATTERSON CASSELLS, M. D., M. R. C. S. In one handsome octavo volume of 800 pages, with 257 original illustrations. Cloth, $5.50. *Just ready.*

The name of Dr. Politzer is indissolubly associated with the progress of aural surgery during this generation. The treatise which he has written on this branch has long been a standard in Germany; and this translation of it, with the author's approbation, and by one of the most eminent aurists of Great Britain, will certainly take rank as a standard work of reference for years to come. The volume begins with a complete exposition of the anatomy of the ear and the physiology of audition.

Then follows a discussion of the diseases of the several portions of the organ, the middle ear, the mastoid process, the internal ear, etc. Injuries of the organ and the relations of ear diseases to the assurance are also treated of. The book closes with chapters on malformations of the ear, deaf-mutism, hearing instruments for the deaf and a satisfactory index. The text is elucidated by more than two hundred and fifty illustrations.—*Medical and Surgical Reporter, Feb. 3, 1883.*

COLEMAN, A., L. R. C. P., F. R. C. S., Exam. L. D. S.,

Senior Dent. Surg. and Lect. on Dent. Surg. to St. Bartholomew's Hosp. and the Dent. Hosp., London.

A Manual of Dental Surgery and Pathology. Thoroughly revised and adapted to the use of American Students, by THOMAS C. STELLWAGEN, M. A., M. D., D. D. S., Prof. of Physiology at the Philadelphia Dental College. In one handsome volume of 412 pages, with 331 illustrations. Cloth, $3.25. *Just ready.*

This volume deserves to rank among the most important of recent contributions to dental literature. Mr. Coleman has presented his methods of practice, for the most part, in a plain and concise manner, and the work of the American editor has been conscientiously performed. He has evidently labored to present his convictions of the best modes of practice for the instruction of those commencing a professional career, and he has faithfully endeavored to teach to others all that he has acquired by his own observation and experience. The book deserves a place in the library of every dentist.—*Dental Cosmos, May, 1882.*

It should be in the possession of every practitioner in this country. The part devoted to first and second dentition and irregularities of the permanent teeth is fully worth the price. In fact, price should not be considered in purchasing such a work. If the money put into some of our worthless standard text-books could be converted into such publications as this, much good would result.—*Southern Dental Journal, May, 1882.*

GROSS, S. D., M. D., LL. D., D. C. L., etc.

A Practical Treatise on the Diseases, Injuries and Malformations of the Urinary Bladder, the Prostate Gland and the Urethra. Third edition, thoroughly revised by SAMUEL W. GROSS, M. D., Surgeon to the Philadelphia Hospital. In one octavo volume of 574 pages, with 170 illustrations. Cloth, $4.50.

For reference and general information, the physician or surgeon can find no work that meets their necessities more thoroughly than this, a revised edition of an excellent treatise. Replete with handsome illustrations and good ideas, it has the unusual advantage of being easily comprehended by the reasonable and practical manner in which the various subjects are systematized and arranged.—*Atlanta Medical Journal, Oct. 1876.*

ROBERTS, WILLIAM, M. D.,

Lecturer on Medicine in the Manchester School of Medicine, etc.

A Practical Treatise on Urinary and Renal Diseases, including Urinary Deposits. Fourth American from the fourth London edition. Illustrated by numerous engravings. In one large and handsome octavo volume. *Preparing.*

THOMPSON, SIR HENRY,

Surgeon and Professor of Clinical Surgery to University College Hospital, London.

Lectures on Diseases of the Urinary Organs. Second American from the third English edition. In one 8vo. volume of 203 pp., with 25 illustrations. Cloth, $2.25.

By the Same Author.

On the Pathology and Treatment of Stricture of the Urethra and Urinary Fistulæ. From the third English edition. In one volume of 359 pages, with 47 cuts and 3 plates. Cloth, $3.50.

BASHAM ON RENAL DISEASES: A Clinical Guide to their Diagnosis and Treatment. In one 12mo. vol. of 304 pages, with 21 illustrations. Cloth, $2.00.

GROSS, SAMUEL W., A. M., M. D.,
Professor of the Principles of Surgery and of Clinical Surgery in the Jefferson Medical College.

A Practical Treatise on Impotence, Sterility, and Allied Disorders of the Male Sexual Organs. New edition. In one octavo volume. *In a few days.*

A few notices of the previous edition are appended.

The author has devoted much time to the hardest study of this most trying class of diseases; and this labor, together with the fruit of laborious research into the scattered literature of the subject, constitutes the result of his investigations. We can earnestly commend it to the practitioner as the very best work upon the subject in the English language.—*Nashville Journal of Medicine and Surgery*, Oct. 1881.

The author is a clear and concise writer, and every page of his treatise gives evidence of his thorough familiarity with recent research, and with the latest journal literature. The book is a thoroughly scientific exposition of our present knowledge of the subjects treated of: its pages are rich in information of high value to the practitioner, and, once read, will be frequently referred to.—*St. Louis Courier of Medicine*, Nov. 1881.

BUMSTEAD, F. J.,   *and*   TAYLOR, R. W.,
M. D., LL. D.,   A. M., M. D.,
Late Professor of Venereal Diseases at the College of Physicians and Surgeons, New York, etc.   *Surgeon to Charity Hospital, New York, Prof. of Venereal and Skin Diseases in the University of Vermont, Pres. of the Am. Dermatological Ass'n.*

The Pathology and Treatment of Venereal Diseases. Including the results of recent investigations upon the subject. Fifth edition, revised and largely rewritten, by Dr. Taylor. In one large and handsome octavo volume of about 900 pages, with about 150 illustrations. *In press.*

The fifth edition of this standard work, now passing through the press, has been subjected to a thorough revision by Dr. Taylor, and all additions have been made necessary to render it thoroughly representative of the present state of syphilology. Recent advanced theories have been fully discussed; space has been devoted to a detailed account of a newly-discovered agent which has been proved of striking value in the treatment of venereal diseases, and a chapter has been added upon the relation of syphilis to marriage. In addition to the improvements in the text, a series of carefully-executed chromolithographic drawings has been inserted, portraying faithfully those morbid conditions impossible to depict without the use of colors. Every care has been taken with the typography, and it is confidently anticipated that the volume will be found in all respects worthy of the exalted position accorded the previous editions.

CORNIL, V.,
Professor to the Faculty of Medicine of Paris, and Physician to the Lourcine Hospital.

Syphilis, its Morbid Anatomy, Diagnosis and Treatment. Specially revised by the Author, and translated with notes and additions by J. HENRY C. SIMES, M. D., Demonstrator of Pathological Histology in the University of Pennsylvania, and J. WILLIAM WHITE, M. D., Lecturer on Venereal Diseases and Demonstrator of Surgery in the University of Pennsylvania. In one handsome octavo volume of 461 pages, with 84 very beautiful illustrations. Cloth, $3.75. *Just ready.*

The anatomical and histological characters of the hard and soft sore are admirably described. The multiform cutaneous manifestations of the disease are dealt with histologically in a masterly way, as we should indeed expect them to be, and the accompanying illustrations are executed carefully and well. The various nervous lesions which are the recognised outcome of the syphilitic dyscrasia are treated with care and consideration. Syphilitic epilepsy, paralysis, cerebral syphilis and locomotor ataxia are subjects full of interest; and nowhere in the whole volume is the clinical experience of the author or the wide acquaintance of the translators with medical literature more evident than in Chapter X. The anatomy, the histology, the pathology and the clinical features of syphilis are represented in this work in their best, most practical and most instructive form, and no one will rise from its perusal without the feeling that his grasp of the wide and important subject on which it treats is a stronger and surer one.—*The London Practitioner*, January, 1882.

It is with the special purpose of showing the evo-

lution of the disease as indicated by histological changes that the author has prepared this volume. In this respect it is much better than any other we could name, and merits the close reading of syphilologists. The translation is well done, and the reader will not regret the considerable additions which the translators have inserted in the text.—*Medical and Surgical Reporter*, Aug. 5, 1882.

The characteristic feature of M. Cornil's work is the attention paid to the minute anatomy of the syphilitic lesions. The histological evolution of the various phases of the disease, from the initial chancre to the gumma, including the mucous patch, the superficial and deep cutaneous syphilides, the osseous and visceral affections—is considered with a detail that is in striking contrast to that of other works upon the same subject. The translation has been made with his consent and approval, and he is fortunate in the selection of his translators, for they have added materially to the interest and value of the volume.—*Maryland Medical Journal*, Aug. 15, 1882.

CULLERIER, A., & BUMSTEAD, F. J., M. D., LL. D.,
Surgeon to the Hôpital du Midi.   *Late Professor of Venereal Diseases in the College of Physicians and Surgeons, New York.*

An Atlas of Venereal Diseases. Translated and edited by FREEMAN J. BUMSTEAD, M. D. In one imperial 4to. volume of 328 pages, double-columns, with 26 pl containing about 150 figures, beautifully colored, many of them the size of life. St bound in cloth, $17.00. A specimen of the plates and text sent by mail, on receipt of

HILL ON SYPHILIS AND LOCAL CONTAGIOUS DISORDERS. In one handsome octavo volume of 479 pages. Cloth, $3.25.
LEE'S LECTURES ON SYPHILIS AND SOME

FORMS OF LOCAL DISEASE AF PRINCIPALLY THE ORGANS OF G TION. In one handsome octavo volu pages. Cloth, $2.25.

EMMET, THOMAS ADDIS, M. D., LL. D.,
Surgeon to the Woman's Hospital, New York, etc.

The Principles and Practice of Gynæcology; For the use of Students and Practitioners of Medicine. Second edition. Thoroughly revised. In one large and very handsome octavo volume of 879 pages, with 133 illustrations. Cloth, $5.00; leather, $6.00; very handsome half Russia, $6.50.

No gynæcological treatise has appeared which contains an equal amount of original and useful matter; nor does the medical and surgical history of America include a book more novel and useful. The tabular and statistical information which it contains is marvellous, both in quantity and accuracy, and cannot be otherwise than invaluable to future investigators. It is a work which demands not careless reading but profound study. Its value as a contribution to gynæcology is, perhaps, greater than that of all previous literature on the subject combined.—*Chicago Medical Gazette*, April 5, 1880.

In no country of the world has gynæcology re-ceived more attention than in America. It is then, with a feeling of pleasure that we welcome a work on diseases of women from so eminent a gynæcologist as Dr. Emmet. The work is essentially clinical, and leaves a strong impress of the author's individuality. To criticise, with the care it merits, the book throughout, would demand far more space than is at our command. To particularize we can say that the work teems with original ideas, fresh and valuable methods of practice, and is written in a clear and elegant style, worthy of the literary reputation of the country of Longfellow and Oliver Wendell Holmes.—*British Medical Journal*, Feb. 21, 1880.

DUNCAN, J. MATTHEWS, M. D., LL. D., F. R. S. E., etc.
Clinical Lectures on the Diseases of Women; Delivered in Saint Bartholomew's Hospital. In one handsome octavo volume of 175 pages. Cloth, $1.50.

They are in every way worthy of their author; indeed, we look upon them as among the most valuable of his contributions. They are all upon matters of great interest to the general practitioner. Some of them deal with subjects that are not, as a rule, adequately handled in the text-books; others of them, while bearing upon topics that are usually treated of at length in such works, yet bear such a stamp of individuality that, if widely read, they certainly deserve to be, they cannot fail to exert a wholesome restraint upon the undue ingenuity with which many young physicians seem bent upon following the wild teachings which so infest the gynæcology of the present day.—*N. Y. Medical Journal*, March, 1880.

GYNÆCOLOGICAL TRANSACTIONS.
Being the Transactions of the American Gynæcological Society for the Year 1881.

VOLUME VI. *Now ready.* Contains Essays by Doctors W. H. Byford, S. C. Busey, H. J. Garrigues, G. H. Lyman, Nathan Bozeman, E. Van de Warker, L. E. Taylor, W. Goodell, H. F. Campbell, T. G. Thomas, T. A. Reamy, A. H. Smith, A. D. Sinclair, J. W. Underhill, E. W. Jenks, LL. D., W. M. Polk, W. R. Gillette, G. C. Lee, F. P. Foster, E. W. Sawyer and B. B. Browne.

With Indexes: (a) of Vol. VI., (b) of the Gynæcological and Obstetric Literature of Countries for the year 1880, (c) of Obstetric and Gynæcological Journals, and (d) of Obstetric and Gynæcological Societies.

The six volumes completing the series will be sent by mail postpaid on receipt of $30; or, if single copies are desired, they will be furnished at the rate of $5 each, excepting Vol. II., for the year 1877, the price of which is $6.50.

HODGE, HUGH L., M. D.,
Emeritus Professor of Obstetrics, etc., in the University of Pennsylvania.

On Diseases Peculiar to Women; Including Displacements of the Uterus. Second edition, revised and enlarged. In one beautifully printed octavo volume of 519 pages, with original illustrations. Cloth, $4.50.

By the Same Author.
The Principles and Practice of Obstetrics. Illustrated with large lithographic plates containing 159 figures from original photographs, and with numerous woodcuts. In one large quarto volume of 542 double-columned pages. Strongly bound in cloth, $14.00.

. Specimens of the plates and letter-press will be forwarded to any address, free by mail, on receipt of six cents in postage stamps.

RAMSBOTHAM, FRANCIS H., M. D.
The Principles and Practice of Obstetric Medicine and Surgery; In reference to the Process of Parturition. A new and enlarged edition, thoroughly revised by the Author. With additions by W. V. KEATING, M. D., Professor of Obstetrics, etc., in the Jefferson Medical College of Philadelphia. In one large and handsome imperial octavo volume of 640 pages, with 64 full-page plates, and 43 woodcuts in the text, containing in all nearly 200 beautiful figures. Strongly bound in leather, with raised bands, $7.

ASHWELL'S PRACTICAL TREATISE ON THE DISEASES PECULIAR TO WOMEN. Third American from the third and revised London edition. In one 8vo. vol., pp. 520. Cloth, $3.50.
CHURCHILL ON THE PUERPERAL FEVER

AND OTHER DISEASES PECULIAR TO WOMEN. In one 8vo. vol. of 464 pages. Cloth, $2.50.
MEIGS ON THE NATURE, SIGNS AND TREATMENT OF CHILDBED FEVER. In one 8vo. volume of 346 pages. Cloth, $2.00.

AN AMERICAN SYSTEM OF GYNÆCOLOGY.

A System of Gynæcology, in Treatises by Various Authors. *In active preparation.*

THOMAS, T. GAILLARD, M. D.,
Professor of Obstetrics, etc., in the College of Physicians and Surgeons, N. Y.

A Practical Treatise on the Diseases of Women. Fifth edition, thoroughly revised and rewritten. In one large and handsome octavo volume of 810 pages, with 266 illustrations. Cloth, $5.00; leather, $6.00; very handsome half Russia, raised bands, $6.50.

The words which follow "fifth edition" are in this case no mere formal announcement. The alterations and additions which have been made are both numerous and important. The attraction and the permanent character of this book lie in the clearness and truth of the clinical descriptions of diseases; the fertility of the author in therapeutic resources and the fulness with which the details of treatment are described; the definite character of the teaching; and last, but not least, the evident candor which pervades it. We would also particularize the fulness with which the history of the subject is gone into, which makes the book additionally interesting and gives it value as a work of reference.—*London Medical Times and Gazette,* July 30, 1881.

The determination of the author to keep his book foremost in the rank of works on gynæcology is most gratifying. Recognizing the fact that this can only be accomplished by frequent and thorough revision, he has spared no pains to make the present edition more desirable even than the previous one. As a book of reference for the busy practitioner it is unequalled.—*Boston Medical and Surgical Journal,* April 7, 1880.

It has been enlarged and carefully revised. The author has brought it fully abreast with the times, and as the wave of gynæcological progression has been widespread and rapid during the twelve years that have elapsed since the issue of the first edition, one can conceive of the great improvement this edition must be upon the earlier. It is a condensed encyclopædia of gynæcological medicine. The style of arrangement, the masterly manner in which each subject is treated, and the honest convictions derived from probably the largest clinical experience in that specialty of any in this country, all serve to commend it in the highest terms to the practitioner.—*Nashville Jour. of Med. and Surg.,* Jan. 1881

That the previous editions of the treatise of Dr. Thomas were thought worthy of translation into German, French, Italian and Spanish, is enough to give it the stamp of genuine merit. At home it has made its way into the library of every obstetrician and gynæcologist as a safe guide to practice. No small number of additions have been made to the present edition to make it correspond to recent improvements in treatment.—*Pacific Medical and Surgical Journal,* Jan. 1881.

EDIS, ARTHUR W., M. D., Lond., F. R. C. P., M. R. C. S.,
Assist. Obstetric Physician to Middlesex Hospital, late Physician to British Lying-in Hospital.

The Diseases of Women. Including their Pathology, Causation, Symptoms, Diagnosis and Treatment. A Manual for Students and Practitioners. In one handsome octavo volume of 576 pages, with 148 illustrations. Cloth, $3.00; leather, $4.00.

It is a pleasure to read a book so thoroughly good as this one. The special qualities which are conspicuous are thoroughness in covering the whole ground, clearness of description and conciseness of statement. Another marked feature of the book is the attention paid to the details of many minor surgical operations and procedures, as, for instance, the use of tents, application of leeches, and use of hot water injections. These are among the more common methods of treatment, and yet very little is said about them in many of the text-books. The book is one to be warmly recommended especially to students and general practitioners, who need a concise but complete résumé of the whole subject. Specialists, too, will find many useful hints in its pages.—*Boston Med. and Surg. Journ.,* March 2, 1882.

The greatest pains have been taken with the sections relating to treatment. A liberal selection of remedies is given for each morbid condition, the strength, mode of application and other details

being fully explained. The descriptions of gynæcological manipulations and operations are full, clear and practical. Much care has also been bestowed on the parts of the book which deal with diagnosis—we note especially the pages dealing with the differentiation, one from another, of the different kinds of abdominal tumors. The practitioner will therefore find in this book the kind of knowledge he most needs in his daily work, and he will be pleased with the clearness and fulness of the information there given.—*The Practitioner,* Feb. 1882.

It is an excellent manual—clear, decided, sufficiently comprehensive for a beginner, extremely handy for any practitioner, safe, cautious and precise. The book reminds us constantly of Thomas' treatise, on which it seems to have been somewhat modelled. As a summary of existing knowledge, empirical and other, it is really to be commended —*Archives of Medicine,* June, 1882

BARNES, ROBERT, M. D., F. R. C. P.,
Obstetric Physician to St Thomas' Hospital, London, etc.

A Clinical Exposition of the Medical and Surgical Diseases of Women. In one handsome octavo volume, with numerous illustrations. New edition. *Preparing.*

GUSSEROW, A.,
Professor of Midwifery and the Diseases of Children at the University of Berlin.

A Practical Treatise on Uterine Tumors. Specially revised by the Author, and translated with notes and additions by EDMUND C. WENDT, M. D., Pathologist to the St. Francis Hospital, N. Y., etc., and revised by NATHAN BOZEMAN, M. D., Surgeon to the Woman's Hospital of the State of New York. In one handsome octavo volume, with about 40 illustrations. *Preparing.*

CHADWICK, JAMES R., A. M., M. D.
A Manual of the Diseases Peculiar to Women. In one handsom 12mo. volume, with illustrations. *Preparing.*

WEST, CHARLES, M. D.
Lectures on the Diseases of W men. Third American from the

A System o   ery, including the **Diseases of Pregnancy** and t
Puerperal State. Third American edition, revised by the Author, with additions
John S. Parry, M. D., Obstetrician to the Philadelphia Hospital, etc. In one large :
very handsome octavo volume of 740 pages, with 205 illustrations. Cloth, $4.50; leath
$5.50; very handsome half Russia, raised bands, $6.00.

The author is broad in his teachings, and discusses briefly the comparative anatomy of the pelvis and the mobility of the pelvic articulations.
The second chapter is devoted especially to
the study of the pelvis, while in the third the
female organs of generation are introduced.
The structure and development of the ovum are
admirably described. Then follow chapters upon
the various subjects embraced in the study of midwifery. The descriptions throughout the work are
plain and pleasing. It is sufficient to state that in
this, the last edition of this well-known work, every
recent advancement in this field has been brought
forward.—*Physician and Surgeon,* Jan. 1880.

We gladly welcome the new edition of this excellent text-book of midwifery. The former editions have been most favorably received by the
profession on both sides of the Atlantic. In the

preparation of the present edition the author
made such alterations as the progress of obste-
rical science seems to require, and we cannot
admire the ability with which the task has been
performed. We consider it an admirable
book for students during their attendance
lectures, and have great pleasure in recomm-
ing it. As an exponent of the midwifery of
present day it has no superior in the English
guage.—*Canada Lancet,* Jan. 1880.

To the American student the work is
must prove admirably adapted. Complete in all
parts, essentially modern in its teachings, and
demonstrations noted for clearness and prec-
It will gain in favor and be recognized as a
of standard merit. The work cannot fail t
popular and is cordially recommended.—N
Med. and Surg. Journ., March, 1880.

SMITH, J. LEWIS, M. D.,
Clinical Professor of Diseases of Children in the Bellevue Hospital Medical College, N. Y.

A Complete Practical Treatise on the **Diseases** of Children. F
edition, thoroughly revised and rewritten. In one handsome octavo volume of 836 p
with illustrations. Cloth, $4.50; leather, $5.50; very handsome half Russin, raised bands

That a book professing to treat of diseases of
children should have reached a fifth edition is in
itself fair evidence of its worth, the more especially
as it has not the field to itself, but has to compete
with several other excellent manuals. The chapter
on Rachitis is excellent and well up to the day—a
remark which may with equal justice be applied to
the chapter on Scrofula, which is one of the best
we remember to have read. The diseases of the
nervous system are well described, and so, for the
most part, are those of the lungs. Dr. Smith would
appear to be quite au courant with the work done
on this side of the world, and refers freely to English and foreign authors, as well as to particularly
especially devoted to children's diseases.—*British
Medical Journal,* May 6, 1882.

There is no book published on the subjects of
which this one treats that is its equal in value to
the physician. While he has said just enough to

impart the information desired by general pr
titioners on such questions as etiology, patho-
prognosis, etc., he has devoted more attentio
the diagnosis and treatment of the ailments wi
he so accurately describes ; and such informs
is exactly what is wanted by the vast majori
"family physicians."—*Va. Med. Monthly,* Feb.

It is a pleasure to peruse such a work as the
before us, and we moreover we have but one
culty—there is but little to find fault with.
author understands what he writes about fr-
practical acquaintance with the diseases inci-
to infancy and childhood, and also thorou
comprehends their pathology and therapeu
The work is full of original and practical rem-
which will be particularly acceptable to the stu-
and young physician; but at the same time we
with great sincerity commend it to the notic
the profession in general.—*Edinb. Med. Jl.,* May

KEATING, JOHN M., M. D.,
Lecturer on the Diseases of Children at the University of Pennsylvania, etc.

The Mother's Guide in the Management and Feeding of Infants.
one handsome 12mo. volume of 118 pages. Cloth, $1.00.

Works like this one will aid the physician im-
mensely, for it saves the time he is constantly giving his patients in instructing them on the subjects here dwelt upon so thoroughly and practically. Dr. Keating has written a practical book,
has carefully avoided unnecessary repetition, and
successfully instructed the mother in such details
of the treatment of her child as devolve upon her.
He has studiously omitted giving prescriptions,
and instructs the mother when to call upon the
doctor, as his duties are totally distinct from hers.
—*American Journal of Obstetrics,* October, 1881.

Dr. Keating has kept clear of the occasion
of works of this sort, viz., mixing the dutie
the mother with those proper to the doctor. T
is the ring of common sense in the remarks a
the employment of a wet-nurse, about the pr
food for a nursing mother, about the tonic eff
of a bath, about the perambulator saves the nur
arms, and on many other subjects concer-
which the critic might say, "surely this is c
on," but which experience teaches us are ex-
the things needed to be insisted upon, with the
as well as the poor.—*London Lancet,* January

WEST, CHARLES, M. D.,
Physician to the Hospital for Sick Children, London, etc.

Lectures on the Diseases of Infancy and Childhood. Fifth Ameri
from the sixth revised and enlarged English edition. In one large and handsome oct
volume of 686 pages. Cloth, $4.50; leather, $5.50.

By the Same Author.

On Some Disorders of the Nervous System in Childhood. In one sm
12mo. volume of 127 pages. Cloth, $1.00.

SMITH'S PRACTICAL TREATISE ON THE
WASTING DISEASES OF INFANCY AND
CHILDHOOD. Second American from the
second English edition. In one octavo volume
of 266 pages. Cloth, $2.50.

CONDIE'S PRACTICAL TREATISE ON
DISEASES OF CHILDREN. Sixth edition, revised and augmented. In one octavo volum
719 pages. Cloth, $5.25; leather, $6.25.

TIDY, CHARLES MEYMOTT, M. B., F. C. S.,
Professor of Chemistry and of Forensic Medicine and Public Health at the London Hospital, etc.

Legal Medicine. VOLUME I. Embracing Evidence, The Signs of Death, Identity, The Causes of Death, The Post-mortem, Sex, Monstrosities, Hermaphrodism, Expectation of Life, Presumption of Death and Survivorship, Heat and Cold, Burns, Lightning, Explosives, Starvation. Making a very handsome imperial octavo volume of 664 pages, with 2 beautifully-colored plates. Cloth, $6.00; leather, $7.00. *Just ready.*

He whose inclinations or necessities lead him to assume the functions of a medical jurist wants a book encyclopædic in character, in which he may be reasonably sure of finding medico-legal topics discussed with judicial fairness, with sufficient completeness, and with due attention to the most recent advances in medical science. Mr. Tidy's work bids fair to meet this need satisfactorily.

The fact that the very numerous illustrative cases are drawn from many sources, and are not limited, as in Casper's Handbook, to the author's own experience, and the additional fact that they are brought down to a very recent date, give them, for purposes of reference, a very obvious value.—*Boston Medical and Surgical Journal*, Feb. 8, 1883.

TAYLOR, ALFRED S., M. D.,
Lecturer on Medical Jurisprudence and Chemistry in Guy's Hospital, London.

A Manual of Medical Jurisprudence. Eighth American from the tenth London edition, thoroughly revised and rewritten. Edited by JOHN J. REESE, M. D., Professor of Medical Jurisprudence and Toxicology in the University of Pennsylvania. In one large octavo volume of 937 pages, with 70 illustrations. Cloth, $5.00; leather, $6.00; half Russia, raised bands, $6.50.

The American editions of this standard manual have for a long time laid claim to the attention of the profession in this country; and the eighth comes before us as embodying the latest thoughts and emendations of Dr. Taylor upon the subject to which he devoted his life with an assiduity and success which made him *facile princeps* among English writers on medical jurisprudence. Both the author and the book have made a mark too deep to be affected by criticism, whether it be censure or praise. In this case, however, we should

only have to seek for laudatory terms.—*American Journal of the Medical Sciences*, Jan. 1881.

This celebrated work has been the standard authority in its department for thirty-seven years, both in England and America, in both the professions which it concerns, and it is improbable that it will be superseded in many years. The work is simply indispensable to every physician, and nearly so to every liberally-educated lawyer, and we heartily commend the present edition to both professions.—*Albany Law Journal*, March 26, 1881.

By the Same Author.
The Principles and Practice of Medical Jurisprudence. Third edition. In two handsome octavo volumes, containing 1416 pages, with 188 illustrations. Cloth, $10; leather, $12. *Just ready.*

The revision of the third edition of this standard work has been most happily confided to a gentleman who was during fourteen years the colleague of the author, and who therefore is thoroughly conversant with the methods of thought which have everywhere gained for the book an exalted position as a work of reference. The present edition, though not so large as its predecessor, contains a large amount of new matter which has been accommodated by a careful condensation wherever it was compatible with clearness. The chapters on poisoning have been in some parts entirely rewritten, a change demanded by the recent advances in this department of Forensic Medicine, and many illustrative cases have been added throughout the entire work. In its present form the work is the most complete exposition of Forensic Medicine in the English language.

By the Same Author.
Poisons in Relation to Medical Jurisprudence and Medicine. Third American, from the third and revised English edition. In one large octavo volume of 788 pages. Cloth, $5.50; leather, $6.50.

LEA, HENRY C.
Superstition and Force: Essays on The Wager of Law, The Wager of Battle, The Ordeal and Torture. Third revised and enlarged edition. In one handsome royal 12mo. volume of 552 pages. Cloth, $2.50.

This valuable work is in reality a history of civilization as interpreted by the progress of jurisprudence . In "Superstition and Force" we have a philosophic survey of the long period intervening between primitive barbarity and civilized enlightenment There is not a chapter in the work that

should not be most carefully studied, and however well versed the reader may be in the science of jurisprudence, he will find much in Mr Lea's volume of which he was previously ignorant The book is a valuable addition to the literature of social science — *Westminster Review*, Jan 1880.

By the Same Author.
Studies in Church History. The Rise of the Temporal Power—Benefit of Clergy—Excommunication. New edition. In one very handsome octavo volume of 605 pages. Cloth, $2.50. *Just ready.*

The author is pre-eminently a scholar. He takes up every topic allied with the leading theme, and traces it out to the minutest detail with a wealth of knowledge and impartiality of treatment that

primitive church traced with so much and with so definite a perception of conflicting sources. The fifty pages of the papacy, for instance, are adv

INDEX TO CATALOGUE.

Books marked * are also bound in half Russia.

HENRY C. LEA'S SON & CO., Philadelphia.